Essential Surgery

FIFTH EDITION

PROBLEMS, DIAGNOSIS AND MANAGEMENT

Clive R. G. Quick

MB, BS(London), FDS, FRCS(England), MS(London), MA(Cambridge)

Consultant General and Vascular Surgeon, Hinchingbrooke Hospital, Huntingdon and Addenbrooke's Hospital, Cambridge; Associate Lecturer in Surgery, University of Cambridge; Former Examine and current Examiner in Basic Sciences and Clinical Surgery for MRCS(England), Royal College of Surgeons of England, London, UK

Joanna B. Reed

BMedSci(Hons), BM BS(Nottingham), FRCS(Eng)

Clinical Director for Surgery and Consultant Laparoscopic and Upper Gastrointestinal Surgeon, Hinchingbrooke Hospital, Huntingdon, UK

Simon J. F. Harper

MB, ChB, BSc, FRCS, MD

Consultant Hepatopancreatobiliary and Transplant Surgeon at the University of Cambridge and Addenbrooke's Hospital, UK

Kourosh Saeb-Parsy

MA, MB, BChir, FRCS, PhD

University Lecturer and Consultant Transplant Surgeon, Department of Surgery, University of Cambridge, UK

Illustrations by

Philip J. Deakin

BSc(Hons), MBChB(Sheffield)

General Medical Practitioner, Sheffield, UK

Foreword by

Andrew T. Raftery

BSc, MB, ChB(Hons), MD, FRCS(Eng), FRCS(Ed)

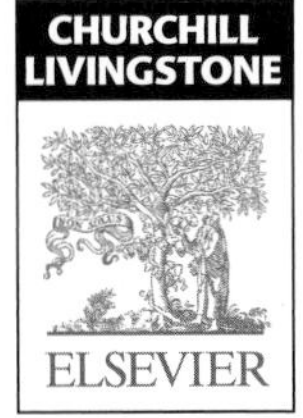

EDINBURGH LONDON NEW YORK OXFORD PHILADELPHIA ST LOUIS SYDNEY TORONTO 2014

CHURCHILL
LIVINGSTONE
ELSEVIER

First edition 1990
Second edition 1996
Third edition 2002
Fourth edition 2007
Fifth edition 2014

ISBN 978-0-7020-4674-2
International ISBN 978-0-7020-4675-9
e-book ISBN 978-0-7020-5483-9

British Library Cataloguing in Publication Data
A catalogue record for this book is available from the British Library

Library of Congress Cataloging in Publication Data
A catalog record for this book is available from the Library of Congress

Notices

Knowledge and best practice in this field are constantly changing. As new research and experience broaden our understanding, changes in research methods, professional practices, or medical treatment may become necessary.

Practitioners and researchers must always rely on their own experience and knowledge in evaluating and using any information, methods, compounds, or experiments described herein. In using such information or methods they should be mindful of their own safety and the safety of others, including parties for whom they have a professional responsibility.

With respect to any drug or pharmaceutical products identified, readers are advised to check the most current information provided (i) on procedures featured or (ii) by the manufacturer of each product to be administered, to verify the recommended dose or formula, the method and duration of administration, and contraindications. It is the responsibility of practitioners, relying on their own experience and knowledge of their patients, to make diagnoses, to determine dosages and the best treatment for each individual patient, and to take all appropriate safety precautions.

To the fullest extent of the law, neither the Publisher nor the authors, contributors, or editors, assume any liability for any injury and/or damage to persons or property as a matter of products liability, negligence or otherwise, or from any use or operation of any methods, products, instructions, or ideas contained in the material herein.

Printed in China

Foreword

It is a pleasure and a privilege to be asked to write the foreword to the Fifth Edition of *Essential Surgery*. The fact that there is a Fifth Edition attests to the popularity of this excellent textbook of surgery. It is over 20 years since the First Edition appeared and the book has maintained its impact in subsequent editions. It is hardly surprising that the Fourth Edition won first prize in the British Medical Association Surgical Book Awards in 2008. When the First Edition appeared in 1990 it was particularly impressive, in that at the time, only the senior author (Clive Quick) was a consultant surgeon while two other authors were junior hospital doctors. Dennis Gatt retired from the Third Edition and now George Burkitt, another founding author, has retired from the Fifth Edition. Clive Quick remains as managing author, bringing with him years of experience as an outstanding clinical teacher and examiner who for many years was a colleague of mine on the Court of Examiners of the Royal College of Surgeons of England. Joanna Reed, a Consultant Surgeon with a particular expertise in minimally invasive surgery also remains from the Fourth Edition and has been joined by two new authors, Simon Harper and Kourosh Saeb-Parsy, both newly appointed consultant surgeons who bring with them a more recent perspective on surgical training and education. The line-up is completed by Phil Deakin, a family practitioner and one of the founding authors, who combines his medical knowledge with considerable artistic skills to produce outstanding diagrams which are easy to interpret and understand, providing one of the great strengths of the book.

Although written primarily for medical students, who will appreciate its clarity and style, the authors have ensured that there is more than enough in the present edition for the basic surgical trainee (to whom I would strongly recommend this book in preparing for the MRCS examination) and indeed some of the chapters will also provide excellent revision material for the higher surgical trainee sitting the UK Intercollegiate FRCS examination in general surgery. *Essential Surgery* is written in a different way from other standard surgical textbooks, describing sound principles of surgery on which to expand one's learning and presenting material in a problem-orientated style. In the Fifth Edition, much of the text has been updated and sections added on ethics, audit and research, orthopaedic surgery, the use on monoclonal antibodies in surgical oncology and damage control surgery in trauma management. The clinical photographs and images throughout the book are of extremely high quality and well labelled to aid interpretation. In Chapter 1 Harold Ellis reminds us of our surgical heritage, commenting on the introduction of the application of basic sciences to surgery in centuries past. This is a ready reminder of their importance today, demonstrated throughout this book in places where the pathophysiological basis of disease is presented in a way that bridges the gap between basic medical science and clinical surgery.

The authors are to be congratulated on the production of this Fifth Edition. This book continues to go from strength to strength and I believe that the reader will enjoy the style of presentation and find it easy to read and to assimilate knowledge. This book has much in it for both undergraduate and postgraduate alike. I wish it the success that it deserves.

Andrew T. Raftery
BSc MB ChB(Hons) MD FRCS(Eng) FRCS(Ed)
Clinical Anatomist. Honorary Teaching Fellow Hull York Medical School. Formerly Consultant Surgeon, Sheffield Kidney Institute, Sheffield Teaching Hospitals NHS Foundation Trust, Northern General Hospital, Sheffield; Member (formerly Chairman), Court of Examiners, Royal College of Surgeons of England; Formerly Member of Panel of Examiners, Intercollegiate Speciality Board in General Surgery; Formerly Member of Council, Royal College of Surgeons of England; Formerly Honorary Clinical Senior Lecturer in Surgery, University of Sheffield, UK

Sheffield
2014

Preface

When we first set about writing this book, we felt we had something worthwhile to say about how surgery worked. If readers could acquire this knowledge and implement it, we believed surgical practice would improve, as would outcomes for patients. We wrote the book in an entirely different way from most medical books, determined to avoid propagating myths and giving inadequate explanations. To achieve this, the authors discussed each topic in depth before writing an agreed version. Many original ideas came in the form of diagrams from Dennis Gatt. We have continued this method for each new edition, and now have the advantage of rapid internet access to check facts and investigate trends. We believe our approach has helped us understand the subjects better and put them across with exceptional clarity.

The original authorship was unusual in that only Clive Quick was a consultant surgeon: George Burkitt was a junior doctor-cum-medical author; Dennis Gatt was a junior surgical trainee (later consultant surgeon); whilst Phil Deakin was a family practitioner. This mix enabled us to address surgical problems from the viewpoint of the student and junior doctor and to this end, trainee doctors have assisted in every edition (Emma McGrath, on the Fourth Edition; Olivia Will and Antonia Wells on both the Fourth and Fifth editions; and Kasra Saeb Parsy on this Fifth edition).

For this edition, Clive Quick has continued in his role as managing author. Joanna Reed is once again an author, giving the fresh perspective of the younger consultant, and one with a particular interest in minimally invasive surgery. Two other authors have joined the author team for this edition, both from Addenbrooke's Hospital: Kourosh Saeb Parsy brings a broad experience of teaching and training and Simon Harper has a personal perspective on surgical training, having recently completed his higher surgical training.

Our overall concept has always been to produce an authored rather than an edited book, so as to retain control over content, to give uniformity of style and apply our own high standard of elucidation so readers could grasp the main ideas easily and effortlessly in one reading. Nevertheless, an enormous amount of help has been generously given over the years by colleagues in specialist areas. Their invaluable contributions have been integrated and edited to emphasise lucidity and fluency (see detail in the Acknowledgements section).

Finally, when complete, the whole text is re-read several times by the authors and given a concluding 'polish'. Writing in this manner is time consuming but if the text proves enjoyable to read and draws the reader in as we intend, we feel it will have been worthwhile.

The book covers general surgery, trauma, orthopaedics, cardiothoracic surgery and urology in detail, with sufficient basic science for modern clinical courses, and we have endeavoured to present sometimes complex ideas in ways accessible to anyone with a moderate understanding of human biology, and yet still prove valuable to readers at more advanced levels.

Changes for this edition

The continuing enthusiasm of students and teachers for this book has highlighted the need for this updated edition which was written for clinical medical students seeking a comprehensive understanding of surgical principles and practice as well as for junior surgical trainees (particularly those preparing for MRCS examinations). We have tried to build on the quality and content of the original without increasing its length. The content of each chapter has been carefully revised, often with input from colleagues with some sections relocated to facilitate navigation. At the same time, we have used the opportunity to match the book's content with the UK Intercollegiate MRCS examination curriculum, rendering the book appropriate for junior surgical trainees. Other major changes represent the evolution and refinement of surgery and our approach to it over the five or so years since the previous edition.

All of the text has been brought up to date, adding new concepts where medical understanding has advanced, for example monoclonal antibodies in surgical oncology and damage control surgery in trauma management. Covering the MRCS curriculum has required adding several new sections including surgical ethics, audit and research, and orthopaedic surgery. New consensus guidelines for managing common disorders have been incorporated where appropriate. We believe that *Essential Surgery* will continue to have the greatest appeal for readers who want to understand surgery rather than merely pass examinations.

Previous editions have demonstrated a broad appeal beyond medical students and junior surgeons, from surgical nurses and trainees in professions allied to medicine, to dentists. In addition, the book was designed to be a continuing reference text for doctors in other specialties, including family practice. We have employed a problem-solving approach to diagnosis and treatment where practicable, believing that understanding how diagnoses are made and why particular treatments are used is more memorable than rote learning. With this in mind, we have tried to view the practical management of patients through the eyes of the trainee or student. In particular, the pathophysiological basis of surgical diseases and management is presented to bridge the gap between basic medical sciences and clinical problems.

Throughout the book we have used original illustrative material to emphasise important concepts, avoid unnecessary text and assist revision for exams. This includes photographs of clinical cases, operations and pathological specimens, radiographs, anatomical and operative diagrams, and tables and box summaries of the text. We believe the illustrations are one of the particular strengths of the book, and have all been reviewed and updated or replaced as necessary. The clinical material is largely drawn from our day-to-day practice and we have generally chosen typical rather than gross examples so the reader can see how patients present most commonly. We have tried to teach in a problem-oriented way where possible, but we believe descriptions of individual diseases are also required and these have been covered in a more conventional manner.

Operative surgery

We make no apology for including outlines of common surgical operations. This is to enable students and trainee surgeons to explain operations to patients, to participate intelligently in the operating department, to understand and thereby prevent complications, as well as to help them perform certain operations themselves.

We hope our readers will continue to enjoy the book and will appreciate the continuing efforts we have made to keep pace with change. Above all, it remains our ambition to stimulate the reader to a greater enjoyment and understanding of the practice of surgery.

C. R. G. Q.
J. B. R.
K. S. P.
S. J. F. H.

Acknowledgements

As in all previous editions, the authors are deeply indebted to contributing authors for helping us keep the book up-to-date and accurate. Some have contributed a large amount of material and others in lesser ways, but without them all, the book would not be what it is.

A continuing debt of gratitude is owed to all who have contributed to each of the editions of *Essential Surgery*, including of course, any whose names are not mentioned here. A substantial part of the book's success is due to them.

In previous editions: we gratefully acknowledge the huge contributions made by Dennis Gatt, now a surgeon in Malta, the late Leonard Beard, medical photographer, Dr Graham Hurst, radiologist, Michael Williams, oncologist and the late Andrew Higgins, urologist. We also owe a tremendous debt to Jane Hailey, then a junior trainee and now a paediatrician in Canada, who helped turn our first edition prose into accessible and fluent text. We owe grateful thanks for contributions from Prof Ted Howard, Stephen Large, Grant Williams, Mark Farrington, Richard Miller, John Benson, Neville Jamieson, Jeffrey Brain, Madan Samuel, Nimish Shah, Sue Clark, Paul Perkins, Adrian Harris, Dr Anita Gibbons, Dr Suzanna Lishman, Dr Helen Smith, David Adlam, Nick Skelton, Paul Hayes, Roger Gray and Elizabeth Ambler.

For this edition we are once again grateful for the substantial and unstinting help we have received from colleagues and friends. Most are based at Hinchingbrooke Hospital, Huntingdon or Addenbrooke's Hospital Cambridge.

We would particularly like to thank Prof Harold Ellis for his contribution 'A brief history of surgery', Mr William Hage for his contribution on 'Elective orthopaedics' and Ms Melanie Sharp and Mr Robert Macfarlane for their contribution on 'Elective neurosurgery' and head injuries.

We would also like to thank the following colleagues and friends for their help with reviewing chapters for the Fifth Edition:

Dr Donald Bermingham, consultant psychiatrist (Breaking bad news in Surgery);

Dr Hemantha Alawattegama, consultant anaesthetist, Addenbrooke's Hospital (Managing physiological change in the surgical patient; Shock and resuscitation);

Dr Andreas Karas, consultant microbiologist, Addenbrooke's Hospital (Immunity, inflammation and infection);

Dr Tony Booth, consultant radiologist, Hinchingbrooke Hospital (Imaging and interventional techniques in surgery);

Dr Catherine Hubbard, consultant radiologist, Hinchingbrooke Hospital (Imaging and interventional techniques in surgery);

Dr Claire Cousins, consultant radiologist, Addenbrooke's Hospital (Imaging and interventional techniques in vascular surgery);

Dr Paul Siklos, consultant physician, West Suffolk Hospital (Medical problems in Surgical Patients);

Dr Katy Hoggarth, consultant haematologist, Hinchingbrooke Hospital (Blood transfusion);

Dr Natalie Cook, consultant oncologist, Addenbrooke's Hospital (Principles of cancer management);

Dr Antonia Wells, specialist registrar in surgery Addenbrookes Hospital (Major trauma);

Mr Aman Coonar, consultant thoracic surgeon, Papworth Hospital (Thoracic surgery);

Prof Peter Brennan, consultant Oral and Maxillofacial Surgeon at Portsmouth Hospitals NHS Trust and Chair of RCS Eng Court of Examiners (Head and maxillofacial injuries; Lumps in the head and neck and salivary calculi; Disorders of the mouth);

Mr George Lamberty, consultant plastic and reconstructive surgeon, Addenbrooke's Hospital (Soft tissue injuries and burns);

Dr Adrian Bomford, reader in hepatology, King's College Hospital (Tumours of the pancreas and hepatobiliary system);

Dr Olivia Will, specialist registrar, Addenbrooke's Hospital (Colorectal carcinoma; Chronic inflammatory disorders of the bowel; Anal and perianal disorders);

Mr Paul Toomey, consultant colorectal surgeon, Epsom and St Helier University Hospitals NHS Trust (Colorectal carcinoma; Anal and perianal disorders);

Mr Kasra Saeb-Parsy, Specialty Registrar in Urology, Addenbrooke's Hospital (Disorders of the male genitalia; Symptoms, signs and investigation of urinary tract disorders; Disorders of the prostate; Tumours of the kidney and urinary tract; Stone disease of the urinary tract; Urinary tract infections; Congenital disorders and diseases secondarily involving the urinary tract)

Mr Patrick Coughlin, consultant vascular surgeon, Addenbrooke's Hospital (Pathophysiology, clinical features and diagnosis of vascular disease affecting the limbs; Managing lower limb arterial insufficiency, the diabetic foot and major amputations; Aneurysms and

other peripheral arterial disorders; Venous disorders of the lower limb);
Mr Stephen Tsui, consultant cardiac surgeon, Papworth Hospital (Cardiac surgery);
Ms Liz Ball, consultant breast surgeon, West Suffolk Hospital, Bury St Edmunds (Disorders of the breast);
Dr Cedric Banfield, consultant dermatologist, Peterborough Hospitals (Disorders of the skin);
Mr Daniel Carroll, consultant paediatric surgeon, Addenbrooke's Hospital (Acute surgical problems in children; Non-acute abdominal and urological problems in children)

Special thanks also to Dr Tony Booth and Dr Catherine Hubbard, consultant radiologists, Hinchingbrooke Hospital for the images they have contributed to the book.

Contents

SECTION 1 Principles of Surgical Care

SECTION 2 Perioperative Care

SECTION 3 Principles of Accident Surgery

SECTION 4 Symptoms, Diagnosis and Management

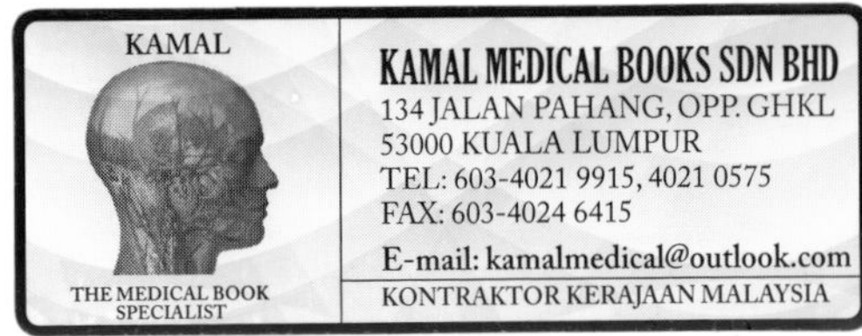

Principles of surgical care

Mechanisms of surgical disease and surgery in practice

1

A SHORT HISTORY OF SURGERY

Prof. Harold Ellis CBE MCh FRCS

There is no doubt that the first surgeons were the men and women who bound up the lacerations, contusions, fractures, impalements and eviscerations to which man has been subject since appearing on Earth. Since man is the most vicious of all creatures, many of these injuries were inflicted by man upon man. Indeed, the battlefield has always been a training ground for surgery. Right up to the 15th century, surgeons dealing with trauma were surprisingly efficient. They knew their limitations—they could splint fractures, reduce dislocations and bind up lacerations, but were only too aware that open wounds of the skull, chest and abdomen were lethal and were best left alone, as were wounds involving major blood vessels or spinal injuries with paralysis. They observed that wounds would usually discharge yellow pus for a time; indeed this was regarded as a good prognostic sign and was labelled 'laudable pus'.

The 15th century heralded a new and dreaded pathology—the gunshot wound. These injuries would stink, swell and bubble with gas. There was profound systemic toxicity and a high mortality. Of course, we now know that this was the result of clostridial infection of wounds with extensive anaerobic tissue damage caused by shot and shell. The surgeons of those times were shrewd clinical observers but surmised that these malign effects were due to gunpowder acting as a poison, for it was not until centuries later that the bacterial basis of wound infection became evident. At that period the remedy was to destroy the poison with boiling oil or cautery. Boiling oil was the more popular since it was advocated by the Italian surgeon Giovanni da Vigo (1460–1525), the author of the standard text of the day, *Practica In Arte Chirurgica Compendiosa*. These treatments not only produced intense pain but also made matters worse by increasing tissue necrosis.

The first scientific departure from this barbaric treatment was by the great French military surgeon Ambroise Paré (1510–1590) who, while still a young man, revolutionised the treatment of wounds by using only simple dressings, abandoning cautery and introducing ligatures to control haemorrhage. He established that his results were much better than could be achieved by the old methods.

Ignorance of the basic sciences behind the practice of surgery was slowly overcome. The publications of *The Fabric of the Human Body* in 1543 by Andreas Vesalius (1514–1564) and of *The Motion of the Heart* by William Harvey (1578–1657) in 1628 were two notable landmarks.

Surgical progress, however, was still limited by two major obstacles. First, the agony of the knife: patients would only undergo an operation to relieve intolerable suffering (for example from a gangrenous limb, a bladder stone or a strangulated rupture) and, of course, the surgeon needed to operate at lightning speed. Second, there was the inevitability of suppuration, with its prolonged disability and high mortality, often as high as 50% after amputation. Amazingly, both these barriers were overcome in the same couple of decades.

In 1846, William Morton (1819–1868), a dentist working in Boston, Massachusetts, introduced ether as a general anaesthetic. This was followed a year later by chloroform, employed by James Young Simpson (1811–1870) in Edinburgh, mainly in midwifery. These agents were taken up with immense enthusiasm across the world in a matter of weeks.

The work of the French chemist Louis Pasteur (1822–1895) demonstrated the link between wound suppuration and microbes. This led Joseph Lister (1827–1912), then a young professor of surgery in Edinburgh, to perform the first operation under sterile conditions in 1865. This was treatment of a compound tibial fracture in which crude carbolic acid was used as an antiseptic. The development of antiseptic surgery and, later, modern aseptic surgery progressed from there.

So at last, in the 1870s, the scene was set for the coming enormous advances in every branch of surgery whose breadth and successes form the basis of this book.

APPROACHES TO SURGICAL PROBLEMS

WHAT DO SURGEONS DO?

Surgeons are perceived as doctors who do operations, i.e. cutting tissue to treat disease, usually under anaesthesia, but this is only a small part of surgical practice. The range individual surgeons undertake varies with the culture, the resources available, the nature and breadth of their specialisation, which other specialists are available, and local needs. The principles of operative surgery—access, dissection, haemostasis, repair, reconstruction, preservation of vital structures and closure—are similar in all specialties.

A **general surgeon** is one who undertakes general surgical emergency work and elective abdominal gastrointestinal (GI) surgery. In geographically isolated areas, such a surgeon might also undertake gynaecology, obstetrics, urology, paediatric surgery, orthopaedic and trauma surgery and perhaps basic ear, nose and throat (ENT), and ophthalmology. Conversely, in developed countries, there is a trend towards greater specialisation. GI surgery, for example, is often divided into 'upper' and 'lower' and upper GI surgery may further subdivide into hepatobiliary, laparoscopic, pancreatic and gastro-oesophageal cancer surgery.

Surgeons are not simply 'cutting and sewing' doctors. The drama of surgery may seem attractive but good surgery is rarely dramatic. Only when things go wrong does the drama increase, and this is uncomfortable. Surgery is an art or craft as well as a science, and judgement, coping under pressure, taking decisive action, teaching and training and managing people skilfully are essential qualities. Operating can be learnt by most people, but the skills involved in deciding when it is in the patient's best interests to operate are essential and must be actively learnt and practised.

Surgeons play an important role in diagnosis, using clinical method and selecting appropriate investigations. Many undertake diagnostic and therapeutic endoscopy including gastroscopy, colonoscopy, urological endoscopy, thoracoscopy and arthroscopy. Indications for laparoscopic surgery, supported by good quality clinical trials, continue to broaden as equipment and skills become more sophisticated.

What sort of patients come to surgeons?

Different types of surgeon practise in very different ways. In the UK, most patients are referred by another doctor, e.g. GP, accident and emergency (ER) officer or physician. The exceptions include trauma patients who self-refer or arrive by ambulance. In some countries, patients can self-refer to the specialist they consider most appropriate. Regardless of the route, surgical patients fall into the following categories:

- **Emergency/acute**, i.e. symptoms lasting minutes to hours or up to a day or two—often obviously surgical conditions such as traumatic wounds, fractures, abscesses, acute abdominal pain or gastrointestinal bleeding
- **Intermediate urgency**—usually referrals from other doctors based on suspicious symptoms and signs and sometimes investigations, e.g. suspected colonic cancer, gallstones, renal or ureteric stones
- **Chronic conditions** likely to need surgery, e.g. varicose veins, hernias, arthritic joints, cardiac ischaemia or rectal prolapse

The diagnostic process

To manage surgical patients optimally, a **working diagnosis** needs to be formulated to guide whether investigations are necessary and their type and urgency, and to determine what intervention is necessary. The process depends upon whether immediate life-saving intervention is required or, if not, the perceived urgency of the case. For example, a patient bleeding from a stab wound might need pressure applied to the wound immediately whilst resuscitation and detailed assessment are carried out. At the other end of the scale, if symptoms suggest rectal carcinoma, a systematic approach is needed to obtain visual and histological confirmation of the diagnosis by colonoscopy and radiological imaging. **Tumour staging** (see Ch. 13, p. 178) aims to determine the extent of cancer spread to direct how radical treatment needs to be. Treatment may be **curative** (surgery, chemotherapy, radiotherapy) or **palliative** if clearly beyond cure (stenting to prevent obstruction, local tumour destruction using laser, palliative radiotherapy).

Formulating a diagnosis

The traditional approach to surgical diagnosis is to attempt to correlate a patient's symptoms and signs with recognised sets of clinical features known to characterise each disease. While most diagnoses match their 'classical' descriptions at certain stages, this may not be so when the patient presents. Patients often present before a recognisable pattern has evolved or at an advanced stage when the typical clinical picture has become obscured. Diagnosis can be confusing if all the clinical features for a particular diagnosis are not present, or if some seem inconsistent with the working diagnosis.

This book seeks to develop a more logical and reliable approach to diagnostic method than pattern recognition, by attempting to explain how the evolving pathophysiology of the disease and its effect on the anatomy bring about the clinical features. The overall aim is to target investigations and management that give the best chance of cure or symptom relief with the least harm to the patient.

PRINCIPAL MECHANISMS OF SURGICAL DISEASE

Surgical patients present with disorders resulting from inherited abnormalities, environmental factors or combinations in varying proportions. These are summarised in Box 1.1, as a useful 'first principles' framework or *aide-mémoire* upon which to construct a differential diagnosis. This is useful when clinical features do not immediately point to a diagnosis. This approach is known as the 'surgical sieve'; however, it is not a substitute for logical thought based on the clinical findings.

Box 1.1 The surgical sieve

When considering the causes of a particular condition, it may be helpful to run through the range of causes listed here. This should only be a first step and not a substitute for thought. This approach gives no indication of the likely severity, frequency or importance of the cause.

Congenital

- Genetic
- Environmental influences in utero

Acquired

- Trauma—accidents in the home, at work or during leisure activities, personal violence, road traffic collisions
- Inflammation—physical or immunological mechanisms
- Infection—viral, bacterial, fungal, protozoal, parasitic
- Neoplasia—benign, premalignant or malignant
- Vascular—ischaemia, infarction, reperfusion syndrome, aneurysms, venous insufficiency
- Degenerative—osteoporosis, glaucoma, osteoarthritis, rectal prolapse
- Metabolic disorders—gallstones, urinary tract stones
- Endocrine disorders and therapy—thyroid function abnormalities, Cushing's syndrome, phaeochromocytoma
- Other abnormalities of tissue growth—hyperplasia, hypertrophy and cyst formation
- Iatrogenic disorders—damage or injury resulting from the action of a doctor or other health care worker; may be misadventure, negligence or, more commonly, system failure
- Drugs, toxins, diet, exercise and environment
  - Prescription drugs—toxic effects of powerful drugs, maladministration, idiosyncratic reactions, drug interactions
  - Smoking—atherosclerosis, cancers, peptic ulcer
  - Alcohol abuse—personal violence, traffic collisions
  - Substance abuse—accidents, injection site problems
  - 'Western diet'—obesity, atherosclerosis, cancers
  - Lack of exercise—obesity, osteoporosis, aches and pains
  - Venomous snakes, spiders, scorpions and other creatures—local and systemic toxicity
  - Atmospheric pollution—pulmonary problems
- Psychogenic—Munchausen syndrome leading to repeated operations, problems of indigent living, ingestion of foreign bodies, self-harm
- Disorders of function—diverticular disease, some swallowing disorders

CONGENITAL CONDITIONS

The term **congenital** defines a condition present at birth, as a result of genetic changes and/or environmental influences in utero such as ischaemia, incomplete development or maternal ingestion of drugs such as thalidomide. Congenital abnormalities of surgical interest range from minor cosmetic deformities such as skin tags through to potentially fatal conditions such as congenital heart defects, urethral valves and gut atresias.

Congenital abnormalities become manifest any time between conception and old age, although most are evident at birth or in early childhood. Some are diagnosed *antenatally*, for example, fetal gut atresias with grossly excessive amniotic fluid (polyhydramnios). There are expanding specialist areas involving *intrauterine* or fetal surgery, for example, for urinary tract obstruction. During *infancy*, conditions such as congenital hypertrophic pyloric stenosis come to light. In *childhood*, incompletely descended testis may become evident. Finally, some disorders may present at *any stage*. For example, a patent processus vaginalis may predispose to an inguinal hernia even into late middle age.

Whilst many congenital abnormalities give rise to disease by direct **anatomical effects**, others cause disease by **disrupting function**, with the underlying disorder revealed only on investigation. For example, ureteric abnormalities allowing urinary reflux predispose to recurrent kidney infections.

ACQUIRED CONDITIONS

Acquired surgical disorders result from trauma or disease or from the body's response to them, or else present as an effect or side-effect of treatment. For example, bladder outlet obstruction may result from prostatic hypertrophy, from fibrosis after gonococcal urethritis or from damage inflicted during urethral instrumentation. The classification detailed here is a framework, but conditions may fit more than one heading, and the mechanism behind some disorders is still poorly understood.

Trauma

Tissue trauma, literally injury, includes damage inflicted by any physical means, i.e. mechanical, thermal, chemical or electrical mechanisms or ionising radiation. Common usage tends to imply blunt or penetrating mechanical injury, caused by accidents in industry or in the home, road traffic collisions, fights, firearm and missile injuries or natural disasters such as floods and earthquakes. Damage varies with the causative agent, and the visible injuries may not indicate the extent of deep tissue damage.

Inflammation

Many surgical disorders result from inflammatory processes, most often stemming from infection. However, inflammation also results from physical irritation, particularly by chemical agents, e.g. gastric acid/pepsin in peptic ulcer disease or pancreatic enzymes in acute pancreatitis.

Inflammation may also result from immunological processes such as in ulcerative colitis and Crohn's disease. Autoimmunity, where an immune response is directed at the body's constituents, is recognised in a growing number of surgical diseases such as Hashimoto's thyroiditis and rheumatoid disease.

Infection

Primary infections presenting to surgeons include abscesses and cellulitis, primary joint infections and tonsillitis. Typhoid may cause caecal perforation, and abdominal tuberculosis may be discovered at laparotomy. Amoebiasis can cause ulcerative colitis-like effects. Preventing and treating infection is an important factor in surgical emergencies such as acute appendicitis or bowel perforation. Despite the rational use of prophylactic and therapeutic antibiotics, postoperative infection remains a common complication of surgery.

Neoplasia

Certain **benign tumours** such as lipomas are common and are excised mainly for cosmetic reasons. Less commonly, benign tumours cause mechanical problems such as obstruction of a hollow viscus or surface blood loss, e.g. gastrointestinal stromal tumours (GIST). Benign endocrine tumours may need removal because of excess hormone secretion (see *Endocrine disorders* later). Finally, benign tumours may be clinically indistinguishable from malignant tumours and are removed or biopsied to obtain a diagnosis.

Malignant tumours may present with signs and symptoms from the primary, the effects of metastases ('secondaries') and sometimes, systemic effects such as cachexia. Malignant tumours are responsible for a large part of the general surgical workload.

Vascular disorders

A tissue or organ becomes **ischaemic** when its arterial blood supply is impaired; **infarction** occurs when cell life cannot be sustained. **Atherosclerosis** progressively narrows arteries often resulting in **chronic ischaemia**, causing symptoms such as angina pectoris or intermittent claudication. It also predisposes to **acute-on-chronic ischaemia** when diseased vessels finally occlude. Other common causes of acute arterial insufficiency are thrombosis, embolism and trauma. Arterial embolism causes acute ischaemia of limbs, intestine or brain; emboli often originate in the heart. If blood supply is restored after a period of ischaemia, further damage can ensue as a result of **reperfusion syndrome**.

When a portion of bowel becomes strangulated, the initial mechanism of tissue damage is venous obstruction and this progresses to arterial ischaemia and infarction.

An **aneurysm** is an abnormal dilatation of an artery resulting from degeneration of connective tissue. This may rupture, thrombose or generate emboli.

Chronic **venous insufficiency** in the lower limb causing local venous hypertension is responsible for the majority of chronic leg ulcers in the West.

Degenerative disorders

This is an inhomogeneous group of conditions characterised by deterioration of body tissues as life progresses. In the musculoskeletal system, **osteoporosis** decreases bone density and impairs its structural integrity, making fragility fractures more likely. Spinal disc and facet joint degeneration is common, causing back pain and disability, and osteoarthritis is widely prevalent in later life: the almost universal musculoskeletal aches and pains are probably caused by degeneration of muscle, tendon, joint and bone.

Other degenerative disorders include age-related retinal macular degeneration, glaucoma, the inherited disorder retinitis pigmentosa, and certain neurological disorders (Alzheimer's, Huntington's and Parkinson's disease, bulbar palsy). Atherosclerosis and aneurysmal arterial diseases are often non-specifically labelled degenerative.

Metabolic disorders

Metabolic disorders may be responsible for stones in the gall bladder (e.g. haemolytic diseases causing pigment stones) or in the urinary tract (e.g. hypercalciuria and hyperuricaemia causing calcium and uric acid stones, respectively). Hypercholesterolaemia is a major factor in atherosclerosis and hypertriglyceridaemia is a rare cause of acute pancreatitis.

Endocrine disorders and hormonal therapy

Hypersecretion of hormones, as in thyrotoxicosis and hyperparathyroidism, may require surgical removal or reduction of glandular tissue. Endocrine tumours, benign and malignant, may present with metabolic abnormalities such as hypercalcaemia caused by a parathyroid adenoma, Cushing's syndrome resulting from an adrenal adenoma or episodic hypertension caused by a phaeochromocytoma.

Diabetes mellitus, particularly when poorly controlled, causes a range of complications of surgical importance, e.g. diabetic foot problems, retinopathy and cataract formation, as well as predisposing to atherosclerosis.

Hormone replacement therapy in postmenopausal women brings mixed benefits: it slows osteoporosis and reduces colorectal cancer risk whilst slightly increasing risk of breast and endometrial cancer. There is also evidence of an increased rate of thromboembolism, as with higher oestrogen-containing oral contraceptive pills.

Other abnormalities of tissue growth

Growth disturbances such as **hyperplasia** (increase in number of cells) and **hypertrophy** (increase in size of cells) may cause surgical problems, in particular benign prostatic hyperplasia, fibroadenosis of the breast and thyroid enlargement (goitre).

In surgery, the term **cyst** imprecisely describes a mass which appears to contain fluid because of characteristic fluctuance and transilluminability. A cyst is defined as a closed sac with a distinct lining membrane that develops abnormally in the body. A variety of pathological processes produce cysts. Most are benign but some cysts may have malignant change in the wall.

Iatrogenic disorders

Iatrogenic damage or injury results from the action of a doctor or other health care worker. It may be an unfortunate outcome of an adequately performed investigation or operation, e.g. perforated colon during colonoscopy or pneumothorax from attempted aspiration of a breast cyst. These are termed **surgical misadventure**. However, if the damage results from a patently wrong procedure, e.g. amputation of the wrong leg or removal of the wrong kidney, then **negligence** is likely to be proven. Such wrong site surgery is easily avoided by preoperative site marking. Other potentially negligent actions include retained surgical swabs after laparotomy, or vascular trauma during central venous line insertion. Complications of bowel surgery such as anastomotic leakage may result from poorly performed surgery but can occur in expert hands; only audited results can demonstrate whether the surgeon is proficient. Wrong drugs or doses are usually iatrogenic. It is unusual for iatrogenic problems to be due simply to one person's failure. More often it is a **system failure**, with inadequate checks and balances in the system.

Drugs, toxins and diet

Problems with prescribed drugs include unavoidable **toxic effects** of certain chemotherapeutic agents, e.g. neutropenia, and the **side-effects** of drugs such as non-steroidal anti-inflammatory drugs (NSAIDs) causing duodenal perforation, or codeine phosphate causing constipation. Drug **allergy, idiosyncrasy** or **anaphylaxis** may result from individual responses to almost any drug, and **interactions** between drugs cause adverse effects; in this respect warfarin is a prime culprit. Maladministration of drugs may also cause problems with, for example, the wrong drug given for intrathecal chemotherapy causing paralysis.

In many countries, venomous creatures such as spiders, snakes or scorpions cause toxic and sometimes fatal harm.

Cigarette **smoking** is the biggest single preventable cause of death and disability in developed countries. Cigarette smoke is highly addictive and contains an array of carcinogens in the tar, the vasoconstrictors nicotine, and carbon monoxide that binds preferentially to haemoglobin. Not surprisingly, smoking is a powerful factor in a huge range of diseases including cardiovascular disorders of heart, limbs and brain, dysplasias and cancers of lung, mouth and larynx, respiratory disorders such as pneumonias, chronic obstructive pulmonary disease (COPD) and emphysema via small airways inflammation, stillbirth and peptic ulcer disease. Smoking compounds the atherogenic effects of diabetes and is also strongly associated with premature skin ageing. Environmental pollution adversely affects health: for example, micro-fine particles produced by diesel engines cause pulmonary inflammation.

Alcohol and substance abuse may have a surgical dimension: alcohol can lead to personal violence or road traffic collisions; cannabis smoke is carcinogenic and causes dysplasias and premalignant lesions of the oral mucosa as well as contributing to mental health problems. Misdirected injection of opioids and other drugs may cause abscesses, false aneurysms and even arterial occlusion.

The so-called 'Western diet', rich in fat and calories and low in vegetables, fruit and fibre, is linked with a range of diseases including colorectal and breast cancers, obesity, dyslipidaemias, diabetes and hypertension. This is particularly so when combined with a lack of exercise. Dietary fibre protects against colorectal adenomas and carcinomas as well as diverticular disease.

Psychogenic disorders

Psychogenic disorders are not often a source of surgical disease but Munchausen syndrome patients may present with abdominal pain and become subjects of repeated laparotomies, psychiatric patients living rough may suffer from exposure and frostbite, and others may repeatedly cause self-harm or swallow foreign bodies, even such items as razor blades or safety pins.

Disorders of function

A range of common disorders are defined by the functional abnormalities they cause, although their pathogenesis often remains ill understood. The gastrointestinal tract is particularly susceptible, with conditions such as idiopathic constipation, irritable bowel syndrome and diverticular disease.

MEDICAL ETHICS AND CONFIDENTIALITY

The term *medical ethics* refers to the universal principles upon which medical decisions should be based, and governs the beliefs and actions that influence the day to day judgements of doctors. Whilst benevolence should govern all medical practice, other factors such as self-interest, money, the distribution of resources and individual technical skills are important motivating factors.

To some extent, the practice of surgery is influenced by the need for self-protection but in trying to avoid litigation, a surgeon may over-treat or over-investigate in ways that are unnecessary and may even be unethical. A degree of self-interest is inevitable but the guiding principle should be that the patient's interests are paramount. Desirable attributes in a surgeon are listed in Box 1.2.

Surgeons generally aspire to practise their craft in line with the principles of the **Hippocratic Oath**. This originated from the Greek School of Medicine around 500 BC and its essence is as follows:

- Doctors must be instructed and then registered to protect the public from amateurs and charlatans
- Medicine is for the benefit of patients, and doctors must avoid doing anything known to cause harm

Box 1.2 Desirable attributes in a surgeon

After Professor George Youngson, Emeritus Prof. of Paediatric Surgery, University of Aberdeen.

- Technical knowledge and clinical experience
- Listening and communication skills with patients, secretary, colleagues and managers
- Qualities of leadership and the ability to work in a team
- Personal attributes—kindness and empathy
- The ability to make reasoned judgements and decisions under pressure, often with incomplete information
- Situation awareness—the ability to collect and synthesise information rapidly
- Problem solving ability—often in situations not previously encountered
- Insight into one's own practice and a willingness to change plans or behaviours if shown to be incorrect. Being prepared to listen and to learn from constructive criticism
- Organisation and planning ability to cope effectively with a heavy workload
- Professional integrity and honesty
- A genuine desire to continue learning and professional development
- Reliability in fulfilling responsibilities and commitments
- The ability to recognise one's own values and principles and understand how they differ from others

- Euthanasia and abortion are prohibited
- Operations and procedures must be performed only by practitioners with appropriate expertise
- Doctors must maintain proper professional relationships with their patients and treatment choices should not be governed by motives of profit or favour
- Doctors should not take advantage of their professional relationships with their patients
- Medical confidentiality must be respected (see below)

Confidentiality

Patients allow the NHS to gather sensitive information about their health and personal matters as part of seeking treatment. They do this in confidence and legitimately expect staff will respect this trust.

In the UK, patient information is held under legal and ethical obligations of confidentiality. This information must not be used or disclosed in a way that might identify a patient without their consent. *Caldicott Guardians* are senior staff in the NHS and social services appointed to protect patient information locally. The doctor's duty of confidence is a legal obligation derived from case law and is a requirement in professional codes of conduct. Even if a patient is unconscious, the duty of confidence is not diminished.

Whilst cases are often discussed over lunch and elsewhere with colleagues, this should not be done in a public place. When patients are discussed at meetings, identification data should be concealed and written notes about patients should not be left lying around or taken from the hospital except using official channels, for example, during patient transfer.

Do not resuscitate (DNR) orders

A DNR order on a patient's file means that doctors are not required to resuscitate a patient if their heart stops. It is designed to prevent unnecessary suffering and potential side-effects such as pain, broken ribs, ruptured spleen or brain damage. The British Medical Association and the Royal College of Nursing say that DNR orders can be issued **only** after discussion with patients or family, difficult though this may be. Decisions should not be made by junior doctors alone but in consultation with seniors. The most difficult cases are those involving patients who know they are going to die and are suffering pain or other severe symptoms but who could live for months.

Guidelines for when a DNR may be issued:

- If a patient's condition is such that resuscitation is unlikely to succeed
- If a mentally competent patient has consistently stated or recorded they do not want to be resuscitated
- If an advance notice or living will says the patient does not want to be resuscitated
- If successful resuscitation would not be in the patient's best interest because it would lead to a very poor quality of life

In the UK, NHS Trust Hospitals must agree explicit resuscitation policies that respect patients' rights and are readily available to patients, families and carers; policies must be regularly monitored.

COMMUNICATION

WITH PATIENTS

Doctor–patient relationships are best learnt by following good examples in the clinic and ward in an apprenticeship model. Patients are vulnerable, often with unpleasant symptoms and usually with little understanding of anatomy, physiology or pathology. They rarely understand the likely progress of a disease or its treatment and may have been conditioned by the media to expect miracle cures or to believe that the latest technology is what they need. Patients take in only about 10% of what is said during a consultation, but this can be improved in the right setting and with reinforcement. Important messages need to be given in comfortable surroundings, without giving the impression the doctor is in a rush, perhaps with family present and with a nurse who can later ensure messages have been understood.

Doctors are in a privileged position, able to make decisions on a patient's behalf that can have dramatic effects on their life and that of their family. Patients these days generally wish to know more about their condition, but can then take greater responsibility for it than in the old days of the paternalistic doctor. Thus an effective doctor–patient relationship involves not only taking an accurate history but also intelligent listening to discover what patients know, or think they know, about their health and likely treatments, and responding to their concerns in ways they can understand. A good interview also involves imagining 'the third eye', how both sides of the consultation might appear to an observer. Patients frequently complain, with good reason, that they 'don't know what is going on'. They pick up bits of information that may be inaccurate, so doctors should anticipate what they should explain to patients and families and give information in a timely fashion.

During the process of diagnosis and treatment, there is often uncertainty and incomplete information, so it is valuable to explain at intervals the stage reached, both to the patient and, with the patient's permission, to relatives. Where there are different treatment options, a balanced view of the alternatives should be given, perhaps with some statistics, but when the doctor has reason to prefer one approach, this should be explained too, and then the patient can make a considered choice. It can be easy to persuade patients to undergo treatment—after all, you are the expert in their eyes—but trust, respect and empathy teach that patients may wish to reflect at leisure. Except in emergencies, patients should be able to go away and consider options rather than have to sign a consent form just before treatment. They may even wish to take a second opinion if choices are uncertain or potentially life-changing; this should be welcomed rather than discouraged. By helping patients understand their condition, their self-management will be more effective. Similarly, key factors such as diet or smoking habits can be discussed in an atmosphere of trust with more hope of success.

Palliative care

Sometimes cure is not possible. Then quality of life may become the goal, with palliative treatment being offered. Patients generally want to know what will happen, including their mode of dying. Whilst this can be hard to predict, they need to know their symptoms, particularly pain, will be managed effectively and that they will be looked after. Experience teaches it is usually impossible to say with accuracy when a patient will die except a few days before it will happen, so it is unwise to predict life span except in general terms.

Breaking bad news

All doctors in clinical practice experience the need to break bad news, such as an unfavourable outcome, unsatisfactory care, a cancer diagnosis or a poor prognosis. It is an event doctors tend to remember and a moment in the patient or relative's life they will never forget.

Ideally, bad news should be conveyed by the most senior member of the team but in reality, bad things often happen at night, often in the A&E department, and the most junior doctor is the one on the spot. Discuss what is to be said with your seniors even under these circumstances wherever possible. The following general points apply:

- Bad news is private. Find a quiet space, preferably an office with chairs (you don't need a desk)
- Avoid hiding behind jargon: 'the metastatic nature of the neoplasm makes it inoperable' is useless. 'I'm sorry to say that the cancer has spread and an operation won't help' is better
- Give time and space; turn off pagers and phones if possible
- Don't be defensive and don't be afraid to express regret
- Avoid filling the silence of grief with continuous chatter
- Allow time for questions. If you don't know the answer, say so and try to find out
- Always offer another meeting, ideally with the head of the team
- Many patients/families will wish to discuss what has been imparted with their family doctor, so it is vital that you get all information to the GP before that visit

COMMUNICATING WITH COLLEAGUES

Communicating with colleagues involves speaking, both face to face and on the telephone (Box 1.3), and writing (handwriting, dictating, typing, emailing) patient notes, information letters to patient or family practitioners, e.g. after an outpatient consultation, referral letters, discharge summaries, reports and presentations for local or larger-scale medical meetings. All of these need to be honest, accurate and timely, particularly when communicating patient information. Remember, recipients are entitled to rely on what you have written in their later treatment of a patient. Also, any written information may be called in evidence in a court of law should something go wrong later. Patient notes must *never* be altered later, although rarely, amendments may be *added* provided they are signed and dated.

Hospital doctors work in teams where it is important to know one's responsibilities and those of everybody else, and to understand when to call for help in good time. Changes in a patient's condition usually need to be passed on to other team members. If you have made a mistake, admit it early and do everything you can to mitigate it.

Box 1.3 Effective telephone consultation and handover

When you need to consult a consultant or colleague by telephone about a patient, particularly during unsocial hours, you must clarify details yourself before phoning. Think through the case, pinpointing key elements listed below:

- On phoning, state your name and status (on-call SpR for instance) and say at the outset what you think you want—whether advice or for the consultant to come in
- Summarise the case succinctly, visualising how your description appears to the listener
- When did the problem start (day, time)?
- What circumstances necessitated the patient coming to hospital?
- What was the patient's state on arrival (conscious/unconscious; wounds or bleeding; level of pain; resuscitation status)?
- Did you examine the patient and establish the signs or were they reported to you?
- Is there any relevant past history?
- What has progress been since arrival?
- What investigations have been ordered and what results do you have so far?
- Are any other specialists involved, e.g. plastics or orthopaedics?
- Finally, indicate again what you want the consultant to do

With diminishing junior doctors' hours, it is vital to have structured *handover* of patients to the incoming team at the end of shifts and at weekends and holidays, including especially details of ill patients and those with complex management problems and any agreed plans for them.

Communication via the clinical record

Reduced junior hospital doctors' hours make it imperative to keep the written records for every patient up to date, including management plans and what to do if predictable changes occur. Date and legibly sign each entry giving your name in capitals and grade, record important test results and write instructions for antibiotic and DVT prophylaxis. In high operative risk patients, seniors should document discussions before surgery. After operation, write or type an operation note with clear postoperative instructions so these are immediately available to recovery and ward staff.

Document details of any discussions with patient and relatives—particularly about poor prognosis or withdrawal of active treatment and who has been told about this or about a diagnosis of malignancy. Regarding a discharge summary, ensure all investigation results have been checked and the diagnosis and future plans have been recorded and send it immediately on discharge. If the patient died, record the cause of death in the notes as it is written on the certificate and inform the family doctor.

EVIDENCE-BASED MEDICINE AND GUIDELINES

History

Evidence-based medicine (EBM) as now understood really began when Professor Archie Cochrane, a Scottish epidemiologist, published his book *Effectiveness and Efficiency: Random Reflections on Health Services* in 1972 and continued with his later advocacy of its principles. EBM has gradually gained political support and acceptance within the medical profession. EBM calls into question the traditional belief that 'we've always based our practice on science'. Cochrane's work has been recognised by the proliferation of Cochrane Centres and the international Cochrane Collaboration, all devoted to meticulously evaluating evidence and promoting its use.

The aim of evidence-based medicine (EBM) is to apply best scientific evidence to clinical decision making. It relies on critical assessment of published evidence about risks and benefits of treatments (or lack of treatment) and of diagnostic tests. Only between 50% and 80% of the volume of medical treatments are evidence based, with better evidence available for more common treatments. Statements by medical experts are seen as the least valid form of evidence, but evidence-based practice is not relevant where imponderables such as quality of life judgements are involved. **Evidence-based guidelines (EBG)** have an appeal to health economists, policymakers and managers as they help to measure performance and perhaps justify rationing or centralising resources.

Austin Bradford Hill, the grandfather of modern medical research, who was fundamental in discovering the link between smoking and lung cancer, produced a set of guidelines, as given in Box 1.4, for assessing *causality*, i.e. the relationship between an exposure and an outcome, and these remain the foundation of evidence-based medicine today.

Cherry-picking the evidence versus systematic review

Cherry-picking is a dubious means of reinforcing what you already believe, the very opposite of systematic review. It involves relying only on published work that supports your view and finding reasons to ignore what goes against it. The solution is a process of systematic review as conducted by the Cochrane Collaboration. Their methodologies were largely established at McMaster University. The term EBM first appeared in 1992 and now journals devoted to the subject include the BMJ's *Clinical Evidence*, the *Journal of Evidence-Based Healthcare* and *Evidence Based Health Policy*, all co-founded by Anna Donald, an Australian pioneer.

Evidence-based medicine encourages clinicians to integrate valid and useful scientific evidence into their clinical expertise. Using systematic reviews, meta-analyses, risk-benefit analyses and randomised controlled trials (RCTs), EBM aims that health professionals make 'conscientious, explicit, and judicious use of current best evidence' in everyday practice. Systematic review of published research studies is a very important method of evaluating treatments. An explicit search strategy is used finding relevant data, both published and raw and unpublished. The methodological quality of each study is evaluated, ideally blind to the results. Alternative treatments are compared, and then a critical, weighted summary is given. This thorough sifting of information often reveals large knowledge gaps and sometimes grossly flawed 'best practices'; it has saved numerous lives without undertaking new research studies. Muir Gray has commented 'advances will be made through clean, clear information'.

The Cochrane Collaboration is perhaps the best known, most rigorous and respected organisation providing systematic reviews. Once the best evidence has been assessed, treatment is rated as 'likely to be beneficial', 'likely to be harmful', or 'evidence did not indicate benefit or harm'. A 2007 analysis of 1016 systematic reviews from all 50 Cochrane Collaboration Review Groups found 44% of the interventions beneficial, 7% harmful and 49% where the evidence did not support benefit or harm. 96% recommended further research.

When it comes to new or radical ideas, well-trained experts using clinical common sense should be able to make rational judgements about what is likely to be true; the more unlikely the claims for a new treatment, the higher must be the standard of proper evidence.

Box 1.4 Guidelines for assessing the relationship between an exposure and an outcome

- A strong and consistent association, specific to the problem being studied
- The supposed cause must come before the possible effect
- There should ideally be a biological gradient or dose-response effect
- The association should be consistent with what is already known or at least not completely at odds with it
- It should be biologically plausible

Longitudinal or cohort studies

For predicting prognosis, the highest level of evidence is a systemic review of *inception cohort studies*, i.e. groups of patients assembled near the onset of the disorder. These groups are followed over years to determine how variables such as smoking habits, exercise, occupation and geography may affect outcome. Prospective studies take years to perform but are valued more than retrospective studies which are more likely to generate bias.

Ranking the quality of evidence (Box 1.5)

The strongest evidence for therapeutic interventions is by systematic review of randomised, double- or triple-blind, placebo-controlled trials with allocation concealment and complete follow-up, in a homogeneous patient population and medical condition. In contrast, patient testimonials, case reports, and even expert opinion have lesser value because of the placebo effect, biases inherent in observation and reporting, and personal and institutional biases.

A series of classifications of the strength of different types of evidence have been fashioned, grading them according to their freedom from biases that plague medical research; all are based around the same descending hierarchy:

Box 1.5 How Cochrane Centres evaluate evidence

Note that the hierarchy of evidence relates to the strength of the literature and not necessarily to its clinical importance.

1. Strength of evidence

a. *Level of evidence*: i.e. is the evidence a true measure of the benefit of an intervention? In descending order of reliability:
   - — Cochrane (or equivalent quality) systematic reviews of all relevant randomised controlled trials
   - — At least one well-conducted randomised controlled trial
   - — A non-randomised trial assigning participants to a treatment group alternately or by date or time of arrival, for example
   - — Non-randomised studies where a control group ran concurrently with an intervention group
   - — Non-randomised studies where intervention effects are compared with historical data
   - — Single case studies
   - — Opinion of experienced experts—'conventional wisdom'

b. *Quality of evidence*: determined by how well the study methods minimise bias

c. *Statistical precision*: the degree of certainty about whether a measured effect truly exists

2. Size of effect

For clinically relevant benefits or harms, how far away is the outcome of the intervention from 'no apparent effect'?

3. Relevance of the evidence

How appropriate is the outcome for the health care problem studied, and how useful is it for measuring the benefits (or harms) of the treatment? To which groups or subgroups of patients may the results apply?

4. The likely range of the true effect

Studies that are well designed and carried out can show unreliable results because of chance. **Confidence interval** (CI) describes the likely range of the true effect. For example, a study may show that 40% (95% CI 30% to 50%) of people appear to be helped by a treatment; we can thus be 95% certain the true effect lies between 30% and 50%.

- Systematic reviews of randomised controlled trials (RCTs)
- Individual RCTs
- Controlled observational studies—cohort and case control studies
- Uncontrolled observational studies and case reports
- Established practice and expert opinion (not to be confused with personal experience, sometimes dubbed eminence-based medicine). Expert opinion may be the best guide in the absence of good research evidence

Other classifications of quality of evidence

For a review of classifications of evidence, see:
http://www.patient.co.uk/doctor/Different-Levels-of-Evidence-%28Critical-Reading%29.htm

For a detailed discussion of the quality of evidence for different purposes, see:
www.nice.org.uk/niceMedia/docs/grading_evidence.pdf

Quality and limitations of clinical trials

Trials must now be registered in advance: the Declaration of Helsinki 2008 requires that every clinical trial be registered in a publicly accessible database before recruitment of the first subject. The International Committee of Medical Journal Editors refuses to publish clinical trial results if the trial was not recorded in this way. This should eliminate the bias inherent in the failure to publish negative trials.

In 1993, 30 medical journal editors, clinical trialists, epidemiologists and methodologists met in Ottawa to develop a new scale to assess the quality of randomised controlled trial (RCT) reports. This eventually resulted in the Consolidated Standards of Reporting Trials (CONSORT) Statement, published in 1996 and now largely adhered to by respected medical journals (http://www.consort-statement.org/home/). Cochrane adheres to similar standards and employs software 'RevMan' to help reviewers evaluate published studies.

RESOURCES

- Cochrane Library: http://www.thecochranelibrary.com/view/0/index.html
- UK National Institute for Health and Clinical Excellence (NICE): http://www.nice.org.uk/
- NHS search engine for Evidence in Health and Social Care (from NICE): https://www.evidence.nhs.uk/

Guidelines

Clinical guidelines, practice policies, protocols and codes of practice are locally or more widely published mechanisms aimed at harmonising processes of care using best practice. Some are produced by surgical societies such as the Association of Surgeons of GB &I (ASGBI). Guidelines should be just that—providing a structure rather than absolute ways to proceed in every case; they may be varied if clinical conditions dictate. Guidelines should have an evidence basis or be of proven clinical effectiveness and need regular review as evidence accumulates. Local guidelines are a natural outcome of clinical audit studies (see p. 13 below).

KEEPING UP TO DATE: CONTINUING MEDICAL EDUCATION

Clinicians are quite properly expected to keep up with current developments and to demonstrate this to be revalidated. Surgical knowledge and wisdom can be acquired by reading, from seniors in clinic and on ward rounds, by discussion at local and regional meetings and by attending courses. Meetings may include journal clubs, case presentations, reviews of specific topics, and presentation of research or audit projects. Broad national update meetings are valuable and in the UK, include the ASGBI and speciality meetings such as the Vascular Society and the British Orthopaedic Association. Meetings are a forum for trainees to present their work, learn from other presentations and find out what is current from colleagues. Surgeons in the UK are required to keep a log-book record of their educational activities to demonstrate their continued learning and this document forms part of regular appraisal and revalidation.

CONSENT TO TREATMENT

Treatment against a patient's will is only rarely justifiable. Clearing the airways of someone about to choke to death who is irrational because of impaired consciousness can easily be justified on the grounds that the patient would have wanted it if fully rational. UK common law holds that an adult of sound mind has the right to determine what is done with his body and a surgeon who performs an operation without consent commits an assault in the eyes of the law.

When is consent necessary?

Ideally, medical treatment should not proceed without first obtaining the patient's consent. Consent may be *expressed*, or it may be *implied*, as when a patient presents for examination and acquiesces in the suggested procedure. Expressed permission can be based on an oral or a written agreement. Most invasive investigations (such as upper GI endoscopy or arteriography) and any surgical operation should be preceded by written consent, ideally well in advance to give the patient time to think it over. If oral consent alone has been obtained, then a note should be made in the patient's record.

A doctor may proceed without consent if the patient's balance of mind is disturbed or if the patient is incapable of giving consent because of unconsciousness. The same principles apply if the patient is a minor, but it is sensible to seek consent from responsible relatives or to check with colleagues that the planned action is in the patient's best interest. Opinions should be recorded in the notes before action is taken.

The unconscious patient

Under the *necessity principle*, a surgeon is justified in treating a patient without expressed consent if what he seeks to protect is more valuable than the wrongful act, i.e. treating without consent, provided there is no objection to treatment. Treatment must be no more extensive than is essential and procedures not needed for the patient's survival must not be performed. For example, a diseased testis could be removed during a hernia repair but sterilising a patient during a Caesarean section without consent constitutes assault.

Ambiguous wording on consent forms requiring a patient to agree to any operation the surgeon considers necessary is regarded by the courts as completely worthless. For this reason a model consent form was produced by the NHS Executive in 1990 to be used throughout the health services.

Practical aspects of consent for treatment

In British law, there is no such thing as informed consent. Surgeons like to feel they obtain informed consent after explaining to the patient in non-technical language the nature, purpose and risks of the proposed investigation or treatment, together with alternatives and the likely outcome of treatment. The patient must be capable of understanding the explanation and if this is not the case then informed consent has not been obtained. It follows that consent cannot be obtained from patients who are unconscious or of unsound mind.

Box 1.6 The informed consent process

The informed consent process should include:

- A description of the procedure or operation and anaesthetic
- Why the procedure is recommended and the risks and benefits
- The degree of severity and likelihood of complications
- Treatment alternatives with related risks and benefits
- Probable consequences of declining the recommended or alternative therapies
- Name of doctor conducting the procedure and the anaesthetic
- Other doctors performing tasks related to the procedure

Obtaining consent (Box 1.6)

Consent should be obtained by a doctor sufficiently knowledgeable to explain the treatment, any alternatives, the likely outcome and any significant risks. Sometimes trained nurses obtain a first stage consent which is confirmed by a doctor later.

The types and level of risk that have to be discussed are not well defined, but a risk of complication or potential failure to treat the condition of 5–10% should certainly be discussed. Operation-specific or disease-specific risks must be explained (e.g. facial nerve damage in parotid surgery, hypoparathyroidism following thyroid surgery) and the discussion detailed in the records. General risks such as DVT or pneumonia are not usually discussed but this does place doubt on whether such consent is truly informed.

Discussion prior to consent should occur in an unhurried manner, giving the patient time to absorb the information, to question the doctor obtaining consent and to indicate treatments he does not want. The patient may wish to discuss aspects of what is proposed with family or friends before consenting. In patients incapable of giving consent it is customary to obtain consent from a near relative. Whilst not essential in law, this represents good practice.

Most patients do not read the forms they sign before undergoing treatment; more than half do not understand them; and only a quarter of forms include all the data needed to make an informed decision. The US Department of Veteran's Affairs has adopted an electronic informed-consent software program with a digital pad to sign, with details stored in their medical record. The program, known as iMedConsent, includes a library of anatomical diagrams and explanations at easy reading level for 2000+ procedures in 30+ specialties. The process was initially slow to perform but soon became quick. Patients having elective procedures could now gain all the information they needed in advance and it was easy to check they had understood it. The main disadvantage is that these privately produced programs are expensive.

Consent in children

Consent can be obtained from children aged 16 and over and occasionally in those under 16. It is always sensible to liaise with parents wherever possible in young people aged 17 and 18. In the absence of parents, another relative or person 'in loco parentis' can give consent for children.

For children in care, the local authority usually has full parental rights and the director of social services or deputy needs to sign the consent form. If the child is in voluntary care, the parents still act as guardians and their consent should be obtained.

Jehovah's Witnesses

Adult Jehovah's Witnesses usually refuse blood or blood product transfusion even in an extreme emergency because of their interpretation of part of the Bible. If permission to transfuse is withheld then blood should not be given. Failure to respect the patient's wish may result in an accusation of battery. The moral dilemma of allowing a patient to die when blood transfusion is likely to prevent death is uncomfortable but the law is clear. General advice is that a surgeon cannot refuse to treat simply because the patient imposes conditions on that treatment, although it may be possible to transfer the patient to a compliant surgeon's care. In these circumstances, it is wise to interview the patient in the presence of a witness and explain the risks. The discussion should be noted and the witness should sign the hospital record.

In children of Jehovah's Witnesses the position is different. If a blood or blood product transfusion is needed to save the life of a child or to prevent harm, the transfusion can be given and defended in law by claiming that the decision was taken in the best interests of the child. If parental consent is withheld and there is ample time, the child can be made a ward of court, but this is not essential to obtain consent. If the decision to give blood is made, a second medical opinion confirming the need should be obtained if time allows. It is important to realise that a child subjected to transfusion against parental wishes may be rejected by the parents.

CLINICAL GOVERNANCE AND CLINICAL AUDIT

Clinical governance is a systematic approach to preserving and advancing the quality of patient care within a health system. Since the 1970s, there has been a growing realisation that looking critically at the way we run our clinical practice and then taking active steps to move ahead is much more effective than simply following time-honoured practices or even opening new avenues of research. In the UK, this movement is now universal but with varying degrees of success. Clinical governance starts with the mindset that the *quality of care* matters; it embodies a range of activities described here and elsewhere in this chapter. See also NHS Scotland clinical governance: http://www.clinicalgovernance.scot.nhs.uk/section1/introduction.asp.

Management attitude to quality of care

Health service managers have to keep quality of care high on their long list of priorities and facilitate clinicians' initiatives.

Education and training of clinical staff

Thorough and well-rounded teaching in medical and nursing school, including anatomy and surgery, is the starting point. Training posts then need to offer a wide range of experience in an apprenticeship model, including step-by-step learning of procedures to back up continuing medical education as well as specific courses such as Advanced Trauma Life Support (ATLS). During training, good behaviours, attitudes and judgement can be acquired (see attributes of a good surgeon earlier). All clinicians need to remain open-minded to change and remember it is their professional duty to remain up to date.

Clinical audit

Clinical audit reviews clinical performance against agreed standards, refining clinical practice and then re-auditing—a cyclical process of improving quality.

Clinical effectiveness

Clinical effectiveness studies evaluate the extent to which an intervention works, its efficiency, safety, appropriateness and value for money. Studies of this type can be instructive and worthwhile for trainees to undertake.

Research and development

Professional practice can change in the light of good research evidence, provided it can be implemented effectively. Evidence-based medicine involves critical appraisal of the literature and development of evidence-based guidelines, protocols and implementation strategies from research.

Clinical performance

Poor performance and poor practice often thrive behind closed doors but can be revealed by a local climate of openness; this also demonstrates the organisation meets the needs of its population. In surgery, trouble may come to light through morbidity and mortality meetings, clinical audit, via patient complaints or by 'whistle blowing', and these should provide the motor for change. Critical incident meetings, for example, can thoroughly examine particular adverse events and recommend change.

Nationally in the UK, the National Patient Safety Agency (http://www.npsa.nhs.uk/) 'informs, supports and influences healthcare organisations and individuals' by handling patient safety incidents, by running national independent Confidential Enquiries (NCEPOD in surgery and anaesthesia), by encouraging ethical research, and by developing and implementing safety recommendations, advice and strategies. Through the National Clinical Assessment Service (http://www.ncas.npsa.nhs.uk/), it endeavours to solve concerns about the performance of health practitioners short of referral to the General Medical Council.

Risk management

This is a prospective process to identify hazards that could cause harm, decide who might be harmed and how, then evaluate the risks and decide on precautions. Risks in a health service include: risks to patients, risks to practitioners and risks to the organisation itself. Recognising in advance where particular risks lie is the first step to minimising those risks. Areas of potentially high risk include:

The elderly: surgeons deal with an increasingly elderly population. The likelihood of co-morbid disease is higher, although chronological age by itself is less important than biological age

Emergency surgery: this carries a higher risk of complications and death than elective surgery. Patients may be more physiologically disrupted or not fully resuscitated, intervention may be required out-of-hours when the ideal mix of staff is not available; investigations such as CT scanning may also not be available

Day surgery: preoperative assessment can preselect patients for day surgery and minimise risk

Critically ill patients: these patients need optimising before surgery, often with shared care with a senior anaesthetist, physician or other specialist. More preoperative investigations and resuscitation may be needed, perhaps in an ICU or HDU. The initial surgical approach may become a damage limitation exercise with more realistic expectations about outcome

Operative risk assessment: the American Association of Anaesthesiologists (ASA) grade scheme gives anaesthetist and surgeon a subjective idea of how sick the patient is and the likely outcome.

Information management

Information management is vital to facilitate good, effective and economical practice. For example, high quality and available patient notes, systems for ordering laboratory and imaging tests and receiving results, accurate and prompt discharge summaries, easy outpatient booking, good feedback to family practitioners and reliable A&E systems. Hand-written methods have been employed for many years, with recent attempts to employ computers to streamline processes. These have been successful in countries such as Denmark, but in the UK, system design has largely been driven by computer companies rather than clinicians, so systems are often unfriendly and ineffective. However, the use of individual smart cards for patients to hold their own records, and easily portable devices such as the iPad hold promise for the future, provided clinicians take sufficient interest in their development.

Surgical (clinical) audit

'Research is concerned with discovering the right thing to do; audit with ensuring that it is done right.'
Richard Smith BMJ

There is a tendency to be over-optimistic or even defensive about one's own practice. Yet patients, referring doctors, medical defence organisations (who defend the professional reputations of members when their clinical performance is called into question) and those paying for health care (governments and their agents and private insurers) are entitled to know that the quality of care provided in a given unit is up to standard. Examining morbidity and mortality at regular meetings within a unit ('significant event' reviews) are important but suffer from inherent weaknesses such as defensiveness, incomplete data and rivalry. These meetings usually fail to address overarching problems such as wound infection rates or aspects of care from the patient's point of view, such as delayed treatment, off-hand consultations, poor pain control and failure to give explanations. It is well established that medical errors are generally more likely to be due to a system failure than an individual error and system errors are unlikely to be discovered by these morbidity and mortality meetings.

Clinical audit is a means by which clinicians can be collectively accountable for the care they provide and demonstrate its quality to outsiders. It requires a mechanism for scrutiny of each other's work in a non-threatening and constructive manner or else it would not function. In brief, a group of clinicians examines a topic of concern and agrees in advance what are acceptable standards of practice or outcomes, ideally based on published norms. In other words, they establish and sign up to a set of standards for **indicator based audit**. The process embodies specific objectives, accepting peer review and being committed to change should weaknesses be revealed.

Once a topic is agreed, an **audit cycle** can begin with a pilot project on a small number of subjects, perhaps 20. A questionnaire is designed which ideally is capable of being completed retrospectively by non-clinical staff from hospital notes. With the pilot results, methods are refined and a larger scale project undertaken. Results are analysed by the group and necessary changes, and how these should be implemented, agreed. This is the most thorny aspect of clinical audit and the most difficult to achieve. Once the necessary changes have been implemented, the same audit needs to be repeated after a defined interval (completing the audit cycle) to bring the process up to a quality assurance mechanism.

Clinicians do need to be trained in audit methods and helped to design audits that are useful and sound. It is best to start with a simple project, such as, for example, what proportion of the entries in the notes is clearly signed.

Medical research versus medical audit

Medical research is employed on a one-off basis to determine scientifically how interventions affect outcomes. Clinical audit measures how effectively aspects of good health care are put into practice. Every doctor can improve the way patients are cared for by critically examining local practices against current standards using audit methods.

Clinical audit and research share common features including defining explicitly what is to be measured and analysing and interpreting the data without bias. Audit can improve understanding of system failures, help develop guidelines and identify areas for education and training.

Carrying out an audit (Box 1.7)

Selecting topics for audit means taking into consideration how frequent the condition or treatment is, how high the risk to patients is, whether there is doubt about which treatment is the best, where care crosses specialty boundaries and finally, any topics of particular concern to clinicians or professions allied to medicine.

Single subject audits usually require no more than 50 patients to reveal problems and plan improvements. Subjects focus on aspects of the process of care (including resources employed), appropriateness of tests or treatments or outcomes of treatment. They may include subjects such as adequacy of pain relief from the patient's point of view or,

Box 1.7 Key elements of criterion-based or indicator-based audit

- Looks in a structured way at a small problematic aspect of care
- Criteria need to be agreed in advance by all clinicians involved
- Time is needed to plan and pilot the audit, discuss the results, implement change then re-audit after a period
- Whether criteria have been met must be reliably retrievable by non-medical audit officers
- Recognition that there may be more than one valid way of achieving a solution

from the family doctor's point of view, how long a discharge summary takes to be received.

The group then develops an audit indicator which has objective, measurable standards of care and specifies a percentage of cases expected to reach the standard. For example, perhaps 100% of patients referred for palliative radiotherapy for lung cancer should receive their first treatment in less than 10 days after referral, or wound infection rates after appendicectomy should be no more than 3%. These indicators (known as **criteria**) can be based on published results, on previous local results or on standards the group hopes to achieve after running a pilot study.

Deficiencies usually turn out to be due to **system failure** such as poor coordination between departments (e.g. pre-assessment between anaesthesia and surgery) or poor communication between clinicians, with people not being informed about what is happening when. These factors are usually more important than lack of resources or personnel or poor individual performance. Improvements may result from simple organisational changes.

Peer group review of medical audit data

Using audit indicators has advantages over raw data analysis or informal morbidity meetings. As standards have of necessity been agreed, any numbers of cases can be screened to select out for further discussion only those that vary from the standard. In itself, the process of refining and employing audit indicators is an educational experience that encourages self-analysis by individuals, departments, units or regions.

Examples of how clinical audit can improve the quality of care:

- Reduction of risk of morbidity or mortality
- Improved effectiveness of care such as streamlined processes of treatment
- Improvement in diagnosis—availability, appropriateness or quality
- Improved timing of care—reduced delay, better planning, efficient use of facilities
- Better use of resources—equipment, beds, support services, money
- Consumer satisfaction—patients and referring doctors
- Access to care—availability of diagnostic services and treatment
- Documentation and records—improved recording of the process of care
- Identifying educational needs by audit activity—e.g. pain management

Confidential enquiry into perioperative deaths (CEPOD)

The pilot study was designed in 1983 jointly by the ASGBI and the Association of Anaesthetists to examine perioperative deaths and the delivery of surgical and anaesthetic care in Britain. This was followed by a review of all deaths within 30 days of surgery (all specialties) in three English Regions for the whole of 1986: 500 000 operations were reviewed with 4000 deaths (0.8%); 79% of deaths occurred in patients over 65 years of age. More information is available from: http://www.ncepod.org.uk/, including all published reports from 1987 onwards.

Educational lessons from CEPOD

Many of the substandard practices identified could be put down to a lack of education or training in particular fields. These included:

- When and how to investigate
- When to give prophylaxis against infection and thromboembolism
- When to delay operation in order to resuscitate
- When not to operate
- When to call the consultant
- Management of head injuries
- Managing co-morbid disease and the elderly
- Keeping accurate records
- Safe use of local anaesthetics
- Local protocols for referral, handover and transfer
- Organising effective audit or morbidity and mortality meetings

RESEARCH IN SURGERY

How are potentially improved methods evaluated?

When new surgical techniques appear they must be dispassionately evaluated and compared with existing practices, ideally by people with no vested interest. For a new technique to be introduced, it must be at least as good as existing methods or better in some way, for example, in achieving oncological clearance. New methods should be easily and quickly learnt—an operation that requires a learning curve of 500 patients is little use to those 500. Methods need to be reasonably economical in equipment and in operating time and high-level hazards should be no greater than existing operations. While this may seem utopian, 'the greatest uncontrolled medical experiment of all', namely the introduction of laparoscopic cholecystectomy, was undoubtedly at the expense of a massive increase in common bile duct injuries. The proper view should be that the safety of the many outweighs the foibles of the few.

It was encouraging that laparoscopic hernia repair was not allowed to escape peer review in the same way, with multicentre trials comparing the existing standard of Lichtenstein open repair with the prospective standard of laparoscopic repair. However, laparoscopic colorectal surgery is in danger of escaping proper scrutiny, being carried along by enthusiasts and even NICE. There is no evidence that the operations are being more thoroughly performed, little evidence of reduced pain and rather soft evidence of more rapid discharge from hospital.

Design of research and experiments

All British health authorities have to establish an Ethics Committee charged with examining and sanctioning each research project before it is launched. They help ensure that all projects are ethical and can be justified and that the methodology is sound. Among medical members, these committees generally include lawyers, ethicists, statisticians and lay members.

Clinical trials

Drug trials

Once a potential drug has been identified, say from a likely plant molecule, a cell receptor that might be influenced or a modification of an old drug, it is tested for toxicity in animals and to see if it works. Then Phase I trials 'first in man' are performed on a few healthy young people. This is for toxicity, excretion rates and pathways, etc. If this works, Phase II trials in perhaps 200 people with the relevant illness are performed as 'proof of concept' to see if the drug is effective and to work out the dose. Many drugs fail at this point. Then Phase III trials are performed in hundreds or thousands of patients. These are randomised, blinded trials comparing the new drug against placebo or comparable treatments. More data on efficacy and safety is collected. Once successful trials are complete, the company applies for a licence to sell the drug. After it reaches market, the company and others usually conduct further trials and studies to look out for unnoticed side-effects. However, trials do not tell the whole story: in the 1960s thalidomide, a very effective drug for morning sickness, had not been tested in pregnancy, and this led to many avoidable birth deformities in countries where it had been licensed.

Trial design and conduct

For a surgical trial, background work establishes the depth of current knowledge and the need for a trial. The hypothesis to be tested should be defined before designing the study and perhaps the need for a pilot study.

Generally, *prospective studies* ensure that data are accrued chronologically and that patients are entered into the trial as they become available. However, it may take months (or even years) to recruit enough patients to make the data meaningful.

Retrospective analyses of previously recorded data are open to criticism because of the lack of an appropriate control group and the difficulty of extracting complete data from case notes. Despite flaws, a retrospective study may show the need for a prospective study, give some idea of the likely results and allow the trial design to be streamlined.

Longitudinal studies examine the effects of therapy on a predetermined population or epidemiological changes in a population.

Cross-sectional studies take a 'snap shot' at a particular time and place; these are most commonly used to monitor the incidence and location of diseases and treatment.

For most trials, computer randomisation removes the natural tendency for bias to affect results and is particularly relevant when comparing new treatments with tried and tested techniques. This is often 'blinded' such that only the patient (single blind), or neither the patient nor the investigator (double blind), knows which arm an individual has been allocated to. Any therapeutic effect of placebos is maximized if patients are unaware of the nature of their treatment. The double blind technique attempts to eliminate personal preferences of the doctor for a particular treatment. To study the effects of a treatment in a particular environment, like must be compared with like and a case control study employed. Matching of individuals for characteristics such as weight, sex, age and disease severity allow comparisons to be made when looking for small differences between groups.

Once the study design has been established, an achievable cohort size must be identified which has sufficient power to show differences between treatments and organise data collection, storage and analysis. After that, it is necessary to establish inclusion and exclusion criteria, the population size and characteristics to be studied and then to determine how the data will be analysed and presented statistically.

Specialised personnel, equipment and training must be funded. Worthwhile research is expensive and should not be undertaken simply for the sake of the CV.

PATIENT SAFETY

Dealing with an adverse event

- Apologise to the patient for the failure as soon as the error is recognised
- Report to your consultant and other responsible people
- Take steps to correct the error and make sure you see the patient often
- If an official complaint is made, patient letters are usually sent to the hospital manager then to a complaints officer
- If asked to comment, provide full and honest detail
- If legal action is threatened, contact your medical insurance society
- Adverse outcomes should be discussed at local meetings to seek system problems

Introduction

'First do no harm', an aphorism attributed to Thomas Sydenham, an English physician in the mid-1600s, is sound advice for surgeons too. All surgical treatments should be thought of in terms of their potential harm as well as benefit.

Some hazards are intrinsic to the surgical procedure or disease and are unavoidable. Other hazards are avoidable, and systems need to be designed to assist. Furthermore, the surgeon's prime responsibility is to the patient so, for example, prioritising an operation should be based on need not on financial or managerial grounds, although surgeons have responsibilities to balance demands as far as possible.

To Err is Human is an influential report published by the US Institute of Medicine in 1999 that is well worth reading. It called for a national effort to make health care safer.

General hazards

The two most common sources of error leading to patient harm are communication failures and drug prescribing errors. Some 26% of 100 consecutive cases referred to the Medical Protection Society resulted from communication failure. There need to be explicit systems for dealing with risky situations, for example, informing seniors about sick patients, handing over properly to staff coming on duty, knowing who to call about patients that have 'gone off' during unsocial hours. This applies especially to anyone not familiar with the patient's current state, particularly locums, who are unlikely to be familiar with how things work locally.

Drug prescribing is fraught with dangers: illegible prescription, wrong drug, wrong dose, unexpected drug interactions or failure to elicit a history of allergy or idiosyncrasy. Electronic prescribing systems with built-in warnings of interactions help, but so does the regular presence of a ward pharmacist.

Theatre safety

The period between a patient entering the operating department and leaving the recovery unit is potentially hazardous for both the patient and the staff (Boxes 1.8 and 1.9). A fully conscious patient has automatic defence mechanisms to avoid injury but when anaesthetised or recovering, relies on the care of trained staff.

All operating theatres have safety protocols, with patients' identities, nature and type of operation, allergies, etc. being repeatedly checked—but errors still occur. The World Health Organization (WHO) has developed a well-tested tool for minimising errors using a simple three-stage checklist for each case: before induction of anaesthesia (with at least nurse and anaesthetist), before the skin incision (with nurse, anaesthetist and surgeon) and before the patient leaves the operating room (with nurse, anaesthetist and surgeon). This is now used extensively around the world; see Box 1.8 and: http://www.who.int/patientsafety/safesurgery/en/

Anaesthetic incidents can be substantially reduced by good anaesthetist training, by having trained anaesthetic assistant staff so that more than one pair of hands is available, by standardised patient monitoring including pulse oximetry, and by 'pre-flight' checking of anaesthetic equipment. Professional recovery nurses and equipment further increase safety.

Surgical mishaps

Surgical mishaps in the operating theatre range from dramatic uncontrolled haemorrhage to the harder to define inadequate surgery leading to complications, slow recovery or avoidable recurrence of cancer. Surgeons have long had clear evidence of poor results of surgical treatment and at last, improvements are occurring with audit, specialisation, training and continuing medical education after specialist accreditation. Governments eager to save money sometimes mandate excessively short training and this is likely to impair outcomes and in the end do more damage and cost more.

Box 1.8 World Health Organization Surgical Safety Checklist 2009 (Revised 1/2009 © WHO, 2009)*

Checks before induction of anaesthesia (with at least nurse and anaesthetist)

- Has the patient confirmed his/her identity, site, procedure, and consent? Yes
- Is the site marked? Yes/ Not applicable
- Is the anaesthesia machine and medication check complete? Yes
- Is the pulse oximeter on the patient and functioning? Yes
- Does the patient have a known allergy? No / Yes
- Difficult airway or aspiration risk?
  — No
  — Yes, and equipment/assistance available
- Risk of >500 ml blood loss (7 ml/kg in children)?
  — No
  — Yes, and two i.v.s, central access and fluids planned

Before skin incision (with nurse, anaesthetist and surgeon)

All team members:

- Confirm all team members have introduced themselves by name and role
- Confirm the patient's name, procedure, and where the incision will be made
- Has antibiotic prophylaxis been given within the last 60 minutes? Yes / Not applicable
- Anticipated critical events

To Surgeon:

- What are the critical or non-routine steps?
- How long will the procedure take?
- What is the anticipated blood loss?

To Anaesthetist:

- Are there any patient-specific concerns?

To Nursing Team:

- Has sterility (including indicator results) been confirmed?
- Are there equipment issues or any concerns?
- Is essential imaging displayed? Yes / Not applicable

Before patient leaves operating room (with nurse, anaesthetist and surgeon)

Nurse verbally confirms:

- The name of the procedure
- Completion of instrument, swab/sponge and needle counts
- Specimen labelling (read specimen labels aloud, including patient name)
- Whether there are any equipment problems to be addressed

To Surgeon, Anaesthetist and Nurse:

- What are the key concerns for recovery and management of this patient?

*http://www.who.int/patientsafety/safesurgery/en/

Box 1.9 Avoidable hazards in the operating theatre

- Wrong procedure (including wrong side)
- Anaesthetic mishaps
- Surgical mishaps
- Handling injury (patient or staff)
- Equipment failure
- Cross-infection (patient or staff)

Injuries and hazards of moving and positioning patients

Damage to the cervical spine may occur if the unsupported head is allowed to fall backwards or sideways in unconscious patients, particularly those with rheumatoid arthritis of the cervical spine

Falls to the floor usually occur only if several things go wrong simultaneously

Damage to upper limbs can occur during transfer and positioning, and lower limb damage can occur when placing diseased hips into flexed abduction

Traction on infusion lines, tubes and catheters can cause tissue injury or interfere with monitoring or intravenous therapy, or both

Drains and catheters are at similar risk. *Chest drains* require special attention as detachment allows air to enter the pleural cavity causing pneumothorax

Peripheral nerve injuries

Peripheral nerve injuries after anaesthesia are probably caused by nerve ischaemia and can occur after as little as 30 minutes in an adverse position. Examples include:

Ulnar nerve compression at the elbow, facial nerve damage from face mask pressure, radial nerve injury from a post clamped to the operating table. The brachial plexus is vulnerable to traction. If the arm is to be placed at right angles, the hand should be *pronated* and the patient's head turned towards the arm.

Eye injuries

Irritant fluids such as antiseptics, sprays or gastric acid may be spilled on the cornea causing chemical injury. The eyelids are usually taped gently shut during operation to prevent direct trauma and drying which causes damage after 10 minutes.

Direct pressure effects

Under anaesthesia, the weight of parts of the body may cause pressure necrosis of skin over the occiput, sacrum and heels. The heels of patients with lower limb ischaemia are particularly at risk.

Pressure on calves on the operating table may cause deep venous thrombosis by compression of veins, trauma to the vein wall and stagnation of blood. Elevation by pads under the ankle, graduated compression stockings and pneumatic compression devices all reduce the risk.

Burns

Burns on the operating table are often due to faulty positioning. Diathermy burns occur if the patient comes into contact with bare metal of the operating table. Other diathermy burns result from poor earth plate contact.

Hypothermia

Unintentional hypothermia is a danger to children and to adults undergoing prolonged surgical procedures and is largely avoidable. Reduced core temperature causes changes in drug metabolism, impaired coagulation and an increase in tissue oxygen requirement during the postoperative period and consequent acidosis. This has been shown to predispose to serious postoperative complications. Maintaining normothermia is a mainstay of enhanced recovery protocols.

Infection risks

These are dealt with in Chapter 3.

Hazards during immediate postoperative recovery

20% of all deaths and serious neurological damage due to anaesthesia are believed to occur in the recovery room, and full monitoring and observation needs to be continued in the recovery area.

Radiation hazards

In the UK, all health care workers who use or prescribe X-irradiation undergo mandatory radiation protection training courses to learn the risks and safeguards needed.

Managing physiological change in the surgical patient

2

SYSTEMIC RESPONSES

FACTORS RESPONSIBLE FOR SYSTEMIC RESPONSES (Box 2.1)

Surgical patients are subject to a variety of major injuries and catastrophes that make massive demands on the body's ability to sustain life and maintain physiological equilibrium. Examples of such stressors include:

- **Major operations**—anaesthesia (particularly head-down + pneumoperitoneum for laparoscopic surgery), tissue trauma, blood and fluid loss, healing and repair
- **Major trauma** including fractures and burns; head, abdominal and chest injuries
- **Major cardiovascular events,** e.g. myocardial infarction, pulmonary embolism, stroke
- **Haemorrhage and fluid infusion** including blood; fluid and electrolyte abnormalities
- **Infection, inflammation and sepsis**
- **Hypoxia**

The way the body responds to major systemic insults depends on several factors—the **physiological reserve** of the patient's chief organ systems (i.e. basic fitness), the nature of the injurious process, the severity of physiological disruption, the duration of delay before resuscitation, and the virulence of any microorganisms involved. Most patients are remarkably resilient given good basic care but in a deteriorating patient, several physiological systems are likely to be impacted upon simultaneously, evoking a range of complex homeostatic mechanisms.

MANAGEMENT OF THE DETERIORATING PATIENT

The aim is always to recognise problems early by regular clinical observation, and to correct abnormal physiology rapidly and accurately in order to prevent intrinsic compensatory mechanisms becoming overwhelmed. If this happens in one organ system without correction, snowballing decompensation of other systems follows.

Management requires careful monitoring, often in a high-dependency or intensive care unit, and repeated checks on organ function and dysfunction. In most elective operations, many of the responses discussed below can be mitigated by good preoperative preparation, accurate fluid replacement, ensuring oxygenation, adequate analgesia, reducing psychological stress, preventing infection and using careful operative technique to minimise tissue trauma, blood loss and complications. **Enhanced recovery programmes** are gradually being introduced which give special attention to these factors before, during and after operation (see: NHS Enhanced Recovery Partnership Programme document: *Delivering enhanced recovery—Helping patients to get better sooner*). The individual variables responsible for potentially excessive systemic responses to severe injury or major surgery are summarised in Box 2.1.

STRESSORS IN THE SURGICAL PATIENT

Direct and indirect tissue trauma

Tissue disruption (whether surgical or traumatic) leads to activation of local cytokine responses more or less in proportion to the damage. Responses are exaggerated if wounds are contaminated (e.g. debris, foreign bodies, faeces) or associated with tissue **ischaemia**.

Fall in intravascular volume

This is a key factor in initiating systemic responses. Hypovolaemia results from:

- **Excess fluid loss** (see Box 2.2)
- **Interstitial sequestration** of fluid as oedema in damaged tissues and generally as a result of systemic

hormonal responses. This process is amplified in systemic sepsis
- **Restricted oral intake** during any perioperative period or whilst in intensive care

Falling intravascular volume stimulates sympathetic activity by removing baroreceptor inhibition in an attempt to maintain blood pressure by increasing cardiac output and peripheral resistance. This also explains the mild tachycardia commonly seen in postoperative patients. Compensation is most effective in young fit individuals, but decompensation is often sudden and rapid. **Catecholamines** also have profound metabolic effects, increasing the turnover of carbohydrates, proteins and lipids. Falling renal perfusion activates the **renin–angiotensin–aldosterone system**, increasing renal reabsorption of sodium and water. A centrally mediated increase in antidiuretic hormone (ADH) secretion promotes further conservation of water.

Reduced cardiac output and peripheral perfusion

Circulatory efficiency may be impaired by hypovolaemia, and myocardial contractility may be depressed by anaesthetic agents and other drugs. Anaesthetic drugs generally cause peripheral dilatation and positive-pressure ventilation impairs venous return. Head-down positioning and artificial pneumoperitoneum for laparoscopic surgery further stress cardiovascular physiology. Major events such as sepsis (septic shock), pulmonary embolism or myocardial infarction may precipitate cardiovascular collapse.

Box 2.1 Factors responsible for systemic responses to severe injury or major surgery

- Direct and indirect tissue trauma
- Fall in intravascular volume, leading to a fall in cardiac output and reduced peripheral perfusion and hypoxia
- Excess intravenous fluids, particularly 0.9% NaCl, causing interstitial oedema
- Local and spreading inflammation and infection
- Systemic inflammatory responses and sepsis
- Pain
- Psychological stress
- Excess heat loss
- Secondary effects on the blood
- Starvation

Box 2.2 Sources of excess fluid loss in surgical patients

- **Blood loss**—traumatic or surgical
- **Plasma loss**—burns
- **Gastrointestinal fluid loss**—vomiting, nasogastric aspiration, sequestration in obstructed or adynamic bowel, loss through a fistula or an ileostomy, diarrhoea
- **Inflammatory exudate into the peritoneal cavity**—generalised peritonitis or acute pancreatitis
- **Sepsis syndrome (septicaemia)**—massive peripheral vasodilatation and third space losses due to increased capillary permeability causing relative hypovolaemia
- **Abnormal insensible loss**—fever, excess sweating or hyperventilation

Systemic inflammatory responses and sepsis

(see Ch. 3)

Pain

Pain causes increased catecholamine and adrenocorticotrophic hormone (ACTH) secretion. Perioperative blockade of pain (e.g. by regional anaesthesia) greatly reduces the adverse systemic effects.

Stress

Psychological stress associated with injury, severe illness or elective surgery has an effect similar to pain on sympathetic function and hypothalamic activity.

Excess heat loss

This can occur during long operations and after extensive burns. Heat loss imposes enormous demands upon energy resources; if body core temperature falls, physiological processes such as blood clotting are impaired. Small babies are very vulnerable to heat loss. Heat loss in the operating theatre is counteracted as far as possible by raising the ambient temperature, insulating exposed parts of the body, using warm water underblankets or warm air 'bear-huggers' and by warming fluids during intravenous infusion.

Blood coagulation changes

General metabolic responses to injury activate thrombotic mechanisms and initially depress intrinsic intravascular thrombolysis. Thus the patient is in a **prothrombotic state** and may suffer intravenous thrombosis and consequent thromboembolism.

If substantial haemorrhage occurs, clotting factors eventually become exhausted, causing failure of clotting. The systemic inflammatory response syndrome (SIRS, see Ch. 3, p. 51) may initiate widespread intravascular thrombosis, using up clotting factors and precipitating **disseminated intravascular coagulation (DIC)**, with failure of normal clotting.

Starvation and stress-induced catabolism

Patients with major surgical conditions are often malnourished before operation (see *Nutritional management*, below). Most are starved for 6–12 hours preoperatively and often do not start eating for 12–24 hours after surgery. After major GI surgery, food may be withheld for several days, or much longer with complications such as anastomotic breakdown or fistula formation.

METABOLIC RESPONSES TO PATHOPHYSIOLOGICAL STRESS

In severe trauma or extensive operative surgery, particularly if complicated by sepsis, the key factors in the systemic response

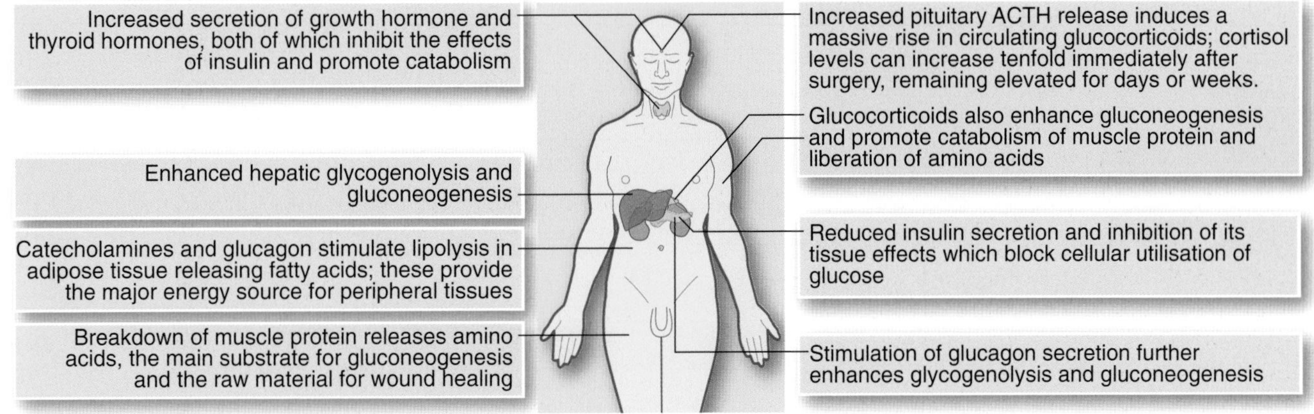

Fig. 2.1 Metabolic responses to major systemic insults

are **increased sympathetic activity** together with increased **circulating catecholamines** and **insulin**. Cytokine responses signal other cells to prepare for action (e.g. polymorphs, T and B cells), to compensate for starvation, provide additional energy and building blocks for tissue repair, and conserve sodium ions and water.

Glucose production is massively increased by **gluconeogenesis** under the influence of catecholamines. There is also enhanced secretion of ACTH, glucocorticoids (cortisol), glucagon and growth hormone, all contributing to the general **catabolic response**. **Insulin** acts as an antagonist of most of these and is secreted in increased amounts from the second or third day after injury.

The sum of these factors is to cause inevitable catabolism and potentially extreme changes in fluid balance and electrolytes. These metabolic changes are shown in Figure 2.1.

Effects on carbohydrate metabolism

The overall effect is rising blood glucose (levels may reach 20 mmol/L), often resulting in **hyperglycaemia** and a **pseudodiabetic state**, and glucose may appear in the urine. This is in marked contrast to simple fasting, in which glucose levels are normal or low and glycosuria does not occur.

Effects on body proteins and nitrogen metabolism

In the normal healthy adult, **nitrogen balance** is constantly maintained. Protein turnover results in daily excretion of 12–20 g of urinary nitrogen which is made good by dietary intake. In a hypercatabolic state, nitrogen losses can increase three- or four-fold. Most importantly, the metabolic environment prevents proper utilisation of food or intravenous nutrition. There is therefore huge destruction of skeletal muscle. This state of **negative nitrogen balance** contrasts markedly with simple starvation in which body protein is preserved.

Effects on lipid stores and metabolism

The effects of major body insults on lipid metabolism are little different from simple starvation; most of the energy requirements are met from fat stores.

Surgical catabolism reverses only as the patient recovers from the illness and therefore early parenteral nutrition has little effect, although carbohydrate administration may spare some protein loss.

Note that when patients have been severely ill, carbohydrate metabolism is minimal and energy comes from catabolism of protein and fat. Once feeding recommences, there is a danger of **refeeding syndrome** which must be anticipated (see below).

FLUID, ELECTROLYTE AND ACID–BASE MANAGEMENT

INTRODUCTION

Fluid, electrolyte and acid–base derangements can be minimised if high-risk patients are assessed before operation and closely monitored before, during and after operation. If abnormalities do develop, the diagnosis and management can be worked out with reasoning and common sense. Plasma urea and electrolytes should be checked at least daily in patients undergoing major surgery or those receiving intravenous fluids.

Severely ill patients with abdominal infection, sepsis and fistulae and patients with severe burns are likely to suffer major problems of fluid balance (and nutrition, see below). These are best managed with the help of experienced anaesthetists in intensive care or high-dependency units, where monitoring and therapy can be rigorously managed.

NORMAL FLUID AND ELECTROLYTE HOMEOSTASIS

The body of an average 70 kg adult contains 42 litres of fluid, distributed between the intracellular compartment, the extracellular space and the bloodstream (see Fig. 2.2). Fluid input is mainly by oral intake of fluids and food but about 200 ml/day of water is produced during metabolism. Normal adult **losses** are between 2.5 and 3 litres/day. About one litre is lost

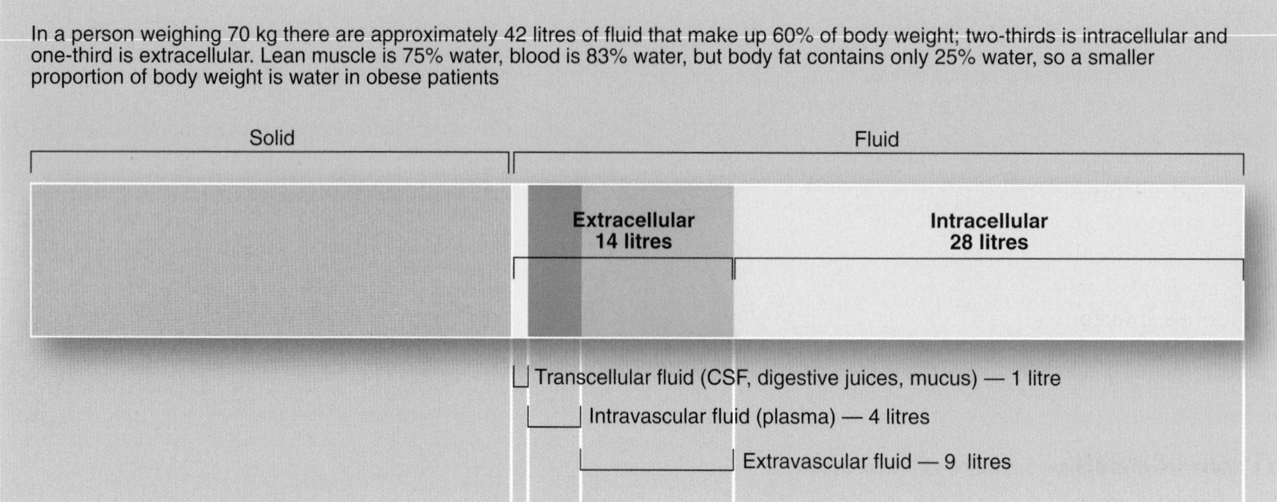

Fig. 2.2 Distribution of fluid content in the body compartments

Table 2.1 Summary—normal daily fluid and electrolyte input and output

Normal daily intake	Normal daily output
Water	
Diet 2300 ml Metabolism 200 ml	Urine 1400 ml (minimum obligatory volume=400 ml) Skin loss 500 ml (obligatory diffusion and vaporisation) *Note: sweating in pyrexia or a high ambient temperature can cause several litres extra loss each day* Lung loss 500 ml (obligatory) Faecal loss 100 ml
Sodium	
Diet 150 mmol/day (range 50–300 mmol)	Stool 5 mmol/day Skin transpiration 5 mmol/day (in the absence of sweating) Urine 140 mmol/day (can fall down to 15 mmol/day if required)
Potassium	
Diet 100 mmol/day (range 50–200 mmol)	Stool 10 mmol/day (obligatory) Skin <5 mmol/day Urine 85 mmol/day (rarely falls below 60 mmol/day)

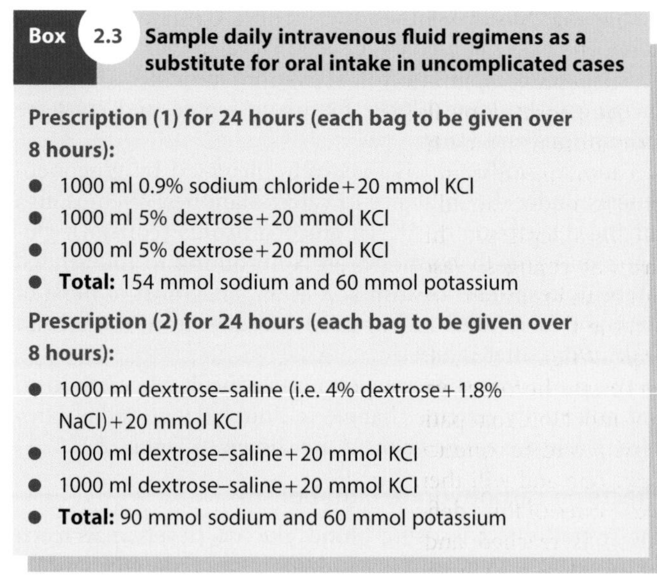
Box 2.3 Sample daily intravenous fluid regimens as a substitute for oral intake in uncomplicated cases

Prescription (1) for 24 hours (each bag to be given over 8 hours):

- 1000 ml 0.9% sodium chloride+20 mmol KCl
- 1000 ml 5% dextrose+20 mmol KCl
- 1000 ml 5% dextrose+20 mmol KCl
- **Total:** 154 mmol sodium and 60 mmol potassium

Prescription (2) for 24 hours (each bag to be given over 8 hours):

- 1000 ml dextrose–saline (i.e. 4% dextrose+1.8% NaCl)+20 mmol KCl
- 1000 ml dextrose–saline+20 mmol KCl
- 1000 ml dextrose–saline+20 mmol KCl
- **Total:** 90 mmol sodium and 60 mmol potassium

insensibly from skin and lungs, 1300–1800 ml are passed as urine (about 60 ml/hour or 1 ml/kg/hour) and 100 ml are lost in faeces. About 100–150 mmol of sodium ions and 50–100 mmol of potassium ions are lost each day in urine and this is balanced by the normal dietary intake (see Table 2.1).

MAINTENANCE OF WATER AND SODIUM

For most patients, the daily water and sodium requirements are best met by using appropriate quantities of **normal saline** solution (0.9% sodium chloride) and **5% dextrose** (glucose) solution. Normal saline contains 154 mmol each of sodium and chloride ions per litre. One litre will thus satisfy the daily sodium requirement of uncomplicated patients. The additional requirement for water is made up with 2–2.5 litres of 5% glucose (see Box 2.3). The small amount of glucose this contains contributes little to nutrition but renders the solution isotonic. This prescription is altered for patients with electrolyte abnormalities by varying the volume of normal saline given.

Note that **Hartmann's solution** (or similar balanced electrolyte solutions such as Ringer's lactate) is often used as the sole fluid for intravenous infusion. This is more physiological and contains less chloride (111 mmol/L), some potassium (5 mmol/L) and insignificant amounts of calcium and lactate.

In children, water excretion is markedly reduced in the postoperative period as a result of increased ADH secretion. Maintenance fluids requirements are based on published guidelines and formulae (see: http://www.nda.ox.ac.uk/wfsa/html/u19/u1914_01.htm).

MAINTENANCE OF POTASSIUM

Basic potassium requirements are met by infusing 60–80 mmol of potassium chloride in divided doses over each 24-hour period. Premixed intravenous fluids are generally available with 20 or 40 mmol of potassium chloride per 1000 ml infusion bags. If concentrations of potassium chloride greater than 40 mmol in 500 ml are required, they should be given via a central venous infusion in a critical care unit, with cardiac monitoring. Bolus injections of KCl must *never* be given because rapid increases in plasma potassium can cause cardiac arrest.

LIMITS OF COMPENSATORY MECHANISMS

Healthy kidneys are normally able to maintain fluid and electrolyte homeostasis in spite of large variations of fluid intake. The same also applies to fluid and electrolytes given intravenously.

The total blood volume in an adult male is about 5 litres, of which about 55–60% is water (about 3.5 litres). Falls in blood volume which are not too rapid or extensive can be compensated by fluid movement from the extracellular compartment which has a volume of more than 10 litres. A deficit of more than 3 litres in whole body fluid volume cannot be sustained and intravascular volume inevitably becomes depleted. This is reflected in compensatory cardiovascular changes. Vasoconstriction causes cold peripheries: this is an important warning sign of hypovolaemia and more reliable than the early mild tachycardia, particularly in children. When overall fluid deficit reaches about 3 litres, the pulse rate becomes very rapid and **hypotension** and shock develop. Note that patients on beta-adrenergic blocking drugs or with cardiac conduction defects may not be able to increase heart rate and will therefore decompensate earlier. With 4 or more litres of fluid deficit, the limit of cardiovascular compensation is reached and the patient develops **hypovolaemic shock**. Note that fit young people are able to sustain normal vital signs longer but when they do decompensate, they do so abruptly.

In neonates, children, the elderly and the chronically ill, cardiovascular compensation capacity is greatly reduced. A relatively small fluid and electrolyte imbalance may cause life-threatening complications.

PHYSIOLOGICAL CHANGES IN RESPONSE TO SURGERY AND TRAUMA

The stresses of trauma or surgery cause a rise in circulating **catecholamines**. Stress also stimulates the hypothalamo-pituitary–adrenal axis, which increases secretion of **cortisol** and **aldosterone**. These hormones promote renal conservation of sodium and water and cause a reduction in urine volume and urine sodium concentration.

Effects of a fall in renal perfusion

Any substantial reduction in effective circulating volume may cause a fall in renal perfusion. In addition, aortic surgery involving aortic clamping may alter the dynamics of renal artery flow, whilst raised intra-abdominal pressure (see *Abdominal compartment syndrome*, below) disrupts renal blood flow.

A fall in renal perfusion activates the renin–angiotensin–aldosterone mechanism to sustain the blood pressure. As glomerular filtration falls, **renin** release is stimulated from the renal juxtaglomerular apparatus and this catalyses the conversion of **angiotensin I** to **angiotensin II** in the lungs. Angiotensin II has a powerful pressor effect on the peripheral vasculature, counteracting hypotension, as well as stimulating **aldosterone** release from the adrenal cortex. Aldosterone promotes active **reabsorption of sodium** ions from the distal convoluted tubules of the kidney, accompanied by passive reabsorption of water. Sodium reabsorption is linked to increased excretion of potassium and hydrogen ions.

The net effect is that in conditions causing renal perfusion to fall, the urine output falls by several hundred millilitres per day, and the urine that is produced is low in sodium (less than 40 mmol/L), high in potassium (greater than 100 mmol/L) and acidic. The loss of hydrogen ions causes a degree of **metabolic alkalosis**.

Other factors in water conservation

Water conservation is further enhanced by stress-mediated secretion of **antidiuretic hormone** (ADH), also known as vasopressin, from the posterior pituitary (neurohypophysis). Loss of water alone increases the plasma osmolality, stimulating ADH release, mediated by osmoreceptors in the hypothalamus. ADH binds to receptors in the distal renal tubules and promotes reabsorption of water. Release of ADH is also stimulated by falls in blood pressure and volume, sensed by stretch receptors in the heart and large arteries. Changes in blood pressure and volume are not nearly as sensitive a stimulator as increased osmolality, but are potent in extreme conditions (e.g. loss of over 15% volume in acute haemorrhage). Stress and pain probably also promote ADH release via other hypothalamic pathways.

Postoperative situation

At the site of trauma or major surgery, fluid is effectively removed from the circulation in the form of inflammatory oedema (isotonic local third space losses). This displaced volume is compensated by fluid retained by the hormonal changes described above. More potassium is released from damaged cells than the excess lost by exchange in the kidney. Thus, the postoperative plasma **potassium level tends to rise** in the first day or two. This is particularly true if stored blood has been transfused as this releases potassium from elderly red cells, so potassium supplements are not usually needed for the first few days after operation provided preoperative plasma potassium is normal and potassium-losing diuretics are not prescribed.

It is important to recognise the normal **phase** of **relative oliguria** and **sodium retention** that inevitably occurs for up to 48 hours after major injury or surgery as this influences fluid management. Like surgical catabolism, these effects are resistant to external manipulation but resolve with recovery of the patient.

Abdominal compartment syndrome

(see http://www.ncbi.nlm.nih.gov/pmc/articles/PMC137242/)

Abdominal compartment syndrome, with the adverse effects it can have on organ systems, is now recognised as an entity. Intra-abdominal pressure is normally less than 5 mmHg, but after surgery or trauma it may rise as high as 15 mmHg. Cardiac output begins to fall off at 10 mmHg, and hypotension and oliguria are likely between 15 and 20 mmHg. Anuria occurs with pressures over 40 mmHg.

The causes of abdominal compartment syndrome are often multifactorial and include **fluid accumulating** as a result of retroperitoneal haemorrhage, e.g. in ruptured abdominal aortic aneurysm, postoperative haemorrhage (particularly if clotting is disordered), organ trauma, pancreatitis, and interstitial oedema in sepsis or zealous fluid resuscitation. When abdominal pressure exceeds the capillary pressure perfusing abdominal organs, dysfunction and eventually infarction of these organs becomes likely.

Adverse effects include:

- Oliguria due to renal hypoperfusion and collapsed renal veins
- Respiratory embarrassment due to restriction and elevation of the diaphragm, and compression of alveoli. This results in increased peak airways pressure, decreased tidal volume, hypoxaemia and hypercarbia
- Decreased venous return leading to falling cardiac output and hypotension
- Bowel ischaemia causing gastrointestinal bleeding

In patients with a distended and taut abdomen, measuring abdominal compartment pressure can help early recognition. Treatment involves reopening the abdomen and leaving it open until the risk of rising pressure subsides.

PROBLEMS OF FLUID AND ELECTROLYTE DEPLETION

Loss of whole blood or plasma

Rapid and copious blood loss in traumatic injury or operative surgery initially depletes the intravascular compartment and loss of only 1 litre may cause hypotension or even hypovolaemic shock. When haemorrhage is less rapid, there is time to replace fluid loss from the extracellular compartment, so greater volumes can be lost before the cardiovascular system becomes compromised, although losses still need to be restored physiologically or by transfusion.

If blood loss has ceased, the need for transfusion is based on estimated or measured volume lost and on known haemoglobin concentration. Acute blood loss of 500–1000 ml is usually treated by transfusing crystalloids. Larger volume losses are best replaced by transfusion of whole blood or packed red cells supplemented by normal saline. Slow chronic blood loss, e.g. from a peptic ulcer or hookworm infestation, does not cause fluid balance problems but may cause symptoms and signs of anaemia; transfusion is not usually required.

In **severe burns**, the amount of plasma likely to be lost is easily underestimated and should be calculated using a standard formula based on the burnt area to guide fluid replacement (see Ch. 17).

Gastrointestinal fluid loss

Between 5 and 9 litres of electrolyte-rich fluid is normally secreted into the upper GI tract each day as saliva, gastric juice, bile, pancreatic fluid and succus entericus (small bowel secretions; see Table 2.2). Most of the fluid is reabsorbed in the large intestine.

Huge volumes of water and electrolytes may be lost as a result of vomiting, nasogastric aspiration, diarrhoea, sequestration of fluid in obstructed or adynamic bowel or drainage to the exterior via a fistula or an ileostomy. If there is widespread **bowel inflammation** causing diarrhoea as in gastroenteritis or ulcerative colitis, inflammatory exudate may greatly increase the total fluid lost.

Cholera and other infective diarrhoeal diseases can cause the loss of up to 10 litres of electrolyte-rich fluid in one day and this fluid loss is a frequent cause of death, particularly in children.

Abnormal fluid losses in hospital must be measured or estimated accurately and recorded on a fluid balance chart. In addition, observations should be regularly made for signs of fluid depletion including pulse rate, blood pressure, periodic urine output and, if necessary, central venous pressure (CVP). These measures enable intravenous replacement to be predicted and the adverse consequences of fluid and electrolyte depletion to be prevented.

Table 2.2 Daily gastrointestinal secretions and electrolyte composition

Secretion	Volume (L)	Na^+ (mmol/L)	K^+ (mmol/L)	Cl^- (mmol/L)	HCO_3^- (mmol/L)
Saliva	1–1.5	20–80	10–20	20–40	20–160
Gastric juice	1–2.5	20–100	5–10	120–160	Nil
Bile	Up to 1	150–250	5–10	40–60	20–60
Pancreatic juice	1–2	120	5–10	10–60	80–120
Succus entericus (small bowel secretions)	2–3	140	5 (increases up to 40 in inflammatory diarrhoea)	Variable	Variable

From Table 2.2, it can be seen that **vomitus**, nasogastric aspirate and diarrhoea are variably rich in sodium and potassium. As a general rule, GI fluid losses should be replaced by an equivalent volume of normal saline, with potassium chloride added as needed. In intestinal obstruction or adynamic ileus, fluid sequestrated in bowel is replaced in a similar manner, although volume requirements have to be estimated. Fistulae and overactive ileostomies cause chronic loss of fluid that is high in chloride and bicarbonate.

Intra-abdominal accumulation of inflammatory fluid

Severe intra-abdominal inflammation may cause several litres of fluid rich in plasma proteins and electrolytes to be lost into the peritoneal cavity. This typically occurs in peritonitis or acute pancreatitis and often in the context of the **systemic inflammatory response syndrome** (SIRS). This is best replaced (as well as can be estimated) by physiological saline or other suitable crystalloids.

Systemic sepsis (SIRS and multiple organ dysfunction syndrome)

Systemic sepsis is associated with widespread endothelial damage and a large increase in capillary permeability mediated by a range of cytokines and other circulating mediators. The result is extensive loss of protein and electrolyte-rich fluid from the circulation into the extravascular space ('third space loss'), which, combined with loss of peripheral resistance, results in cardiovascular collapse and shock.

The required fluid volume is difficult to estimate and replacement is usually given so as to maintain cardiovascular stability (pulse rate and blood pressure) and urinary output (at least 0.5 ml/kg body weight/hour) whilst avoiding fluid overload and cardiac failure. In the severely ill patient, in whom the volume requirements are particularly difficult to judge, a central venous pressure line or transoesophageal Doppler provide a more accurate method of assessing precise fluid replacement needs (see *Enhanced recovery programmes*, below).

Abnormal insensible fluid loss

Abnormal insensible fluid loss can greatly increase overall fluid loss, particularly in the seriously ill or elderly patient and must be included in the fluid balance equation. **Pyrexia** increases insensible loss by approximately 20% for each degree Celsius rise in body temperature, mainly in the form of exhaled water vapour. A pyrexia of 38.5 °C for 3 days would therefore cause an extra litre of fluid loss. **Sweating** causes loss of sodium-rich fluid which can be easily overlooked in patients with fever and when the ambient temperature rises.

Preventing acute renal failure

Maintaining fluid balance in surgical patients depends on anticipating problems before they cause adverse effects and risk acute renal failure. Acute renal failure is a serious complication with a high mortality in surgical patients. Prevention involves similar strategies in all patients at risk, namely:

- Observing changes in vital signs—pulse rate, blood pressure and CVP if appropriate
- Checking hourly urine output is adequate
- Measuring fluid losses to guide replacement
- Seeking clinical signs of fluid imbalance (both dehydration and overload)
- Regularly estimating plasma urea and electrolytes

In patients with cardiac failure or shock, monitoring and treatment is best carried out in an intensive care or high-dependency/critical care unit, using invasive monitoring to help determine the required volume of fluid replacement.

COMMON FLUID AND ELECTROLYTE PROBLEMS

INTERMEDIATE ELECTIVE OPERATIONS AND UNCOMPLICATED EMERGENCY OPERATIONS

Most operations fall into this category. Patients are generally in fluid and electrolyte equilibrium before operation, although diuretic therapy (for cardiac failure, hypertension or chronic renal failure) may cause problems. For these, plasma urea and electrolytes should be checked before operation. Note that loop and thiazide diuretics may cause **hypokalaemia** whilst potassium-sparing diuretics such as spironolactone may cause **hyperkalaemia**. If serious abnormalities are found, operation must be postponed until the problem is corrected. Hypokalaemia can usually be treated by oral potassium supplements or by adding a potassium-sparing diuretic. Hyperkalaemia is usually corrected by substituting a loop or thiazide diuretic.

Mild renal dysfunction (plasma urea up to about 15 mmol/L and creatinine up to about 170 mmol/L) is not usually a contraindication to surgery. These patients tend to be mildly dehydrated, however, and oral fluid intake should be strongly encouraged.

INTRODUCTION TO MANAGEMENT

For elective surgery, the patient is often kept 'nil by mouth' for 6–12 hours before operation, although most can take clear fluids by mouth up to 3 hours before operation. The patient is likely to take very little oral fluid for up to 6 hours after operation and a fluid deficit of 1000–1500 ml is therefore common. Mild fluid deficits can usually be quickly made up once the patient is drinking normally and intravenous fluid replacement is rarely required. For patients with **mild renal failure**, an infusion should be set up at the outset of the 'nil by mouth' period to prevent acute-on-chronic renal failure. Occasionally, and despite the use of anti-emetics, patients vomit after operation and intravenous fluids should be employed if vomiting is prolonged.

Children and especially infants and neonates are much more vulnerable to fluid deprivation because of their small total body fluid volume and disproportionate insensible losses.

Even relatively minor operations can cause dehydration and intravenous fluids may be necessary, with the rate and volume calculated according to body weight and measured blood loss.

As a rule, the sooner the body can assume control over its own fluid and electrolyte homeostasis the better. Intravenous fluids should be discontinued as soon as normal oral intake has been resumed and urine output is satisfactory.

MAJOR OPERATIONS

Major elective or emergency operations, especially those involving bowel, pose particular problems with fluid management. The principal reasons are:

- Patients are often elderly and are likely to have a diminished cardiovascular reserve. They may have pre-existing fluid and electrolyte abnormalities
- Preoperative vomiting and restricted fluid intake may have caused dehydration and electrolyte abnormalities
- Blood loss during and after operation may be substantial
- Operations may take several hours with consequent insensible losses from the open wound
- Third space losses of 500–1000 ml can occur after major surgery or trauma as a result of systemic responses to trauma
- The recovery period when oral intake is nil or restricted may become extended—several days following complicated bowel surgery or peritonitis (e.g. perforated diverticulitis or an anastomotic leak)

Careful pre- and postoperative assessment of patients is crucial so problems can be anticipated. This should include clinical examination for **dehydration** (dry mouth and loss of normal skin turgor) or **overhydration** (elevated jugular venous pressure or cardiac failure). Plasma urea and electrolytes, creatinine and full blood count should be measured daily. Elevated urea concentration with little elevation of creatinine is characteristic of dehydration. An abnormally high haemoglobin concentration (providing polycythaemia is not present) also indicates dehydration, especially if it was normal beforehand.

ENHANCED RECOVERY PROGRAMMES

In recent years, clinicians in surgery have been attempting to shorten hospital stays and reduce complication rates by developing structured systems that reduce the stress response to enhance recovery. These involve attention to all facets of surgical care, so-called '**multimodal optimisation**' or '**fast track recovery**'. This includes special attention to perioperative fluid management, the use of minimal access surgical techniques and mechanisms to preserve postoperative organ function, including:

- Preoperative assessment and improved education and preparation of patients so that they understand what will happen and cope with planned early discharge
- Home care arrangements to cope with early discharge
- Improved methods of calculating fluid replacement that ensure the patient remains normovolaemic within narrow limits, preventing central hypovolaemia and fluid overload. NICE have recommended the use of transoesophageal Doppler ultrasound monitoring of left ventricular stroke volume to enable intraoperative assessment of fluid status and provide **individualised goal-directed fluid therapy**. Trials have shown this can reliably shorten hospital stays and reduce complication rates
- Planned and assisted early postoperative mobilisation
- Early enteral nutrient challenge and the use of gut-specific nutrients such as glutamine, antioxidants and synbiotics (nutritional supplements that improve the balance of intestinal microflora). Methods that enable earlier return of gut function may be fundamental to rapid recovery. Gastrointestinal gut-associated lymphoid tissue (GALT) forms more than half the body's immunological cell mass and is believed to play a key role in stress responses to surgery. Sustaining nutrition of the small bowel wall from within the lumen may prevent breakdown of intestinal barrier function. Healthy bowel function enables earlier tolerance of food, less postoperative ileus and less postoperative nausea and vomiting
- Avoiding opiates by using epidural or regional analgesia
- Delivering high concentrations of inspired oxygen

ABNORMALITIES OF INDIVIDUAL ELECTROLYTES

(see Table 2.3 for a summary of causes and effects)

Abnormalities of plasma sodium concentration

Plasma sodium abnormalities are usually discovered incidentally on regular measurement of electrolytes.

Hyponatraemia

A low plasma sodium level may be real or spurious. Spurious results commonly arise when blood is taken from an arm receiving an intravenous infusion; less commonly, false laboratory results can occur if there is **lipaemia** resulting from parenteral nutrition. If in doubt, the test should be repeated with appropriate precautions.

In hyponatraemia (except in severe hyperglycaemia or infusion of mannitol), the plasma becomes **hypotonic**. This causes cellular overhydration which in severe cases results in cerebral oedema. Mild hyponatraemia is symptomless but when the plasma sodium falls below about 120 mmol/L, patients often become confused. Convulsions and coma occur when concentrations fall below about 110 mmol/L. If hyponatraemia is confirmed biochemically, the next step is to clinically assess the **state of hydration** (i.e. the extracellular fluid volume) and this will guide therapy.

There are three possibilities:

- **Water deficit with a larger sodium deficit** (clinical signs—dry mouth, poor skin turgor, poor urine output, high urine osmolality): sodium insufficiency is usually due to diuretic therapy, vomiting, diarrhoea or other excessive losses of body fluids with inadequate replacement. Treatment involves rehydration with appropriate sodium-containing intravenous fluids
- **Sodium normal with a larger water excess** (clinical signs—weight gain, ankle swelling, raised jugular venous pressure): this usually results from organ dysfunction.

Table 2.3 Causes and effects of sodium and potassium deficiency and excess

Electrolyte abnormality	Causes	Adverse effects
Hyponatraemia	Diuretics (especially thiazides) Water excess (ingested or intravenous) Diarrhoea Vomiting Losses from intestinal fistula Renal failure Syndrome of inappropriate antidiuretic hormone secretion (SIADH) Addison's disease Nephrotic syndrome Liver failure	Confusion Seizures Hypertension Cardiac failure Muscle weakness Nausea Anorexia
Hypernatraemia	Fluid loss without water replacement, e.g. diarrhoea, vomiting, burns Saline excess (usually iatrogenic) Diabetes insipidus Diabetic ketoacidosis Primary aldosteronism (Conn's syndrome)	Thirst Dehydration Confusion Coma Seizures
Hyperkalaemia	Sampling artefact (haemolysis of sample or delayed processing) Drugs, e.g. ACE inhibitors, spironolactone, suxamethonium Digoxin poisoning Excess potassium chloride (iatrogenic) Massive blood transfusion Burns Rhabdomyolysis Tumour lysis syndrome Renal failure Aldosterone deficiency Addison's disease Metabolic acidosis	Cardiac arrhythmias Sudden death
Hypokalaemia	Vomiting Diarrhoea Losses from intestinal fistula Diuretics Purgative abuse Renal tubular failure Cushing's disease, exogenous steroids or ACTH Metabolic alkalosis Primary hyperaldosteronism (Conn's syndrome) Secondary hyperaldosteronism	Cardiac arrhythmias Muscle weakness Hypotonia Muscle cramps Tetany

Cardiac failure is the most common cause, followed by renal, liver and respiratory failure. Overhydration is compounded by excessive intravenous fluid administration. Management is based primarily on treating the organ failure, e.g. diuretics for cardiac failure

- **Water excess**: this is uncommon and is usually due to **inappropriate antidiuretic hormone (ADH) secretion**. This is rare on a surgical ward except for TUR syndrome in which excess fluid is absorbed during transurethral resection of the prostate. It can also occur following head injury or neurosurgery, or may occur in pneumonia, empyema, lung abscess or oat-cell carcinoma of the lung. Excess ADH increases water reabsorption by the renal tubules independently of sodium. The result is water overload and dilutional hyponatraemia. Inappropriate ADH secretion is the most likely diagnosis if the urine osmolality is found to be high and the plasma osmolality low. Hyponatraemia caused by inappropriate ADH secretion is managed by restricting fluid intake to 1 litre per day

Hypernatraemia

This is uncommon and is often iatrogenic in the surgical patient. The usual cause is either excess administration of sodium via intravenous fluids or inadequate water replacement. Hypernatraemia is more likely to occur after operation because increased aldosterone secretion causes sodium to be conserved by the kidney. Very rarely, hypernatraemia is caused by **Conn's syndrome** (primary hyperaldosteronism).

Treatment involves encouraging the patient to drink more water, or infusing fluids with a low sodium content.

Abnormalities of plasma potassium concentration

Acid–base abnormalities (see below) can have a profound effect on plasma potassium concentration but are likely to correct spontaneously as the acid–base problem is treated.

Hypokalaemia

In the preoperative patient, hypokalaemia usually results from poor dietary intake, diuretic therapy, chronic diarrhoea, losses from a malfunctioning ileostomy or, rarely, excess mucus secretion from a rectal villous adenoma. Rarely, hypokalaemia may be caused by **primary hyperaldosteronism** (Conn's syndrome).

Postoperatively, hypokalaemia is usually caused by inadequate potassium supplementation in intravenous infusions. The lack of intake is compounded by increased urinary losses from stress-induced **secondary hyperaldosteronism**.

Hypokalaemia causes skeletal muscle weakness and reduces GI motility, with paralytic ileus in extreme cases. When severe, there is also a risk of sudden cardiac arrhythmias or even cardiac arrest. Hypokalaemia can usually be corrected with oral potassium supplements (effervescent or slow-release tablets). For patients on intravenous fluids, potassium supplements are added as appropriate. The infusion rate should not generally exceed 15–20 mmol per hour, but larger quantities may be required following operations involving cardiopulmonary bypass.

Hyperkalaemia

This is less common than hypokalaemia in surgical patients but may require urgent correction. In the preoperative patient, it is most commonly caused by chronic renal failure, high doses of ACE inhibiting drugs or potassium-sparing diuretics. Occasionally, non-steroidal anti-inflammatory drugs cause hyperkalaemia. Postoperative hyperkalaemia is usually iatrogenic, caused by excessive intravenous potassium administration, although it may be associated with acute renal failure or blood transfusion.

Hyperkalaemia is asymptomatic in its early stages but there is a high risk of sudden death from asystole when plasma potassium concentration reaches about 7.0 mmol/L. The emergency management of hyperkalaemia is shown in Figure 2.3.

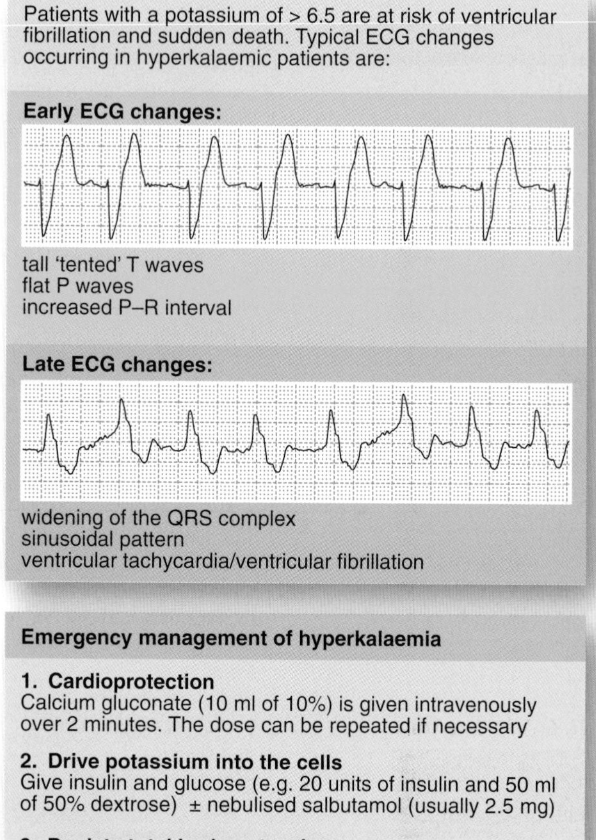

Fig. 2.3 Emergency management of hyperkalaemia

ACID–BASE DISTURBANCES (see Fig. 2.4 and Table 2.4)

Major acid–base abnormalities are rare in uncomplicated surgery and usually arise in seriously ill patients. In a nutshell, when breathing is inadequate, carbon dioxide builds up and combines with water to produce carbonic acid ('respiratory acid') which contributes to an acidic pH. Treatment is to lower the PCO_2 by assisted breathing. In addition, when normal metabolism is impaired, oxidative metabolism declines and lactic acid accumulates. Treatment is directed at the cause of metabolic impairment, e.g. sepsis, together with organ support therapy, e.g. oxygen, intravenous fluids and antibiotics.

Metabolic acidosis

Metabolic acidosis usually follows an episode of severe tissue hypoxia resulting from hypovolaemic shock, myocardial infarction or systemic sepsis. The most common cause is inadequate tissue oxygenation leading to accumulation of lactic acid. In surgical patients, the onset of metabolic acidosis is often an indicator of serious intra-abdominal problems such as an anastomotic leak. Metabolic acidosis is also seen in acute renal failure and uncontrolled diabetic ketoacidosis. Clinically, patients have rapid, deep, sighing 'Kussmaul' respirations as they hyperventilate to blow off carbon dioxide (a respiratory compensatory mechanism). Arterial blood gas estimations show the characteristic picture of raised hydrogen ion concentration and low standard bicarbonate with a low arterial PCO_2. Plasma potassium concentration is elevated because of a shift from the intracellular compartment to the extracellular compartment. Treatment is directed at the underlying cause.

Respiratory acidosis

This results from carbon dioxide retention in respiratory failure. The usual causes in surgical patients are underlying chronic respiratory disease made worse by postoperative chest complications or prolonged respiratory depression due to sedative, hypnotic or narcotic drugs. Plasma hydrogen ion concentrations and PCO_2 are elevated but standard bicarbonate is initially normal. A degree of metabolic compensation may occur as the kidneys excrete excess hydrogen ions and retain bicarbonate. Treatment is directed at the underlying cause and to providing assisted ventilation.

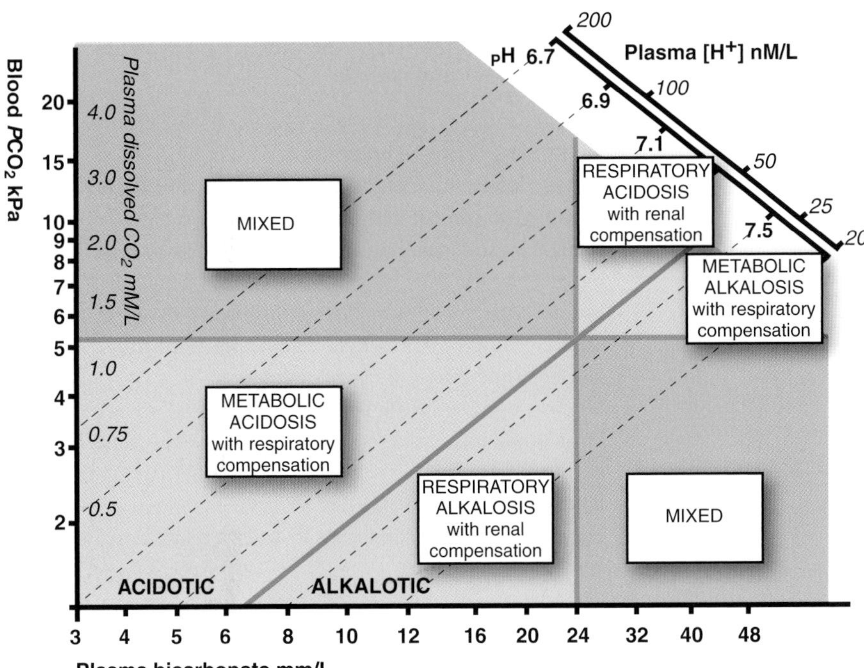

Fig. 2.4 Interpretation of blood gas analyses in the patient with acid–base disturbances

Table 2.4 Acid–base disorders

Acid–base status	Blood gas analyses		
	pH	PCO_2	HCO_3^-
Respiratory acidosis	↓ or normal (if compensated)	↑↑	↑ (if compensated)
Respiratory alkalosis	↑ or normal (if compensated)	↓↓	↓ (if compensated)
Metabolic acidosis	↓ or normal (if compensated)	↓ (if compensated)	↓↓
Metabolic alkalosis	↑ or normal (if compensated)	↑ (if compensated)	↑↑

Metabolic alkalosis

Metabolic alkalosis is usually caused by severe and repeated vomiting or prolonged nasogastric aspiration for intestinal obstruction. The latter classically occurs in pyloric stenosis with gross loss of gastric acid. The patient becomes severely dehydrated and depleted of sodium and chloride ions; the condition is thus known as **hypochloraemic alkalosis**. The kidney attempts to compensate by conserving hydrogen ions but this occurs at the expense of potassium ions lost into the urine. Patients become hypokalaemic not only from excess urinary loss but also because potassium shifts into the cells in response to the alkalosis. Treatment of hypochloraemic hypokalaemic alkalosis involves rehydration with normal saline infusion including potassium supplements; large volumes (up to 10 litres) are often required. Renal excretion of bicarbonate ions eventually corrects the alkalosis.

Respiratory alkalosis

This occurs when carbon dioxide is lost via excessive pulmonary ventilation. The usual cause in surgical practice is prolonged mechanical ventilation during general anaesthesia or in the intensive care unit without adequate monitoring.

NUTRITIONAL MANAGEMENT IN THE SURGICAL PATIENT

ESSENTIAL PRINCIPLES

Malnutrition is a wasting condition resulting from deficiencies in energy (i.e. calorie), protein and sometimes vitamins and trace elements. Recognising and treating pre-existing malnutrition and preventing postoperative starvation are important aspects of surgical management that are often neglected. Basic evaluation for malnutrition should be a standard part of assessing surgical patients (see Box 2.4) because untreated malnutrition predisposes to a range of problems that substantially increase morbidity and mortality rates and delay recovery (see Box 2.5).

Causes of malnutrition include **reduced food intake** (anorexia, fasting, pain on swallowing, physical or mental

Box 2.4 Assessing patients for malnutrition

Clinical assessment

- Lack of nutritional intake for 5 days or more
- Clinical appearance ('end-of-bedogram')—does the patient look malnourished?
- Unintentional weight loss of more than 10% from usual body weight within previous 6 months indicates malnutrition. More than 20% is likely to represent severe malnutrition
- Body mass index (BMI)—less than 18.5 suggests malnutrition

Anthropometric assessment

- Triceps skin fold thickness—technically difficult to perform but provides a good proxy for body density and hence overall fat content
- Mid arm circumference—unreliable because of technical measurement artefact and lack of dependable data upon which to base measurements
- Hand grip strength—easy to perform but lack of reproducible baseline data limits application to research projects

Blood indices

- Reduced plasma albumin, prealbumin or transferrin. In critically ill patients, plasma albumin of less than 35 g/L is associated with a five-fold increase in complications and a 10-fold increase in death rate. Note that low plasma albumin alone is not an accurate marker of malnutrition but may be caused by other metabolic abnormalities
- Reduced lymphocyte count. If plasma albumin and lymphocyte count are both low, there is a 20-fold increase in death rate

impairment), **malabsorption** (impaired digestion or absorption, or excess loss from gut) and **altered metabolism** (trauma, burns, sepsis, surgery, cancer cachexia). Patients with any of these predisposing factors need to be scrutinised more thoroughly for malnutrition.

In practice, most surgical patients have no special nutritional requirements and easily withstand the short period of starvation associated with their illness and operation. All hospitalised patients should be screened using a recognised screening tool and their nutritional state optimised preoperatively as far as is feasible. In any case, optimal nutritional support should be provided after operation.

Nutritional support in hospital is usually provided by a dedicated team and input ranges from encouraging the patient to eat regularly through offering easily prepared but tasty oral diets (e.g. liquidised normal food), through concentrated **sip feeds** (e.g. Fortisip) and various types of supplementary **enteral nutrition** given via tube, to managing long-term **total parenteral nutrition (TPN)** for patients unable to absorb nutrients from the gastrointestinal tract.

Box 2.5 Adverse effects of protein/calorie depletion in surgical patients

- Protein deficiency leads to impaired wound healing and higher rates of wound breakdown
- Protein depletion seriously impairs immune function and the ability to combat infection
- Skeletal muscle mass is lost, reducing muscular strength and general physical activity as well as causing fatigue. This increases the risk of thromboembolism and pressure sores
- Thoracic muscle mass depletion depresses respiratory efficiency and increases risk of pneumonia
- Albumin becomes depleted leading to generalised oedema
- Small bowel mucosal atrophy reduces its ability to absorb nutrients and may lead to bacterial translocation into the bloodstream because of loss of mucosal integrity
- Impaired mental function leads to apathy, depression and low morale
- Postoperative complication rates are higher—twice the rate of minor complications, three times the rate of major complications and three times the mortality compared with well-nourished patients
- Combinations of these factors lead to prolonged recovery times and longer hospital stays

RECOGNISING THE PATIENT AT RISK

Malnutrition is common in surgical patients and often goes unrecognised. Studies have shown that as many as 50% of surgical inpatients suffer from mild malnutrition and 30% from severe malnutrition. Simple clinical assessment is the best determinant of the state of nutrition, although other indices can also be used (see Box 2.4).

For patients found to be malnourished, studies have shown that simple pretreatment with regular proprietary sip feeds can stave off postoperative muscle weakness, reduce fatigue and markedly lessen complication rates. However, the evidence of clinical benefit is weak for more complex and prolonged endeavours to improve nutrition by the parenteral route (for example, in oesophageal cancer). Even if it is impracticable to improve the preoperative nutritional state, malnutrition still needs to be recognised and attention given in the postoperative period. The duration of starvation should be kept as short as possible and appropriate nutrition provided. This contributes to healing, improves resistance to infection and reduces complications caused by muscle weakness (see Box 2.5).

EFFECTS OF STARVATION

Simple starvation

During simple starvation (i.e. in the absence of illness or trauma), blood glucose concentration is maintained by lowering of insulin secretion and increasing glucagon production. Liver glycogen becomes exhausted within 24 hours but

gluconeogenesis in liver and kidneys is enhanced, utilising amino acids from protein breakdown and glycerol from lipolysis as substrates. Much of the glucose thus produced is used by the brain, as most other tissues are able to metabolise fatty acids and ketones derived from adipose tissue. Overall energy demands fall in simple starvation and energy is obtained largely from body fat. Protein is conserved until a late stage.

Trauma, surgery or sepsis

In severe trauma or major surgery, and particularly in sepsis, energy requirements increase by 20–100% of normal. As in simple starvation, lipid becomes a major fuel source; this decreases glucose utilisation, but fatty acids other than glycerol cannot be used for glucose synthesis. Hepatic glucose production increases, but peripheral glucose utilisation is impaired, often leading to hyperglycaemia.

Skeletal **muscle proteolysis** and urinary nitrogen excretion increase enormously compared with the fasted state. Protein from skeletal muscle is catabolised to release amino acids (particularly alanine), lactate and pyruvate. The stimulus for proteolysis is likely to be macrophage cytokines (e.g. IL1, IL6, TNF). IL1 reduces hepatic albumin synthesis in favour of more urgently needed **acute-phase proteins** and gluconeogenesis. Amino acids are also used directly in wound healing and in haemopoiesis.

In **sepsis**, there is a progressive inability at mitochondrial level to fully oxidise substrates for energy generation, leading to a fall in oxygen consumption as sepsis worsens. Fatty acids are increasingly mobilised from adipose tissue, manifesting as hypertriglyceridaemia; mobilisation is governed by raised levels of glucagon, catecholamines, cortisol and TNF. Fatty acids are oxidised for adenosine triphosphate (ATP) production in order to fuel synthesis of new glucose and proteins. If liver failure develops, amino acid clearance deteriorates and plasma concentrations rise. Some amino acids are then metabolised into false neurotransmitters which promote the vasodilatation and hypotension seen in sepsis and cause septic encephalopathy.

SUPPLEMENTARY NUTRITION

Supplementary nutrition other than liquidised diets and sip feeds is a complicated and sometimes expensive process with distinct risk of complications. It should not be undertaken without proper assessment. Deciding whether a patient is likely to benefit from supplementary nutrition depends on determining:

- That the patient is malnourished or will be deprived of nutrition for at least 5 days
- That the patient is likely to benefit—certain conditions make supplemental nutrition ineffective (e.g. enteral feeding in high output enterocutaneous fistula)
- Whether there is an appropriate route for administration, e.g. suitable gut function

Nutritional support is generally recommended in well-nourished patients who are unable to tolerate oral feeding for 7–10 days, or 5–7 days if already malnourished.

Methods of giving supplementary nutrition

Box 2.6 summarises the range of nutritional regimens and their main surgical indications. The gastrointestinal tract should be used whenever possible because any form of enteral feeding is intrinsically safer than parenteral nutrition and is much cheaper. In addition, the small intestinal mucosa tends to atrophy when not used. Enteral feeding supports the **gut-associated immunological shield** and prevents microorganisms translocating into the circulation, reducing the chances of blood-borne infection. Contraindications to enteral feeding include intestinal obstruction, high-output intestinal fistula, intractable vomiting or diarrhoea, and severe malabsorption.

Sip feeds

If the patient is able to eat, fluid diets (total or supplementary) can be given orally. Proprietary sip feeds containing easily absorbed calories, protein, minerals and vitamins are available in a variety of formulations and flavours and are well tolerated.

Box 2.6 Special methods of nutrition and their indications

1. **Selective diets for specific indications**, e.g. diabetic, low-protein (renal and liver failure), low-fat (gallstones), high-fibre (constipation, diverticular disease) or weight reducing (obesity)
2. **Liquidised normal diet**—for patients with partial oesophageal obstruction (e.g. stricture, tumour or oesophageal intubation for cancer)
3. **High-protein, high-calorie dietary supplements 'sip diet'**—for chronically malnourished patients capable of a normal diet or debilitated convalescent patients
4. **Polymeric liquid diet** via tube—short chain peptides, medium chain triglycerides and polysaccharides plus vitamins and trace elements These contain the full range of nutritional requirements often including fibre. Used for nutritional support of patients unable to eat or drink such as the unconscious, ventilated and seriously ill patient in intensive care or patients unwilling to take adequate nutrition following major surgery or trauma
5. **Elemental diet** via tube, containing L-amino acids and simple sugars requiring no digestion and minimal absorptive capacity—for patients with minimal remaining bowel after massive resection. These are expensive and unpalatable and the high osmolarity can cause diarrhoea
6. **Peripheral parenteral nutritional support** for patients unable to have tube feeding but needing specific energy or protein supplementation
7. **Total parenteral nutrition (TPN)**, i.e. comprehensive intravenous nutrition—for patients with prolonged ileus or a very proximal fistula

Tube feeds

Certain patients are unsuitable for sip feeding but can be fed by one of several tube feeding routes. Indications include patients with swallowing difficulties (including overspill and lack of cooperation), anorexia, lack of palatability of liquid feeds, the need for a higher volume of feed than the patient can comfortably manage and anticipated substantial delay in resuming oral feeding after operation.

Even if the patient is unable to swallow (for example, because of bulbar palsy, unconsciousness or facial fractures), complete enteral nutrition can be delivered by means of a **fine-bore nasogastric** or **nasojejunal tube**, the latter for those who require post-pyloric enteral feeding, e.g. in acute pancreatitis). An individual fluid diet is formulated and is delivered at a controlled rate using a pump, often overnight.

Feeding tubes can also be placed percutaneously into stomach or jejunum, either at operation (if feeding problems are anticipated) or with endoscopic or laparoscopic help. Gastrostomies are often employed in patients after stroke or in those with upper gastrointestinal anastomoses or obstructing lesions. The usual technique nowadays is by **percutaneous endoscopic gastrostomy (PEG)**, combining gastroscopy and percutaneous placement. PEG tubes are contraindicated in peritonitis, ascites and prolonged ileus.

For **jejunostomy** placement, the tube is tunnelled submucosally for a distance before entering the bowel lumen using a wide-bore needle; this minimises the risk of leakage. Jejunostomy tubes must be placed under direct vision at operation or laparoscopically.

Certain patients not requiring full enteral or parenteral feeding may benefit from vitamin supplements, for example, folic acid and thiamine for alcoholics, or vitamin K injections for patients on prolonged antibiotic therapy where disturbed gut flora may impair absorption of vitamin K.

TOTAL PARENTERAL NUTRITION (TPN)

Parenteral nutrition should be reserved for appropriate cases of intestinal failure (see below) and should not be embarked upon lightly.

TPN formulations principally contain a mixture of glucose, amino acids, lipids, minerals and vitamins. Non-nitrogenous sources of energy in the form of glucose and lipids have a **protein-sparing** effect and minimise the consumption of amino acids as energy.

The osmolality of the mixture is usually high so that administration needs to be via a dedicated central venous line to minimise the risk of venous thrombosis; formulations for peripheral infusion are available but the technique is losing favour. The usual aim of TPN is to provide sufficient nitrogen and energy to offset the catabolic demands of surgery and/or trauma and their complications and, if possible, compensate for any pre-existing malnutrition.

In calculating requirements, protein intake should be matched to estimated nitrogen losses; this can be calculated by measuring urinary nitrogen losses as urea or else a standard formula (which also estimates other requirements) can be employed. For example, basic adult daily requirements are 100 g protein (as amino acids), 350 g glucose and 50 g lipid to provide energy. These quantities need to be adjusted according to individual requirements.

Excessive nutrition can be a problem. Hyperglycaemia can be corrected with modest doses of insulin but in the longer term disturbances of liver function may reflect intrahepatic cholestasis caused by fatty infiltration. In intrahepatic cholestasis blood tests show elevated plasma alkaline phosphatase and gamma glutaryl transferase.

Indications for TPN

Parenteral nutrition should be reserved for patients who are already malnourished (or are likely to become malnourished), in whom the GI tract is not functional or is inaccessible and is likely to remain so for a substantial period of days or weeks. Note that in major sepsis, the metabolic changes described earlier mean that TPN brings little benefit.

Indications may include:

- Enterocutaneous fistula
- Intra-abdominal infection
- Short bowel syndrome where there is insufficient residual absorptive capacity after massive small bowel resection
- Multiple injuries involving viscera

Methods of giving TPN

Parenteral nutrition is usually delivered into the superior vena cava via the internal jugular or subclavian vein. This is so that high venous flow rapidly dilutes the hyperosmolar solution, minimising thrombosis risk. If long periods of nutritional support are anticipated, a designated **tunnelled line** is usually employed, with the skin access point remote from the venous entry point to minimise risk of line infection.

The choice and quantity of nutrients starts from a standard baseline for body weight and is varied (with specialist advice) according to individual needs.

Parenteral nutrition is costly in materials and staff time and is prone to complications; it should be discontinued as soon as nutrition can be supplied by an enteral route. Patients on TPN need close and regular monitoring for a range of problems including line problems, local and systemic infection, fluid balance and deficiencies of electrolytes (see Box 2.7). Complications of TPN are detailed in Box 2.8.

REFEEDING SYNDROME

Refeeding syndrome was first described in prisoners in the Far East after the Second World War who developed cardiac failure when starting to eat after prolonged starvation. With reduced carbohydrate intake, insulin secretion falls and fat and protein are catabolised in place of carbohydrate. This results in loss of intracellular electrolytes, particularly phosphate, which becomes depleted. Phosphate is essential for generating adenosine triphosphate and for other vital phosphorylation reactions.

When enteral or parenteral feeding is restarted after starvation, there is sudden reversion from fat to carbohydrate metabolism. Insulin secretion rises and cellular uptake of glucose, phosphate, potassium and water increases. This can lead to profound hypophosphataemia, often with hypokalaemia and hypomagnesaemia. Note that all extracellular fluid is

Box 2.7 Monitoring of parenteral nutrition

8-hourly

- Blood glucose (finger-prick sticks) 2–4 times daily
- Temperature and pulse rate

Daily

- Fluid balance charts and body weight
- Inspection of line entry site (blood cultures on any sign of local or systemic infection)
- Plasma urea, electrolytes until stable

Twice-weekly

- Creatinine and liver function tests

Weekly

- Plasma calcium, phosphate, magnesium (if risk of refeeding syndrome, should be measured daily until stable)
- Zinc and selenium can be measured initially and then every 2–4 weeks

affected by declining levels of these electrolytes. In the starved state, there is total body depletion of electrolytes but plasma concentrations can be misleadingly normal because of renal compensation.

Refeeding syndrome occurs when plasma phosphate falls to less than 0.50 mmol/L. Clinical features include **cardiac and respiratory failure, arrhythmias, rhabdomyolysis, white cell dysfunction, seizures, coma and sudden death**. Early signs may go unrecognised; the plasma phosphate may not be measured or the significance of grossly abnormal results not appreciated.

Malnourished patients at risk of refeeding syndrome should start artificial feeding with a quarter to half of the expected calorie requirements. Plasma phosphate, magnesium, calcium, potassium, urea and creatinine concentrations should be measured daily and deficiencies corrected. If required, 50 mmol of intravenous phosphate is given over 24 hours and may need repeating. Thiamine must also be replaced in these patients.

Box 2.8 Complications of parenteral nutrition

Catheter problems (10% of central lines develop substantial complications)

- Central venous line placement problems, e.g. failure to cannulate, trauma to great arteries or veins, pneumothorax, haemothorax, brachial plexus injury, loss of Seldinger wire into vein
- Line infection—a common cause of fever and tachycardia likely to progress to systemic sepsis. If suspected, blood cultures should be taken from the line. If positive, line must be removed and tip cultured
- Blockage, breakage or leakage of catheter
- Air embolism
- Central venous thrombosis

Metabolic problems (5% develop metabolic derangements)

- Hypophosphataemia (PO_4 < 0.5 mmol/L)
- Hypernatraemia (Na > 150 mmol/L)
- Hyponatraemia (Na < 130 mmol/L)
- Hyperglycaemia
- Overnutrition
- Long-term—fatty degeneration of the liver
- Trace element and folate deficiency
- Deranged liver function tests
- Linoleic acid deficiency

3 Immunity, inflammation and infection

IMMUNE RESPONSES

INTRODUCTION

The **innate immune response** constitutes the first line of defence against invading microorganisms. The key mechanism is recognition of pathogen-derived molecules by Toll-like receptors (TLRs) found on the surface of dendritic cells, which triggers inflammatory responses to limit infection. The **adaptive immune system**, involving T and B cells, is much more organism specific. During the course of an infection, it evolves to deal optimally with the microorganism(s) involved. Once created, memory T and B cells remain, priming the body for any later attack by the same organism. Vaccines operate by promoting this adaptive system.

INNATE IMMUNITY

The innate system produces a semi-specific response to newly encountered organisms. It is also essential to triggering adaptive responses via signalling cytokines. **Macrophages** and **dendritic cells** patrol the tissues for foreign proteins likely to indicate infection. Invaders bearing foreign proteins are engulfed and destroyed by antimicrobial molecules and the **complement system** is activated. Once engaged, the Toll-like receptors prompt the cells to unleash particular suites of cytokines which recruit additional macrophages, dendritic cells and other immune cells to contain and destroy the infecting organisms. **Dendritic** cells containing engulfed protein then transit to lymph nodes where they present fragments of the pathogen's protein to an array of T cells and release more cytokines. **Lipopolysaccharide** (LPS) produced by Gram-negative bacteria is a particularly powerful immune stimulator. It prompts inflammatory cells to release **tumour necrosis factor alpha (TNF-alpha), interferon** and **interleukin -1 (IL1)**. These cytokines are probably the most important in controlling the inflammatory response, and also, if unchecked, in causing autoimmune disorders, e.g. rheumatoid arthritis.

At least 10 human varieties of TLRs are known. They act in pairs and each pair binds to a different class of protein characteristic of a type or group of organisms, e.g. Gram-negative bacteria, single-stranded DNA viruses or flagellin. The released cytokines generate the typical symptoms of infection—fever and flu-like symptoms.

Overactivity of this innate system can lead to potentially fatal **sepsis**. TLRs may also be implicated in **autoimmunity** by responding inappropriately, for example to damaged cells. A range of **drugs** that activate particular TLRs are in advanced stages of testing, e.g. as vaccine adjuvants or antiviral agents. Inhibitors are also under development for treating sepsis, inflammatory bowel disease and autoimmune diseases, so far with limited success.

ADAPTIVE IMMUNITY

Macrophages and other antigen-presenting cells, having 'processed' a pathogen, display fragments on their surface. This ultimately activates B and T cells that recognise that fragment to proliferate, and initiate a powerful and highly focused immune response. Activated B cells secrete antibody molecules that bind to unique antigen components and destroy the target or else mark it for destruction. T cells recognise antigens displayed on cells. Some activate more B and T cells whilst others directly attack infected cells. Following the initial infection, enough memory T and B cells remain to deal effectively with the organism, should it return. This can occur so quickly that inflammation may not occur.

INFLAMMATION

ACUTE INFLAMMATION

Introduction

Acute inflammation is the principal mechanism by which living tissues respond to injury. The purpose is to neutralise the injurious agent, to remove damaged or necrotic tissue and to restore the tissue to useful function. The central feature is formation of an inflammatory exudate with three principal components: **serum**, **leucocytes** (predominantly neutrophils) and **fibrinogen**.

Formation of inflammatory exudate involves local vascular changes collectively responsible for the four '**cardinal signs of Celsus**'—rubor (redness), tumor (swelling), calor (heat) and dolor (pain)—as well as loss of function. These vascular phenomena are described in Figure 3.1. The outcomes of acute inflammation are summarised in Figure 3.2.

Resolution

If tissue damage is minimal and there is no actual tissue necrosis, the acute inflammatory response eventually settles and tissues return virtually to normal without evidence of scarring. A good example is the resolution of mild sunburn.

Abscess formation (Fig. 3.3)

An abscess is a collection of pus (dead and dying neutrophils plus proteinaceous exudate) walled off by a zone of acute inflammation. Acute abscess formation particularly occurs in response to certain **pyogenic** microorganisms that attract neutrophils but are resistant to phagocytosis and lysosomal destruction. Abscesses also form in response to localised tissue necrosis and to some organic foreign bodies (e.g. wood splinters, linen suture material). The main pyogenic organisms of surgical importance are *Staphylococcus aureus*,

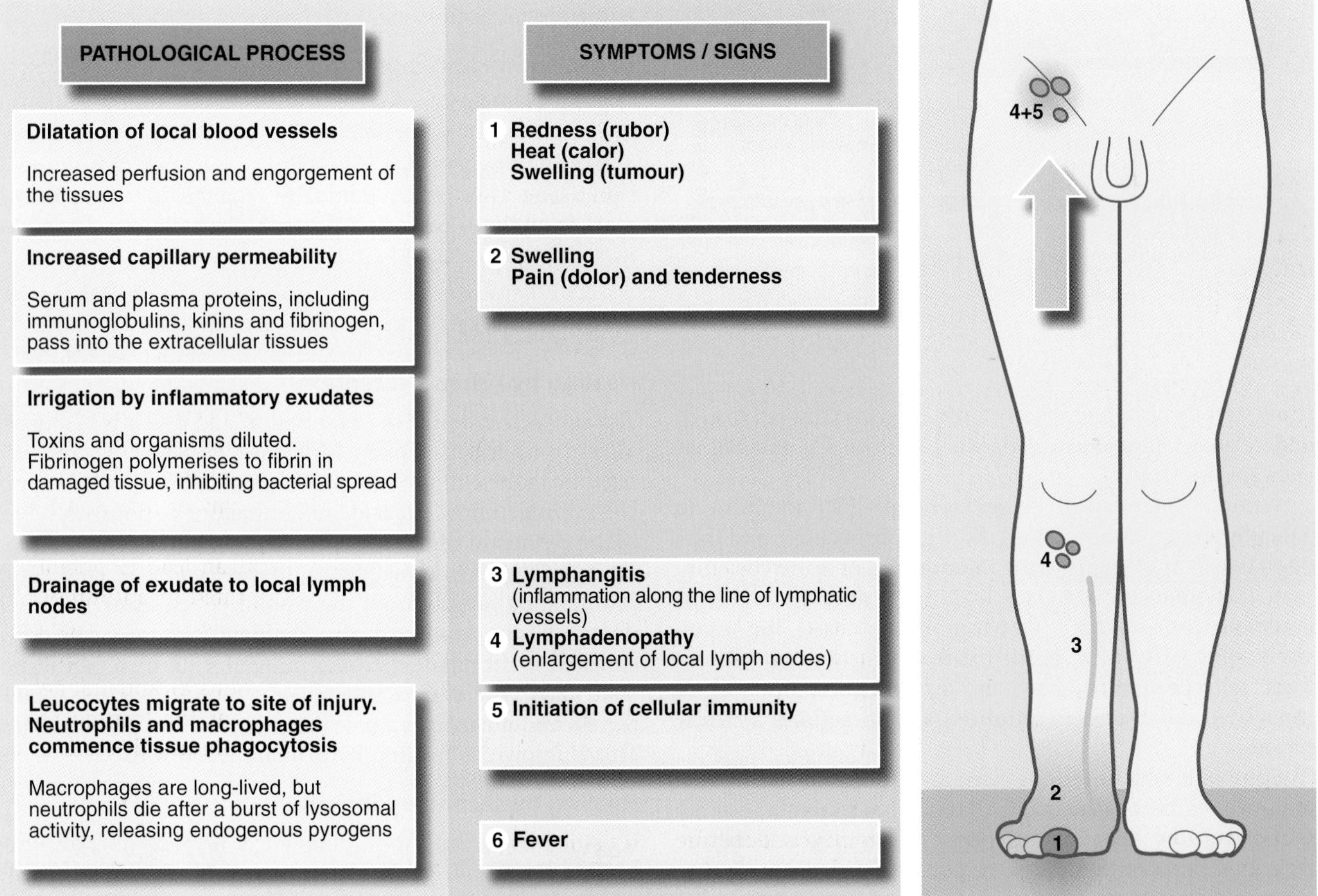

Fig. 3.1 Acute inflammation—pathophysiology and clinical features

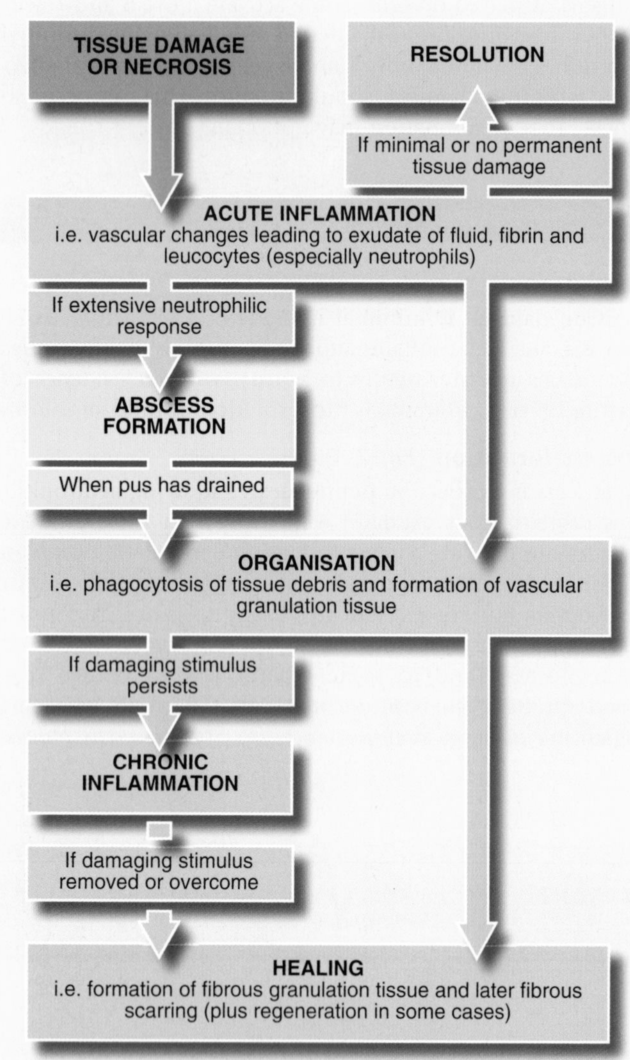

Fig. 3.2 Acute inflammation and its sequelae

some streptococci (particularly *Strep. pyogenes*), *Escherichia coli* and related Gram-negative bacilli ('coliforms'), and *Bacteroides* species (spp.).

Without treatment, abscesses eventually tend to '**point**' to a nearby epithelial surface (e.g. skin, gut, bronchus), and then discharge their contents. If the injurious agent is thereby eliminated, spontaneous drainage leads to healing. If an abscess is remote from a surface (e.g. deep in the breast), it progressively enlarges causing much tissue destruction. Sometimes local defence mechanisms are overwhelmed, leading to runaway local infection (**cellulitis**) and sometimes systemic sepsis.

Even with small, well-localised abscesses, showers of bacteria may enter the general circulation (**bacteraemia**) but are mopped up by hepatic and splenic phagocytic cells before they can proliferate. This is responsible for the **swinging pyrexia** characteristic of an abscess. The abscess site may not be clinically evident if deep-seated (e.g. subphrenic or pelvic abscess) and the patient may be otherwise well. In the presence of an abscess, circulating neutrophils rise dramatically as they are released from the bone marrow; thus, a marked **neutrophil leucocytosis** (i.e. WBC greater than 15×10^9/L with more than 80% neutrophils) usually indicates a pyogenic infection. Severe infection causing excessive cytokine responses spilling over into the systemic circulation causes **systemic sepsis** and rapid clinical deterioration (see p. 51).

The chronic state

(see *Chronic inflammation*, p. 37)

The essence of managing any abscess is to establish complete **drainage**, usually by incision or aspiration. Any residual necrotic or foreign material needs to be eliminated by curettage or excision. If drainage of an abscess does not eliminate the injurious agent, the neutrophil response persists and pus continues to be formed, resulting in a **chronic abscess**.

Antibiotics and abscesses

If appropriate antibiotics are given early enough, organisms can be eliminated before abscess formation. In surgical operations with a particular risk of infection, therefore, **prophylactic antibiotics** dramatically reduce abscess formation and other infective complications. However, once an abscess has fully formed, antibiotics seldom effect a cure because pus and necrotic material remain and the drug cannot gain access to the bacteria within. Nevertheless, antibiotics may halt expansion or even sterilise the pus; the residual sterile abscess is known as an **antibioma**.

Organisation and repair

The most common sequel to acute inflammation is **organisation**, in which dead tissue is removed by phagocytosis and the defect filled by vascular connective tissue known as **granulation tissue**. This tissue is gradually 'repaired' to form a **fibrous scar**. Sometimes the original tissue regenerates, i.e. rebuilds its specialised cells and structure.

WOUND HEALING

Healing by primary intention

The simplest example of organisation and repair is healing of an uncomplicated skin incision (see Fig. 3.4). There is no necrotic tissue and the wound margins are brought into apposition with sutures. An acute inflammatory response develops in the vicinity of the incision, and by the third day granulation tissue bridges the dermal defect. In the meantime, epithelium proliferating rapidly from the wound edges restores the epidermis. Fibroblasts invade the granulation tissue, laying down collagen so the repair is strong enough for suture removal after 5–10 days. The scar is still red but blood vessels gradually regress and it becomes a pale linear scar within a few months. This is known as **healing by primary intention**.

Healing by secondary intention

If tissue loss prevents the wound edges from coming together, healing has to bridge the defect, which is initially filled with blood clot. This later becomes infiltrated by vascular granulation tissue from the healthy wound base. Inflammatory

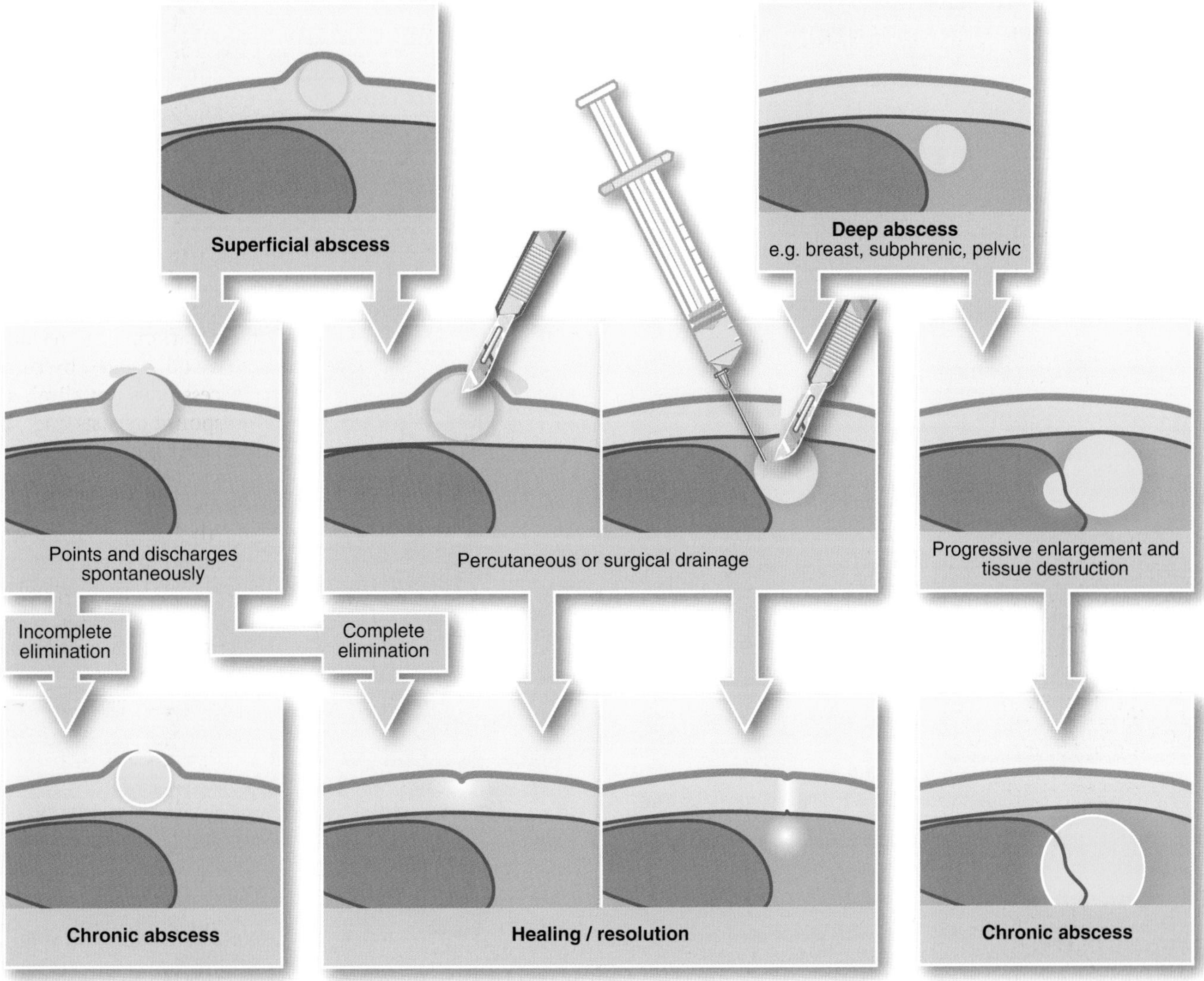

Fig. 3.3 Outcomes after abscess formation

exudate solidifies, forming a protective scab. Fibroblasts invade and lay down collagen in the extracellular spaces; after about a week, some fibroblasts differentiate into **myofibroblasts** and contraction of their myofibrils eventually shrinks the wound defect by 40–80%, beginning about 2 weeks after the injury. Over the weeks and months, blood vessels regress and more collagen is formed, leaving a relatively avascular scar; gradual contraction of the mature collagen (cicatrisation), combined with wound contraction, ensures the final scar is much smaller than the original defect. The epidermal defect is gradually bridged by epithelial proliferation from the wound margins. Epithelial cells slide over each other beneath the edges of the scab on the granulation tissue surface and the scab is eventually shed. This whole process is known as **healing by secondary intention** (see Fig. 3.4).

Factors impairing wound healing

The rate and success of wound healing may be impaired by a variety of local, regional and systemic factors (see Fig. 3.5).

CHRONIC INFLAMMATION

Sometimes an injurious agent persists over a long period causing continuing tissue destruction. The body attempts to deal with the original and the continuing damage by acute inflammation, organisation and repair, all at the same time. The damaged area may display several pathological processes at once, i.e. tissue necrosis, an inflammatory response, granulation tissue formation and fibrous scarring. This is known as chronic inflammation and is characterised histologically by a predominance of **macrophages** (sometimes forming giant cells), responsible for phagocytosis of necrotic debris. Lymphocytes and plasma cells are also present, indicating immunological involvement in chronic inflammation.

Chronic inflammation represents a tenuous balance between a persistent injurious agent and the body's reparative responses. Healing only occurs if the injurious agent is removed and then proceeds in the usual manner but often with much more scarring.

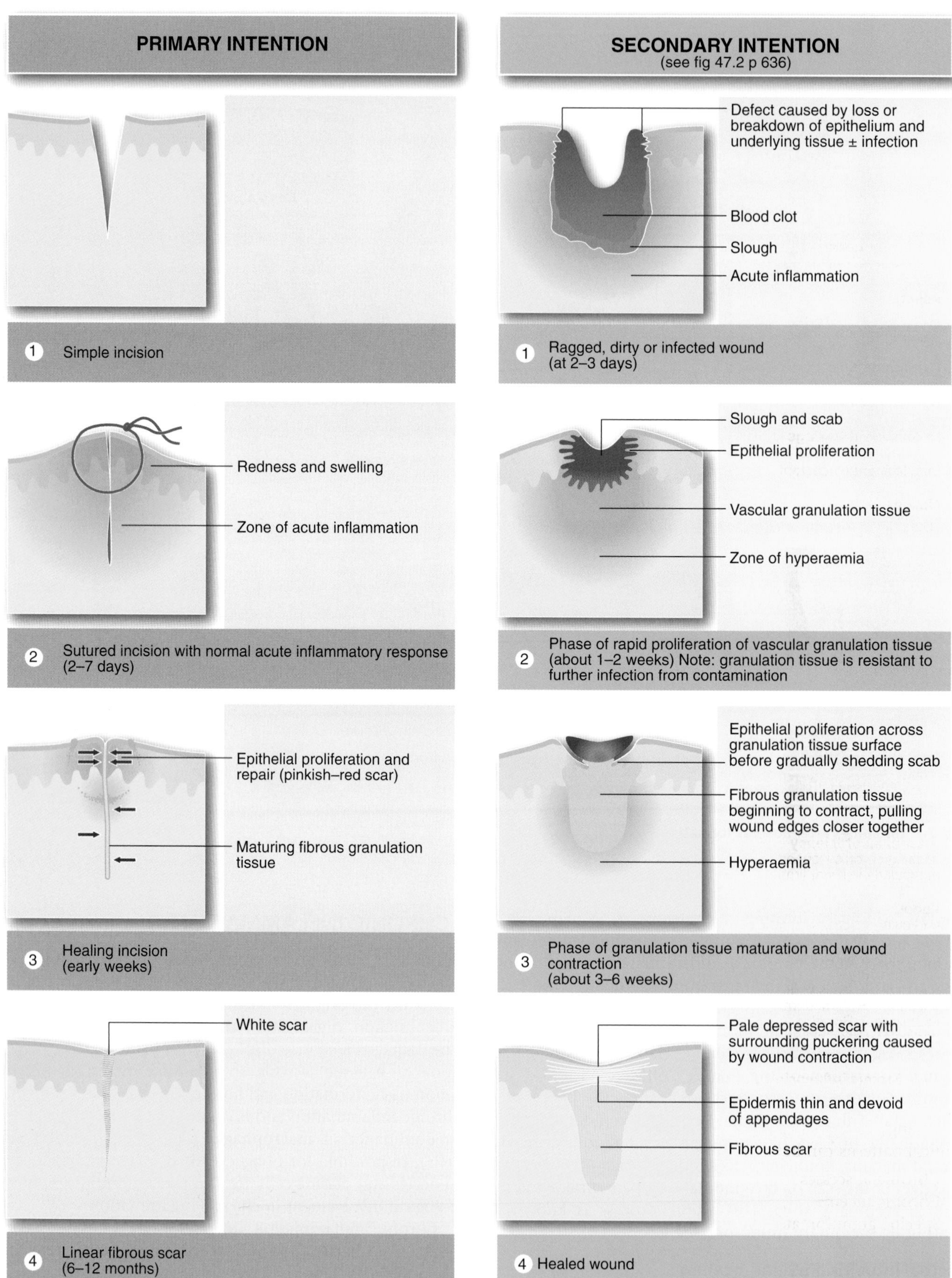

Fig. 3.4 Wound healing by primary and secondary intention

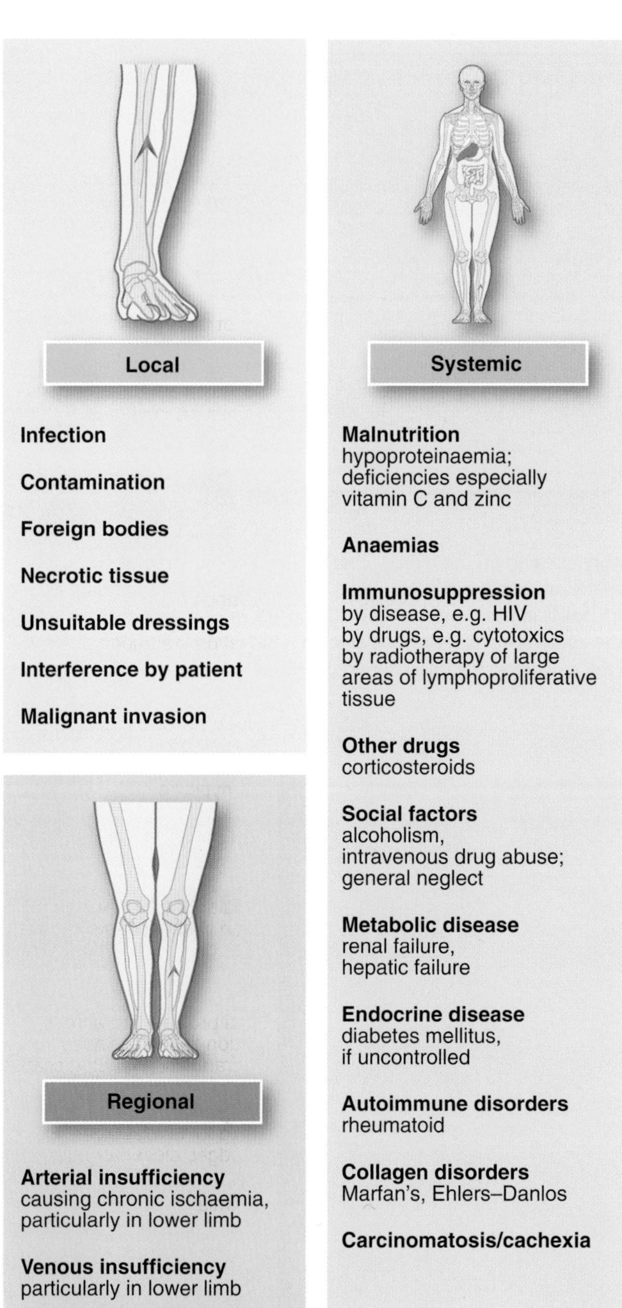

Fig. 3.5 Factors influencing wound healing

A range of agents can lead to chronic inflammation. The clinical patterns can be grouped into three categories:

- Chronic abscesses
- Chronic ulcers
- Specific granulomatous infections and inflammations

CHRONIC ABSCESSES

A chronic abscess arises if the agent causing an acute abscess is not fully eliminated. Pus continues to be formed and the abscess either persists, discharges continuously via a **sinus** or else 'points' and discharges periodically with the sinus healing over between times. A chronic abscess wall consists of fibrous scar tissue lined with granulation tissue.

Causes of chronic abscesses include:

- **Infected foreign bodies** are probably the most common cause in modern surgical practice. Foreign bodies implanted deliberately may become infected (e.g. synthetic mesh for inguinal hernia repair, prosthetic hip joint); others become embedded during trauma (e.g. glass fragments)
- **Dead (necrotic) tissue** can act as a foreign body, forming a nidus for infection. For example, diabetes may be complicated by deep foot infections with necrosis of tendon and bone leading to chronic abscesses and ulcers. Hairs deeply implanted in the natal cleft skin may cause a pilonidal sinus or abscess. An infected dead tooth or root fragment may intermittently discharge via an associated 'gum boil' (see Fig. 3.6). Chronic osteomyelitis is associated with remnants of dead bone known as **sequestra**
- **Deep abscesses**. A chronic abscess can arise without a foreign body if the acute abscess is so deep as to prevent spontaneous drainage. The best example is a subphrenic abscess

CHRONIC ULCERS

An ulcer is defined as a persistent defect in an epithelial or mucosal surface. Except for malignant ulcers, ulceration usually results from low-grade mechanical or chemical injury to epithelium and supporting tissue, together with an impaired reparative response. For example, elderly debilitated patients are susceptible to **pressure sores** ('bed sores') which develop over bony prominences such as the sacrum and heels. In these cases, immobility or diminished protective pain responses prevent the patient regularly shifting position to relieve the pressure of body weight. Tissue necrosis results and healing is impaired by the presence of necrotic tissue and continuing pressure ischaemia. Other contributing factors may include poor tissue perfusion (from cardiac or peripheral vascular disease) and malnutrition.

Another common ulcer is the longstanding leg ulcer in chronic venous insufficiency; this fails to heal because of local nutritional impairment induced by high venous pressure and oedema and is often exacerbated by secondary infection. Ischaemic leg ulcers fail to heal because of insufficient arterial blood flow.

In summary, a chronic ulcer represents an unresolved balance between persistent damaging factors and inadequate reparative responses. The principle of managing ulcers is to remove damaging factors and promote healing mechanisms.

SPECIFIC GRANULOMATOUS INFECTIONS AND INFLAMMATIONS

Certain microorganisms excite a minimal acute inflammatory response whilst stimulating a chronic inflammatory response almost from the outset. These include *Mycobacterium tuberculosis*, *Mycobacterium leprae* and *Treponema pallidum* (causing tuberculosis, leprosy and syphilis, respectively). Lesions are

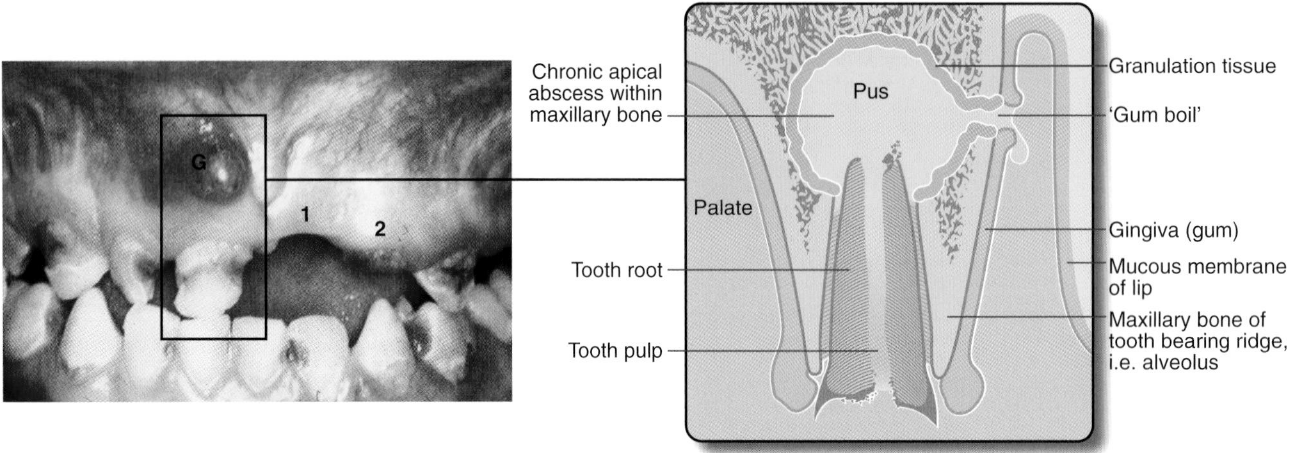

Fig. 3.6 'Gum boil' as an example of a chronic abscess
Grossly neglected mouth showing widespread dental caries. There is an inflammatory swelling on the buccal (cheek) aspect of the alveolus **G** caused by a chronic apical dental abscess on the upper right incisor. Note the left central incisor 1 is missing and the left lateral incisor 2 has fractured at gum level because of caries. Sagittal section through gum boil of upper incisor tooth. The gum boil is in fact a sinus on the gum which discharges either chronically or intermittently. Exposed to infection, the tooth pulp has become necrotic while the apical abscess is slowly expanding due to the continued presence of infected necrotic tissue (i.e. the tooth pulp). The tooth root is all that remains after the crown has fractured due to dental caries

CASE HISTORY

Fig. 3.7 Tuberculous ulcer

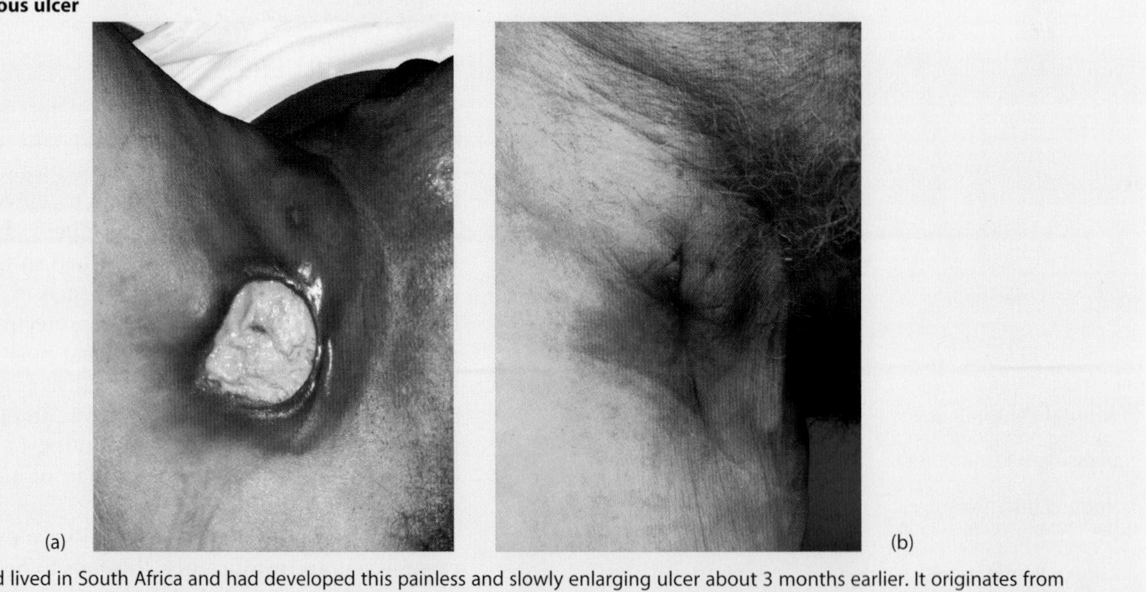

(a) (b)

(a) This patient had lived in South Africa and had developed this painless and slowly enlarging ulcer about 3 months earlier. It originates from nearby infected lymph nodes and shows the typical appearances of a 'wash leather' base and an undercut edge. Diagnosis was based on a biopsy and treatment involved draining the involved lymph nodes visible above the ulcer and a course of antituberculous chemotherapy. **(b)** The healed lesion 2 months later

characterised by accumulation of macrophages forming **granulomas**, and the diseases are known as **granulomatous infections**.

A tuberculous **cold abscess**, now rare in developed countries, is a pus-like accumulation of liquefied caseous material containing the occasional mycobacterium. In contrast to a pyogenic abscess, the lesion is cold to the touch since there is no acute inflammatory vascular response. Cervical lymph node tuberculosis ('scrofula') often produced a 'collar-stud' abscess, i.e. a superficial fluctuant abscess communicating with a deep (and often larger) lymph node abscess via a small fascial defect. Tuberculosis of the thoracolumbar spine causes local destruction and deformity and may track down beneath the inguinal ligament within the psoas sheath, presenting as a '**psoas abscess**' in the groin. A tuberculous ulcer overlying tuberculous inguinal nodes is shown in Figure 3.7.

Certain extremely fine particulate materials such as talc and beryllium produce similar granulomatous reactions known as **foreign body granulomas**. Talc was traditionally used as a lubricant powder in surgical gloves and sometimes caused severe peritoneal granulomatous reactions. For this reason, when body cavities are opened, best practice is to use gloves without powder.

INFECTION

GENERAL PRINCIPLES

It is important to distinguish between colonisation, infection and sepsis:

- **Colonisation** is when bacteria are present in or on a host but do not cause an immune response or signs of disease
- **Infection** occurs when microorganisms provoke a sustained immune response and signs of disease, for example, when normal commensal bacteria in the colon such as *E. coli* contaminate the peritoneal cavity
- **Sepsis** (systemic sepsis) is the result of an excessive and inappropriate production of cytokines in response to severe infection or tissue necrosis (e.g. a gangrenous limb) that causes organ dysfunction and progressive organ failure

Clinically significant infection arises when the size of an inoculum or the virulence of a microorganism is sufficient to overcome the innate and adaptive immune responses and lead to symptoms. The **virulence** of an organism depends on its qualities of adherence and invasiveness and its ability to produce toxins. **Tissue invasion** of microorganisms may be enhanced by their secretion of enzymes (e.g. hyaluronidase and streptokinase), by mechanisms to avoid phagocytosis (e.g. encapsulation or spore formation), by inherent resistance to lysosomal destruction or by their ability to kill phagocytes. Toxins may be secreted by the organism (**exotoxins**) or released upon the death of the organism (**endotoxins**). In either case the toxin may produce local tissue damage (e.g. gas gangrene), cause distant toxic effects (e.g. tetanus), or activate cytokine systems to cause systemic sepsis, sometimes including disseminated intravascular coagulopathy.

Infections may be **community-acquired** (e.g. pneumococcal lobar pneumonia in a fit young adult) or **hospital-acquired**. The latter are also known as **nosocomial** infections and are defined as infections not present or incubating at the time of admission. A third category is health care-associated infection (HCAI) in patients making frequent contacts with health care institutions or in long-term care. Nosocomial infection may be acquired by cross-infection from infected patients, from contaminated furnishings, or from '**carriers**' among staff by inhalation, ingestion or through contamination of medical equipment and devices such as intravenous cannulae or urinary catheters. These infections are often caused by antibiotic-resistant bacteria such as meticillin-resistant *Staphylococcus aureus* (**MRSA**). Risk of such infections can be drastically reduced by the simple measure of everyone in contact with patients cleansing their hands with alcohol-based gel between **every patient contact**. Known MRSA-infected patients or carriers should be isolated when in hospital. Patients having operations where infection carries very high risk should ideally be treated in areas separated from sick patients, especially emergency admissions from long-term care institutions. Particular risk is associated with eye surgery, joint replacements and prosthetic vascular grafts.

Postoperative patients are at particular risk of nosocomial infections (e.g. pneumonias, urinary tract infections) as host defences are impaired by the surgical assault, and physiological **protective mechanisms** are disrupted allowing infection to gain ascendancy. For example, neutropenia predisposes to infection, and smokers are more liable to develop bronchopneumonia following general anaesthesia. The surgical patient's **general resistance** may be further impaired by malnutrition, malignancy, rheumatoid disease, corticosteroids or other immunosuppressive drugs.

In **post-surgical** ('surgical site') infections, organisms enter the tissues via an abnormal breach of epithelium. This may be surface damage (such as a surgical or traumatic wound or an injection) or result from a perforated viscus. The infecting organisms are often part of the patient's normal skin, bowel or respiratory tract flora or are normally present in the external environment. For example, *Staph. epidermidis* is commonly present on skin but causes serious chronic infection of implanted arterial grafts.

METHODS OF CONTROL OF NOSOCOMIAL INFECTION

Environment

Patient areas in hospitals must be clean and free from contaminating bacteria, including MRSA, especially where invasive procedures occur such as operating theatres and high-dependency units. Special precautions are taken in theatres (see Ch. 10, p. 124).

Staff

Staff must be vaccinated against hepatitis B. HIV-positive individuals should not undertake invasive procedures. Open wounds must be securely covered and staff with infective skin lesions should avoid patient contact. Universal blood and body fluid precautions should be taken to prevent viral transmission (see below) and guidelines followed for dealing with needle-stick injuries. Risk of MRSA and other infections can be drastically reduced by the simple measures such as washing hands with alcohol-based gel between **every patient contact**.

Patients

Bacterial swabs should be taken for MRSA from patients before admitting them to hospital and MRSA-positive patients should receive topical eradication therapy and have follow-up bacterial screening cultures to assess MRSA status before major surgery, e.g. hip replacements, arterial grafts. Patients known to have transmissible infections or to be carriers, e.g. of MRSA, should be nursed in isolation. Surgery should ideally be deferred on patients with acute respiratory or urinary tract infections.

Procedures

Equipment—including instruments, needles, theatre gowns and drapes—must be sterile, in secure packaging or as single-use disposable items.

UNIVERSAL BLOOD AND BODY FLUID PRECAUTIONS

Increasing awareness of blood-borne viral infections such as hepatitis B and C and the prevalence of HIV led to the concept of **universal blood and body fluid precautions** in combating cross-infection between patients and staff. Staff often try to be vigilant with high-risk patients but relax at other times. However, this extra care soon lapses. For this reason, every patient should be assumed to be a potential carrier of blood-borne infection and precautions employed whenever skin is likely to be breached and whenever instruments contaminated with blood or other body fluids are handled. Transmission of infection occurs in obvious situations such as needle-stick injury (see below) and with less obvious events such as splashes of infected material into the eye.

Disposable gloves should be worn for all medical procedures and physical examinations except for palpating skin with no obvious open lesion in patient or examiner. Staff with broken skin should apply occlusive dressings. Protective **eyewear** should be worn during invasive procedures to prevent conjunctival splashes.

Hepatitis B vaccination

Staff directly involved in patient care should be vaccinated against hepatitis B. Hepatitis B serology should be checked 2 months after completion of vaccination. Around 5% of healthy young people fail to seroconvert and should be revaccinated. Half of these will seroconvert and the remainder are genetic non-responders.

Needle-stick and other penetrating injuries

Sharps injury, especially from a contaminated hollow needle (needle-stick injury), may lead to transmission of infection if the patient carries a blood-borne virus. Such injuries are capable of transmitting hepatitis B and C but the risk for HIV is much lower because the viral concentration in HIV-positive fluids is much lower and the volume transmitted is small.

Needle-stick injury is common but is largely avoidable: resheathing of used needles causes about 40% of needle-stick injuries and should be avoided. Venepuncture is a high-risk procedure and should be performed with caution. Needles, scalpel blades and other disposable instruments contaminated with blood should be handled with care and disposed of immediately into special plastic 'sharps' containers.

Viral infection following sharps injury

If a definite sharps injury has occurred that involves blood being transmitted from an infected person, the risk of hepatitis B infection to the recipient is about 25%. For hepatitis C the risk is 2% and for HIV 0.5%. There is also a very high risk after sharps injury in a recreational environment (e.g. needles left on the beach by intravenous drug users) since hepatitis B and HIV survive well in warm, moist conditions, especially in serum and tissue debris. Thus all sharps injuries should be treated with the utmost concern. A recommended protocol is shown in Box 3.1.

After a significant exposure to HIV, antiretroviral drugs should be given promptly for post-exposure prophylaxis, ideally within 24 hours. A combination of antiretroviral drugs is given for 4 weeks. Side-effects are often very unpleasant and include bone marrow suppression, nausea and other gastrointestinal symptoms, and headache. For health care workers exposed to hepatitis C, no vaccination or preventative treatment can yet be recommended. Guidelines for post-exposure management are to enable early identification of infection and specialist referral.

Box 3.1 Protocol for managing 'sharps' injuries

1. Wash injured area immediately and encourage blood to flow from wound
2. Record names of people involved and all details of incident
3. Test injured person (the recipient) serologically for HIV, hepatitis B and hepatitis C
4. Test person whose blood/body fluids contaminated the sharp (the donor) for HIV, hepatitis B and hepatitis C
5. If hepatitis B status of recipient or donor is uncertain and cannot be determined reliably within 48 hours of injury (e.g. over a weekend), administer the following to the recipient as soon as possible:
   - hepatitis B immunoglobulin (0.06 ml/kg body weight)
   - hepatitis B vaccine—first dose
6. The immune status of donor and recipient dictates further management as follows:
   - recipient hepatitis B immune—no further action (or may give hepatitis B booster)
   - recipient hepatitis B non-immune (or non-responder) and donor positive or unknown—give hepatitis B immunoglobulin and start course of hepatitis B vaccination
   - recipient hepatitis B non-immune and donor negative—start course of hepatitis B vaccination
   - donor HIV antibody positive or in high-risk group (e.g. homosexual, intravenous drug user, prostitute, heterosexual patients from high HIV incidence countries)—consult infectious diseases physician for post-exposure prophylaxis
   - counsel recipients on safe sex procedures to prevent possible infection of their sexual partners
7. Follow up recipients with serological testing after 3 months (hepatitis B, hepatitis C, HIV), 6 months (hepatitis B and C) and 12 months (hepatitis C); ensure completion of hepatitis B vaccination courses instituted earlier

USE OF MICROBIOLOGICAL TESTS IN MANAGING SURGICAL INFECTIONS

Surgical infection should be diagnosed clinically and the lab used to define its nature and guide antibiotic therapy. Inexperienced junior staff often take swabs which grow organisms in the lab, without realising this may be from **colonisation** and not a clinically important infection. The clinical picture should always determine decisions to treat, although organisms such as *Strep. pyogenes* may require treatment to prevent cross-infection even if the lesion is mild.

Results of specimens from contaminated sites must be interpreted with caution. Superficial slough or discharge often contains only colonising organisms. For example, in *Staph.*

aureus osteomyelitis, the sinus opening may be colonised by *Proteus* or *Pseudomonas* spp. The infecting organism may not be grown unless the wound is cleaned with saline and then swabbed deeply. If possible a syringe of pus or excised infected tissue should be sent for culture. Samples should ideally be taken before antibiotics are given.

For best results, microbiological specimens should be transported to the lab within 2 hours or kept at 4 °C. Blood culture specimens should be incubated at 35 °C.

New technologies are becoming a reality: MALDI-TOF (Matrix Assisted Laser Desorption/Ionisation—Time of Flight) enables same day microbe identification, and molecular techniques such as 16S PCR allow identification of microbes from culture-negative samples.

PRINCIPLES OF TREATMENT OF SURGICAL INFECTION

Removal of infected foci

A poorly vascularised infected area is effectively isolated from humoral and cellular defence mechanisms and from circulating antibiotics. Retained infected material may overactivate cytokine mechanisms and thus precipitate systemic sepsis. A vital first step is to remove infected necrotic tissue and drain collections of pus. This applies even if the patient appears too ill for operation because the very ill patient may recover dramatically after this type of surgery. Common examples include draining abscesses, amputating infected necrotic limbs, removing infected foreign bodies (e.g. cannulae, prostheses, trauma debris) and draining the infected contents of hollow viscera such as bile ducts, kidneys and ureters.

Antibiotic therapy (see Table 3.1)

Empirical antibiotic therapy

If treatment is urgent, antibiotics are chosen according to the most likely pathogens and local antibiotic sensitivity profiles. A Gram stain on material from a usually sterile site can guide initial therapy until detailed results are available. In abdominal wound infections where hollow viscera have not been opened, *Staph. aureus* is the likely organism and flucloxacillin can be commenced. If the patient is a known MRSA carrier, vancomycin may be indicated. If bowel has been opened, Gram-negative organisms including anaerobes are likely and an antibiotic regimen is chosen to include these.

Specific antibiotic therapy

Once microbiological results are available, therapy is modified to deal with the organisms and their sensitivities. 'Narrow-spectrum' therapy is more effective with fewer side-effects than broad-spectrum 'empirical' therapy. It also minimises superinfection with organisms such as *Clostridium difficile* and yeasts. *C. difficile* infections have become a major scourge of hospitals in North America and Europe, mainly due to an ageing population more susceptible to infection and the emergence of a highly virulent clone. Extreme measures to control its spread have been required including strict isolation of patients, high level environmental cleaning and strong antibiotic controls.

Nutritional support

Major infection and sepsis result in severe catabolism (see Ch. 2, p. 29), often associated with hypoalbuminaemia and malnutrition. In these cases nutritional support such as nasogastric tube feeding or parenteral nutrition may be appropriate.

Table 3.1 The main surgical infections, their common microbial causes and suggested empirical therapy

Clinical condition	Common pathogen	Commonly used antibiotics
Gastrointestinal tract		
Gastroenteritis	**Bacterial:** *Campylobacter* *Salmonella* *Shigella and others* **Viral:** SRSV Adenovirus Rotavirus **Travel associated:** *Entamoeba histolytica*	Antibiotics not normally required If severe or lasting >48 h, give ciprofloxacin Metronidazole
Pseudomembranous colitis (hospital-acquired)	*Clostridium difficile*	Metronidazole orally Vancomycin orally second line
Peritonitis Biliary tract	Coliforms Anaerobes *Enterococcus* spp. *E. coli* *Klebsiella* *Bacteroides* *Enterococcus* *Pseudomonas* Clostridia	Co-amoxicillin-clavulanate (ciprofloxacin + metronidazole for peripancreatic infections) or ampicillin + gentamicin + metronidazole

Table 3.1 Continued

Clinical condition	Common pathogen	Commonly used antibiotics
Gastrointestinal tract		
Oesophageal perforation	*Candida*	Fluconazole or itraconazole + Co-amoxicillin-clavulanate
Superficial and wound infections		
Breast abscess or mastitis	*Staphylococcus aureus*	Flucloxacillin or cefradine or erythromycin
Carbuncle, furunculosis	*Staphylococcus aureus*	Avoid antibiotics unless signs of systemic infection Flucloxacillin or cefradine or erythromycin If recurrent, mupirocin/Naseptin nasal cream
Cellulitis	*Staphylococcus aureus, Streptococcus pyogenes* (group A Strep.)	Flucloxacillin or cefradine or erythromycin. If diabetes mellitus, add ciprofloxacin or gentamicin
Gas gangrene	*Clostridium perfringens* and other spp. *Bacteroides spp.* and other anaerobes Coliforms	Surgery essential Penicillin + clindamycin
Infected surgical wound 6–72 hours 3–7 days >7 days	*Streptococcus pyogenes* (group A) *Clostridium* *Staphylococcus aureus* *Streptococcus pyogenes* (group A) *Pseudomonas aeruginosa* *Coliforms*	Surgery essential Co-amoxicillin-clavulanate Co-amoxicillin-clavulanate Drainage/debridement if necessary. Antibiotics if spreading infection
Infected traumatic wound	*Staphylococcus aureus* *Streptococcus pyogenes* (group A)	Cefradine or erythromycin
Necrotising fasciitis	*Streptococcus pyogenes* (group A) Mixed infection with anaerobes and coliforms	Surgery essential Piperacillin-tazobactam + clindamycin
Bites (cat, dog, human)	Anaerobes *Pasteurella spp.* *S. moniliformis*	Co-amoxicillin-clavulanate or doxycycline
Lungs		
Pneumonias Community-acquired	*Staphylococcus* *Pneumococcus* *Chlamydia psittaci* *Mycoplasma* *Legionella*	Co-amoxicillin-clavulanate + clarithromycin + Rifampicin if *Legionella* suspected

BACTERIA OF PARTICULAR SURGICAL IMPORTANCE

STAPHYLOCOCCI

Pathophysiology

Staphylococci are **Gram-positive cocci**, and *Staph. aureus* is the main pathogenic species. It is part of normal human bacterial flora, with about 30% of the population being nasal carriers and 10% carrying it on perineal skin. *Staph. aureus* typically produces pustules, boils, breast abscesses, wound infections and osteomyelitis. Its virulence is partly due to the enzymes and toxins it produces. A few patients harbour virulent strains that produce the **toxic shock syndrome** toxin (TSST-1). Infection produces toxic shock syndrome with serious systemic effects such as hypotension, shock and multi-organ failure. *Staph. epidermidis* (formerly *Staph. albus*), a **coagulase-negative** staphylococcus, is a universal skin commensal rarely causing significant infection and meriting antibiotics only when it causes infections of exogenous materials such as prosthetic implants and intravenous cannulae.

Some strains, including MRSA, can be passed from patient to patient on staff hands if care is not taken with hand washing after every patient contact.

Antibiotic sensitivities

Most strains were sensitive to penicillin but more than 85% are now resistant in family practice and hospital. Resistance is largely due to production of the enzyme beta-lactamase (also known as **penicillinase**). Most strains remain sensitive to a range of common antibiotics, e.g. **flucloxacillin**, **erythromycin** and some **cephalosporins**. **Gentamicin** is also active.

MRSA

Some strains of *Staph. aureus* are resistant to flucloxacillin, cephalosporins, gentamicin, erythromycin and chloramphenicol and are sensitive only to the glycopeptide antibiotics, **vancomycin and teicoplanin**, given parenterally; these are **meticillin-resistant *Staph. aureus* (MRSA)**. Meticillin is employed in the lab to predict flucloxacillin and cephalosporin resistance. MRSA now accounts for about half of all *S. aureus* isolates in hospitals and is also a problem in the community with community-acquired MRSA (CA-MRSA). Ward areas at greatest risk are burns units, intensive care units and cardiothoracic, neonatal, orthopaedic and geriatric wards. It is often erroneously believed that MRSA is more pathogenic than other strains. In fact, the organisms excite similar inflammatory responses but MRSA infections are more difficult to treat. In some cases, oral treatment with **tetracycline**, **co-trimoxazole** or a **combination of rifampicin and fusidic acid** is appropriate; the combination prevents rapid development of resistance to each agent alone.

A worrying development is the emergence of vancomycin-insensitive *Staph. aureus*, **VISA**. Inappropriate use of vancomycin must be avoided to prevent selection of such mutants. New antibiotics active against MRSA and VISA have been developed, including linezolid (which can be given orally), daptomycin and tigecycline.

STREPTOCOCCI

Pathophysiology

Streptococci are **Gram-positive** coccoid organisms first described in infected surgical wounds by Billroth in 1874. They are classified by their oxygen requirements into **aerobic**, **anaerobic** and **microaerophilic** and subdivided by their **haemolysis** patterns on blood agar culture plates. **Alpha-haemolytic streptococci** cause partial haemolysis with green discolouration; important pathogens include the ***viridans*** group and *Strep. pneumoniae*. **Beta-haemolytic streptococci** produce complete haemolysis and can be grouped serologically into **Lancefield groups** A to O. The important human pathogens are group A (*Strep. pyogenes*—of major surgical importance) and group B (*Strep. agalactiae*—a common cause of serious neonatal sepsis). Group C and G streptococci are occasional causes of cellulitis and bacteraemia. Microaerophilic streptococci such as *Strep. milleri* carry a group F antigen.

Streptococci of particular surgical significance

Strep. pyogenes (group A *Strep.* and other beta-haemolytic streptococci)

This is the main human pathogenic streptococcus and is carried in the upper respiratory tract by about 10% of children but less often by adults. It can cause cellulitis and is a common cause of sore throat as well as post-streptococcal syndromes such as rheumatic fever (which predisposes to cardiac valvular damage and risk of infective endocarditis).

Acute **cellulitis** is a locally spreading infection of dermis and hypodermis, facilitated by production of hyaluronidase and streptokinase. In limb infections, organisms draining towards lymph nodes can produce perilymphatic inflammation and painful red streaks along the limb, i.e. **lymphangitis**. Regional nodes react vigorously, becoming enlarged, painful and tender, i.e. **lymphadenitis**. This may also occur in staphylococcal infections.

Highly invasive strains of *Strep. pyogenes* may cause **necrotising fasciitis,** a deep-seated infection of subcutaneous tissue that progressively destroys fascia and fat. Exotoxins produced by certain strains can lead to a life-threatening **streptococcal toxic shock syndrome**, with fulminant soft tissue infection, shock, acute respiratory distress syndrome and renal failure; 30–70% of patients die in spite of aggressive modern treatments.

Viridans streptococci

The *viridans* group are oral commensals of low virulence but are the most common organisms causing infective endocarditis. The subject is described in Chapter 8, p. 106.

Strep. pneumoniae (pneumococcus)

This is the most common cause of lobar pneumonia and can cause bronchopneumonia in susceptible post-surgical patients, as well as middle ear infections (otitis media) and acute exacerbations of chronic bronchitis. Pneumococcal meningitis may occur in the young and elderly and may complicate head injury. Severe pneumococcal sepsis is particularly likely after splenectomy but may be prevented by vaccination and penicillin prophylaxis.

Strep. milleri (*anginosus* group)

Many of the *Strep. milleri* group have microaerophilic culture requirements. They are often found in abscesses in the appendix area, the liver, lung and brain.

Anaerobic streptococci

These are bowel commensals and may form part of the mixed flora in intraperitoneal abscesses or infections associated with necrotic tissue, e.g. diabetic foot ulcers.

Antibiotic sensitivities

Penicillin is the drug of choice for most streptococcal infections. In seriously ill patients, **benzylpenicillin** is given parenterally. For less serious infections in patients able to tolerate oral therapy, **penicillin V (phenoxymethylpenicillin)**, **ampicillin** or **amoxicillin** are the drugs of choice. Many streptococci are also sensitive to **macrolides** (e.g. **erythromycin**, **clarithromycin**). Some pneumococci are now partially resistant to penicillin. Most infections, however, are still cleared with high-dose penicillin although meningitis needs alternative antibiotics such as ceftriaxone or vancomycin.

ENTEROCOCCI

Pathophysiology

The enterococci are **Gram-positive cocci** closely related to streptococci. *E. faecalis* (formerly *Strep. faecalis*) is the most common species. Enterococci are part of the normal bowel flora and may cause infection where bowel has been opened or else infect urinary or genital tracts.

Antibiotic sensitivities

Penicillin, **ampicillin**, **amoxicillin** or **vancomycin** are used for enterococcal infections. In serious infections such as endocarditis, a combination of high-dose penicillin and gentamicin ensures bactericidal activity. The cephalosporins are all ineffective. In hospitals where broad-spectrum cephalosporins are used empirically for bowel-related infections or septicaemia, enterococci are a frequent cause of nosocomial (hospital-acquired) infection. **Vancomycin-resistant enterococci (VRE)** are now being found. They are usually low-grade pathogens infecting intravascular lines in transplant and haematology patients and on ICUs. VRE endocarditis is difficult to treat, but newer antibiotics linezolid, daptomycin and quinupristin/dalfopristin are active against most strains.

ENTEROBACTERIACEAE

Pathophysiology

The Enterobacteriaceae are a large family of **Gram-negative bacilli** (rods) and usually make up about 1% of intestinal flora (see Table 3.2); they are known as **coliforms** and can be cultured under aerobic and anaerobic conditions and, like other bowel flora, grow in bile salt-containing media such as MacConkey or CLED agar; this helps identification.

Infections of surgical importance are usually opportunistic with the bacteria originating from the patient's bowel. Infection results from direct contamination (perforated or surgically opened bowel), perineal spread (to nearby wounds or urinary tract) or haematogenous spread. These and other Gram-negative organisms contain the sugar **lipopolysaccharide** (LPS), a powerful stimulator of inflammation and macrophage production of TNF-alpha and interleukin-1 cytokines.

Escherichia coli is the most common pathogen of the group and causes many surgical infections, often in synergy with other bacteria. *E. coli* causes **Gram-negative sepsis** and about 80% of urinary tract infections. Coliform bronchopneumonia occasionally occurs in debilitated, immunosuppressed or seriously ill patients. *Klebsiella*, *Enterobacter* and *Serratia* are found more often in surgical bowel-related infections. *Proteus* is a common cause of urinary tract infections but occasionally causes other surgical infections, usually originating from the urinary tract.

Table 3.2 Bacteria of the family enterobacteriaceae

Organism	Clinical infection
Primary gut pathogens	
Salmonella, e.g. *S. typhi*, *S. enteritidis* *Shigella*, e.g. *S. dysenteriae*, *S. sonnei* Some *Escherichia coli* strains, e.g. O157:H7	Typhoid fever Gastroenteritis Dysentery Traveller's diarrhoea Haemolytic uraemic syndrome
Gut colonisers that can cause infections	
Escherichia coli *Klebsiella* *Proteus* *Enterobacter* *Morganella* *Citrobacter*	Peritonitis and intraperitoneal abscesses (usually mixed infection with anaerobes) Septicaemia Urinary tract infections Ascending cholangitis (May also cause hospital-acquired infections, e.g. after instrumentation, central venous catheters, pneumonia in intensive care)
Gut colonisers that rarely cause infection	
Enterobacter *Serratia* *Morganella* *Citrobacter*	Usually hospital-acquired infections, e.g. after instrumentation, central venous catheters, in intensive care

Antibiotic sensitivities

Many coliforms are now resistant to ampicillin (and amoxicillin) and first-generation cephalosporins, e.g. cefalexin, but most are sensitive to **second- and third-generation cephalosporins**, e.g. **cefuroxime**, **cefotaxime**. Gentamicin is still a very effective and cheap agent. Many are sensitive to fluoroquinolones (ciprofloxacin, levofloxacin, moxifloxacin) but resistance is emerging. For prophylaxis in bowel and biliary tract surgery and for related local and systemic infections, gentamicin or an amoxicillin–clavulanate combination (co-amoxiclav) is recommended for its additional anaerobe activity. Antibiotic and beta-lactamase inhibitor combination antibiotics such as co-amoxiclav or piperacillin–tazobactam are very active against bowel flora with good activity against anaerobes. Anaerobes are the main colonisers of the bowel and often accompany Enterobacteriaceae in infections.

Resistant strains of Enterobacteriaceae are much more frequent in hospitals (often on ICUs) than in the community. They often cause urinary tract infection in catheterised patients after repeated courses of antibiotics. Multi-drug resistant strains of *E. coli* and *Klebsiella* spp. have emerged in hospitals all over the world since the 1980s. They produce enzymes (extended spectrum beta-lactamase enzymes or ESBL) that destroy second- and third-generation cephalosporins, and are often resistant to quinolones and most aminoglycosides. The only active antibiotics are the **carbapenems** (meropenem, imipenem, ertapenem) and amikacin. The carbapenems are very broad spectrum, but expensive and must be given parenterally. Hospital use is restricted to prevent development of resistance. The emergence of carbapenemase-producing Enterobacteriaceae (called KPC or NDM) is a growing problem as treatment is largely limited to old and toxic antibiotics such as colistin. Resistant bacteria have now spread around the world and pose the greatest current infection threat to patients in hospital.

'Non-surgical' Enterobacteriaceae

Other members of the family cause primary bowel infections. *Salmonella typhi* causes **typhoid** which may cause bowel perforations and *Shigella* causes **bacillary dysentery**. Rarely, *Salmonella* is incriminated in acute appendicitis and primary 'mycotic' aneurysms. An increasingly important cause of **acute haemorrhagic colitis** is *E. coli* O157:H7 and other verotoxin-producing *E. coli*. This is indistinguishable from acute haemorrhagic ulcerative colitis and should be sought bacteriologically in all cases. These strains have also caused large outbreaks of food-borne disease and produce a verotoxin (Shiga-like toxin) responsible for haemolytic uraemic syndrome (HUS) resulting in acute renal failure. *Yersinia* sometimes produces an acute ileal inflammation which may mimic acute appendicitis and has a similar appearance to Crohn's disease at laparotomy. *Campylobacter jejuni*, the most common cause of food-borne infection, can also cause a pseudo-appendicitis by initiating terminal ileitis and mesenteric lymph node inflammation.

PSEUDOMONAS

Pathophysiology

The main pathogen in this group of **aerobic Gram-negative rods** is *Pseudomonas aeruginosa*, an uncommon cause of surgical infection except in debilitated, hospitalised patients. It is found in a wide variety of habitats including soil, water, plants and animals, reflecting its predilection for moist environments. It is commonly found on hospital and cleaning equipment and even in chemical disinfectants and antiseptics. In about 10% of the population, *Ps. aeruginosa* is a normal intestinal commensal and is primarily an in-hospital (nosocomial) pathogen. The organism is resistant to many antibiotics and so tends to proliferate when other flora are suppressed by broad-spectrum antibiotics.

Pseudomonas is a common colonising organism in long-standing wounds such as compound fractures, chronic leg ulcers and indwelling urinary catheters but its presence is not always clinically significant. In wounds and ulcers, it can be recognised by its characteristic blue-green discharge. It colonises burns and may become pathogenic with extensive burns, giving rise to fatal sepsis. *Pseudomonas* infection can be serious in ophthalmic surgery and may lead to loss of the infected eye and is often responsible for chronic and recurrent external ear infections (otitis externa). Finally, *Ps. aeruginosa* may be responsible for hospital-acquired pneumonias in ventilated patients or for fatal systemic sepsis in terminally ill patients.

Antibiotic sensitivities

True infection must, as ever, be distinguished from colonisation where treatment is not indicated and would encourage development of resistance. *Ps. aeruginosa* is intrinsically resistant to most antibiotics; those that have activity include the **aminoglycosides (gentamicin** and **tobramycin)**, some extended-spectrum beta-lactam antibiotics (**ceftazidime** or **cefepime**), the combination of **piperacillin** and **tazobactam** and the carbapenems (**imipenem** or **meropenem**). The quinolones, **ciprofloxacin** and **ofloxacin**, are the only orally effective anti-pseudomonal agents.

ACINETOBACTER

These are Gram-negative coccobacilli that are strictly aerobic non-fermenters and are generally not pathogenic to healthy individuals. Their importance lies in causing infections in vulnerable patients, especially on ICUs, and their high rate of intrinsic antibiotic resistance, including to carbapenems; treatment options are usually limited to amikacin or colistin. The most commonly identified species is *A. baumanii*.

ANAEROBES

Anaerobic bacteria form a major part of the GI tract flora, outnumbering *E. coli* and related coliforms by 1000 to 1. Many parts of the body are colonised by anaerobes, even those exposed to air, including skin, mouth, upper respiratory tract, external genitalia and vagina. These colonising organisms become important because surgery disrupts anatomical barriers to allow contamination and infection. Other important factors that promote anaerobe growth include intestinal obstruction, tissue destruction and hypoxia (as in burns and vascular insufficiency), and foreign bodies. Anaerobic infection can be life-threatening and surgical management is often required. Some anaerobes cause toxin-related diseases including tetanus. The most commonly encountered anaerobes are:

- **Gram-negative bacilli**—*Bacteroides fragilis* and other *Bacteroides* species (spp.), *Porphyromonas* spp., *Prevotella* spp., *Fusobacterium* spp. and *Bilophila wadsworthia*
- **Gram-positive cocci**—*Peptostreptococcus* and microaerophilic streptococci
- **Gram-positive bacilli**—*Clostridium* spp. (spore forming), *Actinomyces* spp., *Propionibacterium* spp. and Bifidobacterium spp.

Antibiotic sensitivities

Most anaerobes are highly sensitive to **metronidazole**. Metronidazole can be given orally, intravenously or rectally, with the rectal route resulting in plasma levels equivalent to intravenous administration. Metronidazole is standard prophylaxis before appendicectomy and large bowel surgery, and has dramatically reduced peritoneal and wound infections. Other antibiotics with broad anaerobic activity are **co-amoxiclav** (Augmentin), piperacillin/tazobactam (Tazocin), the carbapenems (imipenem and meropenem) and chloramphenicol.

BACTEROIDES

Pathophysiology

Bacteroides cause pyogenic infections after faecal contamination of the peritoneal cavity, along with other gut commensals, and occasionally cause sepsis in debilitated patients.

Bacteroides were not identified as pathogens until the early 1970s because their strict anaerobic culture requirements were unrecognised. Indeed *Bacteroides* spp. were probably responsible for many so-called 'sterile' intra-abdominal abscesses. The importance of *B. fragilis* as a cause of surgical infection is probably still underestimated.

CLOSTRIDIA

Clostridia are Gram-positive rods widely distributed in soil and as intestinal commensals. Clostridia form **spores** resistant to drying, heat and antiseptics and can survive for long periods. They are mostly **obligate anaerobes** which can only proliferate in the absence of oxygen; they cause much of the putrefaction and decay of animal material in nature. The main pathological effects are caused by powerful **exotoxins**. Those of surgical importance are **gas gangrene**, **tetanus** and *C. difficile* **pseudomembranous colitis**.

Gas gangrene

Gas gangrene results when *Clostridium perfringens* (formerly *C. welchii*) and other anaerobes (e.g. *Bacteroides* spp. and streptococci) proliferate in necrotic tissue, secreting powerful toxins. Toxins spread rapidly and destroy nearby tissues, generating gas which causes the characteristic sign of crepitus ('crackling') on palpation and the typical X-ray appearance (Fig. 3.8). Deep traumatic wounds involving muscle, and wounds contaminated with soil, clothes or faeces are most susceptible. The condition is very common in battle wounds—gas gangrene was responsible for vast numbers of deaths during the First World War.

In surgical practice, the highest risk of gas gangrene is in **lower limb amputations** for ischaemia (infection from the patient's bowel) and in high-velocity **gunshot wounds** (from perforated bowel or by external contamination). Gas gangrene occasionally occurs in surgical wounds when ischaemic tissue is contaminated with bowel flora. The area of muscle necrosis may initially be small. Gas gangrene is recognised when the overlying skin turns black and spreads at an alarming rate. Within hours, necrosis rages along muscle planes. Later the skin breaks down and a thin, foul-smelling purulent exudate leaks out. Toxins are absorbed and cause rapid clinical deterioration and death within 24–48 hours unless the process can be halted by timely and vigorous intervention.

C. perfringens is very sensitive to **benzylpenicillin** which should be given prophylactically by injection as soon as possible after a traumatic injury involving muscle, or less than an hour before ischaemic limb amputation (metronidazole is suitable for patients allergic to penicillin). In the surgery of contaminated wounds, preventing clostridial infection requires meticulous excision of all necrotic tissue followed by packing of the wound rather than suturing. Further excisions are likely to be needed and delayed primary closure performed when risk of infection is over, a few days later.

CASE HISTORY

Fig. 3.8 Gas gangrene

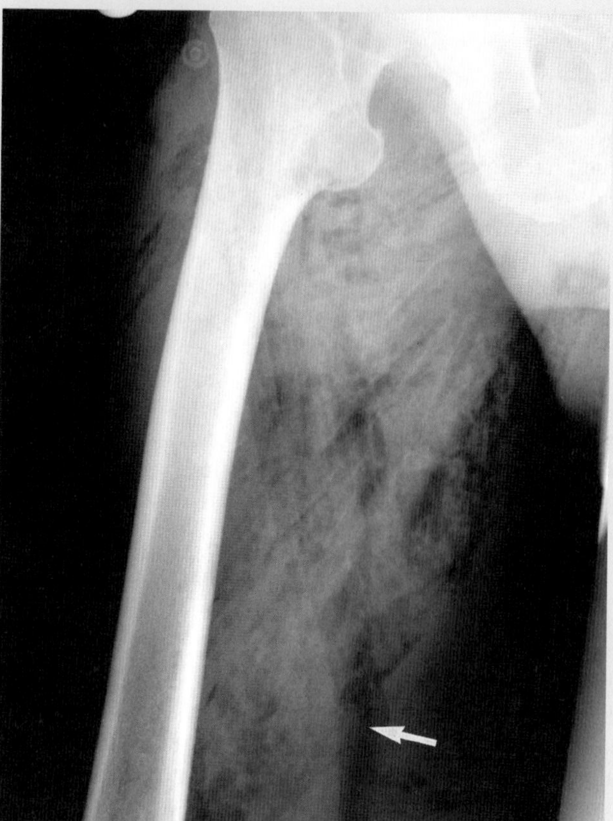

This 46-year-old man sustained extensive contaminated lacerations of the medial right thigh (arrowed) in a road traffic collision. Gas gangrene developed, rapidly involving all the muscles of the thigh because the condition was not recognised early and necrotic muscle was not excised immediately and completely. Note the widespread streaks of radiolucent gas bubbles tracking along the muscle planes. This patient died of toxaemia despite antibiotics, surgery and hyperbaric oxygen therapy

Treatment of gas gangrene

Treatment of established gas gangrene is urgent and must proceed vigorously for any hope of survival. Treatment is with high doses of intravenous penicillin to kill organisms in viable and vascularised tissue, and emergency radical excision of all necrotic tissue. This involves carving back the necrotic muscle to healthy bleeding tissue; affected muscle is recognised by its brick-red colour and failure to contract on cutting. In the surgery of contaminated wounds, preventing clostridial infection requires meticulous excision of all necrotic tissue followed by wound packing rather than suturing. Further excisions are likely to be needed and delayed primary closure performed a few days later.

Hyperbaric oxygen therapy can raise oxygen tension in necrotic tissues, inhibiting organism growth. The patient is placed in a high-pressure chamber with pure oxygen at about 3 atmospheres for several hours daily. However, gas gangrene may still spread, necessitating further heroic surgical interventions. Even with intensive treatment, the prognosis for established gas gangrene remains bleak.

Tetanus

Tetanus is caused by *Clostridium tetani*, which also infects dirty wounds. The entry wound may be minute, perhaps caused by a rose thorn or splinter. The organism produces an **exotoxin** with little local effect but, even in minute quantities, with powerful neuromuscular effects causing widespread muscular spasm. The first signs are often **acute muscle spasms** and **neck stiffness** or **trismus ('lockjaw')**. If untreated, these progress to **opisthotonus** (arching of the back due to extensor spasm), generalised convulsions and eventually death from exhaustion and respiratory failure several days later.

Tetanus is now rare in developed countries because of immunisation with **tetanus toxoid** during childhood, followed by boosters at 10-year intervals. In the UK, boosters are no longer needed if an initial five-dose vaccination schedule has been completed. In Australia and New Zealand a single booster is recommended at age 45–50. In developed countries, the annual incidence of tetanus is about one per million and is most common following trivial gardening injuries in the elderly. If the immunisation status following a major contaminated injury is unknown, **benzylpenicillin** should be given plus passive immunisation with **tetanus immune globulin**. Treatment of established tetanus usually requires artificial ventilation with drug paralysis, antibiotics and passive immunisation. Mortality remains high, especially in the elderly.

Globally, tetanus after trauma remains a massive problem. In some developing countries, neonatal tetanus results from the practice of applying cow dung as a dressing to the umbilical stump.

Pseudomembranous colitis

Pseudomembranous colitis can be the most serious form of **antibiotic-associated diarrhoea** (see Ch. 12) and is caused by overgrowth of a toxigenic *Clostridium difficile*. The organism gets its name from the difficulty of growing it in culture. Infection produces a thick fibrinous 'membrane' on large intestinal mucosa, within which the organism proliferates. Its toxins cause a profound watery and sometimes bloody diarrhoea, leading to dehydration and electrolyte loss.

Pseudomembranous colitis may develop after only a single dose of any antibiotic. Cephalosporins and ciprofloxacin are now the most common cause. Diagnosis can be made by sigmoidoscopy and biopsy in the 50% of patients with left-sided colonic involvement. Cases of pseudomembranous infection are increasingly recognised in patients after total colectomy and *C. difficile* should be suspected in cases of large unexplained stoma output and rising white cell count. Diagnosis is best made by **detecting the specific toxin in the stool** and looking for a cytopathic effect on cells cultured in vitro. *C. difficile* can also be cultured from the stool. Although the organism is sensitive to penicillin, this fails to penetrate the pseudomembrane. **Oral metronidazole** is usually effective but takes at least 2 days before clinical response is observed. Relapses are common in the elderly and oral **vancomycin**, which is not absorbed from the GI tract, can be employed or when metronidazole fails. Oral vancomycin should also be used if severe disease is suspected; the intravenous formulation can be given by rectal tube in patients unable to take oral treatment, especially on intensive care units. A new antibiotic, fidaxomicin, has recently been licensed for *C. difficile* infection and appears to have a lower relapse rate than traditional treatment.

VIRUSES OF PARTICULAR SURGICAL IMPORTANCE

The chronic blood-borne viral infections **hepatitis B** and **C** and **human immunodeficiency virus (HIV)** are important in surgical practice because of the risk of virus transmission from patient to surgeon during operation and vice versa, as well as cross-infection between patients. Patients may also need surgical intervention for complications of hepatitis or HIV infection.

HUMAN IMMUNODEFICIENCY VIRUS (HIV)

Classification of HIV infections

The human immunodeficiency virus causes a chronic infection that usually progresses to the **acquired immune deficiency syndrome (AIDS)** over 7 or more years. The illness evolves through several stages or groups, classified by the US Centers for Disease Control, in 1986, as:

- (Group I) the **acute seroconversion illness**. Seroconversion occurs as long as 3 months after infection, and as many as 70% of infected patients are asymptomatic at the time of seroconversion. Patients usually test negative for antibodies against HIV before and during the seroconversion illness
- (Group II) the **asymptomatic period** during which patients usually feels completely well
- (Group III) as the disease progresses, the patient may develop generalised lymphadenopathy and wasting **(AIDS-related complex)**
- (Group IV) **AIDS** is manifest by development of unusual opportunistic infections (e.g. *Pneumocystis* pneumonia, cytomegalovirus (CMV) infections, cerebral toxoplasmosis, atypical mycobacterial infections), certain malignant diseases (Kaposi's sarcoma, generalised or cerebral lymphoma, aggressive invasive uterine cervical cancer) and neurological disease **(AIDS dementia complex)**

The use of combinations of antiretroviral drugs ('high activity antiretroviral therapy') has dramatically affected the natural history, with a large sustained drop in mortality from opportunistic infections.

Surgical involvement in HIV cases

Surgeons may be involved in diagnosing bowel-related problems (e.g. oesophageal candidiasis) by oesophago-gastro-duodenoscopy (OGD). In late-stage disease, cytomegalovirus (CMV) infection may involve any part of the GI tract, ranging from mouth ulcers, to ulcers in the jejunum that may perforate, to colitis. For AIDS colitis, colonoscopy and biopsy are often required for diagnosis. Treatment involves intravenous antiviral drugs.

AIDS patients may develop severe perianal herpes with secondary anal fistula or abscess formation. In a patient with known AIDS, perianal lesions should be assumed to be herpes until proven otherwise as the presentation is often atypical. Kaposi's sarcomas (see Ch. 46, p. 575) may require local excision. Other examples of surgical involvement with HIV-infected patients include insertion of long-term central venous catheters (e.g. Hickman line), insertion of percutaneous endoscopic gastrostomy (PEG) tubes for feeding, or joint replacements in HIV infected haemophiliacs.

VIRAL HEPATITIS

Viral hepatitis manifests with anorexia, nausea and sometimes abdominal discomfort in the right upper quadrant followed by jaundice. Many viruses cause hepatitis, often with different modes of transmission, incubation times, prognosis and complications. These include CMV, Epstein–Barr virus (EBV) and the hepatitis viruses.

Hepatitis A

Hepatitis A is transmitted by the faecal–oral route and has an incubation period of 2–6 weeks. It rarely causes fulminating disease and never leads to chronic hepatitis or cirrhosis. Its only surgical importance is in the differential diagnosis of jaundice. A vaccine for hepatitis A is available.

Hepatitis B

Hepatitis B is transmitted by blood or body fluids, including sexual intercourse, or from mother to fetus or baby (termed **vertical transmission**). Incubation is 6 weeks to 6 months. Hepatitis B infection leads to chronic hepatitis and cirrhosis in 5–10%; this variety of cirrhosis commonly progresses to **hepatocellular carcinoma** (the most common cause world-wide). Hepatitis B is preventable by vaccination and this is indicated for neonates of mothers who carry the virus, all health care workers and people living in high-risk areas.

Exposure to hepatitis B virus has several possible outcomes:

- Acute fulminant hepatitis—rare but fatal
- Acute hepatitis—clearing of the virus leads to lifelong immunity
- Chronic infection—may lead to chronic hepatitis/cirrhosis (and hepatocellular carcinoma)
- Chronic carrier state—mainly due to infection at birth but can occur later with development of immune tolerance and no obvious active disease

Diagnosis of hepatitis B

The hepatitis B surface *antigen* **(HBsAg)** can be detected in blood in the early stages. Patients later develop *antibodies* to the viral core **(anti-HBc)** which is a marker of exposure to the virus but does not confer immunity. Later still, with clearance of the virus, patients develop surface *antibodies* **(anti-HBs)** which confer lifetime immunity. Patients who do not clear the virus remain surface *antigen* (HbsAg) positive and may become **chronic carriers**, i.e. remain infectious to other people and prone to risk of complications themselves.

HBsAg-positive patients may transmit the virus if there is recipient exposure to sufficient material, e.g. by blood transfusion. The special case of **e antigen positivity** (HBeAg) indicates patients with high infectivity.

Hepatitis B vaccines contain recombinant inactivated surface *antigen* and induce immunity by stimulating production of surface *antibody*; this is the only positive serological marker in vaccinated people.

Treatment of hepatitis B

Hepatitis B DNA can now be detected in blood, giving a definitive diagnosis and an estimate of the quantity of virus in the bloodstream (viral load) to guide treatment. Therapy with interferon and lamivudine has been partially successful in treating chronic infections, reducing infectivity and the risk of hepatocellular carcinoma. Chronic carriers failing therapy should be monitored for hepatocellular carcinoma by annual estimation of **serum alpha-fetoprotein** and undergo liver ultrasound scanning every 2 years, as partial hepatectomy can sometimes cure early cases.

Hepatitis C

Hepatitis C is transmitted via the same routes as hepatitis B but sexual transmission is believed to be less common. The incubation period is approximately 2 months. Chronic liver disease develops in a higher proportion of cases (30–50%) but is often of low grade. Hepatitis C is also an important cause of hepatocellular carcinoma world-wide.

Serological diagnosis is troublesome because HCV antibody tests often give false positives. Seroconversion occurs late, often weeks to months after the acute illness. Definitive diagnosis is made by detecting hepatitis C RNA in serum. As in hepatitis B, viral load assays are used to monitor response to therapy and infectivity, and treatment with interferon and ribavirin has also been partially successful. In most cases a positive hepatitis C antibody test is likely to mean continuing infection.

Hepatitis D

This is a defective virus that requires hepatitis B surface antigen for full expression; it occurs only as a co-infection with hepatitis B and can be prevented by vaccination for hepatitis B.

Hepatitis E

Hepatitis E is transmitted by the faecal–oral route and is usually self-limiting.

SEPSIS (see also http://www.survivesepsis.org/)

MULTIPLE ORGAN DYSFUNCTION AND THE SYSTEMIC INFLAMMATORY RESPONSE SYNDROME

Multiple organ dysfunction syndrome or MODS (multi-organ failure or MOF) was recognised as a clinical entity in the mid-1970s when it became recognised that any major physiological insult could lead to failure of organs remote from the initiating disease process. Later, the underlying condition was found to be an unrestrained systemic inflammatory response (**systemic inflammatory response syndrome, SIRS**), initiated by adverse events such as trauma, infection, inflammation, ischaemia or ischaemia–reperfusion injury. MODS is the most common reason for surgical patients to stay longer than 5 days in intensive care (see Box 3.2).

Sepsis (also known by or incorporated in the terms **septic shock**, **systemic sepsis**, **septicaemia** and **sepsis syndrome**) describes the clinical features when infection is the initiating factor of MODS. Early on, the condition may be reversible. Note that sepsis is *not* synonymous with infection. In MODS, the sequence of individual organ failure often follows a predictable pattern with **pulmonary failure** first, followed by hepatic, intestinal, renal and finally cardiac failure. Pulmonary failure is associated with acute (formerly 'adult') respiratory distress syndrome (**ARDS**). In hepatic failure, patients have a rising bilirubin, serum glutamic oxaloacetic transaminase (SGOT) and lactate dehydrogenase (LDH). Intestinal failure is recognised by **stress bleeding** requiring transfusion, renal failure by rising plasma creatinine and low urine output, and cardiac failure by low cardiac output and hypotension. Altered mental states such as confusion also occur (cerebral failure), as may disseminated intravascular coagulopathy (DIC).

The mortality of MODS is related to the number of failing organs: mortality is 40% with one organ; 60% with two; and more than 90% with three.

Box 3.2 Definitions of SIRS, MODS and sepsis

Systemic inflammatory response syndrome (SIRS)

Present if two or more of the following are present:

- Temperature > 38°C or < 36°C
- Heart rate > 90 beats/min
- Respiratory rate >20 breaths/min or $PaCO_2$ < 4.3 kPa
- White cell count > 12 000 or < 4000 cells/mm^3 or more than 10% immature forms
- Serum lactate >4 mmol/L

Multiple organ dysfunction syndrome (MODS)

Present if SIRS is associated with organ dysfunction, e.g. oliguria, hypoxia

Sepsis (or systemic sepsis)

Defined as SIRS in association with bacterial infection proven by culture

Severe sepsis

Defined as sepsis associated with signs of organ dysfunction, e.g. renal failure

Septic shock

Defined as SIRS associated with hypotension refractory to volume replacement and requiring vasopressors

Pathophysiology of SIRS and MODS

SIRS involves widespread changes, including inflammatory cell activation leading to cytokine release, endothelial injury, disordered haemodynamics and impaired tissue oxygen extraction. It thus represents grossly exaggerated activation of innate immune responses intended as host defences. An unregulated release of inflammatory mediators causes widespread microvascular, haemodynamic and mitochondrial changes that eventually lead to organ failure.

Following initial tissue injury, a local inflammatory response occurs with cytokine induction (see *Immunity* at the start of this chapter). The response to this is mobilisation of inflammatory cells including macrophages and neutrophils which diapedese into the tissues. In addition, cytokines provoke systemic elements of inflammation, including activation of endothelium, the complement system and blood coagulation, amplifying the primary inflammatory response. This sequence is part of the normal and appropriate inflammatory response. However, if the injury is severe or persistent, the local reaction may extend excessively into the systemic circulation producing a systemic inflammatory response, or if initiated by infection, the sepsis syndrome.

Mediators of SIRS and MODS

SIRS and MODS involve complex interactions of endogenous and sometimes exogenous mediators. A range of cytokines is released from activated macrophages and from endothelial and other reticulo-endothelial cells. The suite of cytokines released depends on the nature of the provoking agent and is governed by the specific type of Toll-like receptor that recognises the aggressor. Cytokines released include **tumour necrosis factor-alpha** (TNF-alpha), the **interleukins** (particularly IL1 but also IL2, IL6) and platelet activating factor. Pharmacological attempts to suppress excess cytokine responses have thus far been ineffective.

Sepsis

The classic septic response, with a hyperdynamic circulation, systemic signs of inflammation and disrupted intermediary metabolism, can be induced in healthy volunteers by injecting **lipopolysaccharide** (from the cell walls of Gram-negative bacteria) or the cytokines TNF-alpha or IL1. In Gram-negative sepsis, the lipopolysaccharide component of the organisms powerfully activates Toll-like receptors on dendritic cells and hence the whole inflammatory cascade. This results in endothelial activation which increases vascular permeability and neutrophil–endothelial interaction. The final common pathway may involve activated neutrophils migrating into the interstitial space of the affected organ and tissue hypoxia. In sepsis, these and other circulating factors working in synergy bring about the devastating effects of MODS.

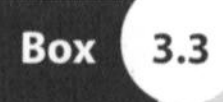

Box 3.3 Prevention and early treatment of multiple organ dysfunction syndrome

General prevention

- Rapid resuscitation and early definitive treatment of major injuries
- Good surgical technique
- Appropriate use of prophylactic and therapeutic antibiotics
- Early diagnosis and treatment of infective surgical complications, e.g. leaking anastomoses
- Early and thorough excision of necrotic and infected tissue

Prevention for at-risk patients and treatment of early signs

- Rapid cardiovascular resuscitation and prevention of shock (minimise splanchnic ischaemia)
- Optimisation of oxygen delivery (measure arterial PO_2 and pH and correct metabolic acidosis)
- Nutritional support via an enteral route (to nourish enterocytes)

The Sepsis Six (http://www.survivesepsis.org/)

All within 1 hour:

1. Give high-flow oxygen via non-rebreathe bag
2. Take blood cultures and consider source control
3. Give i.v. antibiotics according to local protocol
4. Start i.v. fluid resuscitation with Hartmann's or equivalent
5. Check lactate
6. Monitor hourly urine output; consider catheterisation

CLINICAL CONDITIONS LEADING TO SIRS AND MODS

These include infection and endotoxaemia (Gram-negative sepsis) in 50–70% of cases, retained necrotic tissue and shock. Any of these can initiate distant organ failure by the following mechanisms:

- Inducing excessive release of endogenous cytokines
- Disrupting oxygen delivery to the tissues
- Impairing intestinal barrier function allowing **translocation** of intestinal bacteria and endotoxin to the portal and systemic circulations
- Damaging the reticulo-endothelial system

Organ failure induced by acute pancreatitis is caused by a combination of these factors.

Infection

The infection source that leads to MODS may be **acquired** (e.g. intra-abdominal abscess) or **endogenous**, i.e. from the patient's bowel. Local infection, especially with Gram-negative bacteria, stimulates the release of inflammatory cytokines. A similar response is provoked by a substantial volume of necrotic tissue, e.g. gangrenous leg, and is worse if the tissue is infected. These **paracrine responses** are beneficial in a local sense, combating infection by increasing blood flow and vascular permeability to allow influx of dendritic cells and macrophages, and activating neutrophils to degranulate and release cytotoxic oxygen radicals. If the stimulating factor is great, a cascade is initiated which leads to sepsis and MODS. Superoxide radicals and other circulating factors then damage cells elsewhere, causing widespread vasodilatation and increased vascular permeability leading to hypotension and circulatory collapse. The myocardium is depressed and cellular metabolic functions are disrupted.

Endogenous sources of infection

Large bowel is a reservoir for bacteria and endotoxin which are normally safely contained. If the **intestinal barrier** is breached by splanchnic ischaemia, impoverished luminal nutrition of enterocytes or altered intestinal flora, **translocation** of bacteria into the portal circulation can occur in as little as 30 minutes. If the liver Kupffer cells are also impaired, intestinal bacteria and endotoxin are not prevented from reaching the systemic circulation in the normal way. This may explain the potential for renal failure in jaundiced patients undergoing operation (hepatorenal syndrome). This endogenous source probably explains the 30% of patients who suffer organ dysfunction without an obvious source of infection. Typically, such patients become affected after prolonged hypotension (hypovolaemic or cardiogenic shock) or hypoxaemia (e.g. multiple trauma victims), or as a result of direct visceral ischaemia (e.g. prolonged aortic clamping and hypotension in a patient with a ruptured aortic aneurysm).

Prevention of sepsis and MODS

Prevention and early treatment of MODS is summarised in Box 3.3.

Surgical aspects

In surgical patients, multiple organ dysfunction often results from a complication such as a bowel anastomotic leak or from severe acute pancreatitis (which may be sterile but becomes devastating if infected). Tissue necrosis following trauma, or death of an ischaemic limb may also precipitate the syndrome.

Organ dysfunction often begins insidiously. At an early stage, dysfunction can be confirmed by investigation and active resuscitation and treatment of causative factors are likely to have beneficial effects. By 7–10 days without effective treatment, pulmonary failure (ARDS) and hepatic and renal failure appear; MODS is now present and the prognosis becomes substantially worse.

Preventing sepsis and early management of major gut-related infection before it provokes the SIRS–MODS cascade is vital. Appropriate use of **prophylactic antibiotics** in bowel surgery or trauma helps, but intraoperative and postoperative **errors in technique** or clinical judgement are major factors in more than 50% of patients with multiple organ dysfunction. Good clinical judgement, effective resuscitation, good operative technique, effective excision of necrotic tissue, minimising bacterial contamination and preventing accumulation of postoperative fluid collections (serum or blood) are all necessary for prevention. The purpose is to eliminate environments in which bacteria multiply and improve the delivery of host antibacterial defences.

Surgical complications with septic potential should be treated early, usually by definitive surgery, e.g. removal of necrotic tissue, drainage of abscesses and control of peritoneal contamination by exteriorising leaking anastomoses. This helps reduce the circulating level of inflammatory mediators and limits the period of stress. It is often better to perform a laparotomy on suspicion and find it normal than to 'wait and see' and risk rapid deterioration and death.

Other preventive factors in at-risk patients

Adequate and early **fluid resuscitation** is vital in patients with hypovolaemia, including in trauma victims, acute pancreatitis or bowel obstruction, because the loss of intravascular volume leads to deficient tissue perfusion (i.e. shock) and splanchnic ischaemia. Maintaining tissue oxygenation is also vital; at-risk patients must have arterial blood gases and pH estimated and receive supplemental oxygen or assisted ventilation as required. To help prevent intestinal bacterial translocation, enterocytes and colonocytes are best supported by **enteral feeding**, if necessary by a feeding jejunostomy or a fine-bore nasogastric tube. Glutamine, arginine and omega-3 fatty acids are believed to be important.

4 Shock and resuscitation

THE PATHOPHYSIOLOGY OF SHOCK

The term 'shock' can be defined as **acute circulatory failure of sufficient magnitude to compromise tissue perfusion**, which if untreated, proceeds rapidly to irreversible organ damage and death of the patient.

Hypoxia in the shocked patient compounds the problem of cellular oxygen delivery. It may be caused by mechanical airways obstruction, impaired gas exchange (e.g. pneumonia or pulmonary embolism) or hypoventilation (e.g. respiratory depression due to opioids) for example.

There are several mechanisms of shock:

- **Hypovolaemic shock**
- **Cardiogenic shock** occurs when the pump function of the heart is impaired
- **Septic shock** arises as a result of microvascular changes and cardiac depression caused by systemic inflammation
- **Anaphylactic shock** is an acute hypersensitivity reaction to an allergen

The classical symptoms and signs of shock include hypotension, hyperventilation, a rapid weak pulse, cold clammy cyanotic skin and oliguria. Mental changes also occur, most commonly anxiety, confusion and combativeness. Investigations reveal metabolic acidosis, low oxygen saturation and low central venous pressure. Notably, in **septic shock** there is peripheral vasodilatation rather than vasoconstriction.

Shock has been described as progressing through three stages. In stage I, there are attempts at **compensation** with skin and splanchnic vasoconstriction. Symptoms and signs are minimal but recognisable. In stage II, **decompensation** occurs, with body mechanisms unable to sustain tissue perfusion despite working at full capacity. Urgent intervention is needed at this stage. By stage III the changes are essentially **irreversible**, with prolonged shock having caused severe damage to major organs. Successful treatment depends crucially on **early recognition** of shock and its precursors, prompt diagnosis and treatment of the underlying cause and effective support of vital organ function.

EARLY RECOGNITION OF SHOCK

When surgical patients deteriorate catastrophically, it is often found on retrospective examination of charts that vital signs had been deteriorating for some time, but that clinical staff had failed to respond. Early recognition and intervention is crucial because failure of one organ leads to synergistic failure of other organs and an escalating risk of irreversible damage and death.

To help recognise these patients early, structured scoring systems have been developed, seeking to emulate the simplicity, reliability and clinical value of the Glasgow Coma Scale (Table 16.1, p. 219). These generally employ routinely recorded physiological data and most are modifications of the **Early Warning Score** (Table 4.1). These have proved extremely useful for spotting those at risk of deterioration needing urgent medical attention and have become part of standard care for surgical patients.

TYPES OF SHOCK

Hypovolaemic shock (preload insufficiency)

Preload is defined as the rate of venous return of blood to the heart. Preload insufficiency reduces the diastolic filling pressure and volume and leads to low cardiac output. The underlying problem may be inadequate total blood volume and underfilling of the venous compartment, i.e. **absolute hypovolaemia** (hypovolaemic shock) or else may be **relative hypovolaemia** (distributive shock) caused by an increase in capacity of the venous compartment or capillary beds relative to blood volume. Hypovolaemia is responsible for the majority of cases of shock encountered in hospital. Figure 15.1 (p. 200) shows the changes in vital signs associated with increasing amounts of blood loss.

The main causes of fluid loss leading to hypovolaemic shock are:

- 'Revealed' haemorrhage, e.g. massive haematemesis from peptic ulcer, deep lacerations, large haematemeses

Table 4.1 Modified Early Warning Score (MEWS)*

Score	3	2	1	0	1	2	3
Respiratory rate (bpm)		<9		9–14	15–20	21–29	≥30
Heart rate (bpm)		<40	41–50	51–100	101–110	111–129	≥130
Systolic blood pressure (mmHg)	<70	71–80	81–100	101–199		≥200	
Temperature (°C)		<35		35–38.4		≥38.5	
AVPU score				**A**lert	Reacting to **V**oice	Reacting to **P**ain	**U**nresponsive

*MEWS is one form of bedside scoring that can help early identification of patients likely to need urgent assessment (score 3 or more). A score of 5 or more indicates that the patient is likely to require critical care, usually in a high-dependency or intensive care unit

(vomiting of blood), continued loss from a wound drain indicating internal bleeding

- 'Concealed' haemorrhage, e.g. intra-abdominal bleeding from ruptured spleen or aortic aneurysm, haemorrhage from a duodenal ulcer into small intestine, intramuscular blood loss from fractures
- Extensive burns, resulting in massive loss of serum into blisters or from the skin surface
- Severe vomiting or diarrhoea, or prolonged fluid loss from a small bowel fistula or ileostomy
- Excessive urinary fluid loss, e.g. diabetic ketoacidosis, recovering acute tubular necrosis
- Sequestration of fluid in bowel caused by bowel obstruction
- Massive loss of fluid into interstitial tissues ('third space losses') as occurs in sepsis
- Major accumulation of fluid in the peritoneal cavity, e.g. acute pancreatitis

Distributive shock

Relative hypovolaemia occurs if there is inappropriate expansion of the circulatory capacity in relation to blood volume; it may result from failure of normal peripheral resistance and/or venodilatation of large veins. Peripheral resistance normally maintains cardiac afterload and is controlled by the tone of smooth muscle arteriolar and capillary sphincters. About 80% of capillaries are normally closed, and any mechanism that causes inappropriate opening greatly expands circulatory capacity. In septic shock, both arteriolar dilatation and an increase in venous volume play a part.

Septic shock

Septic shock is impaired tissue perfusion in the context of an inflammatory response. The aetiology is frequently infective but not always; it may be traumatic or surgical, or it may involve local inflammation, infection, severe burns or the presence of necrotic tissue, e.g. a gangrenous leg. If immune responses escape local control, this spill over provokes a complex cellular response and mediator cascade that leads to progressive clinical manifestations including the **systemic inflammatory response syndrome (SIRS)** and, later, **multiple organ dysfunction (MODS)**. Mediator responses involve the complement system, acute phase proteins and cytokines (particularly TNF-alpha and the interleukins IL1-beta and IL6); once triggered, the inflammatory response cascade is difficult to control or suppress.

Septic shock is a combination of distributive shock and organ dysfunction induced by mediators of the host inflammatory response (e.g. cytokines, complement) and sometimes directly by bacterial toxins, especially certain staphylococci or Gram-negative bacilli, e.g. from a colonic anastomotic leak. Bacterial toxins and cell wall components activate defensive mechanisms and the net result of this **immune burst** is that oxygen usage declines, metabolic acidosis develops and multiple organ dysfunction ensues. Failure of oxygen usage is the result of cardiorespiratory impairment, microcirculatory imbalance and, at cellular level, mitochondrial dysfunction.

Septic shock itself can be thought of in three phases. Initially there is extensive vasodilatation, causing relative hypovolaemia. In phase 2 there is widespread endothelial damage causing greatly increased capillary permeability and massive fluid leakage into the interstitial space. This manifests clinically as inadequate blood pressure in the presence of normal or increased cardiac output; until phase 3, when depression of myocardial contractility ensues.

The inflammatory burst also upsets normal blood coagulation by downregulating normal anticoagulants such as alpha-1-antitrypsin, and stimulating procoagulants such as **tissue factor** as well as inhibiting fibrinolysis. The result may be **disseminated intravascular coagulation** with microvascular occlusion, large vessel thrombosis and ischaemia, all contributing to organ dysfunction.

Toxic shock syndrome is a particular form of septic shock associated with staphylococcal or streptococcal infection associated with the use of super-absorbent tampons.

Pump failure (cardiogenic shock)

Cardiogenic shock describes a drastic reduction in cardiac output resulting from any form of 'pump failure' caused by direct myocardial damage, mechanical abnormality or malfunction of the heart. This most commonly arises from an **acute myocardial infarction** or an **acute ventricular arrhythmia**. Myocardial infarction may cause ischaemia or infarction of papillary muscles which produces acute mitral regurgitation. Another cause is when a large **pulmonary embolus** obstructs blood flow through the lungs and causes secondary cardiac failure. Other causes include cardiac (pericardial) tamponade and tension pneumothorax.

Anaphylactic shock

Anaphylactic shock is a generalised form of type I hypersensitivity reaction. The stimulatory antigen binds with antibodies attached to the surface of mast cells, triggering degranulation and release of histamine and other vasoactive amines. The predominant effect is extensive **dilatation of the venous compartment** and rapid movement of fluid into the tissues. The systemic effects are compounded by hypoxia due to bronchoconstriction and often laryngeal oedema.

In surgical practice, anaphylactic shock usually results from drug administration, particularly via the intravenous route. **Antibiotics**, particularly penicillins, and radiological contrast are the most common culprits. Anyone administering a drug must ensure the patient is not sensitive. Anaphylactic reactions may also occur after intravenous injections of **radiological contrast media**. Insect bites (wasps, bees and hornets) and ingested nuts are also important causes and may be encountered in the emergency department.

CLINICAL FEATURES OF SHOCK

The essential feature of any type of shock is a **precipitate fall in arterial blood pressure** with systolic pressure dropping by at least 40 mmHg from usual levels. The immediate homeostatic response is **intense sympathetic activity** and catecholamine release. The heart rate increases dramatically in an attempt to increase cardiac output. Except in septic shock, there is intense cutaneous and visceral vasoconstriction to restore intravascular volume by increasing peripheral resistance. Sudomotor activity causes profuse sweating. Hypoxic tissues revert to anaerobic respiration, producing lactic acid sufficient to cause a metabolic acidosis and compensatory tachypnoea. The clinical picture is a cold, pale, clammy, hypotensive patient with a rapid thready pulse and increased respiratory rate.

Septic shock presents a contrasting clinical picture in which cytokine-mediated peripheral vasodilatation is unresponsive to circulating catecholamines. The patient's skin is flushed and hot and cardiac output is increased to fill the dilated periphery. The pulse is typically 'bounding' in quality. Temperature may be above normal or below normal ('cold sepsis').

In all forms of shock, the circulatory system cannot support the main organ systems without treatment, and organs fail (i.e. decompensate) one by one in a synergistic manner. Pulmonary failure leads to **acute respiratory distress syndrome** (ARDS), and cerebral hypoxia soon causes confusion and eventually coma. Inadequate renal perfusion causes oliguria which, if not rapidly corrected, leads to acute tubular necrosis and renal failure. Cerebral ischaemia causes confusion and, if shock persists, reduced coronary flow and heart failure cause death. In septic shock, organ damage is exacerbated by an intense inflammatory burst and deterioration is inevitable unless the source of infection can be rapidly eliminated and effective support instituted.

SPECIFIC TREATMENTS FOR SHOCK

Hypovolaemic shock

Identifying the cause of the fluid loss is the top priority. Immediate measures should be taken to control blood loss, e.g. pressure on a swab over a bleeding wound, endoscopic injection of bleeding peptic ulcer. Fluid replacement should be equivalent to estimated fluid loss but adjusted according to the response of pulse rate, blood pressure, observed JVP (or central venous pressure) and urine output. If available, trans-oesophageal ultrasound helps assess stroke volume and hence preload adequacy. Small falls in stroke volume of 15–20 ml can radically affect splanchnic flow. Where possible, fluids of similar composition to those lost should be used: whole blood for haemorrhage, colloids after major burns. Fluids should be titrated in rapid boluses, e.g. 250 ml at a time, and the response observed.

Cardiogenic shock

The management of cardiogenic shock is best reviewed in a medical textbook; the management of pulmonary embolism (which may present as cardiogenic shock) is discussed in Chapter 12, p. 168. Fluid overload is a significant hazard in cardiogenic shock.

Septic shock

(see SIRS and MODS, Ch. 3, p. 51)

Systemic sepsis leading to septic shock usually originates from a specific focus of infection or bacterial translocation from the patient's own intestine. In general surgical practice, septic shock most commonly results from **faecal peritonitis** following large bowel perforation or **anastomotic breakdown**. Infection in sites unrelated to the primary surgical pathology, such as bladder, chest or 'line' (usually central venous cannula) infection, are often the cause. Debilitated patients, uncontrolled diabetics and infants are particularly vulnerable to acute sepsis; a clear source of infection is less often found. Gangrene of a leg is also a potent cause. The damaging effects of the underlying poor organ perfusion are increased by direct and indirect bacterial exotoxic and endotoxic tissue damage.

Treatment of septic shock is urgent and involves fluid resuscitation, oxygenation, administration of appropriate antibiotics and the tracing and eliminating of the source of infection. Blood cultures must be taken and intravenous broad-spectrum antibiotics administered on a 'best-guess' basis. Because of interstitial losses, plasma expanders are often needed in large volumes, but should still be titrated against clinical parameters (e.g. pulse, CVP). Volume expansion helps to sustain cardiac output and tissue perfusion but addition of inotropes which induce peripheral vasoconstriction, in particular noradrenaline (norepinephrine), may be required. Corticosteroids are known to stabilise cell membranes and low dose administration has been shown in some clinical trials to prolong survival in patients with refractory shock.

If the diagnosis of septic shock is correct, resuscitative measures should produce dramatic improvement in the patient's condition within 1–2 hours. By that time, the patient should be ready for immediate operation if an abscess, bowel perforation or other surgically remediable cause needs treatment. It is important to emphasise that the source of infection must be urgently eliminated if the septic cascade is to be reversed.

Disseminated intravascular coagulation

A major problem in sepsis is generalised activation of the clotting cascade causing disseminated intravascular coagulation (DIC). This exhausts the supply of platelets and clotting factors V, VIII and fibrinogen (**consumption coagulopathy**) and activates intrinsic fibrinolytic mechanisms. DIC manifests as spontaneous bleeding or bruising and uncontrollable haemorrhage from operation sites. Diagnosis is made by finding low **fibrinogen** levels and high levels of **D-dimers**, cleaved from fibrin by plasmin and providing evidence of fibrin lysis. Treatment includes managing the initiating cause, giving intravenous heparin to arrest the coagulation process and transfusing appropriate clotting factors, e.g. fresh-frozen plasma, cryoprecipitate.

Anaphylactic shock

Immediate treatment of anaphylactic shock includes securing the airway and giving oxygen, laying the patient flat and raising the feet and administering 500 mg of intramuscular adrenaline (epinephrine), i.e. 0.3 ml of 1 : 1000 solution. This dose may be repeated at 5 minute intervals if necessary. An antihistamine (e.g. chlorphenamine 10–20 mg) should be given by slow intravenous injection and continued for up to 48 hours to stabilise mast cells. Hydrocortisone 100–300 mg should also be given intravenously but takes several hours to block histamine receptors and so should not be regarded as contributing to emergency treatment. Intravenous fluids may also be needed to treat hypovolaemia.

RESUSCITATION OF THE 'COLLAPSED' NON-TRAUMA PATIENT

Principles of managing shock by resuscitation

In the collapsed trauma patient, initial resuscitation focuses on the airway and replacement of blood loss. In contrast, shocked non-trauma patients often have multiple co-morbidities, both medical and surgical, which combine to produce the similar clinical picture of shock. Whatever the cause, the aim is to restore tissue perfusion and oxygenation by resuscitative measures while making the diagnosis and before specific treatment begins.

Early management, ideally within 24 hours of acute deterioration, can be summarised as follows:

- **Clinical volume assessment**—dryness of mouth, peripheral perfusion, pulse rate, blood pressure (compared with normal), jugular venous pressure observation, peripheral and pulmonary oedema (lung bases), measured urinary output, fluid balance charts and trends in body weight
- **Treat the cause of shock**—this can shut down the inflammatory response. Treatment may mean an operation to exteriorise a leaking anastomosis (i.e. bring the bowel ends to the skin surface) or to excise infected and necrotic tissue or drain pus
- **Treat infection**—if infection is apparent or suspected, institute antibiotic therapy using potent agents chosen on clinical suspicion until definitive microbiological results
- **Support vital organs** during the time it takes surgery or antibiotics to work. Airway and breathing support (e.g. oxygen administration, intubation, ventilation) benefits most patients, but the critical concern is to optimise the cardiovascular and haemodynamic system, aiming for a central venous pressure between 8 and 12 mmHg, a mean arterial pressure over 65 mmHg and a urine output of at least 0.5 ml/kg/hour
- **Monitor and assess the response**—clinically, by urine output and, ideally by transoesophageal Doppler assessment of stroke volume

A SCHEME FOR MANAGING THE ACUTELY ILL OR SHOCKED PATIENT

This scheme is given in note form as an *aide-mémoire* for clinicians.

RECOGNITION OF THE ACUTELY UNWELL PATIENT

(see Table 4.1)

The cardinal signs in a patient likely to need critical care in a high-dependency or intensive care unit include:

- Substantially increased or decreased respiratory rate
- Bradycardia or tachycardia
- Low blood pressure (compare with usual BP)
- Hypo- or hyperthermia
- Decreased level of consciousness

SEQUENCE FOR ACTION IN THE PATIENT AT RISK

In summary this includes the following steps, which are detailed below:

A. Initial assessment
B. Broad diagnosis
C. Immediate care
D. Monitoring and reassessment
E. Investigation to narrow the diagnosis
F. Definitive treatment

A. Initial assessment

The aim is rapidly to establish the urgency and severity of the situation. If vital signs are unsatisfactory and the patient unresponsive, a cardiac arrest or 'crash call' may be needed to bring more hands to assist. If an early warning score (EWS) is above a predetermined threshold, consultation is needed to arrange transfer to a critical care unit.

History

As much history should be gleaned as time permits, e.g. the context of the acute deterioration, medical state before deterioration, past medical history including allergies, and recent treatments including operations. Check drug charts.

Vital signs

Nurses can help gather information while assessment continues; vital signs should be monitored at frequent intervals. Observations include respiratory rate, temperature, pulse rate, systolic blood pressure and level of consciousness (the AVPU descending scale is simple and reproducible—A means the patient is fully **a**lert, V means responds to **v**oice, P means responds to **p**ain and U is **u**nresponsive).

Initial tests include oxygen saturation, blood glucose estimation, blood gas analysis and ECG for evidence of myocardial infarction. Note that new onset atrial fibrillation or flutter on ECG is often an indicator of sepsis. A bounding pulse and flushed extremities may suggest septic shock.

Examination—the initial survey

General impression including skin

- Intravenous lines and fluids, drug treatments being given via syringe driver, catheters, etc.
- Peripheral perfusion, hydration, oedema, anaemia, jaundice, bruising, rashes, nutritional state

Head and neck

- Stridor—obstruction of upper airway, e.g. bleed into thyroid lesion/mediastinal mass (?metastases); inhaled foreign body; inhaled vomitus
- Mouth and throat—evidence of abscess, e.g. peritonsillar abscess (quinsy), Ludwig's angina

Chest

- Localised poor air entry—infection, atelectasis, pneumothorax
- Generalised poor air entry—asthma, large pleural effusions
- Expiratory wheeze—anaphylaxis or cardiac failure
- If acutely breathless, consider thromboembolism

Heart

- New onset chest pain—myocardial infarction (MI)
- Cardiac murmurs—infective endocarditis, MI, acute valve prolapse
- Elevated jugular venous pressure—acute cardiac failure due to MI
- If cardiac problem suspected, check ECG for changes of ischaemia, arrhythmias

Abdomen including rectal and/or vaginal examination if necessary

- Localised tenderness—localised intra-abdominal infection, renal colic (loin)
- Generalised tenderness—peritonitis
- Distension—bowel obstruction, intraperitoneal or retroperitoneal bleed, ascites
- Melaena or fresh blood per rectum—gastrointestinal bleed
- Lump—strangulated hernia, intra-abdominal mass

Limbs

- Unilaterally (or bilaterally) pale and cold with or without necrosis—acute ischaemia
- Globally pale, cold—peripheral shutdown due to shock
- Swollen and blue—deep venous thrombosis (in patient with suspected pulmonary embolism)
- Red—cellulitis, diabetic foot infection with systemic sepsis

Neurology

- Conscious level
- Signs of unilateral palsy—stroke

B. Broad diagnosis

Priorities for immediate treatment and further investigation need to be decided following initial assessment, if necessary from a single major finding. Priorities change as evidence is collected and depending on the response to treatment.

Examples are:

- ***Respiratory***—upper airways obstruction, e.g. thyroid enlargement/haemorrhage into nodule
- ***Vascular events***—abdominal aortic aneurysm rupture, aortic dissection, pulmonary embolism, acute coronary syndromes including MI, stroke and lower limb gangrene (usually causes insidious rather than acute development of shock)
- ***Abdominal problems***
  a. **blood loss**—upper or lower gastrointestinal bleeding, intra- or retroperitoneal bleed
  b. **gastrointestinal obstruction including strangulation**—gastric, small bowel or large bowel, hernia, volvulus
  c. **generalised peritonitis**—perforation of an abdominal viscus (appendix, peptic ulcer, diverticular disease); acute pancreatitis
  d. **abdominal colic**—ureteric, biliary, intestinal
  e. **intra-abdominal infection**—gastroenteritis, acute appendicitis, diverticulitis, cholecystitis; urinary tract infection
  f. **obstetric and gynaecological**—ruptured ectopic pregnancy/ovarian cyst/pregnancy/salpingo-oophoritis
- ***Other infections***—infected central venous line, abscesses, cellulitis, diabetic foot, limb gangrene, gastroenteritis including antibiotic-associated colitis
- ***Metabolic***—surgical disease can precipitate or be complicated by hypoglycaemia in diabetics; consider Addison's disease (adrenal insufficiency) if the patient is hypotensive

C. Immediate care

Inform a senior doctor about the urgency of the case if appropriate.

Oxygen

Immediately secure a mask delivering 100% oxygen. The comatose patient may need to be intubated and positive pressure ventilation commenced.

Fluid management

Haemodynamic optimisation is very important and is based on clinical signs and monitoring of central venous pressure and urine output.

- Take **venous blood** for haemoglobin, haematocrit, urea and electrolytes, glucose, amylase and blood grouping/ordering of blood for transfusion if necessary. Take an arterial sample for blood gas estimation and acid–base status; get blood cultures if septic shock is suspected
- Set up an **intravenous infusion** and administer i.v. fluids/drugs, guided by vital signs and findings. For example, if the patient is hypotensive, give crystalloid or colloid solutions (at least 1 litre rapidly); if cardiogenic shock is likely, the circulating volume must not be expanded rapidly
- Blood transfusion if necessary
- Urinary catheter to monitor hourly output; urine dipstick

Drugs

- Analgesia if in pain—i.v. morphine
- Infection—antibiotics
- Low blood glucose—dextrose

D. Monitoring and reassessment

Monitoring

The most useful guides to the success of resuscitation are respiratory rate (unless ventilated), central venous pressure (CVP), hourly urinary output and plasma lactate.

- Central venous line—often required to monitor central pressure and response to fluids
- Arterial line if necessary
- Nasogastric tube if vomiting; include fluid aspirated on the fluid balance chart
- Request a cardiac ECG monitor if a cardiac problem is suspected

Reassessment

Check the response to therapy: respiratory rate, pulse rate, blood pressure, CVP and plasma lactate. Consider moving the patient to a critical care bed and surgical intervention if the response to therapy is inadequate.

E. Investigation to narrow the diagnosis

Consider the most likely diagnosis and quickest route to confirming the initial 'best guess':

- Check blood results
- If there is infection: blood culture, sputum culture
- Chest problems: chest X-ray, CT pulmonary angiogram if pulmonary embolism is suspected
- Cardiac problems: troponin blood levels, echocardiogram
- Abdomen: plain X-ray/ultrasound or CT scan/endoscopy if the clinical diagnosis is equivocal

F. Definitive treatment

Give definitive treatment as required according to the diagnosis.

5 Imaging and interventional techniques in surgery

INTRODUCTION

This chapter gives an overview of imaging and endoscopic procedures used for investigation (including biopsy) and treatment. **Interventional radiology** describes minimal access procedures using image guidance to treat conditions whilst causing least trauma. It is usually performed by radiologists, although other clinicians may be involved. Examples include ultrasound or CT-guided biopsy and endoscopic placement of biliary stents.

PLAIN RADIOLOGY

Body tissues absorb X-rays proportionate to the density (atomic number) of their elements, e.g. calcium in bones absorbs a great deal of X-irradiation so bones are displayed white on radiographs or computed tomography. Contrast media also absorb X-rays well as they usually contain iodine or barium, both large atoms with many electrons. Low-density tissues made up of atoms with a low atomic number, such as air in lungs, absorb few X-rays and hence display as black. Intermediate densities such as water in muscle or organs are displayed as grey. Remember, fat floats on water because it is less dense, demonstrating its electron density is less than water, so fat is displayed darker than muscle but not as dark as air. This varied absorption of X-rays results in differential penetration and exposure of traditional **X-ray films** or activation of sensors in a filmless rig. A radiograph is in effect a 'shadow' picture of electron density.

Some **foreign bodies** in wounds are radiopaque, including metal and most glass fragments, but wood and plastic are radiolucent and invisible. Gauze swabs used in operating theatres are radiolucent but have a radiopaque strand allowing them to be located radiographically if left in a wound (Fig. 5.1).

CASE HISTORY

Fig. 5.1 Plain abdominal X-ray showing retained surgical swab

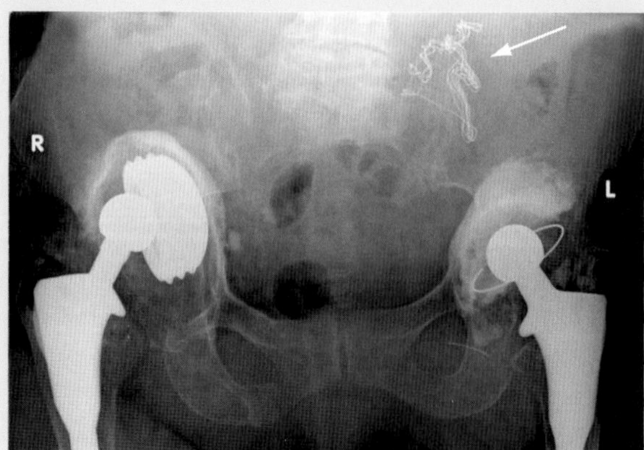

This 83-year-old woman had persistent pain in the left iliac fossa after a left hip replacement. This pelvic X-ray was taken to investigate the new joint. However, a radiopaque marker was spotted (arrowed) indicating a surgical swab that had been left in the abdomen after a laparotomy for perforated duodenal ulcer 8 years previously. The swab was removed uneventfully at a second laparotomy

PERSONAL RADIATION PROTECTION

Ionising radiation is both mutagenic and carcinogenic and irradiation of patients and observers must be minimised. This is achieved by:

- Giving training in radiation protection to all staff using and working near X-ray equipment
- Ensuring every investigation helps with management and none is performed merely as 'routine'
- Improving design of X-ray equipment to minimise radiation dose whilst preserving diagnostic detail. X-ray **scatter** is minimised and unwanted types of radiation removed by filters
- Physical barriers are built into radiology suites or provided to protect staff. These include barium plaster in walls, lead-glass windows and lead-rubber aprons
- Workers involved in X-rays should keep away from the direct beam line and maintain a good distance from the X-ray source during exposure. Note the inverse square law determines the fall-off of radiation with distance
- All involved in radiography should wear X-ray-sensitive **film badges** which need to be regularly monitored for excess radiation

GENERAL PRINCIPLES OF RADIOLOGY

These factors are involved in producing a useful radiographic image:

- **X-ray power and exposure time**—chosen to give a diagnostically useful exposure without excess dosage. Good quality images have a range of densities appropriate to the anatomical area. For example, thoracic spine views require a larger dose than lungs
- **Different projections (views)** produce different views of the same subject. The X-ray tube is effectively a point source with a diverging beam (see Fig. 5.2), so the subject is magnified. The distortion least affects the body part closest to the film, which is thus shown most clearly. The beam direction should be recorded on the film as it has consequences for interpretation, e.g. a frontal chest film might be PA (postero-anterior) or AP (antero-posterior). With lateral exposures, the side nearest the film is indicated, e.g. a 'Rt' lateral chest X-ray (CXR) has the right side nearest the film
- **Patient position** during exposure (i.e. supine, prone, oblique or erect) affects the image because of gravity affecting organs, gas or fluid. Most films are taken with the patient lying supine with the X-ray beam aimed vertically downwards. A horizontal beam can demonstrate fluid levels in a cavity or bowel (lateral decubitus), or free gas under the diaphragm

ELECTRONIC RECORDING TECHNIQUES

X-ray, magnetic resonance (MRI), ultrasound and isotope scan images are increasingly being recorded **digitally** rather than in **analogue** form. Digital images can be manipulated to optimise available information-enhancing contrast between tissues, magnifying areas of interest and abstracting the relevant parts from image series. Electronic **storage** has a number of advantages over conventional film:

- Substantial cost saving on film and processing chemicals
- Reduced physical space needed for storage
- Reduced staff costs—no need to file or retrieve films
- Better availability of images—no need to obtain physical films; several viewers can see the same images simultaneously in their place of work
- Substantially reduced numbers of missing examinations
- Easy transmission of images from one institution to another—by portable storage media (CD-ROM) or electronic links

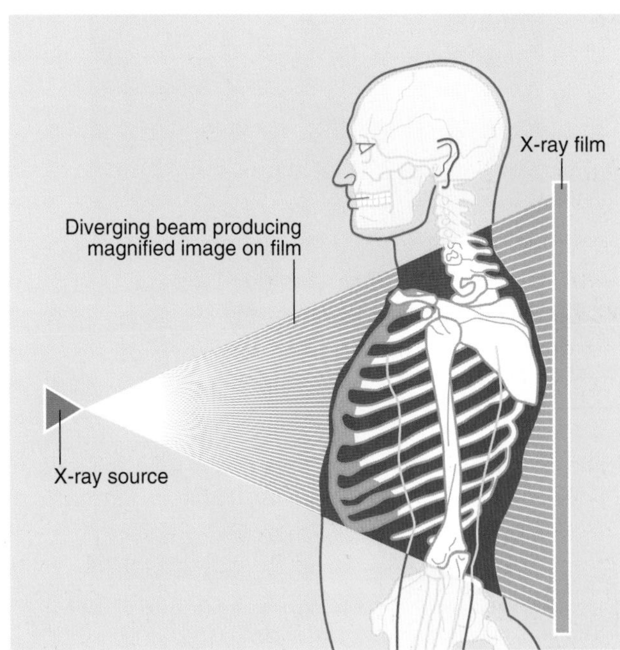

Fig. 5.2 Radiological projection

'Filmless' X-ray departments are becoming the norm, with images displayed on terminals dispersed around the hospital. Images can be accessed remotely by family practitioners and clinicians at home or in other hospitals.

PLAIN RADIOLOGY

Chest X-ray

Interpreting plain chest X-rays requires a methodical approach. Several learned documents have been written on the subject (see e.g. http://student.bmj.com/student/view-article.html?id=sbmj04018), and no attempt will be made to produce an incomplete version here.

Plain abdominal radiology

Most abdominal films are taken with the patient supine. Bowel is visible when it contains gas (Figs 5.3 and 5.4); normal **small bowel** is less than 3 cm wide and tends to occupy the centre of the abdomen. When dilated, it shows transverse folds (**plicae circulares**) which completely cross the lumen. The colon usually lies peripherally and has **haustrations**; these folds only partly traverse the lumen (Fig. 5.3). Normal colon is less than 6 cm wide and often contains faecal lumps with a mottled appearance. Further reading about this topic is available from: http://www.studentbmj.com/topics/clinical/imaging_techniques.php.

The kidneys may be outlined by a border of perinephric fat but outlines are often obscured by bowel gas and faeces. After nephrectomy, the 'renal outline' may persist and the kidney appears to be present. Small urinary tract stones are easily obscured and the liver may be visible but its size cannot be estimated.

When examining an abdominal X-ray, important features to look for are:

- Calcification in areas prone to stone formation, e.g. kidney, ureters, bladder or biliary tree (see below, *Urography*, Fig. 5.8a)
- Dilated bowel (stomach, small or large bowel)
- Free intraperitoneal gas indicating bowel perforation
- Gas in abnormal places (e.g. biliary tree or urinary tract) suggesting a fistula with bowel
- Non-biological objects, e.g. foreign bodies, surgical tubes or pieces of metal
- Pathological calcification, e.g. aortic aneurysm, pancreas, adrenals or uterine fibroids

The limitations of plain abdominal radiography are summarised in Box 5.1.

Free intraperitoneal gas

Free gas is diagnostic of **bowel perforation** except after recent laparotomy. A horizontal beam chest or upper abdominal X-ray with the patient **erect** is the most useful method of demonstrating it as a radiolucent layer beneath the diaphragm (see Fig. 19.8, p. 275). The layer can be very small but is often obvious. Perforation can also be confidently diagnosed when the inside and outside of the bowel wall are both outlined by radiolucent shadows, but this is rare (Rigler's sign, Fig. 32.7, p. 413). Where the result is doubtful or the patient too ill to sit or stand, he or she should be placed in the **right-side raised lateral decubitus position** (i.e. lying on the left side)

CASE HISTORY

Fig. 5.3 Abdominal X-ray

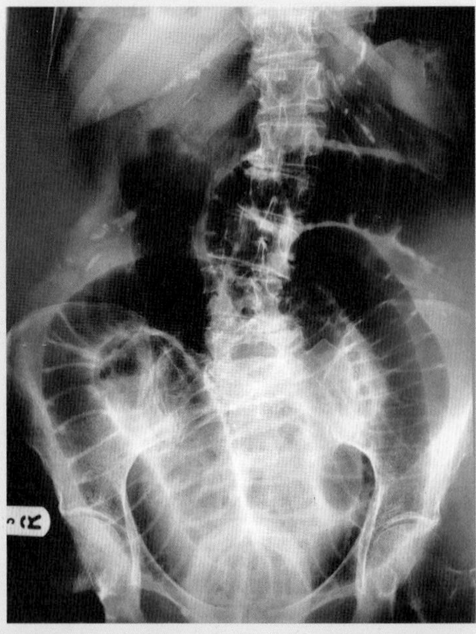

Supine plain abdominal film showing gross small bowel dilatation. At laparotomy, the cause proved to be an obstructing carcinoma of the caecum

Fig. 5.4 Abdominal X-ray

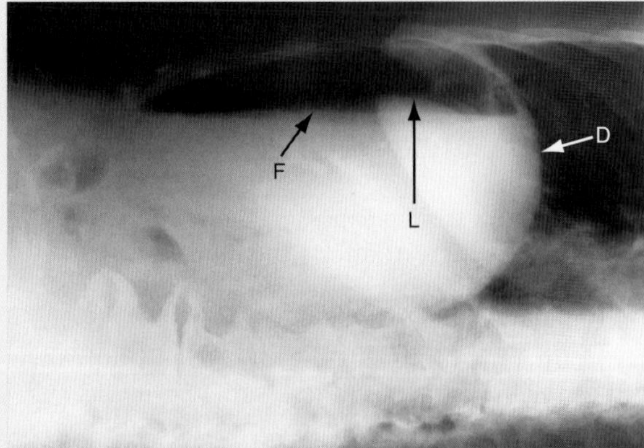

This 78-year-old woman presented with a sudden onset of severe abdominal pain. Erect chest X-ray failed to show free abdominal gas but a perforation was clinically suspected so this lateral decubitus X-ray was performed. The right side is raised and the head is to the right of the picture; the X-ray beam was horizontal. Free intraperitoneal gas is seen above a fluid level **F** beneath the diaphragm **D** and 'floating' over the liver **L**. At laparotomy, the cause proved to be a perforated duodenal ulcer

Box 5.1 Limitations of plain abdominal radiography

- Intraperitoneal structures are not visualised unless they contain gas themselves, displace gas-filled bowel or indent structural fat
- Stones that are not calcified (90% of gallstones, 10% of urinary tract stones) are not visible
- Bowel gas and faeces easily obscure stones
- Phleboliths, calcified abdominal lymph nodes and costal cartilages readily mimic stones
- Liver and spleen size cannot be estimated accurately
- Free intraperitoneal gas is not usually visible on a supine film (a horizontal beam film is needed)

for 10 minutes. A horizontal beam X-ray taken across the table can then reveal as little as 2 ml of gas above the lateral liver border (Fig. 5.4).

Bone X-rays

Conventional radiographs of bones continue to play an important role in diagnosis of bone disease, particularly fractures, but also infection, neoplasia and degenerative conditions. Other investigations including bone scintigraphy, CT, MRI and ultrasound are often used, particularly if conventional X-rays are normal. If in doubt it is best to discuss with a radiologist.

CONTRAST RADIOLOGY

When plain radiography is inappropriate, a highly X-ray-absorbing **contrast medium** may be employed. Contrast media outline structures either **directly**, or **indirectly** by being concentrated in the target organ. Contrast studies can still be helpful when supervised by trained and experienced personnel but are increasingly being replaced by other tests. For example computed tomography (CT) instead of barium enema or intravenous urography (IVU), duplex ultrasound instead of venography and some arteriography, and magnetic resonance angiography (MRA) instead of conventional angiography.

Direct studies include contrast material swallowed, instilled into body orifices, sinuses (sinogram) or fistulae (fistulogram), or injected into blood vessels or hollow viscera. Examples are barium enema for large bowel and arteriography for the arterial system. **Indirect contrast studies** include IVU where contrast injected intravenously is excreted in urine to display the urinary tract.

Contrast materials

Barium sulphate is the best agent for directly outlining the GI tract. It is insoluble in water and is not absorbed. An aqueous suspension is non-irritant and very radiodense. Barium investigations of the upper and lower gastrointestinal tracts have been largely superseded by endoscopy or cross-sectional imaging but are still occasionally employed.

Water-soluble **iodinated benzoic acid derivatives** can be injected into arteries or veins to opacify them (arteriography or venography). Injectable contrast media have improved over the years to make them safer but they remain potentially nephrotoxic in patients with renal impairment.

Direct venography has largely been replaced by colour duplex ultrasound, and CT or MR angiography is used more than direct studies for diagnosis.

Examples of contrast radiology

Bowel contrast radiology

Any part of the gastrointestinal tract can be demonstrated using contrast. Most barium studies use a **double contrast** method. Following barium, air or carbon dioxide is used to distend the bowel and separate the barium-coated bowel walls. An anticholinergic agent such as hyoscine butylbromide (Buscopan) is sometimes given at the same time to abolish spasm, further improving the image.

If substantial peritoneal spillage is likely, as in possible perforation or when checking a recent rectal anastomosis, barium should be avoided as it causes peritonitis. In these, a water-soluble contrast medium is best given initially, and barium substituted if no leak is detected.

Preparation for bowel contrast studies

For upper gastrointestinal studies, patients should be fasted overnight except for water. For a barium enema, bowel preparation is performed with laxatives (e.g. sodium picosulphate) and sometimes bowel washouts, so artefacts are removed (faecal lumps look similar to polyps) and small mucosal defects are not obscured.

Upper gastrointestinal tract

For examining the upper GI tract, barium suspension is given orally (**barium swallow** for oesophagus and **barium meal** for stomach and duodenum. Progress of contrast is observed by **screening**, with a moving image displayed on a screen. The radiologist usually selects representative **spot films** to summarise the examination. Screening is useful to study rapid GI motility as in swallowing; images can be studied later in slow motion.

Large bowel

The **large bowel** is examined by means of contrast material given rectally (**barium enema**). The lower rectum is often poorly shown so prior rectal examination and sigmoidoscopy is best to ensure low lesions are not missed.

With improved technology, **CT** is increasingly used for large bowel examination. It can be performed without laxative preparation where it would be acceptable to miss small polyps, for example in suspected obstructing lesions. CT can be useful in the frail elderly when a right-sided colonic cancer is suspected because of anaemia or a palpable mass. For a more complete examination, **CT colonography** (also known as CT coloscopy or virtual colonoscopy) requires full bowel cleansing. During the procedure, air or carbon dioxide is insufflated into the colon; the technique is sensitive enough to detect lesions larger than 1 cm. The investigation is quicker and less unpleasant than barium enema and has replaced it altogether in some units. Hundreds of images are produced and the best are viewed on workstations along with reconstructed axial and 3D images of the bowel lumen (see Fig. 5.5).

Small bowel

For **small bowel** examination, a barium meal may be 'followed through' into the small bowel, or contrast can be

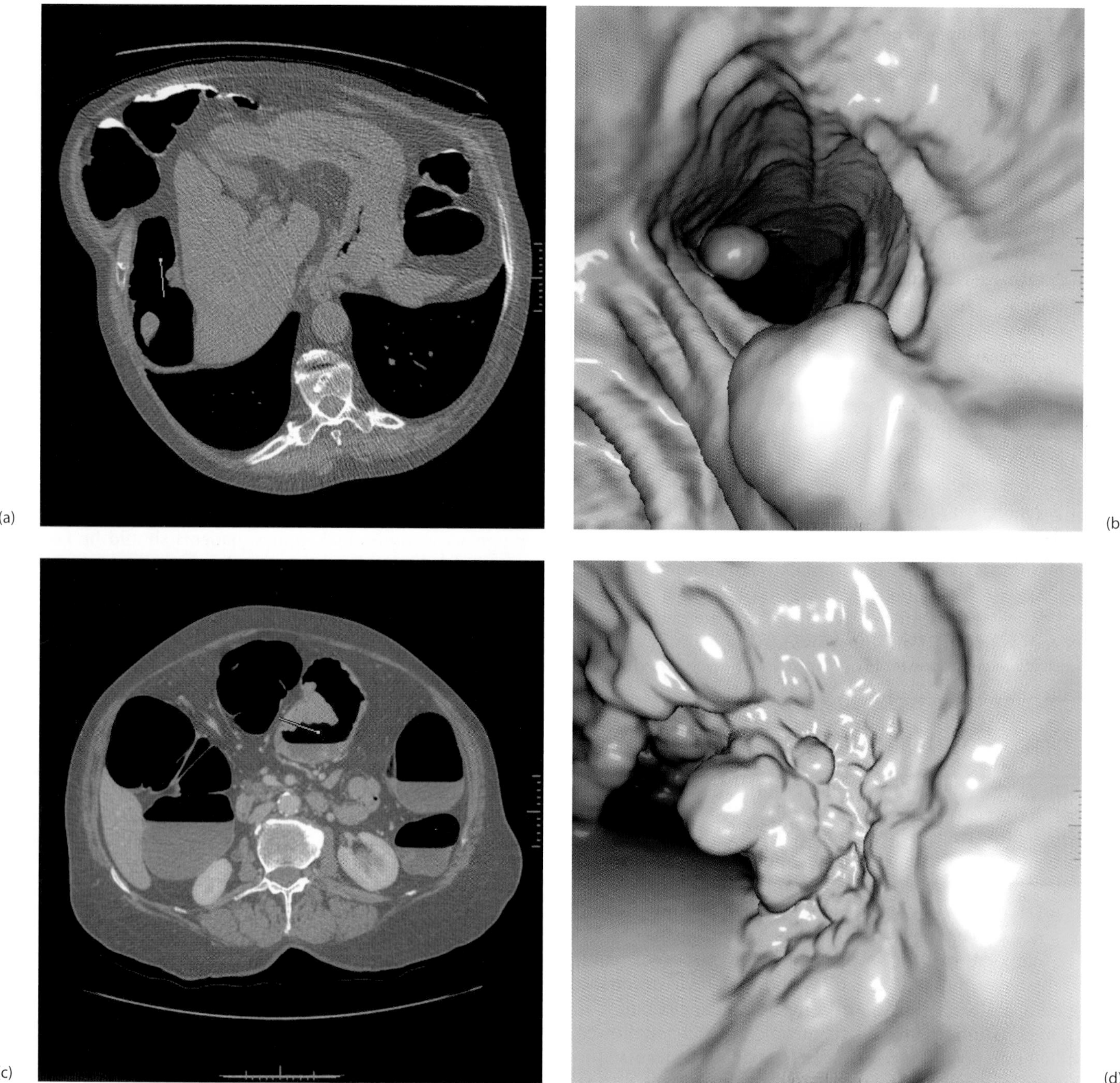

Fig. 5.5 Examples of CT colonography (a) Prone. One of the axial CT images used to reconstruct the 3D image showing an adenomatous polyp in **(b)**. **(c)** One of the axial CT images used to reconstruct the 3D image showing a transverse colon carcinoma in (**d**)

instilled directly into the proximal jejunum via a nasal or oral tube. In either case, the diagnostic yield is poor and these techniques are likely to be replaced by CT or MR studies of the small bowel or **capsule endoscopy** (see below).

Complications of barium contrast studies

The limitations of barium contrast studies are summarised in Box 5.2. There is a risk that contrast material may be aspirated into the bronchial tree, causing aspiration pneumonitis, so care must be taken when giving oral barium to patients with swallowing difficulties. CT scanning is safer and more likely to provide useful information such as the level and cause of obstruction, and associated pathology such as lung or liver metastases.

BILIARY RADIOLOGY

Some biliary investigations described in previous editions of this book (e.g. oral cholecystography and intravenous cholangiography) have been superseded by ultrasound and increased availability of endoscopic retrograde cholangio-pancreatography (ERCP, p. 65) and magnetic resonance cholangio-pancreatography (MRCP).

Box 5.2 Limitations of barium contrast studies

- It is often impossible to distinguish between different types of pathological lesion, e.g. between malignant and inflammatory colonic stenosis, or between malignant and peptic ulcer of the stomach
- Fine mucosal detail is not shown, e.g. gastric lesions such as inflammation, shallow ulceration or early cancer, or angiodysplasias of the colon. In acute gastrointestinal bleeding, barium meal may miss the bleeding lesion
- Small bowel is difficult to examine in detail because of contrast dilution by bowel contents and loops of bowel overlying each other
- The luminal outline of obstructed bowel cannot be satisfactorily demonstrated with contrast; barium in a follow-through does not reach the site of complete obstruction. 'Instant' or unprepared barium enema examination is useful in distinguishing mechanical large bowel obstruction from pseudo-obstruction but does not demonstrate the bowel proximal to an obstruction
- Barium taken orally may turn an incomplete colonic obstruction into complete obstruction, as may barium given rectally
- Major abnormalities may be concealed because of tissue overlap. Multiple projections, double contrast techniques and tube angulation reduce this deficiency

Magnetic resonance cholangio-pancreatography (MRCP) (Fig. 5.6 e and f)

MRCP now produces images that rival the quality of ERCP. MRI differentiates tissues and organs by their varying water content. Bile and pancreatic juice are mostly water, hence MRCP gives clear images of bile in the gall bladder and ducts and outlines the pancreatic duct. It reveals filling defects caused by stones or tumours. MRCP can identify bile leaks, gallstones in the bile ducts, and duct obstruction from any cause. There are no known hazards. MRCP is increasingly used prior to ERCP for pancreatico-biliary investigation to reduce the number of patients requiring the more invasive investigation.

Indications for MRCP include:

- Suspected bile duct stones, especially within the liver and for seeking retained stones after operation
- Bile duct strictures, particularly within the liver—post-surgical, cholangiocarcinoma
- Suspected sclerosing cholangitis
- Acute pancreatitis of unknown aetiology—MRCP reveals anatomical duct abnormalities
- Biliary-type pain with abnormal liver function tests in patients without stones on ultrasound
- Choledochal cysts
- Patients unsuitable for ERCP because they are intolerant of the procedure or have had previous gastrectomy

Percutaneous transhepatic cholangiography (PTC)

Percutaneous cholangiography is rarely used for diagnosis but has occasional therapeutic indications. A long fine (22 G) 'Chiba' needle is passed percutaneously, directly into dilated intrahepatic ducts, and contrast injected to display the duct system (see Fig. 5.6c). This shows the configuration of extra-hepatic duct obstruction from the proximal direction.

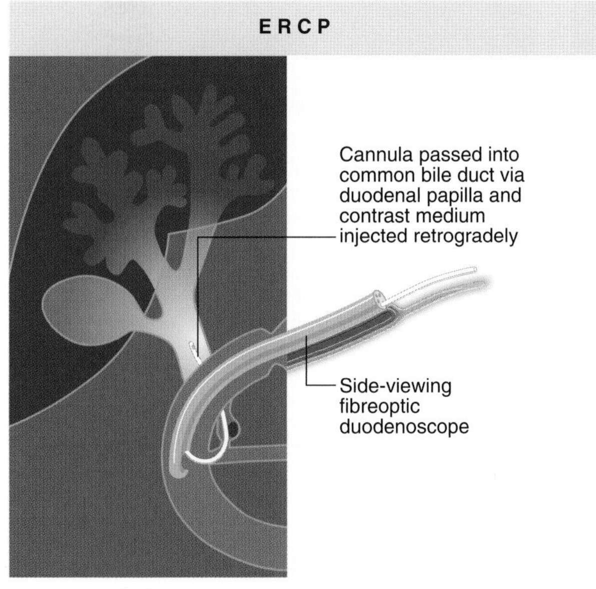

(a)

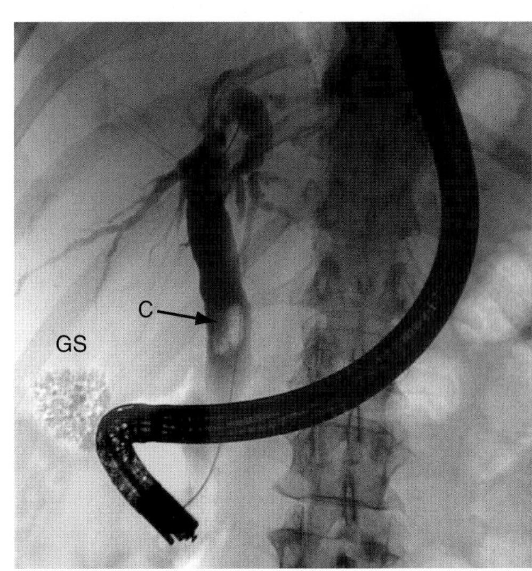

(b)

Fig. 5.6 Some techniques for demonstrating the biliary system
(a) and **(b)** Endoscopic retrograde cholangiography
The patient is sedated and a side-viewing gastroscope passed down so the tip reaches the second part of the duodenum. The ampulla of Vater is cannulated under direct vision and contrast medium injected to outline the bile ducts. **(b)** A large gallstone **C** is seen within the dilated common bile duct and a collection of radiopaque gallstones **GS** is seen in the gall bladder

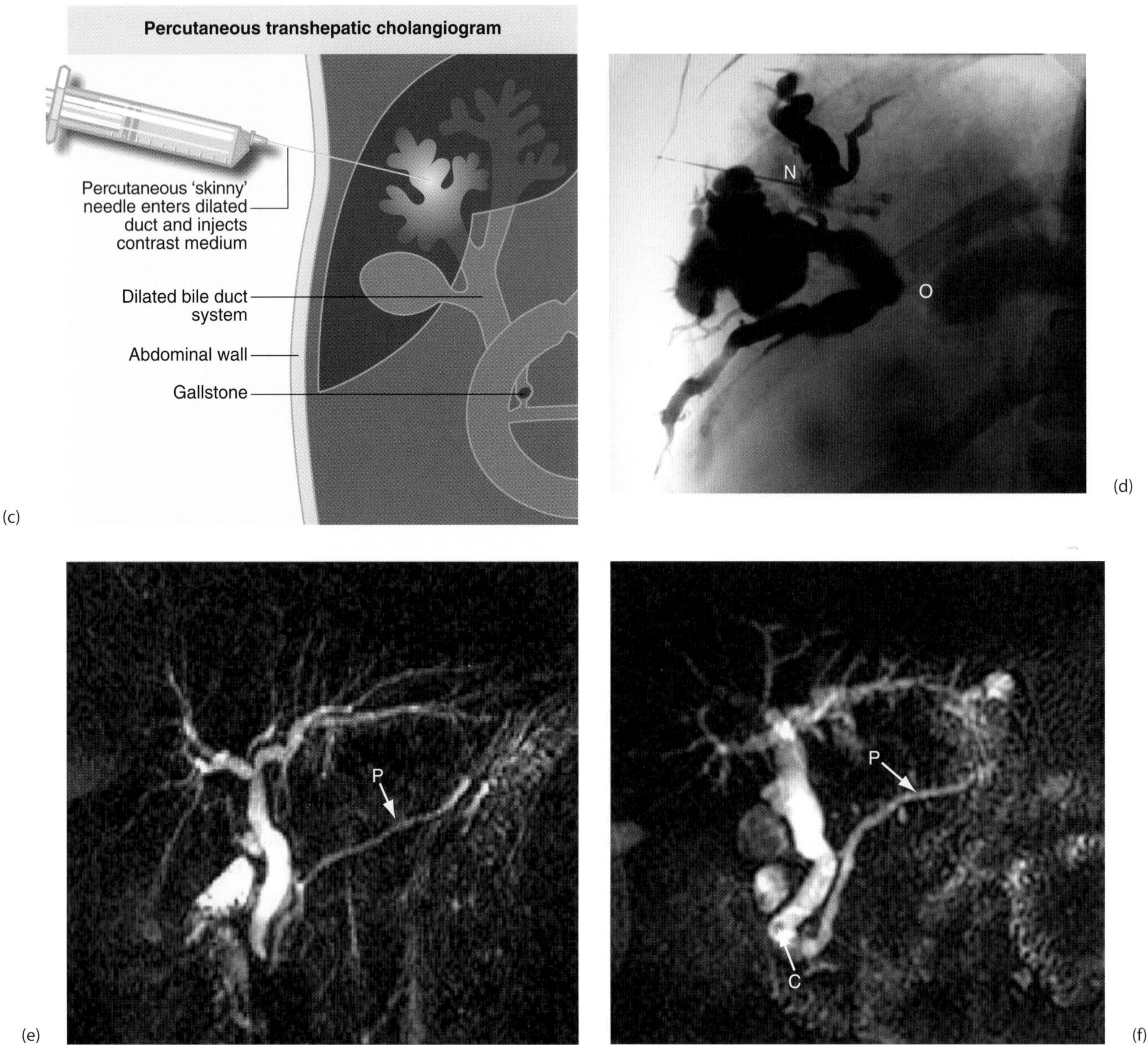

Fig. 5.6, Continued (c) and **(d)** Percutaneous transhepatic cholangiography

A needle **N** is passed into the liver until it encounters a dilated duct. Contrast medium is then injected to outline the ducts. (d) Case study—this deeply jaundiced 57-year-old woman has grossly dilated intrahepatic ducts and complete obstruction of the proximal common bile duct in the porta hepatis at **O**. This was due to lymph node metastases from carcinoma of stomach. This method is employed less often nowadays because of the superior safety of other methods described here

(e) and **(f)** Magnetic resonance cholangio-pancreatography (MRCP)

The technique produces images of static fluid, thus the images are of native biliary and pancreatic secretions. Each image was obtained in one second using a thick slab 'projection' method that generates images very similar to ERCP. The pancreatic duct in each image is labelled **P**. **(e)** An example of normal biliary and pancreatic duct systems. **(f)** A small calculus, **C**, in the distal common bile duct. There is also mild dilatation of the pancreatic duct with some side branches visible

Occasionally, PTC is employed to drain obstructed ducts after failed endoscopic placement of a drain or stent. In jaundiced patients, disordered blood clotting is likely so a **clotting screen** and platelet count should be performed before PTC, and any clotting disorder corrected.

Endoscopic retrograde cholangio-pancreatography (ERCP)

This is described below (see *Diagnostic and therapeutic duodenoscopy*); its use in obstructive jaundice is described in detail in Chapter 18. The basic technique is illustrated in Figure 5.6 a and b.

Operative cholangiography and choledochoscopy

It is standard practice to perform operative cholangiography during open cholecystectomy. For laparoscopic cholecystectomy, some surgeons routinely perform operative cholangiography whilst others prefer no imaging at all for selected cases or else preoperative assessment using MRCP for cases deemed likely to have duct stones.

Operative cholangiography allows the (highly variable) biliary anatomy to be displayed, it demonstrates stones in the bile ducts and it shows whether contrast flows freely into the duodenum. A fine plastic cannula is introduced into a small cystic duct incision and passed into the common bile duct. Water-soluble contrast material is injected to outline the duct system and fluoroscopic images or X-ray films are taken. If duct stones are demonstrated, they are often retrieved surgically at the same operation. At open cholecystectomy, this is via a longitudinal incision in the common bile duct (**exploration of the common bile duct**). At laparoscopic surgery, the same technique is used with a small transverse or longitudinal choledochotomy, depending on the duct size and the stone size to be retrieved. A flexible 5 mm or 3 mm endoscope called a choledochoscope is passed into the bile duct and stones may be retrieved using a range of techniques including snares, baskets, balloons, or they can even be shattered with lithotripsy probes. The choledochoscope enables the bile and intrahepatic ducts to be inspected afterwards to see that all stones have been removed. A further cholangiogram is often done afterwards to ensure the duct is clear. Stone removal may be deferred and performed later at ERCP although it carries risk of complications, including biliary leakage and acute pancreatitis.

T-tube cholangiography

Following exploration of bile ducts for stones, a T-tube is often left in situ to drain the duct. The transverse limb of the T lies in the duct and the long limb drains out through an opening in the duct to the skin where it is connected to a drainage bag. About 1 week after operation, contrast can be injected along the T-tube to outline the biliary tree and show abnormalities such as residual stones, bile leakage and duct stenoses as well as confirming free drainage into the duodenum. If residual stones are still present they can be retrieved either at ERCP or sometimes by the radiologists via the T-tube itself.

VASCULAR RADIOLOGY (ANGIOGRAPHY)

GENERAL PRINCIPLES AND HAZARDS OF ARTERIOGRAPHY AND VENOGRAPHY

Further detail about applications of vascular radiology is given in Chapter 41.

The veins or arteries of an anatomical region can be opacified by intravenous or intra-arterial injection of contrast medium. This is **angiography** and includes arteriography and venography. In **arteriography**, needle puncture of the access artery is followed by guide-wire insertion, needle removal and catheter insertion over the guide-wire. Shaped catheters and wires are used to advance the catheter tip to an appropriate position for arteriography. Favoured access sites are the femoral artery in the groin, the brachial artery above the elbow and, more recently, the radial artery at the wrist using smaller diameter catheters.

If there is suspicion of a bleeding disorder, **clotting studies** should be performed beforehand to anticipate potential haemorrhagic complications from the vessel puncture site.

The contrast medium is the same as that used for computed tomography (CT) and carries similar hazards, i.e. allergic reaction and nephrotoxicity (see *Urography* below). There is also the risk of complications from the cannulation, which may cause bleeding or thrombosis and, for arteries, wall dissection, arteriovenous fistula or false aneurysm formation.

ARTERIOGRAPHY

Digital subtraction is now standard for contrast vascular studies. The unchanging opacities of a plain radiographic image (particularly bone and bowel gas) are **subtracted** from the image after the injection of contrast medium so lower doses produce better images. In some cases, intravenous contrast alone can produce useful images, although this is used less frequently with advances in CT angiography (CTA) and magnetic resonance angiography (MRA).

In **lower limb arteriography**, if the aorto-iliac system is occluded and femoral pulses undetectable, the usual femoral artery access is not accessible, so a catheter can be placed via the radial or brachial artery. However, magnetic resonance angiography (MRA) or CTA is often preferred when available. Arteriography will demonstrate stenoses or occlusions due to thrombosis, atheroma and embolism.

ENDOVASCULAR TECHNIQUES

Percutaneous transluminal angioplasty (PTA) or balloon angioplasty

Angioplasty under local anaesthesia is a less invasive alternative to surgery for treating many peripheral and coronary arterial stenoses. In general, short stenoses in large vessels are most suitable. The method is particularly useful for lower limb atherosclerosis (especially iliac and superficial femoral arteries) and for coronary artery disease and, to a lesser extent, renal artery and mesenteric artery stenoses. Carotid artery disease is also suitable for angioplasty in some cases; filters are usually placed above the stenotic segment before dilatation to reduce the risk of embolism to the brain.

Major complications of angioplasty are rare in experienced hands but there is a small risk of precipitating acute ischaemia due to distal embolisation or dissection. Thus, surgical salvage should be readily available should complications develop. Unfortunately, 25–40% of angioplastied lesions undergo restenosis or occlusion within 1 year, but the process can usually be repeated. Where stenoses fail to remain open at angioplasty, expandable **stents** can be placed within the treated lesion. Peripheral arterial stents are most often used to treat iliac occlusive disease and improve long-term patency. These stents are either mounted on an angioplasty balloon or are self-expanding on withdrawal of the introducer sheath. Stents are being increasingly used in superficial femoral artery stenoses and occlusions. Overall, angioplasty causes minimal interventional and anaesthetic stress to the patient and is often performed on a day-case basis.

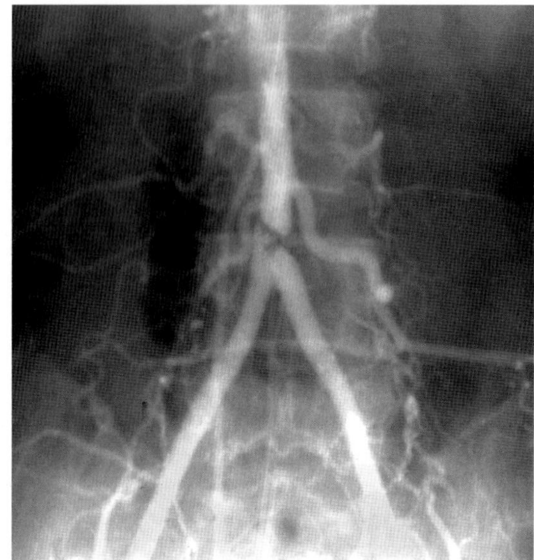

(a)

(b)

Fig. 5.7 Percutaneous transluminal angioplasty
This man of 55 presented with bilateral calf and thigh claudication. **(a)** A localised severe stenosis of the distal abdominal aorta. **(b)** The 'kissing balloon' technique used to dilate the stenosis. Two balloons, shown inflated, are used to prevent asymmetrical dilatation which might compromise the opposite common iliac artery

Techniques of percutaneous angioplasty

Angioplasty is usually performed under local anaesthesia (Fig. 5.7). A needle is first inserted into an accessible artery and a short flexible guide-wire passed through it into the artery and the needle removed. A working sheath with a valved side-arm is passed over the guide-wire and advanced into the artery. A catheter is inserted and a long guide-wire is then substituted for the first and manipulated up to and through the stenosis using contrast injections and fluoroscopic control. An **angioplasty catheter** with a plastic inflatable balloon at its end is then passed over the guide-wire and manipulated across the stenosis. Angioplasty balloons are now no wider than the catheter before inflation, and inflate to a fixed diameter at a given pressure. It is possible to measure the arterial pressure above and below the stenosis to determine the pressure gradient before and after angioplasty, although this is not performed routinely. The balloon is then inflated to a pressure of typically 6 and 15 atmospheres, depending on the balloon type, to dilate the stenosis, then further contrast is injected to check the result. Angioplasty techniques and equipment have progressively improved and many patients now return to near-normal life after minimal intervention.

Many patients with ischaemic legs or coronary heart disease who might not have been suitable for reconstructive surgery can now have angioplasty because of its minimally invasive nature and low complication rates.

Local arterial thrombolytic therapy

An artery freshly occluded by thrombosis and causing ischaemia can be recanalised by local intra-arterial infusion of thrombolytic agents. High local concentrations with limited systemic spill-over were intended to avoid the serious bleeding and allergic complications of systemic thrombolysis. However, experience has shown that the risk of major haemorrhage still exists, some episodes of which have been fatal. Examples include intracerebral haemorrhagic strokes and bleeding from recent surgical wounds or from the gastrointestinal tract. For this reason, the treatment has limited indications, i.e. recently occluded native arteries or bypass grafts. The thrombolytic agent usually used is **recombinant tissue plasminogen activator** (R-tPa). R-tPa acts more quickly and does not have the frequent allergic effects of the older agents, e.g. streptokinase.

For recent acute embolic ischaemia, surgical embolectomy remains the best treatment.

Therapeutic embolisation

Highly vascular lesions that would be difficult or impossible to treat by surgery alone, such as some arteriovenous malformations, can have their arterial supply reduced or obliterated by embolisation. The main supplying artery is identified by selective arteriography and a catheter manoeuvred into it, close to the lesion. The materials chosen for embolisation depend on the nature of the lesion but include **gelatin foam**, **polyvinyl alcohol particles**, **minute steel coils**, **plugs**, **cyanoacrylate glue** or **liquid polymers**. The process can be repeated for all the feeding vessels.

Embolisation is particularly useful in the treatment of gastrointestinal haemorrhage, some pseudoaneurysms, uterine fibroids and internal iliac arteries prior to endovascular aneurysm repair (EVAR). The technique is also used to treat hepatic tumours (primary and secondary) and some bone metastases prior to surgery.

Minimal access graft placement

EVAR is now widely used to treat both abdominal and thoracic aortic aneurysms. There are several different devices available, composed of metal stents and graft material, and technical improvements are continuing. The device is correctly positioned in the aorta, and then deployment consists of unsheathing the device under fluoroscopic guidance. Graft limbs are used to extend the device into the iliac arteries. There are now stent grafts capable of treating more complex aneurysms with side branches/grafts into the renal, mesenteric, internal iliac or arch arteries. One disadvantage of the technique includes **endoleakage**, i.e. continued slow bleeding into the aneurysm sac because of an inadequate seal or, more commonly, from lumbar arteries or the inferior mesenteric artery. Other complications include graft migration, limb occlusion or limb dislocation. Although reintervention rates are higher than with open aneurysm repair, these techniques have allowed many patients to be treated who would never be fit for open surgery. The late complication rate is about 10% per year, considerably greater than for open aneurysm grafting, but rates are falling with improving techniques.

VENOUS TECHNIQUES

Venography

Colour duplex Doppler ultrasound scanning has replaced contrast venography for diagnosing **deep vein thrombosis** (DVT) as well as for demonstrating reflux from deep to superficial vessels in varicose veins. A skilled operator can demonstrate the patency or otherwise of all the lower limb veins and the presence of fresh or old thrombus. Valve competence can be shown in deep and superficial veins and perforating veins. Vein wall irregularity caused by previous DVT can also be displayed. Contrast venography can sometimes be helpful in defining the anatomy of complex superficial varicose veins and very occasionally to diagnose or exclude calf vein DVT where duplex is inconclusive.

Placement of vena caval filters

After venous thromboembolism, a few patients experience **recurrent pulmonary embolism** despite adequate anticoagulation. In others, anticoagulation therapy is contraindicated and other methods of preventing pulmonary embolism must be found, e.g. in pregnancy, after a haemorrhagic stroke, in patients with a high risk of falling or those with certain bleeding disorders. In these groups, the risk of pulmonary embolism can be markedly reduced by placing a filter in the inferior vena cava, above or below the renal veins. This still allows venous blood to return to the heart but traps substantial embolic material in the flowing blood. Since the mid-1960s a range of filtration devices have been developed that can be inserted relatively simply using a catheter via the femoral or jugular vein. Typical examples are the Celect or Optease filter. Some filters can be retrieved by percutaneous techniques if necessary within a limited time period. Complications are uncommon and include caval occlusion, migration and strut fracture.

Minimally invasive treatment of varicose veins

Several methods of ablating the long or short saphenous vein have appeared recently including foam sclerotherapy and laser or radiofrequency ablation. These are described in Chapter 43.

UROGRAPHY

General principles of urography

Urography is a radiological technique for examining the kidneys and urinary collecting systems using intravenous contrast concentrated and excreted by the kidneys. A plain abdominal **control film** is taken beforehand so calcified opacities can be compared with post-contrast images. This helps identify if an opacity lies within the renal tract and hence whether it is likely to be a stone (see Fig. 5.8a).

In intravenous urography (IVU), films are taken at intervals after injection. The renal parenchyma normally opacifies almost immediately and contrast then flows into the renal pelvis, ureters and bladder.

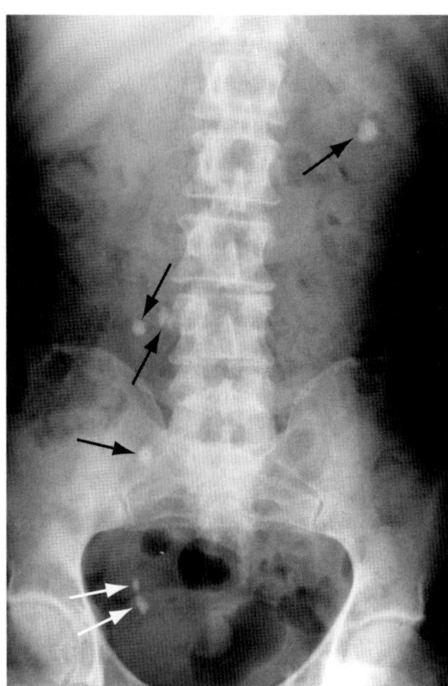

(a)

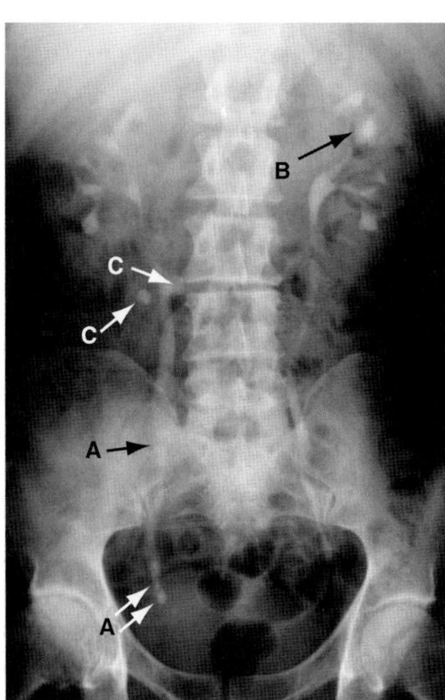

(b)

Fig. 5.8 Plain abdominal X-ray and IVU compared
(a) A plain abdominal film and **(b)** an intravenous urogram (IVU) of the same patient showing urinary tract stones. In the plain film, several calcified opacities (arrowed) are seen. From the IVU, in which the pelvicalyceal systems and ureters contain contrast material, it can be seen that three stones **A** lie within the lower right ureter and stone **B** lies within the upper calyces of the left kidney. On the right side, two other opacities **C** are seen to lie outside the urinary tract, probably representing calcified lymph nodes in the small bowel mesentery

Special precautions with intravenous urography

Intravenous contrast is potentially nephrotoxic in patients with impaired renal function. Risk factors should be specified to help the radiologist plan the safest investigation. Alternatives such as ultrasound, unenhanced CT or occasionally MR may be considered. Important risk disorders are:

- Diabetes mellitus
- Renal insufficiency (add results of renal function tests to request form)
- Multiple myeloma
- Heart failure

CT urography

Unenhanced CT of the renal tract is increasingly used instead of IVU to diagnose renal or ureteric colic. It is more sensitive for detecting stones and is quicker to perform but usually gives a higher radiation dose. CT with intravenous contrast is frequently used to investigate persistent haematuria when other tests are normal; in some centres, it is used earlier in the diagnostic pathway.

Percutaneous therapeutic techniques

The renal pelvis can be punctured percutaneously with a needle guided by ultrasound or CT scanning. The tract is then dilated to allow tubes of various types and sizes to be inserted. Gaining access to the kidney in this way is known as **percutaneous nephrostomy**. It can be employed to remove stones from the renal pelvis, to urgently but temporarily relieve acute distal urinary obstruction and drain the kidney over a few days ahead of a definitive procedure.

MEDICAL ULTRASOUND

Medical ultrasound developed from sonar used for submarine detection in the Second World War. The technology remained an official secret until the 1960s but since then, the principle has found many applications, from identifying shoals of fish to non-invasive imaging of body organs.

Medical ultrasound was pioneered in obstetrics where it has long been an important part of prenatal assessment. Its use in the body is now protean and there is hardly an organ or system where diagnostic ultrasound does not have a role. **Grey-scale ultrasound** displays a whole range of tissue echogenicities rather than just black and white. Interpreting ultrasound depends on the dynamic picture seen during the examination. The film record may mean little to anyone but the operator.

GENERAL PRINCIPLES OF MEDICAL ULTRASOUND

Ultrasound is non-invasive, painless and safe. An ultrasound probe containing the transducer is applied to the skin over the area of interest and the image of deeper structures displayed on a screen. The probe must be 'coupled' to the skin with jelly to exclude an air interface and is moved in different directions and angles to best display the organs of interest and any abnormalities. 'Spot' films are taken to record the examination.

The piezo-electric transducer both transmits and receives ultrasound, and reflections show as bright spots on a dark screen in real time. This is known as **B-mode** (brightness mode) with the intensity of each spot proportional to reflectivity of tissue interfaces.

The length and breadth of organs or lesions can be accurately determined by electronically measuring the image, and the **volume** of some structures such as the urinary bladder or left ventricle can be estimated. This can give functional information such as the volume of residual urine in chronic retention, or the completeness of left ventricular emptying in cardiac failure.

Bone, stones and other calcified tissues cause an abrupt and marked change in acoustic impedance, giving complete reflection of ultrasound. Thus the surface of hard tissue such as gallstones is revealed by the **acoustic shadow** it casts (see Fig. 20.4, p. 285). A smaller change in acoustic impedance occurs at gas/soft tissue interfaces such as bowel wall and its gas-filled lumen.

Minimal patient preparation is needed. For biliary examinations, the patient should be fasted to minimise bowel gas shadows and reduce gall bladder contraction. For pelvic examination, the bladder should be full of urine. This provides a fluid-filled, non-reflective 'window' for ultrasound to reach the pelvic organs.

Duplex scanning is a technological advance for studying blood flow in which 2D imaging and Doppler shifted ultrasound are employed. A further improvement is **colour duplex** in which the image has false colour added to show the direction and approximate volume of flow, with red indicating one direction and blue the opposite.

Special transducers

Probes have been developed for use via different body orifices, and for body cavities via endoscopic instruments, percutaneous cannulae and laparoscopes. These devices are placed closer to the structures being examined than surface probes. This allows higher-frequency sound to be used which has lower penetration but greater spectral resolution and gives a more detailed display. These transducers are often combined with biopsy devices to enable tissue sampling.

Rectal probes are used for examining the rectal wall and prostate gland in detail and **vaginal probes** for investigating the pelvic organs. **Endoscopic probes** (e.g. transoesophageal) can examine and monitor the heart, upper GI organs and adjacent tissues. **Laparoscopic probes** can be applied directly to viscera to seek the extent of tumour spread or metastases, e.g. pancreas, liver. They provide a more reliable diagnosis of liver metastases than percutaneous ultrasound or cross-sectional imaging.

APPLICATIONS OF ULTRASOUND IN GENERAL SURGERY

Ultrasound has replaced cholecystography for diagnosing gall bladder disease and largely replaces IVU for the urinary tract. In children and in women of child-bearing age, ultrasound should be preferred to other tests where appropriate because it avoids potentially damaging ionising radiation.

Ultrasound is useful for:

- Reliably distinguishing **solid** from **cystic** lesions, e.g. a thyroid cyst from solid nodule, renal or pancreatic cyst from solid tumour
- Assessing palpable **abdominal masses** in the upper abdomen or pelvis
- Detecting **abnormal tissues** in a homogeneous organ, e.g. liver metastases or renal adenocarcinoma
- Detecting **damage to solid organs after trauma**, e.g. splenic or liver rupture
- Detecting **abnormal fluid collections**, e.g. pseudocyst of pancreas, ascites, pleural effusions, abscesses
- Assessing the nature of lesions from the way the **echo texture** contrasts with the normal, e.g. distinguishing liver secondaries from benign lesions or normal liver
- Detecting **movement**, such as pulsation of an aneurysm, contraction of the heart (echo shows valve morphology and movement, ventricular wall movement), and fetal anatomy and movement
- Detecting upper urinary tract **dilatation** (hydronephrosis)
- **Measuring physical dimensions**, e.g. the diameter of an abdominal aortic aneurysm or a dilated bile duct, or the volume of residual urine in the bladder after micturition
- Investigating the **biliary system** for gallstones, thickened gall bladder wall, dilated ducts, masses in the head of the pancreas or porta hepatis
- **Guiding percutaneous interventional procedures** for tissue sampling, e.g. aspiration or biopsy of liver metastases, pancreatic tumours or retroperitoneal masses, or drainage of fluid collections
- Investigating **breast lumps**, e.g. distinguishing cystic from solid lesions, suspected malignant lesions, guided cyst drainage, guiding fine-needle aspiration (FNA) for cytology, or core biopsy

The limitations of diagnostic ultrasound are summarised in Box 5.3.

Doppler-shifted ultrasound

Ultrasound can detect and study blood flow by applying the Doppler principle. Simple hand-held equipment is cheap and portable, and is invaluable in the vascular clinic (see Fig. 5.9). Using a probe coupled to the skin with conduction gel, a beam of ultrasound is directed at an artery or vein. Ultrasound reflects from moving red cells and causes a shift in sound frequency related to blood velocity. Reflected ultrasound is used to generate an audible signal (for detecting blood flow) or is processed to reveal information about the nature of flow. The audio pitch is related to blood **velocity** and provides some qualitative assessment of whether flow is normal or abnormal.

Box 5.3 Limitations of diagnostic ultrasound

- Bone almost completely reflects ultrasound and, as a result, obscures any tissues beyond it. Ultrasound is therefore of little use for examining the brain and spinal cord, although it is valuable in examining the heart (echocardiography) and for fluid collections in the chest; special **transcranial** Doppler probes are used for monitoring during neurosurgery and carotid artery surgery
- Bowel gas partly reflects ultrasound, which may prejudice the examination. Starving the patient and giving laxatives may help
- A thick layer of fat degrades the ultrasound image. Thus ultrasound is less accurate (but still the first choice) for investigating suspected gall bladder disease in obese patients
- Ultrasound is unreliable for showing stones at the lower end of the common bile duct

Main applications of hand-held Doppler ultrasound

- Measuring systolic blood pressure when it is low. This includes brachial pressure in shocked patients or in infants, and ankle systolic pressures in lower limb ischaemia. For this, a sphygmomanometer cuff is placed around the arm or ankle and a flow detector is applied to an artery beyond the cuff (Fig. 5.9)
- Detecting fetal heart rate
- Simple detection of venous blood reflux at the sapheno-femoral or sapheno-popliteal junction in varicose veins, particularly if recurrent

Duplex Doppler ultrasound scanning

Duplex Doppler scanning combines frequency spectral analysis of blood flow using Doppler ultrasound with 2D imaging of the vessel. **Colour flow Doppler** adds false colour to show the direction of blood flow and gives qualitative information about flow volume.

Duplex equipment is still expensive, and the diagnostic process is time-consuming and requires special training. However, it has largely superseded established methods in some areas, for example, replacing venography for deep venous insufficiency and arteriography for carotid artery disease. Blood vessels can be imaged in longitudinal or transverse section to reveal the direction of flow, its velocity (which rises as blood passes through a stenosis), and the presence of abnormal vessel walls or mature thrombus in the lumen.

Cardiac echo investigation (transthoracic echocardiography) employs similar instruments and provides comprehensive information about cardiac structure and function. As with ultrasound generally, images are best viewed as moving pictures. Echocardiography allows the study of pathological anatomy, patterns of blood flow, cardiac wall movement, cardiac output and valve movements. The most common reason for requesting an echo is to study **left ventricular function**, particularly when symptoms suggest heart failure. Echo can determine the severity and the underlying cause of heart

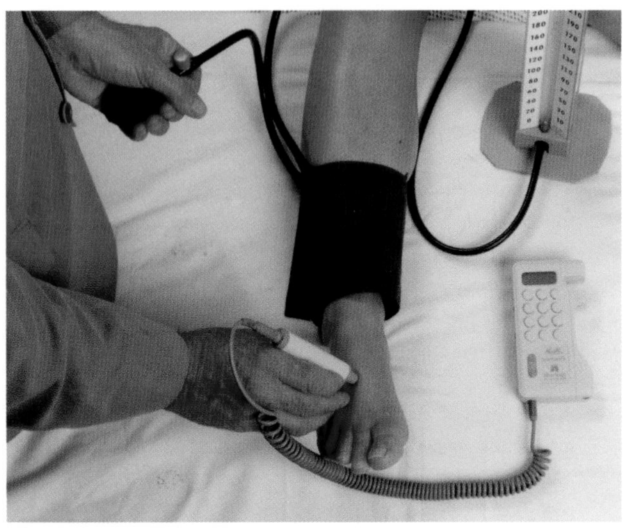

(a)

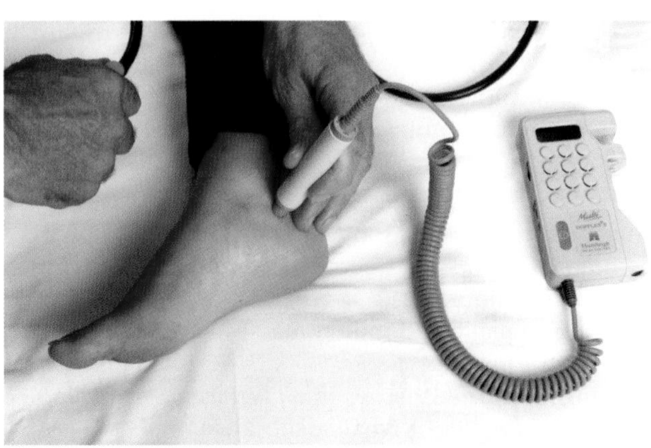

(b)

Fig. 5.9 Measuring ankle systolic pressure using a hand-held Doppler flowmeter (a) A standard sphygmomanometer cuff is placed around the ankle just above the malleoli. Ultrasound conducting gel is applied to the tip of the probe and the probe placed lightly over the likely position of the dorsalis pedis (DP) pulse, between the first two metatarsals. The probe is moved a tiny amount at a time so as to obtain the strongest signal, then the cuff is inflated until the pulse disappears. The cuff is then released gradually and the systolic pressure recorded at the point of return of signal. **(b)** The same process is repeated at the posterior tibial pulse (PT), using the midpoint of a line between the heel and the medial malleolus to find the pulse. Note that accurate measurements require considerable experience, especially when the pressure is low. Headphones are recommended to reduce interference

failure, e.g. ischaemic left ventricular dysfunction, dilated cardiomyopathy, valve dysfunction or right ventricular dysfunction. In addition, ischaemic regional wall movement abnormalities can be identified. These include **hypokinesis** (diminished movement), **akinesis** (absent movement) and **dyskinesis** (passive outward bulging in systole suggesting ventricular aneurysm). The **ejection fraction** (ratio between stroke volume and end-diastolic volume) can easily be assessed.

Echo is the investigation of choice for **valve abnormalities**. It can define the cause of a heart murmur, assess the severity of valvular stenosis or reflux and determine the need for antibiotic prophylaxis in patients with a murmur. In patients with **atrial fibrillation**, echo can detect underlying structural defects and guide the need for anticoagulation or cardioversion. In patients with **systemic embolism**, echo rarely shows intracardiac thrombus but is likely to show any underlying cardiac defect that is the source of embolism such as mitral valve disease or vegetations, left ventricular aneurysm or a patent foramen ovale.

Applications of duplex Doppler

- **Deep vein thrombosis**—this is the method of choice for detecting postoperative DVT. Thrombus more than 24 hours old can be seen and venous flow changes detected. However, the profunda vein and small calf veins are often poorly seen
- **Chronic lower limb deep venous insufficiency**—patency and valvular competence in deep veins (e.g. femoral and popliteal) can be determined dynamically; perforator incompetence can also be detected
- **Varicose veins**—duplex ultrasound is useful for detecting and guiding marking of the short saphenous/popliteal junction before operation and for detecting communications between superficial veins and the sapheno-femoral junction in 'recurrent' long saphenous varicose veins. There are advantages to performing ultrasound in all varicose vein patients before treatment to clarify the diagnosis
- **Carotid artery disease**—duplex has now become the standard test for investigating extracranial vascular disease in preference to carotid angiography (which carries distinct risks). Duplex shows the morphology of diseased arteries and the velocity of flow, allowing the percentage of stenosis to be calculated. The severity of stenosis determines whether operation is required. Duplex is useful for evaluating asymptomatic bruits and following up patients after carotid endarterectomy, including in the early postoperative period
- **Femoro-popliteal bypass grafts**—duplex is used for marking out the saphenous vein graft before surgery and for graft surveillance after surgery to detect remediable vein graft stenoses
- **Aorto-iliac and femoro-popliteal occlusive disease**—duplex is proving valuable for estimating the sites and severity of stenoses and occlusions and replaces arteriography in some circumstances
- **Deeper blood vessels**—these can be imaged for blood flow and obstruction, e.g. superior mesenteric and renal arteries, and renal veins for spread from renal cell carcinoma
- **Cardiac disease**—echocardiography is used for detecting abnormal anatomy and function including heart failure, ventricular dysfunction, valvular abnormalities including stenoses, congenital cardiac defects including septal defects, and intracardiac abnormalities predisposing to embolism

CROSS-SECTIONAL IMAGING

COMPUTERISED TOMOGRAPHY (CT SCANNING)

General principles of CT scanning

Computerised tomography involves X-raying a series of thin transverse 'slices' of the patient's head, body or limbs. A precise fan-shaped beam of X-rays is repeatedly pulsed from successive angles around the circumference of each slice and the transmitted radiation is electronically recorded on the opposite side (see Fig. 5.10).

Since CT was first introduced in the 1970s, the pace of development has been rapid. Modern machines capture images in a continuous spiral around the patient (**spiral CT**), usually as **multislice CT** which enables several slices to be captured simultaneously with each revolution of the X-ray tube. All modern machines now generate at least 64 slices for each turn. The result is rapid image capture of thinner slices at higher resolution. Spiral multislice CT machines can now produce images of both chest and abdomen in less than 1 minute. The data quality also allows images to be accurately reconstructed in three dimensions or in any chosen plane, e.g. sagittal, coronal or oblique, to improve the detection of abnormalities.

Note that the best CT images are obtained in well-nourished patients because some fat lies between the organs, enabling them to be differentiated more precisely than in very thin patients.

Further information can often be gained by performing CT after or during contrast, air or CO_2 enhancement. For example, oral or rectal contrast clearly outlines bowel, whilst intravenous contrast can show blood vessels, kidneys, damage to the blood–brain barrier or areas of absent blood flow in pancreatic necrosis.

CT and MRI are complementary techniques, each having advantages and disadvantages. The decision to use one or

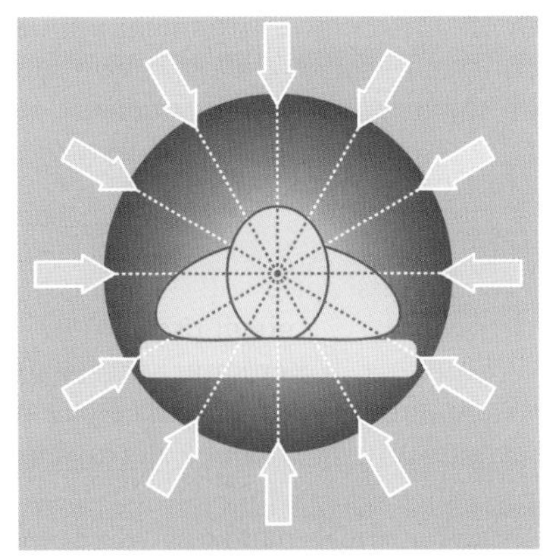

(a)

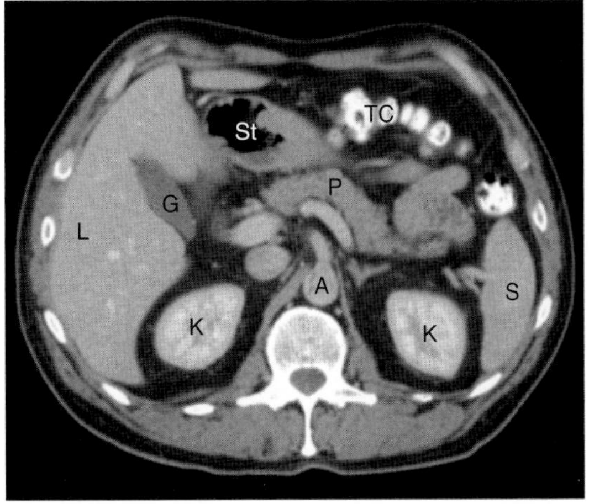

(b)

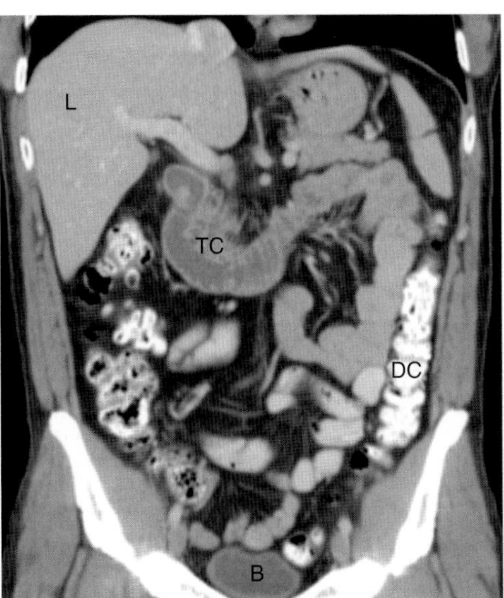

(c)

Fig. 5.10 Computerised tomography
(a) Principle of CT scanning. All images are fed into a computer and a single image of each slice produced. **(b)** Normal transverse CT scan. Liver **L**, gall bladder **G**, stomach **St**, kidneys **K**, aorta **A**, pancreas **P**, spleen **S**. **(c)** Normal CT scan reconstructed in the coronal plane. Liver **L**, bladder **B**, transverse colon **TC**, descending colon **DC**

other depends on patient factors and availability of equipment as well as the suspected disease.

Applications of CT scanning

Pathological anatomy can be studied in great detail and a huge array of information can be obtained non-invasively to assist surgical diagnosis. Often the information is more accurate than could be obtained by exploratory operation. This is outstandingly so in brain injury after trauma where the management of serious head injuries has been transformed by head scanning. The technique enables timely and appropriate surgical intervention and avoids unnecessary exploratory operations.

As CT becomes more available, cheaper and technically better, it is often being used earlier in the diagnostic process, particularly in emergency cases, and for an increasing range of clinical conditions, though it is important to use clinical method and clinical common sense before ordering such tests.

Some indications for CT scanning are:

- Investigating areas difficult to examine by standard radiology or ultrasound. Examples include the retroperitoneal area and pancreas (deep inside the body), the lungs and mediastinum, and the brain and spinal cord (encased in bone)
- Investigating acute abdominal pain—early CT misses fewer serious diagnoses and may reduce mortality and shorten hospital stay (see below)
- Investigating abdominal pathology when ultrasound has proved unsatisfactory or as an alternative to more intrusive investigations such as barium enema for suspected large bowel disorders
- Pretreatment planning and follow-up of malignant tumours being treated with radiotherapy and/or chemotherapy, e.g. for staging lymphomas (replaces laparotomy)
- Planning surgery, e.g. establishing the extent of local invasion of oesophageal carcinoma, identifying the upper level of an aortic aneurysm, investigating the extent of lateral spread in rectal or prostatic cancer, preoperative assessment of intrathoracic tumours including retrosternal thyroid enlargement
- Assessing solid organ damage in abdominal or thoracic trauma
- Guiding needles during biopsy of masses, drainage of fluid collections or obtaining aspiration cytology specimens
- Diagnosis of pulmonary embolism, renal tract calculi and arterial disease. Multislice CT has now also developed to a stage where it can often replace diagnostic coronary arteriography

MAGNETIC RESONANCE IMAGING (MRI)

Principles of magnetic resonance imaging

Magnetic resonance imaging (MRI) was introduced into clinical practice in the early 1980s. MRI involves applying a powerful magnetic field to the body which causes the protons of hydrogen nuclei to become aligned. The protons are then excited by pulses of radio waves transmitted at a frequency that causes them to resonate and emit radio signals; these are recorded electronically. Sophisticated computation then produces images which can be viewed in any plane, transversely, longitudinally or at any obliquity (see Fig. 5.11).

Lipids have particularly high hydrogen content and are clearly seen on MRI. For this reason, the initial applications of MRI were in examining the brain and spinal cord. The technique is increasingly employed for investigating joints such as the knee, shoulder, hip and ankle, and in some cases replaces the need for arthroscopy. Examination times have fallen and good-quality images of chest, abdomen and pelvis can now be obtained. However, MRI is unsuitable for imaging gas-filled organs and dense bone.

Disadvantages of MRI

Some patients are unable to tolerate MRI because of claustrophobia but the main technical drawback is the effect of magnetism on metal. Thus metallic foreign bodies, especially in the eyes, may move in the magnetic field and cause damage. MRI cannot be used with cardiac pacemakers and some metallic implants, and patients being artificially ventilated require machines made of non-ferrous materials. Scanning times are still longer than for CT (though falling) and so MRI is less suitable for young children, the elderly or confused, patients in pain, ventilated patients and emergency patients with active bleeding. The diagnostic applications of MRI continue to expand in parallel with the technical improvements.

Applications of magnetic resonance imaging

General surgical diagnosis

MRI is especially useful for assessing soft tissue tumours, biliary anatomy and pelvic disease. For soft tissue tumours of the extremities, MRI is valuable in planning surgery. It can demonstrate the true extent of the tumour and its relationship to vital structures, so excision margins can be decided before operation.

MRI is useful for imaging the biliary tree as previously discussed. Pelvic MRI is invaluable for assessing the sites and anatomical complexity of **anorectal fistulae** as well as the extent of some **pelvic malignancies**. There is also a role for MRI in **breast cancer**. Contrast enhanced MRI may be shown to have advantages over mammography in distinguishing benign from malignant disease and in assessing multifocal disease. In young women with a strong family history or genetic predisposition to breast cancer, screening needs to begin at an age at which mammography would be unlikely to have sufficient discrimination. MRI may accomplish this screening role without using irradiation.

Blood flow

An exciting development is the ability to demonstrate **blood flow** in the heart and blood vessels, i.e. **magnetic resonance angiography (MRA)**. Blood vessels can be visualised without need for contrast injection and abnormalities detected as in conventional angiography. In addition, volume flow can be calculated in particular vessels. Spatial resolution can be improved by injecting paramagnetic materials such as compounds containing **gadolinium**. MRI is playing an

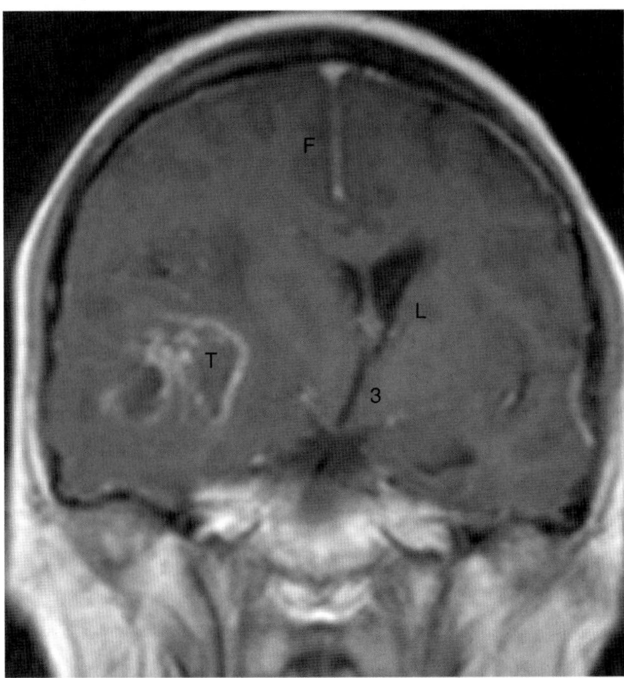

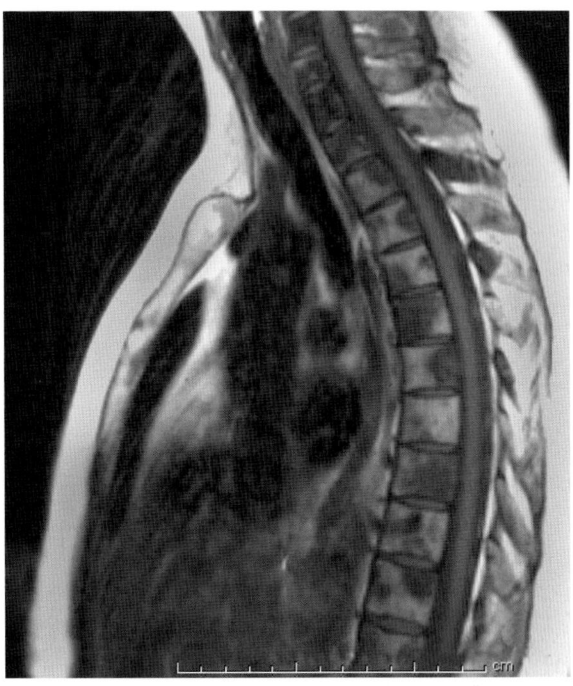

(a) (b)

Fig. 5.11 Magnetic resonance images
(a) Gadolinium enhanced T1-weighted coronal MRI of the brain. Note enhancement of a tumour **T**, midline shift with compression of the right lateral ventricle **L**. The falx **F** and third ventricle **3** are also labelled. **(b)** T1-weighted sequence sagittal MRI of the thoracic spine in a patient with known prostate cancer, back pain and an elevated prostate specific antigen. The image demonstrates bony metastases as dark areas in the vertebral bodies and spines; the white areas are normal fat in the marrow

escalating role in diagnosing cardiac and arterial disease and may in time replace diagnostic coronary angiography.

POSITRON EMISSION TOMOGRAPHY (PET)

PET measures physiological function by looking variously at blood flow, metabolic rates of tissues and the distribution of neurotransmitters and radio-labelled drugs. It depends on detecting radioactivity from the target organ after a small amount of positron-emitting radioactive tracer is injected into a peripheral vein (usually oxygen-15, fluorine-18, carbon-11 or nitrogen-13). PET is usually combined with CT (**PET-CT**) to enable accurate 3D anatomical location of abnormalities discovered.

PET is commonly used to measure the rate of **glucose consumption** in parts of the body. The isotope ^{18}F replaces some of the oxygen in glucose to produce fluorodeoxyglucose (FDG). As this sugar is metabolised, more radioactivity is emitted from more active cells. Cancer cells are often metabolically very active, and this principle enables **FDG-PET** to detect malignancy and differentiate between malignant and benign tissue in many cases. PET can be more sensitive than CT or MRI for detecting cancer. Whole body PET scanning is employed to stage some cancers before attempting curative surgery, e.g. oesophagus and lung, or to distinguish recurrent tumours from radiation necrosis or scar tissue, e.g. following treatment of lymphoma.

Blood flow and oxygen consumption in the **brain** can be examined using PET to help understand strokes and dementias and to track chemical neurotransmitters such as dopamine in Parkinson's disease.

INTERVENTIONAL RADIOLOGY

Many of the conventional X-ray, ultrasound and CT techniques already described have been adapted to guide needles for biopsy, to place drains, to dilate diseased arteries, for example, enabling less invasive therapeutic manoeuvres than formerly. Some techniques have revolutionised treatment and established the interventional radiologist as a front-line clinician, and the field is still growing. Important surgical applications are described in this chapter or in relevant sections elsewhere.

TISSUE SAMPLING

Fine-needle aspiration cytology (FNA) and core biopsy

A fine needle (22 gauge) can be safely passed through most organs or small bowel to aspirate fragments of tissue from a suspicious lesion. Larger-diameter needles can be used for direct core biopsy of masses. The depth and direction of the needle can be accurately guided by ultrasound or CT to ensure a representative sample is taken. For example, pancreatic masses can be reached by transfixing bowel lying in front of the pancreas; this causes remarkably few side-effects. Where practicable, many surgeons and pathologists prefer the larger specimens obtainable with **core biopsy** techniques using special needles such as the **Trucut**, available in various configurations and dimensions.

Minimally invasive applications in breast disease include ultrasound- or mammographically-guided fine-needle aspiration (FNA) or core biopsy of asymptomatic abnormalities detected on mammography, including those found on screening. **Stereotactic apparatus** can be employed to make this process more accurate. Mammographic guidance is also sometimes used to place a hooked wire close to an impalpable abnormality to locate it before surgical excision (**mammographic localisation**).

Guided core biopsy or FNA techniques are also important in the diagnosis of thyroid lumps, for sampling liver nodules and for taking renal biopsies in diffuse renal disease.

DRAINAGE OF ABSCESSES AND FLUID COLLECTIONS

Ultrasound and CT are often used to guide percutaneous drainage of well-defined fluid collections in the abdomen or chest, e.g. pancreatic pseudocysts, or abscesses, e.g. paracolic or subphrenic. Ultrasound or CT can demonstrate the site and the dimensions of the fluid collection and show the least harmful route for drainage. Fluid can be drained via a needle on a once-only basis or else a self-retaining 'pigtail' drain can be placed and drainage allowed to continue. In the first category, a subphrenic or other localised abscess can be drained; in the second, a drain can be placed into a pancreatic pseudocyst or locally to drain a biliary leak after surgery or a gaseous/purulent diverticular perforation. In this way, many major surgical interventions can be avoided.

DILATATION OF GASTROINTESTINAL STRICTURES

Large balloon catheters similar to angioplasty catheters can be used to dilate benign oesophageal strictures caused by oesophagitis. For **achalasia**, balloon dilatation is now a standard technique. Balloon dilatation is sometimes used for benign rectal strictures such as may occur at an anastomosis site, provided they are not caused by recurrent tumour.

Cloth-lined expanding metal stents are now successfully employed, usually after dilatation, for oesophageal, gastric outlet and colonic strictures caused by malignancy. They are usually placed endoscopically, often after contrast radiology. However, stenting is not indicated as a permanent solution for benign conditions.

RADIONUCLIDE SCANNING

PRINCIPLES OF RADIONUCLIDE SCANNING

Radionuclide or isotope scanning is the application of nuclear medicine for diagnosis, by identifying sites of abnormal physiology, e.g. the presence of pus, abnormal phagocytic activity or areas of excessive bone turnover. Isotope scanning, however, gives poor anatomical detail. Suitable tracer agents combine a substance taken up physiologically by the target tissue and a **radioactive label**, usually technetium-99m (^{99m}Tc).

The tracer is concentrated in a specific type of tissue (such as iodine in the thyroid) or else in tissues with similar physiological or pathological activity such as reticulo-endothelial cells or areas of inflammation.

A **gamma camera** consisting of multiple detector units collects and counts the level of radioactivity across the area of interest. This produces a complete image in one exposure (see Fig. 5.12). Several views are taken from different directions (usually anterior, posterior and oblique).

Some pathophysiological functions can be investigated by **dynamic imaging**. For this, detection of isotope continues over a period and the changing level of radioactivity is recorded for later analysis. Examples of this include estimating renal blood flow and studying renal clearance.

APPLICATIONS OF RADIONUCLIDE SCANNING

Lung scanning

Lung scanning was widely used in the diagnosis of pulmonary embolism but is used much less since multislice CT became widely available.

Bone scanning

Phosphate-based agents (phosphates or bisphosphonates) labelled with technetium are usually employed. The tracer is taken up in areas of increased bone deposition and resorption, indicating sites of bone growth and repair (see Fig. 5.13). These include **growth plates, some primary tumours, secondary tumours, foci of bone infection, healing fracture sites, active arthritis** and **Paget's disease**. Bone scanning is highly sensitive but interpretation of the scans requires caution

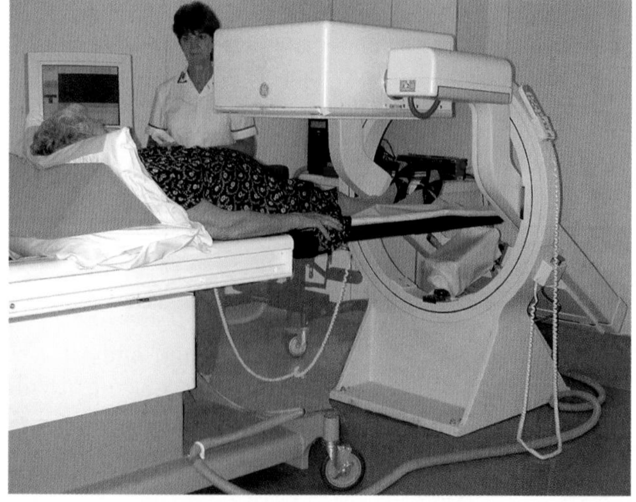

Fig. 5.12 Isotope scanning using a gamma camera
The patient has received an intravenous injection of radiolabelled tracer. The pattern of uptake is imaged by the detector array and transmitted electronically to be displayed on a monitor

because it lacks specificity. They are usually interpreted alongside plain radiographs to improve specificity.

The tracer agent is injected intravenously and becomes distributed throughout all body fluids. The highest concentration collects at sites of osteogenesis about 6 hours later and the patient is then scanned. The tracer is also taken up in areas of **dystrophic calcification** and may sometimes reveal an unsuspected carcinoma of breast, an old myocardial infarction scar or a uterine fibroid.

The main indications for bone scanning are:

- Suspected bone metastases (e.g. staging prostate carcinoma) or investigation of bone pain
- Biochemical abnormalities suggesting bone disease (e.g. hypercalcaemia or raised plasma alkaline phosphatase)
- Suspected occult (stress) fractures of bone
- Suspected osteomyelitis
- Localising abnormalities in unexplained skeletal pain

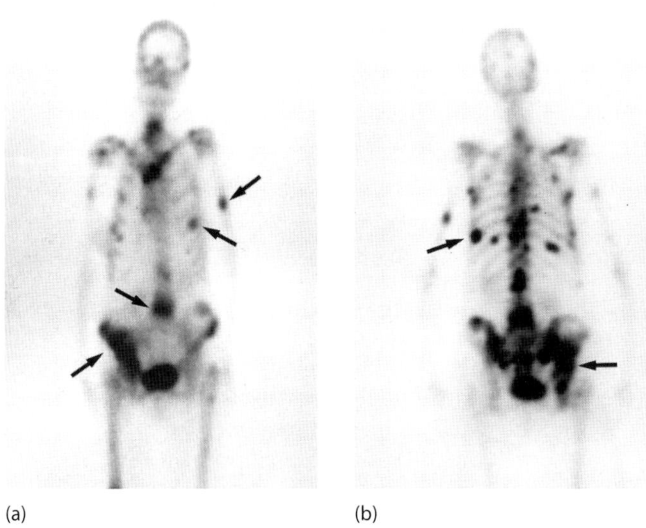

Fig. 5.13 Isotope bone scans
(a) Anterior view of bone scan in a patient with multiple bony metastases (arrowed) from breast cancer. **(b)** Posterior view of bone scan in the same patient

Renal scans

Renal scanning is an important method of investigating the urinary tract. It can obtain information not available from any other source, is quick and simple to perform and allows the function of each kidney to be assessed individually.

There are three main varieties of scan, using different isotopes. DTPA (diethylene tetramine penta-acetic acid) is excreted in the urine like urographic contrast, while DMSA (dimercaptosuccinic acid) and MAG3 remain in cortical tissue. (*Aide-mémoire*: DT 'Pee' A, excreted in urine; D 'Meat' SA, retained in cortical tissue.) Examples are shown in Figure 5.14.

DTPA scanning is used to follow up children with reflux nephropathy. The isotope is instilled into the bladder; the child then voids urine while being scanned and any vesico-ureteric reflux is demonstrated. DTPA is also used to diagnose ureteric obstruction and to distinguish obstructed from merely capacious non-obstructed renal tracts.

When unilateral renal parenchymal disease is being investigated, both DMSA and DTPA can give an estimate of excretory activity. The two agents can be used to estimate differential renal function when investigating renal artery stenosis or the function of a transplanted kidney. DMSA is used specifically to image the renal parenchyma to demonstrate renal scars or tumours.

Scanning for gastrointestinal bleeding

Scanning using the patient's own isotopically **labelled red cells** may be employed to locate a source of continuing or intermittent gastrointestinal bleeding. This is useful where the rate of bleeding is relatively slow or in a patient with recurrent haemorrhage, particularly where a source cannot be identified by endoscopy or arteriography.

The patient's blood is labelled with radioactive technetium and reinjected, then the abdomen is scanned at intervals over the next 24 hours or so for 'hot spots' indicating accumulating gastrointestinal haemorrhage. If the rate of bleeding is more than about 0.1 ml per minute, the scan usually reveals activity concentrated in one part of the bowel. This indicates the general area of haemorrhage and enables the surgical search to be focused, for example on the distal stomach or right side of the colon. Radionuclide scanning can detect blood accumulating over a period, whereas **selective angiography**

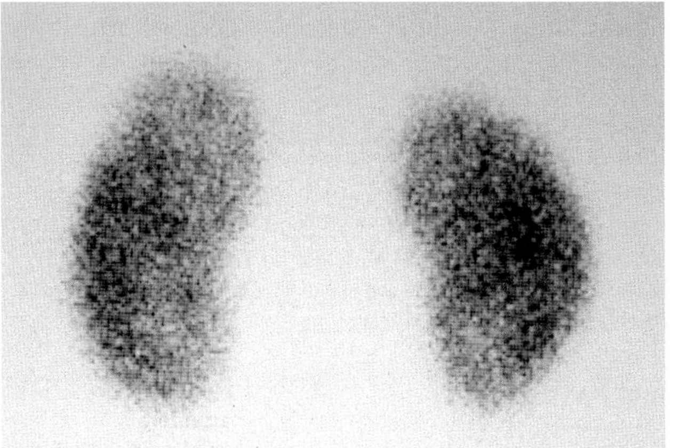

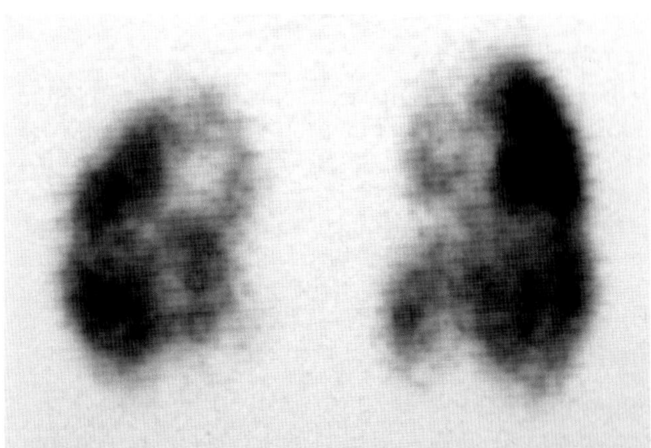

Fig. 5.14 Renal DMSA isotope scans
(a) Normal and **(b)** abnormal showing patchy scarring due to episodes of pyelonephritis. In this case, there had been bilateral reflux of urine in childhood

requires a higher rate of bleeding at the moment of injection; however, it can reveal the site more precisely.

In children, rectal bleeding may be due to bleeding from a Meckel's diverticulum caused by ulceration of ectopic gastric mucosa. A radionuclide compound of technetium concentrated in gastric mucosa may reveal the source.

Leucocyte scanning for inflammation and infection

When an abscess or other infected focus is suspected but cannot be localised, the patient's white blood cells can be labelled with indium-111 or technetium-99m, then reinjected and scanned. Typical indications are patients with a high swinging pyrexia after operation, or with sepsis of unknown origin. The process is expensive but has a high degree of specificity and sensitivity; however, there is a small proportion of false negatives where an occult abscess is not revealed by the scan.

Leucocyte scanning can determine the extent of bowel involvement in inflammatory bowel disease, both ulcerative colitis and Crohn's disease. Tc-hexamethylpropyleneamine oxime (HMPAO)-labelled leucocytes migrate towards areas of inflamed bowel which are then revealed on imaging.

Thyroid scans

Thyroid scanning is described in Chapter 49. Its use is declining in favour of fine-needle aspiration and cytology except in specific disorders of thyroid function.

Cardiovascular imaging

A multiple gated acquisition (MUGA) scan can provide information about ventricular function. This can be useful following myocardial infarction or for patients receiving doxorubicin (Adriamycin) chemotherapy which can damage heart muscle. Radionuclide lymphangiography in chronic lymphoedema can demonstrate the patency and capacity of lower limb lymphatics.

Liver and spleen scans

Hepatobiliary imaging (HIDA scanning)

Technetium-labelled imido-diacetic acid (IDA) derivatives are concentrated by hepatocytes and excreted into bile even in the presence of jaundice. This provides a means of testing the patency of the biliary tree and cystic duct.

Hepatobiliary imaging can be used for:

- Demonstrating cystic duct obstruction in suspected acute cholecystitis
- Demonstrating whether bile ducts are obstructed in jaundiced patients. This is often employed in neonates with jaundice. If there is unequivocal evidence of intestinal excretion of the radiolabel, the patency of the extrahepatic biliary system is confirmed

FLEXIBLE ENDOSCOPY

PRINCIPLES OF FLEXIBLE ENDOSCOPY

Strictly speaking, endoscopy applies to any method of looking into the body through an instrument via an orifice such as nose or mouth, or via an artificially created opening (e.g. laparoscopy, thoracoscopy or arthroscopy). Endoscopy using simple tubular instruments was used for many years and some methods are still in use, e.g. rigid sigmoidoscopy. Developments in fibreoptics first led to improved illumination for rigid endoscopes and later to construction of flexible instruments. These greatly extended the range and sophistication of endoscopic diagnosis and therapy. The unqualified term **endoscopy** now means GI endoscopy using flexible instruments with fibreoptic illumination and video image transmission.

Fibreoptic illumination

Rigid endoscopes and early flexible instruments were illuminated by tiny incandescent bulbs prone to failure. These were superseded by **fibreoptic light guides** in both rigid and flexible endoscopes. Fibreoptic light guides channel light from a powerful, remote fan-cooled light source to the distal end of an endoscope. They are made up of thousands of glass fibres, each with total internal reflection, so very little light is lost and no heat is transmitted. A powerful, cool light beam emerges from the distal end of even the longest endoscope.

Image transmission

The next development crucial to the design of early flexible endoscopes was the invention of **coherent viewing bundles** where the orientation of fibres at the distal end exactly matched the proximal viewing end. Each fibre transmitted a tiny part of the distal scene to the viewing end. The distal end of most endoscopes allowed a viewing angle of over 100°, and lenses gave a remarkable depth of focus. Accurate diagnosis could often be made on inspection alone.

A later development was the charge-coupled device (CCD) **video camera**, a light- and colour-sensitive microchip positioned at the distal end. The image is transmitted to a colour monitor and the system has now replaced the older direct viewing method.

Structure of flexible endoscopes

Most flexible endoscopes include a mechanism to steer the distal end in four directions (except for specialised ultra-slender scopes), a distal imaging chip for video endoscopy, one or two fibreoptic light guides, a suction channel and a channel for inflating the hollow viscus under inspection with air, doubling as a lens washing channel (see Fig. 5.15). The suction channel is also used to pass slender flexible operating tools such as tiny forceps for biopsies, grasping forceps for retrieving foreign bodies, laser guides for therapy (haemostasis or tumour destruction), snares for excision of polyps, diathermy wires, scissors for cutting sutures and needles for injecting haemostatic agents.

APPLICATIONS OF FLEXIBLE ENDOSCOPY

Flexible endoscopes were first used to inspect the stomach in the late 1960s and the range of instruments has progressively expanded since then. There are now instruments available to

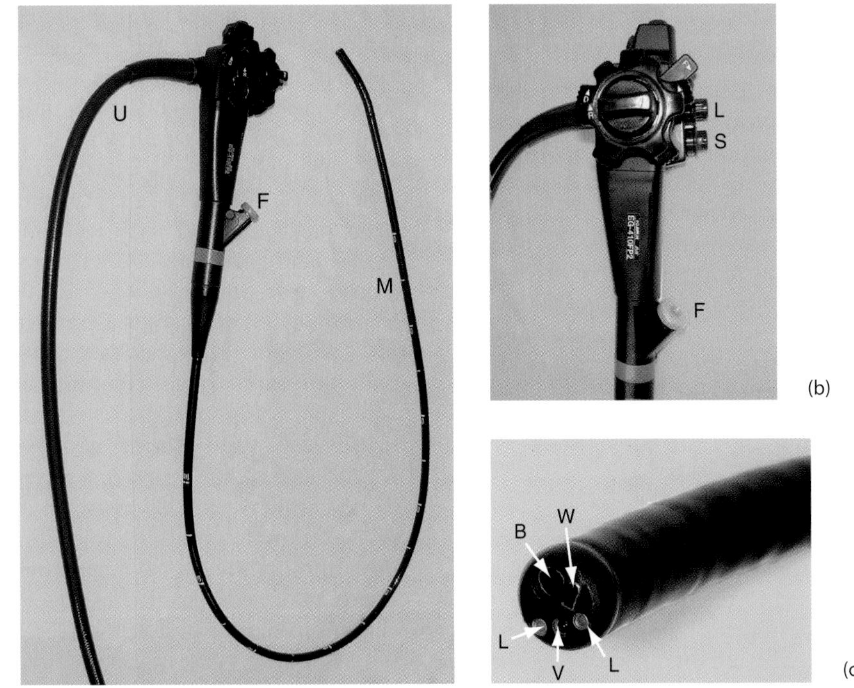

Fig. 5.15 Flexible fibreoptic gastroscope
(a) This end-viewing gastroscope is composed of a flexible main shaft **M** which is 1 m long and marked at 10 cm intervals; the distal 10 cm can be flexed in four directions to steer the instrument in order to advance it and to obtain the best view. There is also an 'umbilical cord' **U** which is plugged into the control box. This carries air to inflate the viscus, water to wash the viewing lens and suction to aspirate fluid from the lumen. There is a flush tube **F**, through which fluid can be injected to wash the stomach wall. The steering controls are better seen in **(b)**. **(b)** The steering controls consist of two concentric wheels labelled respectively **D** and **U** (down and up) and **L** and **R** (left and right). The channel **F** is also used to pass instruments; buttons control suction **S** and air inflation and lens washing **L**. **(c)** shows the tip of the instrument in detail. The two light guides are marked **L**, **V** is the lens for the imaging chip, **W** is the exit for the inflation air and lens washing water and **B** is the channel for passing instruments and for suction. Note that the video image is transmitted up the 'scope and along the umbilical cord to the processor unit, from where it is displayed on a video monitor

inspect and cannulate the duodenal papilla, to examine all or part of the large bowel, to inspect the interior of the bile ducts at operation, to examine bronchi and to examine the bladder interior using only local anaesthesia.

Choledochoscopes are rigid or flexible instruments to inspect the interior of the bile ducts at open or laparoscopic operation to ensure stones are cleared. Their use has improved the rate of clearance during exploration of the common bile duct.

Narrow fibreoptic **bronchoscopes** can be passed under topical anaesthesia. They are used to inspect bronchi for disease and take biopsies and can aspirate mucus plugs responsible for postoperative lobar collapse.

Diagnostic upper gastrointestinal endoscopy

Oesophago-gastro-duodenoscopy, also known as **OGD** or **gastroscopy**, involves inspecting the upper GI mucosa using a steerable, flexible endoscope. It is usually carried out under intravenous sedation and local anaesthetic spray on a day-case basis. Among other applications, gastroscopy enables the whole area prone to peptic ulcer disease and cancer to be directly and comprehensively examined.

Flexible endoscopy has the following advantages over GI contrast radiology:

- Structural abnormalities such as chronic ulcers can be inspected directly whereas radiology provides only a two-dimensional image with little information about surface characteristics
- Benign ulcers and early malignancies are often indistinguishable on radiology whereas at endoscopy, suspicious lesions such as ulcers can be inspected and biopsied
- Shallow mucosal abnormalities invisible on radiology such as superficial ulceration or vascular malformations can be inspected at endoscopy
- Bile reflux through the pylorus may be visible
- Fibrosis and anatomical distortions from previous disease or surgery interfere much less with recognition of what is abnormal on endoscopy than on radiology
- Endoscopy can often identify the exact site of the lesion causing acute upper gastrointestinal haemorrhage and give an indication of the rate of haemorrhage and the likelihood of rebleeding. Tracing the source is often impossible radiologically
- During endoscopy, therapy may be applied during the same procedure, e.g. injection of the source of acute bleeding, retrieving swallowed foreign body, placement of feeding gastrostomy tube

Therapeutic upper gastrointestinal endoscopy

Treatment of upper gastrointestinal haemorrhage

First-line therapy for upper gastrointestinal haemorrhage caused by bleeding ulcers typically involves injection of the ulcer base with adrenaline solution alone or in combination with sclerosants. Other treatments such as laser or direct heat coagulation have proved less effective, but are sometimes used. With these techniques, the need for urgent surgery for bleeding has been substantially reduced. Patients successfully treated for acute haemorrhage from benign lesions can often be managed in the long term without surgery; this subject is discussed in detail in Chapter 19. Haemorrhage due to oesophageal varices is now best treated in most cases by endoscopic band ligation or injection sclerotherapy rather than surgery.

Treatment of oesophageal strictures

Endoscopic methods are often used for dilating benign strictures. The endoscope is passed until the stricture is visible and then a flexible wire is passed through into the stomach. The endoscope is removed, leaving the wire in situ. Plastic or metal dilators of increasing size are then passed over the wire which guides them safely through the stricture until sufficient dilatation is achieved. The technique is relatively safe, can easily be repeated and avoids the need for general anaesthesia. There is a small risk of oesophageal perforation (see Fig. 5.16).

CASE HISTORY

Fig. 5.16 Pneumomediastinum following perforation of an oesophageal tumour during endoscopy

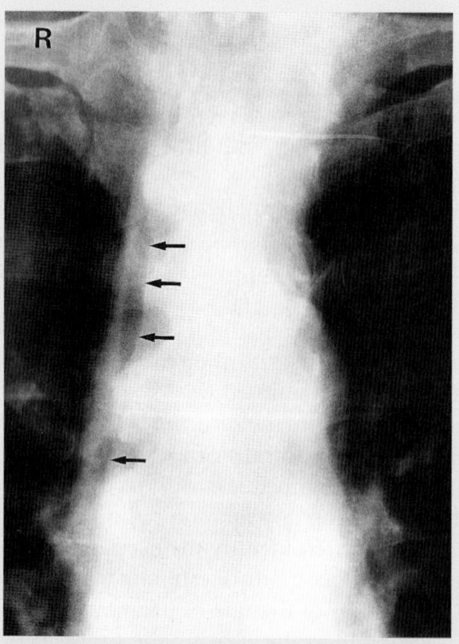

This 56-year-old man who was being investigated for difficulty in swallowing complained of chest pain after the examination. Crepitus was found in the neck due to surgical emphysema resulting from oesophageal air leaking out of the perforation and tracking up the mediastinum into the neck

Dysphagia caused by an inoperable malignant stricture can be improved by creating a pathway through the tumour with endoscopically guided **laser fulguration**. Unfortunately the tumour inevitably recurs and multiple treatments are likely to be necessary, but swallowing can be maintained and the patient's quality of life improved without major surgery. In other cases, a **stent** can be placed endoscopically to keep the oesophagus open. This involves first dilating the stricture, then pushing a collapsed metal expanding stent covered with cloth down until it lies across the stricture. The cover is removed from the stent to deploy it and it expands outwards. This avoids a risky operation and may provide worthwhile palliation for an obstructing tumour.

Diagnostic and therapeutic duodenoscopy

A side-viewing duodenoscope can be used to inspect the duodenal papilla and guide insertion of a cannula or therapeutic tools. Cannulation allows injection of contrast material into the common bile duct and separately into the pancreatic duct. The technique is known as ERCP (**endoscopic retrograde cholangio-pancreatography**) (see Fig. 5.17 and Ch. 11) and is an important part of gastroenterological investigation.

ERCP can be both diagnostic and therapeutic. Indications for diagnostic ERCP may be decreasing as newer and safer techniques such as MRCP (**magnetic resonance cholangio-pancreatography**) become available. Therapeutic ERCP allows many bile duct disorders that would previously have required difficult, time-consuming and dangerous operations to be managed by minimal access techniques, with short hospital stays. For example, bile duct stones can often be removed endoscopically by slitting the sphincter at the lower end (**sphincterotomy**) and retrieving them with a balloon catheter or a Dormia basket. Other therapeutic measures include inserting bile duct stents for palliating malignant biliary obstruction (cancer of pancreatic head, bile duct or duodenum) and for managing postoperative bile leaks.

Enteroscopy

Barium follow-through, CT and MRI have low rates of positive diagnosis in small bowel disorders. Direct small bowel visualisation used to be achieved by 'push' enteroscopy (with a 2 m endoscope that could examine up to a metre beyond the duodeno-jejunal flexure) or by operative enteroscopy via a laparotomy. Later, a technique of double-balloon enteroscopy appeared, with an endoscope passed via the mouth and then coaxed along the small bowel using attached balloons as counter-traction. None of these methods was convenient or reliable.

A newer development for small bowel investigation is **capsule endoscopy**, introduced in 1999. This enables the entire 3–5 metres of small bowel to be visualised with relative ease. The patient swallows a capsule which is propelled through the gastrointestinal tract by peristalsis. An imaging device continually transmits images to sensors on the abdominal wall and the capsule-camera then passes in the stool.

One device, the PillCam SB capsule endoscope, is only 26×11 mm, weighs under 4 g. It contains a battery, light-emitting diodes, an imaging chip camera that captures images at 2 frames a second and a radio transmitter that passes images

Fig. 5.17 Stenting of biliary stricture

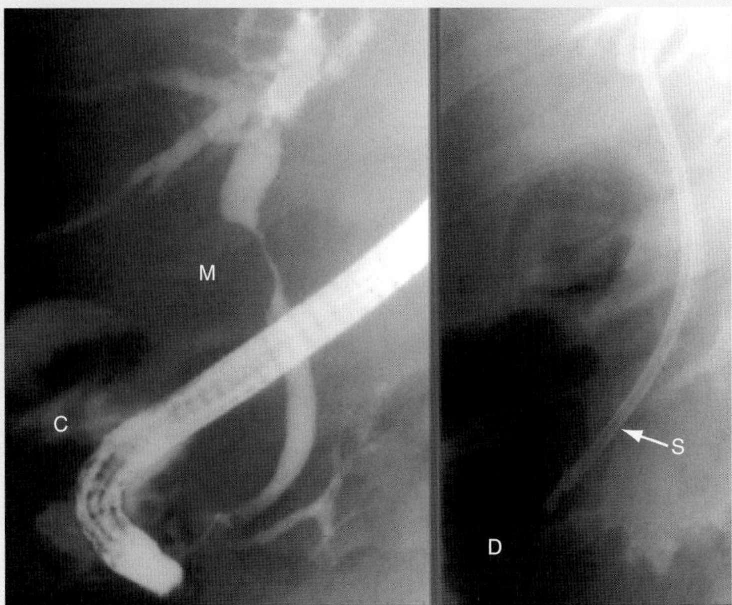

(a) This 54-year-old man developed painless, unremitting obstructive jaundice. This ERCP shows a malignant stricture of the common bile duct **M** due to cholangiocarcinoma. Contrast has been injected to outline the bile ducts and has leaked back into the duodenum **C**. **(b)** A stent **S** was placed endoscopically across the stricture for palliation. The second part of the duodenum is outlined by gas **D**

to a sensor array for up to 8 hours. The camera has an image field of 140°. If obstruction is suspected, a different model with a body made of lactose can be used. This disintegrates in less than 48 hours if arrested.

Capsule endoscopy has a positive diagnosis rate of around 65% compared with around 20% for other methods. In obscure gastrointestinal bleeding, there is a positive diagnostic yield of 45–75% in patients who have already had negative upper and lower GI endoscopy. Typical findings include angiodysplasia, tumours, varices and ulcers. Other indications include suspected small bowel Crohn's disease, particularly in children, assessment of coeliac disease, screening in familial polyposis syndromes and diagnosis of Barrett's oesophagus (by attaching a string). Biopsies cannot yet be taken.

Large bowel endoscopy (colonoscopy)

Flexible endoscopes of different lengths are available for large bowel examination (see Fig. 5.18). The shortest, the **fibreoptic sigmoidoscope**, is about 60 cm long. It is simple to use and allows examination of the rectum, sigmoid colon and descending colon with minimal bowel preparation. Longer colonoscopes enable the entire large bowel to be inspected, and vary in stiffness to assist intubation to the caecum. Other techniques also help reach the caecum, including insufflation with carbon dioxide rather than air, and releasing seed oil from the tip to lubricate the instrument.

Colonoscopy allows inspection of pathological lesions, biopsy of suspicious lesions and resection of lesions such as polyps. Colonoscopy is also employed for surveillance and follow-up of patients treated for colorectal cancer or polyps. New tumours or polyps (metachronous lesions) are looked for and the original site of surgery can be examined. Similar examinations are also used for surveillance of patients with longstanding ulcerative colitis; multiple biopsies are taken to examine for dysplasia, and the entire large bowel is inspected for adenomas or carcinomas. Acutely bleeding angiodysplastic lesions in the large bowel can be treated with diathermy.

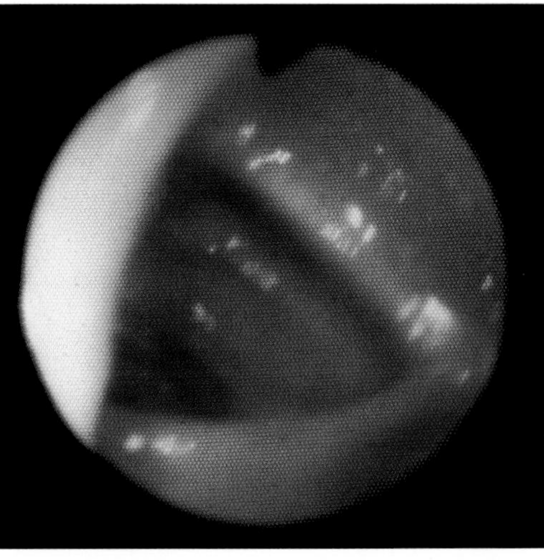

Fig. 5.18 Colonoscopic view of normal transverse colon
When seen colonoscopically, the transverse colon is typically triangular in cross-section; the taenia coli form the apices

Colonoscopy is the most reliable method of screening asymptomatic people for colorectal carcinoma. However, its application is limited by the lack of trained endoscopists, by cost and by lack of patient compliance.

Urological endoscopy

Endoscopic urology is a progressively larger part of urological surgery with flexible instruments used for diagnostic cystoscopy and ureteroscopy.

Cystourethroscopy (cystoscopy) using a rigid instrument is the main diagnostic and therapeutic tool for disease of the urethra, prostate and bladder. Transurethral resection of the prostate has virtually eliminated the need for open retropubic prostatectomy and most early bladder tumours can be treated endoscopically. Laser enucleation of prostatic adenomas is an exciting development. An instrument similar to the cystoscope (but longer), the **ureteroscope**, can now be used to retrieve stones from the lower half of the ureter.

Endoscopic methods of percutaneous stone removal from the renal pelvis have become widely available (**percutaneous nephrolithotomy**). These involve creating a channel from the skin into the renal pelvis and dilating it until an endoscope can be passed. When the stone is seen, various instruments can be used to fragment it and achieve its removal.

Diagnostic and therapeutic laparoscopy

This is covered in Chapter 10.

Screening for adult disease

6

PRINCIPLES OF SCREENING

INTRODUCTION

Medical screening is a public health activity that involves examining or testing asymptomatic, apparently healthy people to detect disease at an early stage. Measures can then be taken to prevent the disease (if there is a precursor stage), treat it early (hoping for improved cure rates), or at least offer treatment to delay advanced disease. For example, colonic screening can detect adenomas and carcinomas; removing adenomas prevents the well-recognised adenoma–carcinoma sequence, and actual cancers detected are often earlier and at a more curable stage. Unfortunately, for cancers without an easily detected early precursor stage such as breast or prostate, beneficial outcomes are elusive.

Screening can detect disorders that predispose to other diseases, for example, hypertension or elevated cholesterol levels, to discover people at increased risk of atherosclerotic heart disease and stroke. Screening is also useful for infection control, e.g. preoperative screening of patients from residential homes for meticillin-resistant *Staphylococcus aureus* (MRSA) carrier status to enable elimination therapy before operation.

An entire population can be screened (**mass screening**) but more usually it is **targeted** at at-risk groups. Selection might be by age, gender or cardiovascular risk factors, for example (Box 6.1). **Opportunistic screening** involves a more random approach, such as screening patients who happen to attend a particular clinic.

ASSESSING THE POTENTIAL BENEFITS OF SCREENING

Many subscribe to the simplistic view that screening must be 'a good thing'. These include the lay public, people associated with distressing diseases, populist politicians and people with vested financial interests. Poorly conceived screening, however, may consume massive resources to identify just a few new cases with little clinical benefit, e.g. CT scanning for lung cancer. Worse still, early diagnosis of a condition where early intervention brings no advantage may cause suffering. These people can be prematurely placed into an anxiety-provoking sick role and given unrealistic expectations. They may also be subjected to unnecessary treatments with potentially severe side-effects, e.g. some breast or prostate cancers that might never progress to invasive disease.

As with any public health measure, medical and social benefits accruing from any screening programme need to be rigorously evaluated and the process separated entirely from the incentive to screen for profit. Whole-body scanning by CT or MRI is currently strongly marketed on the basis that a scan will show unsuspected abnormalities and allow early treatment. Abnormalities are bound to be discovered by such extensive screening, but it is difficult to reliably determine which signify serious disease and which (if any) should be treated. Doctors should not perform unvalidated screening tests any more than they should use unproven drugs, and should resist patient pressure for inappropriate screening.

Premature introduction of screening

Politicians can play a part in initiating inappropriate screening programmes. UK prime minister, Margaret Thatcher sanctioned nationwide breast screening in 1988, 2 weeks before a general election; some believe this was to garner the women's vote. The decision was premature and based on insufficiently validated evidence from the Swedish two counties study and the UK Forrest report. In the 1970s, screening for cancer of the uterine cervix was widely introduced, also before its efficacy had been fully evaluated. Fortunately, it has proved successful despite the difficulty of engaging women at high risk. Sadly, the natural history of untreated dysplastic cervical cellular abnormalities was not properly established before the impact of widespread screening made this ethically impossible. This severely hampered scientific study of the disease, its early diagnosis and best treatment.

Box 6.1 Disorders potentially suitable for adult screening*

Infections

- Tuberculosis
- MRSA

Malignancy and premalignancy

- Cervix; colorectal (current programmes show benefit)
- Breast (doubtful overall benefit)
- Prostate; bronchus (no proven benefit)
- Oesophagus (beneficial in parts of China with a high incidence)
- Stomach (beneficial in Japan with a high incidence)

Cardiovascular disease

- Hypertension (beneficial in preventing future cardiovascular events)
- Cholesterol (beneficial in preventing future cardiovascular events)
- Abdominal aortic aneurysm (proven benefit)
- Ischaemic heart disease; carotid atherosclerosis; peripheral arterial disease (no proven benefit but lifestyle changes likely to bring benefit in subjects with disease detected)

Metabolic disease

- Diabetes (beneficial in population screening and opportunistic screening)
- Retinopathy in diabetes (screening programmes not fully operational but promising evidence of benefit)
- Thalassaemia—successful national premarital screening programme for 3 million couples has reduced the expected birth rate of affected infants by 70%

*This list is not exhaustive and does not include genetic screening or conditions with special risk factors

Box 6.2 World Health Organization guidelines for assessing when screening is appropriate (Wilson and Jungner 1968*)

1. The condition being screened for should be an important health problem
2. The natural history should be well understood
3. There should be a detectable early stage
4. Treatment at an early stage should be of greater benefit than at a later stage
5. There should be a suitable test for the early stage
6. The test should be acceptable
7. Intervals for repeating the test should be determined
8. There should be adequate health service provision for the extra clinical workload resulting from the screening
9. The risks should be less than the benefits
10. The costs should be balanced against the benefits

*Wilson JMG, Jungner G. Principles and practice of screening for disease. Geneva: WHO; 1968.

Criteria for assessing a screening programme

Many years ago the World Health Organization (WHO) realised that even beneficial screening could be expensive, unpleasant, inaccurate and unproductive, and could adversely affect psychological or physical well-being. In 1968, they published a list of criteria for effective screening programmes (Box 6.2) including attributes of the disease, the test and the treatment. These principles are still relevant today and have been added to by the UK National Screening Committee and other groups. Box 6.3 shows a summary of these modified criteria.

Box 6.3 Summary of attributes of a good screening programme

The disease

- Important health problem
- Detectable truly early stage
- Predictable biological behaviour
- Long period between first detectable stages and overt disease

The diagnostic test

- Valid (sensitive and specific)
- Simple and cheap
- Safe and acceptable
- Reliable and reproducible

Diagnosis and treatment

- Effective, acceptable and safe treatment available
- Evidence of better outcomes if treated early
- Benefits of screening must outweigh risks
- Treatment facilities must be adequate
- Screening overall must be cost effective
- Screening must be sustainable

Evolution of screening programmes

Once begun, any screening programme must remain under constant evaluation and modified or discontinued when criteria are no longer being met. For example, in the 1950s and 1960s, screening for pulmonary tuberculosis (TB) by mass miniature chest X-ray was highly successful but it was disbanded in the 1970s when new cases fell below a level at which the unit cost per new case could be justified; interestingly, by then, the yield of new cases of lung cancer from screening began to exceed that of TB, but there was virtually no effective treatment for it at the time.

CRITERIA FOR AN EFFECTIVE SCREENING PROGRAMME

In order to initiate a new national screening programme, certain criteria must be fulfilled. There must be a perceived need in the medical community or in the wider public. Pilot studies are then carried out. If outcomes are promising, large scale **prospective randomised controlled trials (RCTs)** need to be performed, seeking robust evidence for implementation. This is critical because it is politically difficult to stop a screening programme, even when evidence shows little benefit, e.g. breast screening (Nordic Cochrane Collaboration 2001 and 2006).

The disease

The screened condition should be an important health problem either because it is common (such as lung or prostate cancer) or has serious but preventable consequences such as carotid artery disease or abdominal aortic aneurysm (AAA). The **prevalence** (proportion of cases already in a population) and the **incidence** (the proportion of new cases) of the disease in the population at risk are discovered from pilot studies. There should be a truly early stage where treatment outcomes are better than at a late stage. Colorectal adenomas and early cancers are good examples.

The biological behaviour or natural history of the disease should be well understood, including how latent disease progresses to clinical disease, and the disease course should be reasonably predictable. For example, AAAs are known to expand smoothly for the most part and rarely rupture until they are large. The risks of untreated disease also need to be understood and there should be a long period between the first detectable stages and overt disease.

The diagnostic test

The test must be valid, i.e. reliable in detecting the disease. This is defined by **sensitivity** and **specificity**. Sensitivity is the capability of the test to identify affected individuals in the screened population, i.e. the proportion of people who have the disease and are detected. A test with many false negative results is insensitive and unreliable. A UK appeal court ruled that sensitivity is paramount in (cervical) screening and awarded damages to women with missed diagnoses at screening. Specificity is the degree to which a positive test can be relied upon to prove the disease is present; in other words, the higher the false positive rate, the lower the specificity.

The test must be simple and cheap and it must identify the disease by a reliable, validated and reproducible method. The distribution of test values should be understood well enough to define normality or relative risk associated with particular stages, e.g. for an AAA, the diameter with a high risk of rupture. Intervals for repeating the test should be worked out for normal subjects and for those with positive results near the threshold.

The complete screening programme must be clinically safe and acceptable socially and ethically to health professionals and the public. This includes the test and any diagnostic procedures, treatments or interventions screening initiates. For example, if a test is perceived as unpleasant, e.g. colonoscopy, uptake is low and the benefits are proportionately smaller.

The overall benefits should be greater than the risks; this includes any physical and psychological harm caused by the test, diagnostic procedures and treatment.

Diagnosis and treatment

Cases identified by the test must be amenable to effective, acceptable and safe diagnostic procedures and the potential benefits of medical or surgical intervention prompted by earlier diagnosis need to be understood.

There should be clear evidence from high-quality randomised controlled trials (RCTs) that early treatment produces better outcomes than treatment at later stages, i.e. 'cure' should be more likely, survival longer, or earlier treatment easier. Treatment should have minimal side-effects. There also needs to be agreement in advance about who should be offered treatment and its nature; this evidence may emerge from RCTs.

The overall benefits of screening must outweigh the risks. This includes any physical and psychological harm caused by the test, the diagnostic procedures and the treatment. Treatment facilities must be adequate with the capacity to deal with the extra workload from screening.

Screening overall must be cost effective compared with other health care interventions and needs. Costs include the testing, further diagnostics and treatment, administration, staff training and quality assurance. For example, because of its high unit cost, CT screening is unlikely to ever be implemented unless proved extremely effective in early diagnosis of a common, highly remediable life-threatening condition. In a world of competing public health measures, debate continues about what is an acceptable cost per life year saved: £100—£5000—£35 000?

Any screening programme must be sustainable in terms of management, monitoring and quality standards. High-quality, realistic, unbiased information needs to be offered to potential participants about the consequences of testing, investigation and treatment to help them decide whether to go ahead. This is currently a subject of debate regarding breast screening in the UK.

Ideally, any primary prevention interventions for the disease should be implemented before or in parallel with the screening programme.

Limitations of screening

Screening is conceptually and ethically different from usual clinical practice as the process is aimed at the whole population, and achieved by dealing with apparently healthy individuals. Participants expect the diagnosis of the presence or absence of disease will be accurate, and that if disease is found, the outcome will be favourable. However, there is no guarantee of protection because there will always be false positive and negative results, however good the test. Also, the disease may appear or progress unexpectedly rapidly between screenings. This emphasises the importance of good population education and properly informed consent for individuals engaging in the programme. Participating in screening must be a free choice and it may or may not have health benefits and significant adverse effects.

Bias

A number of phenomena can lead to mistaken claims for efficacy of a screening programme:

Lead time bias—screening relies on the principle that a serious or fatal disease can be diagnosed at an early stage, and that doing so will definitively improve morbidity and mortality. However, if it does not alter the disease course, earlier diagnosis gives the statistical illusion of prolonged survival. It also makes affected patients acutely aware of the presence of their disease for longer.

Selection bias occurs if the more health conscious people, often at lower risk of the disease, undergo screening.

Length bias occurs when screening detects less aggressive variants than those the screening programme was set up to discover. Length bias is frequently cited in the context of breast cancer screening.

Participation rates

Universal participation is not usually necessary to achieve measurable community benefit and cost effectiveness. This is because community benefit is the sum of individual benefits (except for infectious diseases such as tuberculosis). If a validated screening programme has low set-up costs, benefits are usually proportional to costs. For colorectal cancer screening, for example, cost effectiveness falls off only at extremely low levels of participation.

Other aspects of screening

Cost effectiveness

Imponderables such as the economic value of saving a life or extending survival need to be considered. All screening studies cost money in detecting and treating cases. The cost effectiveness of a screening programme is usually reported as **cost per life year saved** or the cost of increasing **'quality adjusted life years' (QALYs)**. The acceptable cost per life-year saved is a matter for debate; somewhere between £12 000 and £30 000 is often quoted as acceptable in developed countries.

Research benefits

Screening a population can teach the clinical community and the public much about the natural history and progression of a disease, its aetiology and its various associations, for example the link between abdominal aortic aneurysm and smoking. Different investigations and treatments can be trialled in large groups of affected individuals, to the ultimate benefit of the population at large.

Consent

Organisers are obliged to provide participants with reliable and unbiased information about the benefits and risks of any screening process and its consequences. There must not be any form of coercion to participate. Much current information tends to overemphasise the benefits of screening and minimises the risks, often not indicating that participation is voluntary. Breast cancer screening in the UK has been criticised in this respect.

SCREENING FOR CANCER

EARLY DETECTION OF CANCER

As a principle, the earlier in its natural history that malignancy is diagnosed and treated, the better the prognosis. The ideal would be to detect cancer before invasion or metastasis had occurred, i.e. during the pre-invasive stage. However, many cancers invade and spread before they reach a detectable size or produce tumour markers. Where true early detection is possible, health education can alert the public to early symptoms and warning signs. In skin and testicular tumours, this should include regular self-examination. Self-examination is still promoted for breast cancer but large trials have shown it to be ineffective and that it causes harm with more biopsies.

The common cancer killers are shown in Table 6.1, with bronchus still leading the field. Unfortunately, this disease does not fit criteria for screening, having no detectable early stage; attempts at screening have been uniformly ineffective.

In women, breast cancer is a huge public health problem, followed by carcinoma of the cervix and ovary. In men, prostate cancer is a large and growing problem. Colorectal cancer is common and evenly matched in frequency in both sexes in the UK; 30 000 new cases are detected each year and 16 000 die of it. Gastric and pancreatic cancers are also big killers but screening is of little value except in areas of exceptionally high incidence. In China, high-risk areas for oesophageal cancer

Table 6.1 Most frequent deaths from cancer, UK 2010*

Cancer site	Female	Male
Lung	15 500	19 400
Genital (ovary + uterus in female; prostate + urinary tract in male)	6230	16 500
Breast	11 550	80
Colorectal (inc. anus)	7300	8700
Oesophagus	2500	5100
Pancreas	4030	3900
Stomach	1860	3100
Leukaemia and non-Hodgkin's lymphoma	4050	4900
Other sites*	21 829	20 893

*Note that in males, three cancers—lung, prostate and bowel—account for just under half of all cancer deaths; in females, three cancers—lung, breast and bowel—also account for nearly half of all cancer deaths. Note also a large proportion of deaths occur where the primary has not been identified

have been identified and brush cytology without gastroscopy has proved beneficial.

Several genetic predispositions to cancer have been identified, e.g. polyposis coli for colorectal cancer and *BRCA1* and *BRCA2* for breast and other cancers. Genetic screening is not covered in this chapter but individual disorders are described in other chapters.

CERVICAL CANCER

Poorly organised screening trials using cervical smears and Papanicolaou staining began in the UK in the mid-1960s and national screening started in 1988. Nearly all reports show early detection and treatment prevents 80–90% of invasive cervical cancers and has greatly reduced cervical cancer mortality. The International Agency for Research on Cancer (IARC) indicated that yearly screening between the ages of 25 and 64 reduces invasive cancer by 94%, 3-yearly screening reduces it by 91%, 5-yearly by 84%, and 10-yearly by 64%. These figures are the basis for the present UK policy—that yearly screening is unnecessarily frequent and 3- or 5-yearly screening is best.

In the UK, 4 million women are screened annually and 82% of the 14 million eligible women have been screened over the previous 5 years. The programme costs £150 million a year, amounting to £37.50 per screen. Both the number of invasive cancer cases and deaths from it halved between 1988 and 2005, taking the disease from sixth most common cancer in women to 13th.

British data show that about a quarter of all cervical cancers occur in each of the four age groups 25–39, 40–54, 55–69 and 70+ years but there are problems with recruiting young women and women from lower socio-economic strata. Both groups have been shown to be at higher risk. In a study from Hawaii in 2003, only 1 in 12 eligible women had not been screened in the preceding 5 years, but this small group accounted for two-thirds of the invasive cancers in the community. Thus there are real concerns that those at greatest risk are not being tested. In addition, those with positive results may not be treated effectively. Recent recommendations in the UK are that women should first be invited for screening at age 25. They should then be screened 3-yearly until 49 and 5-yearly from 50 to 64. Women of 65+ only need screening if they have not been screened since age 50 or a recent abnormality has been found.

A recent cost effectiveness study from Peru, India, Kenya, Thailand and South Africa indicates that a single screen (and treatment if necessary), employing testing for human papillomavirus (HPV) in cervical cells or visual inspection of the cervix after swabbing with acetic acid rather than a cervical smear is a cheap and effective way to reduce a woman's lifetime risk by 25–36%. Types 16 and 18 HPV cause most cervical cancer worldwide and effective vaccines are now available. Two rounds of screening at 35 and 40 years could reduce lifetime risk by a further 40%. If screening were introduced across the developing world then the global incidence of cervical cancer could fall by about 50%. Ideally, all young women should be vaccinated against HPV with modern effective quadrivalent vaccines; this would virtually eliminate cervical cancer and the need for screening.

OVARIAN CANCER

Ovarian cancer screening is not yet reliable enough for general use, but a study of 200 000 women aged 50–74 were screened with transvaginal ultrasound (US) alone or with blood testing for the tumour marker CA125. Sensitivity for US+CA125 was 89% and specificity was 99.8%, both better than US alone. Only 84 cancers were detected overall in preliminary screening and 13 interval cancers were detected in the ensuing year.

BREAST CANCER

Mammographic screening for breast cancer was introduced nationally in the UK in the late 1980s following the Forrest report of 1986. Most developed countries followed suit after results from the HIP study of New York, the Swedish two-county study and the Canadian National Breast Screening Study. These appeared to demonstrate a 30% reduction in mortality from breast cancer in screened women. In the Swedish study, there was also a significant 13% reduction in all-cause mortality.

Mammographic screening detects breast cancers of smaller size than those presenting clinically, with around 30% either carcinoma in situ or invasive cancers less than 0.5 cm in diameter. A high proportion are node negative—only about 20% have axillary spread compared with 40% for symptomatic cancer. By detecting small lesions, screening substantially increases the reported incidence of invasive breast cancer. This might be expected to mean fewer new cases in later years, as prevalent cases would disappear from the population. In Norway and Sweden this has proved untrue, suggesting that screening is not detecting most of the clinically important cases that progress to become invasive or metastasise.

In any population of women with breast cancer, lesions will be at different stages of development and pathological potential. These may be grouped as follows:

- **Biologically early cancers**—these include lesions too small to be detectable but with metastatic potential
- **Small cancers and carcinoma in situ**—these predominantly non-aggressive lesions may never metastasise
- **Large or advanced tumours**—these are usually symptomatic and quickly fatal

Large trials have concluded that as many as one-third of cancers detected by screening would never have presented clinically.

The sensitivity of screening for clinically significant cancers is poor; in particular, lobular or mucinous cancers and some rapidly proliferating, high-grade tumours may not be detectable. This is illustrated by the high proportion of **interval cancers** presenting clinically between screening visits. In one representative series, 38% of all breast cancers presented as interval cancers. These tended to occur in younger patients with dense breasts and with a higher usage of hormone replacement therapy (HRT) or the oral contraceptive pill. A study in New South Wales estimated that screening overdiagnosed invasive cancer by 30–42% in women aged 50–69 and other studies have confirmed this. A Dutch study showed that false positives adversely affect quality of life for at least a year.

On the basis of tumour doubling times, breast cancers detected clinically have been present for an average of 8 years, whereas mammographically detected lesions have been present for about 6 years—a long period in which to metastasise. This may explain the failure of screening to increase the cure rate for clinically significant cancers, and also calls into question the political pressure for patients with suspected breast cancers to be evaluated within a very short time.

Effectiveness of mammographic screening

Mammographic screening every 2 years has been estimated to avert only 2 deaths in 1000 women aged between 50 and 59 over a period of 10 years. To achieve this requires 5000 screens and 242 recalls, and for 64 women to have at least one biopsy. Five women will have ductal carcinoma in situ detected, some of which may never progress to invasive cancer. Less than 1% of women invited for screening will benefit; a much larger percentage have to endure false alarms, unnecessary surgery and inappropriate labels of cancer.

In the USA, the independent Health Services/Technology Assessment Texts (HSTAT) reviewed published clinical trials and concluded that 'in absolute terms, the mortality benefit shown with mammography screening was small enough that biases in the trials could erase or create the observed mortality reduction'.

The Cochrane view of breast screening

The Cochrane Collaboration is an international non-profit organisation that rigorously and dispassionately reviews published research evidence and provides up-to-date information about the effects of health care. Over 11 000 articles have been published in 20 years on breast screening. The Nordic Cochrane Centre reviewed all RCTs in 2001 and found that astonishingly few were of sufficient rigour to reliably determine whether screening reduced morbidity and mortality. Only seven RCTs were identified, of which only two were of sufficiently high quality. Evidence from the adequately randomised Canadian and Malmö trials showed screening had no significant effect. The other five trials, in which randomisation was inadequate, found that screening decreased the risk of death by about 25% but showed a slight **increase** in risk for screened women for death from any cause. A further Cochrane review was published in 2006, which reanalysed data from published trials. Both reviews found little benefit from breast screening and in 2006 they stated that the absolute risk reduction for breast cancer from screening was only 0.05%. They also found that screening led to substantial over-diagnosis and over-treatment. They concluded: 'the currently available reliable evidence does not show a survival benefit of mass screening for breast cancer, and the evidence is inconclusive for breast cancer mortality.' These controversial conclusions imply that breast screening does no good, causes actual harm and probably should be abandoned. This, however, is unlikely to happen.

Why breast screening is claimed to improve survival

Several factors could explain how screening could appear to reduce mortality, as follows:

- Lead time bias with over-detection of clinically insignificant lesions increases the apparent number of breast cancers. These cases do well
- Mortality from breast cancer can occur over a very long period; 35 years after treatment, the commonest cause of death in a Cambridge UK series was still breast cancer. Thus screening studies need to be prolonged
- Improvements in breast cancer treatment took place over the period of the main trials. Tamoxifen and perhaps improved chemotherapy undoubtedly extended absolute survival between the early and late 1980s. Over a similar period, other cancer rates fell for largely unknown reasons: thyroid cancer fell by 12%, testis by 17% and melanoma by 23%
- Subjectivity, unrealistic optimism and perhaps vested interests may lead to misleading presentation of statistics and unsustainable claims for the industry of breast screening

Other benefits from breast screening

Experience gained from breast screening and managing patients detected has brought rapid improvements in mammographic equipment, techniques and interpretation as well as a more sensitive approach to patients. It has generated much scientific study of the management of early breast cancer. All of this will eventually bring benefits for women with breast cancer and for people with other types of cancer.

For the future, there is interest in using magnetic resonance imaging (MRI) for screening, particularly among high-risk women, as MRI detects more cancers than mammography and is better able to discriminate between cancer and a scar.

COLORECTAL CANCER

Colorectal cancer is a major health hazard that kills 16 000 people a year in the UK; only about 10% are diagnosed early. Early cancers have survival rates of better than 90% but the all-stage 5-year survival rate of 35% has hardly improved despite treatment advances, because most cases present late. Nine out of 10 cases occur in people over 50.

Screening for colonic cancer has a good chance of being effective. It fulfils many criteria required for a screening programme. In particular there is a clear sequence of adenoma progressing to adenocarcinoma. Also, early cancers are detectable and progress steadily to advanced cancers. About 75% arise sporadically, most likely in pre-existing adenomas. Thus a window of opportunity exists for detecting adenomatous polyps at a premalignant stage or cancers at an early invasive stage (i.e. pathologically less advanced than those with symptoms), where they are potentially curable. The transition phase from benign to malignant is long, shown by the cumulative risk of cancer in polyps 10 mm or larger being only 8% at 10 years.

However, detection methods are the stumbling block. Screening by symptoms alone is very unreliable. The **sensitivity** of guiac faecal occult blood (FOB) testing is no better than 50% and the **specificity** is also low. A new quantitative FOB test, faecal immunological testing (FIT) is much more sensitive and specific and is likely to replace the guiac test. With

2-yearly FOB testing alone, there are many **interval cancers**: 30–60% of cancers and as many as 80% of polyps are missed after three rounds of testing. Sensitivity and interval cancer rates can be improved by adding flexible sigmoidoscopy. A randomised multicentre once-only trial of flexible sigmoidoscopy in 100 000 people found it reduced the rate of colorectal cancer by 33% and deaths from it by 43%. Rectosigmoid cancers were reduced by 50% (Lancet 2010; 375; 1624–1633) but right-sided cancers are not detected. Unfortunately, both faecal occult blood (FOB) testing and flexible endoscopy are distasteful and patient participation is low. Better forms of screening would undoubtedly improve participation.

Despite the drawbacks of FOB testing, meta-analysis of four RCTs has shown that FOB screening can reduce mortality from colorectal cancer by 16% for those allocated to screening and by 23% of those actually screened. On this basis, a 2-yearly FOB screen offered to 10 000 people aged over 40 with two-thirds attending for at least one test would prevent 8.5 deaths (CI: 3.6–13.5) from colorectal cancer over 10 years, a mortality reduction of 23% (RR 0.77, CI: 0.57–0.89); 2800 participants would have a colonoscopy and there would be 3.4 major complications from this, i.e. perforation or haemorrhage (Cochrane). The cost of screening was £5290 per cancer detected and an estimated £1584 per life year gained.

Reports of pilot screening studies suggest screening could improve mortality by 33%, and national screening with FOB testing every 2 years has been approved for implementation in the UK. This started in April 2006 for men and women aged 60–69 (50–74 in Scotland). In addition, large-scale pilots of endoscopic colorectal screening are being trialled in patients in their late 50s.

PROSTATE CANCER

Prostate cancer is the most common cause of cancer deaths in older men and 84% of deaths are in men over 70. Unfortunately, the prospects for prevention remain poor. The problem is not so much in detecting the disease but in avoiding false positives, detecting it early enough and predicting its clinical course. Many cancers remain forever dormant, as shown by post-mortem studies in men who have died of something else: foci of prostate cancer occur in 70% of 70-year-olds, 60% of 60-year-olds and 50% of 50-year-olds. These patients died *with* the disease rather than from it and offering radical treatment for them is clearly inappropriate. Serum prostate specific antigen (PSA) levels increase with the volume of tumour, so high levels indicate extensive disease. In one study the age-specific median concentration was 40 μg/L in men who died within 3 years, 6 in men who died in 3–6 years and 4 in those who died between 6 and 10 years. In another study, using a cut-off level of 10 μg/L, the false positive rate was 4% (similar to breast screening) but 15/16 men with prostate cancer had extra-prostatic disease. Using the common cut-off of 4, false positive rate was 18% and 22/33 had extra-prostatic disease. Thus PSA is a good test only for cancers that cause death within 3 years; after that the common cut-off of 4 detects only half of those that would cause death or serious morbidity. Unfortunately, histological grade only partly predicts clinical outcome.

In the USA, uncontrolled screening using PSA has spawned an apparent epidemic of prostate cancer. The chairman of the UK National Screening Committee stated that 'the scientific evidence is that screening for prostate cancer does not reduce mortality, and causes actual harm by exposing people to a procedure which has side effects of incontinence and impotence and where there is no evidence that they will benefit'.

The UK government sponsored a Health Technology Assessment on prostate screening in 1997, which stated that the criteria for a population screening programme had not been met. Their findings were that:

- The epidemiology and natural history of the disease were ill understood
- Screening tests were inaccurate and staging was unreliable
- There was poor evidence of the effectiveness of treatment
- Little research had been conducted into the complications and quality of life after radical treatment
- On present evidence, there was no justification for PSA testing in primary care and there was insufficient evidence to support national screening
- PSA testing should be limited to symptomatic men, to monitoring prostate cancer treatment and to randomised trials investigating screening

Overall, PSA screening causes harm. Some men receive unnecessary treatment because the cancer is incurable or because it would never have presented clinically, and those treated risk infection (from biopsies), incontinence and impotence.

LUNG CANCER

A Cochrane review of all randomised controlled trials showed that no screening test had an impact on the treatment or deaths from lung cancer, despite early stage cancers being detected and resected (most likely because these would not have progressed). Tests examined include chest X-ray, sputum tests and CT scanning.

SCREENING FOR CARDIOVASCULAR DISEASE

HYPERTENSION

Hypertension is an important cause of myocardial infarction and stroke. Lowering elevated blood pressure substantially lowers the risk. However, blood pressure on its own has proved a poor screening tool; in one large study, the 10% with the highest blood pressures suffered only 21% of the ischaemic cardiac events and only 28% of the ischaemic strokes. Even after adding other risk factors, including low-density lipoprotein (LDL) cholesterol, diabetes and smoking history, the top 5% had only 28% of the deaths from myocardial infarction. Advancing age or a previous cardiovascular event are probably the best predictors of future cardiovascular events, thus all patients with risk factors should receive best advice and appropriate treatment.

ABDOMINAL AORTIC ANEURYSM

INTRODUCTION

Ruptured abdominal aortic aneurysm (AAA) causes at least 6000 deaths each year in the UK and 1.4% of all deaths in men over 65. The peak mortality is between 65 and 85 years and the risk of rupture is roughly proportional to the diameter; when this reaches 6 cm, the risk rises sharply. A ruptured aortic aneurysm is nearly always an acute emergency and carries a very high mortality. About half the cases never reach hospital and die at home or in transit to hospital. Half of the remainder (25%) die without an operation and half undergoing operation die. Thus the true mortality rate is 85–90%. An emergency operation requires a trained vascular surgeon, ties up an emergency team for 3 or more hours, requires an intensive care bed for 3 or more days, uses large quantities of bank blood, and costs 25% more than an elective procedure, whether or not the patient survives. Detecting aneurysms before rupture means that less risky elective interventions, with a mortality of 5% or less, can be employed.

APPROPRIATENESS OF SCREENING FOR AAA

By WHO criteria, AAA is a near ideal candidate for screening. It is an important health problem, the natural history regarding expansion and rupture is fairly well understood, there is an easily detectable early stage, and treatment at an early stage is more beneficial than at a later stage (i.e. ruptured). Ultrasound is a suitable and highly reliable test for the early stage and it is acceptable, with an average of 80% of those invited attending. Appropriate intervals for retesting have been determined by randomised trials. There is adequate health service provision for the extra workload: a screening programme generates approximately 6 extra aneurysm repairs per year per surgeon.

Several trials have shown that the risks are less than the benefits, with up to 75% reduction in rupture rate, a low elective operative mortality, no excess psychological morbidity in those screened, and survival after operation being little different from an unaffected population. Costs appear to be balanced against benefits, with trials estimating the cost per life year saved at between zero (Huntingdon and Danish studies) and £12 500 (2006 figures from the UK Multicentre Aneurysm Screening Study).

TRIALS OF AAA SCREENING

Several large studies have published data, with a remarkable concordance between results. The prevalence of AAA, the age distribution, attendance rates, reduction in AAA mortality and the cost effectiveness calculations from studies in Chichester, Gloucester, Huntingdon, Denmark, Western Australia and the large UK Multicentre Aneurysm Screening Study all concur.

Only one study, from Chichester, has randomised women into screening. The prevalence of AAA was six times lower (1.3%) than in men (7.6%). Over 5- and 10-year follow-up intervals, the incidence of rupture was the same in the screened and the control groups. Screening women for AAA was considered to be neither clinically indicated nor economically viable.

The Danish study

A Danish study randomised 12 500 men of 65 and over to AAA screen or nothing. Of these, 75% attended and 4% had aneurysms. Screening reduced the rate of emergency surgery by 75% (CI: 51–91%); 59 were operated on electively with a 5.1% mortality. As regards cost effectiveness, 352 needed to be screened to save one life, 4 years after screening. The screened population was rescreened after 5 years: 30% of those with aortas 25–29 mm developed an aneurysm but none of those originally less than 25 mm did so. People

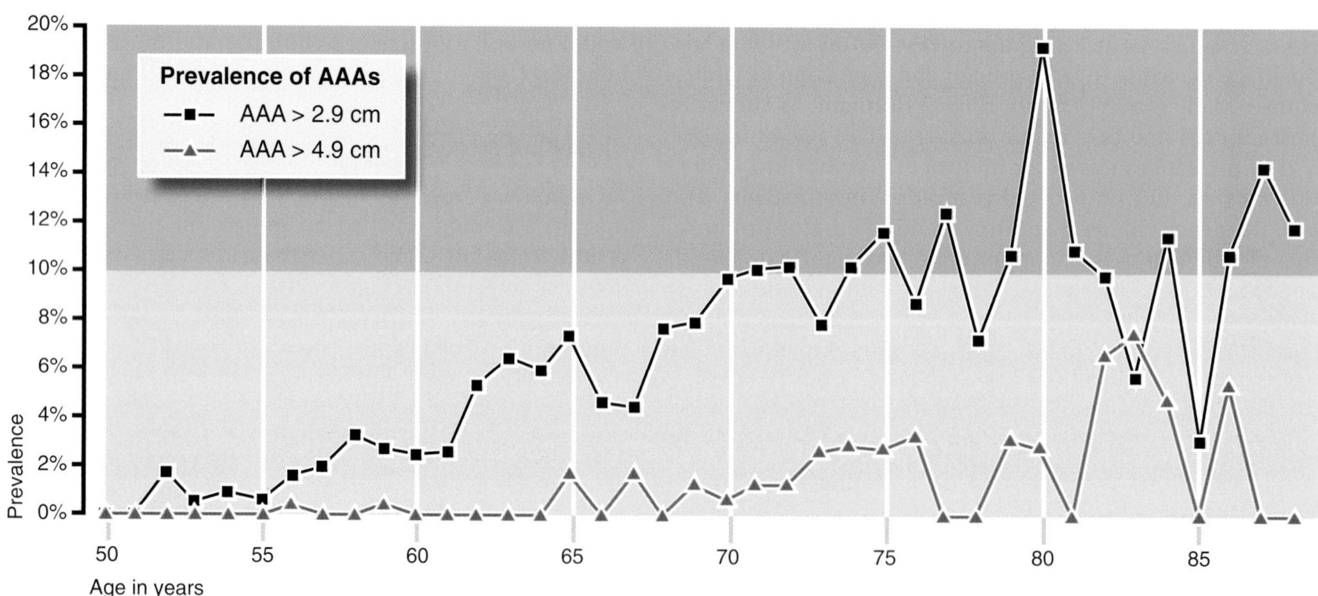

Fig. 6.1 Prevalence of AAA in men over 50 in the Huntingdon Screening Programme
The graphs show the percentage of those screened found to have small aneurysms (black line) and large aneurysms (green line). Note that the lines are approximately parallel, suggesting that small AAAs become large AAAs some years later

with aortas of 25 mm or more diameter need periodic rescreening.

The Huntingdon study

In the Huntingdon study, 15 000 men of 50 and over were screened over 7 years: 540 were found to have an AAA larger than 2.9 cm, and 69 an AAA larger than 4.9 cm (Fig. 6.1). Very few small and no large aneurysms were found under the age of 60, an important factor when planning screening. Over the age of 70, there was virtually a 10% incidence of small AAAs. In this study, AAA mortality also fell by 75% and the number needed to be invited to save one life was 600.

The UK MASS study

Screening was undertaken in four centres and 68 000 people were randomised to screening or not, beginning in 1997. Some 98% of people in both groups were matched with national mortality statistics. After 7 years, 21% of men had died. There was a 76% attendance among those invited (27 147 were screened) and 4.9% had an aortic diameter of 3 cm or greater. All-cause mortality fell by 4% in those invited and there was a 47% risk reduction for AAA deaths in this group. The cost of screening and treating detected aneurysms was £12 500 per life year saved and no adverse effects were found on quality of life. The 30-day mortality for elective cases was 6%; for emergency cases operated upon, mortality was 37%. It was calculated that if screening were offered to a population, only 6% of AAA workload would eventually be on ruptures compared with around 30%. After 10 years, the relative risk-reduction of aneurysm-related deaths was still 49% (CI: 37–57%), the cost per man invited was £100 and the cost per life year gained was £7600. Thus the benefit of a single screen lasted at least 10 years, though the incidence of rupture rose after 8 years.

THE CONSEQUENCES OF SCREENING FOR AAA IN AN AREA

There is a rise in elective AAA surgery during the first 5–7 years, as the existing but undiagnosed cases are progressively detected. This is gradually offset by a fall in rupture rates and a reduction in surgical referrals of symptomatic and incidentally discovered aneurysms. This becomes apparent 4 years after screening starts and continues rising until the entire population has been screened. The cost per life year saved compares favourably with colonic and cervical cancer.

Perioperative care

Preoperative assessment

7

INTRODUCTION

When a patient is admitted for surgical investigation or treatment, a detailed history and examination (**clerking**) should be done and recorded. These patient notes are essential to make information available to other clinicians and also form a permanent record for medico-legal purposes if things go wrong. Notes must be accurate and legible, entries dated and signed, and the doctor's name identifiable.

For *elective treatment*, clerking is often performed at a **pre-assessment visit** by a junior doctor or a surgical or anaesthetic assistant. This is to anticipate potential medical and social complications, and take preventive action (Box 7.1). In patients with significant co-morbidity, a senior anaesthetist (anaesthesiologist) should also make an assessment. This is often performed in specialised clinics, which increasingly have direct access to advanced assessment tools such as cardiopulmonary exercise testing and pulmonary function analysis.

For *emergency admissions*, review is often a layered process, with junior doctors performing initial assessment and then reporting to seniors. The prime purpose is to diagnose the primary disorder, but co-morbidity and complicating factors are also sought. For *major trauma*, senior staff are usually mobilised by phone before the ambulance arrives.

PRINCIPLES OF PREOPERATIVE ASSESSMENT

The essence is careful questioning and examining to foresee anaesthetic and surgical problems, plus any social aspects relevant to the admission. Most surgical cases are uncomplicated but preventable disasters occur unless the approach is systematic. The patient's condition may need optimising, taking the urgency of surgery into account. The assessor aims to answer the questions in Box 7.1. The review may disclose the need for tests or other actions and also identifies patients with medical co-morbidity who have risks of particular perioperative problems. Current treatment of co-morbidity (e.g. diabetes, hypertension) also needs review. Investigations provide baseline information against which later changes can be measured, e.g. echocardiography in heart failure. Common problems of high-risk groups are summarised in Table 7.1.

ESSENTIALS OF PREOPERATIVE ASSESSMENT

Standard preoperative procedures vary in different hospitals but basic steps ensure the greatest patient safety (see Box 7.2). The nature and urgency of the operation and the state of the patient determine what is needed.

EXPLANATIONS TO THE PATIENT AND INFORMED CONSENT

(see Ch. 1 for the legal framework, for further detail and special cases)

In order to make informed choices, patients need to understand the nature of their condition and the range of treatments available, with attendant risks and benefits. Patients often absorb little of what is said initially because most have little understanding of how their body works and what can go wrong. They are often anxious and overwhelmed by the clinic visit and so cannot comprehend the full implications.

For **elective operations**, consent should be in two stages: first an initial explanation and the range of options discussed well in advance, without pressure of an imminent operation. Information leaflets and guidance about accurate internet sites should also be given. Second, before operation, the patient's understanding is checked and consent confirmed. The doctor should adopt a sympathetic and unhurried approach and often needs to explain things more than once. Informed consent also requires an account of potential complications. Generally, complications should be discussed if there is a 5% or greater risk, or if there are rarer but serious procedure-specific risks such as recurrent laryngeal nerve injury in thyroid surgery.

For **emergency surgery**, there may not be time to go through this process, nor may it be clear what might be found at operation, but explanations by the surgeon or a surgeon

Box 7.1 Preoperative assessment and planning

1. Diagnosis
- (Provisional) diagnosis; how confident is it?
- Are any further investigations needed to confirm the primary diagnosis?
- Important aspects of the history?
- Findings on examination?
- Results of investigations already performed?
- If appropriate, have tissue diagnoses been obtained before admission to hospital?

2. Operation
- What operation or procedure is planned?
- Have any circumstances changed relating to the planned operation?
- Has the patient got better or worse?
- Has any new diagnostic information appeared? (e.g. pulmonary metastases on a chest X-ray)
- Is the planned operation still appropriate?
- Any special risks attending this particular operation, intraoperative or postoperative? (e.g. risk of DVT after pelvic surgery)
- Any standard procedures needing to be performed for this operation? (e.g. ordering blood if heavy blood loss anticipated)
- Any operation-specific actions needing to be performed? (e.g. examining vocal cord movement before thyroid surgery, arranging perioperative radiology)

3. Anaesthesia
- What type of anaesthesia is to be employed?
- Can any anaesthetic complications be anticipated? (e.g. risk of postoperative chest infection after thoracotomy or upper abdominal surgery, risk of a patient with bowel obstruction inhaling vomitus during anaesthetic induction)

4. Fitness for operation
- Any intercurrent diseases and are they being appropriately treated, e.g. insulin-dependent diabetes, or any that might pose special problems? e.g. rheumatoid arthritis with cervical spine involvement
- Are any preoperative investigations or treatments needed for intercurrent disease? (e.g. lung function tests and physiotherapy for chronic bronchitis, cervical spine radiology for rheumatoid arthritis)
- Does the surgical condition pose special problems? (e.g. fluid or electrolyte disturbances from vomiting)
- Is the patient taking any drugs which might cause problems with anaesthesia or operation? (e.g. monoamine oxidase inhibitors or corticosteroids)
- Is the patient fit for the planned anaesthetic and operation?

5. High risk
- Is this patient particularly predisposed to anaesthetic or surgical complications (Table 7.1)?

6. After the operation
- Can any special problems be anticipated during the postoperative period and after discharge? (e.g. elderly patients living alone)
- Any problems specific to this anaesthetic or operation regarding recovery and rehabilitation, and is any special planning required? (e.g. prostheses after mastectomy, stoma care, limb fitting and rehabilitation following amputation)

Table 7.1 High-risk groups for perioperative complications

Group	Particular risks	Management
Premature or tiny babies, neonates and infants	Fluid and electrolyte loss Heat loss in operating theatre	Careful measurement and replacement of fluids and electrolytes Warming blanket, temperature monitoring
Patients over 60	Cardiovascular disease	Chest X-ray and ECG preoperatively if indicated by guidelines, and monitoring during operation
Very elderly patients	Confusion Hyponatraemia Immobility	Multifactorial—see Chapter 8 Preoperative electrolyte estimations and correction Good nursing and rehabilitation
Smokers	Postoperative chest infection and atelectasis Increased risk of myocardial infarction	Stop smoking before operation—ideally at least 4 weeks beforehand Preoperative chest X-ray Preoperative and postoperative physiotherapy Preoperative ECG; avoid hypoxia during and after operation; postoperative oxygen therapy
Obese patients	Increased risk of DVT Increased risk of wound infection Reduced mobility	DVT prophylaxis—see Chapter 12 Preoperative counselling during consent process Early mobilisation with assistance Encourage patients to lose weight prior to surgery
Patients with intercurrent medical disease	Depends on medical condition	Early referral to anaesthetist and/or medical specialist

Box 7.2 Essential steps in preoperative assessment and preparation

- History taking
- Physical examination
- Collating pre-admission information about diagnosis
- Arranging any further diagnostic investigations
- Making special preparations for the particular operation
- Investigating any intercurrent or occult illness suggested by medical clerking or enlisting appropriate specialist help
- Discussing the operation and the recovery period with the patient and obtaining signed consent
- Marking the operation site
- Making arrangements with operating theatre staff
- Arranging and informing the anaesthetist
- Prescribing medication, prophylactic antibiotics and thromboembolism prophylaxis, as appropriate
- Planning rehabilitation and convalescence

capable of performing the operation should be given as far as possible, and if necessary include close relatives. Patients trust doctors for the most part and seek their guidance on what should be done. The doctor can be unambiguous about best treatment for many conditions but should be prepared to discuss alternatives, even if it means referral to another specialist. Patients tend to be attracted to treatments perceived as modern, often involving 'keyhole surgery' or lasers, but a balanced view must be presented, with the doctor understanding the risks and benefits of each procedure.

PLANNING THE RECOVERY PERIOD

If the immediate postoperative period is likely to be unpleasant or unfamiliar, such as admission to an intensive care unit, it is prudent to forewarn the patient and arrange a visit beforehand. Patients with learning difficulties and some elderly people have difficulty in adapting to changing circumstances and care should be taken to familiarise them with facilities and staff.

Plans for rehabilitation and convalescence should be discussed with the patient and relatives including the likely rate of recovery and levels of activity possible on discharge, allowing social, business and domestic arrangements to be made early. If necessary, domestic or home nursing help can be arranged. Uncertainty about these matters often causes anxiety and prolongs recovery.

MARKING THE OPERATION SITE

When obtaining final consent, the surgeon should **mark the operation site** on the patient's skin with an indelible pen. This is particularly important if the operation could be performed on either side of the body, for example an inguinal hernia repair or limb amputation. It is even more important if the patient is likely to be turned prone (face down) in theatre as this causes confusion, and failure to mark the site represents a disaster in waiting (and there is no legal defence). This marking procedure also allows the patient to agree which operation is to be done and on which side. Checking processes for identity, type of operation, side and marking should be in place at several stages during the patient's journey to the operating theatre and many units have introduced the World Health Organization checklist (see Ch. 1, Box 1.8). Of course, the surgeon needs to be entirely clear what is to be done on the anaesthetised patient presented to him or her!

IMMEDIATE PREOPERATIVE STARVATION AND FLUID RESTRICTION

Any patient about to undergo general anaesthesia needs an empty stomach to minimise the risk of aspirating gastric contents into the lung on induction of anaesthesia or during early recovery, but efforts should be made to reduce the 'nil-by-mouth' period. Patients can usually eat until 6 hours before operation and clear oral fluids should be allowed until 2 hours before surgery. **Carbohydrate loading** reduces anxiety, improves hydration, reduces insulin resistance and inflammatory responses and improves surgical outcomes. Specially formulated oral fluids containing complex carbohydrates with low osmolality empty rapidly from the stomach and can be given 12 hours before surgery, and up to 2 hours before going to the operating theatre (provided gastric emptying is not impaired). In patients at special risk of inhalation, e.g. gastro-oesophageal reflux, intestinal obstruction, the anaesthetist may prescribe acid suppressing and prokinetic drugs. In day surgery patients, starvation and hydration need to be checked carefully.

LIAISON WITH ANAESTHETIST

For elective cases, the anaesthetist should be informed in advance of the proposed operation or list of operations. For emergency cases, the anaesthetist needs to know which patient is having which operation, how urgent the procedure is, and the condition of the patient and the state of resuscitation. The anaesthetist visits the patient to anticipate problems, discuss the anaesthetic and prescribe premedication. The anaesthetist is responsible for the patient's fitness for operation and often assists in resuscitation.

OPERATING THEATRE ARRANGEMENTS

For any operation, the junior surgeon (intern) is usually responsible for informing the operating department about the operation(s) and any special arrangements needed. A formal **operating list** should be prepared, giving name, age, sex, ward, and proposed operation for each patient. The side of the body to be operated on should be clearly (and correctly!) noted. Any special instruments, intraoperative radiography or patient positioning must be listed. The presence of meticillin-resistant *Staphylococcus aureus* (MRSA) infection or a carrier state should be recorded, as well as any important allergies, e.g. to latex or iodine. In some hospitals, the amount of bank blood ordered for a patient is also noted. If changes are made, a complete new list should replace the old to avoid confusion.

PLANNING THE ORDER OF AN OPERATING LIST

For elective cases, the following order can normally be recommended:

1. **Latex allergy**—the theatre needs to have all latex containing products removed and be 'purged', i.e. pressure ventilated, for several hours beforehand

2. **Paediatric cases**—to minimise the period of starvation and to reduce anxiety
3. **Diabetic patients**—to make perioperative diabetes management as smooth as possible, minimise the period of starvation and return rapidly to normal diet and treatment
4. **Adult day cases**—to maximise the amount of available recovery time before discharge
5. **Inpatients** with no special theatre requirements
6. **Contaminated, infected cases, colorectal cases, gangrenous limbs**—so as not to infect later cases on the list
7. **Patients with transmissible infections**, e.g. MRSA, blood-borne viral infections requiring barrier nursing—non-essential equipment and personnel are removed from theatre; disposable items replace recyclable items of linen, and theatre can be cleaned before next list

PREPARATION FOR MAJOR OPERATION

The following example illustrates the way a patient might be prepared for a major operation and the considerations in preoperative management. This account is typical of what would be recorded in the hospital notes.

HISTORY

James Brown, a 70-year-old retired farmer, with a proven carcinoma at the rectosigmoid junction admitted electively for anterior resection of the rectum.

Presenting complaint

Seen urgently in outpatient clinic 3 weeks ago with a 5-week history of loose stools three to five times a day, without blood or mucus. GP reported three stool specimens positive for occult blood. Lost about 4 kg over the last 3 months, but has been trying to lose weight anyway.

Results of outpatient investigations

- Flexible sigmoidoscopy—obvious fungating tumour of upper rectum. Scope could not be passed beyond it. Biopsies confirmed adenocarcinoma
- Contrast enhanced CT scan of abdomen and pelvis—no other synchronous colonic cancers seen; liver free of metastases
- Chest X-ray—normal, no metastases
- Transrectal ultrasound for local staging—no spread outside bowel wall
- Blood tests: full blood count—haemoglobin 11.6 g/L, otherwise normal. Urea and electrolytes, liver function tests—normal

Systems enquiry

Generally well, but recent onset of shortness of breath after walking 200 metres on flat ground; occasional fast palpitations. No other cardiorespiratory symptoms. Poor stream on micturition. Nil else on systems enquiry.

Past medical history

Appendicectomy aged 14; no anaesthetic complications. Serious farming injury to left elbow aged 20. Jaundiced during the Second World War in Asia, nil since. Hypertensive for 10 years and on drug treatment for 5 years. Diabetes discovered 3 years ago on routine urine testing, controlled by diet alone.

Table 7.2 Example of preoperative assessment of a patient admitted for a major operation (see text, *Preparation for major operation*)

Problem	Surgical significance	Plan of action for each problem
1. 'Mild' diabetes mellitus	No such thing as mild diabetes! Is it under good control?	All urine samples to be tested for glucose Fasting blood glucose estimation and HbA1c May need sliding scale insulin perioperatively
2. Obesity	Multiple potential problems Lifting and handling on the ward and in the operating theatre May make access difficult at operation Predisposes to wound infection Increased risk of deep vein thrombosis or pulmonary embolism	Early referral to anaesthetist Is special bed or operating table required? Availability of hoist postoperatively Ensure adequate theatre time available plus at least two assistants Consider delayed primary closure of wound if contaminated Prophylaxis, e.g. low dose heparin plus graduated compression stockings
3. Hypertension	How well is hypertension controlled on present medication? Is elevated BP on admission just due to anxiety? Are there other complications of hypertension such as ventricular hypertrophy or dilatation?	Monitor blood pressure 4-hourly on admission and then decide about drug therapy Check pulse rate and BP at intervals over several hours Perform (and check) ECG and chest X-ray. Echocardiography if indicated

Table 7.2 **Continued**

Problem	Surgical significance	Plan of action for each problem
4. Recent shortness of breath on exertion and palpitations	Are these merely symptoms of anxiety or significant cardiac or respiratory disease?	Consult cardiologist re palpitations ECG and chest X-ray Possibly lung function tests Recheck Hb—has anaemia worsened?
5. Poor urinary stream and enlarged prostate	Possible carcinoma of prostate Possible difficulty with catheterization required at operation Risk of postoperative urinary retention when catheter removed	Measure plasma PSA Transrectal ultrasound; biopsy if necessary Anticipate—may need suprapubic catheterisation kit in theatre Anticipate
6. Jaundice in the past	History suggestive of hepatitis	Serological tests needed if hepatitis B or C is likely
7. Smoker	Possible occult lung cancer Possible impaired lung function Increased risk of postoperative chest infections Increased risk of myocardial infarction	Chest X-ray Respiratory function tests Preoperative physiotherapy and breathing exercises Postoperative oxygen therapy
8. Left elbow injury	May cause inconvenience during operation	Inform theatre staff about need for careful positioning on the operating table
9. Diuretic therapy	Are electrolytes and renal function normal?	Plasma urea, electrolytes and creatinine estimations
10. Aspirin therapy	Could gastric irritation partly account for mild anaemia? May cause excess bleeding at operation	Use non gastric irritant analgesics Anticipate—stop 10–14 days before surgery if practicable
11. Possible penicillin allergy	A penicillin often used for prophylaxis or treatment of infections	Record possible penicillin allergy; alternative drugs may have to be used
12. Cardiac murmur	Is this clinically significant? Is cardiac antibiotic prophylaxis necessary?	Consult anaesthetist or cardiologist; consider echocardiogram Consult guidelines, e.g. BNF
13. Lives alone, looks after animals	Who will look after him when he returns home? Who will look after animals while he is in hospital?	Discuss domestic arrangements and convalescence plans with medical social worker
14. Low haemoglobin	Not low enough to need preoperative transfusion but there is less reserve for the operation Potentially extensive operation—may have large blood loss	Order at least two units of blood to cover operation Order extra blood, i.e. at least 4 units in all
15. May need temporary or even permanent colostomy	Does he understand about stomas? Will he be able to cope?	Refer to stoma nurse for counselling and possible preoperative 'trial' of colostomy appliance (see Ch. 27)
16. Bowel will be opened during operation	Potential for faecal contamination of abdominal cavity and wound	May need bowel preparation and will need perioperative prophylactic antibiotics
17. Lesion at pelvic brim	Does it involve the ureter?	Consider ultrasonography of kidneys to exclude hydronephrosis
18. Varicose veins	Increases risk of DVT (already high because of major pelvic operation and age 70)	Give prophylaxis—low dose heparin, antiembolism stockings Early mobilisation

Family history
Mother was obese; died age 55 from complications of diabetes (gangrene). Older brother had major stroke at 64 but partially recovered. No family history of bowel cancer.

Social history
Widowed for 2 years, wife died of breast cancer. Has one son and one daughter, both married with young children but living far away. Lives in own house with an upstairs lavatory, on a smallholding with a few stock animals. Lives independently, and uses car for shopping. Smoker—20 cigarettes a day since age 15; alcohol intake averages 4 units a day.

Drug history
Takes atenolol 50 mg (a beta-blocker) and bendroflumethiazide 2.5 mg (a diuretic) once a day in the morning for hypertension. Takes aspirin 75 mg daily 'for his heart'. Told in the past not to have penicillin, but cannot recall why; does not remember when he last had penicillin. Not allergic to iodine.

EXAMINATION

General. Fit-looking man of 70, not obviously anxious. Tanned; not evidently anaemic; no cyanosis, jaundice, lymphadenopathy or clubbing; no thyroid enlargement. Fingers tobacco stained. Not febrile.

Cardiovascular and respiratory system. Pulse 68 beats per minute, regular. BP 150/110 mmHg. Soft systolic murmur at the left sternal edge. No ankle swelling and JVP not elevated. Extensive bilateral varicose veins. Chest examination unremarkable apart from a few crepitations which do not clear with coughing.

Abdomen. Moderately obese. Appendicectomy scar. Soft to palpation. No organomegaly. Possible mass in left iliac fossa—not indentable (i.e. not faeces). No groin hernias. External genitalia normal. Rectal examination—moderately enlarged smooth prostate and normal-coloured stool.

Central nervous system and locomotor system. Fixed flexion deformity of left elbow at 90°, otherwise normal.

SUMMARY

A 70-year-old man with proven rectosigmoid carcinoma without obvious dissemination, admitted for anterior resection of the rectosigmoid.

A problem list was constructed from this information, which led to further investigations and a management plan. The reasoning is shown in Table 7.2.

Medical problems

8

INTRODUCTION

General surgical operations are now performed on patients who are older, more frail and with significant and often multiple (medical) co-morbidities, so it becomes even more important to appreciate and consider these 'medical' conditions. Rates of deaths and complications after abdominal surgery have been the subject of a report by the Royal College of Surgeons of England (at: www.rcseng.ac.uk/publications/docs/higher-risk-surgical-patient). A high-risk patient is defined as one whose estimated risk of mortality is greater than 5%, and includes any patient over the age of 65 years undergoing major gastrointestinal or vascular surgery, and any patient over 50 years with diabetes mellitus or renal impairment. Recommendations include preoperative risk assessment with a tailored management plan directed by consultant surgeons and anaesthetists, and rapid identification and treatment of postoperative infection.

'Medical' disorders appear in surgical practice in four main ways:

- A pre-existing medical condition may precipitate a surgical admission because of exacerbation, progression or complications of the condition: for example, foot problems in diabetes
- A pre-existing medical condition may be made worse by operation. In chronic obstructive pulmonary disease, for example, general anaesthesia and postoperative sputum retention may precipitate life-threatening pneumonia
- A surgical condition may be complicated by an unrelated medical disorder. For example, a patient with rheumatoid arthritis on steroid therapy is vulnerable to impaired healing and recurrent infection
- An occult condition can become manifest under the stress of anaesthesia and operation. For example, perioperative or postoperative myocardial infarction can be caused by occult ischaemic heart disease

CARDIAC AND CEREBROVASCULAR DISEASE

Emergency surgery in patients with cardiac disease is about four times more likely to result in death than the same operation done electively. Thus, preoperative assessment is vitally important in emergency patients so any cardiac condition can be recognised and stabilised, electrolyte imbalances corrected and appropriate anaesthesia, surgical technique, monitoring and aftercare employed to minimise risk.

1. ISCHAEMIC HEART DISEASE

The clinical manifestations of ischaemic heart disease are:

- Chronic stable exertional angina; previous myocardial infarction
- Acute coronary syndrome
- Cardiac failure
- Arrhythmias, e.g. atrial fibrillation
- Asymptomatic atherosclerotic coronary artery disease

Asymptomatic coronary artery disease may progress to infarction under anaesthetic and surgical stresses, including laryngoscopy and endotracheal intubation, pain, hypoxia, rapid blood loss, anaemia, hypotension, hypocarbia and fluid overload. For major operations, general anaesthesia and spinal anaesthesia carry similar risks. Local anaesthesia, when practicable, is much safer.

Clinical problems

a. Stable angina and myocardial infarction more than three months previously

There is usually little increased risk during operation and exercise tolerance is by far the most important indicator of the patient's ability to tolerate anaesthesia and surgery. This can be assessed in the history (remembering that exercise tolerance may be limited by mobility problems rather than cardiorespiratory problems). Formal assessment on a treadmill may be helpful, and occasionally coronary angiography is required to fully assess cardiac risk.

In general, all cardiac medication should be continued perioperatively. Nitrates, which dilate the coronary arteries and reduce preload and left ventricular work, may reduce cardiac ischaemia during general anaesthesia and should not be stopped in the perioperative period. A transdermal nitrate patch is a useful alternative to tablets or sprays. Beta-adrenergic blockers, which reduce cardiac work and oxygen demand, should be continued unless non-ischaemic cardiac failure develops. Most patients will be taking aspirin (and some clopidogrel in addition), and the risks of bleeding have to be weighed against the risks of stopping anti-platelet treatment.

b. Acute coronary syndrome (ACS)

This is a term applied to a spectrum of conditions from unstable angina to non-ST-elevation myocardial infarction (NSTEMI) to ST-elevation myocardial infarction (STEMI). Acute coronary syndrome associated with surgery usually occurs during the first few days after operation, particularly on the second to fourth postoperative nights, rather than during the operation. Typical chest pain is not always a feature and postoperative ACS may present 'silently' (i.e. painlessly) with otherwise unexplained hypotension, cardiac failure, arrhythmias or cardiac arrest, particularly in patients with diabetes. Diagnosis is made on the basis of at least two of the following: appropriate symptoms (particularly typical cardiac ischaemic pain); a significant rise in a cardiac biomarker, usually troponin; and ECG changes consistent with ischaemia (dynamic changes including ST depression, T-wave flattening or inversion) or infarction (ST elevation). It is always helpful to have a preoperative ECG for comparison which should be performed on all patients over 50 years of age and any with cardiac symptoms or signs.

Troponin is a very specific marker of myocardial damage, but be aware that this damage may result from conditions other than ischaemia or infarction due to coronary artery disease, e.g. sepsis, hypotension or heart failure, and therefore the management may differ from that of ACS.

The medical treatment of ACS includes aspirin, clopidogrel (for anti-platelet activity) and fractionated heparin (given subcutaneously). These drugs adversely effect clotting in the perioperative period and the 'harm/benefit' balance requires negotiation between cardiology and surgical teams. Other treatments such as nitrate and beta-adrenergic receptor blockade are less likely to have adverse 'surgical' effects. ST-elevation myocardial infarction is ideally treated by emergency primary revascularisation but this depends on the 'surgical' stability of the patient, and on how close the nearest coronary intervention centre is. Thrombolysis is an option, but the potential salvage of myocardium has to be weighed against the serious risk of major haemorrhage.

2. CHRONIC HEART FAILURE (CHF)

This is a complex clinical syndrome with symptoms and signs resulting from impairment of the heart as a pump due to structural or functional abnormalities. The severity of heart failure correlates poorly with objective measurements of heart function (such as ejection fraction), such that up to 50% of patients presenting with symptoms and signs of heart failure will have 'preserved ejection fraction' (previously called 'diastolic heart failure'). Assessment of severity is based on clinical features, particularly when exercise tolerance is limited (New York Heart Association classification). Patients with renal impairment or electrolyte abnormalities have a poorer prognosis and tend to decompensate more readily with operative stress.

Most patients will be taking diuretics, an angiotensin converting enzyme (ACE) inhibitor and a beta-blocker as first line treatment, and nitrates and digoxin if the condition is more severe, and these treatments should be continued if possible.

Patients with CHF should be optimised before major surgery, but there is still an increased mortality of up to 5%. The causes, symptoms and signs of cardiac failure are shown in Figure 8.1.

Clinical problems

a. CHF before operation

Surgery should be postponed until treatment has been optimised and the clinical condition stabilised. Hasty preoperative diuretic therapy is dangerous because it may provoke intravascular volume depletion, hypotension and electrolyte abnormalities. Patients taking diuretics (and often ACE inhibitors or angiotensin receptor antagonists in addition) may have abnormalities such as:

- Hypokalaemia (usually due to potassium-losing diuretics prescribed without potassium supplements)
- Hyponatraemia
- Raised plasma urea and creatinine with hyperkalaemia (particularly if taking an ACE inhibitor and spironolactone)—the urea is often raised to a greater extent than creatinine indicating intravascular volume depletion
- Postural hypotension

b. Decompensated heart failure developing during or after operation

This problem results from poor tolerance of intravenous fluids, unaccustomed supine posture, myocardial infarction or ischaemia in the perioperative period, or arrhythmias (particularly atrial fibrillation) induced by the stresses of surgery and anaesthesia. Prompt and vigorous diuretic therapy with intravenous furosemide and nitrate is required to prevent worsening cardiac failure, hypoxia, renal failure or other potentially lethal complications. In addition, treatment of any precipitating factors should be instituted such as reducing cardiac stress by giving good pain relief. Postoperative cardiac failure is best managed in an intensive care unit, using a central venous pressure (CVP) line to guide fluid replacement.

Preoperative assessment of cardiac failure

Chest X-ray may demonstrate cardiomegaly and there may be signs of pulmonary oedema including upper lobe diversion, hilar congestion, septal Kerley B lines and pleural effusions

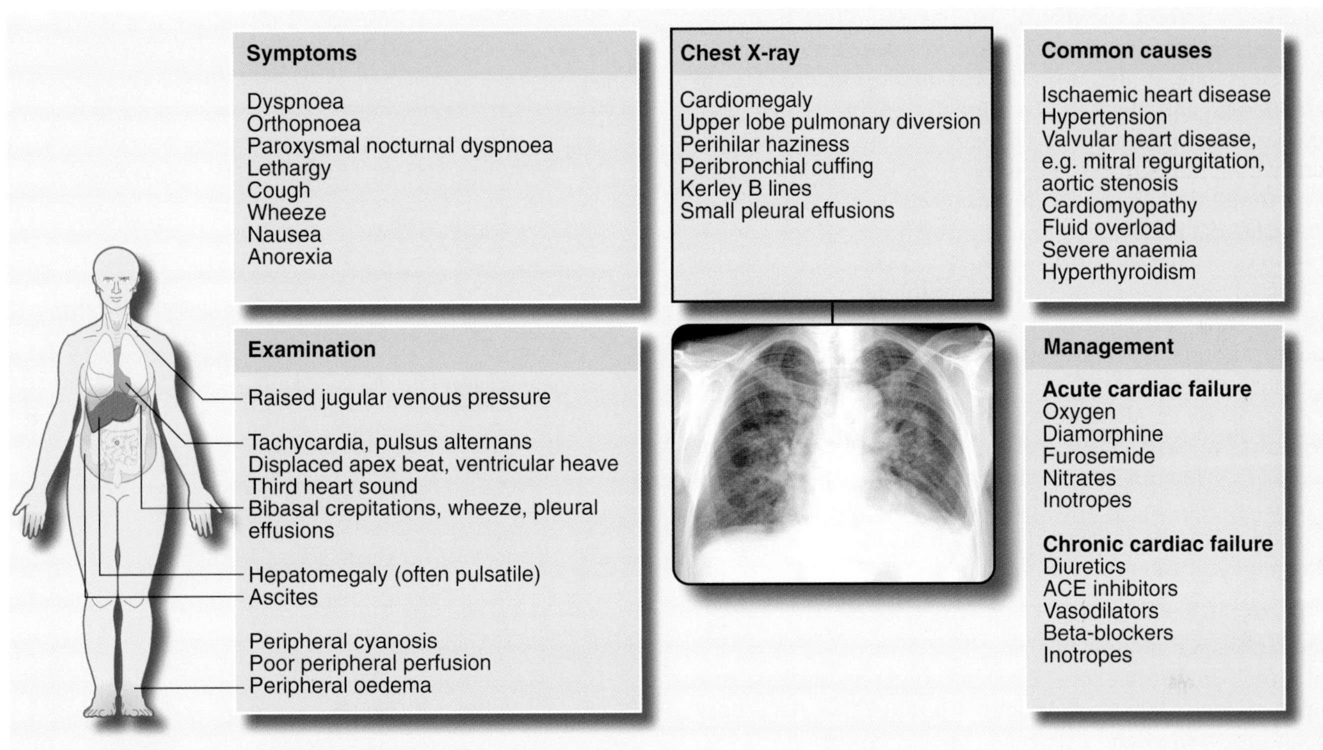

Fig. 8.1 The causes, symptoms and signs of cardiac failure
The chest X-ray is of a 60-year-old woman with a history of ischaemic heart disease. The signs indicate congestive heart failure. *Note*: some of these changes are subtle and do not reproduce well in illustrations

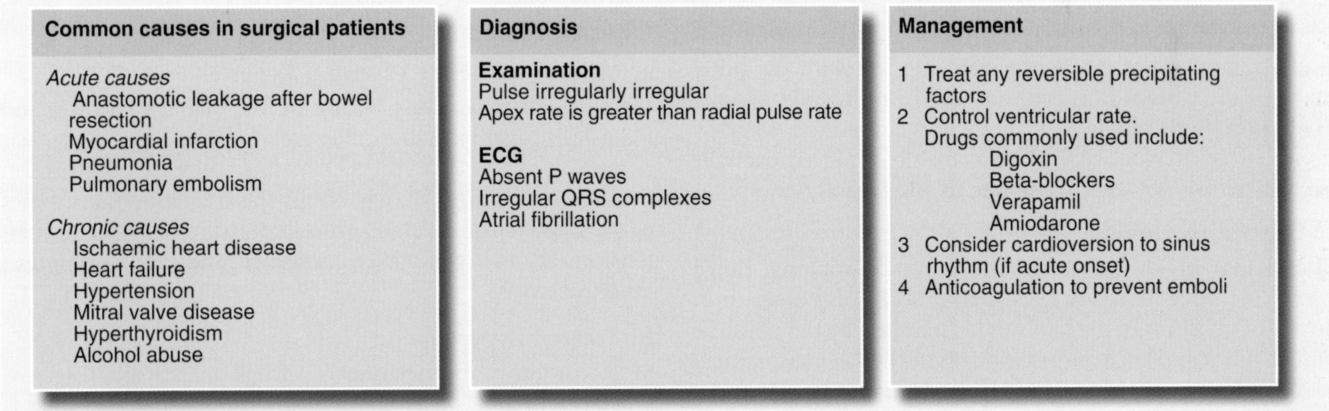

Fig. 8.2 Atrial fibrillation—causes, diagnosis and management

(see Fig. 8.1). ECG may show an arrhythmia, myocardial ischaemia, ventricular hypertrophy, left bundle branch block or loss of R waves.

Left ventricular function can be assessed by echocardiography and documented more precisely by radionuclide studies using multiple gated acquisition (MUGA), but the best assessment is a clinical one based on exercise tolerance. Measurement of blood urea and electrolytes is important as baseline and also indication of severity of the condition.

If there is any doubt about the fitness of a patient for operation, a cardiological opinion should be sought.

3. CARDIAC ARRHYTHMIAS

Clinical problems

a. Atrial fibrillation (Fig. 8.2)

Pre-existing (preoperative) atrial fibrillation is usually secondary to ischaemic heart disease but may be caused by mitral valve disease or thyrotoxicosis. Atrial fibrillation with a controlled ventricular rate (i.e. a pulse rate of less than 90 beats per minute at rest) causes minimal extra risk. An uncontrolled ventricular rate may cause perioperative heart failure. Atrial fibrillation (even with a controlled ventricular response) increases the risk of **arterial embolism** from any thrombus present in the left atrium. Adequate control of ventricular rate should be achieved before operation with beta-blocker and digoxin, occasionally supplemented with verapamil or amiodarone. Digoxin can be given intravenously if rapid control is necessary but potassium levels need to be monitored closely as digoxin given in the presence of hypokalaemia can lead to further arrhythmias. If the patient is anticoagulated with warfarin, there is a small risk of excessive bleeding at operation; stabilising the international normalised ratio (INR) between 1.5 and 2.5 may be the safest option. Another alternative is to stop warfarin and change to heparin.

Acute onset of AF postoperatively may be due to a major surgical (e.g. anastomotic leakage after bowel resection) or medical (e.g. pneumonia) complication (Fig. 8.2). If the onset of atrial arrhythmia (particularly atrial fibrillation) is associated with right bundle branch block on the ECG, this suggests a diagnosis of pulmonary embolism.

b. Bradycardia

Bradycardia is common in young fit athletic patients and is not a problem. In patients taking beta-blockers or digoxin, if the apex rate is below 60 beats per minute, that day's dose should be omitted and the regular dose reviewed.

Bradycardia may be caused by **complete heart block**, which should be easily diagnosed on the ECG. This may require urgent temporary **transvenous pacing**, particularly when there is significant haemodynamic compromise.

If a patient has a **cardiac pacemaker**, it is important to know the reason for its insertion: is the patient pacemaker-dependent, has the pacemaker been checked recently, what type of pacemaker has been inserted? Surgical diathermy, particularly monopolar diathermy, can interfere with the pacemaker if the current flows close to the heart. Ideally, bipolar diathermy should be used if diathermy is required. In addition a strong magnet should be available; if placed over the pacemaker this will return the rate to 100 beats/min.

c. Other arrhythmias

Bifascicular block, in which conduction is impaired down two of the three main fascicles (right bundle plus anterior or posterior divisions of the left bundle, manifest by right bundle branch block and left axis deviation on the ECG), may progress to complete heart block (and low cardiac output) under anaesthesia. For these patients, a prophylactic temporary transvenous pacemaker should be considered before operation.

4. HYPERTENSION

About one in four patients coming to surgery is either hypertensive or is receiving antihypertensive therapy. Most have **'essential' hypertension**, but causes such as renal artery stenosis and phaeochromocytoma must be considered in patients presenting with raised blood pressure which has not been appropriately investigated. (For other causes see Fig. 8.3.) Undiagnosed renal artery stenosis puts the patient at risk of severe acute kidney injury if there is an episode of hypotension, and phaeochromocytoma of potentially fatal hypertensive crisis.

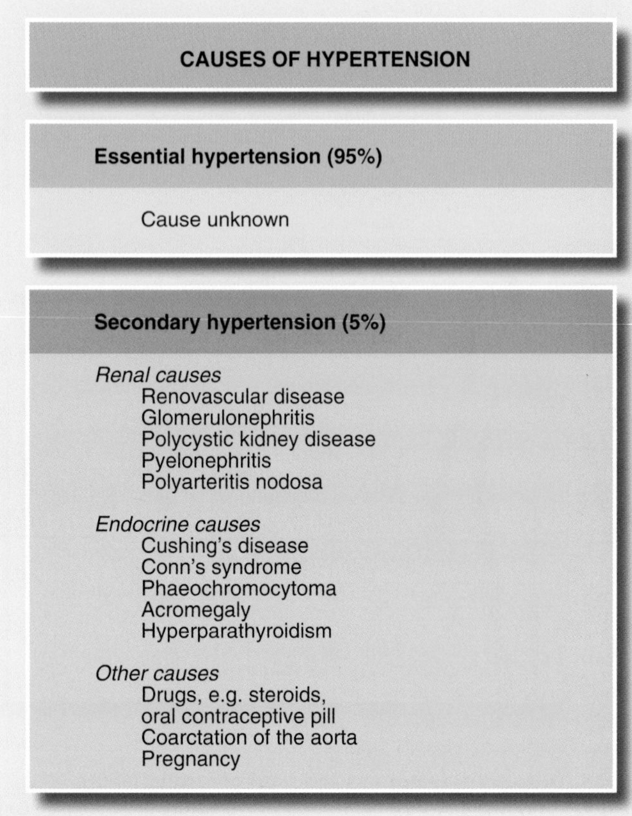

Fig. 8.3 Causes of hypertension

Clinical problems

a. Mild-to-moderate essential hypertension

Patients with a systolic pressure of less than 180 mmHg and a diastolic less than 110 mmHg are at minimal risk of cardiac complications unless there is some other cardiovascular disease. Sometimes, anxiety about the operation contributes to the hypertension. A labile blood pressure or systolic hypertension at any time may, however, indicate widespread atherosclerosis.

b. Treated hypertension

Most common antihypertensive drugs are 'cardioprotective' and should not be stopped prior to general anaesthesia. Despite the patient being 'nil by mouth' in the immediate preoperative period, the normal dose of oral antihypertensive drugs should usually be given with a small amount of water. Sudden withdrawal of antihypertensive drugs may cause rebound hypertension. Withdrawal of beta-blockers may trigger autonomic hyperactivity and lability of blood pressure. Postural hypotension may occur after operation, especially if there is dehydration.

c. Severe or poorly controlled hypertension

If the diastolic BP is > 110 mmHg, then treatment needs to be instituted and any non-urgent operative procedure delayed. During anaesthesia the untreated hypertensive patient has a very labile BP and is at high risk of perioperative myocardial infarction, cardiac failure or stroke.

Preoperative assessment of hypertensive patients

Chest X-ray may identify cardiomegaly or cardiac failure, both of which increase the perioperative morbidity and mortality. An ECG may reveal signs of ventricular hypertrophy and ischaemia. Plasma urea and electrolytes should be measured in all patients taking diuretics or ACE inhibitors and in any patient with suspected chronic renal impairment.

5. CEREBROVASCULAR DISEASE

A patient has cerebrovascular disease if there is a **history of stroke or transient ischaemic attacks (TIAs)**. Cerebral atherosclerosis may render the blood flow to the brain precarious, with an increased risk of perioperative stroke from hypoxia, hypotension or increased blood viscosity resulting from dehydration.

Patients with **ischaemic heart disease** or **peripheral vascular disease** should also be assumed to have cerebrovascular disease and, as a minimum, the carotid arteries should be auscultated for bruits. In high-risk patients, or if a carotid bruit is present, a duplex Doppler examination of the carotid arteries should be performed, and patients with a stenosis greater than 70% considered for carotid endarterectomy before the planned operation if conditions permit. The anaesthetist should be warned of any signs or symptoms suggestive of carotid artery disease so that special care can be taken to avoid hypotension during surgery.

After a **stroke**, operation should be avoided for at least 2 months if practicable. This is because autoregulation of cerebral blood pressure becomes disrupted, so that cerebral arterial pressure becomes directly related to systemic arterial pressure. Brain perfusion thus loses the buffering effect of autoregulation on peaks and troughs of blood pressure that tend to occur during anaesthesia and surgery. If operation cannot be delayed, it is important to prevent hypertension and hypotension in the perioperative period.

There are few other measures likely to reduce cerebrovascular complications in patients with cerebrovascular disease, although there is an argument for prescribing low-dose **aspirin** (75 mg daily) to inhibit platelet aggregation. The surgeon needs to be involved in any decision to stop or start aspirin; in any case, this needs to be stopped at least a week before major surgery to reduce the risk of excessive bleeding.

6. VALVULAR HEART DISEASE

The common valvular abnormalities are mitral regurgitation, aortic stenosis and aortic regurgitation. Any of these may dangerously alter cardiovascular dynamics, but stenotic lesions are more serious than regurgitant ones, as the cardiac output tends to be fixed.

Under perioperative stress, valvular disease may precipitate acute myocardial ischaemia, hypotension, cardiac failure, arrhythmias or thromboembolism. Valvular heart disease also predisposes to infective endocarditis.

Aortic stenosis

Aortic stenosis is potentially the most serious valvular disorder in a surgical patient because it limits the cardiac output and reduces blood flow to the coronary arteries. Indeed, the patient may already be functioning close to the limit with almost no reserve. Perioperative hypotension and tachycardia can be life-threatening in such cases. **Aortic 'sclerosis'** produces a similar ejection systolic murmur and is caused by fixed, rigid valve leaflets, usually with systolic hypertension. The perioperative risk is that of the hypertension and arterial disease.

In a patient with an ejection systolic murmur, any associated **cardiac symptoms** may help identify the murmur as pathological, e.g. a history of syncope, angina or shortness of breath on exertion. Note, however, that any systolic murmur is difficult to categorise clinically, particularly in the elderly, and an **echocardiogram** must be performed to identify the valvular cause and offer an assessment of severity. A specialist cardiology assessment may also be required.

Clinical signs of aortic stenosis are:

- Slow rising upstroke of the carotid pulse
- A harsh ejection systolic murmur radiating into the neck
- Hyperdynamic apex beat indicating left ventricular hypertrophy. (*Note*: the apex beat is only displaced laterally if aortic stenosis coexists with aortic regurgitation or is complicated by cardiac failure)
- Left ventricular hypertrophy on ECG

If aortic stenosis is suspected, an echocardiogram will confirm the diagnosis and aid assessment of severity by measuring the aortic valve area, the gradient across the valve and an estimate of left ventricular systolic function.

Non-urgent surgery may be best delayed until after operative intervention to the aortic valve. This may now be carried out percutaneously in frail or elderly patients in whom previously the risk of valve replacement was prohibitive.

Symptomatic valvular disease is potentially dangerous and requires full preoperative assessment and treatment. Major valvular heart disease may be discovered in recent immigrants from developing countries where **rheumatic heart disease** is prevalent. Patients with valvular heart disease require cardiac monitoring during operation and usually intensive care afterwards.

Patients with mechanical valves are usually maintained on permanent warfarin anticoagulation and it is important to maintain this to prevent valve thrombosis, a potentially fatal condition. Patients with bioprosthetic valves (pig valves) do not usually require anticoagulation.

It should be remembered that warfarin is intended to minimise intravascular thrombosis and does not affect the extrinsic thrombotic mechanisms. For many operations it is safe to continue warfarin therapy as long as the INR is maintained in the lower therapeutic range (INR 1.5–2.5). For major surgery where much bleeding is anticipated, some surgeons prefer to stop warfarin 2 days before operation and substitute subcutaneous heparin or an intravenous infusion. For patients with mitral valve prostheses where the risk of thrombosis is high, full heparinisation must be carefully maintained throughout the perioperative period. However, heparin anticoagulation is more brittle than warfarin and carries a greater risk of over-anticoagulation and potential haemorrhage. For other patients, heparin can be stopped 12 hours before operation and restarted once the danger of bleeding is over. The advantage of heparin over warfarin is that its effects can be quickly

Cardiovascular lesions at risk of infective endocarditis and indications for perioperative antibiotic prophylaxis

High-risk conditions	Low-risk conditions	Minimal-risk conditions
Prosthetic valve or other intracardiac surgery Rheumatic valve disease Congenital heart disease (structural valve defects, atrial and ventricular septal defects) and aortic coarctation, whether or not corrected Degenerative valve disease Previous infective endocarditis	Mitral valve prolapse Haemodialysis shunts Transvenous pacemakers Ventriculo-atrial and ventriculo-peritoneal shunts for hydrocephalus	Coronary bypass grafts Closed patent ductus arteriosus Closed atrial septal defect Established prosthetic arterial grafts

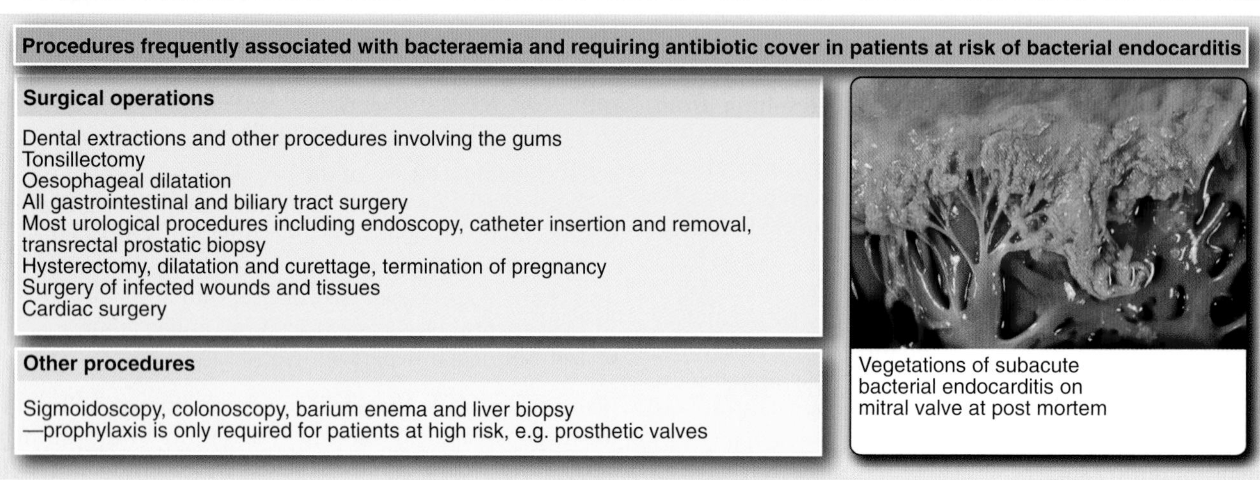

Fig. 8.4 Infective endocarditis

reversed by stopping the infusion or with **protamine** if bleeding is excessive. However, rapid reversal may precipitate thrombosis.

In all cases it is advisable to involve the haematologist in discussion for advice on management, and in anticipation of specific treatment.

Infective endocarditis and indications for antibiotic prophylaxis

Valvular disease, and in particular prosthetic replacement valves, carry a risk of **infective endocarditis**. When blood is forced under pressure through a narrow orifice, laminar flow is disrupted and eddy currents predispose to local thrombus formation and deposition of circulating bacteria. The vegetations of infective endocarditis thus form on the low-pressure side of the jet of blood passing through a damaged valve or a ventricular septal defect. The left side of the heart is more susceptible than the right because of the higher pressures and greater potential for turbulence.

Streptococcus viridans is the most common causative organism of infective endocarditis. Other bacteria, such as coliforms or fungi, e.g. *Candida*, may also be responsible. Many types of operation and some invasive investigations cause transient bacteraemia. Although the incidence of infective endocarditis following such procedures is small, the consequences can be catastrophic. The efficacy of prophylactic antibiotics is not absolutely proven, but they are all that is available. The relative risks associated with various cardiac and valvular lesions are summarised in Figure 8.4. The procedures most likely to cause bacteraemia are also shown in Figure 8.4.

The choice of prophylactic antibiotics and the dose regimen depend on the anticipated organisms, the operative procedure and local protocols.

RESPIRATORY DISEASES

Respiratory complications (mainly atelectasis and pneumonia) occur in as many as 15% of surgical patients and are the leading cause of postoperative mortality in the elderly. The risk of a respiratory complication increases with the increasing duration of anaesthetic and is amplified by pre-existing respiratory disease such as chronic obstructive pulmonary disease, asthma or bronchiectasis. Other important factors include smoking, cardiac failure, obesity, old age and general debility. Good postoperative pain relief allows the patient to breathe deeply and cough, which, along with effective physiotherapy, helps reduce the risk of respiratory complications.

CLINICAL PROBLEMS

a. Chronic obstructive pulmonary disease (COPD)

COPD (smoking-related lung disease—chronic bronchitis and emphysema) is common and strongly predisposes to postoperative respiratory complications, particularly bronchopneumonia, lobar collapse and pneumothorax. There is often a degree of reversible **bronchoconstriction**, and this can be assessed before operation by measuring peak expiratory flow before and after bronchodilator treatment. Many patients will already have had spirometry and vitalography in family practice or in specialist hospital COPD services and their treatment optimised. Otherwise preoperative assessment by the hospital 'chest team' will help bring the patient into optimum health. The forced expiratory volume in 1 second (FEV_1) is perhaps the single most useful assessment of severity of chronic lung disease.

Other chronic lung diseases include bronchiectasis, pneumoconiosis, pulmonary fibrosis, sarcoidosis and pulmonary tuberculosis.

b. Cigarette smoking

Smokers of cigarettes have a five-fold greater risk of postoperative respiratory problems than non-smokers. This is partly due to pre-existing smoking-related respiratory disease but also because smokers have a highly reactive airway. This increases the intraoperative risk of laryngeal spasm and bronchospasm.

Smoking should be stopped at least 4 weeks before operation and ideally 8 weeks before if any early benefit is to be achieved. This gives time for recovery of physiological respiratory functions such as bronchial ciliary activity. Stopping smoking just before surgery may actually be detrimental because it causes an increase in bronchial mucus production.

c. Current respiratory infections

Acute upper respiratory tract infections (usually viral) are common and these patients have reduced resistance to surgical trauma and infection. This alone may be grounds for postponing an elective operation.

Conditions associated with chronic infection such as bronchiectasis and cystic fibrosis are more difficult. Elective operations should be carried out during remissions where possible, with intensive physiotherapy and perioperative prophylactic antibiotics.

d. Asthma

Asthma is common in children and adolescents but may occur later in life, particularly as a component of COPD. The main elements of asthma are airway hyper-reactivity (with constriction), bronchial wall oedema, excessive mucus production and airway plugging. All these factors predispose to atelectasis, infection and hypoxia.

Asthmatic problems can be exacerbated by the following factors associated with general anaesthesia and surgery:

- Endotracheal intubation—increases airways sensitivity
- Increased airways secretions—caused by intubation or the autonomic side-effects of anaesthetic drugs such as muscle relaxants
- Dehydration—increases mucus viscosity
- Limitation of movement and posture because of pain—inhibits coughing to clear secretions
- The direct effects of other drugs, e.g. bronchoconstriction caused by beta-blockers or morphine-associated respiratory depression

In patients with asthma, the usual medication should be continued in the perioperative period, given via a nebuliser if necessary. Operations should be postponed during acute exacerbations.

e. Previous pulmonary embolism or deep venous thrombosis

These patients have a greatly increased risk of recurrent thromboembolism. Prophylactic measures are mandatory for all but the most minor procedures.

PREOPERATIVE INVESTIGATION OF RESPIRATORY DISEASE

A chest X-ray should be performed on any patient with symptoms or signs of chest disease. There is no need for 'routine' chest X-rays on all preoperative patients as undirected screening of asymptomatic patients has a low yield of abnormalities likely to influence surgical outcome.

Appropriate **lung function tests** should be performed in patients with chronic lung disease. Peak flows help evaluate airflow limitation. The reversible element of bronchospasm can be assessed using peak flow measurements before and after bronchodilators. Blood gas measurements are indicated if hypoxaemia or carbon dioxide retention is likely.

PERIOPERATIVE MANAGEMENT OF RESPIRATORY DISEASE AND HIGH-RISK PATIENTS

The following measures will maximise respiratory function and reduce the risk of postoperative complications:

- **Preoperative physiotherapy**—helps prevent postoperative chest complications. Physiotherapy should include teaching the patient breathing exercises and correct posture
- **Drug therapy**—adjust to achieve optimum respiratory function. Theophyllines may be added in patients with asthma, and nebulised bronchodilator drugs (such as salbutamol) may improve the reversible component of COPD and help to prevent a perioperative exacerbation of asthma. Adequate hydration reduces the risk of retained secretions which might cause airways obstruction. Prophylactic antibiotics are not recommended for COPD
- **Encouragement of smokers to quit**—should be started at the time of booking for elective surgery
- **Alternative methods of anaesthesia—local, regional or spinal**—should be considered for patients with chronic respiratory disorders, but are not necessarily the best solution. With the use of newer anaesthetic drugs and techniques, patients may be better off with endotracheal intubation and ventilation using short-acting muscle relaxants. These techniques allow good bronchial toilet at the end of operation. Certain abdominal operations are technically more difficult under spinal anaesthesia, for example if a patient with chest trouble coughs persistently during the procedure; general anaesthesia avoids this
- **Early postoperative physiotherapy**—aims to enhance deep breathing, coughing and general mobility, reducing the incidence of respiratory complications

GASTROINTESTINAL DISORDERS

The main gastrointestinal conditions giving rise to complications in surgical patients are malnutrition, dental problems, peptic ulcer disease, gastro-oesophageal reflux and inflammatory bowel disease. Previous abdominal surgery may also complicate inpatient treatment.

MALNUTRITION

Many surgical patients are malnourished because of reduced food intake, malabsorption and changes in metabolism (in trauma, burns and sepsis). Studies have shown that 50% of patients undergoing gastrointestinal surgery are mildly malnourished and 30% are moderately or severely malnourished. The severity of malnourishment proportionately increases postoperative morbidity and mortality. For example, severely malnourished patients experience eight times the rate of complications and three times the expected mortality following gastrointestinal surgery. Wound healing is delayed, immune resistance is impaired and muscles are weakened.

Nutritional assessment

There is no universal tool for assessing malnutrition but the combination of a BMI of less than 18.5 kg/m^2 with weight loss exceeding 5% of usual body weight over the preceding 1–2 months and a serum albumin level below 35 g/L (in the absence of renal or hepatic disease) indicates significant malnutrition. Other tools include measuring mid-upper arm circumference, skin fold thickness and grip strength.

Indications for nutritional support

If enteral support (i.e. supplemental nutrition into the gastrointestinal tract) is practicable before operation, certain patients benefit from it by reduced mortality and morbidity. Indications published by the British Society of Gastroenterology include patients with severe anorexia, with moderate or severe malnutrition unable to eat or swallow sufficient by mouth, with recent weight loss of 10% or more, or with intestinal failure, and patients not expected to resume oral intake for 10 or more days after operation. Nutritional support is best given as supplements by mouth if possible or else via a fine-bore nasogastric tube.

DENTAL PROBLEMS

Teeth and artificial fixed crowns and bridges are vulnerable to damage during intubation. This causes not only cosmetic and medico-legal problems, but also exposes the patient to the risk of aspirating foreign bodies into the bronchial tree. Similarly, infected material from carious (decayed) teeth or inflamed gums may be aspirated. This causes particularly grave aspiration pneumonia. Dentures must be removed before operation and labelled so the patient can retrieve them afterwards. In unconscious trauma victims, the possibility of aspiration, swallowing or pharyngeal obstruction by a dental prosthesis should always be considered.

PEPTIC ULCER DISEASE

Peptic ulcer disease may be a surgical problem in its own right, but patients admitted for other reasons may have an active peptic ulcer exacerbated by hospital stresses. These include serious illness and trauma, operations, and drugs such as aspirin, NSAIDs and corticosteroids. The result may be a sudden catastrophic **haemorrhage** (presenting as haematemesis or melaena), or occasionally **perforation**. Bleeding may also result from **acute stress ulceration** in the seriously ill patient. Note that stress ulceration is distinct from chronic peptic ulcer disease.

Patients with known peptic ulcer disease or strongly suggestive symptoms should receive perioperative prophylaxis with proton pump inhibitors. NSAIDs and irritant oral drugs should be avoided.

Previous gastrectomy may have a number of long-term side-effects. These include anaemia (deficiency of iron, vitamin B_{12} and occasionally folate) and, rarely, osteomalacia. A full blood count should be included in the preoperative assessment of these patients.

GASTRO-OESOPHAGEAL REFLUX DISEASE (GORD)

Patients with GORD are at risk of aspirating acidic gastric contents during induction of anaesthesia and should receive preoperative treatment with proton pump inhibitors. Aspiration may cause interstitial lung damage which, in its severe form, is known as **Mendelson's syndrome** (chemical pneumonitis).

INFLAMMATORY BOWEL DISEASE

Patients with chronic inflammatory bowel disease may be anaemic or malnourished if the disease is active. Patients may also be **steroid dependent** because of adrenal suppression from long-term steroid therapy, requiring perioperative hydrocortisone. Occasionally immunosuppressive drugs such as azathioprine are being taken and may increase the predisposition to infection.

HEPATIC DISORDERS

Pre-existing liver disease may have important consequences in the surgical patient and generally increases postoperative morbidity and mortality. A history of jaundice must be evaluated as it may be a clue to serious risks for both patient and medical staff.

CLINICAL PROBLEMS

a. History of jaundice

A past history of jaundice raises the possibility that the patient may be a carrier of hepatitis B or C and this can readily be transmitted to health care staff. The main danger is from needle-stick injuries.

Most previously jaundiced patients will have suffered acute infective hepatitis (hepatitis A) and this poses no risk to staff because the infective agent does not cause a chronic carrier state. In contrast, lifetime **chronic hepatitis** develops in 5–10% of those infected with hepatitis B virus (HBV) and in 80% of those infected with HCV. These diseases should be suspected if the illness associated with the previous jaundice was prolonged or serious. Jaundice contracted in developing countries should be regarded with suspicion because hepatitis B and C are often endemic. Hepatitis C causes a high

Box 8.1 CAGE questionnaire for assessing possible alcoholism

- Have you ever felt you ought to **Cut down** on your drinking?
- Have people **Annoyed** you by criticising your drinking?
- Have you ever felt bad or **Guilty** about your drinking?
- Have you ever had a drink first thing in the morning to steady your nerves or get rid of a hangover (**Eye-opener**)?

long-term rate of cirrhosis, although it often develops slowly over many years. Hepatitis B and C are also common among men who have sex with men and intravenous drug abusers who share syringes. The history should include questions to determine whether the patient falls into a high-risk group. Clinical examination should include a search for intravenous injection sites characteristic of drug abuse. In high-risk patients, screening for hepatitis B surface antigen (HBsAg) and hepatitis C antibody should be performed (see Ch. 3).

b. Presence of obstructive jaundice

Surgery in this situation is usually performed to relieve an obstruction in patients where endoscopic stenting of the bile ducts is inappropriate, has failed or is unavailable. This surgery carries a number of special risks and management problems which are described in Chapter 18. These include ascending cholangitis, clotting disorders, deep vein thrombosis and acute renal failure.

c. The patient with known hepatitis

Patients with any form of hepatitis, whether viral or alcoholic, tolerate general anaesthesia and surgery badly and there is a definite mortality risk. Surgery should be avoided unless essential. If alcoholism is suspected, a CAGE questionnaire (Box 8.1) should be completed. Positive answers to two or more of the four questions suggest a drinking problem.

An elevated serum gamma glutaryl transpeptidase level and mean corpuscular red cell volume (MCV) are fairly good indicators of excessive alcohol intake.

d. The patient with known cirrhosis

Patients with cirrhosis have a high risk of perioperative morbidity and mortality. The main factors are:

- Anaemia
- Portal hypertension
- Defective synthesis of clotting factors and thrombocytopenia
- Malnutrition
- Electrolyte disturbances (particularly hyponatraemia)
- Defective energy metabolism (gluconeogenesis and glycogenolysis)
- Abnormal drug metabolism and distribution (due to hypoalbuminaemia)
- Ascites

Box 8.2 Preoperative blood tests for patients with liver disease

Initial tests

- Serological testing for hepatitis B and C
- Consider HIV testing

Further tests

- Full blood count
- Clotting screen
- Consider blood group and cross-match if excess bleeding anticipated
- Plasma urea and electrolytes
- Bilirubin
- Transaminases
- Gamma glutaryl transpeptidase
- Albumin
- Calcium
- Phosphate

The main postoperative complications of cirrhosis are excessive bleeding, defective wound healing, hepatocellular decompensation leading to encephalopathy, and susceptibility to infection.

Excessive bleeding results from several factors:

- Defective synthesis of clotting factors (all but factor VIII are synthesised in the liver)
- Thrombocytopenia (due to hypersplenism and depressed platelet production)
- Abnormal polymerisation of fibrin
- Portal hypertension (greatly expanded intra-abdominal venous network under high pressure). This, together with numerous vascular adhesions, makes dissection in the abdominal cavity tedious, difficult and bloody

Portal hypertension may initially be discovered because of ascites or splenomegaly or an acute upper gastrointestinal haemorrhage from oesophageal varices, gastroduodenal ulcers, Mallory–Weiss tears or gastric erosions. If a patient with known oesophageal varices requires an operation, preoperative endoscopic assessment is important and sclerotherapy or banding may be appropriate.

PREOPERATIVE ASSESSMENT AND MANAGEMENT

Preoperative blood tests for patients with liver disease are listed in Box 8.2. If the prothrombin ratio is prolonged, intravenous vitamin K injections are given for several days before operation. If this fails to correct the abnormal clotting (as in severe hepatocellular impairment), it is important to liaise with a haematologist who may recommend perioperative administration of **fresh-frozen plasma or prothrombin complex concentrate** (e.g. Octaplex or Beriplex), containing factors II, VII, IX, X, protein C and protein S. If the patient is thrombocytopenic, platelet transfusion may also be required.

RENAL DISORDERS

Renal impairment is commonly encountered in general surgical patients. There is impaired homeostasis of fluid and electrolytes and reduced excretion of nitrogenous compounds. The risk of perioperative complications increases with the degree of renal impairment. Patients fall into two groups: mild and severe chronic renal failure (CRF). Acute renal failure (acute kidney injury) is usually a postoperative complication, often with several contributory causes including hypovolaemia, and is described in Chapter 12. Patients with pre-existing renal disease are particularly vulnerable to progress to acute renal failure ('acute-on-chronic renal failure').

CLINICAL PROBLEMS

a. Mild/moderate chronic renal failure (CKD stage 1–3, eGFR >30 ml/min)

This is common in the elderly and often associated with hypertension and diabetes. The main management problems in surgical patients are:

- **Impaired excretion of drugs**—drugs handled by the kidney must be given in smaller doses or less frequently, as documented in official drug formularies. In practice, digoxin and gentamicin pose the main problems
- **Fluid and electrolyte homeostasis**—only becomes a problem if fluid balance is not monitored carefully in the perioperative period. Monitoring should include regular checks of plasma urea, electrolytes and creatinine, especially if the patient is receiving diuretic therapy
- **Reduction in renal reserve**—even a small increase in plasma creatinine implies a significant reduction in renal reserve. For example, major reconstructive surgery to the abdominal aorta in a patient with mild renal impairment may interfere with renal function because of aortic cross-clamping near the renal arteries. This is exacerbated by transient hypotension caused by blood loss. The lack of renal reserve in these patients may then progress to acute renal failure

b. Severe chronic renal failure (CKD stage 4–5, eGFR <30 ml/min)

These patients are usually under the care of specialist physicians who should be involved in perioperative management. Patients may be receiving regular haemodialysis or ambulatory peritoneal dialysis; in such patients, surgery may be for renal transplantation (see Fig. 8.5).

The main perioperative problems of severe CRF are:

- **Fluid overload**—caused by impaired glomerular filtration and may require correction with large doses of diuretics, fluid restriction and haemofiltration if necessary
- **Regulation of plasma osmolality**—this is disordered in patients with severe CRF who are particularly vulnerable to hypo- and hypernatraemia. Care must be taken that the sodium content of intravenous fluids is appropriate
- **Hyperkalaemia**—this is a particular risk in advanced CRF. Patients with lesser degrees of CRF are vulnerable to an increase in potassium load (due to transfusion, tissue damage or hypoxia) or changes in glomerular filtration rate (caused by cardiac failure or hypotension). Hyperkalaemia may cause cardiac arrest and susceptibility to this may be assessed by monitoring the ECG. To minimise this risk, the preoperative plasma potassium level should be stabilised below 5.0 mmol/L, but in chronic hyperkalaemia a plasma potassium up to 6.5 mmol/L rarely causes problems.
- **Metabolic acidosis**—this tends to develop in chronic renal failure but it is usually compensated by respiratory alkalosis. This compensation is disrupted by general anaesthesia and also by additional metabolic acidosis resulting from tissue ischaemia or hypoxia
- **Chronic normochromic normocytic anaemia**—this results from decreased erythropoietin production by the kidney. Cardiovascular function is usually well adapted to this anaemia and preoperative transfusion is unnecessary. If the haemoglobin concentration is substantially below 10 g/dl, the patient is usually treated with **erythropoietin**

Fig. 8.5 Cimino–Brescia arteriovenous fistula

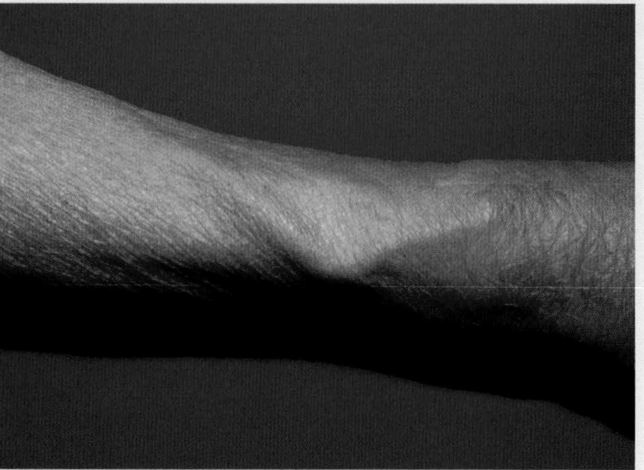

This recently constructed fistula was performed for chronic renal failure in a diabetic woman of 56. It involved dividing the cephalic vein and suturing its proximal end to the side of the radial artery. It was performed under local anaesthesia via the visible incision. The wrist veins are already dilating and will soon be usable for renal dialysis

PREOPERATIVE ASSESSMENT

Patients with severe renal failure should be asked about their daily urine volume, as those who are oliguric are at risk of over-hydration. The state of hydration should be assessed clinically, looking for dehydration or fluid overload (particularly jugular venous pressure). Plasma urea, electrolytes, creatinine and bicarbonate, calcium and phosphate should be checked, and also haemoglobin.

DIABETES MELLITUS

Severe hypoglycaemia and hyperglycaemia are life-threatening conditions. The blood glucose levels of a surgical patient with diabetes need to be closely monitored and treated.

Box 8.3 Specific perioperative problems in patients with diabetes

Predisposition to ischaemic heart disease

- Greater risk of perioperative myocardial infarction, and has a substantially higher mortality, particularly females
- Infarction may be painless or 'silent' (possibly due to autonomic neuropathy)

Increased danger of cardiac arrest

- Due to autonomic neuropathy

Renal problems

- Predisposition to diabetic nephropathy
- Tendency to chronic renal failure

Predisposition to peripheral vascular disease

- Greater risk of perioperative strokes and lower limb ischaemia

Predisposition to heel pressure sores

- Especially if there is peripheral neuropathy and/or ischaemia

Increased incidence of postoperative infection

- In the wound, chest or urinary tract

Obesity

- Particularly common in type 2 diabetes
- Associated with increased operative morbidity

Patients with diabetes are at special risk from general anaesthesia and surgery for the following reasons:

- Some complications of diabetes are associated with a higher perioperative risk. These are summarised in Box 8.3
- Stress (including surgery, trauma and infections) causes increased production of catabolic hormones which oppose the action of insulin (see Ch. 2), making diabetic control more difficult
- General anaesthesia, surgery, deprivation of oral intake and postoperative vomiting disrupt the delicate balance between dietary intake, exercise (energy utilisation) and diabetic therapy
- Diabetic ketoacidosis is a cause of elevated leucocyte count and raised amylase level, which may be confusing in the diagnosis of patients presenting with an acute abdomen. Indeed, ketoacidosis may sometimes present with abdominal pain
- There is a greater risk of hospital-acquired infection, which may be elusive as a cause of deterioration
- Episodes of cardiac ischaemia and infarction may be painless
- There may be reduced renal reserve or more overt evidence of renal impairment

CLINICAL PROBLEMS

Preoperative assessment in patients undergoing major surgery should include evaluation of current diabetic control by serial blood glucose and **glycosylated haemoglobin** measurements. Potential cardiovascular and renal complications should be assessed by performing an ECG (with Valsalva manoeuvre to look for autonomic neuropathy) and measuring plasma urea and electrolytes.

Perioperative management aims to maintain blood glucose between 4 and 10 mmol/L, but hypoglycaemia must be avoided. Above 13 mmol/L, the risk of ketoacidosis or a hyperosmolar non-ketotic state is unacceptable unless surgery is critically urgent. Surgery in the presence of ketoacidosis has a high mortality and should be avoided if possible until the acidosis is under control, i.e. until bicarbonate is greater than 20 or pH >7.3.

For the purposes of perioperative management, patients with diabetes fall into three groups: those who are **insulin dependent**, those taking **oral hypoglycaemic** medication and those who are **diet controlled**. These are general guidelines—there are usually local guidelines and readily available clinical advice (often led by specialist nurse teams).

a. Insulin-dependent diabetes

Insulin-dependent diabetics depend for their metabolism on administered insulin. If the blood glucose level is low, insulin is not withheld but glucose infusion is increased. The general principles of perioperative management are:

- Establish good diabetic control before operation
- Give insulin as a continuous intravenous infusion during the operative period
- Give an infusion of dextrose (glucose) throughout the operative period to balance the insulin given and to make up for lack of dietary intake
- Add potassium to the dextrose infusion
- Monitor blood glucose and electrolytes frequently throughout the operative and early postoperative period

A typical management protocol is given in Box 8.4 and a recommended insulin infusion regimen (a 'sliding scale') in Box 8.5. The key is to adjust the insulin dose hourly according to blood glucose results.

b. Diabetics controlled on oral hypoglycaemic drugs

Many patients are receiving short-acting sulphonylureas such as glipizide. Metformin should be discontinued because of the risk of lactic acidosis. If glycaemic control is difficult then an insulin regimen should be used as above.

On the morning of the operation, the patient is starved in the usual manner and the short-acting sulphonylurea omitted to be reintroduced when oral intake is resumed. Blood glucose should be monitored regularly (at least 4-hourly). If glucose rises above 13 mmol/L, it can be controlled by small subcutaneous doses of short-acting insulin, e.g. 6 units of soluble insulin. If a major operation is planned or if postoperative 'nil by mouth' is likely to be prolonged, it is best to use insulin and glucose infusions as for insulin-dependent diabetes.

c. Diabetics controlled by diet alone

If preoperative control is adequate, these patients require no special perioperative measures; they do not become hypoglycaemic and blood glucose rarely drifts above acceptable levels.

Box 8.4 Perioperative management of insulin-dependent diabetes

Before operation

1. Arrange preoperative outpatient stabilisation of diabetes with diabetes physician and specialist nurse in advance
2. If outpatient preparation is unavailable or unsatisfactory, admit patient at least 1 day before operation
3. Establish optimal preoperative control—may need advice from diabetic management team
4. Monitor blood glucose throughout the day, e.g. before and after meals and at bedtime
5. Check blood glucose and electrolytes before operating list commences—postpone if glucose level greater than 13 mmol/L or electrolyte abnormalities found
6. Arrange for the operation as early as possible in the day

Operation day

1. Starve from midnight and omit first dose of insulin
2. Commence intravenous dextrose and insulin infusions
3. Check blood glucose and electrolytes at conclusion of operation (or at 1–2-hour intervals in a long operation)
4. Adjust concentration of infusions and rate of administration as required

After operation

1. Check glucose hourly initially and electrolytes 6–12-hourly and adjust infusion as indicated
2. Continue infusion until full oral diet is established, then reintroduce subcutaneous insulin, using the preoperative regimen

Box 8.5 Perioperative management of diabetics using insulin infusion

1. Intravenous 5% or 10% dextrose infusion at 125 ml per hour
2. Constant pump-controlled intravenous soluble insulin infusion. This is adjusted according to 2–4-hourly blood glucose estimations
3. If there is a need to limit fluids—use 20% dextrose solution and infuse at 50 ml per hour

Finger-prick blood glucose measurement may be used if there is any doubt.

d. Poorly controlled diabetes on emergency admission

Any diabetic patient may present with uncontrolled diabetes, particularly if admitted as an emergency. This may be due to infection or vomiting. The diabetes must first be brought under control with rehydration and infusions of insulin, glucose and potassium.

Fig. 8.6 Thyrotoxic eye signs

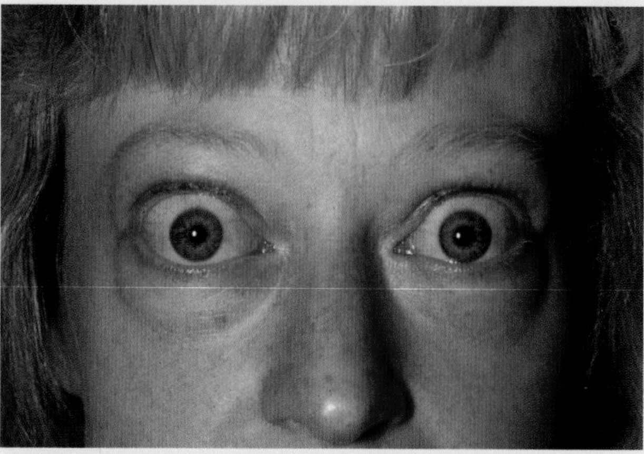

This woman of 36 presented with a typical history of primary thyrotoxicosis (Graves' disease), with weight loss, irritability and menstrual irregularity. In addition her eyesight had become blurred. She had florid exophthalmos with protruding eyeballs (proptosis) and lid lag. She was barely able to close her eyelids and would soon be at risk of corneal drying

THYROID DISEASE

THYROTOXICOSIS (Fig. 8.6)

Thyroid or non-thyroid surgery for a patient with uncontrolled thyrotoxicosis carries a risk of thyrotoxic crisis and this carries a high mortality. Thus any patient with features of thyrotoxicosis should have thyroid function tests (TSH and fT4) included in the preoperative assessment.

In surgery for hyperthyroidism, the patient should be rendered euthyroid before operation using antithyroid drugs (propylthiouracil can be useful as it blocks peripheral conversion of T4 to the active T3) and non-selective beta-blocking drugs.

HYPOTHYROIDISM

Patients with untreated hypothyroidism are at moderately increased risk when undergoing surgery. They are more sensitive to CNS depressants, have a decreased cardiovascular reserve, and are also susceptible to electrolyte disorders (particularly water retention). Severe infection, especially accompanied by trauma, a cold environment or depressant drugs, may precipitate myxoedema coma which, though very rare, is often fatal.

If there is clinical suspicion of hypothyroidism, operation should be postponed and thyroid function checked by measuring free thyroxine (fT4) and thyroid stimulating hormone (TSH) levels. If hypothyroidism is diagnosed, oral replacement therapy is commenced, but it may take several weeks to achieve the euthyroid state. If surgery must be performed urgently, it is usually best to proceed with the operation and begin oral treatment later.

DISORDERS OF ADRENAL FUNCTION

ADRENAL INSUFFICIENCY

The most common cause of adrenal insufficiency is hypothalamo–pituitary–adrenal suppression by long-term corticosteroid therapy. It is occasionally caused by primary adrenal failure (**Addison's disease**) or secondary to pituitary dysfunction (due to tumour or surgery). Very rarely, it results from previous adrenalectomy for treatment for a hypersecretion syndrome or bilateral primary adrenal tumours.

In primary or secondary adrenal failure, the patient is usually already taking oral steroid replacement therapy, but the lack of additional adrenal response to the stresses of trauma, surgery or infection may cause acute postoperative cardiovascular collapse with hypotension and shock (**Addisonian crisis**).

The 'typical' abnormal biochemical profile which should raise concern of the possibility of adrenal insufficiency is hyponatraemia, hyperkalaemia and raised blood urea (intravascular volume depletion). However, these abnormalities are neither sensitive nor specific and a short Synacthen test will be diagnostic.

Perioperative 'steroid cover'

Patients with potential adrenal insufficiency must be given steroid cover during the perioperative period. This is usually in the form of intravenous hydrocortisone, e.g. 25–50 mg prior to the operation and 50 mg daily until recovery. It is better to give prophylactic hydrocortisone in doubtful cases than risk acute hypoadrenalism. For any steroid-dependent patient, a doctor should write clearly in the notes *'Treat any unexplained collapse with hydrocortisone.'*

CUSHING'S SYNDROME

Cushing's syndrome results from excess secretion of cortisol. This may be in response to excess adrenocorticotropic hormone (ACTH) secretion by a pituitary tumour, ectopic ACTH secretion (usually by a malignant tumour) or rarely due to a primary tumour of an adrenal gland. The most common cause of Cushingoid features is long-term steroid therapy for conditions such as polymyalgia rheumatica or asthma. Clinically the patient may be plethoric, 'moon-faced', hypertensive, hirsute and obese with abdominal striae and have a characteristic 'buffalo hump'. The main surgical problems in Cushingoid patients are hypertension, hyperglycaemia, poor wound healing, infection and peptic ulceration. If the condition is due to steroid therapy, there is an additional risk of secondary adrenal insufficiency.

MUSCULOSKELETAL AND NEUROLOGICAL DISORDERS

Musculoskeletal and neurological disorders influence the outcome of surgery in two main ways. First, any condition which hinders mobility predisposes to chest infection, deep venous thrombosis and pulmonary embolism, aspiration pneumonitis and pressure sores. The last is even more likely if there is also sensory impairment due to stroke or diabetic peripheral neuropathy. Second, specific aspects of these disorders must be considered in relation to general anaesthesia, positioning of the patient on the operating table and the use of drugs.

RHEUMATOID ARTHRITIS

Rheumatoid arthritis poses special problems related to chronic anaemia, drug therapy and spinal complications. (*Note that some of these problems are shared by other collagen disorders*):

- **Normochromic normocytic anaemia**—common in chronic inflammatory disorders, including rheumatoid arthritis, although less common now that active inflammation is better controlled with modern drug therapy. The anaemia is refractory to iron therapy and there is no benefit from preoperative transfusion unless haemoglobin concentration is <8 g/dl, or the patient is symptomatic
- **Gastrointestinal disorders**—most will be taking NSAIDs, which together with long-term steroid therapy, predispose to peptic ulceration and perforation. Chronic low-grade bleeding from the upper gastrointestinal tract may exacerbate the existing anaemia in these patients. Operative stress may also precipitate acute gastrointestinal haemorrhage. NSAIDs may contribute to kidney injury
- **Long-term steroid therapy**—may result in adrenal insufficiency under stress
- **Other medications**—powerful drugs now used include chloroquine, methotrexate, sulfasalazine and cytokine inhibitors. Refer to standard formularies for potential problems
- **Odontoid subluxation** (Fig. 8.7)—if rheumatoid arthritis involves the atlanto-axial joint, the transverse ligament may be destroyed, allowing the odontoid process to sublux. During general anaesthesia, the protective reflexes are lost. If the neck is hyperextended during intubation, there is a serious risk of injury to the spinal cord by the unrestrained odontoid

Preoperative assessment of a patient with rheumatoid arthritis

Full blood count is essential to check for non-specific anaemia or iron deficiency anaemia; and plasma urea, electrolytes and creatinine are measured to identify chronic or drug-induced disturbance of renal function; inflammatory markers (ESR and CRP) indicate the activity of the disease. Preoperative assessment must include clinical examination of neck movements and cervical spine X-rays.

HAEMATOLOGICAL DISORDERS

ANAEMIAS

Severe anaemia leads to increased perioperative morbidity and mortality. General anaesthesia poses the greatest risk. For elective surgery, the haemoglobin concentration should be above 10 g/dl before operation but long-standing chronic anaemia probably poses little increased risk.

Management depends on the cause of the anaemia. Whether to transfuse before operation depends on the level

Fig. 8.7 Subluxation of the atlanto-axial joint in rheumatoid arthritis

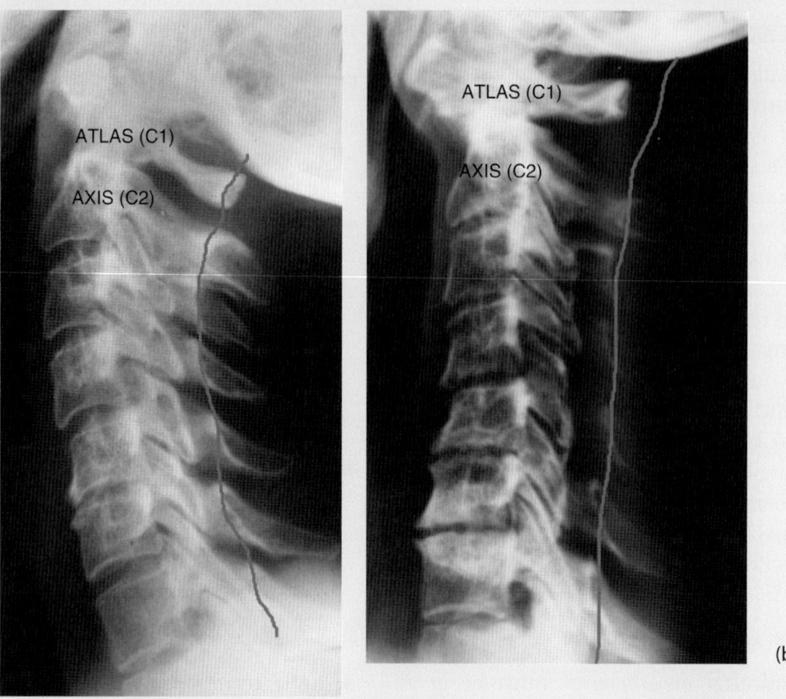

This 62-year-old woman with longstanding severe rheumatoid arthritis required a major abdominal operation. Cervical radiographs were taken before operation to anticipate problems during anaesthesia. (**a**) Cervical spine in extension. (**b**) The same patient in flexion. On each X-ray, a red line is drawn along the posterior limit of the spinal canal. Anterior subluxation (i.e. partial dislocation) is most obvious if the most posterior part of the spine of the atlas is compared with the line and with that of the axis in the two pictures. This mobility is caused by destruction of the transverse axial ligament of the odontoid by pannus (excessive granulation tissue) from the synovial joint. Under general anaesthesia, muscle relaxation may allow exaggeration of the subluxation, causing damage to the cervical cord

of anaemia (trigger levels have come down in recent years as a response to the shortage of blood for transfusion; see local guidelines), whether the anaemia is acute, and the expected operative blood loss. Transmission of human immunodeficiency virus (HIV) and other infective agents by transfusion is a very small risk in developed countries where sophisticated screening of donors is usual, but remains a serious risk in countries without such precautions. Transfusion for anaemia can usually be avoided in young, fit patients but elderly or very ill patients with less cardiorespiratory reserve are more likely to need transfusion. Transfusions should be given at least 24 hours before operation to allow fluid balance to stabilise and ensure optimal red cell function. For diagnosed deficiency anaemias, treatment as appropriate with iron, vitamin B_{12} or folate may be all that is necessary before operation. Treatment with erythropoietin (EPO) for patients with chronic renal failure is expensive but effective.

HAEMOGLOBINOPATHIES

Patients with sickle-cell disease and beta thalassaemia have a high operative mortality and morbidity, particularly if the condition is unrecognised, e.g. in emergencies. They require intensive perioperative management, avoiding hypoxia, infection, acidosis, dehydration and hypothermia. Patients with sickle-cell trait are at much lower risk and develop complications only if they become severely hypoxic. Sickle-cell trait and disease occur amongst black and mixed race people, who should always be asked specifically about a history of sickle-cell disease. A sickle-cell test must be performed before operation on any patient at risk so that the anaesthetist can be prepared.

POLYCYTHAEMIA

Polycythaemia may be caused by a primary myeloproliferative disorder such as **polycythaemia vera** or be secondary to chronic cardiac or pulmonary disease or heavy cigarette smoking. There is an increased red cell mass in primary and secondary polycythaemia producing a high haematocrit and increased blood viscosity. In primary polycythaemia, the platelet count may be increased which, paradoxically, is associated with defective haemostasis as well as the risk of thrombosis.

The main complications of polycythaemia vera are **haemorrhage** and **arterial or venous thrombosis**. The risk increases once the haematocrit rises above 50%. In general, operation should be postponed to allow treatment by venesection or myelosuppression. If possible, the cardiovascular system should be allowed to stabilise for about a month after treatment. In an emergency, the haematocrit may be reduced by preoperative venesection, restoring the volume by colloid infusion.

LEUKAEMIA, LEUCOPENIA AND THROMBOCYTOPENIA

Patients with these haematological disorders may need surgery for unrelated conditions. Prophylactic antibiotics may be required in neutropenia, and haematologists give specific advice in patients on chemotherapy. In thrombocytopenia, haemorrhage can be minimised by transfusing platelet concentrates.

BLEEDING DISORDERS

Bleeding diatheses such as thrombocytopenia, von Willebrand's disease (abnormal platelet function and factor VIII deficiency) and haemophilia are occasionally encountered in surgical practice. Most surgical haematological bleeding problems, however, are caused by poorly controlled anticoagulant therapy, liver disease, aspirin therapy and sometimes vitamin K malabsorption. The last occurs in obstructive jaundice and malabsorption syndromes.

A history of abnormal bleeding or factors which may predispose to abnormal bleeding should be sought from every surgical patient as follows:

- Excessive bleeding from simple cuts, previous surgery, dental extractions or childbirth
- Current use of anticoagulant drugs or anti-platelet drugs (aspirin and clopidogrel)
- A family history of bleeding disorders
- Intercurrent haematological or liver disease, cystic fibrosis or other malabsorption syndromes
- Recent jaundice
- Previous intestinal resection or bypass surgery

Recognising and treating a clotting problem before operation is vital because runaway haemorrhage can easily occur, causing clotting factor depletion. At this point, bleeding may be impossible to control even with transfusion of clotting factors.

If a bleeding disorder is suspected, a **platelet count** and **clotting screen** must be performed. The latter includes prothrombin time or ratio and activated partial thromboplastin time. If an abnormality is found, assays of individual clotting factors may be needed. Operation should be deferred if possible until the problem is overcome.

Clinical problems of bleeding disorders

a. Inherited clotting disorders

Haemophilia occurs in males. The disorder is an X-linked deficiency of factor VIII or, less commonly, factor IX. Specific antihaemophilic factors are administered before operation and for up to 2 weeks afterwards until the danger of secondary haemorrhage is past. **Von Willebrand's disease** is an autosomal dominant condition with abnormalities of both factor VIII and platelet function. It is managed with replacement of the specific factors.

b. Anticoagulant therapy

The management of patients on warfarin and other anticoagulants is described earlier in this chapter and in Chapter 12.

c. Liver disease

Bleeding disorders in cirrhosis are described earlier in this chapter, and disorders in the jaundiced patient are described in detail in Chapter 18.

d. Aspirin and clopidogrel therapy

Aspirin has an irreversible inhibitory effect on platelet aggregation which persists clinically for at least 10 days. The effect is reversed only when the affected platelets have been replaced. Most NSAIDs act on platelets in a similar but less profound way. High doses of intravenous penicillin cause a similar but short-lived effect. Aspirin ingestion, even in low doses, tends to cause oozing during and after operation, although this is rarely serious. For major elective arterial surgery, aspirin should ideally be stopped about 2 weeks before operation.

e. Malabsorption of fat-soluble vitamins

Vitamin K absorption may be impaired in pancreatic dysfunction, after resection of the proximal ileum or in malabsorption syndromes. The problem is readily overcome by preoperative injections of vitamin K.

PSYCHIATRIC DISORDERS

MENTAL ILLNESS AND LEARNING DISABILITY

Antidepressant drugs (tricyclic antidepressants) and antipsychotic (neuroleptic) drugs (such as phenothiazines) have a wide range of interactions (see *British National Formulary*). Plasma urea, electrolytes and thyroid function should be checked in patients taking **lithium** (usually for bipolar disorder), which may cause renal parenchymal damage and disturbed thyroid function.

ALCOHOLISM AND DRUG ADDICTION

Alcoholics are prone to cirrhosis, malnutrition and peripheral neuropathies. Drug addicts are at risk of hepatitis, HIV/acquired immunodeficiency syndrome (AIDS) and other infections. Alcohol acutely potentiates general anaesthetic agents, and an inebriated patient needs smaller doses. In contrast, chronic alcohol abuse induces liver enzymes which break down anaesthetic agents. This also increases tolerance to central nervous system depressants and higher doses of anaesthetics are needed. Similarly, larger doses of sedatives are required for gastrointestinal endoscopy. Opiate addiction leads to similar dosage problems.

Problems of drug withdrawal

Withdrawal symptoms may develop unexpectedly after operation if drug or alcohol addiction has been concealed. Alcohol withdrawal is characterised initially by irritability and tremors. Convulsions may develop after 24–48 hours. Full-scale **delirium tremens** may appear as long as 10 days after alcohol withdrawal. It is characterised by confusion and visual hallucinations accompanied by fever, tachycardia, pallor, vomiting and sweats. Similar symptoms and signs also occur in a range of other postoperative complications and alcohol withdrawal can be overlooked.

Alcoholic cirrhosis may cause episodic hypoglycaemia, the symptoms of which may be confused with those of delirium tremens. Hypoglycaemia should be excluded by measuring blood glucose.

Mild alcohol withdrawal states may be managed with regular oral doses of clomethiazole or benzodiazepines. Parenteral B vitamins are usually given daily. Opiate withdrawal symptoms are broadly similar to those of alcohol. Treatment is usually with a substitute drug such as methadone.

DEMENTIA

Patients with even mild dementia become even more confused when subjected to the strange and ever-changing environment of the surgical ward. They tolerate the stresses of general anaesthesia and operation poorly and so the benefit of any elective procedure should be carefully weighed against the possible adverse effects.

Sudden deterioration in mental state or increasing confusion may be provoked by infection, dehydration, electrolyte disturbances, hypoxia or overdose of drugs such as digoxin, hypnotics and sedatives. All these causes should be considered if a patient's mental state deteriorates in the perioperative

Table 8.1 Surgical complications of obesity

Complication	Factors
Cardiopulmonary complications such as cardiac failure and chest infections	Predisposing factors are atherosclerosis, increased demands on the cardiovascular system, decreased chest wall compliance, inefficient respiratory muscles and shallow breathing
Wound complications such as infection, dehiscence	Poor-quality abdominal wall musculature with fat infiltration. Large 'dead space' in which fat predisposes to haematoma formation
Venous thromboembolism—increased risk of deep venous thrombosis and pulmonary embolism	Poor peripheral venous return; delayed return to normal mobility
General anaesthesia complications	Anatomical problems, e.g. intravenous cannulae difficult to insert and intubation more difficult. Clinical signs of dehydration and hypovolaemia are more difficult to elicit Physiological problems: metabolic, e.g. altered distribution of drugs
Predisposition to various **medical disorders**	Hypertension, ischaemic heart disease, type 2 diabetes, gallstones, gout
Operative difficulties	Operations take longer because of difficult access and obscuring of vital structures by fat. Leads to a higher incidence of anaesthetic and surgical complications, particularly of the wound
Problems of manual handling	Weight and size limitations of standard equipment including CT scanners, operating tables, beds Need for hoists, powered beds Risks to staff involved in lifting and handling

Box 8.6 Potentially dangerous drugs in the surgical patient*

- Glucocorticoids
  - Predispose to peptic ulceration, delayed wound healing and infection
  - Adrenal atrophy caused by long-term steroid therapy may lead to acute adrenal insufficiency causing cardiovascular collapse
- Antihypertensive and anti-anginal drugs
  - Should not be stopped. Hazardous if abruptly stopped, which may cause rebound hypertension or angina
- Antidepressants
  - MAOIs are rarely used but should be stopped 2 weeks before surgery. Tricyclic antidepressants need not be stopped but carry risks of arrhythmias, hypotension and interaction with vasopressor drugs. Selective serotonin reuptake inhibitors should be continued. Stop lithium 24 hours before major surgery but not minor surgery
- Oral contraceptives and hormone replacement therapy (HRT)
  - Mildly increased risk of deep venous thrombosis and pulmonary embolism. HRT should be stopped 2 weeks before major surgery. Stopping OCP risks pregnancy
- Anticoagulants and anti-platelet drugs
  - Predispose to haemorrhage and need careful management
- Diuretics
  - May cause electrolyte abnormalities and dehydration. Potassium-sparing diuretics should be stopped on the morning of surgery

*Note that formularies such as the *BNF* carry details of drug interactions with anaesthetic agents

period. Such deterioration can be assessed using a mini-mental test questionnaire.

OBESITY

Gross obesity carries 2–3 times the risk of perioperative death or morbidity, as outlined in Table 8.1. Whenever possible, weight should be reduced before operation, particularly if it is not urgent. Referral to a dietician may be helpful although self-help groups often provide stronger motivation. Preoperative investigations for obese patients include blood glucose measurement, respiratory function tests and ECG, even if the patient is asymptomatic.

CHRONIC DRUG THERAPY

Many drugs prescribed for long-term treatment of 'medical' conditions can complicate management of the surgical patient. Note that the risk of stopping long-term medication before surgery is often greater than the risk of continuing it throughout. Drugs that should not normally be stopped include anticonvulsants, antiparkinsonian drugs, antipsychotics, anxiolytics, bronchodilators, cardiovascular drugs, glaucoma drugs, immunosuppressants, drugs of dependence and thyroid or antithyroid drugs. The most important of these commonly encountered in practice are summarised in Box 8.6.

9 Blood transfusion

PRINCIPLES OF BLOOD TRANSFUSION

The ability to safely transfuse blood and blood products revolutionised outcomes from major trauma. It also enabled extraordinary advances in areas of surgery involving heavy blood loss such as arterial reconstruction, open-heart surgery and organ transplantation.

Nevertheless, blood transfusion carries a range of potential **hazards**, including transfusion reactions, transmission of infection, clerical errors leading to incompatible transfusion, and potential immunosuppression in cancer patients. For replacing blood loss, stored blood has the advantage over gelatin and electrolyte solutions that it remains within the vascular compartment, although most 'blood' for transfusion consists of concentrated red cells with platelets and clotting factors removed. Potentially lethal side-effects mean that a decision to transfuse blood or blood products must be based on clear indications and after considering alternatives (see *Reducing the need for bank blood transfusion*, p. 120). The types of transfusion components available and the general indications for their use are summarised in Box 9.1.

LABORATORY ASPECTS OF BLOOD TRANSFUSION

BLOOD GROUPING AND COMPATIBILITY TESTING

Transfusion of ABO incompatible blood may be fatal. Transfusion practice aims to minimise this risk and involves two steps: first, determining the patient's ABO and Rhesus groups; second, screening the patient's blood (and each unit of donor blood) for antibodies. Traditionally, each unit of group-compatible donor blood has been directly **cross-matched** against the patient's serum to ensure compatibility. Fortunately, in donor blood shown to be antibody-free, 97% is completely compatible with a group-matched recipient and can safely be transfused without cross-matching. Thus grouped and antibody screened blood can be supplied quickly from a prepared pool, rather than individually cross-matching it. This saves time and money and most hospitals are adopting this practice.

After transfusion of about 10 units of blood, the patient's antibodies are so depleted that group-compatible blood can safely be given safely. In an emergency (e.g. obstetric haemorrhage) where group-compatible blood is unavailable, group O, Rh-negative blood can be given with comparative safety.

STORAGE AND USEFUL LIFE OF BLOOD

Blood and blood products have exacting requirements for preserving their quality. Their usefulness is easily impaired if handled inappropriately.

Packed red cells are stored between 2 °C and 6 °C, and have a shelf life of 35 days. Improved preservative solutions mean red cell quality deteriorates little during storage but pH changes occur and potassium leaches from the cells. The latter is only significant in neonates undergoing exchange transfusion or in patients with renal failure.

To ensure vitality, blood should be retained in the designated blood refrigerator until just before use. Blood removed for more than 30 minutes and not transfused should be returned to the laboratory for disposal because of the risk of bacterial proliferation. As soon as it becomes clear that blood products will not be required, the laboratory should be informed so they can be made available for other patients. Empty blood packs should be retained for 48 hours for examining and testing in the event of a transfusion reaction.

BLOOD TRANSFUSION IN CLINICAL PRACTICE

BLOOD TRANSFUSION AND ELECTIVE SURGERY

Attitudes to transfusion in elective surgery are becoming more conservative. Blood is expensive and its use carries risks. In elective surgery, patients fall into one of three categories: transfusion not anticipated (e.g. hernia repair), transfusion possible but unlikely (e.g. cholecystectomy), and transfusion probable (e.g. major arterial reconstruction). For patients in the second category, blood should be sent for ABO and Rhesus grouping and antibody screening, and serum retained for compatibility testing if required later ('group and save'). For patients in the third category, an appropriate number of units

Box 9.1 Types of transfusion and indications for their use

Whole blood

Very rarely used because of the demand for separate blood components. Whole blood carries greater risks of adverse reactions owing to the presence of leucocytes

Packed or concentrated red cells (the most common transfusion product)

For use in substantial haemorrhage and severe anaemia. Whole blood is collected then centrifuged to separate the red cells (and platelets and plasma). Packed/concentrated red cells are then suspended in a preservative solution ready for reinfusion. A bag of red cells is approximately 300 ml and raises the haemoglobin concentration by approximately 1 g/dl

Human albumin solution, available as 4.5% and 20% solutions

Albumin is expensive and is derived from human donor blood. In terms of efficacy, mortality and cardiorespiratory function, there is little evidence that albumin solutions are better than plasma substitutes or normal saline for resuscitating patients with **traumatic** or **septic shock** or requiring large perioperative volume replacement

Transfusion of albumin solutions should probably be restricted to patients with hypoproteinaemic oedema with nephrotic syndrome or with ascites in chronic liver disease. Other uses are difficult to justify in the absence of scientifically proven benefit

Fresh-frozen plasma (FFP)

Plasma is separated from fresh whole blood and then frozen. FFP contains near normal amounts of all clotting factors and other plasma proteins. It should be blood group compatible when possible and should not be used simply for volume replacement. FFP is often used to replace clotting factors exhausted during major haemorrhage (due to a combination of consumption of clotting factors by attempted haemostasis and the lack of clotting factors in transfused blood). This is likely when blood loss exceeds 1.5 times the blood volume, and the loss has been replaced rapidly with red cells and crystalloids or colloids. Clotting studies usually demonstrate a coagulopathy

FFP is also used to replace deficiencies of coagulation factors when there is continued bleeding and the necessary specific factor concentrates are unavailable. This may occur in liver disease, thrombotic thrombocytopenic purpura (TTP) and acute disseminated intravascular coagulation (DIC)

Platelet concentrates

Used for platelet exhaustion during major haemorrhage (e.g. ruptured abdominal aortic aneurysm) and in thrombocytopenia. Indicated if the platelet count is $<50\times10^9$/L, or massive blood loss is occurring. Platelets should be avoided in autoimmune platelet disorders except in the presence of life-threatening haemorrhage

Cryoprecipitate, fibrinogen and other specific clotting factor concentrates

Used for various specific coagulation deficiencies, e.g. severe hypofibrinogenaemia, haemophilia. These should only be used in consultation with a haematologist

Plasma substitutes

These are solutions of macromolecules with colloid osmotic pressure and viscosity characteristics similar to plasma. Gelatin solutions (e.g. Haemaccel, Gelofusine) and etherified starch solutions (e.g. hetastarch) are used for initial restoration of circulating volume in haemorrhage or burns and to maintain volume, blood pressure and renal perfusion intraoperatively where blood transfusion is not indicated

is requested for the operation; many hospitals operate a maximum blood ordering schedule (MSBOS) to ensure appropriate ordering. The blood is prepared a day or so before operation. If the antibody screen is negative and criteria for electronic cross-match are met, a serological cross-match is unnecessary and group-specific blood can be immediately issued. If a further transfusion is required more than 72 hours later, a new blood sample must be tested for new antibodies.

To prevent the disaster of giving blood to the wrong patient, transfusion blood samples must be scrupulously labelled **in the presence of the patient**. Immediately before transfusion, the label of each unit of blood must be checked against the identity and blood group of the patient (along with any compatibility slip).

VOLUME AND RATE OF TRANSFUSION

The volume of blood required and the rate of transfusion depend on age, the indications for transfusion and the patient's general and cardiovascular condition.

Volume and rate in haemorrhage

Haemorrhage can be classified according to rate and volume of loss. Loss of less than 1500 ml (30% of blood volume) normally requires only crystalloids/colloids except in preexisting anaemia. Loss of 30–40% of blood volume requires red cell transfusion, and more than 40% loss, equivalent to 2 L in an adult, requires rapid volume replacement with crystalloids/colloids followed by urgent provision of blood and blood products according to the local Massive Blood Loss protocol. Massive blood loss is defined as haemorrhage of 2 L blood in 3 hours, 4 L in 24 hours or >150 ml blood per minute. Urgent provision of blood products for life-threatening haemorrhage needs focus and good communication between transfusion laboratory and clinicians.

A sample massive loss protocol is to follow immediate resuscitation with 4 units of red cells via a blood warmer. O-negative blood can be given if the blood group is unknown, followed by group-specific or cross-matched red cells. If bleeding continues, further red cells should be accompanied by fresh-frozen plasma (FFP) to prevent coagulopathy. The ideal ratio of red cells to FFP is unclear but is about 4:4 or 4:3. Platelet concentrates are given to maintain levels at $>100\times10^9$/L. Repeat coagulation screens are needed after every 4 units to determine the need for other blood products, e.g. cryoprecipitate for fibrinogen levels. Hypothermia and hypocalcaemia should be corrected. If bleeding persists despite adequate blood product support, recombinant activated factor VII is occasionally recommended.

Volume and rate in anaemia

In anaemic elective surgical patients, the cause of anaemia should be investigated beforehand and appropriate treatment with haematinics begun. If transfusion proves necessary, it should be given at least 2 days before surgery to maximise its beneficial effects and allow fluid balance to stabilise. Surgery can usually be performed safely on patients with haemoglobin >10 g/dl. In addition, compensated anaemia down to 8 g/dl in a young person may be well tolerated. Older patients are less tolerant of anaemia unless it is chronic and little operative blood loss is expected.

REDUCING THE NEED FOR BANK BLOOD TRANSFUSION

Deaths and serious reactions still occur from incompatible transfusions (particularly when blood products are administered under general anaesthesia). In addition, serious infections such as hepatitis, malaria, HIV and variant Creutzfeldt–Jakob disease (vCJD) can be transmitted despite careful screening of donors and donations. The risk increases proportionate to the number of units transfused and can be reduced by critical scrutiny of the indications for transfusion.

NON-TRANSFUSION METHODS

Preoperative

- Tolerating lower haemoglobin concentration
- Iron therapy for iron deficiency anaemia
- Treatment with erythropoietin before or after operation, using recombinant human erythropoietin (rHuEPO)—this is very expensive

Intraoperative

- Using crystalloid or gelatin solutions for hypovolaemia

AUTOLOGOUS TRANSFUSION

Transfusion methods involve 'recycling' the patient's own blood **(autologous transfusion)** by one of the following methods:

Preoperative autologous donation (PAD)

Pre-deposit programmes where up to 4 units can be collected at weekly intervals from a patient planned for major elective surgery have several drawbacks: the collection, storage and checking system is costly and complicated and patients must be prepared well in advance. In addition, incompatible blood could be transfused because of clerical errors. As a result predonation is now rarely recommended.

Acute normovolaemic haemodilution (ANH)

This involves collecting whole blood from the patient immediately before surgery and replacing it afterwards if necessary. At collection, normovolaemia is restored with colloid or crystalloid. This allows autologous transfusion without the disadvantages of pre-donation or need for expensive intraoperative collecting and cell washing equipment. In adults without cardiac disease, up to 2 litres of blood can safely be removed.

The procedure reduces the venous haematocrit and increases cardiac output. When about 300 ml of low-haematocrit blood has been lost at operation, reinfusion is begun. The procedure is inexpensive, convenient and flexible as regards operation scheduling. The blood is fresh and contains functioning platelets and clotting factors. The collected blood is retained in the operating theatre, minimising the risk of clerical error. The technique has been used extensively in cardiac and vascular surgery but other types of surgery with a potential blood loss of more than 20% of blood volume could benefit.

Intraoperative cell salvage (IOCS)

UK government directives and national guidelines have endorsed intraoperative cell salvage as effective and appropriate in cardiac, vascular and orthopaedic surgery.

Intraoperative cell salvage involves collecting blood spilled at operation by suction, processing and reinfusion. There are two main techniques:

- In **manual** (unwashed) salvage, blood is collected into a reservoir containing anticoagulant before being reinfused via a fine filter
- In **washed** systems, an automated cell saver collects, washes, concentrates and resuspends salvaged red cells in physiological solution. This blood, with a packed cell volume of 50%, is then available for reinfusion. Some Jehovah's Witnesses allow this, as blood is regarded as never having left the body. The technique remains controversial in malignant disease even though clinical studies have not demonstrated dissemination of metastases.

Postoperative cell salvage (POCS)

Blood lost in the postoperative period is collected via a filtered wound drain and transfused via another filter. This is suitable for procedures with an expected and 'clean' postoperative blood loss such as total knee replacements.

HAZARDS AND COMPLICATIONS OF BLOOD TRANSFUSION

FEBRILE NON-HAEMOLYTIC TRANSFUSION REACTIONS (FNHTR)

These are usually caused by leucocyte incompatibility and are rare since universal leucodepletion of blood products. Febrile reactions are more common in multi-transfused or parous women. A temperature rise of greater than one degree and shivering during or after transfusion indicates a FNHTR. Symptoms usually subside after stopping the transfusion for 15–30 minutes and administering antipyretics and

Box 9.2 Clinical features of a haemolytic transfusion reaction

- Rapidly developing pyrexia at onset of transfusion
- Dyspnoea, constrictive feeling in chest, intense headache
- Severe loin pain
- Hypotension
- Acute oliguric renal failure with haemoglobinuria (due to obstruction of tubules with haemoglobin, hypotension causing acute tubular necrosis)
- Jaundice (developing hours or days later)
- Disseminated intravascular coagulation with spontaneous bruising and haemorrhage

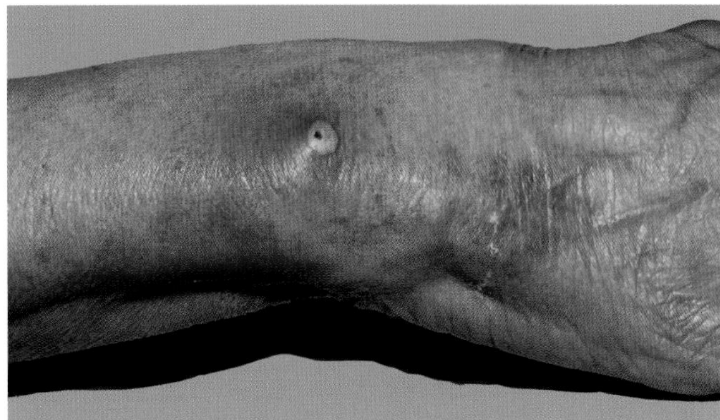

Fig. 9.1 Infected cannula site at the wrist

antihistamines. These reactions are rarely life-threatening, but fever with or without rigors may herald a serious reaction.

HAEMOLYTIC REACTIONS

If there is major ABO incompatibility, massive haemolysis may be fatal. Incompatibility of minor determinants causes a lesser degree of haemolysis. Almost all haemolytic reactions are caused by human error and incompatible transfusion. Clinical features are summarised in Box 9.2. The diagnosis is confirmed by blood tests—finding hyperbilirubinaemia and a positive Coombs' test, and demonstrating a new antibody. With massive haemolysis, haemoglobinaemia and haemoglobinuria may occur. The transfusion must be halted immediately and the patient resuscitated. Oliguria is treated by osmotic diuresis (e.g. mannitol), sometimes aided by a loop diuretic.

ALLERGIC REACTIONS

Allergic reactions to transfusion manifest as fever, pruritus (itching), skin rashes, wheals or angio-oedema (periorbital, facial and laryngeal swelling) and rarely, anaphylaxis. Mild reactions can usually be managed by slowing or stopping the transfusion for 30 minutes and administering antihistamines. Recurrent severe allergic reactions require antihistamine premedication and, occasionally, the use of saline washed cells. Investigation of the cause is required. Note that latex allergy is increasingly common and the effect may be wrongly interpreted as a transfusion reaction.

INFECTION

Infection may arise from three sources: the donor, contamination during blood preparation and storage, or from the giving set or cannula site (Fig. 9.1).

Infections transmitted by donor blood or blood product transfusion

Donated blood can now be screened for most significant transmissible infectious agents. Many tests rely on detecting antibodies to viruses and cannot identify disease acquired too recently for the antibody response to develop.

Donor infections are most likely when a **chronic latent carrier state** exists in the donor. Diseases include:

- **Viral infections**—hepatitis B, C and D; HIV I and II; HTLV I and II; cytomegalovirus; Epstein–Barr virus
- **Bacterial infections**—syphilis; brucellosis
- **Protozoal infections**—malaria; Chagas disease and babesiosis
- **Prions**—variant Creutzfeldt–Jakob disease (vCJD)

The more frequent of these infections are discussed below.

Hepatitis viruses

In carriers or infected individuals, hepatitis B virus is transmitted by any blood product. Donors have been screened for hepatitis B virus (HBV) by all transfusion services in the developed world since the late 1960s and this has dramatically reduced transfusion-related hepatitis B. Despite screening, infections occasionally occur because the surface antigen HBsAg, the first marker to appear, may be absent early after infection. For this reason, patients needing multiple transfusions or blood products should be vaccinated against hepatitis B.

Hepatitis C used to be transmitted via blood transfusion twice as often as hepatitis B. The illness caused by hepatitis C is often mild but up to half of all cases progress to chronic hepatitis (10% for hepatitis B), and 10% develop cirrhosis or hepatoma or both. Since 1991 all UK donations have been screened and the incidence of post-transfusion hepatitis C has fallen from 1.3 per 1000 units transfused to 0.1. However, the 'window' for HCV antigen to appear after infection can be up to 3 months.

Human immunodeficiency virus (HIV)

In 1981, the HIV epidemic and its link with blood transfusion was recognised, with reports of opportunistic pneumonias in haemophiliacs. By the mid-1980s, the risk of HIV transmission via transfused blood in the USA was as high as 1 in 2500. Luckily, transmission via surgical blood transfusion has been rare in the UK. Haemophiliacs were much less fortunate, being infected via clotting factor VIII preparations, often collected abroad.

In the UK, all blood donors and donations have been screened for HIV antibody since 1985. About 5 per million donors in the UK have proved HIV positive. Current HIV antibody detection is very reliable but there is a 'window' lasting 1–3 months after infection when antibody may be undetectable. The most effective method of reducing risk where donors are unpaid is self-exclusion by donors if they have transmissible infections or fall into high-risk categories. When combined with a low prevalence of HIV in the donor pool (as in the UK), the risk of transmitting HIV via a screened blood or blood component donation is small but not negligible.

Cytomegalovirus

Infection with cytomegalovirus is widespread, with the virus remaining latent in leucocytes. The risk of infection is significant only in immature neonates and CMV seronegative immunosuppressed patients. To minimise risk, donated blood for these groups should be screened for CMV-specific antibody. Leucodepletion removes 99.9% of white cells and is as effective in reducing the risk of CMV infection.

Protozoal infection—malaria

Transfusion-transmitted malaria remains rare in developed countries. In endemic areas it is common and most healthy blood donors are potentially infectious. The disease should be considered if a patient becomes ill after transfusion.

Variant Creutzfeldt–Jakob disease (vCJD)

vCJD was first described in the UK in 1996. It differs from the familial forms of CJD and is closely linked to bovine spongiform encephalopathy in cattle (BSE), and is thought to be acquired by ingestion of infected meat. There are currently 12–15 new cases of vCJD per annum in the UK, but the number incubating the disease is unknown.

vCJD is transmissible through blood products. There is currently no screening method, diagnostic tool or treatment for this disease. Avoiding unnecessary blood transfusion is the only way to minimise the risk. Prion filters have been developed and these will probably soon be recommended for transfusion recipients born after 1996.

Contamination of blood or giving sets with microorganisms

Low-grade environmental contamination of blood packs rarely has serious consequences because of the low temperature of blood storage and the self-sterilising properties of blood. However, microorganisms may proliferate if storage conditions are poor.

Transfusion of bacterially infected blood products is rare but can be catastrophic, leading rapidly to death. Platelet transfusions have been incriminated most often. Gram-negative aerobic bacilli, particularly *Pseudomonas* and *Salmonella* species, have been identified. Accumulation of exotoxins or endotoxins may also lead to life-threatening complications.

Giving sets may become contaminated unless strict aseptic technique is maintained during setting-up or changing of any component of transfusion equipment. Finally, peripheral intravenous cannulae, and particularly central venous lines, may become infected by opportunistic skin commensals (e.g. coagulase-negative staphylococci) or contaminating pathogens (e.g. *Staph. aureus, E. coli*) causing local infection (see Fig. 9.1), bacteraemia or even systemic sepsis. Cannula sites should be inspected daily and changed at least every 72 hours. In a patient with a central venous line and pyrexia of unknown origin, the line should be removed and tested bacteriologically.

The clinical result of transfusing a bacterially contaminated donation resembles a haemolytic reaction, with fever, chills, hypotension, nausea and vomiting, oliguria and disseminated intravascular coagulation. If a patient develops these symptoms, investigations should include culture of the patient's blood and the blood product as well as rechecking compatibility.

IMMUNOSUPPRESSIVE EFFECTS OF BLOOD TRANSFUSION

Blood transfusion has a potential for immunosuppression, which may influence recurrence of certain cancers and may increase postoperative infection rates. Nevertheless, data are contradictory in both areas and there is no definite evidence of an important clinical effect. In some patients, the potential immunosuppressive effects of blood transfusion may bring benefit, for example those undergoing renal transplantation.

FLUID OVERLOAD

Fluid overload is rarely a problem of blood transfusion in healthy adults but may readily develop if the cardiovascular system is already compromised or if particularly large volumes are given. Overload is a real risk when transfusing babies and small children.

TRANSFUSION-RELATED ACUTE LUNG INJURY (TRALI)

Transfusion, particularly of a plasma-containing product, may be followed by acute and rapid onset of shortness of breath and cough. There is typically a 'white-out' on chest X-ray. TRALI is treated in the same way as adult respiratory distress syndrome (ARDS) from any cause; it usually requires intensive care and mechanical ventilation. The injury is caused by donor antibodies reacting with the patient's leucocytes. Implicated donors are usually multiparous women and hence FFP is now sourced almost entirely from male donors.

DELAYED TRANSFUSION REACTIONS

Post-transfusion purpura (PTP)

This is fortunately rare as it is potentially fatal. It is more common in females and is caused by platelet-specific alloantibodies. Symptoms usually occur about a week after transfusion, with the patient developing thrombocytopenia and bleeding. PTP is treated with high doses of intravenous immunoglobulins, which gives a favourable response in around 85%.

Transfusion-associated graft versus host disease (Ta-GvHD)

In certain cases, transfused donor lymphocytes recognise the recipient's cells as foreign (even though compatible with the recipient) and initiate **graft versus host disease**. Patients most at risk are those with defective cell-mediated immunity. Irradiation of blood products is needed to inactivate T cells likely to cause GvHD in susceptible patients. The mortality rate of Ta-GvHD is 75–90% as there is no effective treatment.

10 Principles and techniques of operative surgery including neurosurgery and orthopaedics

INTRODUCTION

This chapter describes the operating environment and outlines the principles of operative surgery including those employed in 'minor' surgical techniques. All of these should be understood by all doctors, not just by surgeons, to help them appreciate the scope of surgery, to enable them to give meaningful explanations to patients before and after surgery and to help them assist intelligently at the operating table. Furthermore, most doctors are required to perform minor operations, emergency department procedures or invasive investigations at one time or another and these require knowledge of techniques.

Various suffixes derived from Greek and Latin are used in describing certain surgical techniques; these are summarised in Box 10.1.

PRINCIPLES OF ASEPSIS

INTRODUCTION

The main bacteria and viruses involved in surgical infections have been described in Chapter 3. The chief sources of infection are the patients themselves (particularly bowel flora), less commonly the hospital environment, food or cross-infection from other patients, and occasionally bacteria and viruses carried by ward staff or theatre personnel. Rare sources of infection are contaminated surgical instruments or equipment, dressings or parenteral drugs and fluids. The viruses causing hepatitis B and C and particularly human immunodeficiency virus (HIV) pose sinister risks of transmitting infection from patient to operating staff and vice versa. These risks make it mandatory to observe **universal blood and body fluid precautions** as described in Chapter 3.

The risk of postoperative bacterial infection depends on the extent of contamination of the wound or body cavity at operation or, in the case of intestinal perforation, before operation. Bacteria enter a wound by five possible routes:

- Direct inoculation from instruments and operating personnel
- Airborne bacteria-laden particles
- From the patient's skin
- From the flora of the patient's internal viscera, especially large bowel
- Via the bloodstream

Modern operating theatre design and correctly observed aseptic procedures minimise wound contamination but when infections occur, results can be devastating especially in relation to artificial prostheses, skin grafts, bone and the eye. Furthermore, some patients are particularly vulnerable to infection, notably neonates, the immunosuppressed, the debilitated and the malnourished. Note that treatment of established infection is no substitute for prevention.

The use of preoperative prophylactic antibiotics began in the 1970s and has revolutionised the outcome of certain types of operative surgery in a manner comparable to the changes

Box 10.1 Surgical terminology

- *oscopy*=examination of a hollow viscus, body cavity or deep structure employing an instrument specifically designed for the purpose, e.g. gastroscopy, colonoscopy, laparoscopy, arthroscopy, bronchoscopy. The general term is **endoscopy**
- *ectomy*=removal of an organ, e.g. gastrectomy, orchidectomy (i.e. removal of testis), colectomy
- *orrhaphy*=repair of tissues, e.g. herniorrhaphy
- *ostomy*=fashioning an artificial communication between a hollow viscus and the skin, e.g. tracheostomy, colostomy, ileostomy. The term may also apply to artificial openings between different viscera intra-abdominally, e.g. gastro-jejunostomy, choledocho-duodenostomy (i.e. anastomosis of duodenum to common bile duct)
- *otomy*=cutting open, e.g. laparotomy, arteriotomy, fasciotomy, thoracotomy
- *plasty*=reconstruction, e.g. pyloroplasty, mammoplasty, arthroplasty
- *pexy*=relocation and securing in position, e.g. orchidopexy (for undescended testis), rectopexy (for rectal prolapse)

heralded by Lister's introduction of antisepsis in the late nineteenth century.

THE OPERATING ENVIRONMENT

Modern **operating theatre design** plays a key role in control of airborne wound contamination. This is important mainly for staphylococci carried on airborne skin scales.

The main factors influencing airborne operating theatre infection rates are:

- The concentration of organisms in the air
- The size of bacteria-laden particles
- The duration of exposure of the open wound

The first two are influenced mainly by theatre design and air supply, and the last can be minimised by avoiding unnecessarily long procedures. Operating theatre complexes are laid out so as to minimise introduction of infection from outside via air, personnel or patients. Air is drawn from the relatively clean external environment, filtered and then supplied to the theatres at a slightly higher pressure than outside to ensure a constant outward flow. **Air turnover** is the most important factor; the aim is to ensure 3–15 air changes per hour which 'scrubs out' the theatre air by dilution. Standard air delivery systems aim to achieve a constant flow of clean air towards the operating table, which is then exhausted from the theatre. Despite this, convection currents allow some recirculation of air, which may be contaminated, into the operation site.

The crucial importance of preventing infection in joint replacement surgery led to the development of sophisticated **ultra-clean air delivery systems**. These reduce postoperative infection two- to four-fold in joint replacement surgery, but the cost is very high. Enclosure of the patient in a sterile tent in which the surgeons wear space-type suits can reduce infection rates by a further 5–7.5%.

Minimising infection from operating theatre personnel

Only a modest proportion of wound infections derive from theatre personnel. Bacteria reach the wound via the air or by direct inoculation, often from viscera within the wound. About 30% of healthy people carry *Staphylococcus aureus* in the nose but pathogenic organisms may also be present in axillae and the perineal area, the last probably being the most important source of wound infections from theatre personnel. In addition, skin abrasions are usually infected, as are skin pustules and boils; thus personnel with these lesions must ensure that they are effectively covered with occlusive dressings or else should not enter the operating area.

Airborne, personnel-derived infection is reduced by changing from potentially contaminated day clothes to clean theatre clothes and shoes which should not be worn outside the theatre complex. Trouser cuffs should be elasticated or tucked into boots. Females should wear trousers instead of dresses, in order to reduce 'perineal fallout'. **Face masks** are worn to deflect bacteria-containing droplets in expired air, but most types become ineffective after a very short period, especially when wet. With the exception of nasal *Staph. aureus* (particularly important in prostheses infection), bacteria derived from the head do not generally cause wound infection. The effectiveness of wearing masks and hair coverings to reduce infection is unknown.

Sterile gloves and gowns are worn by surgeons and staff directly involved in the operation to prevent inoculation of bacteria. Gloves are impermeable to bacteria but hands and forearms need washing before gloving and gowning with antiseptics that persist on the skin. This minimises bacterial contamination if a glove is punctured (as often happens) or the sleeve of the gown becomes wet. The traditional ritual of scrubbing with a brush for 3 minutes is actually less effective than washing the hands thoroughly because it causes microtrauma and brings bacteria to the surface.

Despite the protection given by wearing gloves and gown, the less a wound is handled the better. This principle applies particularly when aseptic conditions are less than ideal. On the ward, minor procedures such as bladder catheterisation or chest drain insertion should be performed using sterile precautions and a **no-touch technique**. Catheters, for example, should not be handled directly but only within their wrapper or with instruments.

Minimising infection from the patient's skin

The patient's skin, especially the perineal area, is the source of up to half of all wound infections. These may be minimised by the following measures:

- **Removing body hair**—body hair was thought to be a source of wound contamination but this is no longer believed. Hair is removed only to allow the incision site to be seen and the wound to be closed without including hair. Shaving produces abrasions which rapidly become colonised with skin commensals. Most surgeons now restrict hair removal to clipping away just enough to provide skin access.
- **Painting the skin with antiseptic solutions**—povidone-iodine or chlorhexidine in alcoholic or aqueous solution is applied to a wide area around the proposed operation

site ('skin prep'). In the past, patients were subjected to ineffective applications of antiseptics such as gentian violet for several days beforehand!

- **Draping the patient**—the operating area is isolated by placing sterile, (ideally self-adhesive) drapes made of impermeable paper or coated waterproof material over all but the immediate field of operation.

Reducing infection from internal viscera

The large bowel teems with potentially pathogenic bacteria and the peritoneal cavity inevitably becomes contaminated in any operation where large bowel is opened. Pathogenic bacteria are also found in obstructed small bowel. The same applies to the stomach and small bowel of patients on proton pump inhibitors where the normal bactericidal effect of gastric acid is lost. Great care should be taken at operation to minimise this contamination. Bowel preparation of the colon before operation may help this process. All patients having bowel operations should be given prophylactic antibiotics before operation.

Sterilisation of instruments and other supplies

(see Table 10.1)

In modern surgical practice, infection from instruments, swabs, equipment and intravenous fluids has been virtually eliminated by the use of sterile packs from central sterile supply departments (CSSD). Reusable instruments and drapes are sterilised by high-pressure steam autoclaving according to strict regulations. Most disposable items are purchased in pre-sterilised, sealed packs. Sterilisation in small autoclaves near the operating theatre should only be performed if instruments in short supply are required for successive operations. Sterilisation by any method is ineffective unless all organic material is first removed by thorough cleaning. It is also important to transport soiled instruments promptly to CSSD as proteinaceous material becomes fixed to metal and resistant to removal. This is especially true for small and microsurgical instruments (e.g. in ophthalmology), where channels easily become blocked by organic matter and prevent effective sterilisation.

Instruments which would be damaged by heat, including plastics, cystoscopic lenses, flexible endoscopes and electrical equipment, can be sterilised using a variety of chemical methods such as ethylene oxide gas. The Sterilox method is commonly used for endoscopic instruments that need to be reused several times during a session; the endoscopes are bathed in an electro-chemically activated water system through which an electrical current is passed.

World-wide, many surgical instruments are prepared by boiling water 'sterilisers'. Boiling water is markedly inferior to other methods but is included here as it may be the only practical method in developing countries because of cost and technical difficulties. Boiling water kills most vegetative organisms within 15 minutes but spores are not killed. All organic debris should, as always, be scrupulously removed first, then the instruments immersed in visibly boiling water, returned to the boil and boiled continuously for at least 30 minutes to ensure hepatitis and human immunodeficiency viruses are destroyed.

SURGICAL TECHNIQUE

Surgical technique plays an important part in minimising the risk of operative infection. Non-vital tissue and collections of fluid and blood are vulnerable to colonisation by infecting organisms, which may enter via the bloodstream even if direct contamination has been avoided by aseptic technique. Tissue damage should be kept to a minimum by careful handling and retraction and by avoiding unnecessary diathermy coagulation. Haematoma formation is minimised by careful haemostasis and placing drains into potential sites of fluid collection; **closed-drainage** or **suction-drainage** systems reduce the risk of organisms tracking back into the wound from the ward environment.

During extensive resections of bowel, early ligation of its blood supply allows bacteria to permeate the wall (**translocation**) and this may contaminate the peritoneal cavity.

Faecal contamination is associated with a high risk of infection and great care needs to be taken in operations where bowel is opened. In emergency operations for large bowel perforation, free faecal matter is meticulously removed. A planned **'second look' laparotomy** after 48 hours is advisable to deal with remaining contamination and new abscesses even if the patient appears well.

Prevention of cross-infection (nosocomial infection)

Cross-infection is the term used for infection transmitted from other patients in the nearby hospital environment and should be distinguished from **colonisation** with other patients' bacteria. Cross-infection is mainly spread via staff, medical equipment, food or ward furnishings. Doctors are probably the worst offenders as regards transfer of infection—by removing dressings to inspect wounds in the open ward, by failing to cleanse hands between patients and by careless aseptic technique when performing ward procedures such as bladder catheterisation. Minimising patient

Table 10.1 Time and temperature requirements for sterilisation by different methods

Method	Equipment to be sterilised	Temperature	Time
Steam autoclave	Unwrapped instruments and bowls Instrument sets, dressings and rubber	123°C	10 min
		126°C	3 min
Ethylene oxide gas	Heat-sensitive materials; plastics, endoscopes, electrical equipment	55°C	2–24 h
Liquid glutaraldehyde	Cystoscopes and other urological equipment, plastics and heat-sensitive equipment required urgently	Room temperature	10 min

movements between wards and hospital units also decreases cross-infection rates.

A patient with an infection that is potentially dangerous to other patients, such as meticillin-resistant *Staph. aureus* (MRSA), should be isolated and barrier-nursed in a single room.

Prophylactic antibiotics

Despite using the best aseptic techniques, some operations carry a high risk of wound infection as well as other infective complications; these can be dramatically reduced by using prophylactic antibiotics. The chosen antibiotics should be matched to the organisms likely to occur in the area of the operation and should be bactericidal rather than bacteriostatic (see Table 10.2). The relative risk of postoperative infection in different types of operation is summarised in Box 10.2.

As a general principle, pre or peroperative prophylactic antibiotics are indicated if the anticipated risk of infection exceeds 10%, e.g. all emergency abdominal surgery and all elective colonic operations. Prophylactic antibiotics are also

Table 10.2 Recommended antimicrobial prophylaxis for clinical conditions and surgical procedures

	Likely organisms	Antibiotic
Abdominal surgery		
Severe acute pancreatitis	Coliforms Anaerobes	Ciprofloxacin 400 mg i.v. + metronidazole 500 mg i.v. or meropenem 1 g i.v.
Colonic and other bowel surgery	Coliforms Anaerobes *Staphylococcus aureus* *Streptococcus pyogenes* (Group A Strep.)	Co-amoxicillin-clavulanate 1.2 g i.v.
Appendicectomy	Anaerobes	Rectal metronidazole suppository 1 g or proportionately less in children or co-amoxicillin-clavulanate 1.2 g i.v.
Endoscopic gastrostomy Gastroduodenal surgery Oesophageal surgery	Anaerobes *Staphylococcus aureus* *Streptococcus pyogenes* (Group A Strep.) Coliforms *Candida spp.*	Co-amoxicillin-clavulanate 1.2 g i.v. + fluconazole 50 mg i.v.
Inguinal or other hernia repair with mesh	*Staphylococcus aureus* *Staphylococcus epidermidis (coagulase-negative)* *Streptococcus pyogenes (Group A Strep.)* Coliforms	Co-amoxicillin-clavulanate 1.2 g i.v.
Hernia repair without mesh		Not recommended
Laparoscopic cholecystectomy		Co-amoxicillin-clavulanate 1.2 g i.v. (but little clinical evidence of efficacy)
Orthopaedic surgery		
Total hip replacement or prosthetic knee joint	*Staphylococcus aureus* *Staphylococcus epidermidis* (coagulase-negative) *Streptococcus pyogenes* (Group A Strep.) Coliforms	Co-amoxicillin-clavulanate 1.2 g i.v. for 3 doses If MRSA risk factors or known MRSA: add vancomycin 1 g i.v. 12-hourly for 2 doses
Trauma with contaminated wounds	*Staphylococcus aureus* *Streptococcus pyogenes* (Group A Strep.)	Co-amoxicillin-clavulanate 1.2 g i.v. 3 doses or doxycycline 100 mg orally If heavily contaminated or dead tissue, co-amoxicillin-clavulanate 1.2 g i.v. for 7 days
Elective orthopaedic surgery without prosthetic device		Not recommended

Table 10.2 Recommended antimicrobial prophylaxis for surgical procedures and clinical conditions—cont'd

	Likely organisms	Antibiotic
Vascular surgery		
Lower limb amputation or vascular surgery, abdominal and lower limb	*Staphylococcus aureus* *Staphylococcus epidermidis* (coagulase-negative) *Streptococcus pyogenes* (Group A Strep.) Coliforms	Co-amoxicillin-clavulanate 1.2 g i.v. If MRSA, **add** vancomycin 1 g i.v.
ENT surgery		
Head and neck surgery	*Staphylococcus aureus* *Streptococcus pyogenes* (Group A Strep.) Coliforms Anaerobes	Co-amoxicillin-clavulanate 1.2 g i.v. If MRSA, **add** vancomycin 1 g i.v.
Ear, nose, sinus Tonsillectomy		Not recommended
Urology		
Transrectal prostate biopsy Shock wave lithotripsy Transurethral resection of prostate (TURP) or laser enucleation	Coliforms *Enterococcus*	Amoxicillin 1 g i.v. + gentamicin 120 mg i.v. or ciprofloxacin 200 mg i.v.

Box 10.2 Relative risk of infection in surgical wounds

Risk 2–5%

Clean operations with no preoperative infection and no opening of gastrointestinal, respiratory or urinary tracts (e.g. inguinal herniorrhaphy, breast lump excision, ligation of varicose veins)

Risk less than 10%

Clean operations with gastrointestinal, respiratory or urinary tracts opened but with minimal contamination (e.g. elective cholecystectomy, transurethral prostatectomy excision of un-inflamed appendix)

Risk about 20%

Operations where tissues inevitably become contaminated but without pre-existing infection (e.g. elective large bowel operations, appendicectomy where the appendix is perforated or gangrenous, fresh traumatic skin wounds (except on the face))

Risk greater than 30%

Operations in the presence of infection (e.g. abscesses within body cavities, small bowel perforation, delayed operations on traumatic wounds)

Risk greater than 50%

Emergency colonic surgery (bowel unprepared) for perforation or obstruction

Box 10.3 Principles of antimicrobial prophylaxis

- A single dose of antibiotic is adequate for most purposes
- Never continue prophylaxis for more than 48 hours
- Dose should be administered immediately before the procedure
- If the patient is already suspected of having an infection, go straight to treatment

used by many surgeons for operations in the 5–10% risk category, e.g. cholecystectomy. Prophylactic antibiotics are also indicated for inherently low-risk cases where the consequences of infection would be catastrophic, e.g. operations employing prosthetic implants, or in patients with mitral stenosis or other cardiac defects at risk of infective endocarditis. Prophylactic antibiotics can reduce postoperative infection rates in high-risk cases by 75%, and may almost entirely eliminate infection where the risk is lower.

In most wound-related infections, the organisms are introduced during the operation and become established during the next 24 hours. Thus, for prophylactic antibiotics to be effective, high blood levels must be achieved during the operation when contamination occurs. To achieve this, the first dose should be given 1 hour before operation or preferably intravenously at induction of anaesthesia; prophylactic antibiotics should not be given earlier as this may encourage resistant organisms to proliferate (Box 10.3). A single preoperative dose of antibiotic is generally sufficient if it is rapidly bactericidal and the inoculum of bacteria is small; long operations with heavy blood loss, e.g. ruptured abdominal aortic aneurysm, merit a second perioperative dose of antibiotics later in the operation. Longer courses of prophylactic antibiotics are of no advantage.

In general, intravenous antibiotics give the most predictable blood levels and peak tissue levels are achieved within 1 hour of injection. However, for prophylaxis against anaerobes, metronidazole administered rectally gives blood and tissue levels equivalent to intravenous administration but later, 2–4 hours after administration.

Operations involving bowel and biliary system

Patients having these operations are at risk mainly from a mixture of Gram-negative bacilli (Enterobacteriaceae family), faecal anaerobes (*Bacteroides fragilis*) and *Staph. aureus*. Less commonly, enterococci cause surgical infection, notably *E. faecalis* (formerly *Strep. faecalis*).

The most commonly used prophylactic antibiotic regimens are shown below. A more comprehensive list is given in Table 10.2:

- For biliary surgery—co-amoxicillin-clavulanate
- For colonic and other bowel surgery—either co-amoxicillin-clavulanate or a combination of gentamicin, benzylpenicillin (or ampicillin) and metronidazole
- For appendicectomy—rectal metronidazole alone, given 2 hours before operation; this has proved as effective as any other regimen. The evidence for the beneficial effect of metronidazole in preventing infection after appendicectomy is now so strong that it may be negligent not to use it

The choice of antibiotics for prophylaxis must be kept under review because organisms change their sensitivities. Aminoglycosides such as gentamicin have the important advantage do not alter the bowel flora because their concentration in the lumen is low; this is in contrast to the cephalosporins and ampicillin, which have caused a rising tide of beta-lactam-resistant bowel organisms insensitive to cephalosporins and ampicillin but sensitive to aminoglycosides. If resistant staphylococci are a problem, vancomycin or other newer antibiotics may become necessary for prophylaxis.

Operations involving implantation of prostheses

Vascular grafts and joint replacements are at particular risk from *Staph. aureus* infection. Coagulase-negative slime-forming staphylococci (e.g. *Staph. epidermidis*) are a common source of chronic infection. Coliforms are a very rare cause. Flucloxacillin is the agent of first choice for prophylaxis but gentamicin is usually added for extra protection. Rifampicin can be used to soak vascular grafts as it is effective against *Staph. epidermidis*. Meticillin-resistant *Staph. aureus* (MRSA) is becoming a common cause of prosthetic infection. In areas where the risk is substantial, prophylaxis with vancomycin is appropriate.

Operations where ischaemic or necrotic muscle may remain

Lower limb amputations for arterial insufficiency and major traumatic injuries involving muscle are susceptible to gas gangrene and tetanus. **Clostridia** are highly sensitive to benzylpenicillin and metronidazole, one of which should be given in high dose as early as possible after major trauma, and before major amputations for ischaemia. Co-amoxicillin-clavulanate is a good alternative.

BASIC SURGICAL TECHNIQUES

ANAESTHESIA

General principles

Some form of anaesthesia is needed for almost every surgical procedure, with the aim of preventing pain in all cases, minimising stress for the patient in most, and providing special conditions for some operations, e.g. muscular relaxation in abdominal surgery. The choice of anaesthetic techniques includes **topical (surface) anaesthesia, local anaesthetic infiltration or peripheral nerve block, spinal or epidural anaesthesia** and **general anaesthesia**. Methods other than general anaesthesia may be supplemented with intravenous sedation if the patient is anxious or agitated (e.g. with benzodiazepines). Intravenous sedation with these drugs produces relaxation, anxiolysis and amnesia whilst retaining protective reflexes. However, these drugs can also cause unconsciousness and they must be carefully titrated to produce just the desired effects. Intravenous sedation of this type does not provide pain relief; if needed, this is achieved with local anaesthesia or intravenous analgesics.

Choice of anaesthetic technique

Combining local or regional anaesthesia (for pain relief) with general anaesthesia can minimise postoperative respiratory and cardiovascular depression compared with general anaesthesia alone, reducing morbidity. An example is the use of caudal anaesthesia in perineal operations. Local or regional anaesthesia with bupivacaine or levobupivacaine can also be administered during an operation to provide postoperative pain relief; for example, intercostal nerve blocks during an abdominal operation allow more comfortable breathing and coughing, reducing respiratory complications. Another common example is wound infiltration with the same long-acting local anaesthetics. The main factors influencing choice of anaesthesia are summarised in Box 10.4.

INCISION TECHNIQUE

Choice of incision

The purpose of most skin incisions is to gain access to underlying tissues or body cavities. When planning an incision, the first concern is to achieve good access and also allow it to be extended if necessary. It must also be sited in such a way that it can be effectively closed to give the best chance of primary healing and the lowest chance of an incisional hernia later. Despite patients' impressions, the length of an incision (and the number of sutures) has little bearing on the rate of healing, and the success of an operation should not be put at risk by inadequate access.

Box 10.4 Choice of anaesthetic technique

1. Local anaesthesia

In general, this safest form of anaesthesia is used for calm and rational patients when no autonomic discomfort is anticipated:

- Minor operations, e.g. excision of small skin lesions or dental operations
- Minor but painful procedures, e.g. insertion of chest drain, siting of peripheral venous cannulae
- Unavailability of general anaesthetic expertise, e.g. in developing countries
- Patients unfit for general anaesthesia, e.g. cardiac and respiratory cripples
- Ambulatory ('day case') surgery especially if co-morbidity
- Patients unwilling to undergo general anaesthesia
- Use of combined local anaesthetic and vasoconstrictor to provide a relatively bloodless operative field. (*Note*: this must never be used in the extreme peripheries, i.e. digits, penis, nose)

2. Regional nerve block

- Minor surgery requiring wide field of anaesthesia, e.g. femoral nerve block for varicose vein surgery, pudendal block for forceps delivery
- When it is undesirable to inject local anaesthetic into the operation site, e.g. drainage of an abscess (local anaesthesia works less well in inflamed tissue)
- To avoid tissue distortion from local infiltration in delicate surgery
- Short-lived, wide-field ambulatory anaesthesia for reduction of forearm fractures or hand surgery (Bier's intravenous regional anaesthesia)

3. Epidural and spinal anaesthesia

- Lower limb surgery, e.g. amputations
- Lower abdominal, groin, pelvic and perineal surgery, e.g. Caesarean sections, inguinal hernia repair, prostatectomy, bladder and urethral surgery

4. Intravenous sedation or intravenous analgesia alone

- Short-lived uncomfortable procedures where local anaesthesia is impractical, e.g. gastrointestinal endoscopy, musculoskeletal manipulation

5. Intravenous sedation combined with local anaesthesia

- Potentially unpleasant procedures despite adequate local anaesthesia, e.g. wisdom tooth extraction, toenail operations, siting of central venous lines

6. Regional analgesia with light general anaesthesia

- Caudal epidural plus general anaesthesia for operations in the perineal area, e.g. transurethral prostatectomy or resection of bladder tumours, haemorrhoidectomy, circumcision. This provides perioperative and postoperative analgesia

7. General anaesthesia

- Where all of the above are unsuitable or difficult to achieve
- Severe patient apprehension or patient preference for general anaesthesia
- Major or prolonged operations
- Abdominal or thoracic operations requiring muscle relaxation
- Where it is necessary to secure the airway by intubation
- Special indications, e.g. neurosurgery

Secondary considerations in the choice of incision are as follows:

- **Orientation of skin tension lines (based on Langer's lines) and skin creases**—where possible, incisions should be made parallel to the lines of skin tension determined by the orientation of dermal collagen (e.g. a 'collar' incision for thyroid operations) as the wound is less likely to break down, there is minimal distortion, and healing occurs with little scar tissue to give the best cosmetic result
- **Strength and healing potential of the tissues**—the nature and distribution of muscle and fascia influences the strength of the repair, particularly in different parts of the abdominal wall. For example, a vertical lower midline incision along the linea alba, a strong layer of fascia, is less prone to incisional herniation than a paramedian incision lateral to the midline
- **The anatomy of underlying structures, particularly nerves**—the incision line should run parallel to, but some distance away from the expected course of underlying structures, reducing the risk of damage. For example, to gain access to the submandibular gland, the incision is made 2 cm below the lower border of the mandible to avoid the mandibular branch of the facial nerve
- **Cosmetic considerations**—wherever possible, incisions should be placed in the least conspicuous position, such as in a skin crease or a site that will later be concealed by clothing or hair, e.g. a transverse suprapubic (**Pfannenstiel** or bucket-handle) incision below the 'bikini' line for operations on the bladder, uterus or ovary, or a peri-areolar incision for breast biopsy

Dissection and handling of deeper tissues

The skin consists of thin **epidermis** and dense, somewhat thicker **dermis**, as well as the underlying fatty **hypodermis** which may be 10 cm or more thick in an obese individual.

Once the skin incision has been made, the scalpel is mainly reserved for incising fascia and other fibrous structures such as breast tissue and very fine dissection. Anatomical detail is exposed and displayed by a combination of blunt and sharp dissection. **Blunt dissection** involves teasing or stripping tissues apart using fingers, swabs or blunt instruments, following natural tissue planes. **Sharp dissection** with scissors and forceps or scalpel is used where tissues have to be cut and also to display small structures. Some surgeons prefer sharp to blunt dissection in general, believing it causes less tissue trauma. Most dissection, however, involves a combination of both.

PRINCIPLES OF HAEMOSTASIS

Bleeding is an unavoidable part of surgery. Blood loss should be minimised because bleeding obscures the operative field and hampers operative technique (the finer the surgery, the more bleeding affects visibility and quality of outcome), and because the loss has to be made up later. Excessive bleeding can be averted by judicious dissection with control of bleeding as the operation proceeds, and by minimising the area of raw tissue exposed at the operation site by accurately siting the incision and by avoiding opening unnecessary tissue planes.

Clipping, ligation and under-running

Ligation or specialised bipolar diathermy is obligatory when large vessels are divided and is desirable for vessels larger than about 1 mm calibre (see Fig. 10.1). If the end of a bleeding vessel cannot be grasped by haemostat forceps, a suture can be used to encircle the vessel and its surrounding tissues, a technique often described as **under-running**. It is particularly useful for a bleeding artery in the fibrous base of a peptic ulcer.

Diathermy

Diathermy achieves haemostasis by local intravascular coagulation and contraction of the vessel wall caused by heating (*-thermy*), generated by particular electrical waveforms. However, enough heat is also produced to burn the tissues and these may be needlessly damaged by careless use, particularly near the skin or nerves. Ordinary diathermy is ineffective for large vessels, which should be ligated. There are three main variants of diathermy, illustrated in Figure 10.2, and all three modes are available on modern diathermy machines.

Monopolar diathermy is the most widely used for operative haemostasis but there is wide dispersion of coagulating and heating effects, making it unsuitable for use near nerves and other delicate structures. Since the current passes through the patient's body, there is a risk of coagulating vessels *en passant* (e.g. monopolar diathermy used in circumcision may cause penile thrombosis), as well as provoking arrhythmias in patients with cardiac pacemakers. Monopolar diathermy may also result in skin burns at the **indifferent electrode plate** if skin contact is poor or if the plate becomes wet during operation. To improve contact, hair should be shaved from the skin where the plate is placed.

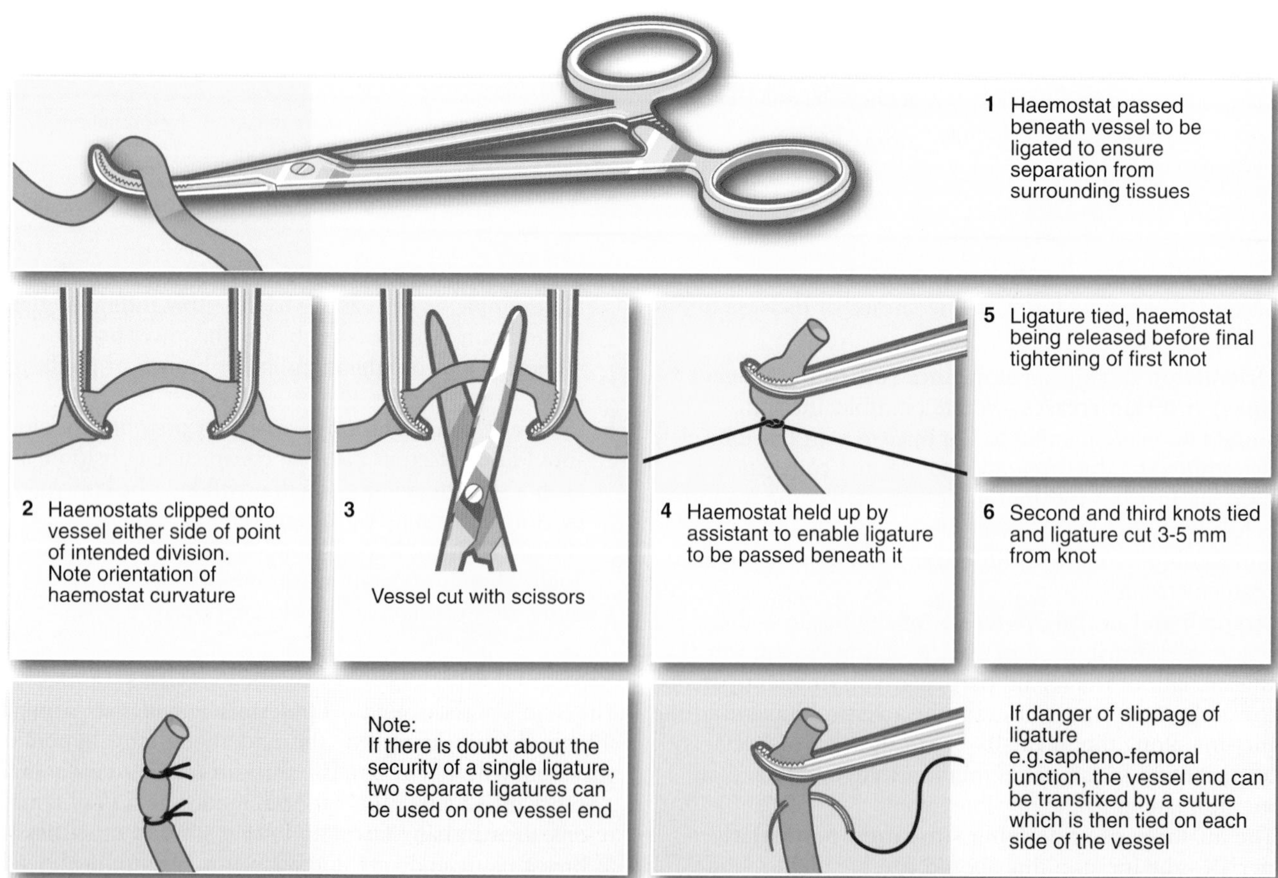

Fig. 10.1 Techniques of haemostasis

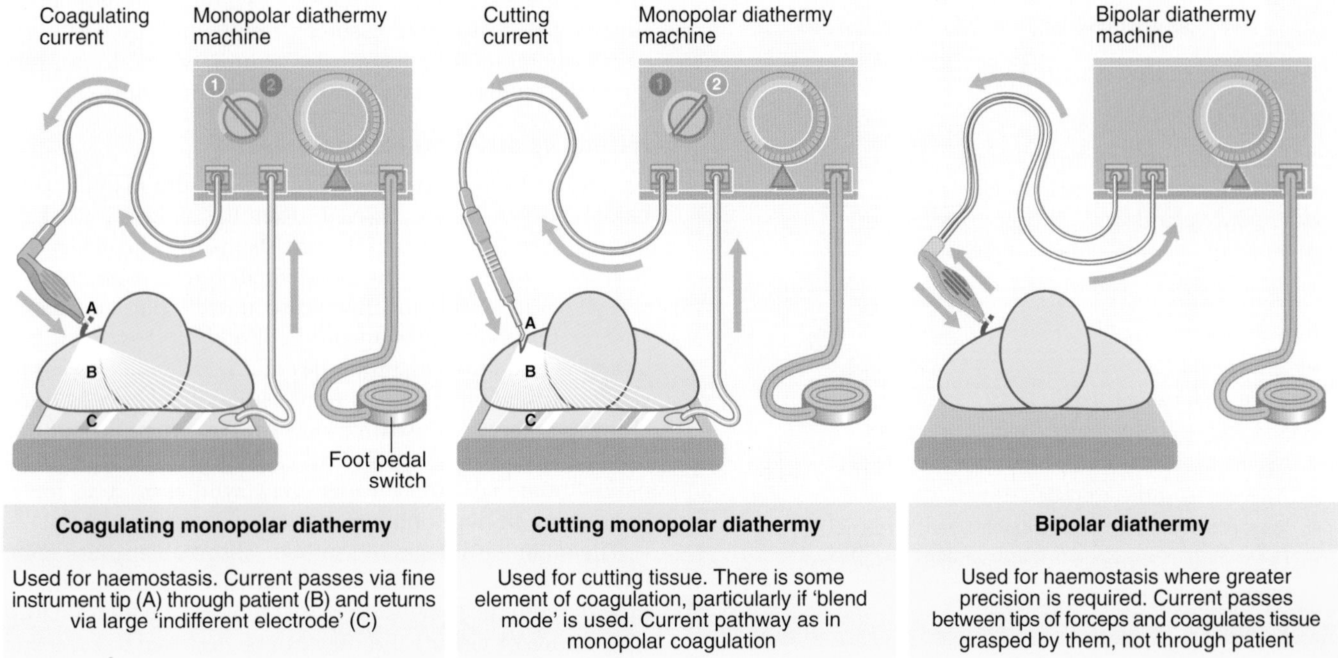

Fig. 10.2 Three modes of diathermy

Bipolar diathermy is used mainly for finer surgery. The current passes only between the blades of the forceps and it requires fairly accurate grasping of the bleeding vessel. It uses low levels of electrical power, there is almost no electrical dispersion from the tip of the forceps and much less heat is generated. The main advantages are minimal tissue damage around the point of coagulation and safety in relation to nearby nerves, blood vessels and cardiac pacemakers. Specialised computer controlled bipolar diathermy is often used for larger vessels during laparoscopic surgery.

Cutting diathermy is mainly used for dividing large masses of muscle (e.g. during thoracotomy or access to the hip joint) and cutting vascular tissues (e.g. breast). The intention is a form of sharp dissection, at the same time coagulating the numerous small blood vessels as the tissue is cut; unfortunately this is not always wholly effective. A blend of cutting and coagulation is sometimes used.

Tourniquet and exsanguination

This technique is used in surgery of the limbs and hands where a bloodless field is desirable. For the whole limb, a pneumatic tourniquet is placed proximally. The limb is exsanguinated by elevation and spiral application of a rubber bandage (Esmark) or a ring exsanguinator from the periphery; the tourniquet is then inflated. Upper limb tourniquets must not be left inflated for more than 30 minutes and lower limb tourniquets for more than about 1 hour to avoid the risk of necrosis.

Pressure

Pressure is a useful means of controlling bleeding until platelet aggregation, reactive vasoconstriction and blood coagulation take over. It can be used for emergency temporary control of severe arterial or venous bleeding but is equally useful for controlling diffuse small-vessel bleeding from a raw area, e.g. liver bed after cholecystectomy. Pressure is usually applied with gauze swabs which must be kept in position for at least 10 minutes. Even if bleeding is not arrested completely, this process usually allows a clearer view and allows haemostasis by standard means.

For intractable bleeding which is not amenable to ligature, diathermy or suture, various resorbable packing materials, e.g. oxidised cellulose, can be left in position until haemostasis occurs, allowing the wound to be closed. If bleeding simply cannot be controlled—for example, after liver injury—the bleeding cavity can be packed with gauze swabs which are left in situ and removed 48–72 hours later at a further operation. Bleeding, once controlled by this method, rarely recurs.

When a raw cavity has been created beneath the skin, external pressure dressings are sometimes a useful method of controlling potential superficial postoperative oozing and minimising haematoma formation.

SUTURING AND SURGICAL REPAIR

Types of suture material and needles

Numerous types of suture are available (see Box 10.5), with the most important distinction being between **absorbable** and **non-absorbable** materials. The groups can be subdivided into **natural** and **synthetic** materials (although natural materials are being phased out) and further subdivided into **monofilament** and **polyfilament** (braided) materials. The choice of suture material depends upon the task at hand, the handling qualities and personal preference.

Box 10.5 Suture materials and their characteristics

Typical brand names are given in parentheses

Absorbable

- Plain catgut—natural monofilament
- Chromic catgut—natural monofilament
- Polyglycolic acid-synthetic braided (Dexon)
- Polyglactin—synthetic braided (Vicryl)
- Polydioxanone—synthetic monofilament (PDS, Maxon)

Non-absorbable

- Silk—natural braided
- Linen—natural braided
- Stainless steel wire—monofilament or braided
- Nylon—synthetic, usually monofilament (Ethilon)
- Polyester—synthetic braided (Ticron, and others)
- Polypropylene—synthetic monofilament (Prolene)
- Polytetrafluoroethylene (PTFE)—synthetic 'expanded' monofilament (Goretex)

Absorbable versus non-absorbable materials

The strength of absorbable sutures declines at a predictable rate for each type of material, although the suture material remains in the wound long after it has any useful ability to hold tissues together.

In increasing duration of useful strength, the main absorbable materials are:

- Plain catgut and chromic catgut—useful strength 3 and 5 days respectively (no longer available in many countries)
- Modified polyglactin (Vicryl Rapide)—useful strength about 6 days
- Polyglycolic acid (Dexon) and polyglactin (Vicryl)—useful strength about 10 days
- Poliglecaprone 25 (Monocryl)—useful strength about 20 days
- Polydioxanone (PDS)—retains its strength for at least 28 days

The eventual elimination of absorbable materials from the body overcomes the problem of a permanent foreign body which can harbour infection. Absorbable sutures are often used in skin to avoid the need for removal; typical applications are minor skin operations, median sternotomies, surgery in children, circumcisions and vasectomies. Polyglycolic acid/polyglactin (undyed) gives good results as the sutures are removed by hydrolysis without inflammation. The modified short-lived polyglactin has ideal properties for skin closure where short suture life is required, e.g. inguinal hernia repair, and the monofilament poliglecaprone 25 (Monocryl) is ideal for situations when longer wound support is required.

Non-absorbable sutures retain most of their strength indefinitely. They are used where the repaired tissues take a long time to reach full strength (e.g. abdominal wall closure) or will be inherently weak (e.g. inguinal and incisional hernia repairs, arterial anastomoses). Non-absorbable sutures are also widely used for skin closure; synthetic monofilament sutures give reasonable cosmetic results and are easily and painlessly removed. Subcuticular sutures, which do not penetrate the epidermis, give excellent cosmetic results.

Natural versus synthetic materials

Catgut has been used as a suture and ligature material since before Roman times, derived from the material used for musical instrument strings. It consists mainly of collagen and is actually made from the dried small bowel submucosa of sheep or cattle. Silk and linen also have a long and distinguished history. Many surgeons believe that silk has the best handling and knotting properties of any material, but it provokes a strong inflammatory response exceeded only by linen. Silk was sometimes used for skin sutures, where its softness means there are no sharp ends to prick nearby skin. In general, natural materials are cheaper than synthetics, a factor of importance in developing countries.

The main advantages of synthetic absorbable suture materials are that they are stronger and provoke little or no inflammatory reaction. There is no risk of biological contamination with prions or viruses and they can be designed to meet specific requirements of absorbability, period of retention of strength, and handling properties.

Non-absorbable synthetic materials, similarly, do not provoke inflammatory reactions. Polyesters, nylon and polypropylene all retain virtually all of their strength over long periods in the tissues; this is particularly important when they are used to suture arterial prostheses where healing alone would not retain the prosthesis.

Monofilament versus polyfilament sutures

Monofilament materials have a smooth surface and can be pulled through the tissues with minimal friction; this makes them easier to insert and remove than polyfilament braided materials. On the other hand, monofilament materials are stiff, springy and more difficult to knot. Braided materials have the best handling qualities, but their interstices are a haven for bacteria. When used at a surface (e.g. skin or bowel wall) they tend to act as a 'wick', drawing infected material in. This problem is partly overcome by the manufacturers' application of surface coatings.

Wire sutures

Metal wire sutures have largely been displaced by non-absorbable synthetics. Stainless steel wire is, however, extensively used in orthopaedic surgery for bone fixation and sometimes for closure of sternotomy wounds in cardiac surgery. It is virtually inert but its main disadvantages are high rates of glove penetration and late breakage due to metal fatigue.

Gauge of suture material

The gauge of suture chosen for a particular task depends largely on practical experience. This takes into account the following factors:

- Strength of repair required
- Number of sutures to be placed—the greater the number, the finer can be the gauge

- Type of suture material used—for a given gauge, the various materials have different strengths
- Cosmetic requirements—multiple fine sutures give a better cosmetic result than fewer heavier sutures

The traditional method of describing suture gauge (US Pharmacopoeia) is confusing for the newcomer and derives from the time when sutures were much thicker than those used today. The finest suture then was designated gauge 1, with gauge 2 and upwards applying to heavier sutures. As finer and finer sutures came into use, the scale had to be taken progressively backwards from 1, i.e. gauges 0, 00 (i.e. 2/0), 000 (3/0) and so on. Nowadays, the finest suture is 11/0, used for extremely delicate surgery such as in the eye. A more rational metric gauge, based on suture diameter, is in use but the traditional gauge is still widely used. A simple guide to the use of different gauges is outlined in Box 10.6.

Types of suture needle

Vast ranges of needles have been designed to accommodate the breadth of different demands of general and specialist surgery and the stringent requirements of microsurgery. Characteristics of needles and broad indications for their use are summarised in Box 10.7 and illustrated in Figure 10.3.

Methods of skin suturing

The objective of skin suturing is to approximate the cut edges so they will heal rapidly, leaving a minimal scar. Edges to be apposed should have been cut in a clean line and perpendicular to the skin surface; ragged or angled edges should be trimmed. The cut edges should be capable of being brought together neatly and without tension; otherwise the wound may break down or the scar slowly stretches, giving an ugly result. To achieve this, it may be necessary to insert a layer of subcutaneous sutures or even mobilise the skin by undercutting in the fatty layer (see Fig. 10.4). Undue laxity should also be avoided by trimming excess skin.

There are many techniques of skin closure, the choice being governed by the nature and site of the operation and by the surgeon's preference. In general, facial wounds are closed with multiple fine sutures removed after 4 or 5 days. Abdominal and chest wound sutures are generally removed after 7 days, while sutures for wounds on the back are best left for 14 days to minimise wound stretching.

Subcuticular sutures, either non-absorbable or absorbable, are often used for longer wounds in cosmetically sensitive areas, provided the risk of infection is low. Elsewhere, the choice is between interrupted and continuous suture techniques. Interrupted sutures are indicated if there is a risk of infection; if infection develops, some sutures can be removed early to facilitate drainage. If the risk of infection is high, e.g. large bowel perforation, skin wounds are better left open and closed 48–72 hours later by **delayed primary closure.** The commonly used methods of skin suturing are illustrated in Figure 10.5.

Clips and staples

Stainless steel clips (e.g. Michel clips) have been used for decades for closing skin wounds and are popular for neck incisions after thyroidectomy as they are haemostatic. As the

Box 10.6 Guide to suture gauges for common procedures

Skin
- Face 5/0 or 6/0
- Hands and limbs 3/0 or 4/0
- Elsewhere 2/0 or 3/0

Abdominal wall
- Two strands of gauge 0 ('loop nylon'), gauge 1 or gauge 2

Gut anastomoses
- 2/0 or 3/0

Arterial anastomoses
- 2/0 down to 7/0 according to size of vessel

Microsurgery (e.g. eyes, microvascular, nerve repair)
- 7/0 down to as fine as 11/0

Box 10.7 Types of suture needle

1. Method of use
- Hand-held needles—routine for skin suturing; sometimes used for abdominal wall closure
- Instrument-held needles—necessary for deeper access and fine control

2. Shape of needle
- Straight—skin suturing
- Curved—half-circle used for most purposes, quarter-circle for microvascular anastomoses, three-quarter-circle for hand closure of abdominal wall

3. Length of needle
- Range from 2 to 60 mm—according to depth of penetration and delicacy of surgery

4. Tissue penetration characteristics
- Round-bodied with smooth pointed tip—most soft tissues, e.g. gut, fat, muscle
- Trocar point (semi-cutting)—moderately tough tissues, e.g. atherosclerotic arteries, fascia
- Cutting point—tough tissues, e.g. skin, breast tissue

5. Means of attachment of suture to needle
- Needles with an eye requiring suture material to be threaded by hand—mainly used in developing countries so that needles can be reused
- 'Atraumatic' needles with suture material already attached (swaged into the end)—this avoids a double thickness of suture material to cause extra drag and trauma as it is pulled through the tissues, and the suture material does not detach from the needle during use

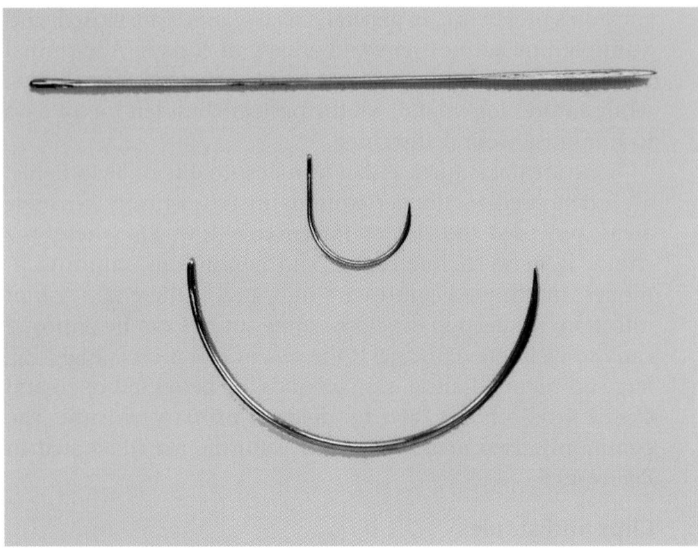
(a)

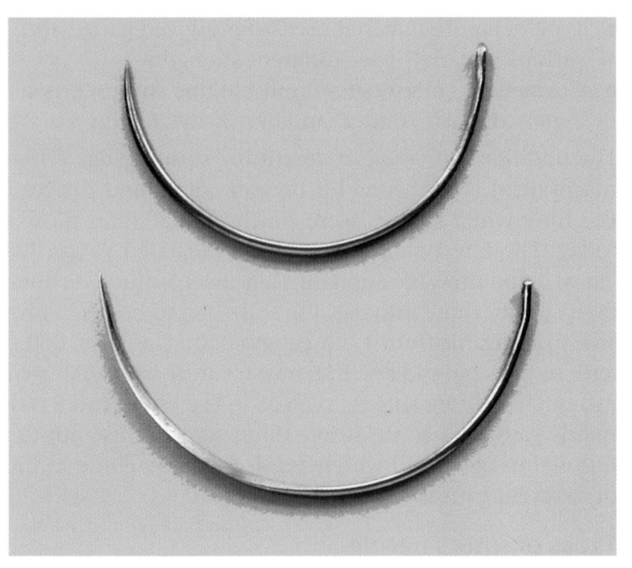
(b)

Fig. 10.3 Various types of surgical needles
(a) Three shapes of needle. The straight needle has a cutting point and is used for skin suturing. The J-shaped needle is used mainly for femoral hernia repairs, and the large half-circle needle is for abdominal wall closure. **(b)** Two large needles showing the difference between 'round-bodied' (above) and 'cutting' ends (below).

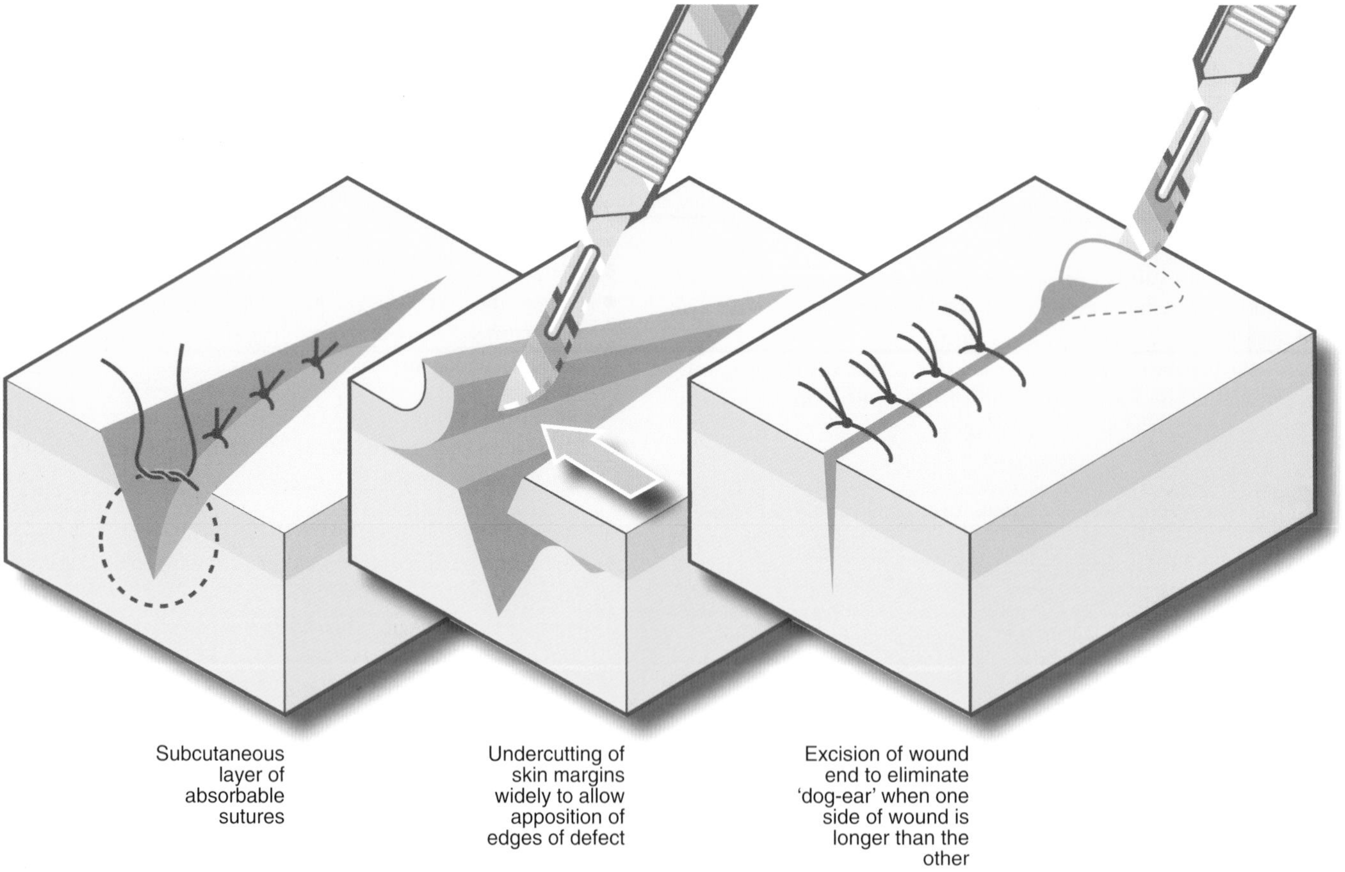

Subcutaneous layer of absorbable sutures

Undercutting of skin margins widely to allow apposition of edges of defect

Excision of wound end to eliminate 'dog-ear' when one side of wound is longer than the other

Fig. 10.4 Methods of approximating skin edges

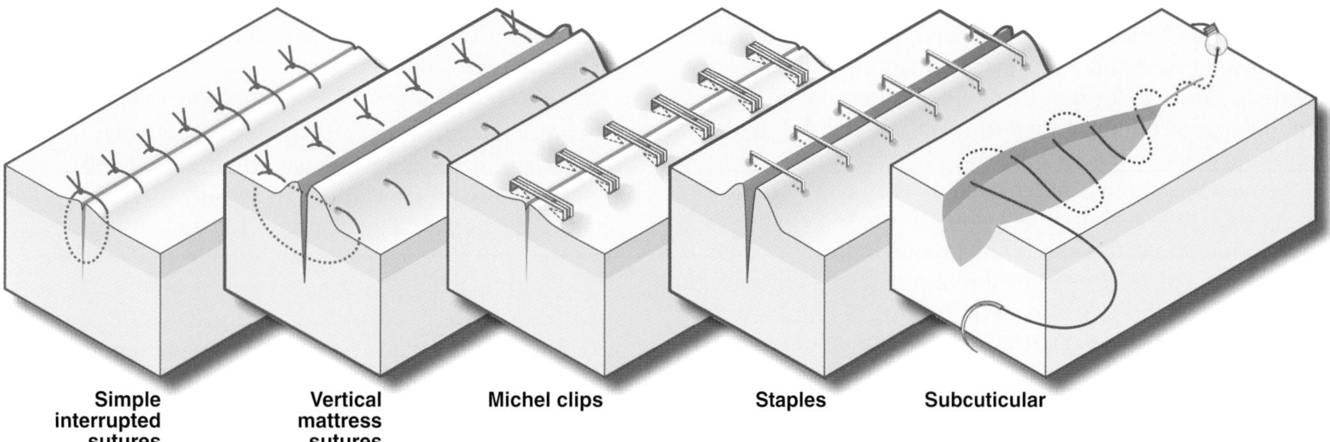

Fig. 10.5 Commonly used skin closure techniques

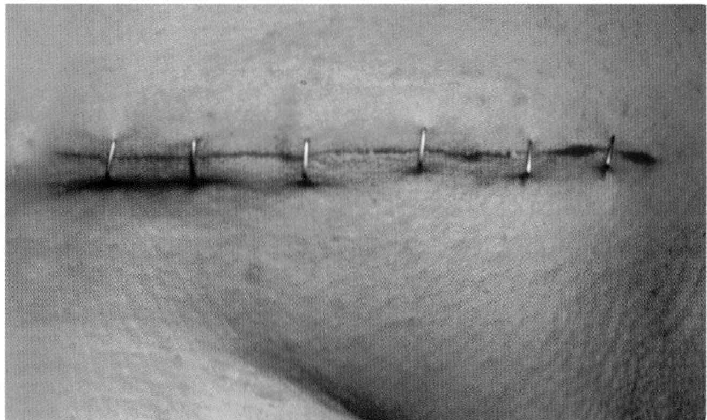

Fig. 10.6 Inguinal hernia wound closed with staples

clips do not penetrate skin yet give good edge apposition, the cosmetic result is excellent. Staples are used for both skin closure and bowel surgery. The skin closure devices are similar in concept to ordinary paper staplers, with staples stored in a magazine and applied singly instead of sutures (Fig. 10.6). More complex devices, which apply multiple staples simultaneously, either in a linear or circular fashion, are available for bowel anastomoses and closure of tubular viscera. Some devices have revolutionised surgical practice, e.g. re-anastomosis of colon to rectum after Hartmann's resection or bronchial stump closure. When used for internal viscera, the staples remain in place indefinitely.

POSTOPERATIVE WOUND MANAGEMENT

Once a wound has been closed, the doctor has three main responsibilities: choosing the dressing, monitoring the progress of healing and deciding when to remove the sutures.

The purposes of dressings for surgical wounds are as follows:

- To maintain the wound in a warm and moist state most conducive to healing
- To absorb or contain any superficial bleeding or inflammatory exudate
- To protect the delicate healing tissue from trauma, bacterial contamination and interference
- To prevent sutures catching on clothing or other objects
- To conceal the wound from view
- To apply pressure to the wound if haematoma formation is likely

Types of wound dressing

For small surgical wounds, particularly on the face, a dressing is often unnecessary as the linear crust of inflammatory exudate performs this task very well. For other simple wounds, plastic spray dressing is suitable, e.g. Opsite. In most other cases, **prepacked adhesive dressings** are used, incorporating an absorbent pad with non-stick film in contact with the wound surface. While convenient, these dressings may conceal accumulations of blood, inflammatory exudate or infected discharge. Wound inspection then requires painful removal of the dressing which can be an opportunity for infection to enter. Transparent **semipermeable plastic film dressings** neatly overcome this problem but are unsuitable for discharging wounds.

A flexible polyamide net coated with soft silicone (e.g. Mepitel) is useful for covering raw areas. This has very low wound adherence and is usually easy to remove. Other dressings include **calcium alginate** (seaweed origin), **hydrocolloids** and **hydrogels**. These dressings offer a better wound environment with increased hydration, fewer dressing changes, easier dressing removal and greater comfort.

Gamgee is a thick cotton wool dressing material enveloped in a thin layer of gauze; this is variously used for padding sites vulnerable to trauma (e.g. amputation stumps) or as pads beneath pressure bandages or as absorbent dressings for leaking wounds. **Dry dressings** are wads of dressing material (e.g. cotton gauze), usually taped or bandaged in place. Dry dressings need regular replacement and may be prevented from sticking by placing a piece of non-adherent dressing (e.g. Melolin, N/A dressing) against the wound.

Removal of dressings and sutures

Provided the dressing remains clean and dry and the patient afebrile and generally well, there is no need to inspect clean surgical wounds until the time of suture removal. If wound complications are suspected, the dressing should be removed and the wound checked and redressed. If infection is apparent, a wound swab should be taken for culture and sensitivity. Localised abscess formation requires suture removal and probing to effect drainage, whilst spreading cellulitis requires antibiotic therapy in addition.

Skin sutures should be removed as soon as the wound is strong enough to remain intact without support. On the back and around joints, this can take 14 days; on the abdomen, it takes about 7 days (longer in the case of steroid therapy or infection). On the face and neck, healing is rapid and less influenced by functional stresses. Here, sutures can be safely removed after 3–5 days, giving a better cosmetic result.

Management of drains in the postoperative period

Abdominal drains provide a potential route for infection to enter, even though the intra-abdominal pressure nearly always exceeds external pressure. The risk can be minimised by ensuring the drain opens into a sterile environment such as a drainage bag (**closed drainage**) and by removing the drain as soon as its task is completed. Decisions about removal of drains should rest with the operating surgeon who will undoubtedly have personal preferences.

The general principles of drain management are as follows:

- Suction drains help to collapse down spaces left in the tissues at operation as well as to drain blood and inflammatory exudate. These are mainly used after extensive surgery where a large covered raw surface remains, e.g. after mastectomy, thyroidectomy or large incisional hernia repair. Suction drains should not be used near bowel for fear of suction perforation. A suction drain is usually retained for only 24 hours unless substantial drainage persists (e.g. >30 ml/24 h)
- Non-suction drains (e.g. large-bore silicone or rubber tubes or corrugated drains) are mainly used for bowel and biliary anastomoses and for abscess drainage. In this case, the drain is left in place for about 5 days. Some surgeons prefer to withdraw the drain in stages so that the deep part of the drainage tract can collapse progressively, reducing the risk of leaving a deep pool of fluid

SOFT TISSUE SURGERY

METHODS OF OBTAINING TISSUE FOR DIAGNOSIS

Open or endoscopic biopsy

If major surgery or other therapy is being considered for a suspected malignant lesion, an accurate **tissue diagnosis** should be made.

Skin lesions can be **biopsied** by incision under local anaesthesia. Rectal lesions can be biopsied without anaesthesia using forceps through a rigid or flexible sigmoidoscope or colonoscope, while gastric and colonic lesions can be biopsied via a flexible endoscope. Breast lumps or suspicious mammographic lesions can be sampled using percutaneous core needle biopsy or by fine needle aspiration cytology (see below). Gastroscopy allows biopsy of upper GI mucosal lesions as well as lesion of the pancreatic head.

Enlarged lymph nodes can often be diagnosed by **incision biopsy** or by removing one or more completely for histological examination (**excision biopsy**), although many units can now obtain satisfactory results by needle biopsy. Lymphadenectomy often requires general anaesthesia, particularly for lumps in the neck.

Biopsy guided by ultrasound or CT scanning

Abdominal masses such as liver metastases or pancreatic lesions can be biopsied percutaneously with the aid of ultrasound or CT scanning. The suspicious lesion is first located as an image and then a biopsy needle is guided into it with the help of further imaging. The technique can be used to sample abdominal masses or suspicious para-aortic lymph nodes in staging lymphomas or following treatment for testicular germ cell tumours.

Cytology

Special staining techniques for malignant cells can be applied to material obtained by fine needle aspiration. Cytological diagnosis requires particular laboratory skills but often permits accurate diagnosis (e.g. of malignancy), which renders more invasive investigations unnecessary. A negative cytological result, however, must be interpreted with great caution because it may be due to sampling error.

Cytological diagnosis can be useful for the following:

- Examining cells aspirated from solid masses. This is particularly useful for thyroid nodules (see Ch. 5, p. 75 and Ch. 49), breast lumps, mammographically detected lesions and pancreatic masses
- Examining ascitic fluid obtained from the abdomen by **paracentesis**, or pleural effusions aspirated from the chest. Fluid may also be sent for microbiological analysis
- Examining cellular material scraped from surfaces, e.g. uterine cervical smears, or fluid obtained from within hollow viscera, e.g. urine, pancreatic secretions, sputum

'MINOR' OPERATIVE PROCEDURES

Many skin lesions are amenable to simple excision or biopsy, often under local anaesthesia. These may be performed in general practice or in dermatological or surgical clinics. Aseptic technique must be employed.

Local anaesthesia for skin lesions

The usual method of administration is by infiltration (injection) of local anaesthetic agents (e.g. lidocaine 0.5% or 1%) into the skin surrounding the lesion. Between 1 and 10 ml of solution is usually required, but care must be taken to remain within maximum safe dosages (see Table 10.3). A vasoconstrictor (e.g. adrenaline (epinephrine) 1 in 200 000) may be incorporated to reduce vascularity in the operative field, but this must **never** be used on the extreme peripheries, i.e. fingers, toes, penis or nose, because of the risk of ischaemic necrosis.

Table 10.3 Maximum safe doses of local anaesthetic agents for infiltration in fit patients

Lidocaine	Bupivacaine (Marcain) or levobupivacaine (Chirocaine)
2% lidocaine is probably no more effective for achieving anaesthesia than 1% or even 0.5% so use lowest concentration needed; 10 ml of 1% lidocaine contains 100 mg	0.5% bupivacaine is probably no more effective than 0.25%; 10 ml of 0.5% bupivacaine contains 50 mg
The maximum safe dose of **plain lidocaine** is 4 mg/kg body weight	The maximum safe dose of **plain bupivacaine** is 2 mg/kg body weight
For a fit 60 kg adult, the maximum safe dose of 1% plain lidocaine is 16–24 ml	For a fit 60 kg adult, the maximum safe dose of 0.5% bupivacaine is 24 ml
With adrenaline (epinephrine), this dose can be increased to 7 mg/kg body weight	Addition of adrenaline (epinephrine) does **not** increase the safe dose of bupivacaine and there is little point in using it for infiltration except to provide vasoconstriction
For a fit 60 kg adult, the maximum safe dose of 1% lidocaine with *adrenaline (epinephrine)* is 30–40 ml	No increase

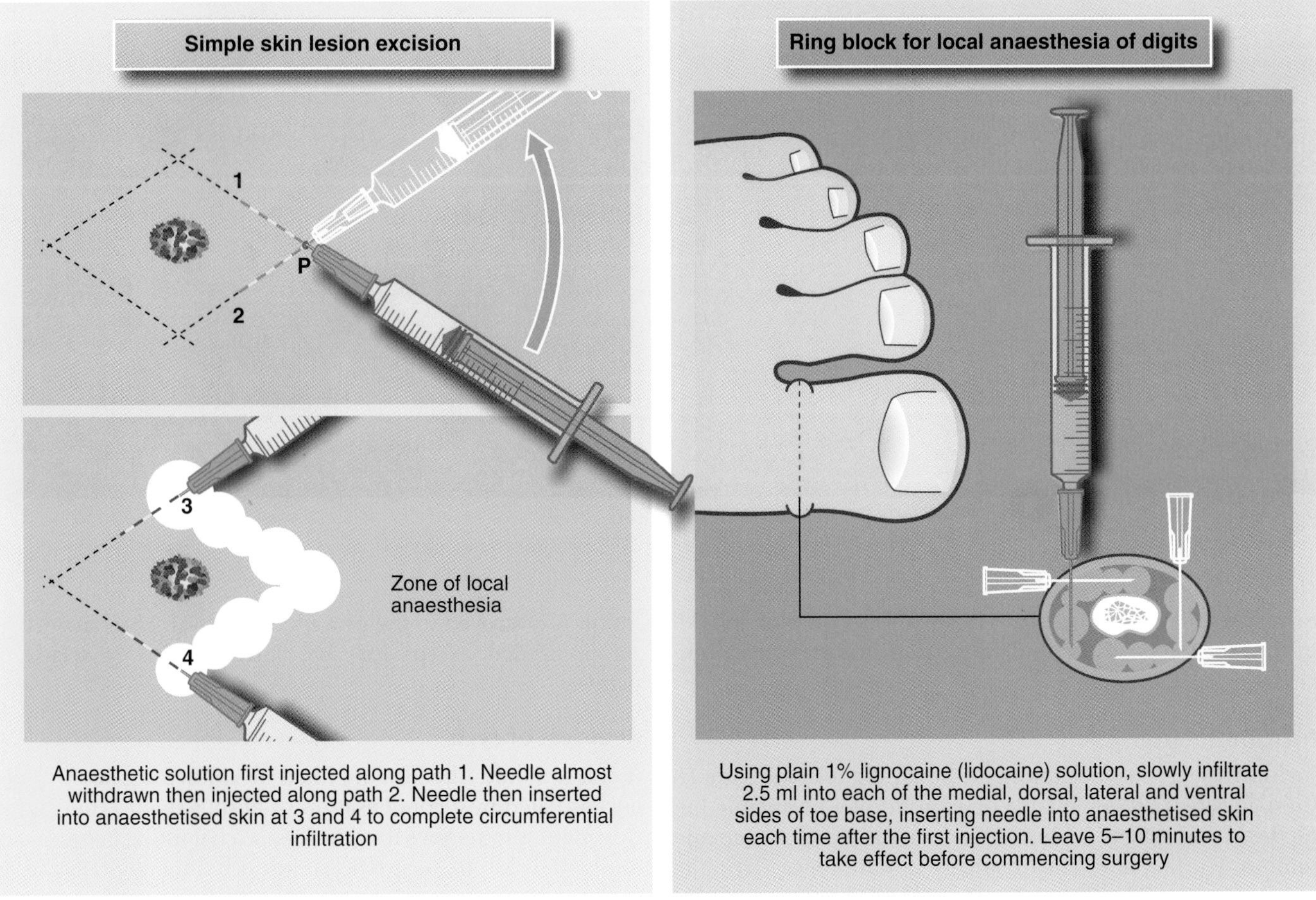

Fig. 10.7 Local anaesthetic infiltration techniques

The injecting needle should be as fine as possible and inserted into the skin as few times as possible to avoid causing unnecessary pain. Before each injection, aspiration is attempted to ensure that the solution is not injected directly into a blood vessel as intravascular injection may cause systemic toxicity. Methods of infiltration of local anaesthetic are illustrated in Figure 10.7.

Biopsy techniques

Excision biopsy

The technique of excision skin or mucosal biopsy illustrated in Figure 10.8 is appropriate for most small lesions not thought to be malignant. The lesion is removed with a fusiform piece of normal skin, with the long axis orientated along skin creases and tension lines. The specimen should include a millimetre or

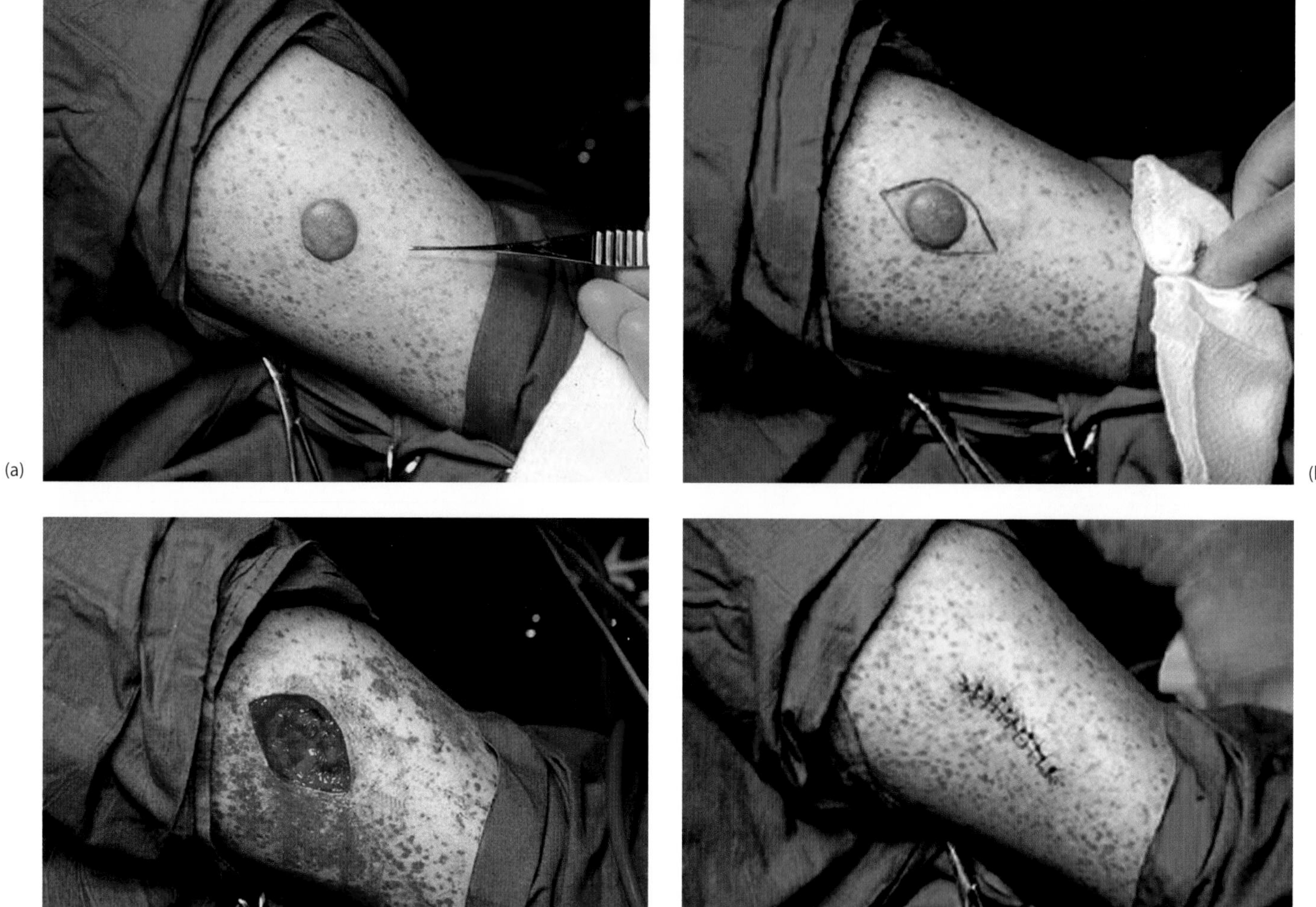

Fig. 10.8 Excision biopsy technique

two of normal skin on either side of the lesion and should include the full depth of the dermis down to the subcutaneous fat.

Incision biopsy

Incision biopsy is a technique of obtaining a tissue sample from a lesion that is too large or anatomically unsuitable for excision biopsy, e.g. a skin rash or a suspected malignant tumour. For the latter, major surgery or radiotherapy should not be performed without histological confirmation of the diagnosis. The biopsy objective is to obtain a representative sample of the full depth of the lesion, including an area of the margin and adjoining normal tissue (see Fig. 10.9).

Destruction of lesions by diathermy, electrocautery, cryocautery or curettage

These techniques are used for small lesions where there is no clinical suspicion of malignancy or for small basal cell carcinomas where a histological diagnosis is not required; the lesion is destroyed in the process of removal. Local anaesthesia is needed except for cryocautery, which is relatively painless.

Removal of cysts

A cyst is a fluid-filled lesion, lined by epithelium and usually encapsulated by a condensation of fibrous tissue. The aim of treatment is to remove the whole epithelial lining because any remnant leads to recurrence. The technique of removal is outlined in Figure 10.10. Ideally, the cyst is dissected out intact without puncturing the cavity. If this occurs, the cyst collapses, making it difficult to identify and remove the epithelial lining. Inflamed cysts are best simply drained and excised later when the inflammation has settled.

Marsupialisation

This is usually employed for cysts or other fluid-filled lesions that are too large, inaccessible or technically difficult to remove. It is rarely appropriate for skin lesions but is

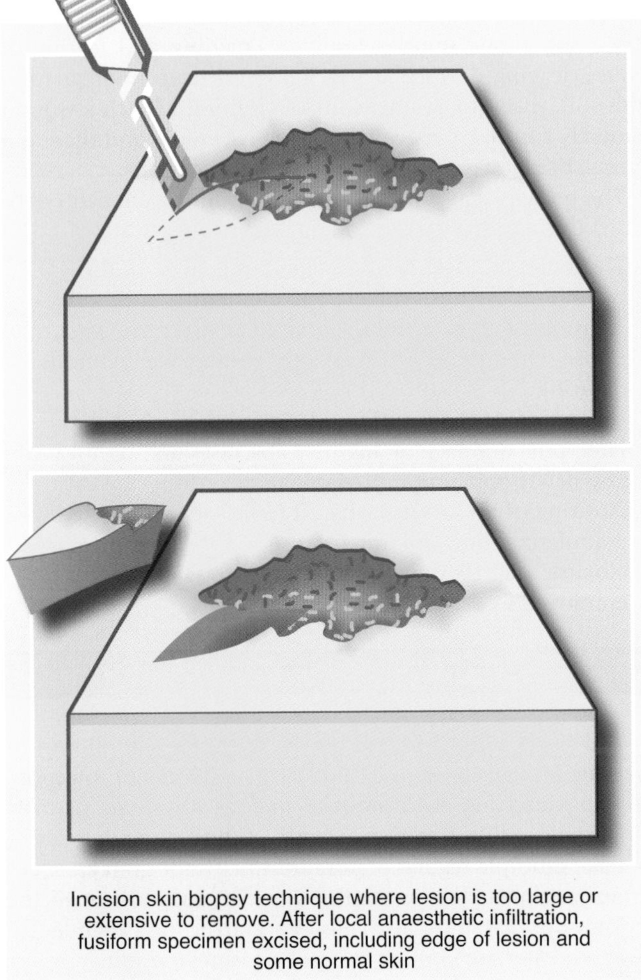
Incision skin biopsy technique where lesion is too large or extensive to remove. After local anaesthetic infiltration, fusiform specimen excised, including edge of lesion and some normal skin

Fig. 10.9 Incision skin biopsy technique

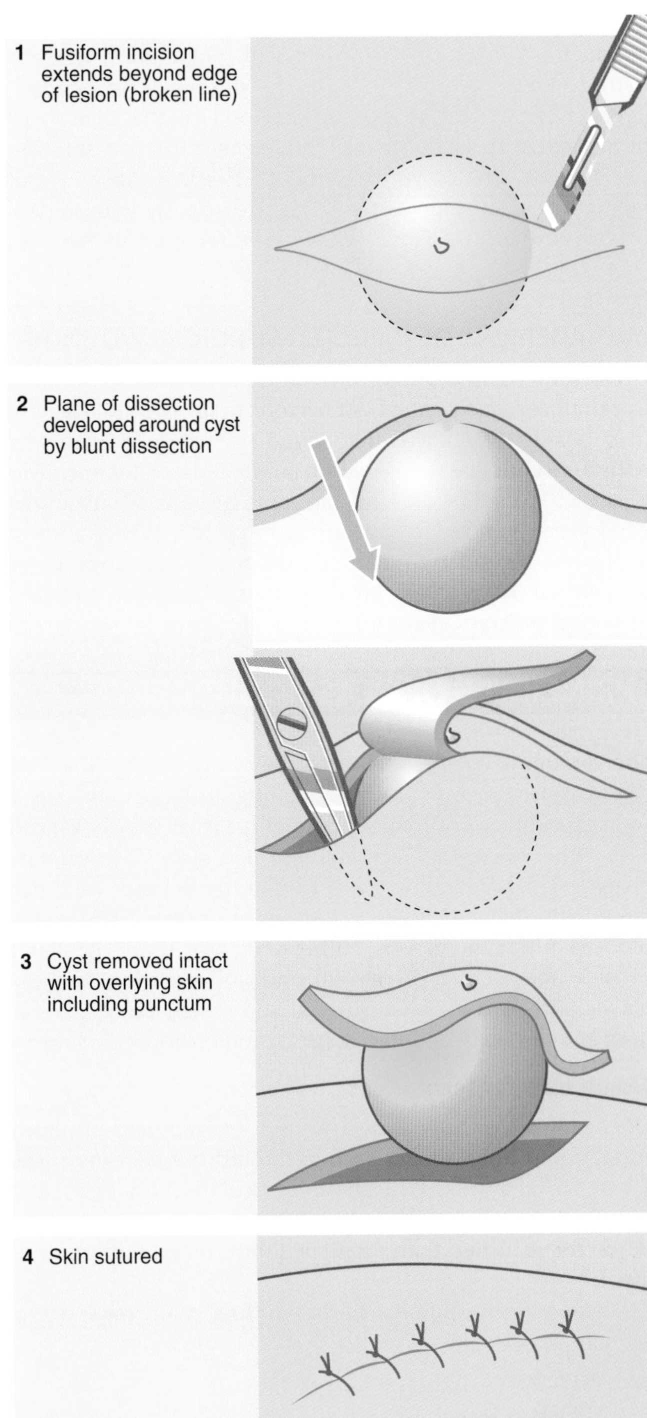

Fig. 10.10 Technique of excision of an epidermal (sebaceous) cyst

often used for large salivary retention cysts in the floor of the mouth, cysts in the jaw and pancreatic pseudocysts. The surgeon usually removes a disc from the wall of the cavity and sutures the lining to the overlying epithelium around the cut edge. This leaves a pouch, which slowly fills in from below once the pressure of the cyst contents has been removed.

SURGERY INVOLVING INFECTED TISSUES

MANAGEMENT OF ABSCESSES

The first principle of managing an abscess is to establish drainage of the pus. When an abscess is 'pointing' to the surface, surgical drainage involves a skin incision at the site of maximum fluctuance followed by blunt probing with sinus forceps or a finger (usually under general anaesthesia) to ensure that all loculi are drained; necrotic material is removed at the same time by curettage.

After drainage, small abscesses need only a dry dressing, the cavity filling in rapidly from beneath. Larger and deeper abscesses need a method of keeping the skin opening patent until the cavity has filled with granulation tissue. A corrugated drain, which is gradually withdrawn ('shortened') over a few days, will achieve this or else the cavity may be packed with ribbon gauze soaked in antiseptic solution, or one of the newer absorbent dressings such as an alginate (e.g. Kaltostat); these packs are usually changed daily or every other day. Good analgesia is required in the early stages.

MANAGEMENT OF INFECTED SURGICAL WOUNDS

Grossly infected surgical wounds must be opened up to ensure free drainage, and cleaned. All necrotic tissue is excised leaving only healthy tissue, and the wound packed daily afterwards with antiseptic-soaked gauze or an alginate or hydrocolloid dressing. Wounds with large amounts of necrotic tissue may need more than one operation. Wounds are usually allowed to heal by secondary intention, although a large wound can be sutured later when infection is no longer a problem ('**delayed primary closure**').

Management of dirty or contaminated wounds

Major soft tissue injuries result in crushing and tearing of tissues, leaving devascularised areas and deep impregnation with soil, road grit or fragments of clothing. If such a wound is merely sutured, pyogenic infection is certain, and there is a serious risk of gas gangrene or tetanus.

The principles of managing these wounds were first established during the First World War, as follows:

- Thorough removal of all foreign material from the wound (sometimes called '**debridement**')
- Excision of all non-viable tissue ('necrosectomy')
- Loose open packing of the wound with gauze without suturing
- Inspection of the wound under anaesthesia 2–4 days later, plus drainage of any new abscesses and removal of any newly apparent non-viable tissue
- Suturing of the wound when it looks clean and granulating, but avoiding tension, i.e. **delayed primary closure**. Alternatively, split skin grafting may be employed without wound closure

PRINCIPLES OF PLASTIC SURGERY

The discipline of plastic surgery was born during the First World War in response to the appalling disfigurement caused by blast injuries, burns and facial trauma from trench warfare. Since then, specialised techniques of skin reconstruction have progressed much further, especially in the fields of axial flap design and microvascular reconstructive surgery. The scope of modern plastic surgery is outlined in Box 10.8. There is a considerable degree of overlap and collaboration between plastic surgery and other surgical specialties, especially ear, nose and throat, maxillofacial, breast and orthopaedic surgery.

Tissue transfer techniques

Obtaining satisfactory skin cover is a key problem in plastic surgery, and other tissues such as fat and muscle cannot satisfactorily be transferred without revascularisation. Free transplantation of full-thickness skin (other than tiny grafts) or any other tissue other than bone without revascularisation is usually unsuccessful.

Tissue transfer can be achieved in three main ways:

- Skin grafts
- Vascularised flaps
- Free flaps

Skin grafts

Split skin (Thiersch) grafting involves transplanting a very thin layer of skin consisting of little more than epidermis, which has no blood supply of its own. It depends on nutrition from the recipient bed for its survival. Split skin grafts are commonly employed for burns and after wide excision of skin lesions, provided there is a recipient base of healthy tissue. The donor site heals rapidly since small islands of epithelium are left behind (see Fig. 10.11). The donor site is potentially more painful than the recipient but pain is well controlled if the donor site is dressed immediately with hydrogel or similar dressings. These are left in position for 7–10 days until the wound has epithelialised. Grafts fail because of sliding or shearing movement, or lifting off by haematoma or infection. Dressings exerting mild pressure such as a 'sponge tie-over' aim to reduce this. Creating a 'mesh' of the graft with a device to make multiple regular perforations helps the graft attach in certain circumstances as it allows free drainage through the perforations. Meshing also allows a graft to be expanded to cover a greater area but gives a poor cosmetic result.

Full thickness (Wolfe) grafts have some advantages for small skin grafts. They do not contract and usually have a better colour match. Donor sites include skin from behind the ear (post-auricular), where the defect can be closed primarily. This can be used for lower eyelid or finger tip reconstruction. However, these grafts pick up blood supply less readily than split skin and so are restricted to reconstructing small areas. See also pinch grafts (Fig. 10.11).

Vascularised flaps

Skin grafts cannot be used where there is a cavity, or bare bone or cartilage and these are absolute indications for flap repair. Flaps can also give good cosmesis, e.g. after skin cancer excision on the face. A flap has a blood supply of its own and is **not** a graft. The blood supply reaches the flap via its base, the vascular pedicle. Flaps can be advanced, rotated or transposed into the defect and this alone may provide sufficient mobility to close a moderate defect. If flap rotation produces a new defect, this clean area can usually be covered with a split skin graft.

The early **random flaps**, devised by Gillies, were limited in scope because there was no dominant blood supply and this prevented construction of a flap longer than 2 : 1 ratio to breadth. Later it was realised that longer flaps could be created by 'axialising' them. Most flaps are now **axial**, using recognised anatomical sites to ensure a blood supply running the full length. An early technique was the **pedicle flap**, a flap

Box 10.8 The scope of plastic surgery

Congenital problems

- Correction of congenital defects, e.g. cleft lip and palate, syndactyly and polydactyly, prominent ears, hypospadias, vascular malformations, craniofacial deformities, congenital skin conditions, e.g. 'port-wine stains'

Trauma

- Reconstruction after mutilating surgery or trauma, e.g. skin cover for compound lower limb fractures, vascularised bone transfer
- Management of facial soft tissue trauma
- Management of burns—grafting, management of scars and deformities
- Hand trauma—tendon repairs, microsurgical nerve and artery repairs, replantation surgery, e.g. digits and limbs

Elective hand surgery

- Dupuytren's contracture, nerve decompressions, joint replacements in rheumatoid disease

Cancer

- Cutaneous malignancies—excision and reconstruction with grafts or local flaps
- Major cancer surgery of the head and neck—excision and reconstruction with free tissue transfer
- Breast reconstruction after mastectomy

Aesthetic (cosmetic) surgery

- Scar removal, breast reduction and augmentation, 'face-lifts', eyelid skin reduction, nasal adjustment including after trauma
- Surgery for obesity, e.g. abdominal skin reduction, liposuction, apronectomy (for pendulous abdomen)

Miscellaneous, including reconstruction of large defects

- Reconstruction for facial palsy, decubitus (pressure) sores, soft tissue sarcoma excision, leg ulcers, reconstruction of skin after radiotherapy, destructive infections, e.g. necrotising fasciitis, compartment syndromes

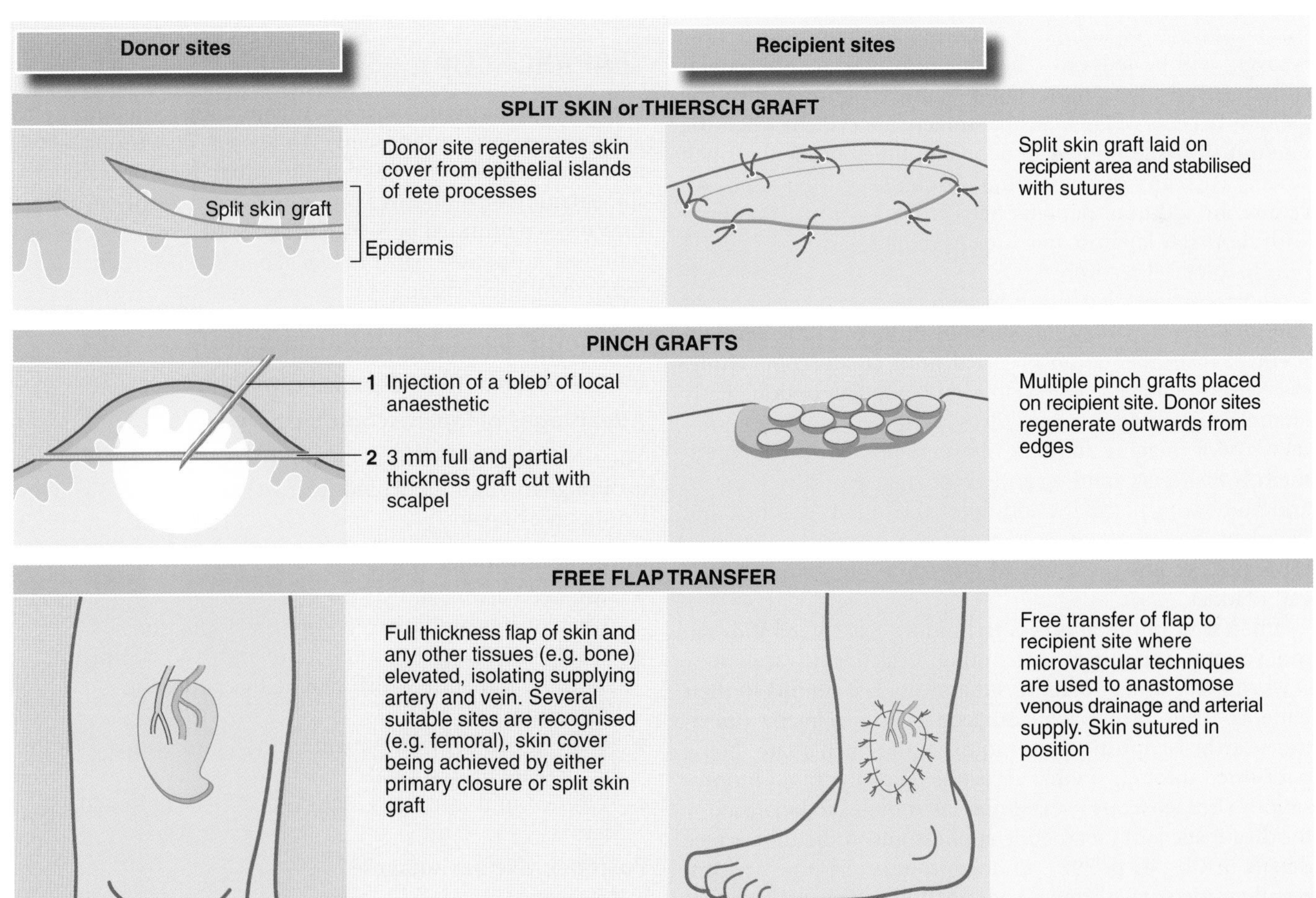

Fig. 10.11 Methods of skin grafting

of skin raised and formed into a tube while initially remaining attached to its site of origin at both ends.

Axial flaps are selected according to the site of the defect and the tissues needed. A series of flaps have now been described, based on detailed anatomical studies of blood supply. Flaps may be **cutaneous** (e.g. forehead flap), **fasciocutaneous** (e.g. the 'Chinese' radial forearm flap), **myocutaneous** (e.g. latissimus dorsi, pectoralis major), **TRAM** (transverse rectus abdominis myocutaneous—often used for breast reconstruction), and **osseous** (e.g. fibula, radius, iliac crest and rib).

Free flaps

In free tissue transfer, a carefully planned piece of tissue is first dissected out, complete with at least one main artery and vein; axial flap sites are often suitable. The whole flap is then relocated to the recipient site where the vessels are anastomosed to a suitable local artery and vein by microvascular anastomoses. The donor site can often be closed primarily or else covered with a split skin graft. Examples are the **radial forearm flap** which supplies bone, muscle and skin (often used for mandibular and intra-oral reconstruction), and the big toe which can be used to replace a lost thumb.

LAPAROSCOPIC SURGERY

INTRODUCTION TO MINIMAL ACCESS SURGERY

The last few decades have seen an explosion of interest and rapid development of techniques to achieve accurate diagnosis and treatment with the least possible tissue injury and trauma. Laparoscopic surgery was among the first to catch surgeons' imagination but other techniques such as lithotripsy, percutaneous stone removal and angioplasty advanced earlier or more or less in parallel. Initially called **minimally invasive surgery**, the principle is that if less tissue is damaged by minimising surgical incisions, then less pain is likely afterwards and the physiological responses to injury which slow recovery will be reduced. The intention is to reduce patient suffering and allow more rapid return to normal life. The greatest benefits of laparoscopic surgery are evident when the amount of tissue injured in accessing the abdomen at open surgery is greater than the surgical trauma of the actual procedure. In addition, patients need to be informed that even with short-stay laparoscopic surgery, there will still be a period of physiological recovery.

Gynaecologists led the way with laparoscopic diagnosis and procedures, particularly tubal ligation, but little development in instrumentation occurred until laparoscopic cholecystectomy emerged as a viable and popular option. Early laparoscopic cholecystectomy was hampered by poor equipment, poor imaging and lack of experience. Now that equipment is first class, training and experience have disseminated and audit is in place, the indications, contraindications and risks have become clear; as a result, laparoscopic cholecystectomy has become the standard procedure for removal of the gall bladder.

Interest in minimal access techniques has spread through the surgical specialties, prompting surgeons to seek new ways of performing operations that cause less trauma to their patients. Thus orthopaedic surgeons perform many operations **arthroscopically** and joint replacements are being performed through smaller incisions, allowing rapid mobilisation. **Thoracoscopy** uses similar instruments to laparoscopy for diagnostic and therapeutic applications in the thorax (see details in Ch. 31, p. 398). Endocrine surgeons now perform parathyroidectomy through very small incisions using special microscopes and retractors. Breast surgeons perform **sentinel lymph node biopsy** for diagnostic purposes using dye or radioactive marker techniques instead of axillary clearance. Many urological procedures such as nephrectomy and ureteric operations are undertaken laparoscopically, and vascular surgeons even perform aortic aneurysm operations laparoscopically. In fact there is probably no abdominal operation that has not been attempted laparoscopically, although the difficulties of many larger procedures make them impractical for standard use. Laparoscopic techniques have proved most useful in areas of the body with limited access, such as the gastro-oesophageal junction, the adrenal gland and the pelvis, allowing delicate instruments to be used in confined spaces with excellent views unhampered by the surgeon's hands.

LAPAROSCOPY

Laparoscopy or peritoneoscopy was in wide use clinically by gynaecologists from the early 1970s for diagnosing pelvic disorders and for sterilisation by tubal ligation. The first therapeutic gastrointestinal procedure was probably an appendicectomy performed by Semm in 1983. In 1987, Mouret first removed a diseased gall bladder laparoscopically in France. Since then, the techniques have been adopted on an increasing scale by general and thoracic surgeons for performing abdominal and thoracic operations via a series of small punctures rather than through large incisions.

Advantages of laparoscopic surgery

The advantages of laparoscopic surgery go well beyond simply avoiding large painful wounds to give better cosmesis and less postoperative pain:

Surgical advantages

- Improved access and vision in difficult areas, e.g. adrenal, pelvic organs and gastro-oesophageal junction
- Avoids handling, exposure, desiccation and cooling of abdominal tissues, which may reduce adhesion formation
- Reduced contact with patient's blood and body fluids for health care professionals
- Fewer wound infections, dehiscences and incisional hernias

Postoperative advantages

- Fewer postoperative chest complications
- Lower analgesia requirements and sometimes shorter hospital stays

Risks and complications

Certain complications are common to open and laparoscopic surgery, but laparoscopic operations carry their own particular risks. Specific problems include:

- Induction of the pneumoperitoneum (inflating the abdomen with gas) may cause subcutaneous emphysema or injury to bowel or major blood vessels and must be performed with care, preferably using an open technique rather than a Veress needle
- Trocar insertion may injure the abdominal wall (including the diaphragm), intra-abdominal organs and blood vessels. It must be performed under direct vision, being alert to structures that could be damaged
- The raised intra-abdominal pressure and head-down position mean that patients have to be ventilated at higher inflation pressures. This reduces venous return and cardiac output and may cause circulatory compromise in patients with cardiac ischaemia. To mitigate this, intra-abdominal pressures should be kept to the minimum necessary for the procedure to be performed safely, i.e. 8–12 mmHg; patients should not be placed in extreme head-up or head-down positions for prolonged periods. Intravenous infusion should be stopped whilst head-down
- The diaphragm is 'splinted' by the pneumoperitoneum and this can precipitate cardiorespiratory complications in patients with respiratory problems. Again, minimising inflation pressures reduces this effect
- The pneumoperitoneum compresses intra-abdominal veins and reduces venous return. This predisposes to thromboembolic complications such as deep venous thrombosis. Patients should receive appropriate prophylaxis at all times
- Inadvertent injury can occur to a range of structures during dissection, diathermy or laser instrumentation, often through excess heating. The damage may go unrecognised if the damage occurs out of the sight of the laparoscope, leading to late complications including haemorrhage and bowel perforation
- Postoperatively, bowel may strangulate through peritoneal defects, and incisional hernias can occur through port sites. The latter should be carefully closed under direct vision to minimise this risk

Technique of laparoscopy

Laparoscopy is usually performed under general anaesthesia, most often with muscle relaxation to allow full and safe insufflation of the abdominal cavity. A **pneumoperitoneum** is first created by introducing carbon dioxide under controlled pressure to lift the abdominal wall away from the viscera, allowing inspection of the peritoneal cavity.

Gas is most safely introduced via a blunt cannula placed by an open technique to enable direct visualisation of the peritoneal contents. The technique has largely replaced 'blind' insufflation via a Veress needle which has a significant risk of vascular injury. The gas pressure should be kept as low as possible while maintaining a satisfactory view, in order to minimise cardiac and respiratory risks. A 5 or 10 mm diameter laparoscope with video camera is then introduced into the abdominal cavity, displaying the image on monitors.

Most laparoscopic procedures need additional cannulae (trocars) through which to pass diathermy hooks, graspers, needle holders, clip appliers and linear staplers. These secondary trocars are inserted through new access points under direct vision from within the abdomen to prevent injury to bowel and other viscera. Different operations each require different port placements. Preferences vary from surgeon to surgeon and port siting also depends on the particular conditions of the operation; for example, cholecystectomy in an obese patient necessitates different port sites from those used in a slim patient.

The laparoscopic operation is performed by an operator and one or more assistants, all observing progress on monitors. Sharp or blunt dissection may be employed as in open surgery. Sharp dissection uses laparoscopic scissors whilst blunt dissection is carried out using fine dissecting forceps ('Petolins' or 'Marylands'), laparoscopic gauze pledgets or the tip of a suction probe. Blunt dissection tears rather than cuts small vessels, deliberately causing minor tissue damage that rapidly activates the coagulation cascade and causes spontaneous cessation of bleeding. This is safer than sharp dissection which may require (potentially excessive) use of diathermy. Haemostasis still requires diathermy and this must be cautiously used to prevent arcing to adjacent organs. Increasingly, safer alternatives are being used such as **bipolar** diathermy forceps or the **harmonic scalpel**, which uses ultrasound to coagulate and cut vessels and tissue.

In laparoscopic-assisted surgery, for example colectomy, a large part of the dissection is performed laparoscopically and then a small abdominal incision is made to deliver the resected specimen.

After operation, patients experience abdominal discomfort at trocar insertion sites and shoulder discomfort from retained gas in the peritoneal cavity. Few restrictions are placed on the patient after discharge; he or she can return to work as soon as comfortable, often after a few days.

Robotic-assisted surgery

Robotically assisted surgical systems are increasingly being used for certain technically challenging operations such as laparoscopic prostatectomy and cardiothoracic operations. These robots are not autonomous but aid the surgeon who sits at a remote console (which may be close to the patient or far away). The surgeon very precisely controls the robotic manipulation of laparoscopic instruments, previously inserted into the anaesthetised patient, via the surgical arm unit. The imaging system provides three-dimensional vision. The da Vinci system allows manipulation of all instruments whilst other simpler systems just control the camera.

Potential benefits include increased precision of movement with 'smoothing' of tremor, prevention of fatigue in long operations and perhaps eventually the need for fewer assistants in the theatre. In the longer term, a surgeon could, at least theoretically, operate on a patient many kilometres away by **tele-surgery**. Disadvantages of robotic surgery include the high capital cost (currently around $1–1.5 million), complete lack of any tactile feedback for the surgeon and long set-up times for individual patients.

APPLICATIONS OF LAPAROSCOPY

Laparoscopy in general surgery has **diagnostic** and **therapeutic applications**. The diagnostic applications are well recognised and are increasingly employed as first-line investigative procedures.

Diagnostic laparoscopy

Diagnostic laparoscopy has long been used by surgeons for assessing chronic liver disease and ascites of unknown origin. Advances in instrumentation and imaging now allow surgeons to perform abdominal exploration almost as thoroughly as is possible via a long laparotomy incision. A key application is for staging gastric or pancreatic cancer to assess operability. This is achieved by inspection, by obtaining peritoneal washings for cytology and by performing biopsies. By this method, patients with incurable disease can be spared the trauma of exploratory open surgery (Box 10.9). Diagnostic laparoscopy is valuable for assessing right iliac fossa pain, particularly in women of menstruating age. The procedure allows more accurate assessment of the gynaecological organs, improves diagnostic accuracy and minimises negative appendicectomy rates.

Therapeutic laparoscopy

Laparoscopic cholecystectomy is already the standard operation for removal of the gall bladder, both in the elective and the emergency situation (described in Ch. 20). Other procedures described below and listed in Box 10.10 are becoming standard operations in the armoury of laparoscopic surgeons.

Laparoscopic appendicectomy

Open appendicectomy for acute appendicitis is one of the most frequently performed operations by general surgeons, and laparoscopic appendicectomy is becoming an operation within the repertoire of surgical trainees. Laparoscopic appendicectomy offers improved diagnostic accuracy with the ability to examine the entire abdomen if the appendix is normal, a lower rate of wound complications, reduced postoperative pain and hospital stay, and perhaps more rapid return to normal activities. Laparoscopic appendicectomy may offer a lower rate of pelvic adhesions because of reduced trauma; this is an advantage in young women.

Laparoscopic inguinal hernia repair

Inguinal hernias can be repaired laparoscopically using a transperitoneal or an extraperitoneal approach. Both techniques involve less dissection than the open approach and are believed to reduce the likelihood of damage to testicular vessels and the ilioinguinal nerve (particularly for recurrent hernias), resulting in a lower incidence of long-term chronic groin pain.

Learning laparoscopic inguinal hernia repair requires a great deal of supervised experience but the procedure is now widely performed, and controlled trials show that it can have results comparable with open hernia repair techniques, including term recurrence rates. Laparoscopic repair is of particular value for recurrent hernias, allowing surgery to be performed in tissue planes free from scarring. It is also recommended for bilateral hernias, when both sides can be repaired through three small incisions.

Laparoscopic fundoplication

Laparoscopic fundoplication can be employed for patients suffering from large hiatus hernias or gastro-oesophageal reflux disease (GORD) resistant to medical management. The technique involves dissecting the gastro-oesophageal junction

Box 10.9 Potential indications for diagnostic laparoscopy

- Evaluation of acute or chronic abdominal pain, e.g. suspected appendicitis, gynaecological pain
- Diagnosis and staging of intra-abdominal malignancies (sometimes with direct ultrasound) (including evaluating the results of chemotherapy or radiotherapy on intra-abdominal malignancies)
- Assessing blunt or penetrating abdominal trauma in stable patients with proven free intra-abdominal fluid
- Evaluation of acute or chronic liver disease
- Diagnosis of ascites of unknown cause
- As a 'second-look' procedure in patients operated on for mesenteric ischaemia
- Exclusion of acute acalculous cholecystitis after major trauma or surgery in intensive care patients

Box 10.10 Current therapeutic applications of laparoscopy

- Cholecystectomy (described in Ch. 20) and common bile duct exploration
- Appendicectomy
- Colonic resections and colostomy formation—benign and malignant disease (although evidence of benefit is scarce)
- Abdominal operations for rectal prolapse
- Division of symptomatic adhesions
- Inguinal, femoral, Spigelian and incisional hernia repairs
- Small bowel surgery—including resection and enteral access procedures
- Peptic ulcer disease (plugging of duodenal perforations)
- Symptomatic hiatus hernias and oesophageal reflux (Nissen fundoplication and other anti-reflux operations)
- Nephrectomy, pyeloplasty and other ureteric procedures
- Splenectomy and adrenalectomy
- Laparoscopic liver biopsy and deroofing of liver cysts
- Distal pancreatectomy
- Laparoscopically assisted oesophagectomy and gastrectomy
- Laparoscopic drainage of pancreatic pseudocysts and pancreatic necrosectomy
- Laparoscopic bypass or banding surgery for obesity
- Laparoscopically assisted total hysterectomy and all tube and ovarian procedures including marsupialisation of ectopic pregnancy

at the hiatus, repairing the crura and wrapping the gastric fundus around the lower oesophagus (Nissen-type wrap). Clinical trials show that it offers rapid return to normal activity and results are as durable as open fundoplication.

Laparoscopic management of duodenal ulcer perforation

Duodenal ulcers usually perforate anteriorly and the perforation can readily be seen with the laparoscope. Under laparoscopic visualisation, the ulcer is closed in the same way as at open operation, with part of the greater omentum secured to the duodenum to seal the perforation with laparoscopically placed sutures. The peritoneal cavity is irrigated with a suction irrigator and the fluid aspirated.

Laparoscopic placement of enterocutaneous jejunostomy tube

In patients requiring long-term enteral feeding in whom a gastrostomy is unsuitable, a fine-bore feeding tube can be placed into the jejunum using laparoscopy, thus avoiding the need for laparotomy.

Laparoscopic splenectomy

Laparoscopic splenectomy has become the gold standard for elective splenectomy, particularly in haematological conditions. Substantially enlarged spleens can be removed laparoscopically but the risk of conversion to open operation rises steeply once the spleen weighs over 1 kg (such spleens usually reach the costal margin). At operation, the patient lies on the right side for best access and vision, and the hilar vessels are divided between clips or with vascular staplers. The spleen is placed in a laparoscopic retrieval bag and broken up or liquidised to enable removal via one of the small port incisions.

Laparoscopic adrenalectomy

Laparoscopic adrenalectomy has proved a highly beneficial procedure, allowing adrenal tumours of all sizes to be removed safely and with much less trauma than the muscle-cutting flank incisions previously employed. It is particularly useful in **phaeochromocytoma** where very delicate handling of the tumour is needed. This includes precise delineation and clipping of the vessels in the appropriate order to avoid catecholamine surges.

Laparoscopically assisted colectomy

Laparoscopic techniques were first used to perform uncomplicated colorectal procedures such as rectopexy and formation of colostomies. Early experience with colorectal cancer showed port site metastases appearing more commonly than wound metastases at open surgery. This led to concern that the cancer was being disseminated by the pneumoperitoneum. However, further research and refinement of 'no touch' techniques have laid these fears to rest. Laparoscopically assisted resection of benign and malignant colonic lesions is becoming more commonplace, and all elective colonic resections can now be undertaken laparoscopically. However, substantial benefits have not yet been demonstrated and there may be a higher rate of anastomotic complications.

Laparoscopic surgery for obesity

(Fig. 10.12)

In recent years there has been a major expansion in laparoscopic surgery for obesity (**bariatric surgery**). The most common technique involves placing an adjustable restrictive silicone band around the upper part of the stomach to create a small proximal pouch that causes early satiety. Results are excellent in carefully selected, well-motivated patients who have good support and follow-up. More radical bariatric operations such as gastric bypass and biliary-pancreatic diversion (BPD) operations are also being performed laparoscopically. These operations achieve greater weight loss and more rapid regression of diabetes but may carry higher rates of morbidity and mortality, largely operator-dependent.

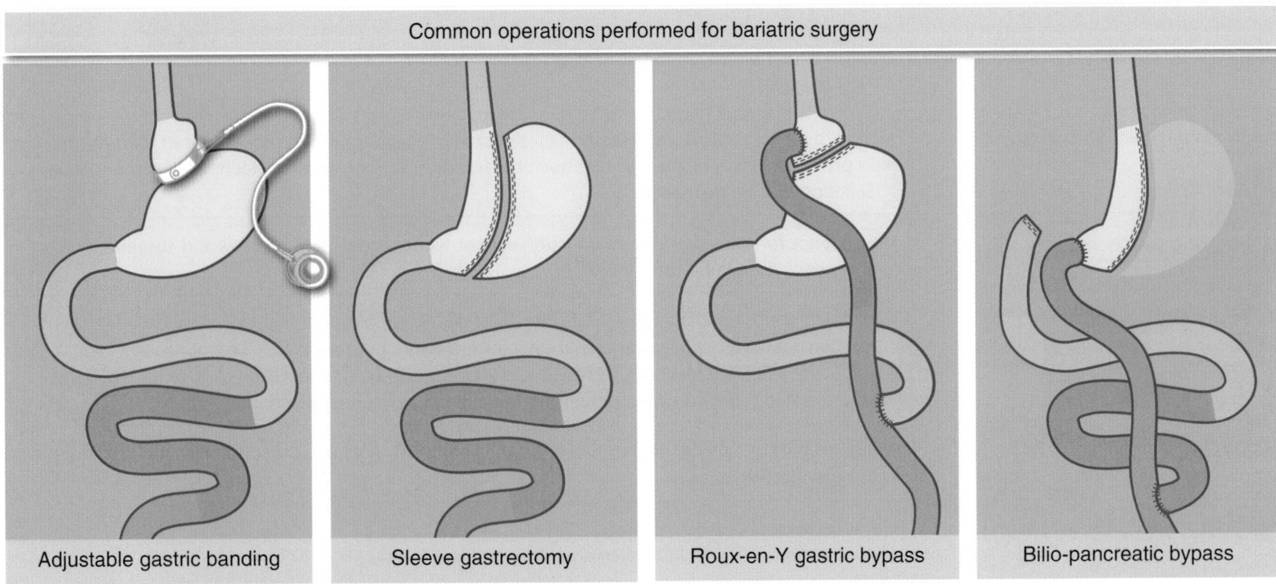

Fig. 10.12 Common operations performed for bariatric surgery

PRINCIPLES OF NEUROSURGERY

Melanie Sharp and Robert Macfarlane

INTRODUCTION

The practice of neurosurgery is evolving rapidly, in much the same way that general surgery did in the 1980s. Neurosurgery is now subdivided into sub-specialities, including head trauma and:

- Vascular (e.g. aneurysm, arteriovenous malformation and stroke)
- Paediatric (e.g. hydrocephalus, tumours and congenital anomalies)
- Spinal (e.g. degenerative disease and tumours)
- Oncology (e.g. glioma, meningioma and metastases)
- Functional (e.g. movement disorders, chronic pain and epilepsy)
- Skull base (e.g. acoustic neuroma, meningioma and chordoma)

Neurosurgery is performed only in specialised centres because the patients present specific challenges that require a multidisciplinary team which includes neuro-anaesthesia, neuro-radiology, neuro-oncology, neuro-intensive care, neuro-rehabilitation as well as specialist nurses/ physiotherapists.

PERIOPERATIVE CONSIDERATIONS

Most neurosurgical units have procedure-specific guidelines for preoperative management including blood ordering. All neurosurgical patients should have baseline neurological assessment recorded and anticoagulants and antiplatelet therapy should be stopped preoperatively. Patients undergoing brain tumour surgery are often on steroids (e.g. dexamethasone) which may cause neutrophilia and adrenal suppression. Angiography and image-guided scanning protocols may be required in some cases.

Intraoperative considerations

Good intraoperative care and attention to detail allows the operation to proceed safely. 'Special considerations' for neurosurgical patients are shown in Table 10.4.

Postoperative considerations

Patients should be recovered in a monitored environment with regular neurological observations. The surgeon should be informed of any neurological deterioration. Depressed consciousness is usually an early sign of rising intracranial pressure. Pupillary dilatation and autonomic changes occur late (e.g. Cushing's reflex).

Postoperative seizures, reduced conscious level or **altered neurology** may herald intracranial complications such as oedema or bleeding. Repeat CT is needed after stabilising blood pressure and oxygenation. Sedating **analgesics** should generally be avoided. Paracetamol and codeine phosphate or small doses of morphine may be appropriate. NSAIDs impair platelet function and should be avoided early on in high-risk patients.

Intravenous fluid needs careful consideration; dextrose may increase cerebral oedema and 0.9% saline or Hartmann's solution is usually administered. Plasma sodium abnormalities are relatively common in neurosurgical patients and need investigation. These include the syndrome of inappropriate antidiuretic hormone hypersecretion (SIADH), which causes

Table 10.4 Specific perioperative considerations in neurosurgical patients

Patient group	Factors to consider
Patients taking anti-epileptic drugs (AEDs)	Measure drug blood levels and check electrolytes. Ensure medications are continued perioperatively
Cognitive impairment and confusion	Mental capacity needs to be assessed before obtaining valid informed consent (See Ethics chapter) New onset confusion needs investigation. It may indicate intracranial or biochemical abnormalities. Sedation may be dangerous.
Hair shaving	No evidence for increased wound infection with or without shaving. Cosmesis and surgeon preference determine the decision
Head positioning	Aim to achieve optimal operating position whilst aiding venous drainage. Avoid excessive neck rotation. Elevation of head reduces intracranial pressure but may risk of air embolism. 3-point clamp fixation stabilises the head and allows table-fixed retraction. During the WHO checklist, the operation side is confirmed against the imaging
Infection prophylaxis	Antibiotic prophylaxis on induction of anaesthetic typically with gram + coccal cover. No further doses in clean elective surgery
Intra-operative measures to lower ICP	Elevation of head (30–45 degrees) Mild hyperventilation to reduce cerebral blood volume Intravenous mannitol

hyponatraemia and sometimes fluid overload, and diabetes insipidus (DI) which causes polyuria and polydipsia by diminishing the ability to concentrate urine.

SURGICAL MANAGEMENT OF HYDROCEPHALUS

Hydrocephalus results from a mismatch between cerebrospinal fluid (CSF) production and reabsorption, leading to raised intracranial pressure. It is classified into **communicating** and **non-communicating** types, depending on whether the obstruction lies within ventricles or the subarachnoid space. Common causes include:

- Congenital (e.g. spina bifida)
- Trauma (blood clot, brain swelling, venous sinus injury)
- Infection (meningitis)
- Vascular (subarachnoid or intracerebral haemorrhage)
- Tumour

Hydrocephalus can be an acute emergency; patients can present to a general hospital with morning headache, vomiting, blurred or double vision and ataxia. Signs include depressed conscious level, papilloedema, cranial nerve IV or VI palsies or nystagmus. An urgent CT scan identifies hydrocephalus or shunt dysfunction. Hydrocephalus in infants may manifest with gradually enlarging head circumference or, in the elderly, with the triad of ataxia, dementia and incontinence ('normal pressure hydrocephalus').

Treatment of communicating hydrocephalus

This can be relieved temporarily via lumbar puncture (but **never** in non-communicating hydrocephalus). Long-term management requires diversion by insertion of a shunt as described below.

Treatment of non-communicating hydrocephalus

If secondary to tumour, this may respond to dexamethasone to temporise before tumour removal. Otherwise the obstruction needs to be bypassed by endoscopic third ventriculostomy, insertion of an external ventricular drain, or creation of a permanent CSF diversion with a shunt. Shunting is usually via a catheter between lateral ventricle and peritoneum with a pressure regulating valve.

BASIC PRINCIPLES OF CRANIOTOMY

Craniotomy is the standard method of accessing the cranial cavity. A bone flap is fashioned which is replaced at the end of the operation. Bevelling the bone edges and using titanium plates and/or screws facilitates closure. If bone is not replaced, this is termed **craniectomy** (the bone forms a template for a titanium or acrylic plate, or is stored for later reimplantation). Indications for craniectomy include raised intracranial pressure refractory to medication, bone infection or osteomyelitis, or infiltration of bone by tumour.

Preparation for operation begins with optimal patient and head positioning. Planning the incision and craniotomy needs to take the following factors into account:

- Cosmesis (e.g. avoiding forehead incisions and excessive hair shaving)
- The scalp blood supply: large arteries include occipital and superficial temporal arteries and these should be preserved. Bleeding from even small scalp arteries can lead to large blood loss
- Avoiding placing implants or foreign material (e.g. screws/plates) directly under wounds
- Location of scalp nerves: damage to temporalis and frontalis nerve branches can cause unsightly forehead muscle asymmetry
- Position of cranial landmarks and underlying structures in relation to the pathology, including major dural venous sinuses, cranial arteries and areas of special importance such as motor and visual pathways. Modern planning includes CT or MR image-guided navigation, but it cannot replace knowledge of anatomy

In elective surgery, craniotomy flaps are 'tailored' to access the operative area, but when an intracranial haematoma needs rapid and safe evacuation after trauma, a standard fronto-temporo-parietal craniotomy is used. Meticulous haemostasis before wound closure is critical in operative neurosurgery.

PRESENTATION OF BRAIN TUMOURS

Brain tumours are primary or secondary. Primary tumours are categorised by histological type, location within the brain and grade. The terms benign or malignant are not normally used because tumours rarely metastasise outside the craniospinal axis, and long-term survival depends on whether tumour growth can be controlled. Glioma is the most common primary brain tumour, whilst meningioma (see Fig. 10.13) is the most common extra-axial tumour. The WHO pathological classification provides a more precise system, encompassing the tissue of origin and its behavioural characteristics. Potential modes of tumour presentation are shown in Table 10.5.

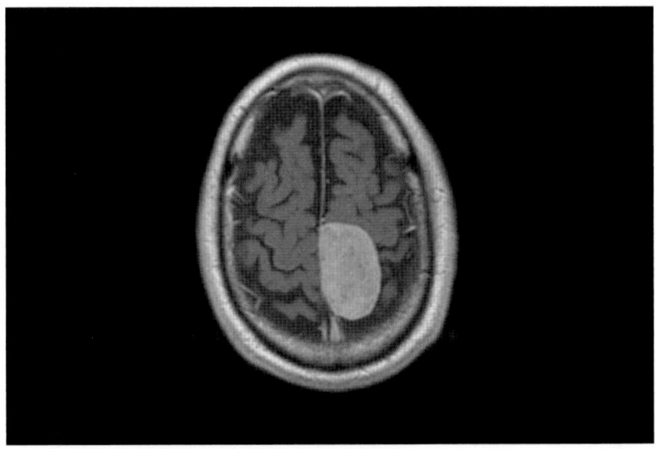

Fig. 10.13 Typical appearance of a meningioma arising from the dura adjacent to the superior sagittal sinus

Table 10.5 Presentation of brain tumours according to site

Mode of presentation	Significance
Incidental finding	Intracranial pathology identified during imaging for another purpose (e.g. sinusitis). A period of active observation may be appropriate
Seizures	**Generalised tonic-clonic seizures**—usually only in supratentorial tumours **Partial sensory or motor seizures**—particularly in tumours around the sensory or motor strip **Complex partial seizures**—particularly in temporal lobe tumours
Raised intracranial pressure	Reduced conscious level, confusion, headache, vomiting, papilloedema, unilateral or bilateral pupillary dilatation
Altered brain function	**Frontal**—altered personality, contralateral face, arm or leg weakness, expressive dysphasia (dominant side), incontinence **Temporal**—upper homonymous quadrantanopia, receptive dysphasia (dominant hemisphere) **Parietal**—lower homonymous quadrantanopia **Occipital**—homonymous hemianopia **Cerebellar**—nystagmus, ataxia, speech disturbance including dysarthria and staccato speech and intention tremor **Brainstem**—vomiting, lower cranial nerve palsies, long tract signs, reduced consciousness, pupil changes, altered eye movements **Hypothalamic/pituitary**—visual deficit (bitemporal hemianopia), endocrine disturbance

ORTHOPAEDIC SURGERY

THE NORMAL LOCOMOTOR SYSTEM

AXIAL AND APPENDICULAR SKELETON

The axial skeleton comprises the skull, spine and rib cage whilst the appendicular skeleton comprises the arms and shoulder girdle, the legs and pelvis. The normal locomotor system relies on a stable skeleton to provide attachment for muscles and a base for positioning the hands and feet in space. Muscles are grouped into bundles or mass-acting units according to function and along embryological lines.

Disease of any part of the control or action mechanism leads to loss of function and requires diagnosis and reversal to restore functional ability. For example, a finger contracture due to Dupuytren's disease limits movement and small items cannot be retrieved from a pocket or purse. Contrast this local problem with a motorbike rider who injures his neck in a collision. The subsequent brachial plexus injury prevents accurate nerve signalling to the hand and he also cannot retrieve his coins. Management of these similar functional disturbances is very different but the aim for both is to recover full functional capability.

STRUCTURE OF BONE AND ARTICULAR CARTILAGE

Bone

Bone is composed of an organic and an inorganic matrix. It undergoes continual adjustment as cells are remodelled and elements refreshed in response to external stimuli. The skeleton is a living organ providing support for muscles and tendons, it has haemopoetic capacity, and it is a calcium reservoir.

Bone structure includes cortical and trabecular components. A solid shell of cortical bone is strong in compression and resists bending forces. Mature cortical bone is arranged in lamellae or layers with vascular channels running through. Its precursor is immature **woven bone**, seen in healing and in the growing skeleton. Its organisation is random without heed to external stresses.

Bone metabolism involves complicated homeostasis of its matrix (governed by physical stresses), plus regulation of minerals and ions, principally calcium and phosphate. The inorganic component is largely crystalline calcium phosphate and hydroxyapatite, and a feedback loop controls mineralisation and turnover, involving serum ion levels, vitamin D_3, parathormone and calcitonin (see Fig. 49.10, p. 611).

The organic matrix of bone is largely composed of type I collagen, with types V and XI in small amounts contributing to flexibility and strength. Also found are bone morphogenic proteins (BMP 1–17), and cytokines and signallers (interleukin 1 and 6 and insulin-like growth factor).

Articular cartilage

Articular cartilage provides a near frictionless interface between bones to facilitate movement. Synovial joints are covered with hyaline cartilage, a special tissue composed of chondrocytes bound in an extracellular matrix. The matrix is layered tangentially and radially throughout the cartilage; 90% of this collagen is type II.

Hyaline cartilage has very poor healing ability. It is aneural, avascular and alymphatic, and derives nourishment by osmosis from synovial fluid. Superficial abrasions or injuries provoke no healing response and result in permanent damage. Deeper injuries that reach the capillary bed of the bone cause clot formation and later repair with fibrocartilage. Healing never perfectly restores the initial hyaline cartilage or its specialised smooth surface.

LIMB COMPARTMENTS

Limb muscles are arranged into compartments during embryological life; grouping those with similar actions limiting friction between them. The compartments have inflexible fascial walls restricting expansion beyond a limited volume so if traumatic swelling occurs, there is a risk of **compartment syndrome** causing ischaemia (see Ch. 17, p. 235).

ORTHOPAEDIC DISORDERS

Mr William Hage

ARTHRITIS

The arthritides are joint disorders leading to pain and dysfunction. They can be grouped into acquired and congenital, inflammatory, infective, autoimmune and degenerative. Anything that alters the low friction surface of a synovial joint leads to pain on movement, and diseases that alter the surface or the synovial envelope can do the same.

Osteoarthritis

Osteoarthritis (OA) is an idiopathic disorder of joint wear. Over the lifetime of a joint, the hyaline cartilage tends to wear out causing pain and stiffness. The process is governed by genetic, developmental and other factors that are not yet completely understood. Some joints such as hip and knee are often affected, whereas others (e.g. ankle) rarely wear out. Some hips wear out because of imperfect articulation or development from birth. It is not yet known why some individuals are plagued by widespread osteoarthritis in their 50s and others have little or none in their 80s. Treatment includes palliative analgesia and often, ultimately surgery.

Post-traumatic osteoarthritis

This is linked to trauma sustained at the joint surface. This may be an intra-articular fracture, a cartilage tear or anything that increases friction at the bearing surface. Post-traumatic OA occurs between 5 and 20 years after the trauma. Heavy impact sport in early life can play a part.

Inflammatory arthropathies

This group includes rheumatoid arthritis (RA) and other joint diseases characterised by a chronic nature and an inflammatory component. Autoimmunity is often involved, and the group should be considered as systemic diseases which often lead to multijoint involvement with symmetrical patterns.

In most inflammatory arthropathies the pathology is synovial, with chronic inflammation and thickening of epithelial layers leading to pain, stiffness and altered blood chemistry. Low-level joint destruction occurs over many years, and secondary osteoarthritis is eventually superimposed. Treatment aims to control or modify the inflammation to prevent progression.

Crystal arthropathies

A subgroup of inflammatory joint diseases occurs in acute episodes and causes painful joints. The most common is **gout**, where monosodium urate crystals enter the synovium and synovial fluid causing profound inflammation. The joint becomes hot, swollen and painful. Initial treatment is analgesia and rehydration with joint splintage. In **pseudogout**, similar problems are caused by calcium pyrophosphate dehydrate.

INFECTION

Orthopaedic infections involve soft tissue and/or bone. Soft tissue infections include those of bursae adjoining joints, in tendons or tendon sheaths of hands and feet, and cellulitis. These are often easy to diagnose, but may be difficult to treat without leaving a functional deficit or stiffness; outcome often depends on the pathogen responsible. Fibrosis of upper limb tendons and sheaths develops quickly even after eradication of infection and can severely limit hand function.

Bone infection is termed **osteomyelitis** and affects cortex or cancellous bone. Joint infection is termed **septic arthritis**. Areas with poor blood supply cannot eliminate infection effectively and antibiotic delivery to these areas is also poor.

Osteomyelitis

Bone infection passes through several stages: an acute inflammatory response with soft tissue swelling, demineralisation and death of bone (sequestrum formation), then, if infection is controlled, new bone (involucrum) formation. Identifying the infecting organism by biopsy, aspirate and culture is critically important before targeted antibiotic therapy. Long courses may be needed to eradicate infection from sites with poor blood supply such as the tibia. Surgical debridement of abscesses and removal of dead bone is also an important step.

Septic arthritis

(Fig. 10.14)

This is an orthopaedic emergency and occurs by traumatic penetration of a joint or by spread from metaphyseal osteomyelitis. Articular cartilage in synovial joints is very easily damaged when a joint fills with pus. Hyaline cartilage breaks down in hours, so treatment is urgent. This means early removal of dead tissue, joint irrigation and targeted antibiotics. Without this, secondary osteoarthritis is inevitable within very few years.

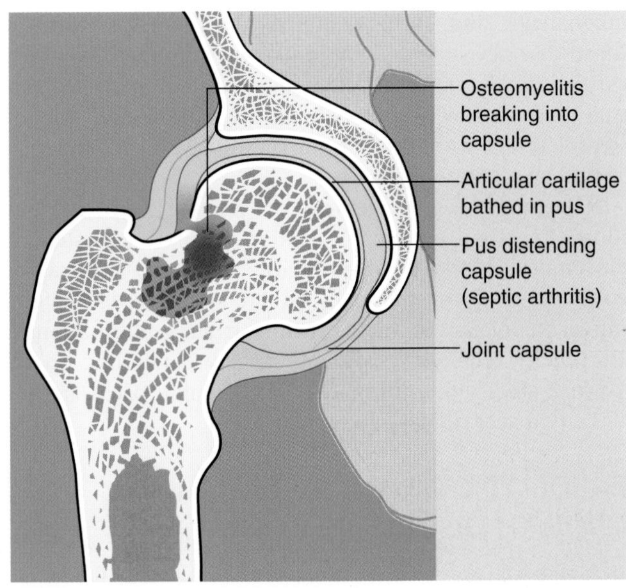

Fig. 10.14 Septic arthritis and osteomyelitis

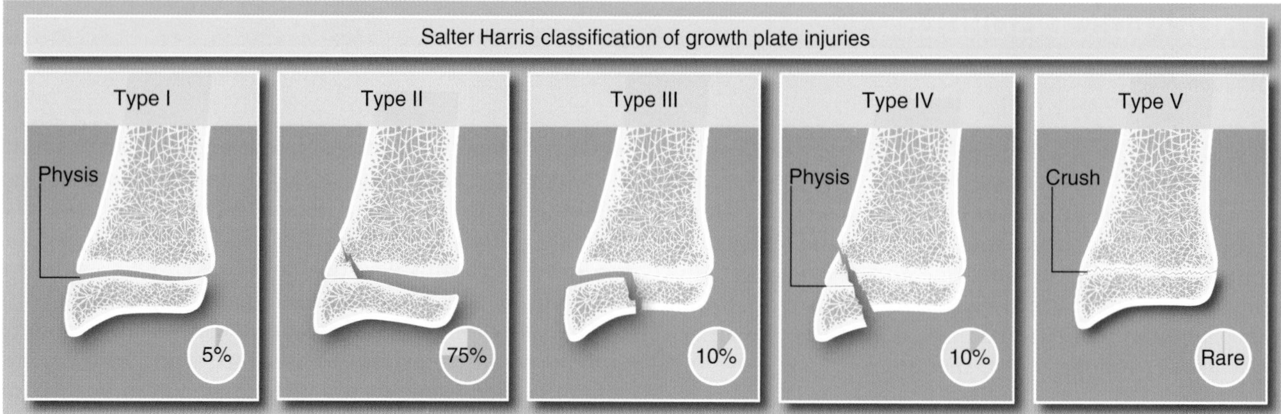

Fig. 10.15 Salter-Harris classification of physis/epiphysis in children

In adults, the usual infecting organism in primary osteomyelitis and septic arthritis is *Staphylococcus* spp., although *Streptococcus* spp., *Salmonella, Pseudomonas* and other rarities occur, usually in immunocompromised patients.

Children also suffer predominantly staphylococcal infection. Widespread immunisation against *Haemophilus* has largely banished it as a cause of bone infection. Yeasts and fungi sometimes infect the musculoskeletal system but viruses do not, although viral influenza can cause multiple painful joint effusions and synovitis.

TUMOURS

Primary bone tumours are rare. Malignant tumours are classified by primary cell type and are staged using the T-N-M system. The neoplastic cell grade gives an indication of aggressiveness.

Bony metastases are much more common than primary malignancies and spring from solid primary tumours or diffuse diseases such as lymphoma or myeloma. The classic primary sources are breast, lung and prostate cancers and the usual presentation is bone pain before pathological fracture. After fracture, the abnormal bone is unlikely to heal and often requires surgical stabilisation.

Diagnosis and management of primary bone tumours follows the usual pattern of detailed history and systematic examination, biopsy for histological diagnosis, and staging. Because of rarity this is usually undertaken in tertiary referral centres. Neoplasms are treated with various combinations of radiotherapy, chemotherapy and surgery depending on cell type and stage. Some primaries, for example osteosarcoma, still carry a very poor prognosis.

PAEDIATRIC ORTHOPAEDICS AND GROWTH DISORDERS

The skeleton begins to form in utero and bones ossify through childhood and teenage years to reach a stable state usually between 15 and 18 years. Most long bones originate with a cartilage shape that gradually transforms to adult-type bone as osteoblasts infiltrate and lay down calcified bone by the process known as enchondral ossification. By contrast, intramembranous ossification occurs without a cartilage model; examples include clavicle and the flat skull bones.

Enchondral ossification proceeds from several ossification centres at varying speeds and with predictable onset. Long bones have one centre in the middle of the diaphysis (main shaft) from where ossification spreads longitudinally, plus centres in the epiphyses (near the ends). The **physis** or growth plate at the bone end is where new bone forms to cause longitudinal growth. Diseases that affect the physis or epiphysis can disrupt bone growth and lead to a range of abnormalities. The Salter-Harris classification (Fig. 10.15) describes fractures at the physis and/or through the epiphysis in children's bones.

Children's bones contain less calcified osteoid (bone matrix) than those of adults; they flex more before they fracture and demonstrate more plastic fracture patterns when they do. Bone healing after fracture is also different: bones heal with callus and re-ossify, but remodel quickly, often smoothing out deformity or malunion. As the bone grows longer, it attempts to return (remodel) to its normal shape; the more growth years left, the more scope there is for remodelling.

Primary bone tumours in children are rare although Ewing's sarcoma must be considered during teenage years. Bone cysts and remnants of ossification errors such as cortical fibromas are often seen incidentally on X-ray. They usually cause no symptoms and need no treatment.

Disorders affecting epiphyseal bone growth can cause dwarfism or short stature and many are effectively uncorrectable. Faults in calcification or generation of bone matrix can lead to weak bone. This is seen in rickets or osteogenesis imperfecta. Cooperative management between endocrinologist, paediatrician and orthopaedic surgeon can limit the functional disturbances.

ELECTIVE ORTHOPAEDICS

INVESTIGATION IN ORTHOPAEDICS

Plain radiology

This is the chief orthopaedic investigation. X-rays have been used for decades and doses and techniques are now refined to minimise ionising radiation. Bones are shown in great detail because of the high calcium content. The usual model is two X-rays at right angles and including nearby joints; both views must be examined for abnormality, fracture or disruption before reaching a diagnosis. Radiology of the skeleton in its loaded state can give more information, e.g. standing or flexed, and X-rays of an arthritic joint are often taken with knees and hips in a standing position.

Ultrasound

Ultrasound is widely used in orthopaedics. It gives a dynamic view of soft tissues and is good at examining liquid filled structures; bones are not seen in useful detail. Cysts, ganglia and tendons are well evaluated and a dynamic picture of a joint is valuable in motion disorders or impingement syndromes.

Magnetic resonance imaging (MRI)

This modality is risk free and is increasingly used to give detail of soft tissues and three-dimensional architecture. Some examples include: nerve roots exiting the spinal cord, menisci and ligaments in the knee joint (with contrast); wrist ligaments and carpal bones can also be examined.

Computed tomography (CT)

CT scans can give detail of bones down to millimetre level. Images can be reformatted into three-dimensional virtual models, e.g. for fractures or to plan complex anatomical reconstructions of acetabulum or spine.

Arthroscopy

Accurate diagnosis of a joint injury often requires internal inspection. Despite accurate history, examination and even MRI, the problem can be missed if it is transient, or only reproduced under conditions of load.

Arthroscopy is often employed for shoulder or knee, less often in the elbow and rarely in the hip. Under anaesthesia, a 5 mm arthroscope (rigid telescope with video camera) is inserted into the joint enabling inspection and, if necessary, probing with another instrument. Abnormalities can often be repaired or material removed at the same time and most procedures take less than 30 minutes so patients can go home the same day and usually recover rapidly. Arthroscopic techniques have been extended over the years to include ligament reconstruction, rotator cuff repair and cartilage repair.

JOINT REPLACEMENT SURGERY

Joint replacement is advocated when pain plus major damage to articular cartilage has exhausted non-surgical options. Replacement of synovial joints can restore anatomical alignment and provide pain-free mobility. Hip replacement was pioneered in Wrightington Hospital, Lancashire, in the 1960s and has taken off world-wide; progress in replacing other large joints proceeds apace. End-stage osteoarthritis remains the most common indication, but replacement is also performed for malalignment, post-traumatic arthritis and revision replacement when primary replacement fails. Joint replacement surgery is a major undertaking; patients are usually in their 60s or 70s and complication rates of 5% are currently unavoidable.

Replacement of the knee, hip, ankle, shoulder, elbow joints and most others relies on surgically excising the diseased, high-friction articular cartilage and resurfacing the bone ends with metal, plastic or ceramic bearing surfaces. Various techniques are used to secure the implant components. Bone cement works very reliably but an alternative method of fixation uses **osseointegration**, encouraging bone growth into a hydroxyapatite-coated metal implant. After joint replacement surgery, pain is markedly reduced but the articulation continues to wear and usually has a finite life with 10–15 years or even more expected for 90% of patients with hip or knee replacement. Revision joint replacement is well established, but success rates drop and functional results are rarely as good.

11 Diagnosis and management of common postoperative problems

INTRODUCTION

Despite good preoperative assessment, surgical and anaesthetic technique and perioperative management, unexpected symptoms or signs arise after operation that may herald a complication. Detecting these early by regular monitoring and surgical review means early treatment can often forestall major deterioration. This chapter uses a problem-orientated approach to help junior (and more senior) doctors deal with such problems. The management of more serious complications is described in the next chapter.

Managing problems such as pain, fever or collapse requires correct diagnosis then early treatment. Determining the cause can be challenging, particularly if the patient is anxious, in pain or not fully recovered from anaesthesia. It is vital to see and assess the patient and if necessary, arrange investigations, whatever the hour, when deterioration suggests potentially serious but often remediable complications. Consider also whether and when to call for senior help.

POSTOPERATIVE PAIN

Some types of wound are more painful, for example vertical abdominal incisions and skin graft donor sites. It is better to prevent pain pre-emptively than react to established pain.

METHODS OF MANAGEMENT

Postoperative pain can be minimised by preoperative counselling, perioperative measures and postoperative analgesia. Counselling lets the patient know the probable extent of pain, the plans for pain relief and the likely degree of mobility after operation. During the operation **pre-emptive analgesia** ensures that pain does not become established.

This may involve:

- Long-acting analgesic drugs given intravenously
- Local anaesthetic infiltration into the wound edges at the end of the operation with a long-acting agent, such as **bupivacaine**
- Regional nerve blocks (e.g. intercostal nerves for upper abdominal surgery using a transversus abdominis plane (TAP) block)
- Epidural analgesia using local anaesthetic and often morphine, during and after abdominal and pelvic surgery. These do not influence the rate of anastomotic leakage
- Non-steroidal analgesics given before the patient awakes by suppository or intravenous injection. These must not be given to patients with known allergy to aspirin or other NSAIDs, a history of severe asthma or angio-oedema, bleeding disorders, renal impairment, hypovolaemia or pregnancy. Mild asthma is not a contraindication. It is also unwise to use these in operations with a high risk of haemorrhage

ANALGESIA FOR MINOR AND INTERMEDIATE SURGERY

Patients vary greatly in their pain tolerance and need for analgesics. For minor and intermediate surgery, pre-emptive analgesia usually means simple analgesic tablets are sufficient. However, anxiety, exhaustion and sleep deprivation may reduce pain tolerance and the amount of analgesia must be adapted to individual need.

ANALGESIA FOR MAJOR SURGERY AND TRAUMA

(see Box 11.1)

Many hospitals now provide an **acute pain service**, run by anaesthetists and specialist nurses. This team can plan individual analgesic strategies and help deal with pain problems as they arise. True objective rating of pain is difficult but some form of visual analogue scale chart can be helpful (Fig. 11.1).

Following major abdominal and perineal operations **epidural analgesia** using local anaesthetic drugs and morphine can be invaluable. A single dose can provide anaesthesia for the operation, e.g. transurethral prostatectomy, plus several hours of complete postoperative analgesia. For more extensive surgery, an epidural cannula can be left in situ to allow

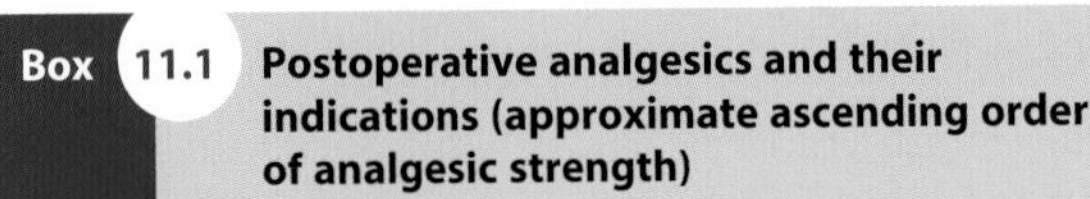

Box 11.1 Postoperative analgesics and their indications (approximate ascending order of analgesic strength)

Mild-to-moderate pain:

- Paracetamol
- Compounds of paracetamol and low-dose codeine, e.g. co-codamol
- Milder non-steroidal anti-inflammatory drugs (NSAIDs), e.g. ibuprofen

Moderate pain:

- Paracetamol
- Codeine or dihydrocodeine 30–60 mg
- Stronger NSAIDs as tablets or suppositories, e.g. diclofenac

Moderate-to-severe pain:

- Other opiate analgesics stronger than codeine, e.g. oxycodone, tramadol
- Non-steroidal anti-inflammatory drugs by intravenous injection, e.g. diclofenac
- Morphine slow-release tablets
- Morphine or diamorphine—patient-controlled intravenous injection

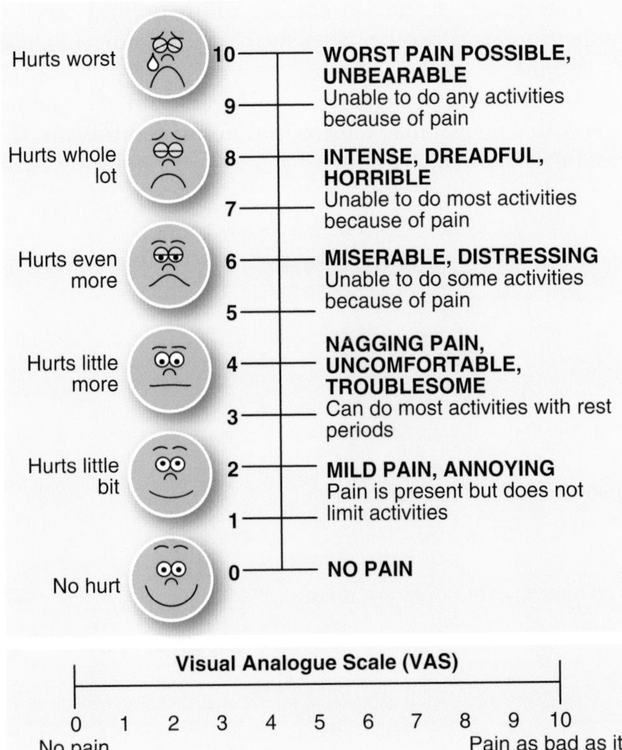

Fig. 11.1 Pain measurement scales

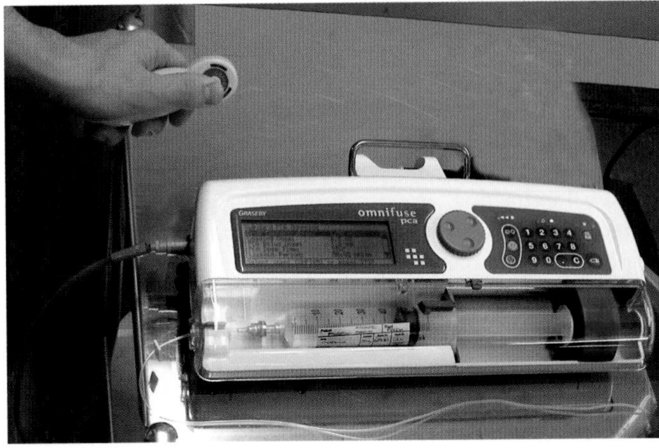

Fig. 11.2 Patient-controlled analgesia
This microprocessor-controlled device prevents overdosage by 'locking out' if used too frequently. The patient's control handset is seen on the left

'topping-up' to extend postoperative analgesia. These patients need careful observation for signs of toxicity, severe hypotension or respiratory depression. Note that moderate hypotension is merely an indication of satisfactory sympathetic blockade.

For major surgery and trauma where epidural analgesia is inappropriate, the analgesic dose needs to be enough to eliminate the pain without causing dangerous side-effects, and to be given often enough for continuous pain relief. Effective pain control can be achieved by allowing patients to give themselves small intravenous increments of opiates using a **patient-controlled analgesia** (PCA) device (Fig. 11.2). This allows presetting of the incremental dose (often 1 mg of morphine), with a 5 minute lockout to prevent it being given too frequently, as well as control of the total dose. Continuous effective pain relief is thus easily achieved and the total dose used is often less than with intermittent injections. This technique causes minimal sedation and respiratory depression whilst maintaining excellent continuous analgesia, although it can cause opiate-induced nausea.

EXCESSIVE POSTOPERATIVE PAIN

If the pain is not controlled by an apparently adequate dose and frequency of analgesia, complications should be suspected. The dose should first be reviewed in relation to the expected severity of pain and the weight of the patient.

- **Local postoperative complications** should be considered. Wound pain may be caused by pressure from a **haematoma**. In limb trauma, bleeding into or inflammatory oedema in a fascial compartment must be diagnosed before ischaemia ensues ('**compartment syndrome**'). Wound pain increasing after the first 48 hours may be caused by **infection**. The wound is unusually tender even before redness and induration develop and there is usually a pyrexia. Other complications with lower limb pain include deep vein thrombosis and acute ischaemia. Lastly, major co-morbid conditions may be the cause of pain, for example myocardial ischaemia, or a fractured neck of femur may follow falling out of bed

- **Major complications** in the operation area. After an abdominal operation, excessive pain can be caused by intra-abdominal complications. These include haemorrhage, anastomotic leakage, biliary leakage, abscess formation, gaseous distension due to ileus or air swallowing, intestinal obstruction, urinary retention and bowel ischaemia, any of which is likely to require reoperation. Constipation may also cause late postoperative pain

As a rule, serious complications cause deterioration in the patient's general condition, whereas the patient remains well with less serious complications such as urinary retention or constipation.

PYREXIA (see Fig. 11.3)

Fever is a common postoperative observation not always caused by infection. Pyrexia within 48 hours is usually caused by basal lung atelectasis and should be treated with physiotherapy and mobilisation. After this period, a search should be made for a focus of infection. The common ones are **superficial** or **deep wound infection, chest infection** (pneumonia), **urinary tract infection** and infection of an **intravenous cannula site**. If there is a central venous line, infection should always be suspected in unexplained pyrexia. Unfortunately, this can only be diagnosed by removing the line and culturing the tip for organisms. Blood cultures alone are often positive but do not reveal the source of infection. Patients usually recover spontaneously once the central line is removed.

Common non-infective causes of pyrexia include **transfusion reactions, wound haematomas, deep venous thrombosis** and **pulmonary embolism**. Pyrexia is sometimes the only sign of an idiosyncratic or allergic **drug reaction**. A rare cause is malignant hyperpyrexia following general anaesthesia.

TACHYCARDIA

Tachycardia (rapid heart rate) may simply indicate **pain** or **anxiety** but it is also a feature of **infection, circulatory disturbances** and **thyrotoxicosis**. Mild tachycardia may be a sign of incipient **hypovolaemic shock** as a result of haemorrhage or dehydration. It may also herald **cardiac failure**. Tachycardia may be a sign of recent onset **atrial fibrillation or flutter**; this is confirmed by electrocardiography, and may indicate the patient has suffered a myocardial infarction. In bowel surgery patients, this is often a sign of **anastomotic leakage**, presumably mediated by cytokines released as a result of the leakage.

COUGH, SHORTNESS OF BREATH AND TACHYPNOEA

These symptoms are often associated with an overt respiratory problem such as **acute bronchopneumonia, aspiration of gastric contents, lobar collapse, pneumothorax** or an exacerbation of a **pre-existing chronic lung disorder**. Clinical examination and chest X-ray will rapidly diagnose most of them.

Shortness of breath and rapid shallow breathing are a feature of alveolar collapse (**atelectasis**), which may not be detected by clinical examination or chest X-ray. Atelectasis usually responds to chest physiotherapy. **Abdominal distension** may also cause rapid shallow breathing by inhibiting diaphragmatic movement. Shortness of breath and tachypnoea may be early features of **cardiac failure** or **fluid overload** but there are usually other clues such as tachycardia and basal crepitations.

A sudden onset of shortness of breath and tachypnoea, often with collapse, may indicate **pulmonary embolism**. This must be recognised, investigated and treated vigorously. **Acute**

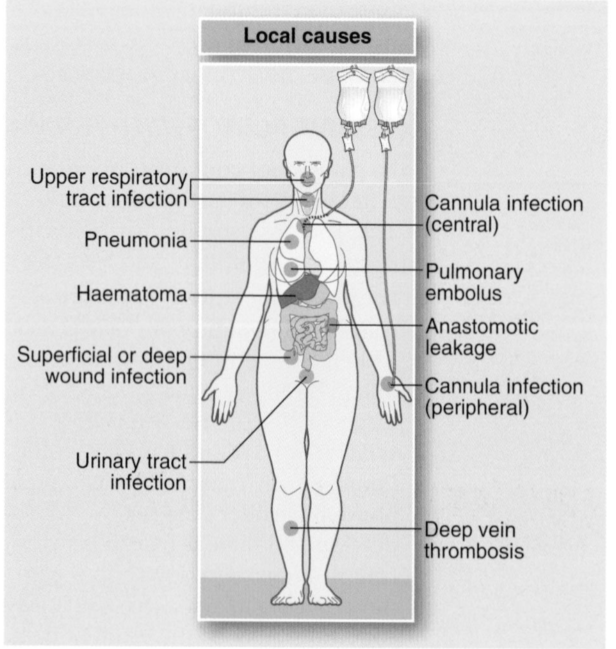

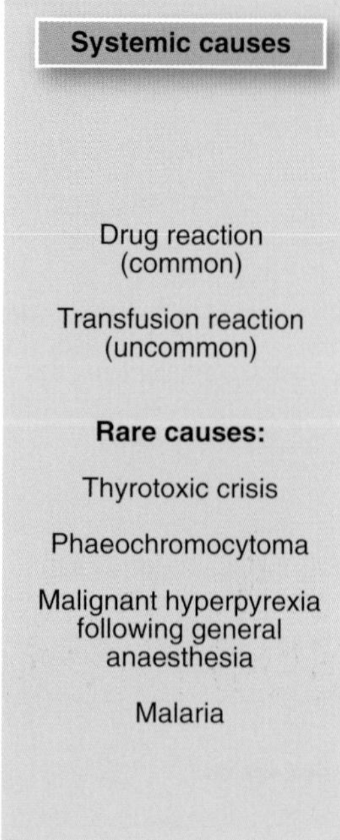

Fig. 11.3 Causes of pyrexia

respiratory distress syndrome may occur in chest trauma, acute pancreatitis or systemic sepsis and should be anticipated in these patients. Finally, respiratory symptoms may be due to **hyperventilation** induced by pain, anxiety or hysteria.

COLLAPSE OR RAPID GENERAL DETERIORATION

The doctor on call is commonly asked to deal with a patient who has 'collapsed' or 'gone off' in a non-specific way. To make matters more difficult, the patient is often under the care of another surgical team. The more serious possibilities are summarised in Box 11.2.

In practice, the problem is tackled in the following order, which usually leads to a logical diagnosis:

- Brief history of the collapse and postoperative course to date.
- Rapid clinical appraisal—check **A**irway, **B**reathing and **C**irculation, then changes in conscious state and neurology
- Chart review reveals changes in temperature, pulse, blood pressure and respiratory rate. Check urinary output and fluid balance
- Review of:
  - Reason for admission and preoperative state
  - Pre-existing co-morbid conditions
  - Nature and extent of surgical operation, including any operative problems
  - Likely extent of perioperative blood and other fluid losses (including sequestration in bowel)
  - Adequacy of fluid replacement
  - Drug therapy—prescribed drugs? Have important drugs been given or omitted?
- Detailed physical examination
- Check blood glucose using reagent strips
- Special tests as suggested by clinical findings, e.g. ECG, chest X-ray, serum electrolyte estimation, arterial blood gas analysis, full blood count, urinalysis

Box 11.2 Important causes of postoperative collapse or rapid deterioration

Cardiovascular
- Myocardial infarction
- Other cause of rapid deterioration of cardiac function, e.g. sudden arrhythmia or fluid overload
- Pulmonary embolism
- Stroke (may be without obvious limb paralysis)

Respiratory
- Failure to reverse anaesthesia adequately (early)
- Drug-induced respiratory depression
- Hypoxia due to a respiratory disorder or respiratory depressant drugs

'Surgical' and infective
- Hypovolaemic shock from acute blood loss, or sudden decompensation in unrecognised hypovolaemia
- Bowel strangulation or obstruction
- Systemic sepsis (often caused by anastomotic leakage)
- Severe localised infection, e.g. chest or operation site

Metabolic
- Electrolyte disturbances, e.g. hyponatraemia
- Hypoglycaemia or hyperglycaemia associated with diabetes
- Adrenal insufficiency, e.g. adrenal suppression by preoperative or earlier corticosteroid treatment; causes hypotension

Drug effects
- Drug reactions, e.g. anaphylaxis

NAUSEA AND VOMITING

DRUGS AS A CAUSE

Nausea and vomiting are common postoperative problems. The usual causes are side-effects from drugs used for general anaesthesia or postoperative analgesia, particularly opiates. Anti-emetics are usually given with opiates 'as required' for the early postoperative period but may have been missed. Nausea and sometimes vomiting later in the postoperative period may be caused by drugs. The worst offenders are erythromycin and metronidazole given orally, and **digoxin** overdosage (particularly in the elderly and in chronic renal failure).

Causes in the immediate postoperative period

- Vigorous handling of the patient in the operating department and in recovery may stimulate vestibular input causing motion sickness
- Oropharyngeal stimulation—caused by a nasogastric (NG) tube or aspiration of secretions
- Hypoxia
- Hypotension
- Pain
- Anxiety

BOWEL OBSTRUCTION CAUSING NAUSEA AND VOMITING

Sustained vomiting 48 hours or more after operation is usually caused by **mechanical obstruction** or by **adynamic bowel** (see Ch. 12, p. 172). Adynamic small bowel (**ileus**) is common after bowel operations and is difficult to differentiate from adhesional obstruction, but if it persists beyond 5 days after surgery, obstruction is more likely than ileus.

Mechanical obstruction, usually of small bowel, can follow any abdominal operation. Early obstruction due to fibrinous adhesions occurs within 4 days of operation and may respond to conservative treatment but often requires a further operation.

Finally, **faecal impaction** is a common problem in the elderly or immobile patient and may cause vomiting.

SYSTEMIC DISORDERS CAUSING NAUSEA AND VOMITING

Electrolyte disturbances, uraemia, hypercalcaemia and other systemic disorders may cause vomiting via central effects. Centrally-mediated vomiting also occurs with raised intracranial pressure. This must be considered following head injuries, neurosurgical operations or in patients with cerebral metastases.

HAEMATEMESIS

Elderly postoperative patients sometimes produce a small quantity of **'coffee ground' vomitus** positive for blood on 'stick' testing. This usually results from trivial bleeding from mild, stress-related gastritis or reflux oesophagitis and rarely indicates major haematemesis. The patient should be closely observed for signs of internal bleeding, and antacid preparations such as a proton pump inhibitor given.

Occasionally, a major upper GI haemorrhage occurs in the postoperative patient. If there has been forceful vomiting, a Mallory–Weiss tear at the oesophago-gastric junction may be the cause. Major bleeding may also arise from exacerbation of a peptic ulcer or even oesophageal varices. Seriously ill patients and the victims of burns and head injuries are susceptible to **acute stress ulceration**, which may cause catastrophic gastrointestinal haemorrhage (see Ch. 21, p. 298).

OTHER DISORDERS OF BOWEL FUNCTION

DIARRHOEA

Transient diarrhoea frequently follows abdominal operations, and should be regarded as normal in the recovery phase following bowel resections or operations to relieve intestinal obstruction, once any ileus has resolved.

Diarrhoea may also complicate **antibiotic therapy**. Several days after starting treatment, loose, frequent stools are passed for a short period, probably as a result of bacterial or fungal overgrowth. Less commonly, **antibiotic-associated diarrhoea** may develop, often due to overgrowth of ***Clostridium difficile*** which can be highly infective. If it progresses to **pseudomembranous colitis** or **toxic megacolon** it can become life-threatening. This is characterised by severe and persistent diarrhoea, sometimes containing blood (see Chs 3 and 12, p. 170).

After surgery of the abdominal aorta, blood-stained diarrhoea may occur a few days postoperatively. This may indicate **large-bowel ischaemia** due to ligation of the inferior mesenteric artery. This is a dangerous complication and requires urgent investigation and surgical exploration.

CONSTIPATION

Constipation is common after surgery. The causes include restriction of oral fluids and fibre, difficulty or reluctance in using a bed pan, slow recovery of normal peristalsis, the use of opiate analgesia and general lack of mobility. **Anal pain** is a powerful disincentive to defaecation following anal surgery. Constipation causes great distress, especially in the elderly. It should be anticipated and prevented if practicable by prescribing **bulk-forming agents** (e.g. methylcellulose or ispaghula husk preparations), **stool softeners** (e.g. docusate), **osmotic laxatives** (e.g. lactulose) or gentle **stimulant laxatives** (e.g. Senokot). Rectal preparations such as glycerine suppositories or enemas can be used if there is still no progress.

Impacted faeces in any patient may result in **overflow incontinence;** thus any patient with abnormal bowel function must undergo digital rectal examination to exclude faecal impaction.

POOR URINE OUTPUT

RETENTION OF URINE

Low urinary output or complete failure to pass urine is a frequent postoperative problem. The most common cause is urinary retention, usually occurring in males. It is readily diagnosed if there is a palpable suprapubic mass which is dull to percussion.

Acute retention needs to be distinguished from true oliguria resulting from poor renal perfusion or acute renal failure; retention can readily be confirmed by ultrasound examination or by passing a urinary catheter.

Pathophysiology

Postoperative retention is much more common in men, particularly when there is prostatic hypertrophy. Patients with bladder outflow obstruction symptoms ('prostatism') are at risk of developing acute retention, although young males can also be affected.

Acute postoperative urinary retention seems to result from a combination of the following factors:

- Pre-existing bladder outlet obstruction
- Difficulty in passing urine in the supine position
- Embarrassment at passing urine without sufficient privacy
- Accumulation of a large volume of urine during the operation and recovery, causing overfilling of the bladder
- Transient disturbance of the neurological control of voiding by general or spinal anaesthesia
- Pain from an abdominal or inguinal wound inhibiting normal contraction of the abdominal musculature and relaxation of the bladder neck
- Problems after certain operations which predispose to acute retention, e.g. abdomino-perineal resection of rectum or (bilateral) inguinal hernia repair
- Constipation—gross faecal loading is common in the elderly in hospital and is probably the most frequent cause of acute retention (and faecal incontinence)

MANAGEMENT OF POSTOPERATIVE URINARY RETENTION

Conservative measures

Most postoperative acute retention can be managed conservatively, bearing in mind the precipitating factors. If the problem is dealt with early, the patient is less likely to require catheterisation, which should be avoided if possible. However, if there is a history suggesting bladder outlet obstruction or previous prostatectomy, catheterisation is more likely to be needed. The first step is to ensure there is adequate **analgesia** and this may be sufficient to enable the patient to pass urine. The next step is to help the patient out of bed to use a commode at the bedside or a urine bottle.

If these measures fail, the patient should be wheeled into a bathroom for privacy and left alone for a while, if fit enough. The familiar sound of a tap left running often encourages micturition. If the patient still does not pass urine, encourage a bowel movement by means of a glycerine suppository. Defaecation is usually accompanied by bladder neck relaxation and micturition.

Catheterisation

If conservative measures fail, catheterisation is usually necessary. In females, bladder drainage and immediate removal of the catheter is done. In males, the catheter is usually left in situ until the following morning or until the patient is well. In patients with prostatic obstruction, a suprapubic catheter is a better option as it avoids urethral trauma and can easily be clamped to check if normal micturition has returned. Recurrent retention is usually caused by bladder outlet obstruction and is managed as described in Chapter 35.

Blocked catheter

If the patient is already catheterised, the catheter may have become blocked. The catheter can be checked for patency and flushed using a bladder syringe or replaced as necessary.

DIMINISHED URINE PRODUCTION

A degree of reduced urine output after operation is normal and results from increased release of ADH and aldosterone caused by surgical stress. **Oliguria** requiring attention in an adult is defined as less than 0.5 ml per kg per hour.

Low urine output is most often caused by **reduced renal perfusion**, resulting from relative hypovolaemia or low cardiac output. This leads to diminished glomerular filtration and enhanced tubular reabsorption. The usual reason is inadequate replacement of perioperative fluid deficit. Potentially more serious causes of reduced renal perfusion include cardiac failure and acute myocardial infarction. Acute renal insufficiency should only be diagnosed if poor renal perfusion (pre-renal failure) can be excluded.

A urinary catheter should be inserted to ensure the bladder is emptying and to enable hourly measurement of output. When retention has been excluded and true oliguria or **anuria** is diagnosed, the problem is to differentiate between acute tubular necrosis and reduced renal perfusion. Poor renal perfusion may be due to **hypotension** during the operation or **hypovolaemia**. If untreated, this may progress to acute kidney injury and in advanced cases, acute cortical necrosis. Renal insufficiency from other causes, in particular systemic sepsis or drug toxicity, should also be considered.

If **hypovolaemia** is suspected, an intravenous **fluid challenge** of 250 ml of crystalloid solution should be given over 15 minutes or so, while monitoring JVP and urine output (Fig. 11.4). This can be repeated after 30 minutes. If this restores output, under-hydration is confirmed and fluid balance corrected to prevent acute tubular necrosis.

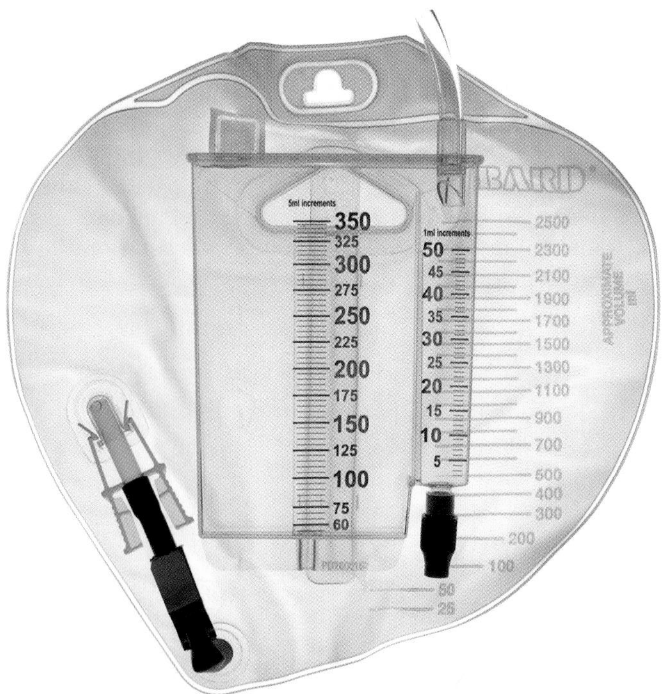

(a)

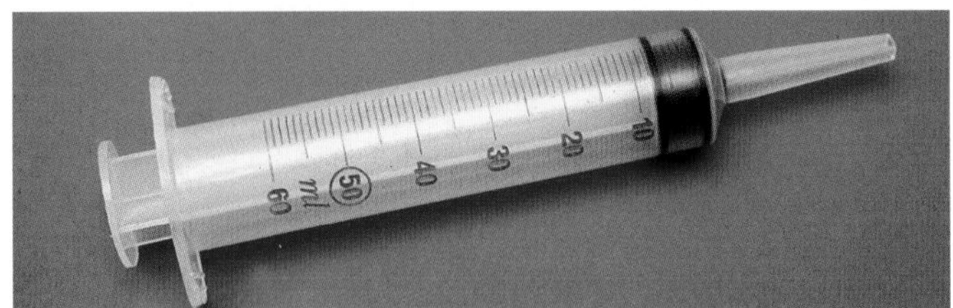

(b)

Fig. 11.4 Urine burette and bladder syringe
(a) Urine burette for precise measurement of urine output. Urine first enters the narrow compartment on the right to enable small quantities to be measured. It is then tipped into the main container to measure running totals. **(b)** Bladder syringe to flush urinary catheters suspected of blockage with debris. The nozzle is shaped to fit the end of a Foley urinary catheter. Note that full sterile precautions must be employed to reduce the risk of urinary infection

If the patient is **hypotensive**, the cause (cardiac failure or hypovolaemia, for example) must be identified and treated. A bladder ultrasound scan will show urine is being produced; a urinary catheter may be needed. If urine output is still poor, an oesophageal Doppler should be placed for monitoring stroke volume to allow goal-directed fluid therapy. Failing this, a central venous line can be used to monitor CVP. If simple measures fail, acute kidney damage must be suspected and investigated.

Lastly, bilateral ureteric obstruction should be considered (or unilateral if only one kidney is present). This is rare as a cause of postoperative low urine output. It can be diagnosed by renal ultrasound which will reveal bilateral hydronephrosis and an empty bladder.

CHANGES IN MENTAL STATE

Marked mental changes may occur early after operation and are most common in older patients. These changes are loosely called 'confusion'. The elderly are vulnerable to dementia and cerebrovascular insufficiency so may have a low tolerance of systemic insults that interfere with cerebral equilibrium. Common phenomena include clouding of consciousness, perceptual disturbances, incoherent speech and agitation or destructive behaviour, such as pulling out cannulas or catheters. Other features are loss of orientation, apathy and stupor, and stereotypical movements such as plucking at the bedclothes.

Factors which predispose to postoperative mental changes in the elderly include:

- Disorientation brought about by rapid changes of environment (from ward to operating theatre or ward to ward for example)
- Dehydration
- Hyponatraemia
- Hypoxia (e.g. from pneumonia or cardiac failure)
- Infection (especially of the urinary tract)
- Drugs (particularly opiates and hypnotics)
- Uraemia
- Hypoglycaemia

In addition, pain, anxiety and sleep deprivation may precipitate confusion.

Other causes

Pronounced alterations in behaviour, particularly in younger patients, may indicate alcohol withdrawal or craving for drugs such as cocaine or heroin. The history is concealed at admission. Patients with a recent history of head injury may behave abnormally if hypoxic, or if intracerebral bleeding develops.

JAUNDICE

GENERAL CAUSES

Jaundice may develop several days after operation in a patient with no history of biliary disease. In these patients, the cause is usually a prehepatic or hepatic disorder. Causes of **prehepatic jaundice** include large blood transfusions, absorption of large haematomas or emergence of a haemolytic disorder such as thalassaemia or sickle-cell trait (exacerbated by postoperative hypoxia, dehydration or hypothermia).

Hepatic causes are less common. They include cholestasis (caused by infection near the liver or drug idiosyncrasy), hepatitis and liver cell toxicity from drug idiosyncrasy and visceral ischaemia caused by shock.

CAUSES RELATED TO BILIARY OR LIVER SURGERY

Patients having biliary tract or liver surgery may become jaundiced after operation. The most likely cause is **obstruction** of the extrahepatic bile ducts due to retained stone, unrecognised surgical trauma or inadvertent duct ligation. Other causes include **infection** such as ascending cholangitis, and systemic absorption of an intra-abdominal collection of bile (biliary peritonitis).

Complications of surgery

12

INTRODUCTION

Any operation, major trauma or other surgical admission may be attended by complications, many of which are preventable. Complications cause added pain and suffering and may even put the patient's life at risk. Also, an anastomotic leak or a wound dehiscence can double the cost of an elective colonic resection.

While some complications are to some extent inherent in the condition being treated (e.g. deep venous thrombosis following lower limb fractures) or arise from some co-morbid (pre-existing) condition such as myocardial ischaemia, others arise from failure to visit or examine a patient when called, errors of judgement (e.g. misdiagnosis), poor nursing practice (e.g. allowing pressure sores to develop) or even frank negligence (e.g. operation on the wrong side). **Poor communication** between hospital staff is a frequent cause of avoidable complications, for example failing to record important events in the patient's treatment (and the date or name of the doctor), or to record a drug allergy in the case record, or neglecting to inform the operating department about a late change to an operating list.

A large proportion of complications can be prevented or minimised by anticipation, by taking prophylactic measures, by attention to detail and by early recognition and treatment of problems as they develop. With potentially serious complications (e.g. bowel anastomotic leak), early diagnosis and reoperation is crucial, as delay often leads to catastrophic 'snowballing' sepsis and multi-organ failure. Once two or more body systems become impaired, survival falls to only about 50%. If, for example, acute respiratory distress syndrome (ARDS) and renal failure complicate an operation for obstructive jaundice in a patient with liver impairment, the odds are heavily stacked against survival.

In operative surgery, complications can be either those of any operation or **specific** complications of individual operations. Both groups can be subdivided into **immediate** (during operation or within the next 24 hours), **early postoperative** (during the first postoperative week or so), **late postoperative** (up to 30 days after operation) and **long-term**.

Surgical complications fall into the five broad categories listed in Box 12.1. 'Medical' complications are discussed in Chapter 8. Complications of specific operations are discussed in Chapters 18–51, as appropriate.

COMPLICATIONS OF ANAESTHESIA

The main complications of anaesthesia are summarised in Box 12.2.

GENERAL COMPLICATIONS OF OPERATIONS

The main complications of any operation are: inadvertent trauma to the patient in the operating department, haemorrhage, surgical damage to related structures, inadequate operation, infection and problems with wound healing.

Box 12.1 Principal categories of surgical complications

1. Complications predisposed to by co-morbid 'medical' disorders, whether symptomatic or occult, e.g. ischaemic heart disease, chronic respiratory disease or diabetes mellitus (Ch. 8)
2. Complications of anaesthesia
3. General complications of operations, e.g. haemorrhage or wound infection
4. Complications of any surgical condition, e.g. pulmonary embolism, pneumonia or urinary tract infection
5. Complications of specific disorders and operations

INADVERTENT TRAUMA IN THE OPERATING DEPARTMENT

Patients are at risk of injury during transport or transfer in the operating department, especially when under anaesthesia. Staff involved in handling patients are also at risk of injury, for example to the back.

The most common causes of trauma in the operating theatre are:

- Injuries resulting from falls from trolleys or from the operating table during positioning
- Injury to diseased bones and joints from manipulation or positioning. These include dislocation of rheumatoid atlanto-axial joints and dislocation of a prosthetic hip joint
- Ulnar, lateral popliteal and other nerve palsies resulting from pressure
- Electrical burns from wet or poorly contacting diathermy pads or misuse of the diathermy probe
- Excess pressure on the calves causing deep venous thrombosis
- Excess heel pressure causing pressure sores
- Cardiac pacemaker disruption by diathermy equipment

HAEMORRHAGE

PERIOPERATIVE HAEMORRHAGE

Haemorrhage occurring during an operation (**primary haemorrhage**) should be controlled by the surgeon before the operation is completed.

EARLY POSTOPERATIVE HAEMORRHAGE

Haemorrhage immediately after operation usually indicates inadequate operative haemostasis or a technical mishap such as a slipped ligature or unrecognised blood vessel trauma. Occasionally it is due to a bleeding disorder.

If an operation involves major blood loss and large volume transfusion of stored blood, haemorrhage may be perpetuated by **consumption coagulopathy**, in which platelets and coagulation factors have been 'consumed' in a vain attempt at haemostasis. **Disseminated intravascular coagulopathy** (DIC) can be one facet of the systemic inflammatory response syndrome (SIRS) with widespread intravascular thrombosis and exhaustion of clotting factors. Occasionally bleeding results from preoperative use of aspirin or aspirin-like drugs (responses vary greatly between patients), uncontrolled anticoagulant drugs or, less commonly, a pre-existing but unrecognised bleeding disorder. Any patient giving a history of excess bleeding should have a platelet count and coagulation screen checked before operation.

Operations at particular risk of early postoperative haemorrhage include:

- Major operations involving highly vascular tissues such as the liver or spleen
- Major arterial surgery, especially ruptured aortic aneurysm (large volume blood loss may occur, and the patient may be heparinised during operation)
- Operations which leave a large raw surface such as abdomino-perineal excision of rectum

This type of postoperative haemorrhage has been traditionally described as **reactionary** in the belief that it was a 'reaction' to the recovery of normal blood pressure and cardiac output. This concept is probably misleading and should now be discarded, especially since it may hinder the decision to reoperate urgently.

Management of early postoperative haemorrhage

This is really a form of primary haemorrhage and, if substantial, the patient must be surgically re-explored and the source treated as at the original operation. It is wise to perform a clotting screen (including platelet count) and order bank blood as a preliminary measure. Good intravenous access should be ensured. If heparin was used at the original operation, **protamine** can reverse any residual activity. If the clotting screen is abnormal, infusions containing clotting factors may be needed, as advised by a haematologist. Many patients will stop bleeding with supportive measures and blood transfusion but re-exploration must be seriously considered at every stage.

LATER POSTOPERATIVE HAEMORRHAGE

Haemorrhage occurring several days after operation is usually caused by infection eroding blood vessels near the operation site; this is known as **secondary haemorrhage**. Treatment involves managing the infection, but exploratory operation is often required to ligate or suture the bleeding vessels.

SURGICAL INJURY

UNAVOIDABLE TISSUE DAMAGE

Anatomical structures, particularly nerves, blood vessels and lymphatics, may be **unavoidably damaged** during operation. This is particularly true in cancer surgery, illustrated by facial nerve excision during total parotidectomy. If anticipated, the probability must be discussed with the patient beforehand (ideally by the surgeon performing the operation) and accepted as part of the operative risk. Sometimes the integrity or location of vulnerable structures can be established before operation, allowing better planning of the operation. For

Box 12.2 Complications of anaesthesia

Local anaesthesia

- Injection site—pain; haematoma; delayed recovery of sensation (direct nerve trauma); infection
- Vasoconstrictors—ischaemic necrosis (if used in digits or penis)
- Systemic effects of local anaesthetic agent
  - Toxicity due to excess dosage (see Ch. 10, p. 136) or inadvertent intravenous injection. Same effect produced by premature release of a Bier's block cuff
  - Toxic effects include: dizziness, tinnitus, nausea and vomiting, fits, central nervous system (CNS) depression, bradycardia and asystole
  - Idiosyncratic or allergic reactions (very rare)

Spinal, epidural and caudal anaesthesia

- Failure of anaesthetic—anatomical difficulties or technical failure
- Headache after operation—loss of cerebrospinal fluid because of dural puncture
- Epidural or intrathecal bleeding—increased risk if patient on anticoagulants
- Unintentionally wide field of anaesthesia
  - In **epidural** anaesthesia, injection into wrong tissue plane may give a spinal anaesthetic
  - In **spinal** anaesthesia, respiratory paralysis occurs if the anaesthetic agent flows too far proximally
- Permanent nerve or spinal cord damage—injection of incorrect or contaminated drug
- Paraspinal infection—introduced by the injection
- Systemic complications—autonomic block may cause severe hypotension or postural hypotension

General anaesthesia

Postoperative nausea and vomiting

- Usually a response to anaesthetic or analgesic drugs. Individual sensitivity varies. Antiemetics usually administered before end of anaesthesia

Pain

- Analgesics usually administered during operation (e.g. intravenous opiates or paracetamol, diclofenac suppositories) plus local/regional anaesthetic techniques

Problems with drugs and fluids

- Fluid and electrolyte imbalance—too little, too much or inappropriate intravenous infusion
- Inappropriate choice of drugs or dosage in relation to age or the requirements of day surgery
- Idiosyncratic or allergic reactions to anaesthetic agents
  - Minor effects, e.g. nausea and vomiting
  - Major effects, e.g. cardiovascular collapse, respiratory depression, halothane jaundice
- Unexpected drug interactions—a wide range of adverse effects may occur
- Inherited disorders
  - Malignant hyperpyrexia (MH): any inhalational anaesthetic or suxamethonium may trigger MH
  - Pseudocholinesterase deficiency produces prolonged apnoea after succinylcholine
- Slow recovery from anaesthetic—many reasons including inadequate reversal
- 'Awareness' during anaesthetic—effective paralysis but ineffective anaesthesia (medico-legally very expensive!)

Cardiovascular complications

- Myocardial ischaemia/infarction/failure, arrhythmias, hypo/hypertension, tachy/bradycardias

Respiratory complications

- Laryngospasm/bronchospasm, atelectasis, upper or lower respiratory tract infections

Renal complications

- Particularly in patients with co-morbid renal impairment—pre-renal, renal or post-renal

Hypothermia (Note: neonates and small infants are especially vulnerable to hypothermia)

- Long operations with extensive fluid loss
- Large-volume transfusion of cold blood

Inadvertent trauma

- Dental problems and prostheses
  - Teeth (particularly decayed or loose), crowns and bridges are vulnerable during intubation. Damage risks aspirating a foreign body into a bronchus and causes cosmetic and medico-legal problems
  - Infected material from carious (decayed) teeth or inflamed gums may be aspirated and cause a particularly grave aspiration pneumonia
  - Dentures must be removed before operation and labelled. Unconscious accident victims may aspirate or swallow a dental prosthesis or obstruct the pharynx with it
- Corneal abrasions
- Pressure injury to nerves (especially ulnar, radial and lateral popliteal)
- Diathermy pad burns
- Initiation of pressure sores

example, indirect laryngoscopy may be done to assess vocal cord integrity prior to thyroid surgery.

INADVERTENT TISSUE DAMAGE

Structures may be **inadvertently damaged** during operation. Examples include recurrent laryngeal nerve damage during thyroidectomy, or trauma to bile ducts during laparoscopic cholecystectomy. The main factors are inexperience, anatomical anomalies, attempts at arresting precipitate haemorrhage and tissue planes obscured by inflammation or malignancy. Signs of damage to structures at particular risk should be sought in the postoperative period; for example, hoarseness after thyroidectomy or jaundice after cholecystectomy.

INFECTION RELATED TO THE OPERATION SITE

MINOR WOUND INFECTIONS

The most common infective complication is a superficial wound infection within the first postoperative week. This relatively trivial infection presents as localised pain, redness and a slight discharge. Organisms are usually staphylococci derived from skin and the infection usually settles without treatment. The exception is the patient into whom a prosthesis such as an arterial graft or artificial joint has been inserted. For these, antibiotics must be given to prevent the devastating consequences of infection around the prosthesis.

WOUND CELLULITIS AND ABSCESS

More severe wound infections occur most often after bowel-related surgery, when staphylococci (meticillin-sensitive or resistant varieties) or faecal organisms are usually incriminated. Most present in the first postoperative week but they may occur as late as the third week, sometimes after leaving hospital. These infections commonly present with a pyrexia; wound examination reveals spreading **cellulitis** or localised **abscess formation** (Fig. 12.1).

Cellulitis is treated with antibiotics after taking a wound swab for culture and sensitivity, whereas a wound abscess is treated by surgical drainage. This may simply involve suture removal and wound probing, but deeper abscesses may need re-exploration under general anaesthesia. In either case, the wound is left open afterwards to heal by secondary intention (see Fig. 12.2).

Intra-abdominal infection is discussed under complications of abdominal and bowel surgery later in this chapter.

GAS GANGRENE

Gas gangrene is an uncommon acute, life-threatening wound infection in which the anaerobic organisms multiply in necrotic tissue, particularly muscle (see Ch. 3, p. 48).

LATE INFECTIVE COMPLICATIONS

A late infective complication of surgery is a chronically discharging **wound sinus** emanating from a deep chronic abscess. It usually relates to foreign material such as a non-absorbable suture or mesh or sometimes necrotic fascia or tendon. These sinuses commonly follow wound infections where healing is delayed and incomplete. Wound sinuses occasionally appear after apparent normal healing, particularly after insertion of a prosthesis.

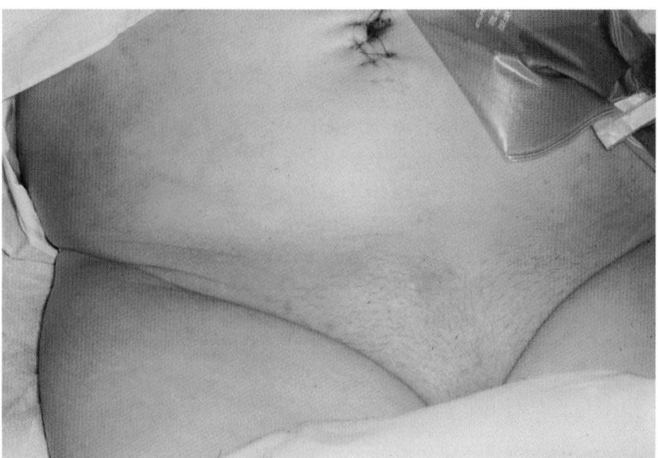

Fig. 12.1 Abdominal cellulitis
This woman of 73 presented with faecal peritonitis caused by a diverticular perforation of the sigmoid colon. She was resuscitated and underwent a laparotomy and sigmoid loop colostomy (note bag), without resection of the perforation. She remained toxic with a high fever and tachycardia, and developed spreading cellulitis in the right groin and flank. This proved to be due to continuing leakage from the perforation. Nowadays, a Hartmann's operation or resection and primary anastomosis is performed so there is no longer a perforation leaking faecal matter into the peritoneal cavity

Sinuses rarely heal spontaneously unless the foreign material is discharged, and the usual treatment is therefore wound re-exploration and removal of the offending substance. In groin sinuses following aortofemoral bypass grafts, removal of the graft would impair the arterial supply of the lower limb and the infected graft must be replaced or bypassed.

IMPAIRED HEALING

FACTORS RETARDING WOUND HEALING

Nearly all wounds heal without complication. It is untrue that wounds heal slowly in the elderly; this is so only when there are specific adverse factors or complications. Wound healing in general is retarded if blood supply is poor (as in lower limb arterial insufficiency) or if the wound is under excess tension. Other retarding factors are infection, long-term corticosteroid therapy, immunosuppressive therapy, previous radiotherapy, severe rheumatoid disease, smoking, global malnutrition and specific vitamin and mineral deficiency, especially of vitamin C and possibly zinc.

WOUND DEHISCENCE ('BURST ABDOMEN')

Wound dehiscence, i.e. total wound breakdown, is uncommon. It affects about 1% of abdominal wounds, usually about 1 week after operation, and is preceded by profuse serosanguinous fluid discharge from the wound. The sudden bursting open of the abdomen revealing coils of bowel is alarming but is remarkably pain-free. Infection and other factors already described may play a part but the usual cause is inadequate abdominal wall repair, often in the presence of infection or

Fig. 12.2 Deep wound infection drained and allowed to heal by secondary intention

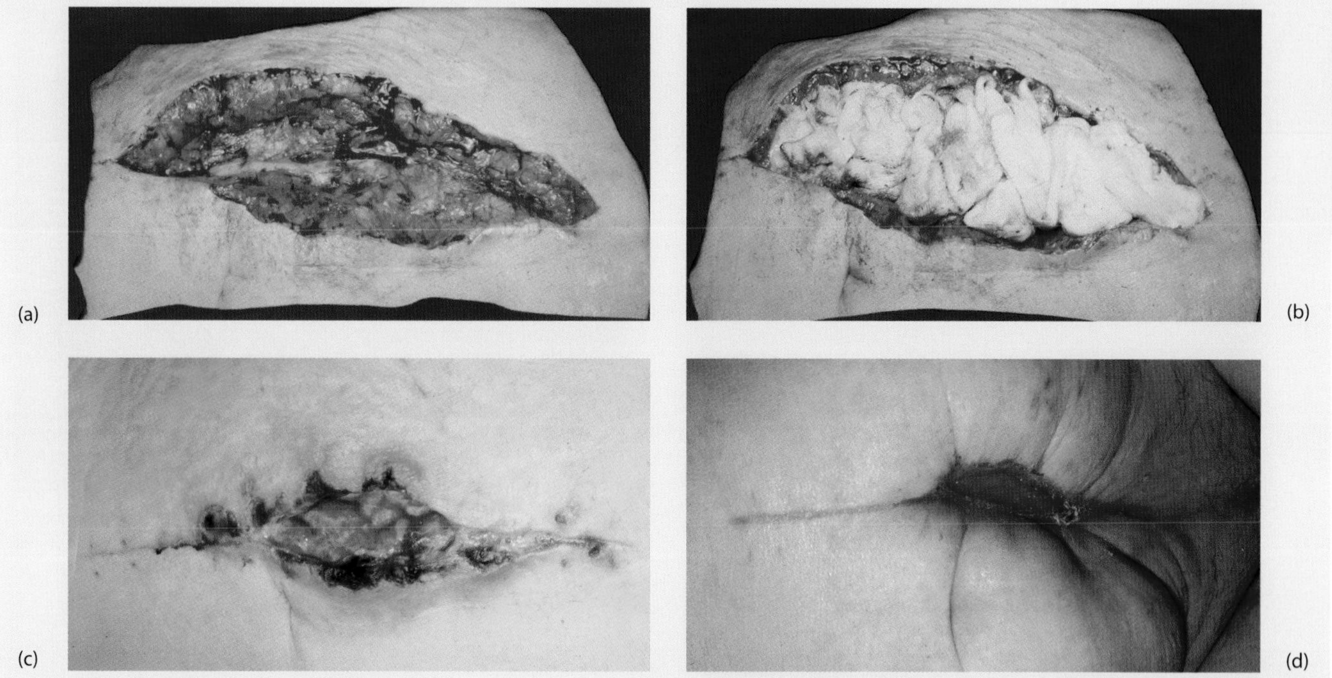

This 80-year-old diabetic woman underwent laparotomy and the wound became infected with *Staphylococcus aureus*. This resulted in a wound abscess and necrosis of the wound edge. **(a)** The wound after all necrotic tissue has been excised. **(b)** The wound packed with gauze and allowed to heal by secondary intention. **(c)** and **(d)** The wound at 3 weeks and 8 weeks. It was completely healed after 2 further weeks. Note the degree of wound contraction, which played a major part in overcoming the tissue defect

malnutrition. This may be compounded by mechanical disruption caused by coughing or abdominal distension.

The wound should be covered with sterile swabs soaked in saline and the patient returned to the operating theatre within a few hours for repair. This usually involves placement of **tension sutures** incorporating large 'bites' of the whole thickness of the abdominal wall (see Fig. 12.3).

INCISIONAL HERNIA

Incisional hernia is a late complication of abdominal surgery. These usually become apparent within the first postoperative year but sometimes develop as long as 15 years later; the overall incidence is about 10–15% of abdominal wounds. The hernia is caused by breakdown of the abdominal wall muscle and fascial repair. Predisposing factors are abdominal obesity, diabetes, smoking, abdominal distension and poor muscle quality, poor choice of incision, inadequate closure technique, postoperative wound infection and multiple operations through the same incision.

An incisional hernia usually presents as a bulge in the abdominal wall near a previous wound. They are usually asymptomatic but occasionally a narrow-necked hernia presents with pain or strangulation. Once an incisional hernia has appeared, it tends to enlarge progressively and may become a nuisance cosmetically or for dressing (see Fig. 12.4). Repair is indicated for strangulation, pain or inconvenience and usually involves placing a synthetic mesh at open operation or laparoscopically.

COMPLICATIONS OF ANY SURGICAL CONDITION

RESPIRATORY COMPLICATIONS

Up to 15% of patients having major operations and general anaesthesia suffer from respiratory complications. The most common are **atelectasis** and **pneumonia**. Pre-existing lung disease greatly increases the risk. Severely ill patients, including those with acute pancreatitis, and burns or trauma victims, are susceptible to **acute respiratory distress syndrome**.

EFFECTS OF ANAESTHESIA AND SURGERY ON RESPIRATORY FUNCTION

Anaesthesia and surgery predispose to postoperative complications by altering lung function and compromising normal defence mechanisms, as follows:

- **Lung tidal volume**—may be reduced by as much as 50%, depending on the incision site; thoracic, upper

Fig. 12.3 Burst abdomen and repair with tension sutures

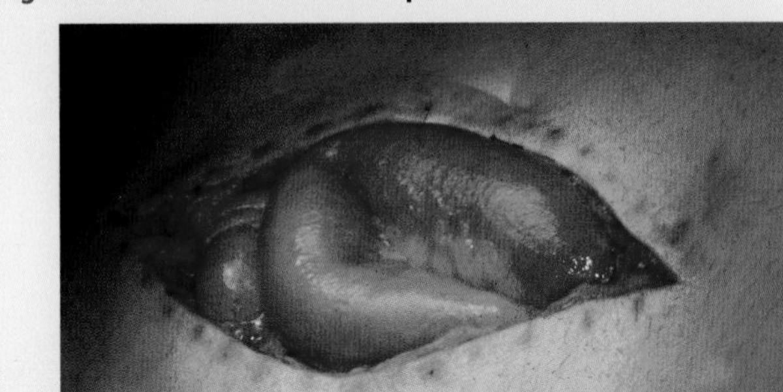
(a)

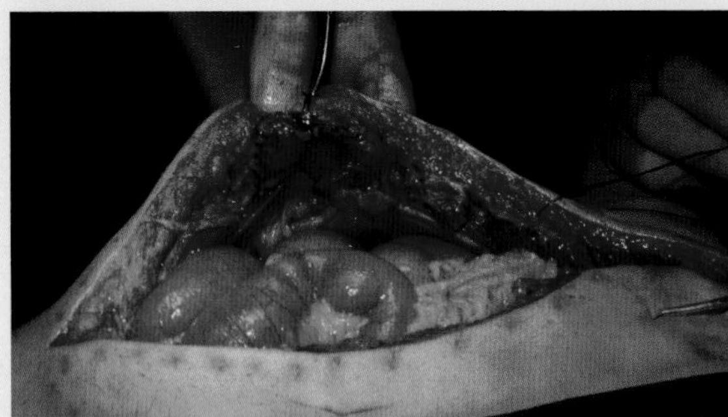
(b)

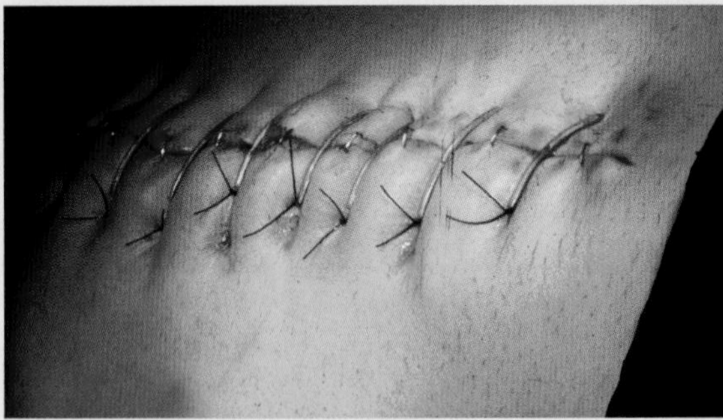
(c)

(a) Complete wound dehiscence 6 days after laparotomy for peritonitis. Note the exposed bowel spilling out of the wound. The patient had no particular risk factors so the cause was probably a poor technique of wound closure. **(b)** Operative photograph showing insertion of 'tension sutures' through the whole thickness of the abdominal wall. **(c)** The completed wound repair

CASE HISTROY

Fig. 12.4 Incisional hernia

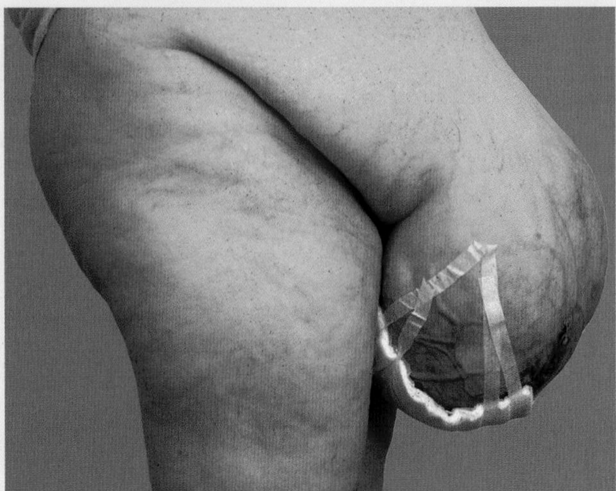

This 55-year-old woman presented with a massive incisional hernia through an old umbilical hernia repair scar. Her only complaint was of skin breakdown at its lowermost extent. Repair presented a huge challenge but was achieved using mesh

abdominal and lower abdominal incisions reduce lung volume in decreasing order of effect

- **Lung expansion**—reduced by the **supine position** during and after operation, pain, abdominal distension, abdominal constriction by bandages and the effects of sedative drugs
- **Ventilation rate**—usually increases and there is loss of normal periodic hyperinflation
- **Diminished ventilation and pulmonary perfusion**—result in reduced gaseous exchange
- **Airway defences**—compromised by loss of the cough reflex and diminished ciliary activity, which both lead to accumulation of secretions
- **Problems associated with laparoscopic abdominal surgery**—the pneumoperitoneum and head-down position lead to diaphragmatic splinting, a reduction in functional residual capacity and changes in intrathoracic blood volume. These lead to atelectasis, pulmonary shunting and hypoxaemia. Raised ventilatory airways pressure may lead to pulmonary barotrauma

ATELECTASIS

Pathophysiology and clinical features

Atelectasis or alveolar collapse occurs when airways become obstructed and air is absorbed from air spaces distal to the obstruction. Bronchial secretions are the main cause. Predisposing factors include shallow ventilation, loss of periodic hyperinflation, inhibition of coughing and pooling of mucus. All of these are greater problems after thoracic and upper abdominal surgery. The resulting **ventilation/perfusion mismatch** produces a degree of right-to-left shunting of blood, which causes a fall in PaO_2. If obstructed airways are small, causing minor segmental collapse, localising signs are minimal and X-ray appearance is unremarkable. Despite this, the overall extent of collapse may be large and cause significant hypoxaemia.

Obstruction of a major airway causes collapse and consolidation of a whole lobe, resulting in the typical signs of dullness to percussion and reduced breath sounds or **bronchial breathing**. Chest X-ray shows the lobe is contracted and opacified, with mediastinal shift and compensatory expansion of other lobes.

Most cases of atelectasis are mild and pass undiagnosed, although the patient may be slow to recover from operation. The patient may be cyanosed, resulting from mild hypoxaemia, and have a mild tachypnoea, tachycardia and low-grade pyrexia, which all resolve spontaneously within a few days. Sputum culture (if any is produced) is usually negative but infection may complicate severe cases.

Prevention and treatment of atelectasis

In patients undergoing major surgery, atelectasis is best prevented by preoperative and postoperative physiotherapy. This includes deep breathing exercises, regular adjustments of posture and vigorous coughing. During physiotherapy, wounds should be supported with the patient's hand. Effective analgesia, e.g. infiltration of the wound with local anaesthetic or epidural analgesia, facilitates physiotherapy and mobility. Nebulised bronchodilators such as salbutamol may assist the patient to cough up secretions. Severe cases of diffuse atelectasis may require non-invasive positive-pressure ventilation. Lobar or whole lung collapse requires intensive physiotherapy and sometimes **flexible bronchoscopy** to aspirate occluding mucus plugs.

PNEUMONIAS

Bronchopneumonia is often seen in surgical patients. It occurs secondarily to chronic lung disease, smoking or following atelectasis or aspiration of gastric contents. *Haemophilus* and *Streptococcus pyogenes* are the common infecting organisms but coliforms may be responsible in elderly, debilitated or seriously ill patients. *Pseudomonas* bronchopneumonia occurs in patients on ventilators or with bronchiectasis.

Infection is manifest by pyrexia, tachypnoea, tachycardia and a raised leucocyte count. The mucopurulent sputum is thick, copious and green. Antibiotics, usually amoxicillin or co-trimoxazole, are given on a 'best-guess' basis until sputum culture and sensitivities are available. Physiotherapy, mobilisation and encouragement to cough are all important for recovery.

Aspiration pneumonitis

Aspiration pneumonitis (Mendelson's syndrome) is a sterile, chemical inflammation of the lungs resulting from inhalation of acidic gastric contents. There is often a clear history of vomiting or regurgitation, followed by a rapid onset of breathlessness and wheezing. This may later become complicated by infection, i.e. bronchopneumonia, with typical symptoms and signs. Chest X-ray shows characteristic 'fluffy' opacities, particularly in the lower lobes, which for anatomical and postural reasons are most affected.

Aspiration occurs when protective laryngeal reflexes are suppressed or when there is intestinal obstruction and regurgitation. Laryngeal suppression may be due to impairment of consciousness (e.g. during recovery from general anaesthesia or in alcoholic intoxication) or loss of consciousness after head injury.

Emergency anaesthesia in the non-starved patient poses special risks. Whenever possible, anaesthesia should be postponed for 4–6 hours after the last food or drink other than water. In accident victims, it is important to note the time of last eating with respect to the accident, and to remember that stress and anxiety may greatly delay gastric emptying., Gastric emptying is also much slower in pregnancy.

A patient with **intestinal obstruction** is at risk of inhalation of gastric contents. Ideally, the stomach should be emptied by nasogastric tube. If general anaesthesia must be performed on the non-starved or otherwise at-risk patient, a **rapid sequence induction** is employed: as the patient loses consciousness, an assistant applies **cricoid pressure** to flatten the oesophagus against the cervical spine, preventing reflux. The airway is then secured with a cuffed endotracheal tube before cricoid pressure is released. Oral antacids may be given beforehand to neutralise acidity. Metoclopramide by injection may also be used to hasten gastric emptying.

Mortality from aspiration pneumonitis approaches 50% and urgent treatment must be started should it occur. This involves thorough bronchial suction via an endotracheal tube (or bronchoscope if necessary), followed by positive-pressure ventilation and prophylactic antibiotics. Intravenous steroids are usually given to limit the inflammatory process, but their efficacy is unproven.

Aspiration pneumonia

Aspiration pneumonia may complicate aspiration pneumonitis, but more often it develops insidiously, following chronic aspiration of infected food and oropharyngeal secretions. In the surgical context, debilitated, confused or elderly patients are the usual victims, but aspiration pneumonia is also seen in alcoholics, drug addicts and stroke patients. Achalasia of the oesophageal cardia and large hiatus hernias can lead to chronic aspiration, particularly at night. The clinical features are of infection and lobar consolidation (usually of the lower lobe) progressing to **lung abscess** formation. Organisms are usually mixed oral anaerobes sensitive to penicillin, but prognosis depends more on the patient's general condition and is usually poor.

ACUTE RESPIRATORY DISTRESS SYNDROME (ARDS)

This syndrome of acute respiratory failure, formerly known as adult respiratory distress syndrome, is characterised by rapid, shallow breathing, severe hypoxaemia, stiff lungs and diffuse pulmonary opacification on X-ray. It develops in response to a variety of systemic and direct insults to the pulmonary alveoli and microvasculature.

Acute respiratory failure has long been recognised in many disparate conditions and has been given names such as shock lung, wet lung, post-traumatic respiratory insufficiency, Da Nang lung (Vietnam war) and white lung (after the X-ray appearance). Box 12.3 lists the main conditions with which ARDS is associated.

Pathophysiology of ARDS

The lung insults causing ARDS all have the effect of increasing the pulmonary capillary permeability, leading to leakage of protein-rich fluid into the alveolar interstitium. This causes interstitial oedema which in turn **reduces lung compliance** and causes 'stiff lungs' and reduced alveolar ventilation. Release of inflammatory mediators cause these effects.

The alveolar lining cells (**type I pneumocytes**) are also damaged. This damage, combined with the increased interstitial hydrostatic pressure, causes leakage of fluid into alveolar spaces until they are filled. The result is disruption of the lung ventilation to perfusion ratio (V/Q ratio), in effect causing **right-to-left shunting** of blood. The intra-alveolar fluid later condenses to form a **hyaline membrane** which lines the alveoli. This is histologically similar to the neonatal form of the disease.

Box 12.3 Conditions associated with acute respiratory distress syndrome (ARDS)

Direct insults to the lung
- Lung contusion
- Near-drowning
- Aspiration of gastric acid
- Inhalation of smoke and corrosive chemicals, e.g. chlorine, phosgene, nitrogen dioxide or ammonia
- Radiation pneumonitis

Systemic insults to the lung
- Multiple trauma with shock
- Systemic sepsis, e.g. after a colonic anastomotic leak
- Severe acute pancreatitis
- Major head injuries ('neurogenic pulmonary oedema')
- Fat, air and amniotic fluid embolism
- Major blood transfusion reaction or massive blood transfusion
- Disseminated intravascular coagulation
- Cardiopulmonary bypass
- Eclampsia
- Severe allergic reactions
- Drug overdose or sensitivity, e.g. heroin, barbiturates, paraquat, bleomycin

The full clinical syndrome often takes 24–48 hours to develop after the initial insult. If the patient eventually recovers, the interstitial damage may result in diffuse **interstitial fibrosis**. It is important to note that cardiac failure is not involved in causing ARDS, but cardiac failure may later complicate it.

Clinical features of ARDS

The main finding is rapid shallow respiration with only scattered crepitations on auscultation. There is usually no cough, chest pain or haemoptysis. Blood gas analysis reveals low PaO_2 but the $PaCO_2$ remains normal except in the most severe cases. Chest X-ray may be normal in the early stages, progressing rapidly through increased interstitial markings to complete or partial 'white-out' (see Fig. 12.5). ARDS may be difficult to distinguish from cardiac failure except that cardiac diameter is normal in ARDS, and cardiac failure usually responds to diuretic therapy.

Treatment of ARDS

The objective is to maintain respiratory function and cardiovascular stability while the underlying cause (e.g. sepsis) is brought under control. This should be carried out in intensive care. The sooner treatment is begun, the greater the chance of recovery.

Most patients require mechanical **ventilation** with **positive end-expiratory pressure (PEEP)** to achieve adequate oxygenation and to try to reverse alveolar oedema and collapse. Fluid balance is complex and requires monitoring of **right atrial pressure** using a central venous line. Cardiac output can be measured using transoesophageal ultrasound. One of the treatment aims is to produce a negative fluid balance and thus minimise fluid accumulation in the lung and interstitial tissue. Loop diuretic infusions or continuous veno-venous haemofiltration can be used to achieve this. Renal insufficiency is a common association, and can also be treated by haemofiltration. Diuretics do not control pulmonary oedema but instead aggravate the hypovolaemia and shock linked with the underlying cause. The mortality rate for complicated cases of ARDS approaches 90%.

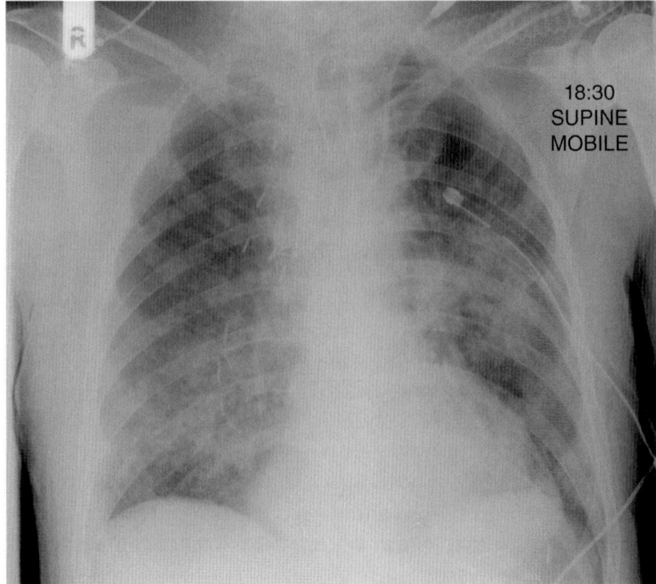

(a)

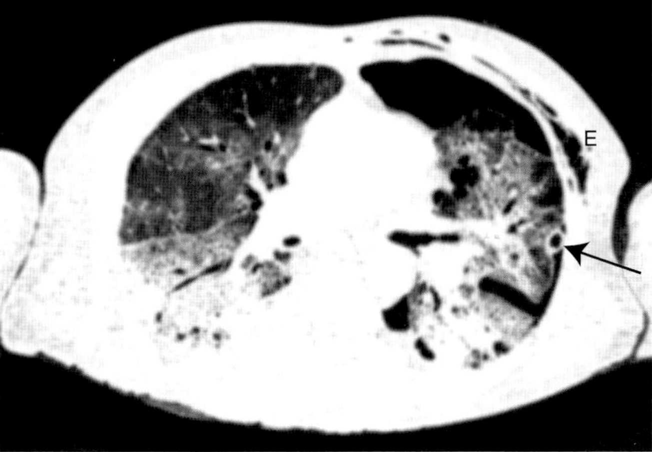

(b)

Fig. 12.5 Acute respiratory distress syndrome (ARDS)
(a) This middle-aged man underwent an oesophagectomy for carcinoma, with the proximal stomach anastomosed to the oesophageal remnant in the chest. He developed ARDS in the early postoperative period. The chest X-ray shows ill-defined alveolar opacification in the lung mid zones. Note the metallic vascular clips on the right side, the chest drain on the left side and the endotracheal tube and central venous line. **(b)** The CT scan shows bilateral consolidation in the dependent portion of both lungs with 'ground glass' opacification in the upper zones. There is a left pneumothorax with a chest drain in situ (arrowed); subcutaneous emphysema **E** resulting from the thoracotomy is also visible

VENOUS THROMBOEMBOLISM (VTE)

PATHOPHYSIOLOGY

Venous thromboembolism is a major cause of complications and death after surgery or trauma and much of it is preventable. Venous blood is normally prevented from clotting within veins by a series of mechanisms that include local inhibition of the clotting cascade, prompt lysis of small clots that do form, and the flushing effect of a continuous flow of blood. In 1856, **Virchow** proposed in his '**triad**' that venous thrombosis was caused by abnormalities in the vein wall (trauma, inflammation), alterations in blood flow (stasis) and changes in the blood (hypercoagulability); this explanation largely holds good today.

The normal antithrombotic balance within veins can be upset by local and/or systemic factors, resulting in thrombus formation in venous sinuses within calf muscles and sometimes primarily in pelvic veins. About 90% of deep vein thromboses (DVTs) start in the calf and about a quarter propagate proximally, usually within a week of presentation, to involve femoral and pelvic veins. Calf vein thrombosis alone is rarely symptomatic yet it predisposes strongly to proximal propagation, and 80% of symptomatic DVTs involve proximal veins. Calf vein thrombi themselves rarely cause substantial embolism but those in larger, more proximal vessels are likely to detach and migrate proximally to impact in pulmonary arteries as pulmonary emboli.

The main **predisposing factors** to venous thromboembolism (VTE) are summarised in Box 12.4, but thromboembolism can occur in healthy individuals without evident predisposing factors. A proportion will have a **prothrombotic disorder** and investigation for these should be performed later. Note that patients may have been ill and dehydrated at home for some time before hospital admission and venous thrombosis may have begun before admission.

The risk of thromboembolism increases incrementally with the number and severity of local and systemic risk factors; this is neatly illustrated in Table 12.1. The impact of many predisposing factors can be minimised by **prophylactic measures against venous thromboembolism** in *all* hospitalised patients.

Box 12.4 Predisposing factors for deep vein thrombosis and pulmonary embolism

- Previous venous thromboembolism
- Trauma and surgery (complex systemic effects)
- Increasing age
- Direct trauma to the pelvis and lower limbs, especially fractures
- Pre-existing lower limb venous disorders causing stasis
- Venous stasis during general or regional anaesthesia (loss of calf muscle pump and postural pressure on the calves)
- Malignant disease
- Immobility, e.g. bed-bound patients after operation or stroke
- Cardiac failure
- High-oestrogen oral contraceptive pill, oestrogen treatment, hormone replacement therapy
- Pregnancy
- Pelvic masses causing venous obstruction
- Groin masses obstructing femoral vein, e.g. femoral aneurysm, malignant lymph nodes
- Obesity
- Dehydration
- Blood disorders, e.g. polycythaemia, thrombocythaemia and prothrombotic disorders

DEEP VEIN THROMBOSIS (DVT)

Lower limb deep vein thrombosis is often silent, with classic clinical features in only a quarter of cases. These include leg swelling, calf muscle tenderness and increased leg warmth; calf pain on passive foot dorsiflexion (**Homans' sign**) is unreliable.

Iliofemoral vein occlusion tends to cause diffuse and sometimes massive swelling of the whole lower limb (see Fig. 12.6a). In addition, there may be tenderness over the femoral vein in the groin. In severe cases (rare nowadays), the limb becomes painful and white, and boggy with oedema; this is known as **phlegmasia alba dolens** (painful white leg). In more extreme cases, the limb becomes more painful and blue, with incipient venous infarction (**phlegmasia caerulea dolens**).

Asymptomatic DVTs have the same potential as symptomatic venous thromboses for causing both pulmonary embolism and long-term chronic venous insufficiency (see Ch. 43), thus emphasising the importance of prophylaxis for all patients at increased risk. To complicate the problem, as many as half the patients who develop swelling and pain in the calf after operation do *not* have deep vein thrombosis.

Diagnostic tests for DVT

Colour duplex ultrasound is now the standard technique for investigation of cases where DVT is suspected. In surgical patients, scanning is the preferred investigation as D-dimer blood tests can be misleading after an operation. Colour

Table 12.1 Factors affecting the risk of deep vein thrombosis after operation

Age	Grade of surgery	Other risk factors	Risk of DVT (%)
20	Minor		1
40	Minor		3
60	Minor		10
60	Major		20
60	Major	Previous DVT	50
80	Major		40
80	Major	Previous DVT + infection or malignancy	96

Fig. 12.6 Clinically obvious deep vein thrombosis

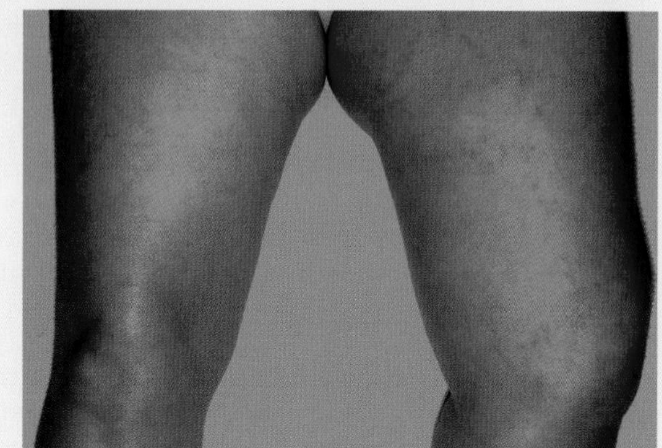

(a)

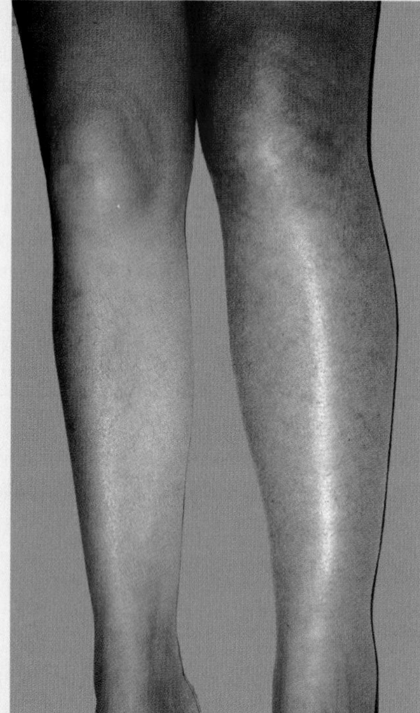

(b)

This woman of 45 underwent radical surgery for ovarian cancer. She suffered swelling and bursting pain in the whole of her left leg 5 days after operation. The left thigh **(a)** and leg **(b)** are both visibly swollen and blueish. On palpation, the limb felt warm. A massive iliofemoral venous thrombosis was diagnosed on venography and the patient was anticoagulated. Luckily she did not suffer a pulmonary embolism and the limb returned to a normal diameter over 6 months. She will be at lifetime risk of post-thrombotic deep venous insufficiency

duplex allows scanning of all the major lower limb deep veins for blood flow and contained thrombus, and when the scan is normal, can reliably exclude the diagnosis.

PULMONARY EMBOLISM

The classic clinical picture of pulmonary embolism (PE) is sudden dyspnoea and cardiovascular collapse, followed by pleuritic chest pain, development of a pleural rub and haemoptysis. In hospital, this is often heralded by physical collapse whilst seated on the toilet. Ten percent of PEs are estimated to be fatal within the first hour. The electrocardiogram (ECG) may show evidence of right heart strain (S wave in lead I, Q wave and inverted T wave in leads III—'S1, Q3, T3'). This presentation, however, is uncommon and occurs only when 50% or more of the pulmonary arterial system is occluded. More extensive occlusion usually results in sudden death.

Small pulmonary emboli are common and are often 'silent', presenting as non-specific episodes of general deterioration, confusion, breathlessness or chest pain. Note that the patient suffering small embolic events is greatly predisposed to a massive or fatal embolus; it is essential to recognise the condition and to treat it seriously. The patient often has a tachycardia and low-grade fever but there are no diagnostic changes on ECG. Deterioration may be attributed to chest infection, atelectasis or cardiac failure unless pulmonary embolism is considered. There are sometimes more specific diagnostic symptoms of small emboli, including localised **pleuritic chest pain** and small **haemoptyses** in the form of blood-streaked sputum.

Venous thromboembolism is most common from about the fourth to the seventh day after major surgery but may present any time during the next month or so, sometimes after the patient has left hospital.

Diagnosis of pulmonary embolism (PE)

In suspected pulmonary embolism, chest X-ray and ECG changes are non-specific and of little value. The choice of investigation depends on the level of clinical probability. Several clinical scoring schemes have been used to categorise patients to low (~10%), intermediate (~25%) or high (~80%) risk of pulmonary embolism. Categories are based on the sum of points allocated to **predisposing factors** (past history of venous thromboembolism, immobility, malignancy) and the **presence of signs** of DVT, tachycardia or an alternative diagnosis.

Blood tests for D-dimers have a high negative predictive value for pulmonary embolism (D-dimers are formed when cross-linked fibrin is lysed by plasmin), although levels are elevated anyway after operation and therefore misleading. The quickest and most reliable method of confirming the diagnosis is by dynamic spiral or multislice CT pulmonary angiography (CTPA) using intravenous contrast (Fig. 12.7a). Where available, this has largely superseded radioisotope ventilation/perfusion scanning (V/Q scanning).

MANAGEMENT OF VENOUS THROMBOEMBOLISM

For most patients, removing or lysing limb thrombus or pulmonary embolus is impracticable. The usual objective in managing thromboembolism is to halt the coagulation process by systemic anticoagulation. This prevents established thrombi from propagating and new thrombi from forming. Thrombus is then gradually removed by the normal body processes of lysis.

Most lower limb thrombi eventually become organised and firmly attached to the vein wall, posing no further risk of embolisation. Thrombus is later invaded by granulation tissue and veins eventually recanalise, restoring blood flow. In the process, valves are often destroyed, leading to **chronic venous**

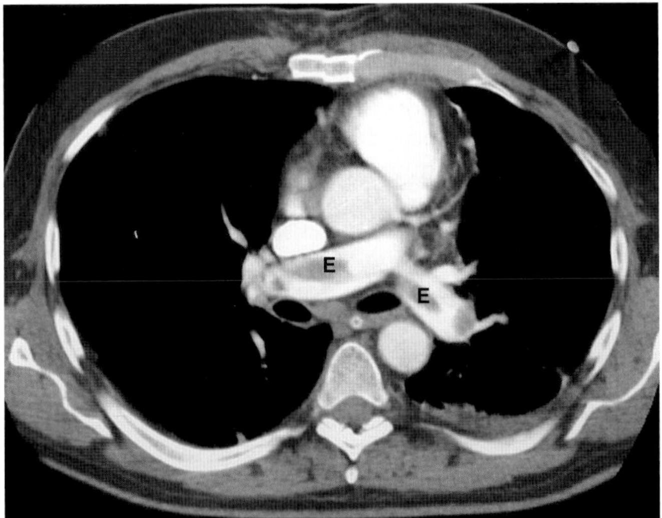

(a)

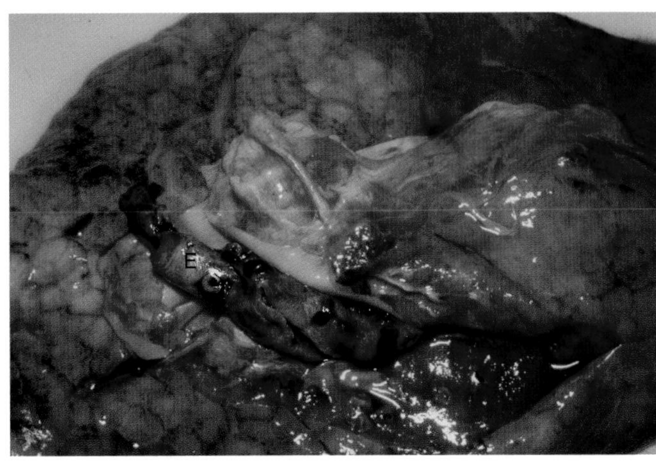

(b)

Fig. 12.7 Pulmonary embolism
(a) Thoracic CT pulmonary artery scan (CTPA) with intravenous contrast showing large emboli **E** in the pulmonary arteries. This is the investigation of choice where there is a high suspicion of PE. **(b)** Post-mortem specimen of lung from a patient who died of massive pulmonary embolism. Embolic material has been removed, but some remains in the pulmonary arteries **E**

insufficiency (see Ch. 43), often many years later. After pulmonary embolism, if the patient survives the initial episode, emboli are efficiently removed by local thrombolysis, leaving little functional deficit.

For treatment, anticoagulation is initially achieved with therapeutic subcutaneous **heparin**. Heparin anticoagulation takes effect immediately and is continued for about 5 days, by which time acute symptoms have usually subsided. In the meantime, oral **warfarin therapy** (which takes several days to become fully effective) is begun. Warfarin is continued for 3–6 months, the period of highest risk of recurrent thromboembolism. It is likely that oral agents like rivaroxaban (see below) will replace both heparin and warfarin in the future for this purpose.

Untreated, about 50% of patients with proximal DVT or PE will have a further thromboembolic event within 3 months. Patients who suffer repeated thromboembolic episodes when taken off anticoagulation may need maintaining on warfarin or an alternative for life. For these patients, a **filter** may be placed in the inferior vena cava via a percutaneous route to trap emboli migrating from leg and pelvic veins towards the pulmonary arteries (see Ch. 5, p. 68).

In the rare case of sub-massive non-fatal pulmonary embolism with evidence of right ventricular dysfunction, surgical **embolectomy** may be appropriate. This is performed under cardiopulmonary bypass and is a major undertaking. An alternative is **systemic thrombolytic therapy**, but this has a high rate of serious bleeding and has largely been abandoned. However, the technique of manipulating a pulmonary artery catheter into the embolus and instilling high doses of **local thrombolytic drugs** or performing **clot suction** has occasionally been successfully employed.

PREVENTION OF VENOUS THROMBOEMBOLISM

The importance of **general measures** in preventing venous thrombosis needs to be emphasised. These include **early postoperative mobilisation**, **adequate hydration** and **avoiding pressure on the calves**. In addition, patients on oestrogen-containing oral contraceptives should ideally stop taking them (using replacement contraceptive methods) at least 6 weeks before major operations, as should patients on hormone replacement therapy (HRT). If these preparations are not to be stopped, consideration should be given to employing heparin prophylaxis for any operation.

For these and for any patients at risk (shown in Box 12.4), specific prophylactic measures should be taken to reduce the risk. Prophylactic measures include the following:

- **Low-dose subcutaneous heparin**—unfractionated heparin (UFH) and low molecular weight heparin (LMWH) both inhibit the activity of factor Xa indirectly by binding to circulating antithrombin III. Both types are as effective for preventing thromboembolism but LMWH has the advantage that it is given only once a day instead of two or three times. Low-dose heparin is currently the most effective method of reducing thromboembolism in at-risk patients. It has been shown to reduce the rate of postoperative DVT by 70% in general surgical, urological, gynaecological, orthopaedic and trauma patients. Similar reductions are achieved in pulmonary embolism rates. The beneficial intravascular antithrombotic effect is not due to anticoagulation, but arises from stimulation of platelet factor antithrombin III; there should be no detectable in vitro anticoagulant effect nor any significant effect on haemostasis during or after operation, although patients on low-dose heparin probably bleed about 10% more at major surgery
- A new class of **orally active direct factor Xa inhibitor anticoagulants** has become available. Rivaroxaban, an oxazolidinone derivative, has shown greater efficacy than enoxaparin (LMWH) in preventing thrombosis after hip and knee replacement, and with a similar safety profile, although the cost is higher. Maximum effect is

reached after 4 hours and lasts 8–12 hours, tapering off afterwards so a once-daily dose of 10 mg is practicable. The drug does not inhibit thrombin (activated factor II), and has no effect on platelets. It has predictable activity across a wide range of age and body weight and has a flat dose response across a range of 5–40 mg. It enables predictable anticoagulation without need for dose adjustment or coagulation monitoring but is irreversible if haemorrhage occurs. The drug is approved widely for hip and knee replacement prophylaxis and further clinical trials are under way
- **Calf compression devices**—several pneumatic and electrical devices are available for intraoperative calf compression to simulate muscle pump activity. These are non-invasive and easily applied to all patients, even those at low risk, but their effectiveness is less than low-dose heparin
- **Graduated compression 'anti-embolism' stockings**—using these stockings is simple and widely practised. Provided they are correctly fitted, stockings offer a suitable level of prophylaxis for patients at low or moderate risk. The stockings must be worn during operation as well as during the early postoperative period
- **Warfarin anticoagulation**—warfarin is an orally active vitamin K antagonist that decreases hepatic synthesis of several coagulation factors. Warfarinisation is one of the best methods of prophylaxis for elective operations and is widely used in the Netherlands. It is considered impractical by many surgeons, not least because of the supposed risk of incidental and operative haemorrhage. In addition, providing an effective service requires a great deal of resources

FLUID AND ELECTROLYTE DISTURBANCES

Fluid and electrolyte disturbances such as **dehydration** or **fluid overload**, **hyponatraemia**, **hypokalaemia** and **hyperkalaemia** frequently develop in the postoperative period. Fluid and electrolyte abnormalities are particularly common after major bowel surgery, especially if there have been massive fluid losses through vomiting, diarrhoea or sequestration in obstructed or adynamic bowel, or surgical complications. These problems are discussed in Chapter 2.

ANTIBIOTIC-ASSOCIATED COLITIS

PATHOPHYSIOLOGY AND CLINICAL FEATURES

Colonic inflammation and other diarrhoeal disorders may be side-effects of almost any antibiotic treatment. The conditions are largely due to selective overgrowth of intestinal organisms which then produce toxins that cause the damage. The clinical picture ranges from a mild attack of diarrhoea to profuse, life-threatening, haemorrhagic colitis.

Antibiotic-associated colitis may develop suddenly or gradually and occasionally becomes chronic or relapsing. Surgical patients are most likely to be affected after operation. *Clostridium difficile* is responsible for many of these cases, and in severe form the full picture of **pseudomembranous colitis** may develop. This can take a particularly virulent form. **Staphylococcal enterocolitis** is less common.

Stool specimens should be examined by microscopy and culture and by measuring levels of *Clostridium difficile* toxin. Sigmoidoscopic inspection and biopsy of the rectum should also be performed. Treatment is based on the results of these tests. If *Clostridium difficile* infection is diagnosed, it is treated with oral metronidazole or, in resistant cases, with oral (non-absorbed) vancomycin and the patient must be isolated and barrier nursed (see Ch. 3).

ACUTE RENAL FAILURE (INSUFFICIENCY)

Acute renal failure is defined as the abrupt onset of oliguria or anuria, associated with a steep rise in blood urea concentration. This is caused by failure to excrete nitrogenous waste products. The usual cause is **acute tubular necrosis**, but acute renal failure is sometimes caused by nephrotoxins. These include the **aminoglycoside antibiotics** gentamicin and tobramycin, myoglobin (released in the crush syndrome) and the 'hepatorenal syndrome' associated with obstructive jaundice (see Table 18.2, p. 262). Acute renal failure is also a particular complication of abdominal aortic surgery, in which the renal arteries may become occluded by inadvertent damage or unrecognised embolism.

PATHOPHYSIOLOGY

Renal tubules are acutely sensitive to a variety of metabolic insults, particularly hypoxia and certain toxins. Hypoxia readily occurs if renal perfusion falls substantially; the usual surgical cause is an episode of severe or prolonged **hypotension**. This may result from hypovolaemic shock (haemorrhage or dehydration), cardiovascular collapse (postoperative cardiac failure or myocardial infarction) or septic shock. In the last, endotoxic and cytokine-initiated renal cell damage is also an important factor. Pre-existing **chronic renal disease** increases a patient's susceptibility to acute renal failure.

If the renal tubular insult is not overwhelming, tubular cell damage is confined to disruption of cellular metabolism rather than tissue necrosis. This is potentially reversible, provided the patient can be maintained in good general condition while tubular recovery takes place. The usual sequence of recovery is that poor urine output continues for a period (**oliguric phase**), followed by **spontaneous diuresis** of large volumes of unconcentrated urine consisting of unmodified glomerular filtrate (**diuretic phase**). Urinary concentrating power then slowly improves as tubules recover normal metabolic function. In contrast, when tubular damage is more extensive, the patient remains anuric or severely oliguric.

PREVENTION AND MANAGEMENT OF ACUTE RENAL FAILURE

Acute renal failure is largely preventable by careful attention to preoperative assessment, fluid balance, and prevention and prompt management of hypotension and sepsis, as well as dose monitoring of potentially nephrotoxic drugs. When acute renal failure is mild, simple conservative measures such as fluid restriction may sustain the patient until tubular function recovers. When complete (oliguric) renal failure occurs, plasma urea, creatinine and potassium concentrations rise inexorably and the patient usually requires **haemofiltration** or **renal dialysis**. Fortunately, many of these patients recover renal function gradually over a few weeks or months and do not require permanent renal support.

PRESSURE SORES

PATHOPHYSIOLOGY

Elderly, debilitated and other bed-bound patients are extremely susceptible to pressure sores ('bed sores'), particularly over bony prominences such as the sacrum and heels (see Figs 12.8 and 12.9). Pressure sores occur because the frequent spontaneous adjustment of position that normally occurs in bed is lost through obtunded sensation and immobility. Diminished protective pain response plays an essential part. Patients with diabetes may have a sensory neuropathy so they are unable to sense the damaging effects of prolonged pressure on a bony prominence. Tissue necrosis and any subsequent failure to heal result from a combination of factors including recurrent pressure ischaemia, poor tissue perfusion (from cardiac or peripheral vascular disease) and malnutrition. Note that patients who have experienced substantial weight loss and patients with relatively ischaemic lower limbs are at particular risk.

PREVENTION AND MANAGEMENT OF PRESSURE SORES

Once established, pressure sores are difficult to eradicate so prevention must be given high priority in patients at risk. Relatively hard surfaces such as accident and emergency department trolleys and operating tables may initiate pressure sores in susceptible patients in less than an hour. Likewise, pressure sores can develop in a remarkably short time in a hospital bed, particularly if the patient is incontinent of urine or faeces. Prevention of pressure sores on the ward is mainly a nursing responsibility; indeed, the incidence of pressure sores is a good indicator of the quality of nursing care.

Prevention of pressure sores involves the following procedures:

- **Special bed surfaces to spread the load**—these include (in ascending order of cost and complexity) pressure-relieving foam mattresses, electric ripple mattresses, water beds, suspended net beds and sophisticated low pressure continuous airflow beds
- **Relieving pressure on the heels**—use of ankle rests while on the operating table, use of heel pads, orthopaedic foam gutters and 'bean-bags' on return to the ward
- **Regular change of posture**—for most patients, this involves encouragement to get out of bed, at least into a bedside chair, and to mobilise beyond the chair as much as possible. A bed-bound patient requires regular turning so that the same skin area is not subject to constant pressure
- Regular checking of pressure areas and local massage
- Management of incontinence

Treatment of established pressure sores is unsatisfactory unless causative factors can be eliminated. This is often impossible in the permanently disabled patient. Avoiding pressure is the mainstay of treatment, supplemented by local cleansing and dressings designed to remove necrotic tissue and control secondary infection. For a deep sacral sore, major plastic surgery involving a rotational buttock flap is occasionally justified.

CASE HISTROY

Fig. 12.8 Typical heel pressure sore

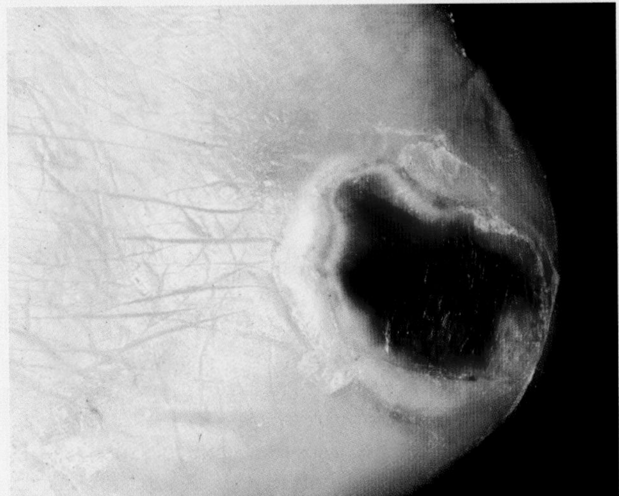

This elderly man presented with a ruptured abdominal aortic aneurysm and had a stormy postoperative course. At some stage, this heel was allowed to remain too long in one position, resulting in deep necrosis. He had no evidence of occlusive peripheral arterial disease

CASE HISTROY

Fig. 12.9 Osteomyelitis of the ischial tuberosity secondary to pressure ulceration

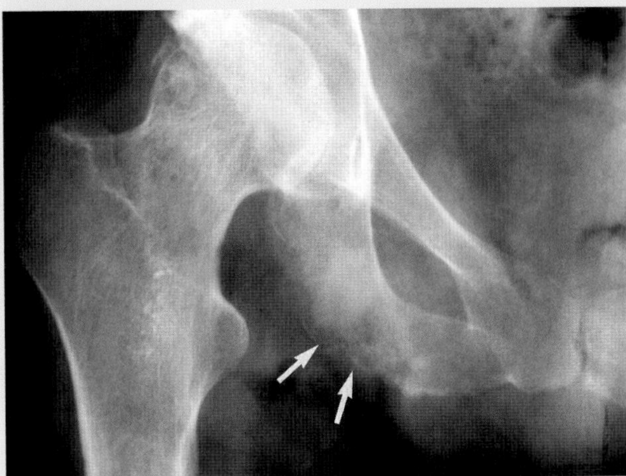

X-ray of the pelvis in an elderly bed-bound woman showing osteomyelitis of the ischial tuberosity (arrowed) underlying a deep, long-standing sacral pressure ulcer

COMPLICATIONS OF OPERATIONS INVOLVING BOWEL

These include delayed return of bowel function, mechanical bowel obstruction, anastomotic failure, intra-abdominal abscesses, peritonitis, bowel fistula and acute bowel ischaemia.

DELAYED RETURN OF BOWEL FUNCTION

TEMPORARY INTERRUPTION OF PERISTALSIS

Any abdominal operation may temporarily disrupt peristalsis. This is particularly true where the operation is for peritonitis, an abscess or intestinal obstruction, or if the operation involves extensive handling of the bowel. Operations involving the retroperitoneal area such as aortic surgery may also disrupt peristalsis, probably via a disturbance of parasympathetic activity. The problem mostly affects the small intestine. Patients may complain of nausea, anorexia and vomiting after oral fluids are reintroduced early in the postoperative period. This condition is often loosely described as **ileus** and is cited as a reason for gradual reintroduction of fluids, followed by solids after abdominal operations. However, if ileus is prolonged, another cause such as intestinal obstruction or an intraperitoneal collection of pus should be sought.

ADYNAMIC BOWEL DISORDERS

Occasionally, a much more prolonged and extensive form of functional adynamic bowel disorder occurs. This presents with vomiting and protracted intolerance to oral intake. Adynamic disorder must be distinguished from true mechanical obstruction, which may require reoperation. Adynamic bowel problems may be a response to local factors (e.g. bowel handling, a bowel wall haematoma or a collection of pus in contact with bowel) or to systemic abnormalities, particularly hypokalaemia.

Acute gastric dilatation

Occasionally, adynamic disorder involves the stomach, causing acute gastric dilatation and accumulation of large volumes of gastric and duodenal reflux secretions. The warning feature is when the patient suddenly vomits a large volume of fluid which may, even on the first occasion, result in fatal bronchial aspiration. Preventing acute gastric dilatation is the main reason nasogastric tubes are used after upper gastrointestinal surgery or after relief of mechanical bowel obstruction. If acute gastric dilatation is suspected, the abdomen should be examined for a **succussion splash**, and a nasogastric tube passed if the result is positive. If present, immediate nasogastric intubation is necessary; two or more litres of fluid that might otherwise be vomited and inhaled may need to be aspirated. Aspiration of gastric contents can cause mild or severe aspiration pneumonia (Mendelson's syndrome).

'Pseudo-obstruction'

Adynamic disorder involving the large bowel is conventionally but inaccurately described as **pseudo-obstruction**, as there is in fact no obstruction present. It may follow any abdominal operation, especially if the retroperitoneal area has been disturbed, as in nephrectomy or aortic surgery. Pseudo-obstruction is also a recognised complication of non-abdominal operations such as fractured neck of femur, especially in frail patients. It may even occur without operation as a complication of severe hypokalaemia, trauma involving the lower spine and retroperitoneal area, or anti-Parkinsonian and other drugs. The diagnosis can rapidly be made on an 'instant' unprepared water-soluble contrast enema by excluding mechanical causes of obstruction. Treatment involves identification and treatment of the underlying cause, together with supportive measures such as an indwelling flatus tube or deflation via colonoscopy until function returns.

MECHANICAL BOWEL OBSTRUCTION

EARLY POSTOPERATIVE MECHANICAL OBSTRUCTION

Postoperative mechanical obstruction of the bowel is uncommon. It may be caused by a loop of bowel becoming twisted or trapped in a peritoneal defect, unwittingly created at open operation or laparoscopy. **Fibrinous adhesions** may also cause obstruction, and these usually develop about 1 week after operation. In both cases, the obstruction may be transient and settle with conservative measures (nasogastric aspiration and intravenous fluids), or may progress to full-scale intestinal obstruction requiring laparotomy. If tenderness and systemic signs of toxicity appear, reoperation becomes urgent to exclude strangulation. Obstruction occurring after gastrectomy or gastroenterostomy may be due to oedema of the mucosa surrounding the anastomosis; this usually settles eventually with conservative measures, although reoperation may be required.

LATE POSTOPERATIVE MECHANICAL OBSTRUCTION

Fibrinous adhesions may organise and persist as broad **fibrous adhesions** between adjacent loops of bowel or as isolated fibrous bands traversing the peritoneal cavity. These are a common cause of an isolated episode of small bowel obstruction or even infarction. Adhesions may also cause recurrent bouts of bowel obstruction months or years after abdominal operations. Most episodes resolve spontaneously with conservative treatment, but failure of resolution or signs of strangulation (tenderness, toxaemia) necessitate laparotomy.

Adhesive obstruction has become less common since talc powder on surgical gloves was discontinued in the 1970s and possibly even less common since the declining use of starch on gloves. However, patients with recurrent intestinal obstruction due to adhesions present a serious surgical challenge. Each laparotomy becomes more difficult and hazardous for the patient. Therapeutic agents to prevent adhesions forming in the form of films are showing promise for high risk cases.

ANASTOMOTIC FAILURE

Anastomotic leakage or breakdown is a major cause of postoperative morbidity after bowel surgery. Inadequate or delayed diagnosis and delayed surgical intervention may lead to multiple and cumulative complications including fistulae, sepsis, multi-organ dysfunction and failure, and death. There should be a low index of suspicion for leaks and a readiness to undertake reoperation if leakage is suspected.

Small anastomotic leaks are relatively common and lead to small **localised abscesses** which are walled off by surrounding gut and omentum. Small leaks manifest clinically by delayed recovery of bowel function resulting from local peristaltic dysfunction. Usually, the problem eventually settles with continued intravenous fluids and delayed reintroduction of oral intake. Reoperation, however, should be repeatedly considered if recovery is slow.

Major anastomotic breakdown results in generalised peritonitis, large abdominal abscesses, progressive sepsis and fistula formation.

INTRA-ABDOMINAL ABSCESSES

ABSCESS ASSOCIATED WITH BOWEL ANASTOMOSIS

An anastomotic leak from any part of the bowel may be walled off by small bowel and omentum in a vigorous intraperitoneal response (see Fig. 12.10). This results in an abscess forming near the anastomosis. The patient will either be non-specifically unwell with delayed recovery, a swinging pyrexia and signs of local peritonitis, or more seriously ill with early signs of sepsis.

Early reoperation is usually necessary to drain the abscess and prevent continued peritoneal contamination. Where the anastomosis has broken down, both ends of the bowel should be brought out to form temporary stomas, since re-anastomosis will almost certainly fail. The bowel can often be rejoined once the local infection and metabolic disruption have resolved.

OTHER INTRA-ABDOMINAL ABSCESSES

Intra-abdominal abscesses may also develop at sites remote from an anastomosis—for example, in the pelvis (**pelvic abscess**) or beneath the diaphragm (**subphrenic abscess**). These occur most often as a complication of treated peritonitis, particularly faecal peritonitis. They may also develop because of contamination of the operative site by faeces or other infected material, or by 'tracking' of an anastomotic abscess within the abdomen. Abscesses of this type usually produce a less severe illness than do those in direct communication with the bowel.

If an abscess is suspected, ultrasound or CT scanning may help to identify its location and guide needle aspiration or

CASE HISTROY

Fig. 12.10 Intra-abdominal abscess following appendicectomy

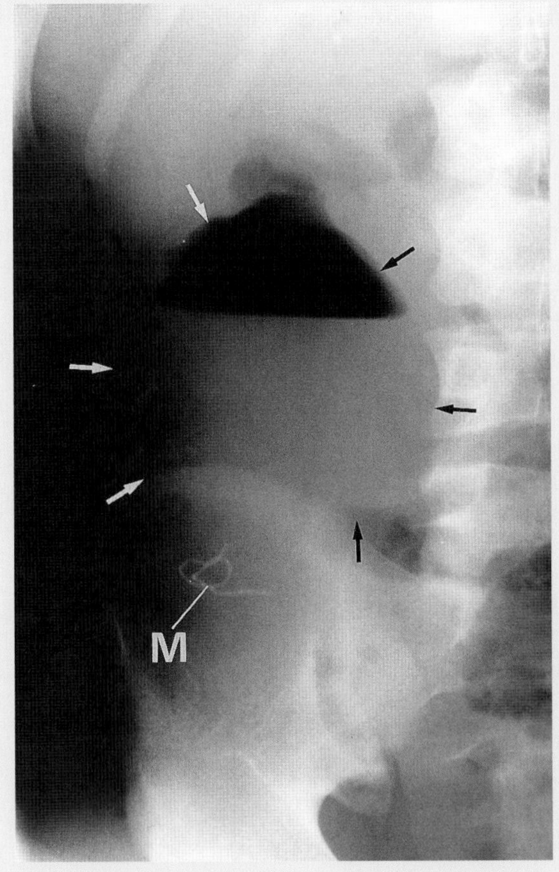

(a)

(b)

(a) This 16-year-old boy had an operation for removal of a perforated gangrenous appendix. He remained ill with anorexia and intermittent vomiting, general malaise and a swinging pyrexia. A large mass was palpable in the right side of the abdomen. Erect abdominal X-ray shows a huge abscess cavity (outline arrowed) with a gas bubble above a fluid (pus) level. Note the radiopaque marker **M** in a gauze swab packed into the open abdominal wound. **(b)** At operation, the abscess was surrounded by adherent small bowel, shown here

placement of a percutaneous drain if appropriate. Surgical exploration may, however, be necessary.

PERITONITIS

Postoperative peritonitis usually results from a major anastomotic breakdown causing extensive peritoneal contamination. In other cases, the cause is perforation of **obstructed or ischaemic bowel** or perforation of an incidental **peptic ulcer**. The clinical picture may develop rapidly over a few hours or, if infection spreads from an intraperitoneal abscess, more gradually over a few days. The patient is systemically ill with severe, generalised abdominal pain; the abdomen is tender and rigid to palpation (see Ch. 19, p. 272 for more details). *Note*: elderly patients with peritonitis may have surprisingly little tenderness. Generalised peritonitis progresses to sepsis and multiple organ failure unless promptly treated.

The patient is resuscitated and commenced on intravenous antibiotics and then returned to theatre for laparotomy. The abdomen is explored, the underlying cause is treated and peritoneal toilet is carried out. Early and vigorous treatment will usually save the patient's life.

BOWEL FISTULA

Fistula formation as a complication of surgery usually results from an anastomotic leak or infarction of a segment of bowel. A local abscess first develops then discharges to the surface via the wound or along the track of an abdominal drain. Anastomotic breakdown is more likely when there is obstruction of bowel beyond the anastomosis; the fistulous tract then provides a means of drainage for obstructed bowel contents. With time, the drainage tract slowly becomes lined with epithelium from the bowel and the skin surface and the fistula becomes permanent. Occasionally a fistula develops in a patient after an operation for **bowel cancer**. In this case the fistula may become lined with malignant cells. Proximal small bowel fistulas result in loss of large volumes of intestinal secretions containing digestive enzymes. This rapidly leads to dehydration and major electrolyte disturbances and usually causes gross intra-abdominal inflammation and skin destruction. The more proximal the origin of the fistula, the greater the volume of fluid and electrolyte loss and the more damaging its consequences.

The general state of the patient with a fistula depends on the extent of intra-abdominal infection. If this is minimal and there is no distal obstruction, the fistula usually closes spontaneously within weeks or months, provided the patient can be sustained in the interim. Proximal small bowel fistulas require **total bowel rest** (i.e. nil by mouth and a nasogastric tube) with full **parenteral fluid replacement and nutrition.** Somatostatin analogues may be given to substantially reduce the volume of secretion into the small bowel. Distal small bowel or large bowel fistulas may be managed with **enteral feeding** using low-residue elemental or semi-elemental fluid diets. These are often given via a fine-bore nasogastric tube.

When a fistula is associated with intra-abdominal infection, the patient is desperately ill, septic and hypercatabolic. These patients need intensive care management and reoperation. Laparotomy is required to bring the disrupted bowel ends to the surface as stomas and to drain the gross foci of infection; further laparotomies, even daily, may still be required before the intra-abdominal infection is brought under control. Mortality from these complicated fistulas is high.

ACUTE BOWEL ISCHAEMIA

Acute bowel ischaemia is an uncommon postoperative complication, usually occurring after abdominal aortic surgery. Infarction of the sigmoid colon follows inferior mesenteric artery ligation (usually a necessary part of the operation) if the collateral blood supply is compromised by obliterative atherosclerosis of the remaining mesenteric arteries. Fortunately, this is rare. The patient has usually progressed well at first then deteriorates unexpectedly several days after operation, often passing fresh blood per rectum. If untreated at this stage, the patient later collapses with peritonitis due to colonic necrosis and perforation.

Clinical signs of acute bowel ischaemia are non-specific, but often the degree of pain and collapse is out of proportion to the minimal abdominal signs. Plain abdominal X-ray may show 'thumb printing' of the affected bowel or the characteristic appearance of gas in the bowel wall. If acute bowel ischaemia is suspected, laparotomy must usually be performed urgently as perforation will soon occur and is nearly always fatal. Even with timely surgery, the prognosis is bleak.

Principles of cancer management

13

INTRODUCTION

Malignant disease afflicts about a third of all people at some time and about one in four die from it. Cancer patients are a major part of the general surgical workload and use as much as 40% of surgical bed occupancy. They place disproportionate demands on services, as operations are often extensive and patients are usually older, slower to recover and more prone to complications. Although rates of many malignancies are falling, the total numbers are rising because of increasing life expectancy. In younger age groups, surgical workload from cancer is growing because of earlier detection, increasing technical capabilities and greater patient expectations. The incidence of common malignancies in Western countries is shown in Table 13.1.

Screening for malignancy (see Ch. 6), notably cervical, breast and colorectal cancer, has so far produced only a modest impact on mortality, because of poor patient compliance (in cervical and colorectal cancer) and because detecting biologically early disease (in breast cancer) is elusive.

Whether curative treatment can be offered depends on location and nature of the primary cancer (i.e. tissue type, metastatic potential) and the extent of spread. Management of particular cancers is becoming more protocol-driven as good randomised trials have identified the most effective treatments. These treatments increasingly involve surgery combined with other treatments, particularly radiotherapy, chemotherapy, and for certain cancers, hormone manipulation. **Targeted therapies** are also starting to play a role, in particular trastuzumab (Herceptin®) in HER2-positive breast cancer.

Whilst the detection and treatment of many types of cancer is improving, a universal preventative or cure for 'cancer' is unlikely ever to appear.

NEOPLASIA

The main characteristic of all neoplasms is uncontrolled growth that persists even after the initiating stimulus has been removed. The p53 protein is a vital cell cycle regulator and has been called the 'guardian of the genome' for its role in preventing genome mutation and stabilising cells in the face of pathological onslaughts. Abnormalities of p53 have been found in over 50% of all cancers and strenuous research efforts are continuing to modify its behaviour.

Most neoplasms can readily be categorised as **benign** or **malignant** according to histological pattern, and for most malignancies, it is possible to predict the likelihood of invasion or of metastasis. Sometimes this is difficult; for example, distinguishing between leiomyoma and leiomyosarcoma may only be achieved by following its long-term behaviour. Neoplasms may also be difficult to distinguish clinically from other **tumour-like disorders** such as **hyperplasia** (e.g. parathyroid adenoma from hyperplasia) or a **hamartoma** (a benign growth composed of a mixture of tissues normally found in that area of the body).

BENIGN NEOPLASMS

Benign neoplasms usually grow slowly. They are typically well demarcated and often encapsulated, with a histological appearance closely reminiscent of the tissue of origin. Benign tumours present to the surgeon in a variety of ways summarised in Box 13.1.

MALIGNANT NEOPLASMS

Malignant neoplasms or tumours are typically non-encapsulated with a poorly defined, irregular outline due to local invasion. They usually grow progressively and often

Table 13.1 The 10 most commonly diagnosed cancers in males and females in the UK (from Cancer Research UK, 2008)*; figures have been rounded

Males		Females	
Prostate	37 000	Breast	47 700
Lung	23 000	Lung	18 000
Colorectal	22 000	Colorectal	17 900
Bladder	7400	Uterus	7700
Lymphoma	6300	Ovary	6500
Melanoma	5600	Melanoma	6200
Oesophagus	5500	Lymphoma	5500
Kidney	5400	Pancreas	4000
Stomach	4900	Kidney	3400
Leukaemia	4400	Leukaemia	3200

* See also Table 27.1 (p. 354)

Box 13.1 Principal modes of presentation of benign tumours

- Lesion suspected by the patient to be malignant, e.g. breast lump
- Overt bleeding or occult blood loss causing anaemia, e.g. bowel polyps
- Local obstructive effects, e.g. leiomyoma of small intestine
- Pressure causing pain or dysfunction, e.g. neurofibroma
- Unacceptable cosmetic appearance, e.g. subcutaneous lipomas
- Production of excessive amounts of hormone by endocrine neoplasms, e.g. parathyroid adenoma, insulinoma, phaeochromocytoma

rapidly. Histologically, the cells range from well differentiated to **anaplastic** (i.e. little or no resemblance to parent tissue), with the aggression of the neoplasm increasing as differentiation decreases.

The cells of malignant neoplasms as well as their nuclei often vary widely in shape and size. The extent of this **pleomorphism** also tends to correlate with the degree of malignancy and the future clinical behaviour of the tumour. The supporting tissue **stroma** of some malignancies may undergo fibrous hyperplasia, which accounts for some of the characteristic clinical features; these include hardness to palpation (induration), intestinal obstruction caused by annular carcinomas of the large bowel, and retraction and dimpling of skin overlying breast cancers. On the other hand, in highly aggressive tumours, the supporting tissue stroma may be inadequate for nutritional support, leading to necrosis and patchy haemorrhage within the tumour. This often presents as a sudden onset of pain and a mass.

Malignant tumours present in a variety of ways as summarised in Box 13.2.

CARCINOGENESIS

Multiple primary lesions and recurrences

Most cancers are probably caused by environmental factors plus factors intrinsic to the patient. About two-thirds of cancers can be attributed in some way to external environmental factors such as ionising radiation, virus infections and carcinogens in air, food and water. When cancer develops, it is likely that the whole of the affected organ or tissue has already been altered by the carcinogen. Consequently, new primary tumours, as distinct from local recurrences, may develop later. This is a factor in deciding follow-up after treatment, although clearly distinguishing between new primaries and recurrences can be impossible. Certain tissues, particularly those of the bladder, breast, skin, head and neck, and large bowel, are at particular risk of new primary carcinomas.

GROWTH AND SPREAD OF MALIGNANT TUMOURS

Malignant tumours spread by local growth and **infiltration** and by **distant metastasis** via lymphatics, the bloodstream and across coelomic cavities. Carcinogenesis, however, is not a single pathological event. Rather, both the onset of uncontrolled proliferation and the capacity for distant spread evolve in a series of mutations over successive cell divisions. Most malignancies probably arise from a single cell line (i.e. are monoclonal) and the initial event is the acquisition of the capability to grow progressively. About 30 cell division cycles are probably needed to produce a clinically detectable lesion of 1 cm diameter containing 1000 million cells. Particular cellular properties, often arising through multiple mutations, enable a tumour to invade surrounding tissues whilst other properties allow invasion of lymphatic or blood capillaries, dissemination and 'taking root' in regional lymph nodes or other distant tissues.

These pathophysiological factors have important clinical consequences. Firstly, the earlier the primary tumour is detected and removed (i.e. the fewer cell division cycles have occurred), the greater the chance of complete cure. Unfortunately, mutations that permit metastasis can appear very early, i.e. by about 20 cell division cycles, when the primary lesion is too small to be detected (about 1 mm diameter).

There are two conflicting theories about the significance of regional lymph node involvement in cancer. Both recognise that lymph node involvement implies a worse prognosis. **Halsted** believed that lymph nodes are important in halting spread, at least for a time, and that radical surgery to remove the nodes offers the best potential for cure. In more than 50% of large bowel cancers, for example, Halsted's view is probably correct and radical surgery remains the treatment of choice. In many other cancers, haematogenous spread is often occult and probably occurs early, rendering the disease incurable by surgery. Unfortunately, identifying which patients already

Box 13.2 Principal modes of presentation of malignant tumours

The primary lesion

- Palpable or visible mass, e.g. breast or thyroid cancer
- Obstruction or other disruption of function of a hollow viscus, e.g. bowel obstruction by colorectal carcinoma, stridor in bronchial carcinoma
- Overt bleeding, e.g. bladder tumour or left-sided large bowel cancer
- Occult blood loss causing anaemia, e.g. carcinoma of stomach or caecum
- Obstructive jaundice, e.g. carcinoma of head of pancreas or extrahepatic bile ducts
- Skin lesion, often ulcerated, e.g. basal and squamous cell carcinomas, malignant melanoma, breast cancer
- Nerve invasion, e.g. facial nerve palsy from parotid carcinoma, recurrent laryngeal palsy from anaplastic carcinoma of thyroid

Note that pain is not a common presenting feature of primary malignancy except in the pancreas, lung and nasopharynx; pain is more often associated with metastases

Metastatic deposits

- Enlarged lymph nodes (nodes tend to be hard, matted and non-tender). Intrathoracic nodes may cause superior vena caval obstruction
- Hepatomegaly, e.g. stomach, large bowel and pancreatic carcinomas
- Obstructive jaundice (usually due to lymph node mass in the porta hepatis compressing the bile ducts, but sometimes extensive liver deposits), e.g. stomach, large bowel and pancreatic carcinomas
- Abnormal masses distant from the primary lesion, e.g. abdomen, pelvis and skin
- Bone invasion causing bone pain or pathological fractures, e.g. prostatic and breast cancers
- Malignant effusions, e.g. pleural effusion in breast cancer, ascites with peritoneal deposits from intra-abdominal malignancies
- Pulmonary metastases—usually asymptomatic and found on chest X-ray
- Brain metastases—behavioural or personality changes, headache, fits, paresis, ataxias, etc.
- Neurological problems—spinal cord lesions caused by spinal fractures or by direct invasion

Generalised systemic manifestations (uncommon except for cachexia)

- Malignant cachexia (severe weight loss and wasting)—probably caused by the production of catabolic cytokines by the tumour
- Fever—characteristic of lymphomas and renal adenocarcinoma; also occurs when there is extensive tumour necrosis
- Migrating superficial thrombophlebitis and chronic disseminated intravascular coagulation (DIC)
- Peripheral neuropathies, myopathies and rare autoimmune neuromuscular phenomena, e.g. myasthenic syndrome
- Other rare autoimmune phenomena, e.g. haemolysis
- Ectopic hormone production, e.g. antidiuretic hormone (ADH), adrenocorticotrophic hormone (ACTH), parathyroid hormone (PTH) and gonadotrophins (all rare in malignancies seen in general surgery)
- Production of fetal and embryonic proteins, e.g. carcino-embryonic antigen (CEA) produced by testicular tumours and colorectal and pancreatic carcinomas; alpha-fetoprotein (AFP) produced by testicular teratomas and hepatocellular carcinomas; prostate-specific antigen (PSA) in prostatic carcinoma—may be useful as **tumour markers** for diagnosis, monitoring treatment and long-term follow-up

have metastatic disease remains difficult, although better imaging, laparoscopy and biopsy techniques are improving pre-treatment staging.

An alternative view about the significance of involved nodes, expressed by **Fisher**, is that any metastases indicate failure of host defences and therefore denote systemic metastasis beyond the nodes. In breast cancer, systemic treatments with cytotoxic and/or hormonal therapy have been developed with the intention of eliminating or suppressing micrometastases. These have improved survival in a small proportion of patients. Nevertheless, local surgery is important in controlling loco-regional disease in the breast, chest wall and axilla.

In practice, when lymph node metastases are present, the probability of surgical cure depends on the point at which the cancer develops its capacity for haematogenous spread. This can be about the same time as lymph node metastases appear, so surgical removal of metastases would be ineffective because haematogenous metastases would already be multifocal. Occasionally blood-borne metastasis appears to be a solitary event and a cure can be achieved—for example, by partial hepatectomy for colorectal cancer or pulmonary lobectomy for renal cell carcinoma, as well as in some paediatric malignancies. The liver, lungs, bone and brain are common organs for haematogenous spread. Multiple metastases often respond temporarily to palliative chemotherapy, radiotherapy or hormone manipulation (e.g. carcinomas of breast, uterus, kidney and prostate), but complete cure is very rarely achieved.

This model of the inception of metastatic potential means that progress in cancer management has to focus on primary prevention, very early diagnosis, and research to find effective non-surgical approaches, e.g. chemotherapy, hormonal manipulation and targeted therapeutic approaches.

TREATMENT OF MALIGNANT TUMOURS

BASIC PRINCIPLES OF CANCER MANAGEMENT

Two broad considerations determine the approach to treatment for any cancer patient. The first is whether an attempt can and should be made to achieve a **cure** or whether **palliation** is more appropriate. This choice depends on the nature of the tumour, the extent of local spread and whether distant metastases are believed to be present. The second consideration is the **prognosis**. This takes further factors into account, including the natural history of the type of cancer and the patient's age and co-morbidity and consequent ability to withstand surgery. Systems of **staging** have been devised for each tumour type, many based on the **TNM system** which scores characteristics of the Tumour, the extent of regional lymph Node involvement and the presence of Metastases. Staging is used in planning treatment, as a guide to prognosis and as a standardised descriptive tool for comparing efficacy of treatment in different patients and in different centres.

Cancer often recurs some time after the primary treatment, and the success of treatment is often described in terms of survival after a given number of years rather than 'cure'. **Five-year survival** is a common yardstick and in many cases can be taken to imply cure. Nevertheless, some tumours, particularly breast cancer, may recur in a disseminated form as long as 30 years after apparently successful eradication. Conversely, colorectal cancer and testicular teratoma and seminoma rarely recur after the patient has survived 7 years.

TEAMWORKING IN CANCER MANAGEMENT

There is a growing trend towards involving a range of specialists working in cooperative teams to manage patients with complex problems. Structured multidisciplinary teams are effective for managing complex cancer cases where the diagnosis needs careful consideration and where the treatment package may involve radiotherapy, chemotherapy or targeted therapy pre- or postoperatively, meticulous planning of an operation, prostheses or reconstructive surgery, stoma care and specialist nursing or physiotherapy, as well as social and psychological support.

The benefits of working in this way stem from the battery of experience brought by experts in different disciplines, particularly in cases where diagnostic and therapeutic options are not clear. Cases can be discussed at any stage in the diagnostic or treatment process and an optimum treatment plan generated; the group has joint responsibility for implementing the plan. Multidisciplinary teams (MDTs) have also been successfully introduced into other areas, for example neck lumps and rheumatoid disease. However, having such teams is expensive and takes staff away from other duties. It is a luxury where health care is less developed or poorly funded.

TREATMENT OPTIONS

The treatment options for malignant disease include **surgical excision, radiotherapy, chemotherapy, hormonal manipulation** and **molecular targeted therapies**, with two or more of these often used in combination. Treatment offered to an individual depends on tumour type and extent, molecular profile, the patient's overall fitness and whether the aim is cure or palliation. A radical or aggressive approach may be recommended where the aim is cure, provided the scientific evidence supports this approach. Where cure is not possible, or where disease has relapsed after radical treatment, the aim is to palliate, i.e. to alleviate the symptoms.

Palliative care focuses on quality of life when cure is not possible and involves weighing up the benefits of treatment against its burdens whilst focusing on what is important to the patient and family. Specialist palliative care teams can offer invaluable outpatient support in difficult matters of symptom control, or psychological, social or spiritual problems. Some patients may need short admissions to specialist units (often called hospices) for symptom control and eventually for terminal care.

Most standard cancer treatments involve unpleasant **side-effects**, easily disregarded by doctor and patient in their enthusiasm for treatment. Patients need to be appropriately informed and involved in treatment decisions, though the amount of information given varies, with some wanting the whole story and others less. How much the patient and the family want to know may differ but a doctor may speak independently to family members with the patient's consent. A diagnosis of cancer should not be concealed from a competent patient as suspicion and fear of the unknown often causes more distress than a frank explanation of the diagnosis and its ramifications. A period of time should be allowed for the patient to formulate further questions and a follow-up consultation arranged in a few days. It often helps to have a friend or relative present. Patients are also helped by well-constructed printed information, by self-help groups and by specially trained cancer nurses who can spend the necessary time and act as an intermediary if necessary.

SURGERY FOR CANCER

GENERAL PRINCIPLES OF CANCER SURGERY (Box 13.3)

The ideal result of cancer surgery is complete eradication of the malignant disease without radically interfering with function. Nearly a third of cancer patients can be cured in this way; these are mainly patients with only primary disease (without nodal or metastatic disease). Decisions about whether to embark on major elective surgery depends on thorough assessment of the nature of the disease and its stage. Modern techniques of cross-sectional imaging, laparoscopy and intraoperative ultrasound greatly assist and may save patients from fruitless radical surgery. Evidence-based reviews of treatments for malignancies at different

Box 13.3 The general principles of cancer management

Note: detection of asymptomatic disease is covered in Chapter 6, including opportunistic screening, screening and surveillance of people with risk factors, and population screening

1. **Pre-referral mechanisms**
- Patient education to recognise danger symptoms and signs
- Self-examination by the patient. e.g. breast, testis
- Education, guidance and post-referral feedback for family practitioners in recognising danger symptoms and signs and reassuring the 'worried well'
- Appropriate referral to specialists, helped by proformas containing indications to refer suspected skin, colorectal, breast, head and neck and upper gastrointestinal cancer
- Ready availability of early assessment and diagnostic tests

2. **Primary diagnosis after referral**—clinical assessment plus investigations, e.g. imaging, endoscopy, biopsy, fine-needle aspiration cytology, laparoscopy
3. **Staging**—additional investigation to evaluate extent of spread:
- Local spread
- Lymph node spread
- Haematogenous spread (bone, lung, liver, brain)
- Peritoneal/pleural spread

4. **Multidisciplinary decision making**—to formulate the aims of treatment and decide optimum treatment:
- Treatment planning and timing of treatment, ideally based on randomised controlled trials (RCTs) but also on experience
- Treatment may involve a single entity, or combinations of surgery, neoadjuvant or adjuvant chemotherapy and/or radiotherapy, postoperative chemo- or radiotherapy, hormonal therapy
- Patients should be entered into clinical trials where best treatment is not established

Note that increasing specialisation and sub-specialisation in the surgical treatment of rarer or more complex cancers produces better outcomes, e.g. sarcoma, oesophageal carcinoma

5. **The treatment**
6. **Repeat staging after operation or other treatment**—with knowledge of operative findings and a review of the histology. This may change the plan for postoperative adjuvant therapy and provide information to calculate the statistical likelihood of survival/cure
7. **Post-treatment surveillance**—for recurrence or appearance of new tumours in the primary field. Guidelines for different cancers are available for the desirability, frequency and duration of clinical assessment, imaging, endoscopy and measuring tumour markers
8. **Audit of local outcomes to improve quality of care. Participation in national audits**

stages also help decide indications for surgery, with level 1 evidence from well-conducted randomised controlled trials being best.

Metastases apparently confined to local lymph nodes are usually excised along with the primary tumour or else at a second operation. In gastric cancer, familiarity with the lymphatic drainage guides excision of defined node groups and this appears to give better long-term cure rates. Even in the presence of incurable metastases, surgical excision of the primary is sometimes required to relieve local effects of the tumour, e.g. bleeding, pain or bowel obstruction. Similar results can often be obtained by radiotherapy, chemotherapy or physical means of destruction such as radiofrequency probes or lasers. Palliative surgery may be required for specific distressing symptoms from locally advanced or metastatic disease (e.g. dysphagia from oesophageal cancer, severe haemorrhage from a bladder tumour) or some emergency problem (e.g. acute bowel obstruction).

Sometimes surgery is used to **debulk** a tumour, usually combined with chemotherapy, to improve its efficacy (as in ovarian carcinoma) or to avoid leaving unstable tissue in abdominal nodes (as in testicular teratoma). Increasingly, chemotherapy and/or radiotherapy is used to 'downsize' a malignant tumour to facilitate excisional surgery, e.g. rectal cancer. This is sometimes inaccurately called 'down-staging', since it has no effect on metastatic disease.

RADIOTHERAPY

GENERAL PRINCIPLES OF RADIOTHERAPY

The value of ionising radiation in treating malignant tumours was recognised soon after the discovery of X-rays in 1895, and radiotherapy is now employed at some stage in about half of all patients with malignant disease. **Orthovoltage** X-rays (up to 250 kV) were the basis of radiotherapy until **megavoltage** irradiation in the late 1950s. Cobalt-60 machines provided more penetrating radiation, but have been superseded by **linear accelerators** which provide photon beams with an energy of 5–20 MeV. With increased energy, the radiation dose peaks deep to the skin, avoiding the former severe skin reactions. Radiotherapy works by the target tissue absorbing radiation, which induces highly reactive free radicals that damage DNA and cause cell death at mitosis. Cancer cells with a high rate of proliferation are particularly sensitive but normal tissues with high rates of cell turnover (e.g. gut mucosa and bone marrow) are also vulnerable. The total dose given depends on the aims of treatment, the site and volume of the tumour and its relationship to important normal tissues. Treatment is by a variable number of sessions or **fractions** over several weeks to allow normal tissues to recover between treatments.

The larger the volume of tumour, the greater the dosage of irradiation required. Since dosage is limited by the tolerance of normal tissues, radiotherapy is more effective for small lesions. Radiation dose is measured in **Gray** (Gy). A common daily dose is around 2 Gy, sufficient to destroy about 50% of viable cells in an average tumour; each subsequent dose destroys 50% of the remainder, causing a logarithmic decline in viable cell numbers as treatment proceeds. Planning radiotherapy for lesions deep within the body has improved as a result of enhanced CT and magnetic resonance imaging (MRI).

Radiation can be directed to a tumour in three ways:

- **External beam irradiation**—this is most commonly employed for skin lesions and deeply located tumours
- **Local application of radioisotopes (brachytherapy)**—this involves placing the radiation source on or in the tissue to be irradiated. **Plaque** sources of radiation can be employed for skin malignancies, and radioactive **iridium wires or caesium needles** can be implanted in the oral cavity, prostate, skin and sometimes breast, giving high-dose local irradiation. Implantation is usually performed under general anaesthesia. For cancer of the uterus and cervix, the radioactive source is placed in a sealed container within the uterine or vaginal cavity; it can be inserted without risk to staff via a flexible tube from the radiation safe using computer control
- **Systemic radioisotope therapy**—radioactive iodine given by mouth or intravenously is a well-established treatment for thyrotoxicosis and can be used for well-differentiated thyroid cancers even if metastases are present, provided the rest of the thyroid has been removed. Attempts are being made to direct radioisotopes precisely to cancer cells by attaching them to tumour-specific markers such as monoclonal antibodies, thus realising the dream of a 'magic bullet', but techniques remain largely in an experimental stage

MAJOR APPLICATIONS OF RADIOTHERAPY

Radiotherapy has three major applications: as a primary cure, as adjuvant treatment to surgery (and/or chemotherapy) or as palliation. The treatment objective must be clearly defined before treatment is begun.

PRIMARY CURATIVE RADIOTHERAPY

Radiotherapy with curative intent is known as **radical**, and is widely used for basal cell and squamous cell carcinomas of skin. Where rates of cure are comparable to surgery, radiotherapy can be used for tumours that are technically difficult to remove or where surgery would be particularly mutilating, as in the head, neck and larynx. Radiotherapy can be directed at the primary lesion and regional lymph nodes if appropriate. In head and neck cancers without distant metastases, cure rates of 50–90% can be achieved with radiotherapy alone, with similar results in carcinoma of the cervix. Radiotherapy is employed in most common solid tumours and in early cases of Hodgkin and non-Hodgkin lymphomas. The efficacy and application of radiotherapy for various tumour types is summarised in Table 13.2. Radiotherapy can also achieve cure in up to 50% of bladder cancers, with salvage cystectomy reserved for recurrence.

ADJUVANT RADIOTHERAPY

The principle underlying **adjuvant therapy**, whether radiological, chemical or hormonal, is to target clinically undetectable micrometastases believed to be responsible for local, regional and systemic recurrence after a primary has apparently been completely removed. Adjuvant radiotherapy can be applied to local tissue and regional nodes before surgery (**neoadjuvant therapy**), after surgery or both. Neoadjuvant therapy, comprising radiotherapy, chemotherapy or both may also be used to 'downsize' a cancer to make surgery practicable, e.g. in locally advanced rectal cancer.

Adjuvant radiotherapy is widely employed for cancer of the breast after removing the primary lesion locally or by mastectomy. If axillary nodes are involved, radiotherapy can be an alternative to radical lymph node clearance; survival rates are comparable to those achieved by surgery. However, the trend of opinion favours radical lymph node clearance for the improved diagnostic accuracy it provides and the prognostic value of knowing the number of nodes involved. The preference for surgery or radiotherapy remains one of local choice. Radiotherapy is also highly effective adjuvant therapy in seminoma of the testis.

PALLIATIVE RADIOTHERAPY

Radiotherapy for palliation is employed for local control of primary or metastatic lesions to treat symptoms whilst causing minimal side-effects. It is also employed to prevent anticipated complications, e.g. spinal cord compression. Much lower total doses are used than for attempts at cure; short courses or **single high-dose fractions** are tolerable and convenient for the patient. Clearly, palliative radiotherapy can only be justified if expert assessment predicts that therapeutic benefit is likely.

Radiotherapy is particularly effective in controlling metastatic deposits in bone and brain. The pain of bone metastases can often be completely relieved by radiotherapy, as can some of the neurological manifestations of brain secondaries.

Radiotherapy is often valuable in providing symptomatic relief in advanced disease. In ulcerating breast cancer, radiotherapy can shrink the primary lesion, permitting healing of overlying skin. Similarly, the distressing symptoms of cough, haemoptysis and pleuritic pain from advanced lung cancer can be eased and symptoms of local recurrence can often be controlled, e.g. pain from rectal cancer. Indications for palliative radiotherapy are summarised in Box 13.4.

COMPLICATIONS OF RADIOTHERAPY

Despite the precise use of high-energy radiotherapy, side-effects and complications still occur; the main early effects are outlined in Table 13.3.

Table 13.2 **Applications of radiotherapy for treating malignant disease**

Tumour type	Radiosensitivity	Indications
Head and neck	Moderate	Highly effective for localised lesions especially larynx
Lung		
Small cell	High (but largely palliative)	Enhances efficacy of chemotherapy but overall cure rate less than 10%
Non-small cell	Low to moderate	Worth a trial in patients with inoperable disease for palliation
Breast	Moderate	Usually as adjuvant to surgery or to treat axillary nodal involvement or advanced local breast cancer
Thyroid		
Well differentiated	High	Low
Poorly differentiated (anaplastic)	High cure rate in combination with surgery (systemic radioiodine therapy)	Rarely useful
Renal cell carcinoma	Low	Rarely appropriate
Transitional cell carcinoma of bladder	Moderate	Good cure rate for localised lesions
Testis	Moderate to high	Good (especially seminoma) but chemotherapy generally better (for teratoma)
Ovary	Very low	Rarely applicable
Uterus		
Cervix	Moderate	High cure rate for localised tumours; also as adjuvant therapy
Body	Moderate	Adjuvant or palliative therapy
Gastrointestinal tract	Low to moderate	Increasingly used for adjuvant therapy in advanced rectal cancers. Definitive treatment for anal carcinomas
Lymphoma		
Hodgkin	High	Excellent cure rate for stage I and II disease
Non-Hodgkin	High	High cure rate when used with chemotherapy
Multiple myeloma	High	Mainly used for palliation
Skin		
Basal or squamous cell carcinoma	High	Highly curable
Melanoma	Low	Used to palliate metastases
Adult central nervous system	Low to moderate	Adjuvant therapy in well-differentiated gliomas Palliation of cerebral metastases
Paediatric malignancies	Variable	Often curative for brain tumours and effective for Wilms' tumour but limited by long-term effects on growth and development

LONG-TERM SIDE-EFFECTS OF RADIOTHERAPY

Modern radiotherapy using high-energy sources with meticulous treatment planning and delivery causes fewer side-effects than the orthovoltage treatment used in earlier days. Side-effects such as **osteoradionecrosis** are rare (see Fig. 13.1), but **endarteritis obliterans** may be a long-term complication affecting any tissue subjected to radiotherapy. The effect is progressive impairment of blood supply, loss of specialised tissues and replacement with fibrosis. In the chest, radiotherapy can cause pulmonary fibrosis and in women treated for left-sided breast cancer, there is an increased risk of cardiac events; techniques have been modified as a result. In

Box 13.4 Indications for palliative radiotherapy

Pain control

- Bone pain (especially breast, prostate and lung metastases)
- Nerve root and soft tissue infiltration (e.g. head and neck, brachial plexus)

Dyspnoea

- Shrinkage of tumour obstructing or compressing a large airway

Ulcerating and fungating lesions

- Breast, skin, head and neck tumours

Haemorrhage

- Haemoptysis
- Haematuria
- Rectal and cervical bleeding

Emergency complications

- Spinal cord compression
- Superior vena caval obstruction
- Raised intracranial pressure
- Obstruction of tubular viscera (e.g. oesophagus, upper gastrointestinal tract, ureters)

Space-occupying lesions caused by symptomatic brain metastases

- Brain metastasis causing hemiparesis

Table 13.3 Early reactions and complications of radiotherapy

Reaction/complication	Management
Systemic side-effects	
Malaise and fatigue—very common	These settle spontaneously with rest
Nausea, vomiting and anorexia	Antiemetics
Effects occurring in irradiated tissues	
Skin (especially axilla, groin and perineum) Redness, itching and mild pain Skin breakdown (in treatment of skin cancers, this heals after 3–4 weeks)	 Mild or moderate-strength topical steroids Moisture-retaining non-adherent dressings Silver–sulfasalazine cream
Abdomen and pelvis Nausea, vomiting, diarrhoea Frequency, dysuria, haematuria (radiation cystitis)	 Antiemetics, antidiarrhoeals Urinary alkalinising agents; exclude infection
Head and neck Dry mouth (xerostomia) due to salivary gland injury Painful mouth, dysphagia and altered taste. This is due to inflammation and atrophy of oral mucosa (mucositis) and may also involve nasal mucosa	 Frequent oral fluids, moist oral swabs, careful attention to oral hygiene Topical steroids for ulcers, topical anaesthetic gels, antifungal agents for candidiasis, artificial saliva
Chest Painful dysphagia (radiation oesophagitis)	 Local anaesthetic gel Compound antacid/alginate preparations, e.g. Gaviscon
Head Hair loss (alopecia)	 Provision of wigs ('wig library')
Bone marrow Myelosuppression	 Discontinue therapy, prophylactic antibiotics, platelet transfusion

the gastrointestinal tract, the effects of radiation on bowel (**radiation enteritis**) can be particularly serious, with continued bleeding (in large bowel) and stricture formation (in small bowel). The same reaction probably accounts for delayed or incomplete healing after surgery with breakdown of intestinal anastomoses or formation of internal fistulae. **Radiation colitis** most commonly results from treatment of uterine cervical cancer.

CHEMOTHERAPY

GENERAL PRINCIPLES OF CHEMOTHERAPY

Success with chemotherapeutic agents in curing many haematological and childhood malignancies encouraged the use of similar drugs for solid tumours previously treated only by surgery or radiotherapy.

Drugs destroy tumour cells by exploiting their increased mitotic and metabolic rates. The main types of chemotherapeutic agent are as follows:

- **Antimetabolites**—analogues of normal cellular nutrients, e.g. methotrexate acts as a substitute for folinic acid
- **Alkylating agents**—these bind to DNA, e.g. nitrogen mustards
- **Drugs which cross-link DNA**, e.g. cisplatin
- **Drugs which disrupt the mitotic spindle**, e.g. vinca alkaloids, taxanes

These cytotoxic mechanisms also affect normal tissues, usually to a lesser extent, and are responsible for most side-effects of chemotherapy. Drug are often used in combination, selected so the toxic effects of each drug impact on a different organ system; this means that each drug can be given in full tumour-toxic dose without excessive damage to normal tissues. The

Fig. 13.1 Osteoradionecrosis after early orthovoltage radiotherapy for breast cancer

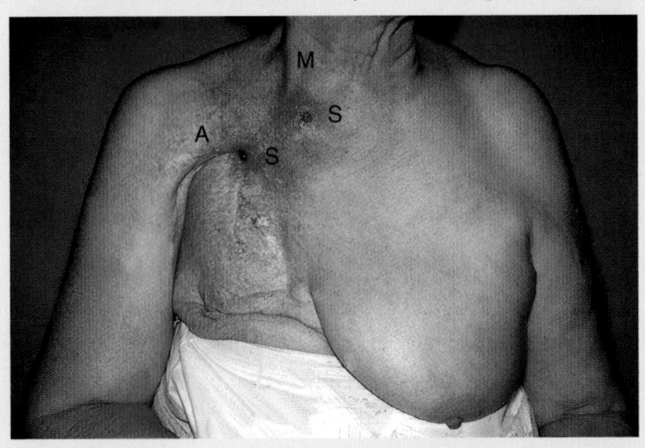

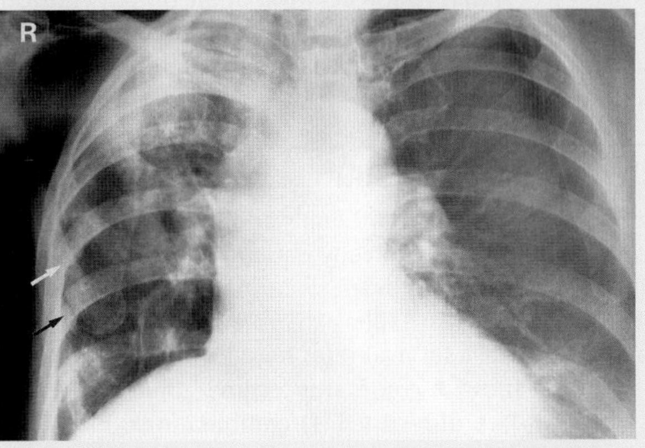

This 75-year-old woman had a radical mastectomy and orthovoltage irradiation for carcinoma of the right breast in 1949, 40 years before this photograph. She presented with two discharging skin sinuses below the clavicles, **S**. **(a)** Gross deformity of chest wall caused by excision of pectoral muscles at radical mastectomy (axilla **A**, sternomastoids **M**). Note sinus openings **S** leading down to sequestra, and widespread telangiectasia, a late result of radiotherapy. **(b)** Chest X-ray showing osteoradionecrosis of the ribs and scapula on the right side. There is typical patchy osteoporosis and osteosclerosis. Several healing pathological fractures are also evident (arrowed). Irradiation has induced lung fibrosis and pulmonary contraction resulting in a shift of the mediastinum towards the right.

Box 13.5 Tumour sensitivity to cytotoxic chemotherapy

Highly sensitive tumours

—reasonable prospect of cure

- Hodgkin's disease
- High-grade lymphomas
- Testicular tumours
- Choriocarcinoma
- Childhood leukaemias
- Wilms' tumour (nephroblastoma)
- Ewing's sarcoma
- Osteogenic sarcoma (lung metastases)

Moderately sensitive tumours

—can increase chances of cure in combination with other treatments

- Breast cancer
- Ovarian malignancies
- Small-cell (oat-cell) carcinoma of lung
- Multiple myeloma
- Acute and chronic leukaemias in adults
- Low-grade lymphomas
- Colorectal cancer

Relatively insensitive tumours

—cytotoxic therapy only indicated in special circumstances or with techniques of regional infusion, or in combination with other treatments

- Carcinoma of lung other than small-cell type
- Squamous carcinomas of the head and neck
- Carcinoma of uterus and cervix
- Melanoma
- Hepatocellular carcinoma
- Osteogenic sarcoma (primary lesions)
- Renal adenocarcinoma
- Bladder carcinoma

most effective combinations and doses for each tumour type have been established mainly by empirical trials. Very good combinations were developed in the 1970s and 1980s, e.g. CMF for breast cancer, CHOP for lymphoma and BEP for testicular cancer, but an increasing range of new chemotherapeutic drugs promise improvements. Drugs are usually given intravenously, often by infusion, in a series of four to six short courses separated by 3–4 weeks to allow recovery of normal tissues.

Experience has revealed a wide spectrum of sensitivities of different malignant tumours to cytotoxic therapy. The sensitivities of different tumour types are summarised in Box 13.5.

MAJOR APPLICATIONS OF CHEMOTHERAPY

Chemotherapy offers substantial benefit and a chance of cure in some well-defined malignancies, as shown in Box 13.5. However, clinicians treating cancer need to be clear whether their objective is cure or palliation, and base decisions on published clinical trials. Given the potential for side-effects and the high cost, there is no place for speculative chemotherapy where evidence shows no benefit.

PRIMARY CURATIVE TREATMENT

This is mainly indicated for highly sensitive **germ cell tumours**, high-grade **lymphomas** and **solid tumours and leukaemias**

of childhood. Chemotherapy may be used alone (e.g. Hodgkin's disease), or it may follow removal of the primary tumour (e.g. teratoma, Wilms' tumour), or it may be used first and then any residual tumour resected (e.g. abdominal para-aortic nodes in testicular teratoma).

ADJUVANT CHEMOTHERAPY

This involves systemic chemotherapy added to local treatment of the primary to destroy already disseminated but undetectable micrometastases. Adjuvant chemotherapy is often used for breast cancer with axillary lymph node involvement, where 5- and 10-year survival rates have both been improved by 5–15%. In cancer of colon and rectum, adjuvant therapy, mainly using 5-fluorouracil (5FU) combinations, has a role in extending recurrence-free survival and life expectancy. Current information on this and other trials is available from Cancer Research UK (www.cancerhelp.org.uk). Chemotherapy plus radiotherapy (**chemo-radiotherapy**) often replaces the need for radical surgery for anal canal, cervical and some head and neck cancers.

GENERAL PALLIATIVE TREATMENT

This is the rationale for chemotherapy in disseminated malignancy of highly sensitive and moderately sensitive tumours. Cure is rare but quality of life may be greatly improved, often through alleviation of specific symptoms (e.g. breast cancer causing lymphatic obstruction) and in some cases, life may be prolonged.

SIDE-EFFECTS OF CHEMOTHERAPY

Chemotherapy is especially toxic to cells with rapid turnover, e.g. bone marrow and gastrointestinal epithelium. Toxic effects are summarised in Box 13.6.

Box 13.6 Toxic effects of chemotherapy

Bone marrow suppression
- Causes anaemia, thrombocytopenia and leucopenia (potentially fatal)

Immunosuppression
- Causes diminished resistance to opportunistic infections

Nausea and vomiting
- Tend to occur within an hour or two of chemotherapy
- Modern antiemetics can usually control these symptoms but delayed nausea over the ensuing days remains a problem

Disruption of gastrointestinal epithelial turnover
- Causes diarrhoea and oral ulceration

Toxicity to hair follicles
- Particularly etoposide, cyclophosphamide and doxorubicin
- Causes hair loss (recovers 6 months after treatment)

Gonadal injury
- Loss of libido, sterility and possible mutagenesis

Long-term risk of inducing other malignancies
- 20–30 times the normal risk (but still low)

Rapid tumour destruction on a massive scale
- Leads to release of purines and pyrimidines (only a problem in leukaemias and lymphomas) which cause hyperuricaemia, presenting as obstructive uropathy and renal failure
- Hyperuricaemia can be prevented by giving prophylactic allopurinol

HORMONAL MANIPULATION

The growth of certain tumours, notably carcinoma of the prostate and some breast cancers, is dependent on sex hormones. Removal of the gonads or use of hormone blocking drugs can have a valuable inhibitory effect on tumour growth. Hormonal manipulation in the treatment of prostatic cancer is covered in detail in Chapter 35, p. 455, and breast cancer in Chapter 45, p. 555.

TARGETED THERAPIES

Oncologists have long dreamed of finding precise ways of delivering cancer-killing drugs to destroy cancer cells without damaging normal cells. This idea of a 'magic bullet' is now becoming real employing **monoclonal antibodies**. The specific antibody recognises certain protein configurations on the surface of cancer cells and 'locks' on to them. The intention is for cells to destroy themselves or trigger the body's immune system to recognise the marked cells as 'non-self' and attack them. So far, this has limited application but much work is continuing in the field.

LYMPHOMA

The antigen CD20 is found on the surface of normal B-cell lymphocytes (but not their precursors) and also on the surface of nearly all abnormal malignant B-cell lymphocytes found in 75% of non-Hodgkin lymphoma. The drug **rituximab** is a genetically engineered chimeric murine/human monoclonal IgG_1 antibody directed against the CD20 antigen. Normal and abnormal B-cells are both destroyed but the body quickly replaces the normal cells, so side-effects from lack of B-cells are minimal. Rituximab combined with chemotherapy has increased response rates in B-cell lymphoma by 20% compared with chemotherapy alone and has become the desirable standard treatment. However, the drug can cause serious adverse effects including mucocutaneous reactions and the rare but fatal **infusion reaction complex** of organ failure.

BREAST CANCER

Human epidermal growth receptor 2 (HER2) is an antigenic protein involved in transmitting growth signals from outside the cell to the nucleus; a strong signal causes the cell to divide. About 20% of breast cancers have excess HER2 (known as HER2-positive tumours). **Trastuzumab** (trade name Herceptin) is a recombinant DNA-derived humanised monoclonal IgG_1 antibody which binds selectively to the surface HER2 receptor (see Ch. 45, p. 556). Its anti-cancer effects are brought about by blocking cell growth and stimulating the immune system to destroy the tumour cells. As with similar drugs, there are potentially serious hazards including severe hypersensitivity reactions, cardiotoxicity and adverse pulmonary events. Herceptin has also recently been approved for the treatment of advance gastric cancers that are HER2-positive.

IMATINIB

In chronic myeloid leukaemia, the Philadelphia chromosome leads to production of an abnormal 'fusion protein' enzyme which continuously activates tyrosine kinase (TK) receptors. This causes uncontrolled cellular proliferation. A similar process occurs in **gastrointestinal stromal tumours (GIST)**, with activation of the **c-kit receptor**. Imatinib preferentially occupies the *TK* active receptor site, thereby decreasing the activity of several oncoprotein TK enzymes. As a result, the drug inhibits cellular proliferation and induces apoptosis (programmed cell death) in malignant cells.

THE FUTURE

Many other monoclonal antibodies as well as other small molecules that interfere with cellular receptors are under development or are in clinical trials for a range of tumour types. Other small molecules approved for use in particular cancer types include:

- Gefitinib and erlotinib (small molecular epidermal growth factor (EGFR) inhibitors, used in EGFR mutation-positive lung cancers)
- Sunitinib, sorafenib and pazopanib (multi-targeted tyrosine kinase inhibitors, approved for renal cell carcinoma)
- Lapatinib (tyrosine kinase inhibitor of HER2 and EGFR approved for use in metastatic HER2-positive breast cancer)

It is likely such targeted therapies will improve the outcome for an escalating range of malignancies. Early stage clinical trials now emphasise the drugs' biological effects, using validated biomarkers as endpoints, and an adaptive approach for analysing results in real time.

PALLIATIVE CARE

PRINCIPLES OF PALLIATIVE CARE

The principles of palliative care are outlined in Box 13.7. The diagnosis of cancer has immense significance to the patient and the patient's family. Areas affected include:

- Psychological—adjustment reaction, anxiety, depression
- Social—loss of role: unable to care for family, no longer viewed as husband/wife/companion
- Financial—loss of job, expense of frequent hospital visits
- Spiritual—patient and family face up to mortality
- Physical—pain, nausea, fatigue, dyspnoea

For specialists, there is a danger of concentrating on the primary disease while failing to treat the patient as a whole. Palliative care is concerned with the problems listed, with the emphasis on the patient's priorities, during and after treatment where complete cure is not possible. As well as trying to bring positive assistance, a doctor's duty includes 'doing no harm' and there is no ethical dilemma in withdrawing treatment unlikely to give benefit.

Increasingly, patients are living longer with a large tumour load. This means they often experience symptoms with multiple aetiologies, resulting in treatment with numerous and often too many drugs. Diagnostic tests should be used only to identify causes likely to be remediable. Time must be made available for clear and honest explanation of proposed treatments with patients and families. Palliative care focuses on **quality of life**, and many clinicians, including family practitioners, are keen to look after their patients at the end of their

Box 13.7 Principles of palliative care

1. Palliative care is not just about dying people. Patients with cancer need to be helped to function as normally as they can for as long as they can. They often contemplate their own mortality and what is important to them
2. Ensure good communication by spending time with the patient and family (empathic listening and giving information according to the patient's needs are crucial). Some patients want more information than doctors give them; some want less. Find out about the patient in front of you. Explore the patient's concerns by asking open questions
3. Anticipate potential problems. Ensure the patient/family know who to call if things go wrong. At an appropriate point, find out where a patient wants to die. Many choose home, some hospital. Hospices are another option. Terminal care at home needs coordinated planning. The family often take most of the burden of care
4. Assess symptoms regularly. Medication may need to be changed frequently as the patient's condition changes
5. Be aware of different cultural practices and religious beliefs when caring for patients and families
6. Be aware of how looking after seriously ill patients can affect health care workers. Working as a team and discussing patients' care regularly helps professionals cope

lives, ensuring a comfortable and dignified demise. Specialist palliative care physicians and nurses can support the primary care team and the patient and family at home and in specialist palliative care units (often called hospices).

APPROACH TO COMMON SYMPTOMS REQUIRING PALLIATION OTHER THAN PAIN

Good communication is the foundation of palliative care. Giving patients and families time to talk about their thoughts and concerns often in itself provides comfort. Palliative pain relief is covered in the next section, and management of other common symptoms is detailed in Table 13.4. Effective management of the symptoms of advancing cancer requires frequent reassessment, and frequent discussion with the patient to assess his or her own priorities.

CANCER PAIN

About three-quarters of patients with advanced cancer have pain at some stage. How individuals perceive pain is influenced by what it means to them (e.g. my cancer is getting worse), as well as other factors in their life, which, if deteriorating, can worsen pain. Addressing these factors is an important way of helping.

Assessment of pain

Patients frequently have more than one source of pain and each must be assessed. Pain measurement tools (e.g. visual analogue or verbal rating scales) and charts can be helpful. In assessing pain, it is useful to use a classification to help plan how to relieve it:

- Visceral pain—a constant 'tumour ache' caused by pressure of cancer or invasion of internal organs. Although severe, it often responds to opioids

Table 13.4 Common symptoms other than pain requiring palliation

Symptom	Causes	Management
Fatigue/asthenia (lack of energy)	Circulating factors released by tumour, chemotherapy, radiotherapy Pain, poor sleep, depression, anxiety	Open discussion with patient and family Encouraging gentle, regular exercise within limitations and a daily routine Address and treat remediable causes—check for anaemia Think of depression which often goes undiagnosed Think of a trial of corticosteroids
Loss of appetite (anorexia) and weight loss	Circulating factors released by tumour, chemotherapy, radiotherapy, chronic pain and nausea, fear, depression, anxiety, 'squashed stomach' syndrome, sore mouth, dysphagia	Explanation to patient and family of known causes Meticulous attention to oral hygiene Correct remediable factors Think of trial of corticosteroids or progestogen to stimulate appetite
Dysphagia	Tumours of pharynx, oesophagus and stomach	Options include insertion of stents, laser ablation, cryotherapy, brachytherapy (local radiotherapy) Radiotherapy, high-dose steroids
	Compression of oesophagus by extrinsic tumour (e.g. mediastinal lymph nodes) Oesophageal candidiasis	Suspect in immunosuppressed patients or patients on steroids; diagnosis may require gastroscopy; may require prolonged treatment with oral antifungal agent
Nausea and vomiting	Drugs: opioids, NSAIDs and others Metabolic causes, e.g. hypercalcaemia, uraemia, liver failure Radiotherapy/chemotherapy	Explanation to allay anxiety; review prescription
	Intracranial lesions causing raised intracranial pressure Gastric outlet obstruction	Antiemetic medication, e.g. haloperidol Antiemetic drugs: cyclizine, short courses of $5HT_3$ antagonist and/or high-dose steroids High-dose steroids reducing to minimal maintenance dose, short course radiotherapy Prokinetic drugs, e.g. metoclopramide or domperidone
	Intestinal obstruction	If not candidate for surgery discuss with specialist. Needs honest discussion with patient—may not be able to stop patient being sick but should be able to reduce it. If incomplete (e.g. no colic and passing wind) may benefit from prokinetic agents If complete, will need anti-secretory drugs (e.g. hyoscine butylbromide or octreotide) as well as antiemetics (e.g. cyclizine or levomepromazine) Should be able to avoid nasogastric tube
	Constipation	Prophylactic laxatives for all patients prescribed opioids; avoid bulk laxatives in preference to softening and stimulant agents

Table 13.4 **Continued**

Symptom	Causes	Management
Breathlessness (dyspnoea), cough, choking	Pleural effusion, cardiac failure, infection, anaemia	Investigate and treat all reversible causes with regard to patient's overall condition
	Laryngeal tumour, pulmonary tumour or major airway obstruction	May require stenting or local treatment, e.g. radiotherapy/laser/cryotherapy
	Lymphangitis carcinomatosa, multiple pulmonary metastases or infiltration	Trial of high-dose dexamethasone 16 mg daily; if beneficial reduce to maintenance dose, e.g. 2–4 mg daily
	Multifactorial: disease and debilitation	Explanation to patient and family Trial of bronchodilator therapy Trial of intermittent oral morphine Trial of oxygen In terminal phase, continuous subcutaneous infusion of diamorphine and/or midazolam may be needed for sensation of breathlessness and associated anxiety Clear explanation, appropriate reassurance
	Anxiety—common in breathlessness	Anxiolytic drugs, e.g. small doses of lorazepam orally/sublingually or midazolam subcutaneously may help
Constipation	There are many factors which make patients more likely to become constipated: immobility, weakness; general debility; poor oral intake; low dietary fibre; hypercalcaemia; hyperkalaemia Drugs, e.g. opioids and tricyclic antidepressants	Discuss nutritional options; encourage increased fluid intake; prescribe antiemetic where nausea contributes to poor intake Laxatives: ● Bulking agents—should be reserved for moderately active patients with good fluid intake who are not on opioid medication ● Osmotic laxatives—lactulose (may cause flatulence and abdominal cramp); magnesium salts (sometimes unpalatable) ● Stimulants—senna, bisacodyl, danthron ● Lubricants—docusate (mainly a softener), liquid paraffin Often necessary to combine softening and stimulant agents Suppositories (glycerol and/or bisacodyl) Enemas sometimes necessary
Confusion	Unfamiliar stimuli Drugs, e.g. opioids, anticonvulsants, tricyclics Metabolic causes, e.g. uraemia, hypercalcaemia, hyponatraemia Cerebral metastases Infection Anxiety Cerebral hypoxia	Explanation and calming reassurance to patient and family Adequate lighting; familiar objects; minimise moving of patient within hospital Investigation and treatment of any reversible causes Medication if necessary: distressed patient may respond to oral or parenteral benzodiazepines, e.g. diazepam 5 mg twice daily, or midazolam by continuous infusion; paranoid or hallucinating patients may require haloperidol orally or subcutaneously, up to 20 mg/24 h
Terminal restlessness (also known as terminal agitation/terminal anguish/terminal distress)	This is a diagnosis made by exclusion and can be distressing for the family	Explanation to family Rule out treatable causes: look for urinary retention; treat pain Sedation; often requires subcutaneous infusion, e.g. midazolam (benzodiazepine) 30–90 mg/24 h ± levomepromazine 12.5–150 mg/24 h
'Death rattle' (i.e. distressing sounds of retained secretions in terminal stage of illness)	Accumulation of bronchial secretions and loss of control of muscles of larynx and pharynx	Explanation to family—more distressing to them than to the patient Positioning of patient often reduces sound and respiratory effort Early and continued use of antisecretory agent, e.g. glycopyrronium subcutaneously in divided doses or continuous infusion up to 1.2 mg/24 h

- Neuropathic pain—caused by pressure or destruction of nerves. Often difficult to describe, this may be a clue to their aetiology. Sometimes words like 'tingling' or 'shooting' are used and pain is in the distribution of a nerve root or peripheral nerve. Such pains are usually only partially responsive to opioids and require the use of adjuvant analgesics such as tricyclic antidepressants (e.g. amitriptyline), anti-epileptics (e.g. gabapentin) or corticosteroids to reduce oedema around tumours
- Bone pain—caused by infiltration of cancer. Clinical features depend on the location, e.g. spinal lesions may cause pressure on the cord causing nerve pain, anaesthesia and weakness. Skull base lesions can lead to cranial nerve palsies

Bony metastases often lead to **incident pain** where pain is tolerable at rest but becomes much worse with movement. This is often difficult to treat and requires local radiotherapy plus bisphosphonate infusions (particularly in breast and prostate cancers and myeloma), together with analgesics. Incident pains are not usually responsive to opioids but adjuvants (mentioned above) may help. It is best to take medication before the activity known to lead to pain.

Principles of cancer pain management

- The aim is to control pain as well as possible, with a balance between analgesia and the side-effects of medication
- Analgesia should be given regularly not just 'as required'
- Analgesics should be titrated against the severity of pain using the three-step analgesic ladder developed by the World Health Organization (Fig. 13.2; see also Table 13.5)

Opioid analgesia

Morphine is generally the opioid of choice. Most patients' pain can be managed with oral morphine, the dose being titrated up or down according to analgesic requirements. Addiction is not a problem amongst cancer patients. If the

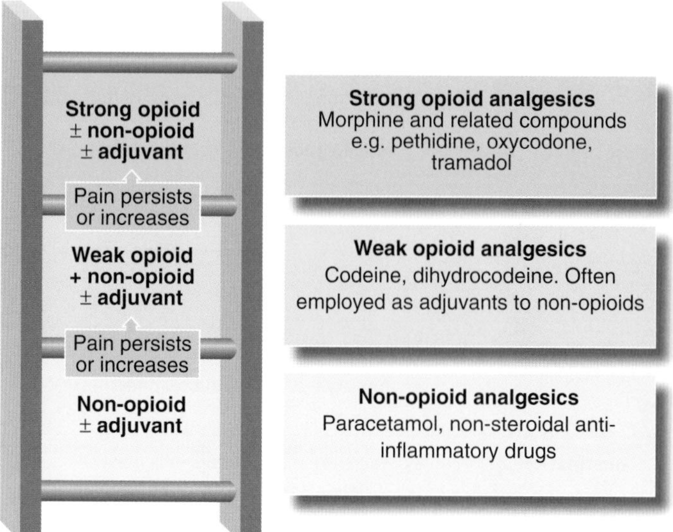

Fig. 13.2 Three-step analgesic ladder for cancer pain control (WHO 1986) (see Table 13.5 for adjuvants)
The World Health Organization has stated that pain relief should be:
(i) by the mouth—oral medication if possible
(ii) by the clock—regularly, not 'as required' (p.r.n.)
(iii) by the ladder—if, after reaching top dose on one rung of the ladder, pain is not controlled, go up the ladder

Table 13.5 Adjuvant analgesics and other treatments for management of cancer pain

Treatment method	Indications
Non-steroidal anti-inflammatory agents—via oral/rectal/transdermal routes	Reduce inflammatory component in pain. Have a role for bony and other musculoskeletal pains and may help neuropathic pains
Tricyclic antidepressants (usually as single evening dose)	Used in treatment of neuropathic pain. Also help patients to sleep. Can help mood as dose is increased
Anticonvulsants (e.g. gabapentin)	Valuable for neuropathic pain
Antispasmodics (e.g. hyoscine butylbromide—Buscopan)	Reduce visceral contractions in colicky visceral pain (intestinal, biliary, ureteric) and overt bowel obstruction
Muscle relaxants (e.g. diazepam)	Relieve muscle spasms
Antibiotics (e.g. metronidazole tablets or gel)	Help treat infected superficial lesions, e.g. ulcerated skin, breast or head and neck tumours (usually involve Gram-negative organisms)
Corticosteroids (e.g. dexamethasone 4–8 mg daily, prednisolone 30–60 mg daily) Dexamethasone causes less fluid retention	Shrink oedema associated with tumour to relieve pressure effects, e.g. cerebral tumours, spinal cord and peripheral nerve compression, liver capsule stretching, tumour swelling causing obstruction to bowel, biliary or urinary tracts
Topical anti-inflammatory agents	For oral and nasal mucositis, ulcerated skin lesions, radiation proctitis
Local palliative radiotherapy	For bone metastases, compressive lesions of brain and spinal cord, large airway and superior vena caval obstruction, fungating or bleeding superficial lesions

Table 13.5 **Continued**

Treatment method	Indications
Bisphosphonates (e.g. pamidronate, clodronate)	Predominantly used for the relief of bone pain in metastatic breast cancer, and multiple myeloma. Can be given parenterally as bolus or continuously as oral therapy
Radioactive isotope therapy	Used for the relief of bone pain due to metastatic disease
Palliative chemotherapy	Sometimes relieves pain by shrinkage of chemosensitive tumours
Nerve blocks (often under radiological guidance)	Very helpful in treating pain in specific areas, e.g. intercostal blocks for chest wall pain, coeliac plexus blocks for pancreatic and other 'foregut' pain. Often reduce the overall requirement for systemic analgesia
Physiotherapy and associated physical modalities (e.g. massage, TENS, hot or cold packs)	Muscle spasm, inflammatory component of pains. Massage for muscle spasms and lymphoedema. TENS may help neuropathic pain
Skeletal immobilisation	Elective internal fixation of long bones for incipient or actual pathological fracture of long bones

Table 13.6 **Opioid drugs used in palliative care**

Analgesic	Equi-analgesic dose of oral morphine	Duration of action	Indications
Codeine 60 mg	6 mg	4–6 hours	Codeine or dihydrocodeine alone or in combination with paracetamol are used to treat mild to moderate pain May cause nausea or constipation
Tramadol 50 mg	5 mg	6 hours	Its effect on monoamine reuptake means that theoretically it may be useful for neuropathic pain
Diamorphine injection 10 mg	20–30 mg	4 hours	Where local regulations permit, it is preferred to morphine if parenteral route required as high solubility means smaller injection volume. Side-effects as morphine
Fentanyl transdermal patch Lowest dose now 12 mg/hour	12 mg/hour equivalent to 30–60 mg of oral morphine in 24 hours	72 hours	Patch works by releasing depot drug into the skin. Takes 12 hours to reach analgesic levels so breakthrough treatment must be available when starting *Contraindicated* in unstable pain Often preferred to oral tablets by patients. Causes less constipation
Fentanyl lozenges Lowest dose 200 mg		1–4 hours	Can start to have its effect after 5– 10 minutes. May be useful for patients with incident pain who can take a lozenge before they want to move
Methadone 5 mg syrup	5–10 mg when given as single dose. Much more potent once drug has accumulated	4–5 hours single dose 6–12 hours after repeated doses	Used in specialist units; initial titration often complex owing to prolonged and variable half-life. Used in low dose, e.g. 2–5 mg nocte, for cough suppression
Oxycodone 5 mg—lowest strength capsule	10 mg	4–6 hours	May be better tolerated in some patients (e.g. elderly) as may cause fewer side-effects, particularly confusion or hallucinations. Should be used only as second-line to morphine

Note: there is no role for meptazinol or pethidine in the long-term treatment of cancer pain as they have limitations, e.g. analgesic ceiling, short duration of action or accumulation of toxic metabolites, which render them unsuitable for regular long-term use.

pain abates, for example after radiotherapy, it is easy to reduce and sometimes to stop morphine. Nevertheless, this should be done gradually. Tolerance and diminishing effectiveness of morphine is uncommon, even among patients who take the drug for months. If a patient on a stable dose requires an increase, this usually reflects disease progression.

Strong opioids are administered parenterally when patients cannot take oral medication because of dysphagia, nausea, vomiting or fatigue. The intravenous route can be used in hospital but the **subcutaneous route** is preferred at home. This route is suitable for single 'breakthrough' doses and for continuous infusion. Infusions are given via an indwelling 'butterfly' needle, usually controlled with a battery-operated syringe driver. In the UK, **diamorphine** is preferred to morphine because smaller volumes provide equi-analgesic doses.

Establishing treatment

The preferred method for establishing dosage is by **titration**. The usual starting dose will be 5–10 mg of immediate-release morphine 4-hourly (or 2.5–5 mg for elderly patients). For those with renal or liver impairment or in the very elderly, 6–8-hourly intervals may be required. In addition to the regular dose, the same dose should be prescribed on an 'as required' basis to treat pain which 'breaks through' before the next dose is due. If morphine relieves the pain, the next day's regular dose (and p.r.n. dose) is ⅙ of the total given over the previous 24 hours, or ½ for slow-release morphine.

Other opioids are used less commonly in palliative care and usually for specific indications. These are summarised in Table 13.6.

Principles of transplantation surgery

14

INTRODUCTION

Many patients face death because a single organ system such as kidney, liver, lungs or heart is failing, but could return to health if organ function could be restored. It is not surprising that physicians have tried over the years to achieve this by transplanting a healthy organ from an animal or another human.

The scene for clinical organ transplantation was set early in the 20th century by Alexis Carrel. He was awarded the Nobel Prize for Physiology and Medicine in 1912 for his pioneering work in vascular surgery and transplantation with Charles Guthrie. Carrel, working with laboratory animals, found that **autografts** (organs removed and reimplanted into the same animal) could be expected to function indefinitely, whereas **allografts** (organs transplanted between animals of the same species) rarely functioned for more than a few days. Early attempts at transplantation in man used **xenografts** (transplantation between different species) to transfer renal tissue from pigs, goats, rabbits and apes; these were uniformly unsuccessful.

The key to organ transplantation lay in the developing field of immunology, first with detection of the mechanisms involved in **graft rejection** and then the elaboration and application of techniques to minimise or prevent it. The first clinically useful transplant for humans involved pig heart valves. These consisted of simple avascular tissue, treated to render it non-immunogenic to avoid rejection. Porcine cardiac valve transplants have been used regularly since the mid 1970s and have advantages over artificial valves in younger people and where anticoagulation must be avoided.

Chemical immunosuppression designed to attenuate graft rejection has continued to advance, leading to improving success rates with transplantation of an expanding range of organs and tissues (see Table 14.1). Human cornea, kidney, liver, pancreas, heart, heart and lung, single or double lung and bone marrow transplantation are all now standard, although not free of rejection or other complications (see: http://www.ctstransplant.org/). Even face transplants are now achieving success.

Promising results are latterly being achieved with small bowel transplantation, in isolation or together with other intra-abdominal organs such as stomach, duodenum, pancreas and liver in **multivisceral transplants**. The ultimate goal of transplant surgeons and immunologists is to generate a state of **tolerance** between graft and the recipient of a transplanted organ.

Organ transplantation already offers improved quality of life to renal transplant recipients and endows life itself to recipients of heart, lung or liver grafts. This surgery is impossible without the generosity of donors and bereaved families in making organs available for transplantation. However, the UK donation rate of 13 donors per million population per year still lags behind the rate of 25–35 per million achieved in comparable European countries such as Belgium, Spain and France. This suggests that many more patients could benefit if the acceptability to the UK community of these innovative procedures could be enhanced. To achieve this, the results of surgery and the ethical basis under which it is conducted need to be promoted more widely.

TRANSPLANT IMMUNOLOGY

MAJOR HISTOCOMPATIBILITY COMPLEX

When transplanted from one individual to another, tissue cells have a number of different surface **glycoproteins** known as **histocompatibility antigens** that are recognised by the recipient's immune system and excite a response. The response involves cell-mediated and humoral mechanisms which cause destruction of the transplanted cells.

Each individual has several histocompatibility antigens, but one group is predominantly responsible for major graft

Table 14.1 Summary of the main immunosuppressive agents used in transplantation

Class of drug	Examples	Mechanism of action	Uses: Induction	Uses: Maintenance	Uses: Rejection	Adverse effects and comments
Biological agents						
Non-depleting antibodies	Basiliximab	Inhibition of IL2-induced T cell activation (mAb)	√			Hypersensitivity and adverse effects are rare
Depleting antibodies	Alemtuzumab (Campath-1H)	Prolonged depletion of B and T lymphocytes (mAb)	√			Cause moderate cytokine release syndrome
	ATG (anti-thymocyte globulin)	Prolonged depletion of T lymphocytes (polyclonal Ab)	√		√	Cytokine release syndrome common
	Rituximab	Depletion of B lymphocytes (mAb)	√		√	Not formally licensed for use in transplantation
Non-biological drugs						
Calcineurin inhibitors (CNIs)	Ciclosporin	Inhibition of calcineurin phosphatase and T cell activation		√		Nephrotoxicity is a significant adverse effect
	Tacrolimus			√		
mTOR* inhibitors	Sirolimus (rapamycin)	Inhibits IL2-induced T cell proliferation		√		Cause impaired wound healing, pneumonitis
Antimetabolites	Mycophenolate mofetil (MMF)	Suppression of B and T cell proliferation		√		Myelotoxicity (pancytopenia) and GI disturbance common
	Azathioprine	Inhibition of DNA synthesis in lymphocytes		√		Generally well tolerated
Corticosteroids	Prednisolone (p.o.)	Suppression of cytokine production, T cell activation and migration		√		Cause the full spectrum of Cushing's syndrome adverse effects
	Methylprednisolone (i.v.)		√		√	

* mTOR: mammalian target of rapamycin; mAb: monoclonal antibody

rejection. These **major histocompatibility antigens** are coded for by a set of genes known as the **major histocompatibility complex (MHC)**. In humans, the MHC gene is located on a segment of the short arm of chromosome 6. It was first discovered in leucocytes and, although now shown to be present in all cells, it is still known as the **human leucocyte antigen (HLA) complex**. Within the human MHC, two major groups of antigens, known as HLA class I and class II, have been described, each with different structures and specificities. The principal class I loci are the **A and B antigens** and the principal class II loci are the **DR antigens**. Since each individual receives one set of genetic information from each parent, there are six principal loci (two each for A, B and DR) and any two individuals can differ at any or all of these loci. Certain HLA types are also associated with particular autoimmune disorders, notably ankylosing spondylitis and coeliac disease, although the reason is unknown.

TISSUE TYPING AND TRANSPLANT SHARING SCHEMES

Methods for determining donor and recipient HLA haplotypes ('HLA typing') are either based on detecting genetic variation in the expressed HLA molecules using antisera (serological typing), or now almost universally, at DNA sequence level (DNA typing). In kidney transplantation, close HLA matching gives significantly better graft survival, i.e. when donor and recipient are identical at all six loci or differ by only one A or B antigen. HLA typing of individuals is therefore used to match the donor and recipient as closely as possible in kidney (and pancreas) transplantation. HLA matching is not currently regularly performed for other organs such as heart or liver transplants, as the number of available organs is too small to allow optimal matching. However, even a fully HLA matched transplant evokes a profound immunological response from the recipient because of differences in other major (non-A, non-B and non-DR) and minor histocompatibility antigens.

Most developed countries have a national transplant sharing mechanism so that donors and recipients can be matched as closely and fairly as possible. Systems are designed to achieve an optimal balance between **utility** (the optimum use of an organ in terms of graft survival) and **equity** of access (the chance that an individual patient will receive a graft within a reasonable period). This typically combines the important matter of tissue matching with other factors such as age and time spent on the waiting list.

ABO blood group compatibility is an obvious prerequisite for organ transplantation which must not be overlooked in the search for ever closer HLA matching.

IMMUNOSUPPRESSION

With any major organ transplant, the recipient's immune response must be suppressed, even with full HLA compatibility, so rejection and graft loss can be minimised. Immunosuppressive therapy needs to be continued indefinitely, although dosage can usually be progressively reduced to maintenance levels after high-dose **induction therapy**. This is because a partly tolerant state is established by diminution of the **alloimmune** response with time. Episodes of **rejection** are often treated with strong or high-dose immunosuppression.

Immunosuppressant drugs are broadly classified into biological (monoclonal or polyclonal antibodies) and non-biological agents; the characteristics of the main examples are summarized in Table 14.1. Immunosuppressive drugs are almost always employed in combination to allow lower doses of individual agents to minimise side-effects. These include infections, impaired wound healing, predisposition to certain malignancies (e.g., skin and Epstein–Barr virus-related lymphoproliferative disorders) and bone marrow suppression. A widely used combination is induction with basiliximab, followed by maintenance on **prednisolone**, **tacrolimus** and **MMF**.

Graft rejection

Graft rejection continues to be a problem despite the increasing range of immunosuppressive agents. It can present in several ways:

Hyperacute rejection

Hyperacute rejection is due to the presence of pre-formed antibodies (e.g. against ABO antigen) in the recipient. It occurs within minutes of reperfusion and is now exceedingly rare owing to improvements in cross-matching techniques.

Acute rejection

Acute rejection occurs in up to 30% of transplants, most commonly during the first 3 months post-transplant. It is predominantly T cell-mediated but can be antibody-mediated in about 10%. It can usually be reversed by a temporary increase in immunosuppression, most often in the form of a short course of high-dose corticosteroids.

Chronic rejection

Chronic rejection occurs months to years after transplantation and is probably the result of antibody-mediated rejection. It is often associated with gradual occlusion of arteries in the graft and can occur even with effective long-term immunosuppression.

PRACTICAL PROBLEMS OF TRANSPLANTATION

SOURCES OF ORGANS FOR TRANSPLANTATION

Organs for transplantation may be procured from living or deceased donors. Deceased donation in the UK can proceed after 'brain death' (donation after brain death—DBD or 'heart-beating') or after 'circulatory death' (donation after circulatory death—DCD or 'non-heart-beating'). Whilst the number of organ transplants from living donors (LD) and DCD donors has increased in the UK over recent years, there has been a slow decline in DBD donors. Consent for deceased organ donation can be given by the donor during his/her lifetime by registration with the Organ Donor Register, or by the donor's next of kin immediately before death (in the case of a DCD donor) or after the diagnosis of brainstem death (DBD donor).

'BRAIN DEATH'

In many countries, criteria have been established for a legal definition of brain death following irreversible brainstem injury (e.g. from head injury or intracranial vascular catastrophe), even in the presence of an intact circulatory system. Once the established criteria have been satisfied and appropriate consent obtained from relatives, the subject becomes eligible for DBD donation and the organ retrieval operation can proceed with the donor ventilated and the organs perfused with oxygenated blood. If brainstem death has not occurred or cannot be confirmed, ventilatory and circulatory support is withdrawn and organ retrieval can only proceed after circulatory arrest and death confirmed by irreversible cessation of neurological (pupillary), cardiac and respiratory activity (DCD donation). These are donor patients with a hopeless prognosis and treatment is withdrawn in an intensive care setting.

The legal criteria for brain death in the UK are summarised in Box 14.1; similar criteria are used in other countries. In the UK, the diagnosis of brain death is made on purely clinical criteria; electrocardiography, cerebral blood flow and other neurophysiological tests are not required. Appropriate clinical examination must be performed by two senior doctors independent of the transplant team and must be repeated at least twice.

Box 14.1 Legal criteria for diagnosis of brain death (UK)

Note: this diagnosis is clinical and does not require special tests

1. There must be a positive diagnosis of severe structural brain damage
2. The condition causing brain damage must be irreversible
3. There must be complete loss of brainstem function—evidenced by fixed pupils, no spontaneous eye movements or response to caloric testing, absent corneal, eyelash and blink reflexes, absent laryngeal and cough reflexes, and no response to deep painful stimuli (*Note*: some spinal reflexes may be retained despite brain death)
4. On removal of ventilatory support, there must be no spontaneous respiratory activity in the presence of a physiologically adequate increase in PCO_2
5. Any possible effects of hypothermia and drugs (e.g. muscle relaxants, respiratory depressants, alcohol) must be excluded

LIVING DONATION

UK law permits kidney transplants from living genetically or emotionally related as well as from altruistic donors. This can only proceed after comprehensive medical and psychological assessment of the donor. Living donor nephrectomy can be performed laparoscopically or through an open (usually retroperitoneal) surgical approach. Laparoscopic nephrectomy results in less wound pain, shorter hospital stay and shorter rehabilitation for the donor. The advantages of living donor transplantation include elective not emergency procedures, better long-term graft outcomes, lower delayed graft function rates, and potentially, pre-emptive (pre-dialysis) transplantation. Living kidney donation has a mortality risk of 1:3000 and a major and minor complication rate of approximately 2% and 20% respectively in the donor.

Living livers donation is also becoming more common. It was introduced to allow donation of a small portion of the left liver from parent to child, but has now expanded to include right liver donation, and allows adult to adult transplantation. The donor risks are greater than in kidney donation. In countries where the availability of cadaveric organs is limited for cultural reasons, such as Japan, these procedures are the mainstay of organ transplantation. The growing shortage of organs for transplantation has led to this being adopted even in countries where cadaveric liver transplantation is well established.

ORGAN PRESERVATION AND TRANSPORT

Donors are often in hospitals many miles from where the recipient operation is to be performed. There may be delay in locating the recipient, and in getting the recipient into hospital and ready for operation. As a result, the organ to be transplanted is usually removed from the donor several hours before transplantation, driving the search for reliable techniques of organ preservation. **Hypothermia** (at 0–4 °C) is the main method of organ preservation by reducing the metabolic demands of the organ. Organs are first flushed with and then stored in preservation solutions which usually have the following components:

- An osmotic agent to provide extracellular oncotic force to prevent cellular oedema
- A buffer to counter intracellular acidosis
- Electrolytes to maintain cellular ionic composition

After retrieval, the bag containing the organ and preservation fluid is usually packed in ice (**static cold storage**) while awaiting transplantation. Alternatively, kidneys may be connected to a machine to continuously circulate cold preservation solution (**machine perfusion**). Machine perfusion is more expensive and cumbersome than static cold storage; its potential advantages include a more physiological environment and the ability to identify and discard non-functioning kidneys with poor perfusion characteristics.

The period of **warm ischaemia** is the time from circulatory arrest to effective cooling of the organ. Warm ischaemia must be minimised to prevent irreversible damage to the organ (less than 40–60 min in kidney transplantation). The period of **cold ischaemia** is from perfusion with cold preservation solution to transplantation. Cold ischaemia time should also be minimized to best preserve graft function and ideally should be less than 24, 12 and 6 hours for kidney, liver and heart transplantation respectively.

SPECIFIC ORGAN TRANSPLANTS

KIDNEY TRANSPLANTS

Kidney transplantation is the longest established and most widely practised of solid organ transplants. It offers a substantial improvement in quality of life for patients with end-stage chronic renal failure who are otherwise faced with twice- or thrice-weekly haemodialysis or a regimen of daily treatment with chronic ambulatory peritoneal dialysis. Donor organs can be obtained from any generally healthy donor up to 70 years of age or even older in certain cases.

The kidney is transplanted into an extraperitoneal location in the iliac fossa and the renal vessels anastomosed to the iliac artery and vein (see Fig. 14.1). The ureter is implanted into the bladder using an intramural tunnel to prevent reflux. Non-functioning kidneys are usually left in situ unless infected or causing unmanageable hypertension.

The signs of **early acute rejection** of the kidney are oliguria, proteinuria, and pain and tenderness of the transplanted kidney. Luckily, this relatively common form of rejection can be usually be reversed easily. Overall results have steadily

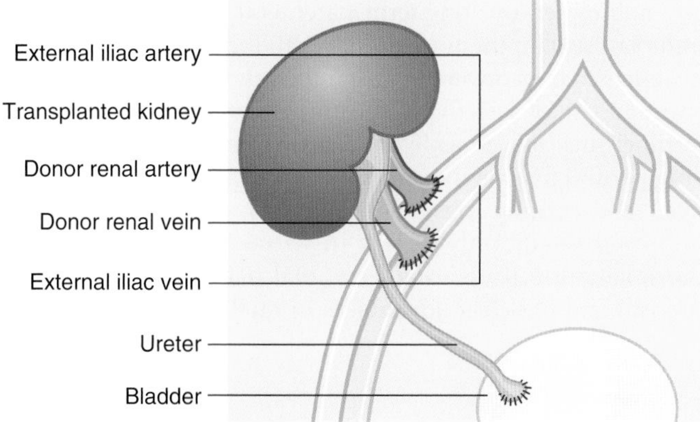

Fig. 14.1 Renal transplantation
The usual site for the transplanted kidney is in the pelvis, with anastomoses being constructed between the donor renal artery and vein, and the recipient iliac artery and vein, and between donor ureter and recipient bladder

improved owing to better tissue matching, more effective and safer immunosuppression, superior organ procurement and preservation, as well as improved surgical technique and peri-operative care of recipients. The survival rate of transplanted kidneys can be as high as 90–95% at 1 year and falls to about 50% at 10 years.

LIVER TRANSPLANTS

Current indications for liver transplantation in adults are end-stage non-malignant parenchymal liver disease (e.g. cirrhosis due to viral hepatitis or alcohol), acute hepatic failure, certain inborn errors of hepatic metabolism and hepatocellular carcinoma (within specific criteria). In children, liver-based inborn errors of metabolism and biliary atresia are the most common indications; the operation often needs to be performed during early infancy.

Rejection in liver transplantation is less of a problem than in kidney transplantation but the operation is more challenging. Most patients have advanced liver disease with disordered coagulation and often severe portal hypertension. A team approach has evolved, with close cooperation between surgeons and specialist anaesthetists. The diseased liver is removed and the new liver placed orthotopically, with vena cava, portal vein and hepatic artery being re-anastomosed in turn. Biliary reconstruction can be performed using a direct duct-to-duct anastomosis or a Roux-en-Y loop. Results have improved greatly since the first liver transplant in 1963 and 1-year patient survival rates of 85–90% and 5-year survival of 70–75% are now standard. For paediatric cases, the problem of an insufficient supply of donor organs has been solved with reduced-size liver grafts. An adult liver can be divided into two to allow a child and an adult to receive grafts from a single organ. The late graft attrition rate appears to be much lower than for kidney grafts even though matching is by blood group without tissue typing. Biliary complications (e.g. strictures) and disease recurrence, particularly when transplantation is for hepatitis C, are important remaining challenges.

PANCREAS TRANSPLANTS

Pancreas transplantation offers the tantalising hope of a cure for diabetes, thus avoiding its many late complications. These include myocardial ischaemia, peripheral vascular disease, peripheral neuropathy, nephropathy leading to renal failure and retinopathy leading to blindness. The pancreas presents particular problems, as the gland combines endocrine and exocrine function. The currently favoured technique involves transplanting the whole pancreas with a small segment of duodenum. The graft is sited in the pelvis and its vessels are anastomosed to the iliac vessels as in a kidney graft. In an early technique, the attached duodenal segment was anastomosed to the bladder, allowing exocrine secretions to drain into the urine. This has been largely replaced by anastomosing the pancreas directly to small bowel or via a Roux-en-Y loop to allow enteric drainage of enzymes. Graft survival rates of 70–80% are now being obtained and there is increasing evidence that the procedure can arrest and sometimes partly reverse the long-term complications of diabetes. Most pancreatic transplants currently performed are in diabetic patients with renal failure and advanced complications of their disease. In these, the pancreatic transplant is performed together with a renal transplant (simultaneous pancreas and kidney transplant—SPK).

A different approach is transplanting pancreatic endocrine tissue alone using **human islet cells** extracted from pancreases by collagenase digestion. The islets are injected into the portal venous system and lodge in liver sinusoids. The extraction yield has improved markedly, allowing a substantial proportion of islets to be recovered from each pancreas. Whilst the success rate is improving, it requires islet cells from more than one donor to achieve euglycaemia, so the procedure is less efficacious than whole pancreas transplantation while organ donors remain scarce.

HEART AND LUNG TRANSPLANTS

Cardiac transplantation has become a standard treatment for patients with ischaemic heart disease not amenable to coronary artery bypass grafting, and for patients with certain cardiomyopathies. A standard operative technique employs **orthotopic** placement, i.e. replacing the diseased organ in the same anatomical location. The donor atria and vessels are sutured directly to those of the recipient. Monitoring for early rejection requires regular right-heart catheterisation and endomyocardial biopsy.

Using immunosuppressive protocols similar to kidney transplantation, results of cardiac transplantation are now excellent, although the shortage of donor organs means cardiac transplantation is unlikely ever to be an option for all those who could benefit.

Combined heart and lung transplants are now accepted as a standard treatment for certain irreversible lung diseases such as cystic fibrosis, and good results are now obtained in specialist centres. Many cases have secondary heart disease and require a combined heart–lung transplant. In other cases the recipient's heart is healthy and can be transplanted into another patient; this is known as the **domino heart** procedure.

Single or even double lung transplants are now also performed successfully in carefully selected patients with chronic respiratory failure.

SMALL BOWEL TRANSPLANTS

Small bowel transplantation is a relatively recent advance. There is a growing number of patients who have lost all or most of their small bowel from vascular problems, volvulus, necrotising enterocolitis, atresias or Crohn's disease, and who are maintained on long-term parenteral nutrition. Specialist units can sustain them in good health for years but treatment is expensive, inconvenient for patients and leaves them at constant risk of infective and thrombotic complications from feeding lines as well as liver disease from parenteral feeding. Small bowel may be transplanted alone or combined with the liver in coexisting irreversible liver disease. Outcomes have improved significantly so that in selected cases, small bowel transplantation rivals long-term total parenteral nutrition in survival and has clear advantages in quality of life.

Principles of accident surgery

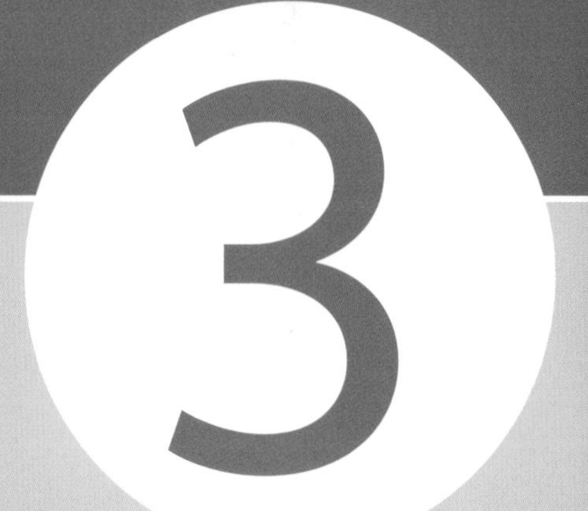

Major trauma

15

INTRODUCTION

Major trauma is a relatively rare event in the UK but much more common in other parts of the world, some with higher rates of road traffic collisions (e.g. Saudi Arabia) and others higher levels of personal violence (e.g. South Africa, parts of the USA). Nevertheless, major trauma is the most common cause of death in young people almost everywhere.

For victims who survive the immediate trauma, there are two periods with a particularly high risk of death. The first occurs during the first or 'golden' hour after the accident and the second over the next few hours. Survival in the golden hour depends on the severity of injury, the competence of immediate care and the speed of transfer to an accident unit (in the UK, the average time to transport a non-trapped trauma victim to hospital is a surprising 57 minutes). Deaths after the first hour are for the most part avoidable, being largely caused by treatable conditions.

PRE-HOSPITAL ASSESSMENT AND INTERVENTION

INTRODUCTION

The golden hour concept comes from US war experience, popularised by Dr R. Adams Cowley. More recently, following the conflict in Afghanistan, this has been expanded to include the 'platinum 10 minutes' during which immediate interventions, particularly in haemorrhage control, may be key determinants of patient survival. Injuries with substantial internal or external bleeding lead to rapid circulatory decompensation; the only effective treatment is expert shock management and surgical arrest of bleeding. Thus, shortening the interval between injury and treatment gives the best chance of survival. The key is rapid essential care at the scene and swift transport to a trauma centre. This strategy is known as **scoop and run**, as opposed to **stay and play,** which is best for less severe cases; in these, the risk of physiological derangement caused during transport may be greater than extending the period before hospital treatment.

ASSESSMENT AT THE SCENE OF A ROAD TRAFFIC COLLISION

'Reading the wreckage' used to foretell patterns and severity of injury to passengers. However, modern cars have sophisticated crumple zones and major vehicle distortion may not cause severe injury, though severe injuries can occur with minor damage. The worst injuries tend to occur in head-on collisions or those affecting the front corners. Some estimate can also be made of whether there was a high- or low-velocity impact. If passengers were killed or thrown out, this indicates a high-velocity impact. Points to check include whether head restraints were in place, whether seatbelts were worn and whether airbags were deployed. For motorcycle crashes, it is best to assume that all victims have pelvic fractures until proved otherwise. When a pedestrian is hit by a car, a 'bullseye' fracture of the windscreen indicates a likely severe head injury.

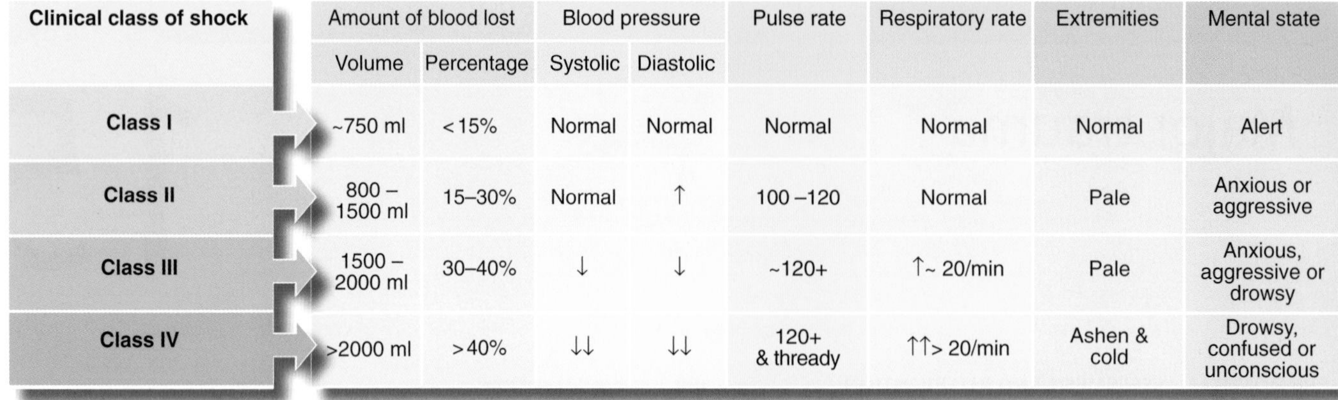

Clinical class of shock	Amount of blood lost		Blood pressure		Pulse rate	Respiratory rate	Extremities	Mental state
	Volume	Percentage	Systolic	Diastolic				
Class I	~750 ml	< 15%	Normal	Normal	Normal	Normal	Normal	Alert
Class II	800 – 1500 ml	15–30%	Normal	↑	100 –120	Normal	Pale	Anxious or aggressive
Class III	1500 – 2000 ml	30–40%	↓	↓	~120+	↑~ 20/min	Pale	Anxious, aggressive or drowsy
Class IV	>2000 ml	> 40%	↓↓	↓↓	120+ & thready	↑↑> 20/min	Ashen & cold	Drowsy, confused or unconscious

Fig. 15.1 Clinical classification of hypovolaemic shock related to probable blood loss

Obvious injuries (e.g. traumatic amputations) are sought in the victims and their level of consciousness and mobility assessed. Trapped wounded need special treatment as they often have long extrication times and need analgesia, intravenous fluids and perhaps sedation to aid release. Trapped patients can quickly become hypothermic and hypovolaemic (see Fig. 15.1).

PREVENTING SECONDARY INJURIES AND DAMAGE

Primary injuries result directly from the trauma. Secondary injuries are an indirect result, e.g. secondary brain damage from hypoxia, fat embolism from fractures, spinal cord damage due to unstable spinal injury. Most are preventable with good immediate care, careful handling, rapid resuscitation and perhaps elective ventilation. Early stabilisation of long bone fractures aids haemodynamic stability, allowing assessment of less urgent head, chest or abdominal injuries.

PRE-HOSPITAL CARE

The guiding principle for the emergency field team is rapid transfer to an appropriate hospital; pre-hospital interventions are limited to essentials. A need for endotracheal intubation is the main intervention to delay transportation but occasionally anaesthetising the patient buys time before direct transfer to a specialised unit.

Airway and breathing

The airway must be assessed and secured first, whilst ensuring the **cervical spine** is immobilised. If the patient can speak, assume the airway is patent, ventilation is intact and the brain adequately perfused. Agitation, however, may be a sign of hypoxia. In an unconscious or semi-conscious patient, the airway can usually be temporarily secured with a jaw thrust. If tolerated, the patient should then have two nasopharyngeal airways and a Guedel oropharyngeal airway placed to maintain airway patency. **Endotracheal intubation** is needed if there is inability to maintain or protect the airway or to provide adequate ventilation (Box 15.1). If this proves unattainable, a useful rescue technique is to insert a laryngeal mask (LMA), as used in general anaesthesia; this may avoid the need for a surgical airway. As a last resort, an airway can be achieved using a needle or surgical **cricothyroidotomy**. In all seriously injured patients, high-flow oxygen therapy (15 L/min) is mandatory.

Box 15.1 Indications for immediate intubation and ventilation following a head injury or multiple injuries

1. Glasgow Coma score <8 or falling score (see p. 219, Table 16.1)
2. Inability to maintain airway
3. Facial trauma or bleeding into the airway
4. Spontaneous hyperventilation causing hypocapnia
5. Inadequate ventilation causing hypoxia and/or hypercapnia
6. Seizures
7. Extreme agitation

Spine

In an unconscious patient after a high-impact collision, a cervical spine fracture should be assumed until disproved. If the patient has multiple injuries, the entire spine must be protected from secondary injury during transfer and assessment. After intubation (if needed), the spine is immobilised in a neutral position on a long spinal board. This requires a semi-rigid cervical collar, side head supports and strapping as a minimum (see Fig. 15.2).

Circulation

Two large-bore intravenous cannulas should be inserted. Initial fluid resuscitation should be based upon injuries

(a)

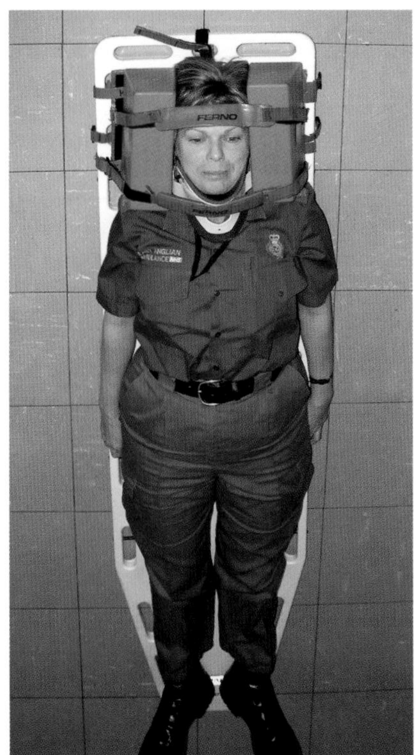

(b)

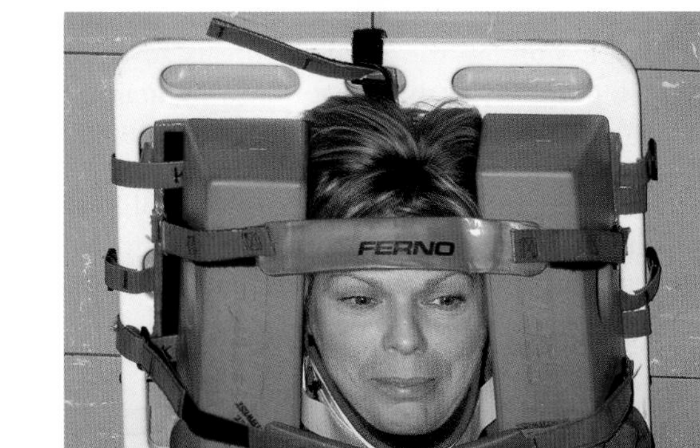

Fig. 15.2 Spine immobilised in a neutral position on a long spinal board

sustained and physiological parameters. More recent studies indicate that **permissive hypotension** is often a better strategy than the previous recommendation of rapid indiscriminate crystalloid infusion. If organ perfusion can be maintained, there are advantages in keeping the pressure low in trauma patients. Physiological compensation is effective at systolic pressures between 70 and 85 mmHg, and cerebral perfusion and urinary output are well maintained. Above this pressure, fresh clot is often dislodged (**'pop a clot'**) and then bleeding recurs. A further disadvantage of unnecessary fluid resuscitation is that infusing just 750 ml of crystalloid activates cytokines and causes dilutional coagulopathy.

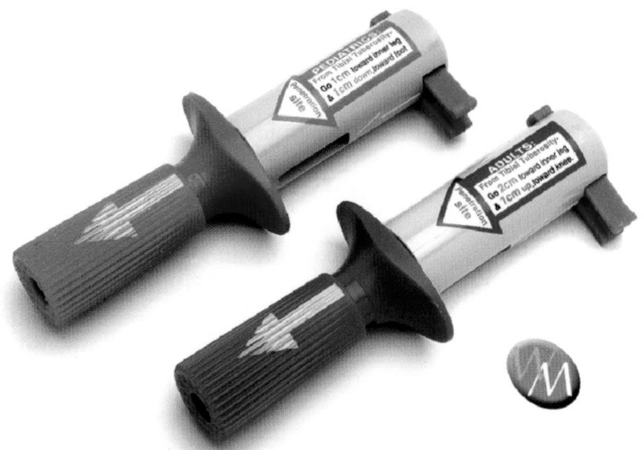

Fig. 15.3 Bone injection gun Photographs courtesy of WaisMed Ltd.

If a patient is **unconscious** without a palpable radial or pedal pulse, 250–500 ml of fluid is given immediately, followed by small boluses, repeated only until the point at which a pulse returns. This is **titration by pulse** and has been successfully employed in major trauma and in military campaigns. If intravenous access is unsuccessful, EZ-IO devices (Fig 15.3) are a quick way of inserting a cannula into bone marrow. Procoagulant agents such as tranexamic acid and activated factor VII are increasingly being used early to reduce blood loss following trauma. If a patient is conscious and orientated or **unconscious** but has a palpable radial pulse, this indicates a systolic of above 90 mmHg and fluid resuscitation is not started.

Wounds

These should be covered with dressings to prevent contamination, or pressure dressings and haemostatic agents (e.g. Celox gauze, a procoagulant derived from crushed shellfish) for bleeding wounds.

Fractured limbs

These should be realigned and splinted. This helps minimise blood loss, aids pain control and may help peripheral perfusion.

TRANSPORT TO HOSPITAL

Injured patients need to be transferred rapidly to an appropriate hospital. Most go by ambulance, but transfer by helicopter can be quicker if the severity of injuries requires a major trauma centre. Note that whilst helicopters can cover great distances quickly, they have inherent disadvantages, namely the risk of secondary injury or displacement of lines or tubes during loading, restricted space for ongoing resuscitation and the risk of pneumothorax associated with changes in altitude.

PRELIMINARY HOSPITAL MANAGEMENT OF MULTIPLE AND SERIOUS INJURIES

ORGANISATION OF THE ACCIDENT DEPARTMENT

Every accident department should have a major disaster plan (Box 15.2). For any major trauma, the field team or ambulance service informs the receiving trauma unit about the impending arrival of seriously injured patients, plus an estimate of numbers and the nature and severity of injuries. This alerts the surgical and anaesthetic teams to be ready when the patients arrive (Box 15.3). Trauma units have a **resuscitation room** (see Fig. 15.4) with all necessary equipment so infusion sets can be prepared and drugs laid out.

Box 15.2 Major disaster planning

Major disaster plan—receiving hospitals need a detailed (and rehearsed) plan for disasters with many casualties (e.g. train or air crashes). Action cards given to nominated staff summarise this when a major disaster is declared.

The plan defines precisely:

- How to recognise a major disaster and how to initiate the process
- The person responsible for each main function (e.g. medical coordinator, field triage officer) and how to contact them
- Their precise duties
- Responsibilities and actions of all other team members

Box 15.3 Major trauma team

Members of a major trauma team

- Team leader
- Senior emergency department doctor
- General surgeons—senior and junior
- Orthopaedic surgeons—senior and junior
- Anaesthetists—senior and junior
- Other specialist surgeons, e.g. cardiothoracic, neurosurgical as needed
- Senior nurses

(*Note*: one junior doctor needs to be 'scribe' to document injuries and sequence of events)

Departments to be notified of impending major trauma incident

- Radiology—on-call radiologist and radiographer
- Blood bank, haematology, biochemistry
- ITU
- Operating department
- Mortuary (in major disasters)

Triage is the process of sorting patients into 'priority of treatment' groups on arrival to enable efficient use of resources. The usual categories are shown in Table 15.1.

Success in managing patients with life-threatening multiple injuries depends on good organisation. It involves concurrent activity between several professionals but with one person, often the surgeon, designated **team leader**. The team leader takes overall medical responsibility as well as coordinating all clinicians.

INITIAL CARE IN THE ACCIDENT DEPARTMENT

When seriously injured patients reach the resuscitation room, the golden hour peak of deaths has passed. The main danger of death is from **hypovolaemia** (intrathoracic or intraperitoneal haemorrhage, blood loss from fractures) or from an expanding **intracranial haematoma**.

Immediate priorities after reaching hospital are:

- Rapid primary assessment combined with resuscitation
- Detailed secondary survey for all injuries
- Prioritisation and treatment of individual injuries

Training has been standardised through **Advanced Trauma Life Support** (ATLS) courses, originally from the American College of Surgeons and now run in many countries. ATLS principles are simple—the greatest threats to life must be treated first. Mortality at this stage following major trauma is now recognised as associated with three key pathophysiological changes termed the 'lethal triad' and comprising coagulopathy, hypothermia and acidosis. Damage control resuscitation has emerged as a means of directly minimising these changes, the key components of which are outlined in Box 15.4.

Assessment of the seriously injured patient

Despite the urgency, primary assessment must be performed systematically as soon as the patient arrives. The **primary survey** includes a rapid evaluation, resuscitation and crucial life-preserving treatment. Priorities are summarised in Figure 15.5. Meanwhile, regular monitoring takes place (Box 15.5).

A rapid history is taken whenever practicable, often alongside the secondary survey. A useful mnemonic for this is **AMPLE**:

Allergies
Medicines and drugs
Past medical history

Table 15.1 Triage priority groups

Category	Definition	Colour	Treatment
P1	Life-threatening	Red	Immediate
P2	Urgent	Yellow	Urgent
P3	Minor	Green	Delayed
P4	Dead	White	

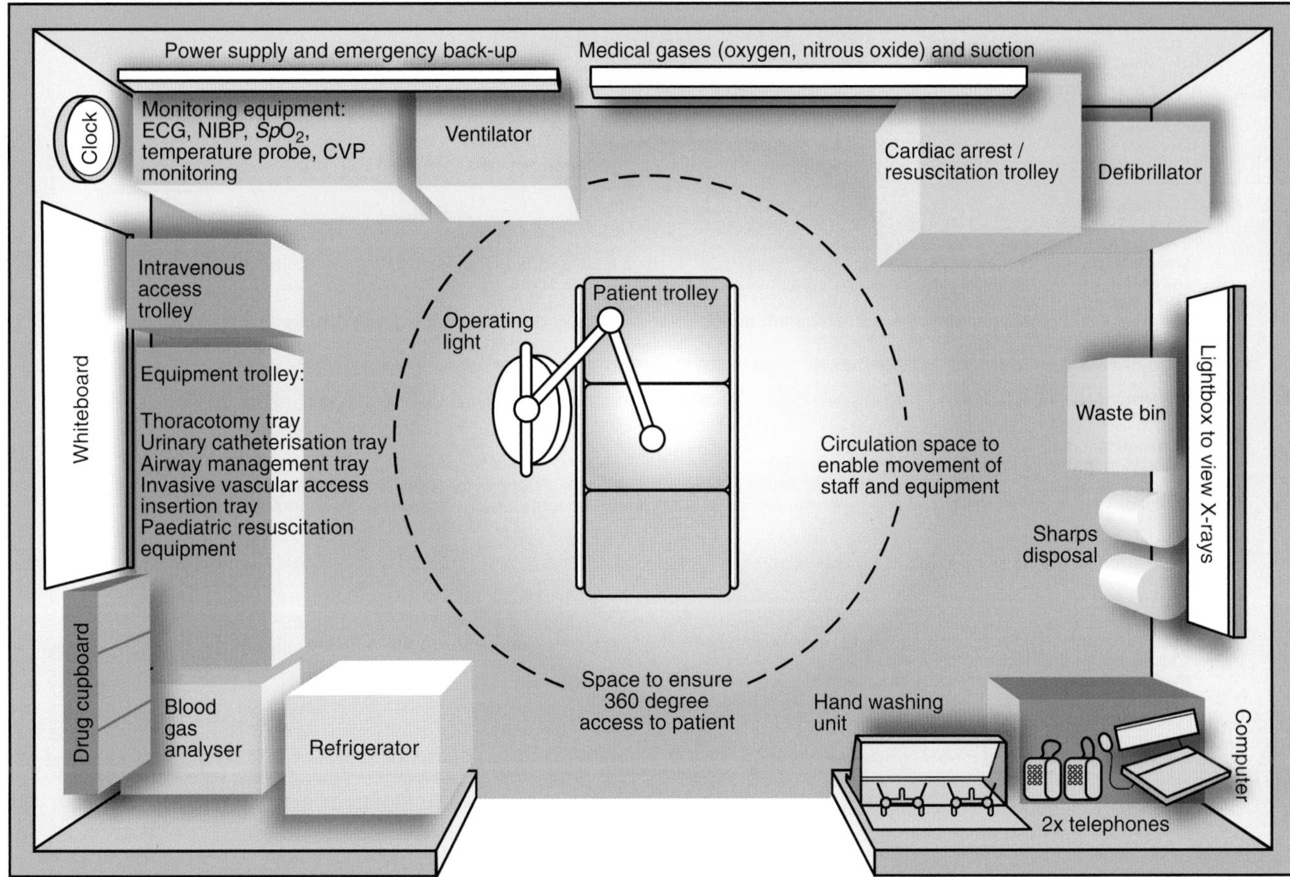

Fig. 15.4 'Bird's eye view' drawing of an ideal resuscitation room

Box 15.4 Damage control resuscitation

- Permissive hypotension
- Early administration of blood products including FFP and platelets
- Close monitoring of coagulopathy/thromboelastography
- Patient warming (bear hugger, forced air blanket, warming mattress)
- Warm fluids (level 1 infuser)
- Early haemostasis; 'turning off the tap' (haemostatic dressing, tranexamic acid, activated factor VII)
- Interventional radiology (covered stents, coil embolisation)
- Damage control surgery

Last meal (including alcohol)
Events leading to accident

Other elements of history come from the field team's notes and include:

- Time of incident
- Conscious level of patient when discovered and later changes

Box 15.5 Monitoring the multiply injured patient

- Glasgow Coma score (see Table 16.1)
- Pulse rate, blood pressure, electrocardiogram (ECG)
- Respiratory rate
- Hourly urine output
- Oxygen saturation by pulse oximetry; blood gases
- Nasogastric aspiration

- Details of drugs, fluids and other treatments administered at scene

Conscious patients with suspected cervical spine injuries should be moved with extreme caution and no passive movements attempted. The patient should perform active movements; spasm or pain restricts movement in significant injury. To examine the back and perform a rectal examination, the patient should be 'log-rolled' by several people.

A **secondary survey** then assesses the potential for life-threatening problems or complications, although urgent initial treatment may delay this. The key clinical features are

1. PRIMARY SURVEY (ABCDE)

A. AIRWAY AND CERVICAL SPINE — is the airway obstructed?

Cervical spine

Cervical spine injury must be assumed in any seriously injured patient

Immobilisation: semi-rigid collar + sandbags or lateral head supports + strapping tape (see Fig.15.2)

Airway management

1. **Airway positioning:** head tilt + chin lift or jaw thrust ± look inside oropharynx if possible for foreign body (teeth, dentures) or other obstruction. Suction if blood/vomitus/secretions.
2. **Oropharyngeal/nasal airways:** Guedel airway + two nasopharyngeal airways or laryngeal mask airway (LMA)
3. **Definitive airway management:** endotracheal intubation if Glasgow Coma Score < 8 or other indication (see Box 15.1) CXR needed to check tube position
4. **Surgical airway management where tracheal intubation impossible, e.g. due to swelling, jaw fractures:** cricothyroidotomy (needle or surgical)

B. BREATHING AND VENTILATION — only assess breathing after airway is secure. Is patient breathing spontaneously and adequately ventilated?

Physical examination

Inspection, palpation, percussion and auscultation:

Observe specifically for injuries (**open wound, flail segment** of chest wall), distended neck veins (**cardiac tamponade**), tracheal deviation and asymmetrical expansion (**pneumothorax/tension pneumothorax**), dull percussion note (**haemothorax**)

Chest X-ray

Assess lungs, pleural spaces, chest wall and diaphragm

Treatment of life-threatening conditions

1. **Open chest wound:** seal with occlusive dressing to limit mediastinal 'flap' movement with each breath + tube thoracostomy
2. **Flail segment:** oxygen, monitoring, analgesia + endotracheal (ET) intubation + assisted ventilation if deterioration
3. **Cardiac tamponade:** pericardiocentesis
4. **Pneumothorax:** may need chest drain/tube thorocostomy if large pneumothorax
5. **Tension pneumothorax:** needle thoracocentesis + tube thoracostomy
6. **Haemothorax:** tube thoracostomy
7. **Diaphragmatic rupture:** repair surgically
8. **Serious head injury:** ET tube + assisted ventilation

C. CIRCULATION — assess circulation only when the patient's airway is secure and the above life-threatening conditions have been excluded, or identified and treatment under way

Physical examination

Assess: pallor, heart rate, blood pressure, temperature, capillary refill time, ECG and urine output. Is there any obvious external haemorrhage?

Management of shock and control of haemorrhage

1. Control external haemorrhage from bleeding open wounds by direct pressure on gauze pack
2. Insert two **wide-bore IV cannulae** into antecubital fossae (or other large veins)
3. If cannulation not possible, **venous cut-down** or **direct bone infusion** may be necessary
4. When venous access achieved, send blood for **urgent cross-matching**, and standard biochemical and haematological analysis
5. In the shocked patient, rapidly infuse two litres of **warmed crystalloid solution** through both peripheral intravenous lines; monitor response of pulse palpability, rate and BP and titrate rate of infusion (note permissive hypotension may be appropriate — see p.223)
6. If the patient fails to improve, consider transfusion of red cells. If the patient is rapidly deteriorating, O negative blood can be given
7. Consider likely causes of significant blood loss in the light of the history and clinical findings: e.g. thoracic trauma, abdominal injury, pelvic fracture, long bone fracture
8. **Catheterise** the bladder to monitor urine production and to provide a guide to renal perfusion
9. **Fracture management** — reduction of fractures may assist in haemostasis, especially femoral shaft fractures and sometimes pelvic fractures (also helps pain relief)
10. Relieve cardiac tamponade by **long needle aspiration**
11. Apply **external cardiac massage** in the case of cardiac arrest

Further management of circulation depends on likely source of blood loss, e.g. if abdominal injury is likely FAST ultrasound confirms and **laparotomy** may be required to control haemorrhage

D. DISABILITY of the central nervous system. Do not move on to assess 'D' until patient's circulatory state is stable

Basic **neurological assessment** is made using the **AVPU score**:

A — Alert
V — responding to Verbal stimuli
P — responding to Painful stimuli
U — Unresponsive

Pupil size, inequality and reactivity to light is also assessed

Estimate Glasgow Coma Scale if practicable and look for other neurological deficits

E. EXPOSURE of the whole patient, **ENVIRONMENT** and **'EXRAYS'** (imaging)

The patient is **fully exposed**, including removal of all clothing, to allow rapid 'top to toe' assessment for external injury and for signs of injury which have not already been recognised and managed. The patient must be kept warm including warming intravenous fluids. Completion of the trauma series **X-rays, CT scans and FAST ultrasound** is performed

Consider the following measures to monitor the patient and aid further assessment, if not already done

Urinary catheterisation
Nasogastric or orogastric tube placement
X-rays of cervical spine (lateral), chest and pelvis (trauma series)
Focused abdominal sonography for trauma (FAST)

Fig. 15.5 Primary survey and initial resuscitation

Management priorities for the patient with multiple injuries. In practice, anaesthetists usually deal with the airway and intravenous access and monitoring while surgeons evaluate the head and neck, chest, abdomen and pelvis for potential life-threatening injuries

given in Figure 15.6; individual systems are described later. Up to 20% of multiple injury patients have injuries missed in the early stages so the secondary survey must be **repeated**.

Recording of events

The time of examination and the clinical findings, plus details of investigations and treatments, must be recorded in the patient's notes, not least for medico-legal purposes.

X-rays and other investigations

In major trauma, the cervical spine (see below, Fig. 15.10), chest and pelvis are X-rayed in the resuscitation room. The chest films must be good enough to exclude major chest wall, mediastinal and lung injuries and provide a baseline if the patient later deteriorates. Polytrauma patients, or patients with serious head injury should have rapid assessment and stabilisation before swift transfer for trauma CT scan. Patients should not be moved to the CT scanner until they are stable—the machine is known as the 'donut of death' in ATLS parlance.

Focused abdominal sonography for trauma, or FAST (see *Abdominal injuries*, below), is performed in the emergency department for suspected abdominal injuries and bleeding. Initial **blood tests** include haemoglobin and group and cross-match or antibody screen and ordering of an appropriate amount of blood. In a desperate emergency, universal donor blood (group O, Rh negative) can be transfused. Evidence from recent conflicts has demonstrated the advantages of early administration of blood products in reducing the risk of haemodilution and coagulopathy. Emergency departments are increasingly using 'blood packs' which include several units of packed red cells, fresh frozen plasma and platelets. These may be transfused in a 1 : 1 : 1 ratio or in a goal-directed manner, guided by coagulation testing and thromboelastography. Plasma electrolytes and glucose are measured, plus arterial blood gases if there is suspicion of respiratory failure.

SECONDARY SURVEY

Head and neck

Look for bruising, soft tissue swelling; signs of basal skull fracture — Battle's sign (bruising over mastoid process), 'racoon eyes'
Lacerations
Depressed vault fractures
Facial and jaw fractures
Pupil size and responsiveness
Range of active neck movements

Chest (front and back)

Signs of respiratory distress — grunting/stridor
Bruising and skin imprinting
Penetrating injuries
Pattern and rate of respiration
Symmetry of chest movement
Gross mediastinal shift
Pattern of air entry throughout lung fields
Crepitus (subcutaneous air)

Abdomen and pelvis

External injuries as for chest (front and back)
Note: buttock injuries may penetrate abdominal cavity
Distension by gas or fluid (including blood)
Tenderness
Presence of palpable or percussible bladder
Pelvic fractures
Bleeding from urethral meatus
PR bruising, palpable pelvic haematoma or loss of anal tone (spinal injury)

Limbs

Neurovascular status of each limb
Lacerations
Deformities
Soft tissue swelling

Further definitive management of lesser injuries

Depends on findings from Primary and Secondary survey
May involve **further imaging** ± **surgery** or **ITU admission**
Before leaving the Emergency Department, **reassessment** is essential to ensure that the patient is safe to be transferred elsewhere

Fig. 15.6 Secondary survey
Special points to note in systematic examination of the seriously injured patient

ABDOMINAL INJURIES

INTRODUCTION

Abdominal and thoracic injuries often coexist, so it is logical to think in terms of **torso trauma**. Major torso injuries are a common cause of death at the trauma scene, for example from avulsion of the thoracic aorta, cardiac injury or massive liver injury. Immediate diagnosis and urgent laparotomy or thoracotomy offers almost the only hope of survival, but the injury is often too extensive or time too short to intervene.

The site and signs of external injury provide clues to internal injuries. This is obvious with penetrating injuries but is also true of blunt injuries. For example, trauma to the left upper abdominal quadrant or lower ribs is often coupled with **splenic rupture**; similarly for the **liver** with right-sided injuries. Lower abdominal injuries may injure the **bladder**, and loin trauma the **kidney**. Central anterior chest trauma can damage the **heart** whilst clavicular area injury may traumatise the **brachial plexus** or **subclavian blood vessels**.

Abdominal injuries are rare compared with head and chest injuries and mortality can be low with prompt and appropriate management. When death occurs, it is usually from massive haemorrhage arising from bursting of liver or spleen or from penetration of major arteries or veins, particularly with gunshot wounds. Note that **unrecognised injuries** are the principal **avoidable** cause of death.

Areas of the abdomen other than the main peritoneal cavity may be wounded; **pelvic** viscera lie within a bony cage but extend low enough to be injured by buttock or perineal wounds. Similarly, **retroperitoneal** viscera may seem protected but are vulnerable to flank or back wounds, or to deep anterior stab wounds or any gunshot wounds. This area is not easily palpated and diagnosis requires cross-sectional imaging.

Overall, 20% of patients with closed abdominal trauma require operation. In penetrating injuries, 30% with stab wounds require operation and close to 100% of those with gunshot wounds.

DIAGNOSIS OF ABDOMINAL INJURIES

Clinical diagnosis is unreliable in blunt injuries because overt signs of bleeding or hollow viscus perforation may not develop until hours after injury. If the patient is stable but the accident involved high energy transfer or other significant injuries are present, early CT scanning should be performed.

Clinical observation

If surgical intervention is not needed, regular nursing observations and serial clinical examination by a doctor should be performed for signs of peritonitis or intra-abdominal bleeding. Note that significant injuries almost always become manifest within 24 hours.

Investigative techniques

Focused abdominal sonography for trauma (FAST)

FAST reliably detects free intra-abdominal fluid and concentrates on five areas, the 'five Ps'—Perihepatic, Perisplenic and Pelvic in the abdomen and Pleural and Pericardial in the chest. It is, of course, user-dependent.

CT scanning for abdominal injuries

CT can identify injuries to all solid abdominal and retroperitoneal organs (liver, spleen, pancreas and kidney), bowel perforations (indirectly by detecting free gas and fluid), diaphragmatic rupture, retroperitoneal blood and pelvic and spinal fractures. This may allow conservative management of less severe splenic and liver injuries. CT is also valuable for defining the extent and configuration of complex pelvic fractures.

PENETRATING ABDOMINAL WOUNDS

STAB WOUNDS AND OTHER SHARP ABDOMINAL WOUNDS

Stab wounds may or may not penetrate the peritoneal cavity. They often cause little damage unless the blade penetrates the retroperitoneal area and injures great vessels or pancreas. It used to be thought that all abdominal stab wounds required surgical exploration but current policy in most cases is more conservative management. A large series from Baragwanath Hospital, Soweto, South Africa, demonstrated that 70% of patients, or more, could safely be managed by observation in hospital for 24 hours, and operated upon only if there were signs of deterioration. However, haemodynamically unstable patients and those with extensive or potentially contaminated penetrating wounds **must** be explored surgically without delay.

For most patients, the first step is to determine whether the peritoneum has been breached, by exploring the wound under local anaesthesia. If it has, then laparoscopy, ultrasonography or CT scanning can be employed to explore intra-abdominal viscera. If the peritoneum is intact and/or imaging is negative (as in most cases), conservative management with careful monitoring is appropriate. However, about one-third who later proved to have significant injury were initially free of signs, emphasising the need for repeated clinical and radiographic reassessment.

BULLET AND OTHER MISSILE INJURIES

The severity of internal injury depends on the path and mass of the missile and especially on its velocity. Low-velocity wounds (e.g. hand-gun bullets) cause damage confined to the wound track, whereas high-velocity (i.e. rifle) bullet wounds injure widely and deeply. This is because the much higher kinetic energy is dissipated in the tissues. In addition, **cavitation** is caused and debris is sucked into the wounds, causing contamination with clothing and soil. If a bullet hits bone, secondary missiles cause further injury. The size of the entry wound is often small because of elastic recoil of the skin and is no guide to the extent of injury. Given the unpredictable extent of injuries, **all** gunshot wounds must be surgically explored to check for visceral organ, intestinal and vascular damage. Buttock wounds should be treated in the same way.

CLOSED (BLUNT) ABDOMINAL INJURIES

Closed abdominal injuries usually result from road traffic collisions, falls, sporting contact injuries and accidents involving horses. Following substantial blunt injury, about 20% will require laparotomy. The **spleen** is the most vulnerable organ, especially in left-sided injuries (see Fig. 15.7). **Liver injury** requires greater impact force, usually from the front or right side. **Pancreatic and duodenal injuries** are uncommon and usually result from a heavy central abdominal impact, transsecting the pancreas or retroperitoneal duodenum across the vertebral bodies. This most commonly occurs in children falling across the handlebars of bicycles. The **kidneys** are vulnerable to punches or kicks in the loins.

Bowel is damaged by rapid deceleration or crushing, and is particularly vulnerable at sites where freely mobile bowel becomes attached to the retroperitoneum, i.e. at each end of the transverse colon, at the duodeno-jejunal flexure and in the ileocaecal area. A full **bladder**, common after a bout of heavy drinking, may rupture into the peritoneal cavity (or sometimes retroperitoneally) after abdominal impact. The **bladder** and **urethra** are also liable to be torn in displaced pelvic fractures. The clinical features and investigation of closed abdominal injuries are shown in Box 15.6.

Box 15.6 Clinical features of closed abdominal injury that suggest visceral injury

1. History

- Substantial trauma to the abdomen or lower chest
- Seatbelt not worn in road traffic collision (especially driver impacting steering wheel)
- Abdominal pain after trauma
- Haematuria, particularly following trauma to the back or loin

2. Physical signs

- Skin bruising immediately after injury—suggests sufficient force to cause internal damage
- Imprinting of cloth pattern on skin (*cloth printing*)—caused by compression of skin against vertebral bodies; implies high energy transfer impact
- Unexplained hypotension—suggests concealed haemorrhage into abdominal cavity or elsewhere
- Abdominal distension, i.e. increasing abdominal girth—from accumulating blood, urine or gas in the peritoneal cavity
- Increasing abdominal tenderness, guarding and rigidity (difficult to assess if abdominal wall bruising)—possible intestinal perforation or intra-abdominal bleeding
- Lateral lower rib fractures—injury to spleen, liver or kidney
- Pelvic fractures, especially 'butterfly' fractures of all four pubic rami—often bladder or urethral injury (especially in males) and pelvic vein injury
- Inability to pass urine and blood at urethral meatus and/or perineal bruising—imply rupture of urethra, usually at pelvic diaphragm, i.e. post-membranous urethra (avoid urethral catheterisation in favour of suprapubic); rectal examination may reveal 'high-riding' prostate
- Damage to anus or rectum may be palpable on rectal examination; presence of blood suggests anorectal injury. If anal sphincter tone low, suggests neurological damage from spinal injury

3. Investigation

- Raised plasma amylase suggests pancreatic injury needing CT scanning
- Chest and plain abdominal X-rays (supine and erect or lateral decubitus) for free intraperitoneal or retroperitoneal gas, rib or pelvic fractures associated with specific visceral injuries and radiopaque missiles such as bullets, shotgun pellets and glass
- Ultrasound and CT scanning—particularly useful for solid organs, i.e. spleen (Fig. 15.7), liver, kidneys, pancreas. Intravenous contrast CT useful for large vessel injuries
- Urethrography—for suspected urethral rupture
- Laparoscopy—increasingly important in closed abdominal trauma in stable patients. Can be performed under local anaesthesia

INJURIES TO SPECIFIC SOLID ORGANS

Spleen (Fig. 15.7)

The spleen is the most commonly injured organ in blunt abdominal trauma. The organ should be preserved wherever possible because of the dangers of post-splenectomy infection and sepsis. In one study, 2.4% of all post-splenectomy patients suffered sepsis and more than 50% of those were fatal.

CT scanning enables accurate assessment and classification of the extent of injury. Haematomas and capsular tears not extending deeply can often be managed conservatively. More severe injuries are treated by urgent laparotomy and where possible, splenic repair (splenorrhaphy) by direct suture, fibrin glue or absorbable mesh bags. Segmental resection or splenic artery ligation can be done, but 50% of splenic substance must be preserved for useful function. Whenever splenic preserving techniques are employed, a period of careful observation for up to 10 days is required as catastrophic secondary haemorrhage can occur.

Liver

Isolated small liver injuries may be treated by surgical repair or local resection but paradoxically, major injuries are often best treated conservatively. This is because control of deep hepatic vessels may prove impossible, particularly bleeding from hepatic veins entering the IVC. Patients with severe liver injuries should be discussed with a regional hepato-pancreatico-biliary (HPB) or liver unit. Conservative management involves large-volume blood transfusions until abdominal tamponade stops the bleeding. If operation is performed and a major liver injury is found and haemorrhage cannot be arrested, the liver should be packed with large pieces of surgical gauze, the abdomen closed and the patient stabilised. Ideally the patient should be transferred to an HPB centre as extensive liver surgery may be necessary when the packs are removed at a 'second look' laparotomy 24–48 hours later.

Other organs

Pancreatic transsection is treated by surgically removing the distal part and oversewing the stump. A crushing pancreatic injury may have to be treated with drainage alone. **Renal injuries** are usually managed conservatively unless nephrectomy is required for uncontrollable bleeding.

BOWEL INJURIES

Injuries to small bowel are dealt with by simple suture or, if mesenteric vascular supply is impaired, by resection and anastomosis. Conventional treatment for right-sided colon injuries is resection and anastomosis of colon to ileum. Localised injuries to other parts of the colon without substantial faecal contamination can usually be resected and joined end to end. After knife or gunshot wounds, simple repair gives good results if there is minimal peritoneal contamination.

CASE HISTORY

Fig. 15.7 Ruptured spleen

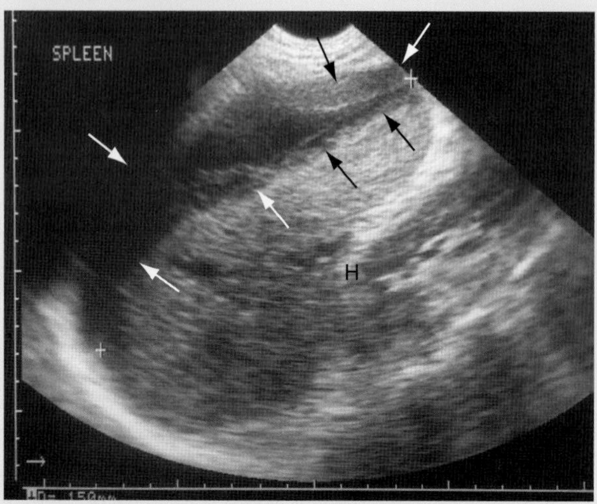

(a)

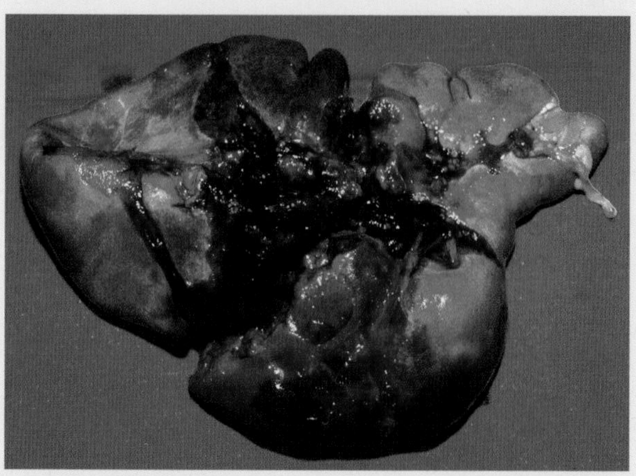

(b)

(a) This 67-year-old woman sustained fractures of the left lower ribs in a fall. Discharged from hospital the next day but re-presented 6 weeks later with abdominal swelling, tenderness and anaemia. This ultrasound scan shows a large subcapsular splenic haematoma (arrowed), which had developed slowly, and intrasplenic haemorrhage **H**. She rapidly recovered after splenectomy. **(b)** This operative specimen comes from a 15-year-old girl who fell off her pony, which then trod on the left chest. She was admitted with bruising over the lower ribs and tachycardia. At laparotomy, her spleen was found to be split completely in half, necessitating removal

Extensive injuries with contamination require **exteriorisation** of the damaged bowel ends to the abdominal wall (see Ch. 27).

High-velocity penetrating injuries wreak havoc on the gut, causing devascularisation and multiple perforations. All necrotic or ischaemic tissue must be excised. The immediate dangers are peritonitis and systemic sepsis from contamination. Exteriorisation of viable bowel ends is mandatory and planned re-exploration usual.

LOWER URINARY TRACT INJURIES

Intraperitoneal rupture of the bladder is treated by laparotomy and suturing, with a urethral catheter left in situ for 5–7 days. **Extraperitoneal** bladder rupture is treated conservatively, with prolonged urethral or suprapubic catheterisation. Urethral tears require specialist urological management. If the urethral wall is partly intact on urethrography, it can be treated, at least initially, by suprapubic catheterisation. Complete urethral avulsion injuries are usually treated by suprapubic catheterisation, with formal repair after inflammation has settled.

DAMAGE CONTROL LAPAROTOMY

Major trauma patients sometimes have extensive and complex intra-abdominal injuries. In an unstable patient, prolonged surgery to manage these definitively greatly exacerbates the lethal triad of coagulopathy, hypothermia and acidosis. Damage control laparotomy can be employed here as a life-saving procedure that should be completed within an hour. Haemorrhage is controlled by temporary clamping, then packing or ligating vessels. Hollow viscus injuries are stapled or resected without anastomosis. The abdomen is temporarily closed and arrangements made for definitive surgery in 24–48 hours following resuscitation.

CHEST INJURIES

The types of chest injury, their clinical features and their treatment are summarised in Table 15.2.

GENERAL PRINCIPLES

Chest injuries are a common cause of death in patients with multiple injuries, although the death rate has fallen dramatically wherever seatbelt wearing is compulsory. Seatbelts, however, often cause typical sash pattern bruising obliquely across the chest, and minor rib and sternal fractures (Fig. 15.8). Serious chest injuries may be present without external injury, particularly tearing of mediastinal contents (aorta, bronchi and oesophagus). Diagnosis goes hand in hand with urgent resuscitation. Good-quality chest X-rays (or CT scans) are essential and usually reveal the diagnosis (see Fig. 15.9).

Mechanisms of chest injury include penetrating trauma, blunt impact and crushing injuries, deceleration injuries and rupture of the diaphragm caused by abdominal compression. Less than 10% of chest injuries require surgical intervention but early recognition of these may be life-saving.

Table 15.2 Types of chest injury and their management

Nature of the injury	Clinical features	Treatment
Sternal fracture	Anterior chest pain and tenderness; 'clicking' on palpation; arrhythmia and ECG changes	Consider cardiac contusion or tamponade; FAST scan; 24h ECG; cardiac enzymes
Rib fractures	Localised pain on respiration or coughing; tenderness over fractures; usually visible on chest X-ray	Analgesia, intercostal blocks, physiotherapy, prophylactic antibiotics in chronic bronchitics
Flail chest, i.e. multiple rib fractures producing a mobile segment	Respiratory embarrassment; 'paradoxical' indrawing of the flail segment on inspiration	Intercostal block analgesia; endotracheal intubation and ventilation if hypoxic
Pneumothorax, i.e. air in pleural cavity causing lung collapse	Unilateral signs: loss of chest movement and breath sounds, percussion note resonant; sometimes chest wall emphysema; confirmed by chest X-ray	Intercostal drain with underwater seal
Sucking chest wound, i.e. open pneumothorax with mediastinum 'flapping' from side to side with each respiration	Gross respiratory embarrassment, audible sucking of air through chest wound	Sealing of chest wound with impermeable dressing; intercostal drainage
Tension pneumothorax, i.e. expanding pneumothorax causing progressive mediastinal shift to the opposite side and tracheal deviation	Signs of pneumothorax with disproportionate and increasing respiratory distress and hypoxaemia	Urgent chest drainage
Lung contusion	Deteriorating respiratory function; opacification of affected lung field on chest X-ray	Oxygenation, physiotherapy, mechanical ventilation if severe
Rupture of bronchus (uncommon)	Respiratory distress, surgical emphysema in the neck; suggested by air in mediastinum on chest X-ray (see Fig. 15.9a); confirmed by bronchoscopy	Operation by thoracic trained surgeon
Rupture of oesophagus (very rare)	May have surgical emphysema in neck and pneumomediastinum on CXR but diagnosis often missed until mediastinitis or empyema develops	Surgical repair if recognised early; surgical drainage and diversion if late
Haemothorax, i.e. blood in the pleural cavity Usually arises from chest wall injury—rib fracture, lung parenchyma or minor venous injury. Most are self-limiting. Arterial injuries less common and likely to need thoracotomy	Dull percussion note, breath sounds absent, tachycardia and hypotension due to blood loss	Most have stopped bleeding by the time of examination and only tube drainage is required Dark, venous bleeding more likely to cease spontaneously than bright arterial bleeding Tube must be large enough to drain without clotting, ideally 32–36°F; placed in sixth intercostal space in mid-axillary line If patient haemodynamically stable, admit and observe. If continuing drainage of 200 ml+ per hour over 4 hours, should undergo thoracotomy
Cardiac tamponade, i.e. bleeding into pericardial cavity (usually penetrating trauma)	Hypotension, inaudible heart sounds, distended neck veins with systolic waves; enlarged, rounded heart shadow on chest X-ray; confirmed with ultrasound	Long needle aspiration via epigastric approach; operation if tamponade recurs
Cardiac contusion	Often arrhythmia or ECG changes similar to myocardial infarction	Conservative management
Rupture of aorta (usually from deceleration injury)—fatal unless false aneurysm develops in mediastinum	Back pain, hypotension; systolic murmur or signs of tamponade in some cases; characteristic widening of mediastinum on chest X-ray; diagnosis confirmed by arteriography	Urgent thoracotomy and Dacron graft or minimal-access stent graft if available
Rupture of diaphragm, linear split usually in left diaphragm with herniation of gut into chest (penetrating or abdominal crush injury)	Respiratory distress, bowel sounds heard in the chest; diagnosis by chest X-ray and confirmed by barium meal; many cases only discovered much later; diagnosis may be made by laparoscopy or at laparotomy	Repair of diaphragm, usually via abdominal approach

CASE HISTORY

Fig. 15.8 Seatbelt injury

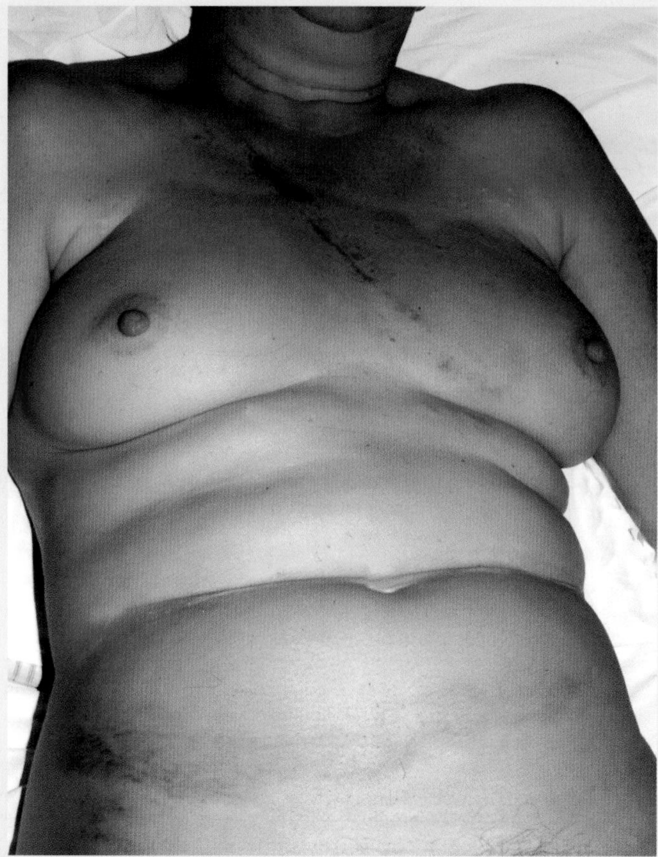

This 60-year-old woman suffered a severe frontal impact whilst driving. The photograph shows typical seatbelt bruising. The body of the sternum had an undisplaced fracture but there were no major injuries; the seatbelt almost certainly saved the patient's life

CASE HISTORY

Fig. 15.9 Serious chest injuries

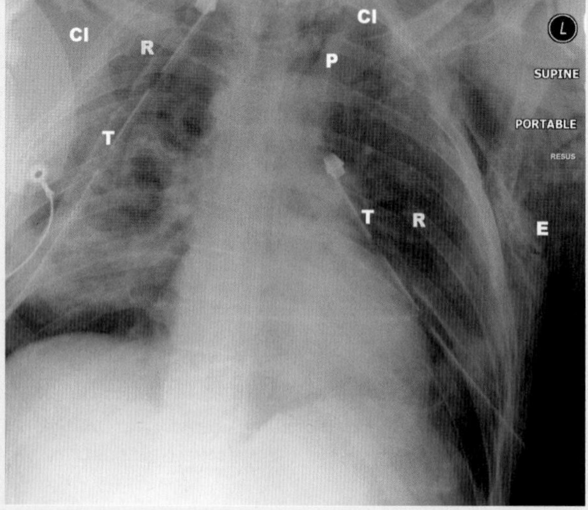

(a)

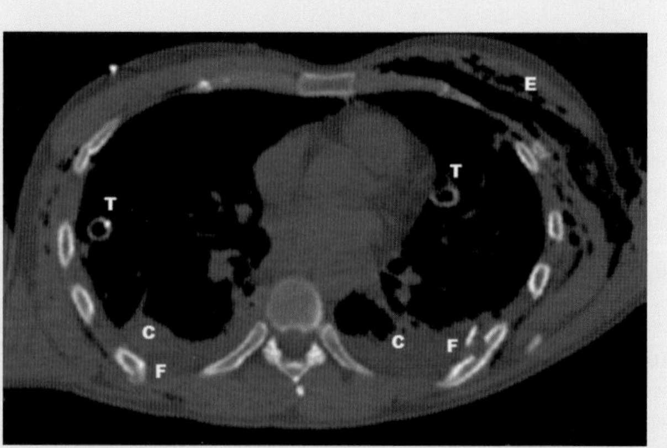

(b)

This 34-year-old male motorcyclist was hit by a car and then by another car whilst lying in the road. His GCS was 12–13 on arrival in the resuscitation room; brain, abdominal viscera and cervical spine were intact on CT. There were multiple fractures of ribs, scapula, clavicle, pelvis, humerus, femur and the chest injuries shown on CT **(b)**. His thoracic injuries were successfully managed conservatively. **(a)** Supine portable chest radiograph taken in the resuscitation room. It is not well centred, reflecting the difficulty in radiographing sick patients being resuscitated. The film shows bilateral clavicle **Cl, Cl** and rib fractures, pneumomediastinum **P**, surgical emphysema **E**, lung contusions and bilateral chest drains **T** inserted for pneumothorax. **(b)** CT on bone window settings showing surgical emphysema **E**, bilateral basal atelectasis of lungs **C, C**, chest drains **T, T**, and bilateral rib fractures **F, F**.

THORACOSTOMY (OPEN AND TUBE)

Following trauma, chest drains are usually placed in the fourth or fifth intercostal space on the mid-axillary line. The technique is shown in Figure 31.6, p. 402. Bilateral open thoracostomy is often used in pre-hospital care in ventilated patients (particularly during helicopter transfer) as a precursor to formal chest drain insertion.

VASCULAR TRAUMA

Veins and arteries may be damaged by penetrating or blunt trauma. Gunshot wounds are more likely to damage vessels than stab wounds, and blunt injuries can damage arterial walls causing occlusion. Iatrogenic injuries are becoming common with the rise in radiological and minimal access procedures, and hip replacements. Damaged vessels bleed or impair distal circulation, or both.

BLEEDING

Bleeding may be revealed (visible), or concealed and the rate of loss determines the presentation and risk of death. Concealed haemorrhage often occurs in the chest, abdomen or pelvis or in limb muscles with fractures; blood from facial fractures may be swallowed and unrecognised.

ISCHAEMIA

Trauma that interrupts arterial flow to a limb or organ causes ischaemia, leading to potential limb or organ loss, stroke, bowel necrosis, and consequent multiple organ dysfunction. Skeletal muscle can survive ischaemia for 3–6 hours and still recover but peripheral nerves are sensitive and deficits can result from brief ischaemia.

If arterial supply is restored after delay, the release of inflammatory mediators, lactic acid and potassium into the circulation can cause **reperfusion syndrome**. In limbs, this can lead to compartment syndrome, and can also initiate a systemic inflammatory response with myocardial and other organ dysfunction.

PATTERNS OF VASCULAR INJURY

Laceration is the most common. Completely severed arteries contract, limiting haemorrhage, but partially transsected arteries continue bleeding. Veins are unlikely to retract.

Blunt trauma causes crushing, stretching or shearing injures to vessels. Intimal flaps can lead to thrombosis or dissection. Thrombosis may propagate down the vessel or embolise distally. Arterial 'spasm' alone does not cause limb ischaemia—the cause is thrombosis or vessel wall damage and requires urgent investigation.

False aneurysm

An arterial puncture (e.g. femoral artery catheterisation or a stab wound) may cause bleeding that is enclosed by connective tissue, forming a pulsatile mass of clot known as a **false aneurysm.** This often presents days or weeks later. Distal flow is usually conserved and diagnosis can be confirmed by duplex Doppler ultrasound. First-line treatment is usually ultrasound-guided compression to cause thrombosis of the leak. If this fails, or for larger defects, suturing or patching may be needed.

Arteriovenous fistula

An injury to an artery and an adjacent vein can cause an arteriovenous (AV) fistula, which may eventually rupture or lead to cardiovascular compromise. These present some days or weeks after the injury. In a limb, the patient complains of a swelling with dilated superficial veins. On examination, there is a machinery-type murmur heard and diagnosis is confirmed by angiography. Treatment is by dividing the fistula and repairing the vein and artery, sometimes with a flap of fascia interposed.

DIAGNOSIS OF VASCULAR INJURY

Clinical signs

Visible bleeding from a traumatic wound with signs of hypovolaemia make the diagnosis obvious. In limbs, palpable distal pulses are the most reliable sign of intact distal circulation. Hand-held Doppler probes can be misleading in detecting distal pulses and in ankle pressure measurement.

The following 'hard' signs of vascular injury indicate a need for urgent operative intervention, often without prior investigation:

- An audible bruit or palpable thrill
- Active, especially pulsatile haemorrhage
- An expanding haematoma
- Distal ischaemia (cold, pale, pulseless limb)

Patients with the following 'soft' signs of vascular injury do not require urgent investigation or exploration; they should be admitted, investigated as needed and observed over 24 hours.

- Haematoma
- History of haemorrhage at the accident scene
- Unexplained hypotension
- Peripheral nerve deficit
- Reduced but definitely palpable pulse
- Injury site near a major artery

Investigation

In expert hands, Duplex ultrasound can detect intimal tears, thrombosis, false aneurysms and arteriovenous fistulae, but **angiography** by direct puncture, CT angiography or on the operating table remains the gold standard for investigation and mapping of vascular injury. Arteriography may be needed to show the extent of injury in a stable patient with equivocal signs; to exclude injury where there are no hard signs but suspicion of vascular injury; in limb fractures with absent pulses; in injury by high-velocity missiles or multiple fragment injuries; and in blunt trauma. Angiography may be used to treat certain injuries by embolisation or stenting where expertise is available.

MANAGEMENT OF VASCULAR INJURY

The priorities in managing vascular injury are arrest of life-threatening haemorrhage and restoration of normal circulation. Temporary bleeding control is usually achievable by pressure over the site of injury, NOT with tourniquets.

Direct exploration of an actively bleeding wound is usually inadvisable because of poor visibility and the technical difficulty of achieving control. Far better to obtain proximal control, if necessary via a separate incision, isolating and clamping the artery before exploring the wound. Sometimes the artery distal to the wound needs clamping remotely too.

With proximal and distal clamps in situ, the wound is explored, debrided and the extent of arterial and venous damage assessed. Generally, large veins should be repaired first to allow drainage as soon as the artery is repaired. A cut or lacerated artery may be amenable to direct repair or to patching, if direct suturing would narrow the lumen. More extensive damage may require an interposition graft, usually autologous long saphenous vein, or sometimes synthetic graft material. Before repair, proximal then distal clamps are released in turn to check for adequate blood flow. If inadequate, a Fogarty balloon catheter is passed to extract thrombus and heparinised saline instilled.

Compartment syndrome

Delayed revascularisation of a limb risks compartment syndrome (see Ch. 17, p. 235). Prophylactic fasciotomy should be performed at the time of repair in these circumstances, particularly if the patient is ventilated or has an epidural, as these mask the symptoms of developing compartment syndrome.

DAMAGE CONTROL IN VASCULAR INJURY

Vessel ligation

In extreme conditions, most vessels can be ligated. The common and external carotid, subclavian, axillary or internal iliac can be ligated with little consequence, but internal carotid ligation carries a 10–20% risk of stroke, and ligation of external iliac, common or superficial femoral arteries has a high risk of causing critical limb ischaemia. Coeliac axis arteries can be ligated, but not the superior mesenteric which would lead to bowel ischaemia. Almost any vein can be ligated, including the inferior vena cava (but this causes lower limb oedema).

Shunting

Where primary reconstruction cannot be performed and where ligation would risk limb loss, stroke or intestinal ischaemia, a temporary intraluminal shunt may be used to restore flow. Purpose-made shunts are available with side arms for flushing but can be constructed from sterile tubing.

Primary amputation

This is usually considered when there is severe injury, including crush injury, with a significant risk of reperfusion injury or when the limb is likely to be painful and useless.

INTERVENTIONAL RADIOLOGY IN VASCULAR INJURY

Interventional radiology is increasingly used in trauma as a means of controlling haemorrhage without need for a surgical procedure. In pelvic fractures, angiography and embolisation has become the gold standard for control of bleeding from iliac vessels; this remains the only firm indication for interventional radiology in unstable patients. In stable patients, embolisation can be used to control bleeding from solid organs (e.g. in splenic laceration) and covered stents can be deployed across major vessel disruptions (e.g. traumatic rupture of the thoracic aorta).

ORTHOPAEDIC TRAUMA

INTRODUCTION

This section contains a brief introduction to the main points of fracture management, followed by detail on spinal and pelvic injuries.

- Pain—major orthopaedic injuries are extremely painful so good analgesia and early reduction is an important part of treatment, contributing to early mobilisation and reducing the potential for deep venous thrombosis (DVT)
- Blood loss—internal blood loss from fractures is often substantial (see Table 15.3), particularly if there are multiple fractures, and blood volume needs to be appropriately replaced. In pelvic fractures, external fixation may reduce blood loss
- Deformity—obvious deformity should be corrected as soon as possible using temporary splinting. This treats pain and may assist vascular supply and limit blood loss
- Vascular and neurological integrity—where limbs are involved, this should be checked and appropriate investigation and intervention arranged
- Definitive fixation of fractures may be needed early or may have to be deferred until other life-threatening injuries have been dealt with

FRACTURES

Introduction

A fracture is when there is a break in continuity of a bone. Fractures are classified so patterns of injury can be recognised,

Table 15.3 Average blood loss from fractures

Site	Average loss (L)
Pelvis	1–4
Femur	1–2.5
Tibia	0.5–1.5
Humerus	0.5–1.5

and the best treatment of any subtype agreed by consensus. Fracture patterns are linked to anatomical location, and mechanism and energy of injury. Eponymous fracture classifications are used in some countries, whereas objective systems such as the Swiss AO system (Arbeitsgemeinschaft Osteosynthesefragen) prevail elsewhere (see Box 15.7).

Bone is strong in compression but weaker in resisting torsional or bending forces. A footballer landing on one foot loads the tibia in compression and this is stable, but with a twisting force in addition, torsion is applied and it fractures. A pure bending force when falling from a height onto a forearm causes fracture, as the energy is applied where the bone is weakest. As velocity increases, **high energy transfer** collisions can fracture the bone in multiple places ($Force = Mass \times Velocity^2$).

Fracture healing

Fractures heal by restoring bone continuity. Cancellous bone heals more quickly than cortical bone and some movement at fracture sites stimulates healing. Healing needs a good blood supply so rates of healing are more rapid in children.

Box 15.7 Classification of fractures

All schemes generally describe fractures along similar lines:

Area of bone involved

- Diaphyseal
- Metaphyseal
- Intra-articular

Configuration of the fracture

- Transverse
- Oblique
- Spiral
- Comminuted (multiple pieces)
- Segmental (two fractures at different levels in the same bone)

Breach of surrounding tissue

- Closed
- Open

Degree of displacement

- Undisplaced
- Displaced
- Angulated
- Translated
- Impacted

Age of patient or existing pathology

- Greenstick fracture (children's bones)
- Osteoporotic (insufficiency) fracture
- Pathological fracture (secondaries)

Pathological fractures occur in abnormal bone, affected by benign, malignant or diffuse disease. The last includes bone affected by disorders of organisation such as osteomalacia or Paget's disease.

Healing can be considered in five stages: first, the bone ends bleed causing a haematoma, and periosteum is stripped from bone. Soft tissues may also be damaged. Second, acute inflammation and cell division begins within 8 hours. Third, osteoblasts proliferate in periosteum and **callus** forms. This is a heterogenous mixture of woven bone (from osteoblasts) and hyaline cartilage from chondroblasts. Osteoclasts resorb dead bone. In stage four, orderly lamellar bone replaces woven bone and the fracture becomes united. Lastly, during remodelling, the bone recovers its normal shape and any medullary cavity is restored.

Principles of fracture management

These include reduction, immobilisation and later, rehabilitation. The need for **reduction** depends on the fracture. Rotational, valgus or varus deformity usually needs correcting and intra-articular fractures need precise anatomical reduction. Reduction can be performed as a closed or open procedure.

Immobilisation by external or internal methods is then needed until fractures unite. External methods include plaster casts, traction and external fixation. Internal methods include plates, intramedullary nails and K-wires.

Initial management of fractures

First aid minimises pain and reduces the risk of secondary damage. Broken bones are usually acutely painful and deviation causes pressure on skin and neurovascular structures. Initial treatment in the field involves assessing overlying wounds and applying dressings, reducing fractures into an immobilising splint or plaster and later, confirming the diagnosis with X-rays. These steps resuscitate the limb and soft tissues. They also reduce pain by limiting movement at the fracture site.

Definitive management of fractures (see Table 15.4)

Fractures were able to heal long before orthopaedic surgery existed, but learning how to restore the anatomy and hold bones immobile while they healed was a major advance. Definitive management nowadays may be operative (open) or non-operative (closed). Operative treatment may not accelerate healing so the extra risks need to be justified. Complications include: infection, non-union, implant failure and refracture.

The main indications for operative treatment are: fracture types that require open reduction, unstable fractures, intra-articular fractures (to stabilise anatomical reduction), multiple injuries, elderly patients (to allow early mobilisation), long bone fractures (tibia, femur and humerus), where blood vessels or nerves need repair (to access and protect the repair), where conservative management has failed, and pathological fractures. A local capability of performing this surgery with low complication rates is also important.

Open (compound) fractures

These must all be assumed to be contaminated. First aid treatment is the same as for closed fracture, but open fractures require early operation, ideally within 6 hours of injury. At operation the wound is cleaned, devitalised tissue is debrided

Table 15.4 Types of limb fracture and their management

Site	Mechanism of injury	Classification (common or important types)	Management	Specific potential complications
Upper limb				
Clavicle	Fall onto outstretched hand	Proximal ⅓, middle ⅓, distal ⅓	Up to 98% of middle third heal with conservative management. Displaced distal may need operation	Plate fixation of middle third fractures threatens underlying neurovascular bundle
Humerus (neck)	Fall onto hand	Neer's	Operate if severe displacement and incongruency	Severely broken humeral heads may need hemiarthroplasty
Olecranon	Fall onto point of elbow		Tension band wire for articular surface reconstruction	
Fracture-dislocations of forearm	Fall onto arm		Accurate reconstruction preserves full range of movement	... but neurovascular structures make operating difficult
Distal radius	Fragility fractures	Smith's, Colles', Barton's	Aim to restore function	Porotic bones makes perfect X-rays difficult
Base of thumb	Forced extension	Rolando's, Bennett's	Accurate fixation to preserve thumb movements	
Metacarpal neck	Punching/fist injuries		Many managed conservatively	
Lower limb				
Neck of femur	Fragility fractures	Garden's, Intra/extracapsular	~100% operation rates to allow early mobilisation	High morbidity and mortality in elderly patients
Tibial plateau	High energy fractures	Schaztker's	Operate to reconstruct vital articular surface	
Tibial shaft	High energy fractures		Conservative and operative methods available	High rates of non-union compared to other bones
Ankle	Low energy fractures	Weber's, AO classification	Operate to restore perfect ankle congruity if casting fails	
Calcaneum	High energy falls	Sanders class		Often lead to hind foot pain or collapse
Forefoot and toes	Low energy falls/trips		Fix and straighten bones, mobilise early	

and the fracture stabilised. Small clean wounds can be sutured but large or dirty wounds should be left open and closed by delayed primary suture after about 5 days.

Pathological fractures

These occur in:

- Generalised bone diseases, e.g. osteoporosis or metabolic bone diseases (osteomalacia, hyperparathyroidism, Paget's disease)
- Localised benign bone disorders, e.g. chronic infection, solitary bone cysts, fibrous cortical defects or chondromas
- Malignant disease: metastatic cancers, myelomatosis, primary malignant bone tumours

Complications of fractures (see Box 15.8)

The likelihood of complications depends on the mechanism of injury and the amount of force through the area at the moment of fracture. Sharp bone ends can perforate or crush nearby structures such as muscles, skin, blood vessels and rarely nerves; hyperextension of the knee can damage popliteal nerves. Prompt recognition and fracture reduction is crucial as fracture deformity continues to provoke inflammation and damage.

Malunion can lead later to disordered mechanical forces in the rest of the limb and back, and may cause osteoarthritis in nearby joints. Displaced intra-articular fractures with an irregular joint surface markedly increases friction, leading

Box 15.8 Complications of fractures

Early complications

Local

- Muscle and tendon injuries
- Nerve injury
- Haemarthrosis
- Vascular injury
- Compartment syndrome
- Infection
- Visceral injuries

Systemic

- Venous thromboembolism (VTE)
- Exacerbation of pre-existing co-morbidity such as respiratory failure or coronary artery disease
- Fat embolism
- Systemic shock
- Acute respiratory distress syndrome (ARDS)

Late complications

Local

- Delayed union
- Non-union
- Malunion
- Volkmann's contracture
- Stiffness and instability
- Avascular necrosis
- Algodystrophy
- Osteomyelitis
- Growth arrest in children
- Complex regional pain syndrome (CRPS)

Systemic

- Overwhelming infection
- Systemic sepsis
- Reduced overall mobility
- Osteoarthritis

to post-traumatic osteoarthritis. **Delayed union** leads to long periods of disuse, and the entire limb can suffer from muscle atrophy, osteoporosis and joint contractures if not treated early. For *Compartment syndrome*, see Chapter 17, p. 235.

SPECIFIC FRACTURES

Common upper limb fractures

The most common and their usual management are:

- Metacarpal neck—often left to heal in mildly angulated position
- Base of thumb metacarpal—fragments accurately reduced and fixed
- Distal radius—deformity reduced and fixed, e.g. Colles type
- Olecranon process—articular process reconstructed and fixed
- Neck of humerus—usually managed non-operatively
- Clavicle—95% heal quickly with only a sling

These fractures each have typical patterns of presentation. For example, distal radius fractures are often in bone weakened by osteoporosis, and a simple fall from standing can cause an angulated and deforming fracture needing surgery. Conversely, entirely normal bone in the metacarpal neck can be fractured in young adults fighting with fists.

Common lower limb fractures

The most common lower limb fractures are:

- Neck of femur
- Ankle
- Forefoot and toes
- Tibial shaft

Fragility fractures due to osteoporosis far outnumber the others and affect a large number of older patients. Femoral neck fracture still carries a high mortality. Operative treatment carries risks but is still the best method of restoring mobility and preventing death from other causes. Nevertheless death rates of 10–30% at 1 year are common.

Dealing with fragility hip fractures presents a challenge. Conservative treatment is rare nowadays, as spending 6 or more weeks in bed leads to high rates of venous thromboembolism, respiratory infection, pressure ulcers and death. These patients are often frail, with impaired cardiovascular and respiratory function, so surgical treatment requires anaesthetic risk assessment and optimising general health. There is a trend in the UK towards involving a dedicated care-of-the-elderly physician in assessing and managing all these patients. This, together with physiotherapists, dedicated theatres to minimise delays, modern surgical stabilisation techniques and skilled anaesthesia, provides optimum care and better outcomes.

Fracturing lower limb long bones in healthy adults requires substantial force. Typical patterns of tibial and femoral shaft fractures occur in motor vehicle accidents, falls from height and high energy collisions on the sports field.

Ankle fractures occur in all age groups, caused by accidental slips and falls. The shape of the talus means that twisting the foot plus body weight exerting downward force can easily break the ankle even with normal bone. Operative or non-operative treatments can be used to fix a broken distal tibia and fibula or ankle joint, depending on the fracture configuration.

Pelvis and spinal fractures

Pelvic fractures

The pelvis is a strong structure and very large forces are needed to fracture it. Most pelvic fractures occur in high energy collisions; if the bony pelvis is disrupted, the soft organs and viscera are also threatened. Pelvic fractures often occur with substantial injuries to the trunk and limbs. The bony pelvis is effectively a ring, and disruption depends on there being at least two fractures or joint separations with consequent instability. The pelvis can be crushed in an antero-posterior, lateral or vertical direction or a combination of all three. Life-threatening internal bleeding from arterial or, most importantly, venous injury to the iliac vessels often accompanies pelvic fractures.

Clinical indications of likely pelvic fracture include:

- Haematuria or in males, signs of urethral injury, e.g. high-riding prostate on rectal examination, scrotal haematoma or blood at urethral meatus
- Rectal bleeding, or a large haematoma or palpable fracture line on rectal examination
- Haematomas of the proximal thigh, above the inguinal ligament, over the perineum or in the flank
- Neurovascular deficits of lower extremities

A plain AP pelvic X-ray reveals 90% of injuries. If a fracture is present or suspected and the patient stable, a pelvic CT scan is the best imaging for pelvic anatomy (including hip dislocation and acetabular fracture) and shows the extent of pelvic, retroperitoneal and intraperitoneal bleeding. Rapid assessment, then temporary stabilisation with a fabric pelvic-binder applied in the accident department may help arrest the bleeding, but transfusion and angiographic embolisation may be needed.

Spinal fractures (Fig. 15.10)

These may be pathological or not. The most common pathological fracture is a fragility (crush) fracture in osteoporotic bone, typically in lumbar spine bodies in older patients. Up to 90% of patients in their 80s are believed to have sustained a vertebral fragility crush fracture. These cause pain and disability but do not benefit from surgical treatment and take time to settle. Pathological fractures through metastatic deposits are a common new presentation of a known neoplasm or of an undiagnosed primary.

Non-pathological spinal fractures usually occur with high energy trauma, but vertebrae can be crushed in healthy adults after a vertical fall from standing height. Any patient suffering sufficient trauma should be assumed to have a spinal injury until proven otherwise. Most attention is directed to the vulnerable cervical spine (see below), but the entire spinal column should be assessed.

The cervical spine may be cleared clinically, without need for radiology, if the following conditions are met:

- Patient alert and orientated
- No head injury
- No drugs or alcohol
- No neck pain
- No abnormal neurological signs
- No significant other injury that may distract the patient from complaining about the spine
- **On examination**: no bruising or deformity around the neck, no tenderness and a normal pain-free range of active movement

A cervical spine CT scan should be performed (usually with a CT head) if the criteria are not met. Thoracolumbar spine imaging is indicated if there is pain, bruising, swelling, deformity or abnormal neurological signs attributable to the region. A fracture anywhere in the spine is an indication for full spinal imaging. Unconscious patients cannot be assessed clinically and require **radiological clearance** of the whole spine (i.e. exclusion of injuries). If in doubt, spinal immobilisation devices are left in place, logrolling for movement and high frequency nursing care is continued while seeking detail about the fracture.

CASE HISTORY

Fig. 15.10 Cervical spine fractures

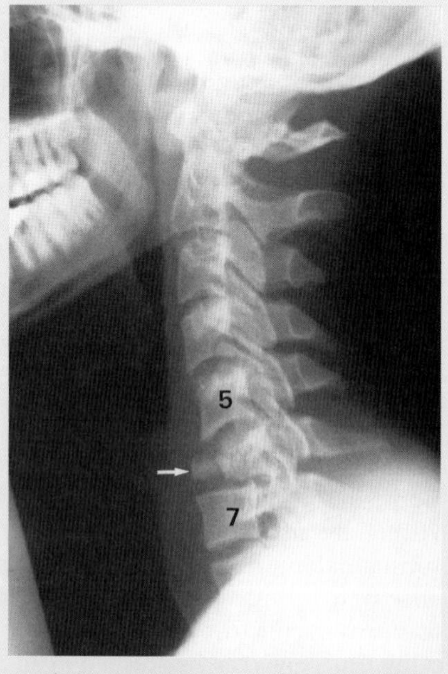

(a)

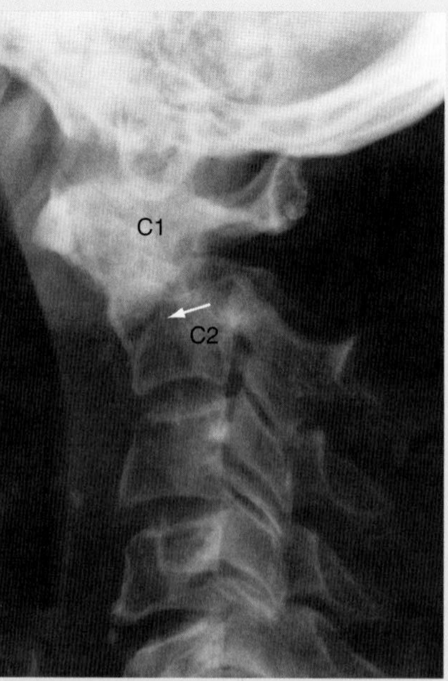

(b)

(a) This 17-year-old boy was admitted semiconscious after crashing his motorcycle and landing head-first in a ditch. On examination he was tetraplegic and unable to move his upper or lower limbs but could shrug his shoulders. This lateral cervical spine X-ray shows a burst fracture of the body of C6 (arrowed) with fragments in the spinal canal; there is also some posterior subluxation of C5. **(b)** Left lateral cervical spine X-ray from another unconscious young patient showing a fracture (arrowed) of the body of C2 and severe anterior subluxation of C1.

The spine has a key role in structural support and fractures are classified to judge stability. Fractures occur in flexion/extension, compression and/or rotation. Understanding altered vertebral anatomy helps decide whether operation is needed. Damage to the spinal cord or peripheral nerves in the vertebral canal causes limb paralysis. This can occur at the moment of trauma and may be an irretrievable neurological injury, no matter what spinal stabilisation is provided. However, the injured spinal cord can enter a period of spinal shock lasting 24–72 hours and sometimes recovery is seen after this. **Spinal shock** is an old term for a period of altered distal function with loss of sphincteric control and reflexes which may result from inadequate tissue perfusion secondary to the spinal injury interrupting autonomic control, leading to bradycardia and hypotension. Management of spinal shock is a period of observation, with protection against pressure ulcers and urinary retention, until the spinal cord settles to a stable state of injury, with neurological deficits at and distal to the level of injury.

COMMON LIGAMENTOUS INJURIES

The notion of a sprain versus a ligamentous tear or rupture is important to clarify. A ligament can be injured but retain its functional length without elongation. This causes an acutely painful inflammatory response known as a **sprain**. Greater energy during injury results in collagen fibre disruption and loss of tensile strength to the point where the ligament tears. Sprains usually resolve without surgical intervention, whereas tears may result in the ligament becoming permanently longer.

Most sprains occur at the ankle and wrist. Both joints have very strong interconnected ligamentous structures. With acute ankle injury, the area rapidly becomes painful and oedematous, but weight bearing may be possible initially as structure remains intact. Later, increasing pain makes weight bearing impossible and medical attention is usually sought. Once a sprain is diagnosed, the management is pain relief, elevation to reduce oedema, initial splintage and rest. Early mobilisation at 1–2 weeks is usually encouraged to prevent stiffness, and movement of the sprained ligament encourages vascularisation and a healing response.

Dislocations

Certain joints can sublux or dislocate after a ligament sprain or rupture. Subluxation is when there is partial loss of congruity between articular surfaces and dislocation is when there is total loss of congruity. Some joints are predisposed to this by their shape and inherent mobility. Sometimes a systemic disease such as the collagen disorder Ehlers–Danlos syndrome, or muscle weakness in muscular dystrophy contributes instability enough for joints to dislocate.

Shoulder dislocation at the glenohumeral joint, and patella dislocation at the patella-femoral joint are common. Both joints have little bony congruity with flat convexities resting in a dish-shaped socket.

Prompt recognition of a dislocation followed by rapid reduction or relocation of joint components is ideal. Reducing the dislocation reduces pain and relieves pressure on nearby structures, including stabilising ligaments and neurovascular structures. Pain usually causes muscle spasm around the site, so good analgesia is needed for reduction in a conscious patient. Skilled emergency room staff can often reduce a dislocated joint if no fracture is present.

DAMAGE CONTROL ORTHOPAEDICS

Advances in understanding physiological responses to severe injury have prompted surgeons to re-examine the management of polytrauma. Long operations soon after a high energy injury definitely increase the threat to life. Open fixation of broken bones causes additional trauma, particularly if there is an enthusiastic desire to fix all fractures in one theatre visit. Such interventions may also cause fat embolism which can lead to respiratory collapse and death. A short surgical intervention after resuscitation could often be justified, but lengthy fixation of all broken bones has been abandoned in favour of temporary stabilisation with external fixators; this is known as damage control orthopaedics. The patient can then be managed or supported for the next 48–72 hours in a high dependency setting whilst the physiological 'storm' is optimised. External fixators can then be exchanged for definitive plates or intramedullary rods between days 3 and 10.

PAEDIATRIC TRAUMA

Paediatric trauma is more complicated to manage because of the physiological differences between adults and children. Airway management and venous access can be challenging and children are more prone to hypothermia, especially if small, so it is important that paediatric specialists form part of the trauma team. Assessment of major trauma still follows ATLS protocols. Children can appear to compensate for profound hypovolaemia without hypotension, but once deterioration occurs, it is often rapid and irreversible. Potential physical and mental effects of trauma in children must be considered as many are left with long-term disability. Child protection may also need to be considered in some presentations of injury.

Patterns of injury are also different from adults because of differences in anatomy (e.g. bladder injury due to shallow pelvis), physiology (e.g. higher risk of secondary brain injury due to greater cerebral blood flow) and mechanism of injury (e.g. duodenal contusion from handlebar impact). In general, children sustain proportionately greater energy in blunt trauma than adults owing to their small size. Bone elasticity and increased visceral mobility means severe soft tissue or solid organ injury can occur without a fracture.

In orthopaedic injury, operative stabilisation of fractures is achieved using special implants and techniques. Interfering with the growth plate (physis) can cause growth arrest, so any metalwork must be placed away from the physis.

16 Head and maxillofacial injuries

HEAD INJURIES

INTRODUCTION

Head injury is a potentially devastating problem with an enormous social and economic cost. Up to a million people attend emergency departments in the UK each year following head injury. Using the Glasgow Coma Scale (GCS, Table 16.1) as a clinical indicator, 90% are classified as mild/minor, with scores of 13–15 respectively, 5% as moderate (score 9–12) and 5% as severe (score 3–8). Head injuries cause approximately 3500 deaths each year in the UK, amounting to about 0.6% of all deaths. Figure 16.1 shows how serious injuries represent the tip of an iceberg of the impact of head injury on health care. The greatest burdens are the acute management of all these cases and dealing with the chronic disability these injuries can cause.

Less than half the head injury patients attending emergency departments require CT scanning or hospital admission and only a small proportion require specialist neurosurgical investigation and care. The difficulty is to recognise those at risk without over-investigating or admitting patients unnecessarily. In order to streamline this process, various triage algorithms have been produced, notably NICE guidelines (http://guidance.nice.org.uk/CG56/Guidance—summarized in Box 16.4, see below). The main focus is detecting clinically important brain injuries (and cervical spine injuries—Box 16.1) whilst avoiding admission of those with low risk of sequelae.

PATHOPHYSIOLOGY OF TRAUMATIC BRAIN INJURY

Traumatic brain injuries can be divided into **primary injury**, from the initial trauma, and **secondary brain injury**, which evolves later. Treatment cannot reverse the primary brain injury but aims to minimise sequelae that add to it. Secondary brain injury is mostly caused by raised intracranial pressure (e.g. from intracranial haematoma or brain swelling), ischaemia or hypoxia, and is amenable to treatment by prophylactic measures and timely intervention. Prospects for improving care of head-injured patients depend on prompt triage, adequate resuscitation, ready access to CT scanning, safe and rapid transfer to neurosurgery units, and the availability of specialist critical care.

At the cellular level, brain injury disrupts the neuronal cytoskeleton, which over a few hours can lead to irreversible axonal injury. High levels of glutamate accumulate extracellularly, damaging neighbouring cells and causing a ripple effect of neuronal death and release of further toxic molecules. Potential neuroprotective agents such as glutamate and calcium antagonists have so far proved ineffective.

The brain has minimal capacity to regenerate after injury but in general, the younger the patient the better the prognosis. Young children may make a remarkable functional recovery despite suffering severe injuries because of the plasticity of the developing nervous system, although some will suffer high level cognitive impairment ('executive dysfunction') in their late teens from failure of frontal maturation. In adults, the primary injury consequences are likely to be more severe with advancing age. One important factor here is that the brain atrophies, allowing greater mobility under impact within the cranial vault.

PRIMARY BRAIN INJURY

CONCUSSION

Concussion is a brain injury associated with brief loss of consciousness, typically for only a few minutes. It causes minor cognitive disturbances such as temporary confusion or amnesia. By definition there are no persisting abnormal

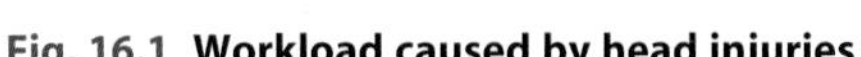

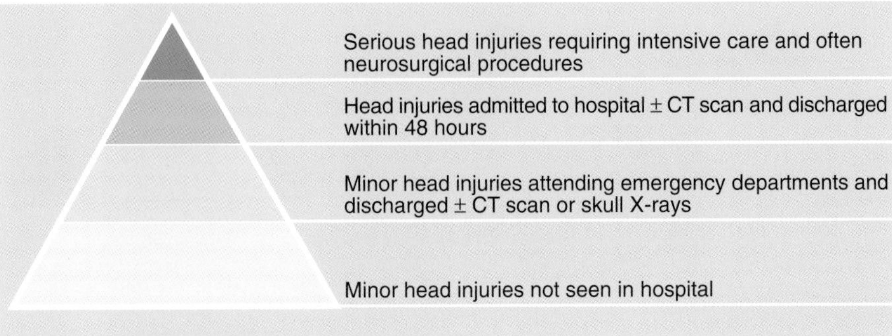

Fig. 16.1 Workload caused by head injuries

Table 16.1 Glasgow Coma Scale (GCS)

Clinical observation	Score*
Eye opening:	
Spontaneous	4
To verbal command	3
To pain	2
None	1
Motor response:	
Obeys commands	6
Localises pain	5
Flexion withdrawal to pain	4
Abnormal flexion (decorticate)	3
Extension to pain (decerebrate)	2
None	1
Verbal response:	
Orientated	5
Confused conversation	4
Inappropriate words	3
Incomprehensible words	2
None	1

*On this scale, a patient's Glasgow Coma score is the sum of the scores from all three sections. The worst total score is 3, the best is 15. After the initial score, the observations and scoring are repeated at intervals to look for deterioration

neurological signs although some patients may report long-term symptoms such as headache, impaired concentration, poor short-term memory and altered affect (the post-concussional syndrome, see below).

DIFFUSE AXONAL INJURY

Diffuse axonal injury (DAI) typically follows significant rotational acceleration and deceleration forces, causing widespread damage to axonal tracts. DAI can be present without abnormal imaging findings. Abnormalities are seen best on MRI, which demonstrates haemosiderin deposition at the junctions of deep grey and white matter, within white matter tracts, or in the basal ganglia. Typically this type of injury does not lead to raised intracranial pressure. Treatment is supportive. Such injuries may result in substantial cognitive impairment and personality change, with or without physical neurodisability.

Box 16.1 National Institute for Health and Clinical Excellence (NICE) guidelines for assessing cervical spine injuries

Indications for immediate CT or 3-view X-ray imaging of cervical spine

- Patient unable to actively rotate neck 45° to left and right
- Not possible to test range of movement in neck
- Patients with neck pain or tenderness aged 65 or more, or who have suffered a dangerous mechanism of injury

Immediate CT imaging of the cervical spine is indicated as follows:

- GCS < 13 on initial assessment
- The patient has been intubated
- The patient is being scanned for polytrauma
- Where X-ray is not possible or technically inadequate
- Where X-ray is definitely abnormal or suspicious
- If clinical suspicion remains despite a normal X-ray study

FOCAL BRAIN INJURIES

Focal injuries are the result of trauma to localised brain areas and are readily visible on CT scanning. The main lesions are cerebral contusion, laceration or haematoma, all of which may act as space-occupying lesions and are liable to result in secondary brain injury. The site and extent of the primary injury depend on the nature of the damaging force (see Fig. 16.2). Contusions may be small or large and occur either beneath the area of impact (**coup**) or contralateral to it (**contre-coup**), caused by rebound of the brain within the skull at the time of impact (Fig. 16.3). The severity of trauma required to cause focal brain injury will usually result in a period of loss of consciousness, followed by confusion.

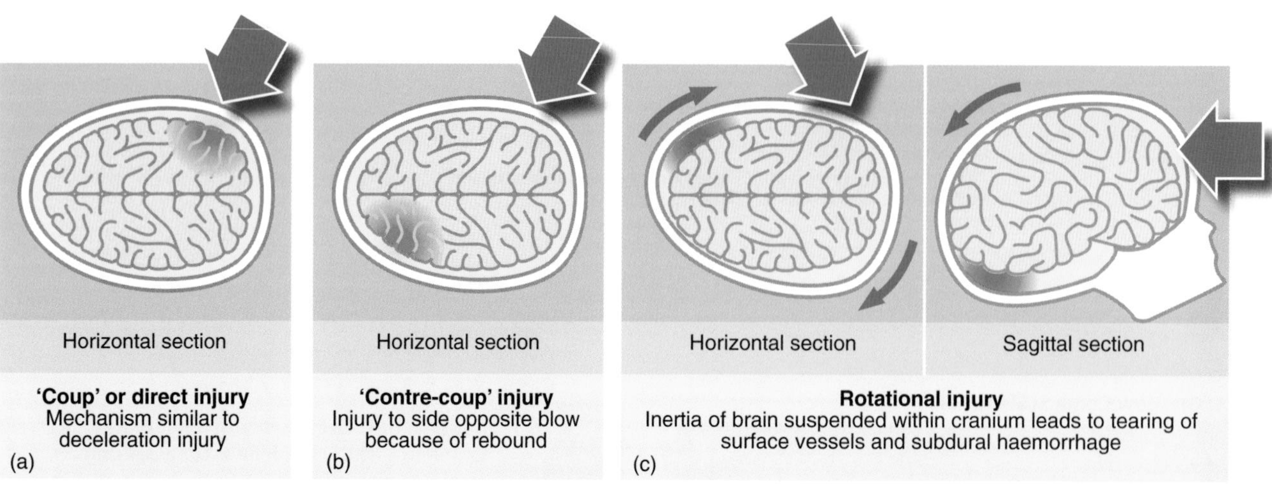

Fig. 16.2 Mechanisms of brain injury
(a) The mechanism of 'coup' or direct injury is similar to a deceleration injury (shown in horizontal section). **(b)** A 'contre-coup' injury affects the side opposite to the blow because of rebound (horizontal section). **(c)** In rotational injury the inertia of the brain suspended within the cranium leads to the tearing of surface vessels and subdural haemorrhage (horizontal and sagittal sections)

CASE HISTORY

Fig. 16.3 Focal brain injury

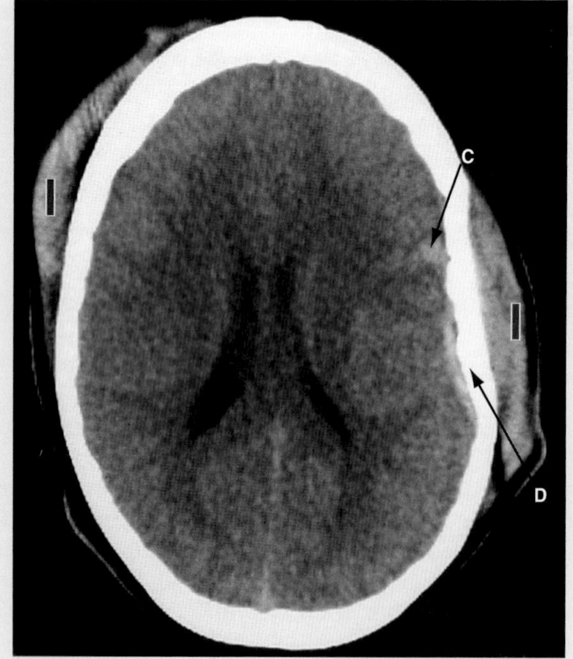

A cyclist was knocked off his bike by a car and suffered a head injury with loss of consciousness of 45 minutes. CT scan of head shows signs of soft tissue injury **I, I** in both left temporal ('coup') and right fronto-parietal regions ('contre-coup'). There is a depressed segment of skull bone in the left temporal region **D** and signs of intracerebral contusion **C** beneath both areas of injury. He gradually recovered without need for operation, but full cerebral functional recovery took several months

SECONDARY BRAIN INJURY

Secondary brain injury can be caused by cerebral hypoxia, intracranial bleeding or infection. These are discussed in detail below.

CEREBRAL HYPOXIA

Central to most mechanisms of brain injury are ischaemia and hypoxia, which lead to **cellular energy failure**. Hypoxia causes cerebral oedema which in turn causes a secondary **rise in intracranial pressure** (ICP) risking further ischaemia. Common causes of hypoxia are airway obstruction, alcohol or drug overdose, chest injury, inhalational pneumonitis, acute respiratory distress syndrome or central respiratory depression. Hypotension due to hypovolaemia also contributes to cerebral hypoxia by reducing cerebral perfusion. Resuscitation aims to prevent or treat hypoxia and hypovolaemia (cerebral perfusion pressure = mean arterial blood pressure – intracranial pressure).

INTRACRANIAL BLEEDING

Post-traumatic intracranial bleeding is classified into **extradural** (epidural), **subdural**, **intracerebral** or **subarachnoid** (see Fig. 16.4). Intracranial bleeding acts as a mass lesion causing a general rise in ICP, whilst local brain compression can cause focal neurological deficit. Untreated, raised ICP may cause 'coning'. One or both **temporal lobes herniate** through the tentorium cerebelli, compressing the third nerve and midbrain, whilst herniation of the cerebellar tonsils through the foramen magnum compresses the medulla, causing neurological deterioration and often death. Rising intracranial pressure manifests initially with deteriorating conscious level. Late clinical signs are:

- An enlarging, unresponsive pupil
- Central respiratory depression
- Falling pulse rate (Cushing's reflex)
- Rising blood pressure (Cushing's reflex)

Extradural (epidural) haemorrhage

Extradural haemorrhage occurs when blood accumulates in the space between dura and calvarium. It is most common in children and younger adults, because their dura is less adherent to the skull. Most have a skull fracture, usually in the temporal region (Fig. 16.5). Almost 90% are due to rupture of an artery,

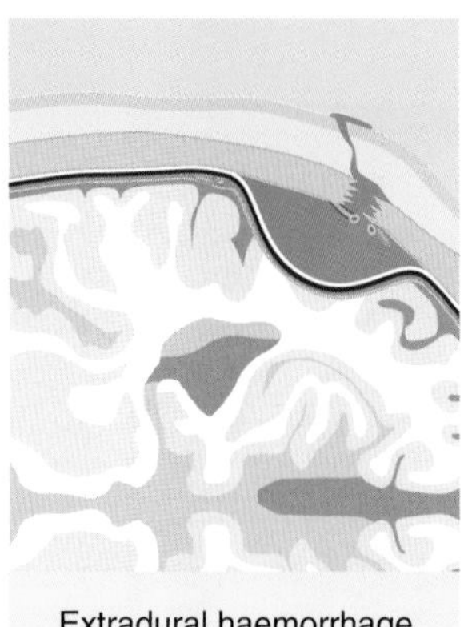

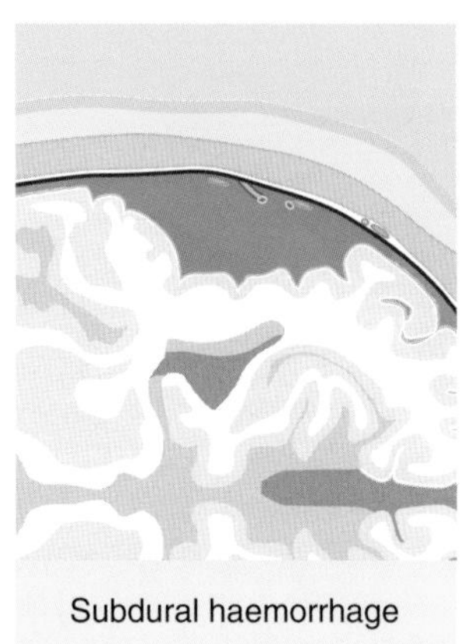

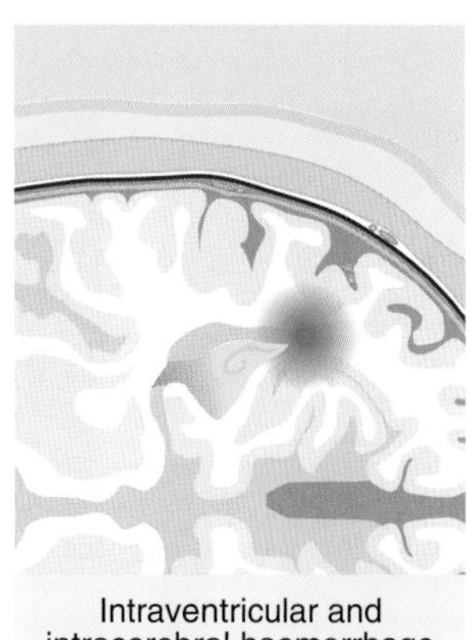

Fig. 16.4 Types of post-traumatic intracranial bleeding

CASE HISTORY

Fig. 16.5 Temporo-parietal fracture with extradural haematoma

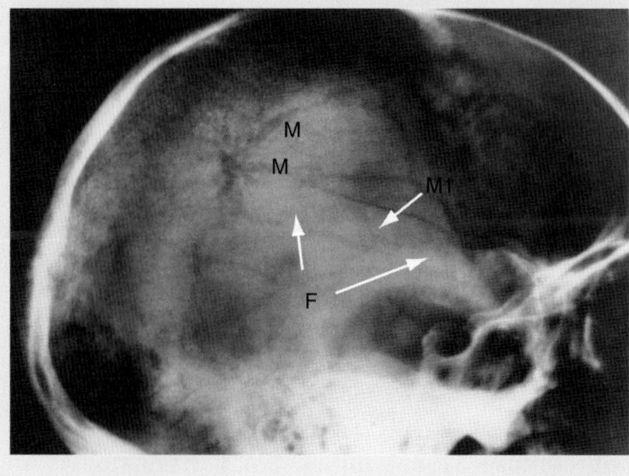

(a)

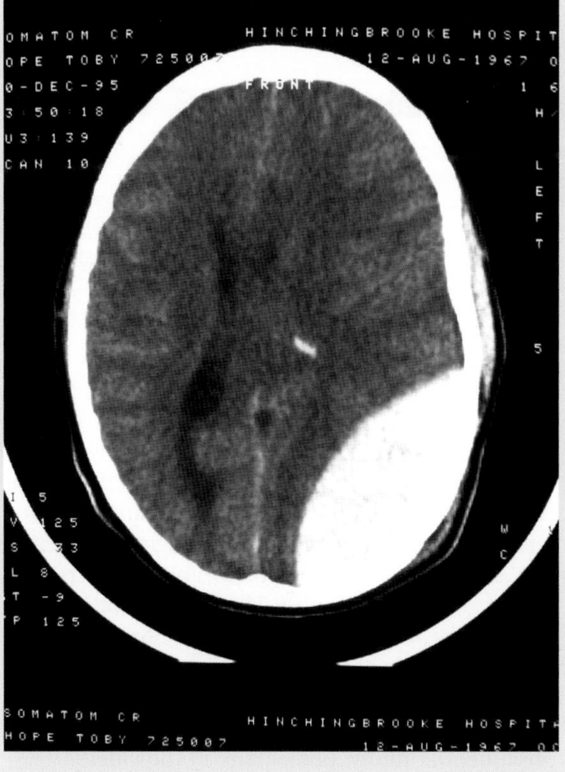

(b)

(a) This 20-year-old man was admitted fully conscious after being knocked off a bicycle but deteriorated rapidly 2 hours later. Lateral skull X-ray showing a linear fracture (arrowed **F**) of the right temporo-parietal bones crossing the course of the anterior branch of the middle meningeal artery **M** on the temporal bone. **(b)** Classical CT appearance of extradural haematoma

usually the middle meningeal or a branch. Immediately after injury causing **loss of consciousness,** in up to half the patients, there will be a **lucid interval**, perhaps with no symptoms other than worsening headache. In either group, this is followed by **deteriorating conscious level**; temporal lobe herniation then leads to compression of the third nerve and **pupillary dilatation**. Death quickly follows unless the haematoma is evacuated rapidly. Emergency CT scanning is indicated to confirm the diagnosis (typically a lentiform-shaped clot—see Fig. 16.5b) and to show its position. With increased awareness of the condition and widespread availability of CT scanning, emergency 'blind' burr hole drainage is almost never appropriate. Urgent transfer to a neurosurgeon for craniotomy is the best course of action, almost without exception.

Subdural haematoma

Subdural haematoma usually results from tearing of veins passing between cerebral cortex and dura, or from injury to vessels on the surface of the brain. Blood accumulates in the large potential space between dura mater and arachnoid mater. The haematoma tends to spread laterally over a wide area (Fig. 16.6). In contrast to extradural haemorrhage, there is usually underlying primary brain injury. Acute subdural

Fig. 16.6 Subdural haematoma

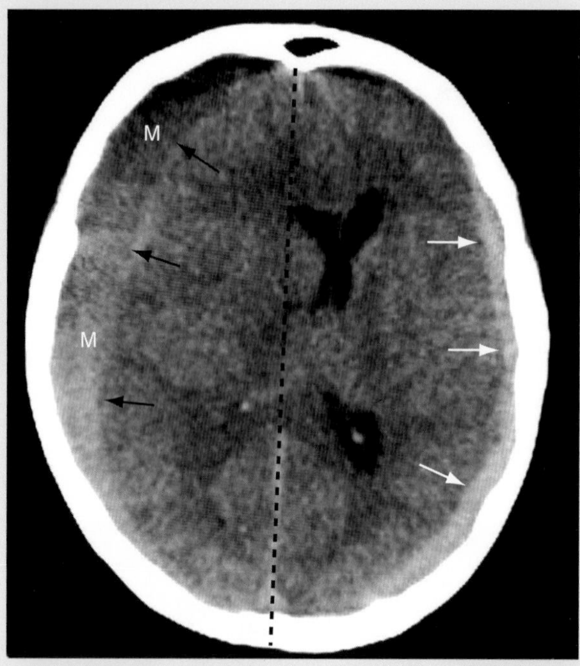

(a)

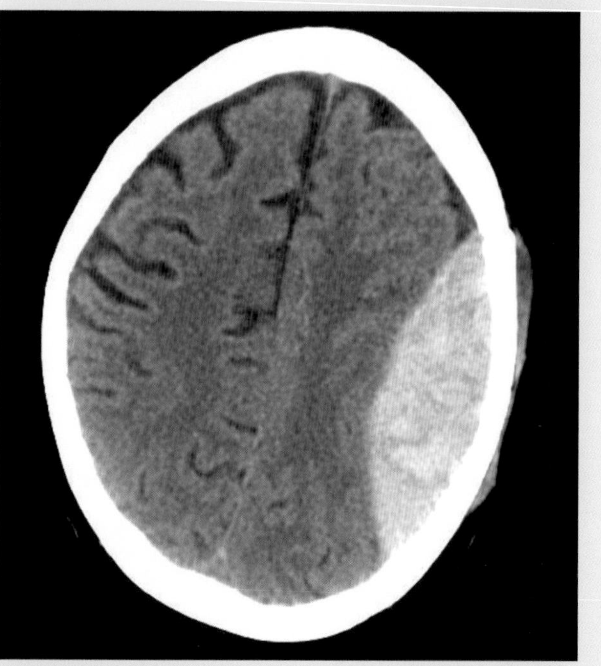

(b)

An elderly man suffered a head injury in a road traffic collision without loss of consciousness 48 hours previously. His conscious level gradually deteriorated and so this CT scan was performed. On the right side, there is a large subdural haematoma of mixed attenuation **M M** (black arrows define the edge of the brain). Such mixed attenuation suggests old liquefying thrombus and is consistent with its origin around the time of the accident. There is a smaller subdural haematoma on the left side (white arrows) of consistent attenuation suggesting that it arose more recently. Note the midline of the brain is shifted to the left by the mass effect of the larger haematoma and there is compression of the lateral ventricles. The patient required neurosurgical drainage

haemorrhage is more common in older adults because the brain is more mobile within the cranial cavity.

In an **acute subdural** haemorrhage, there is usually clinical evidence of brain injury at the outset. A lucid interval between initial loss of consciousness and later deterioration is rare, except where the pathology is tearing of a bridging vein. Evacuation of an acute subdural haematoma cannot be achieved via burr holes because the blood is clotted. Surgical evacuation via craniotomy may halt deterioration but recovery is often incomplete because of the underlying brain injury. With increasing use of anticoagulation and antiplatelet therapy, acute subdural haematoma is seen more commonly after relatively inconsequential injury, particularly in the elderly.

Chronic subdural haematoma

In the elderly, subdural haematomas may develop gradually following trivial, often unrecalled, head trauma. This is due to the relative ease with which their atrophic brains can accommodate blood under venous pressure. Only as the clot lyses and fluid is drawn into the subdural space by osmosis does the condition manifest, some weeks or months later, as non-specific neurological deterioration, chronic headache or coma. At this point the liquid haematoma can be evacuated via burr holes, and the subdural space irrigated with warm saline.

Intracerebral haemorrhage

Haemorrhage into the brain parenchyma is caused by primary brain injury. Multiple small deep lesions are often associated with diffuse axonal injury. Small haematomas should be managed conservatively and monitored for expansion using serial CT scans. A larger haematoma causing 'mass effect' should be evacuated early to prevent secondary brain damage.

INFECTION

Early debridement of compound depressed fractures is important to minimise the risk of infection. Prophylactic antibiotics are not indicated except in contaminated wounds. There is no evidence to support the use of prophylactic antibiotics in cases of cerebrospinal fluid leakage.

SKULL FRACTURES

THE IMPORTANCE OF SKULL FRACTURES (Figs 16.7 and 16.8)

A skull fracture is a measure of impact severity. Consequently, patients with fractures are much more likely to sustain primary brain damage, and are 30 times more likely to suffer secondary brain injury by the mechanisms described earlier. Depressed fractures are often associated with some injury to the underlying brain.

With the advent of NICE guidelines (Box 16.2), CT is the investigation of choice for the diagnosis of clinically significant head injury. Skull radiographs now play little role in the diagnosis, but may be indicated in some instances, for example suspected non-accidental injury in children or lack of access to CT.

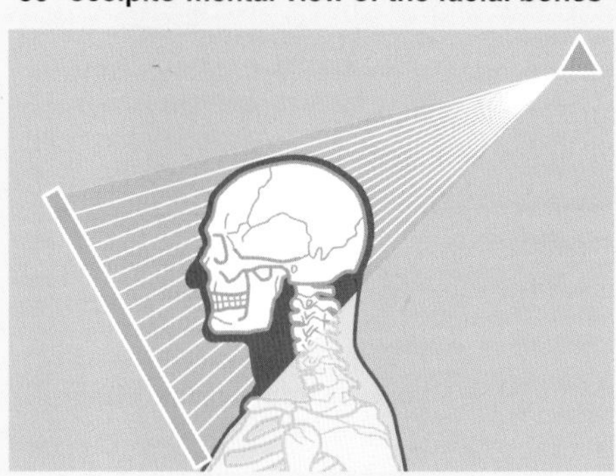

Fig. 16.7 30° Occipito-mental X-ray for facial fractures

TYPES OF SKULL FRACTURE

Linear fractures

These involve mainly the skull vault, often with little external sign of injury, although there may be some overlying scalp bruising or swelling. Linear fractures rarely exhibit displacement unless there are multiple fracture lines.

Depressed fractures

These are usually caused by blunt injuries and the overlying scalp is usually lacerated or severely bruised. Such fractures rarely produce serious primary brain injury unless they are depressed more than the full thickness of the skull vault. Elevation of closed depressed fractures is usually performed for cosmetic reasons.

CASE HISTORY

Fig. 16.8 Standard skull X-ray views and CT scan showing skull fractures

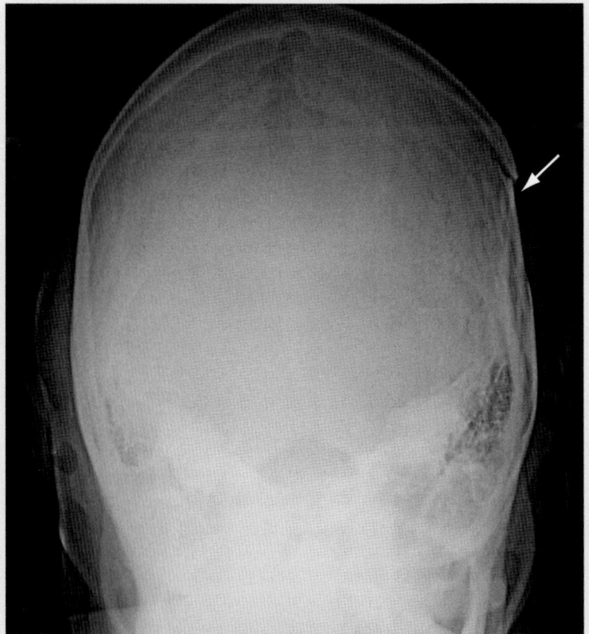

(a)

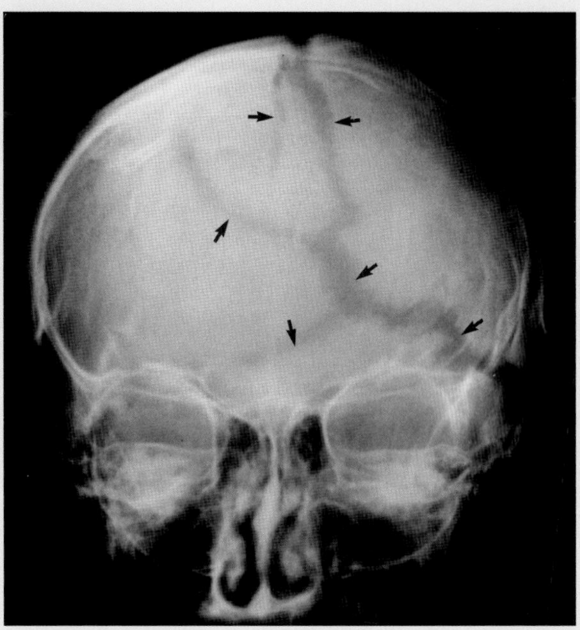

(b)

(c)

(a) Towne's view from a 19-year-old woman after a blunt blow to the side of the head; she was fully conscious. This shows a depressed fracture in the left parietal bone (arrowed). The segment of bone is depressed by more than the thickness of the skull and therefore needed surgically elevating. **(b)** This 24-year-old woman suffered a high impact speed road traffic accident (RTA) and was admitted to hospital deeply unconscious and with deep scalp lacerations. Her GCS was 5. This AP X-ray shows extensive fractures (arrowed) in the parietal, occipital and squamous temporal bones. Because of the lacerations, these fractures were considered compound. **(c)** CT scan of the upper part of the skull vault in a different patient after a road traffic collision showing a normal coronal suture **CS**. There are parietal fractures (arrowed) and diastasis (partial separation) of the lambdoid suture **LS**

Box 16.2 National Institute for Health and Clinical Excellence (NICE) criteria for CT scan

General principles

- First stabilise airways, breathing and circulation (ABC)
- Immediately clinically assess patients with a GCS below 15
- If GCS is 8 or less, involve anaesthetist for airway management and resuscitation
- Perform early CT imaging where appropriate to detect brain and cervical spine injuries (skull X-rays + inpatient observation where CT unavailable)
- Exclude brain injury before attributing depressed conscious level to intoxication
- No systemic analgesia until assessed for conscious level and neurological deficit (local anaesthesia for fractured limbs/other painful injuries)
- Record observations on a standard head injury proforma (paediatric chart for under 16s)

Indications for head CT within 1 hour in adults

- GCS less than 13 at any time since injury
- GCS <15 at 2 hours after injury
- Suspected skull fracture, open or depressed, including signs of basal skull fracture (haemotympanum, 'panda' eyes, cerebrospinal fluid otorrhoea, Battle's sign—Box 16.3)
- Post-traumatic seizure
- Focal neurological deficit
- More than one episode of vomiting
- Coagulopathy

Indications for head CT within 8 hours in adults if the 1 hour criteria do not apply

- Antegrade amnesia (i.e. for events before impact) of more than 30 minutes
- Any loss of consciousness or amnesia plus:
  - — Age 65 years or more
  - — Dangerous mechanism of injury (e.g. pedestrian struck by motor vehicle, occupant ejected from a motor vehicle or fall from more than 1 metre or five stairs)

Box 16.3 Clinical signs of a fracture of the skull base

A basal skull fracture provides a potential route for cerebral infection. Prophylactic antibiotics against meningitis are given for 7 days, or until 7 days after any CSF leak has ceased

Anterior fossa fractures

- Periorbital haematomas (see Fig. 16.13)—usually bilateral 'panda eyes' and limited by the margins of the orbicularis oculi
- Subconjunctival haemorrhage (see Fig. 16.13)—the blood tracks from behind forward and therefore no posterior limit can be seen (unlike localised subconjunctival haematomas that result from direct trauma)
- Cerebrospinal fluid rhinorrhoea—clear fluid running from the nose due to damage to the cribriform plate. Anosmia (loss of sense of smell) is common. Dural repair likely to be required

Middle fossa fractures,

i.e. involving petrous temporal bone

- Cerebrospinal fluid otorrhoea—clear fluid running from the ear via a torn tympanic membrane. Repair not usually required
- Bruising over the mastoid area behind the ear (Battle's sign); may take 24–48 hours to develop

Open (compound) fractures

An open fracture indicates a communication exists between underlying brain and external environment. The communication may be overt (e.g. a penetrating injury), or result from a skull base fracture. Linear and depressed skull fractures can both be compound. There is a high risk of infection in a depressed fracture if the dura is torn, so early debridement and dural closure are indicated. Compound fractures of the base of the skull are diagnosed clinically (Box 16.3) +/- CT. Fluid may be analysed for beta transferrin.

Fractures of the skull base

These usually involve the anterior skull base (frontal/ethmoidal or sphenoidal air sinuses) or the middle cranial fossa (petrous temporal bone). The characteristic clinical features are summarised in Box 16.3.

MANAGEMENT OF HEAD INJURIES

PRE-HOSPITAL MANAGEMENT

Patients with a head injury need a standardised approach as soon as possible after injury such as those outlined in the Advanced Trauma Life Support and Pre-Hospital Life Support courses, both designed to minimise further harm and prevent secondary injury.

Up to the end of the 1990s, triage of head-injured patients was intended to identify those likely to have an evolving intracranial haematoma. The process was based on clinical assessment, with skull X-rays for patients with positive clinical indications. Large numbers of patients had to be admitted for observation because methods were insufficiently reliable. The widespread availability of CT has made it practicable to use this earlier and more often during triage, although there are potential risks of missing early evolving haematomas and some concerns about the radiation dose, especially in children.

A UK National Institute for Health and Clinical Excellence (NICE) committee was charged with evaluating available evidence to construct new guidelines for head injury assessment to reduce delay in detecting life-threatening complications and to ensure better outcomes. The committee concluded that early imaging rather than admission and 'head injury observation' would achieve these aims. The published NICE guidelines use head CT as the primary imaging modality, with **CT diagnosis** replacing **plain X-ray triage**. Skull X-rays plus regular head injury observations should be restricted to infants at risk of intentional injury and where CT is unavailable. The benefits of these new guidelines include early recognition of clinically significant intracranial haematomas and safely avoiding hospital admission where no lesion is found. However, the guidelines specify a short timescale for obtaining CT and this has resource implications. Implementing NICE guidelines increases the head scan rate two- to five-fold (from approximately 2% to 8%), reduces the skull X-ray rate from about 40% to 4%, and reduces hospital admission rates from 10% to 4%. In published studies, the policy change has not resulted in any excess adverse events.

CLINICAL ASSESSMENT

History

The most important factors that indicate potential brain injury and a risk of future complications are **unconsciousness** and amnesia for events before the impact (**retrograde amnesia**). The duration of unconsciousness and amnesia are roughly proportional to the severity of brain injury. If the patient was travelling in a motor vehicle, the extent of injuries to other passengers may give an indication of the energy transfer in the accident. Likewise, knowing the use of seatbelts and helmets can be useful.

Examination

In addition to general examination, a systematic neurological examination must be performed, however trivial the head injury. Particular attention should be paid to:

1. Level of consciousness
2. Pupil size and reactivity
3. Limb movements and responses

The findings should be recorded periodically on a standard head injury proforma, and the Glasgow Coma Scale (GCS) calculated for each set of observations. If there is a deep scalp laceration or a history of penetrating injury, the scalp should be assessed carefully for the presence of a bony defect or step. Because of scalp mobility, any underlying bone injury may not lie directly beneath the scalp wound.

1. Level of consciousness

This is the most important single observation in head injury patients. The GCS (see Table 16.1) is used worldwide to standardise assessment and monitoring of head injuries. Level of consciousness can be categorised simply and reproducibly by this method. Formal assessment should take place after resuscitation and before intubation if possible. Aggressive behaviour in a patient smelling of alcohol or having taken illicit drugs must **not** be assumed to result from intoxication (i.e. removal of social inhibition) because this behaviour can also be a manifestation of brain injury or hypoxia. A thorough examination and CT scan should be performed to exclude significant cerebral injury. In addition to eye opening and verbal responses, the motor response is an important observation. In a patient with impaired conscious level, pressure over the supraorbital nerve at the orbital rim is usually employed to elicit pain. To be scored as being able to localise the pain, the patient's hand should rise above the clavicle.

An assessment of the severity of the head injury can be made on the elicited GCS following resuscitation. The probability of there being an intracranial haematoma likely to need surgery in GCS groups is shown in Table 16.2.

2. Pupil size and reactivity

Pupillary **size** and **response to light** should be assessed, along with the full range of eye movements and, if possible, the visual fields. Normal pupillary size and response to light require the integrity of both 2nd and 3rd cranial nerves. Pupillary changes are a late indicator of developing intracranial hypertension (Table 16.3).

However, benign pupil asymmetry is relatively common in the population and it is important to consider this in conjunction with deteriorating conscious level.

Table 16.2 Probability of intracranial haematoma requiring surgery according to the severity of head injury as assessed by the Glasgow Coma Scale (GCS)

GCS score	Severity of head injury	Probability of haematoma
3–8	Severe	1 in 7
9–12	Moderate	1 in 50
13–14	Mild	1 in 3500

Table 16.3 Significance of pupillary changes in head injury

Pupil finding	Potential significance
Unilateral, dilated pupil	1. Tentorial herniation due to raised intracranial pressure (usually ipsilateral to the side of injury but may be a false localising sign) 2. Direct ocular damage—often associated with hyphaema (bleeding into anterior chamber)
Bilaterally dilated pupil, unreactive to light	Severe brainstem dysfunction
Pinpoint pupils	Primary brainstem injury or drug-induced

3. Limb movements and responses

In a fully conscious patient, tone, power and coordination can be readily assessed. If a subtle abnormality is suspected, the patient should be asked to close the eyes and hold the arms outstretched with palms upwards. Pronation or downward drift on one side indicates brain injury. For the semiconscious or unconscious patient, the pattern of limb response to painful stimuli provides a useful indication of the conscious level, as indicated in the GCS (see Table 16.1).

Ipsilateral hemiparesis may represent Kernohan's phenomenon, also known as the false localising sign. This occurs when an ipsilateral increase in brain pressure pushes the tentorial edge against the opposite cerebral peduncle.

IMAGING FOR SUSPECTED HEAD INJURIES

The published NICE guidelines for head and cervical spine imaging are summarised in Box 16.2.

PRACTICAL MANAGEMENT OF HEAD INJURIES

- Patients with a GCS of 15 and no risk factors demanding inpatient observation (alcohol intoxication, etc.) can be discharged safely to the care of a responsible adult with standard head injury advice. Patients with risk factors requiring admission should be observed in a ward with experience in managing head injuries (Box 16.4)
- Patients with reduced scores require early CT scanning, following NICE guidelines (Box 16.2)
- Patients with normal scans in whom GCS returns to normal can be discharged, unless other injuries or social circumstances make admission necessary (see Box 16.4)
- Patients *admitted* with uncomplicated minor head injuries who are fully alert can safely be allowed to go home after 24 hours of neurological observation
- Severely head-injured patients require urgent discussion with the local neurosurgery unit, resuscitation and transfer once resuscitated and stabilised

Head injury observations

The necessary observations for patients admitted to hospital are shown in Table 16.4. These are sufficiently sensitive to give early warning of developing complications. The frequency of observation depends on the state of the patient. If there is a skull fracture or any suggestion of reduced consciousness, confusion, disorientation, alcohol or drug effects, observations should be made at 30-minute intervals until a GCS of 15 is maintained, then hourly for 4 hours, then 2 hourly after that. Observations are recorded or plotted on a special **head injury proforma** so that deterioration will be immediately obvious and can be reported to medical staff at once. Note that transient unconsciousness or amnesia with full recovery is not necessarily an indication for admission of an adult, but may be so in a child, and patients with head injuries may have other serious internal injuries that are easily overlooked.

Indications for prompt neurosurgical referral after head injury

The care of all patients with new, surgically significant abnormalities on imaging should be discussed with a neurosurgeon and, where possible, the imaging linked electronically. Other criteria for referral include:

- Persisting coma (GCS less than or equal to 8) after resuscitation
- Unexplained confusion for more than 4 hours
- Deterioration in GCS after admission (greater attention should be paid to deterioration of motor response)
- Progressive focal neurological signs
- A seizure without full recovery
- Definite or suspected penetrating injury
- A cerebrospinal fluid leak

Management of moderate and severe head injuries

Most trauma deaths result from head injuries or from multiple injuries involving chest, abdomen and limbs. Some head injuries are so severe as to preclude survival, whilst others require urgent recognition and surgical decompression, e.g. extradural haemorrhage. The report of the Working Party on Head Injuries (Society of British Neurological Surgeons, 1998) recommended a maximum delay of 4 hours between the injury and neurosurgical intervention.

Box 16.4 National Institute for Health and Clinical Excellence (NICE) criteria for admission to hospital following a head injury where CT is available and criteria have been followed

- New and clinically significant abnormalities found on imaging
- GCS has not returned to 15 after imaging, regardless of imaging results
- When CT scanning is indicated but cannot be done within the appropriate period
- Continuing worrying signs, e.g. persistent vomiting, severe headache
- Other sources of concern, e.g. drug or alcohol intoxication, other injuries, shock, suspected non-accidental injury, meningism or cerebrospinal fluid leak from nose or ear

Table 16.4 Essential observations for head injury patients (findings should be recorded on a standard head injury proforma)

Observation	Sign of neurological deterioration
Conscious level (GCS)	Falling score
Pupil size and light response	Dilatation, loss of light reaction or developing asymmetry
Respiratory pattern and rate	Irregularity, slowing or reduced depth of breathing
Developing neurological signs	Focal signs point to localised intracranial damage
Pulse rate	Falling pulse rate (late sign)
Blood pressure	Rising blood pressure (late sign)

Other avoidable deaths from head injury relate to inadequate ventilation and resuscitation. This leads to hypoxaemia, hypercarbia and cerebral swelling, compounding the rising intracranial pressure. If patients are combative or severely agitated, there may be a need for general anaesthesia to enable control of PCO_2.

Initial management

Any patient with focal neurological signs, whose conscious level is moderately depressed (GCS 14 or less) or who is unconscious, must be considered to have a significant head injury. Patients should be resuscitated along ATLS lines, focusing on secondary brain injury prevention, prioritisation of other injuries and the timing of CT scanning. If the receiving hospital does not have CT scanning facilities, the patient may need to be transferred to a regional centre after resuscitation. Patients requiring urgent neurosurgery should be transferred promptly, but only after adequate resuscitation.

Continuing care

Management of severe head injury ideally requires specialist care from neurosurgeons and neurointensivists, and transfer to a neurosurgical unit should be seriously considered. Continuing care of the patient with a stable serious brain injury (usually in a neurological critical care unit) involves some or all of the following procedures:

- **Intensive monitoring** of vital signs and neurological status
- **Endotracheal intubation and artificial ventilation**
- **Nasogastric aspiration** for any unconscious patient to prevent inhalation of gastric contents
- **Monitoring of fluid and electrolyte balance**
- **Monitoring of intracranial pressure** using a surgically implanted ICP monitoring device
- **Measures for control of raised intracranial pressure**— escalating protocols are employed for incremental rises, including controlled hyperventilation (reducing PCO_2 causes cerebral vasoconstriction, reduced cerebral oedema and hence reduced intracranial pressure), CSF drainage, mannitol or hypertonic saline infusion (for its osmotic effect in reducing cerebral oedema), hypothermia, barbiturates and decompressive craniectomy
- **Measures to maintain cerebral perfusion pressure**— (volume expansion and inotropic support)

Rehabilitation

The risk of long-term disability following severe head injury is high, and significant cognitive dysfunction may persist in patients after good physical recovery. Even patients with apparently minor brain injury may be moderately or severely disabled a year after injury (**post-concussion syndrome**). Problems include headache, dizziness, mental deficits, slowness of thought, poor concentration, difficulty communicating, inability to work, poor performance at school and difficulties with self-care.

Potential or actual disability needs to be recognised early, ideally before discharge from hospital. However, no reliable mechanism has been found to exclude patients safely from the need for follow-up. Ideally, all head injury patients should be followed up at least once, and expert and prolonged follow-up is mandatory following severe injuries. Long-term physical and cognitive recovery after serious brain injury is a slow process and involves a multidisciplinary approach, often led by a dedicated rehabilitation team, including physiotherapy, occupational therapy, speech therapy and neuropsychology. Patients can easily languish in the community unless the problems are recognised and supportive measures are put into place.

MAXILLOFACIAL INJURIES

GENERAL PRINCIPLES

Fractures of the facial skeleton are common, particularly after sporting injuries, road accidents and fights. The main fractures involve the mandible, the middle third of the face, the nasal bones, the orbit and the zygoma. Facial fractures rarely pose urgent management problems except for major middle third fractures (in which the upper jaw becomes detached from the base of the skull) and multiple mandibular fractures; both may cause upper airway obstruction, and these patients may require endotracheal intubation or cricothyroidotomy to safeguard the airway. Facial fractures are generally managed by maxillofacial surgeons, who may not be available in smaller hospitals. In most cases, delaying treatment for a few days does not adversely affect the outcome.

EXAMINATION FOR FACIAL FRACTURES

In any facial injury, the contour of the facial bones should be carefully palpated and the eyes examined before oedema develops and obscures underlying bony deformities. The extraocular muscle attachments may be disrupted by orbital wall fractures so the full range of eye movements must be formally examined and the patient questioned about diplopia in all positions. The patient should be asked if 'the teeth bite together normally', and the mouth should be examined for missing or displaced teeth and for the state of dental occlusion. Abnormalities of occlusion are a common and sensitive sign of a jaw fracture that might otherwise be missed. The full range of mandibular movements should also be checked to exclude fractures or dislocations involving the mandibular condyles.

RADIOLOGY

If facial fractures are suspected, X-rays should be taken of the facial bones with views chosen according to the bones under suspicion. Interpretation of facial radiographs can be difficult for the non-specialist but most fractures can be identified if the main bony contours are traced and compared with the opposite side. Opacities or fluid levels in the maxillary sinuses (antra) usually represent haematoma. This commonly follows fractures of the bones surrounding the maxillary sinuses, e.g. zygoma or orbital floor.

MANDIBULAR FRACTURES

The common sites of mandibular fractures are shown in Figure 16.9. Because of the effects of oblique trauma, a fracture on one side is often accompanied by a fracture on the other side in a different position, e.g. body of mandible on one side and condylar neck on the other. Fracture lines tend to occur through points of weakness, e.g. mental foramina, unerupted third molar teeth or condylar necks. Most undisplaced mandibular fractures need no active intervention but displaced fractures require fixation. This can be achieved by wiring the lower teeth to the upper teeth, by direct wiring of the bones or (more often these days) by internal plate fixation (see Fig. 16.10). Any fracture passing through a tooth socket defines the fracture as 'compound' and prophylactic antibiotics should be administered.

FRACTURES OF THE MIDDLE THIRD OF THE FACE

Fractures of the middle third of the facial skeleton range from detachment of the palate and dental arch to complete separation of the middle third complex from the skull base. Diagnosis is based on clinical assessment. A simple test is to grasp the upper teeth or jaw between the fingers and attempt to move them independently of the skull. Treatment may involve disimpaction and usually requires sophisticated external fixation to the skull or internal plate fixation afterwards.

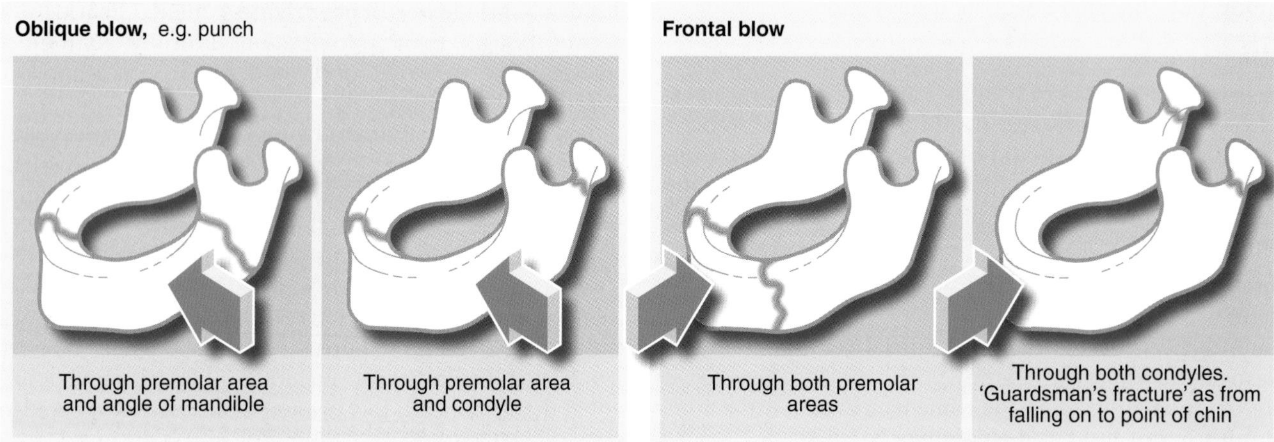

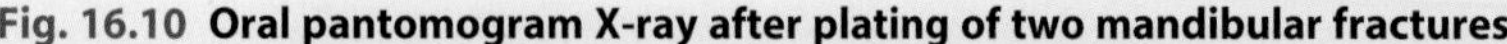
Fig. 16.9 Common sites of mandibular fractures

CASE HISTORY

Fig. 16.10 Oral pantomogram X-ray after plating of two mandibular fractures

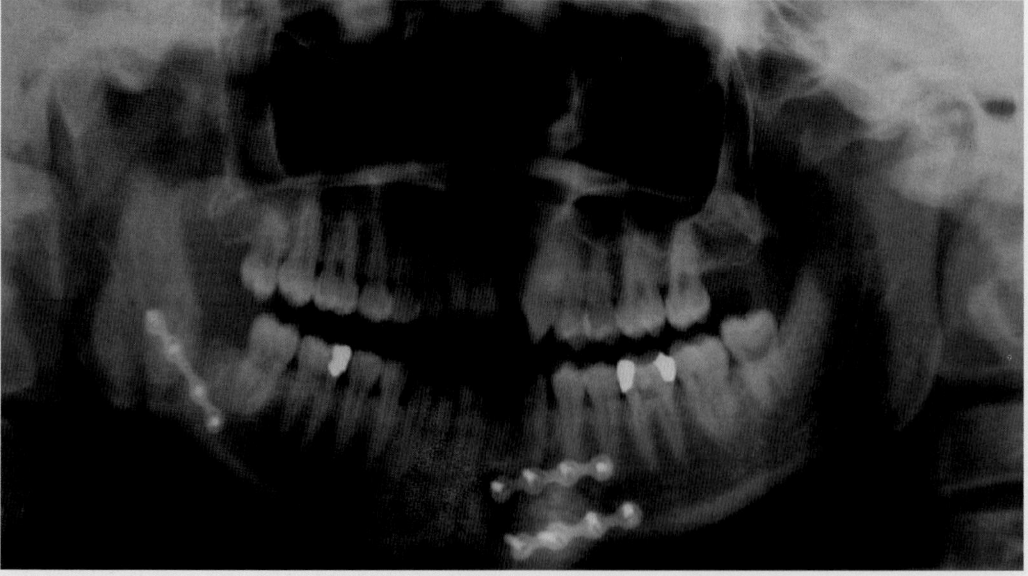

After a blow to the chin, fractures occurred at the angle of the mandible on the right and the anterior body on the left (see **Fig. 16.9**). Both fractures were immobilised by direct bone plating

FRACTURES OF THE NASAL BONES

Trauma to the nose is common and often results in nasal bone fracture. Less often, fracture dislocation of the septum occurs and may interfere with the nasal airway. Diagnosis is made on clinical grounds with the main features being flattening or lateral displacement of the nasal bridge. Bleeding from the nose often indicates a nasal fracture. The fracture is usually reduced several days later by an ENT or maxillofacial surgeon.

FRACTURES OF THE ORBIT AND ZYGOMA

DEPRESSED FRACTURES OF THE ZYGOMA

A depressed fracture of the zygoma (see Fig. 16.11) is the most common orbital fracture and results from a blow to the cheek. The fracture line usually passes through the infraorbital foramen and causes a palpable step in the inferior orbital margin. The infraorbital nerve becomes compressed with any substantial degree of depression, causing paraesthesia or numbness in the upper lip, upper teeth and buccal mucosa on that side. Diagnosis may be suspected by flattening of the cheek contour; this is best seen from above and behind the patient. Overlying oedema may obscure a depressed fracture, and these patients warrant radiological examination. An associated fracture of the lateral orbital wall may produce enough bleeding for it to track forward under the conjunctiva. This type of subconjunctival haemorrhage has no visible posterior limit and is the characteristic sign of an orbital wall fracture (Fig. 16.12).

Treatment is indicated if there is inferior orbital nerve compression or a cosmetically unacceptable deformity. Reduction is usually accomplished via a temporal approach, sliding an elevator under the root of the zygoma, deep to the temporalis fascia.

BLOW-OUT FRACTURES OF THE ORBIT

A direct frontal blow to the orbit from an object about the size of a squash ball (3–4 cm) may act like a plunger, causing a **'blow-out' fracture** of the orbital floor without damaging the orbital margin. Blow-out fractures can also occur after a blow to the inferior orbital rim which then causes a ripple effect, fracturing the orbital floor whilst the rim remains intact. The blow-out most commonly involves the floor of the orbit where the bony walls are thinnest. This causes herniation of peribulbar fat into the maxillary sinus and disrupts the function of the extraocular muscles, causing diplopia and restricted upward gaze (see Figs 16.13 and 16.14). Hence it is important to test eye movements in any patient with a facial injury. Diagnosis is suggested by finding an antral opacity (haematoma) on occipito-mental X-ray, but CT scanning of the orbit is required if the bony defect needs to be demonstrated. Treatment involves exploring the orbital floor and may require a bone graft or silicone implant.

INJURIES TO THE TEETH

Fractures and avulsions of the anterior teeth are common and may require immediate treatment in the emergency department. Correct first-aid treatment may preserve teeth which would otherwise be lost. Fractures involving the loss of more than one-third of the crown should be seen urgently by a

(a)

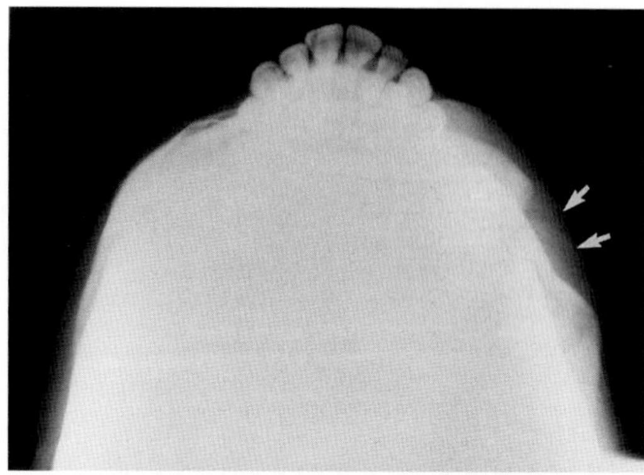

(b)

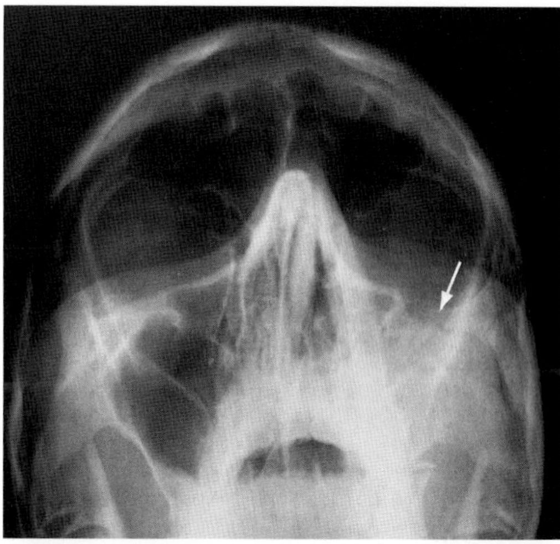

(c)

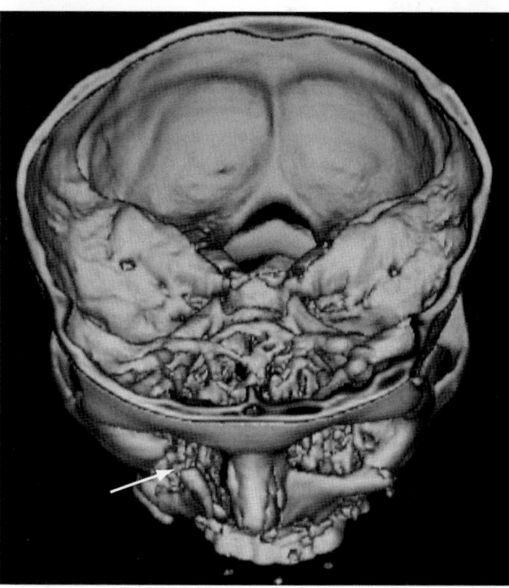

Fig. 16.11 Depressed zygomatic fractures
(a) Submento-vertical projection of a 43-year-old man who had been punched on the left cheek showing a depressed fracture of the zygomatic arch (arrowed). **(b)** 30° Occipito-mental radiograph after a similar injury in a different patient. This patient had a depressed 'tripod' fracture of the zygoma manifest by discontinuity of the lower orbital margin (arrowed). Note that since the roof of the maxilla is involved, the maxillary sinus (the antrum) has typically filled with blood and is rendered radiopaque. **(c)** 3D reconstruction of CT scans showing a severely depressed fracture of right lower orbital rim involving maxilla and zygomatic body (arrowed). The left lower orbital rim is also fractured and displaced

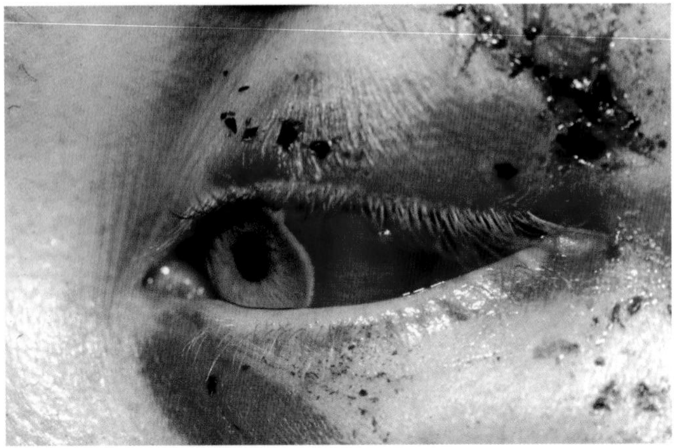

Fig. 16.12 Subconjunctival haematoma following a head injury
This 14-year-old boy fell off his bicycle and momentarily lost consciousness. This photograph shows a subconjunctival haematoma with no posterior limit indicating a fracture of the orbital wall, in this case the petrous temporal bone of the base of the skull

Fig. 16.14 X-ray appearance of blow-out fracture of orbital floor

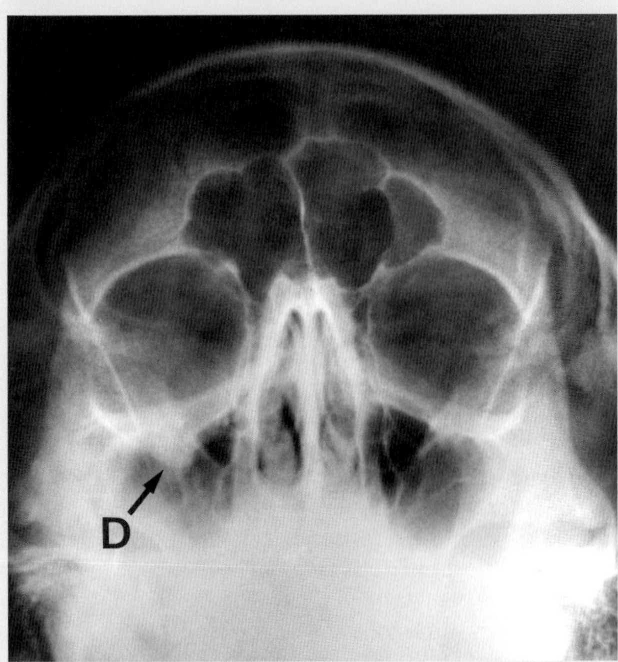

This 30-year-old man was hit on the right eye by a squash ball, causing a blow-out fracture of the orbital floor by hydraulic pressure. Orbital fat and extraocular muscles have been forced into the maxillary antrum and held there by the fractured bone edges. This causes the characteristic 'hanging drop' sign **D**. Upward gaze is restricted, resulting in vertical diplopia

(a)

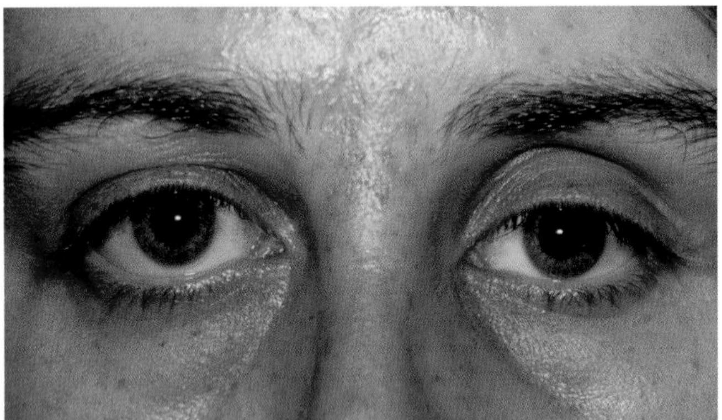

(b)

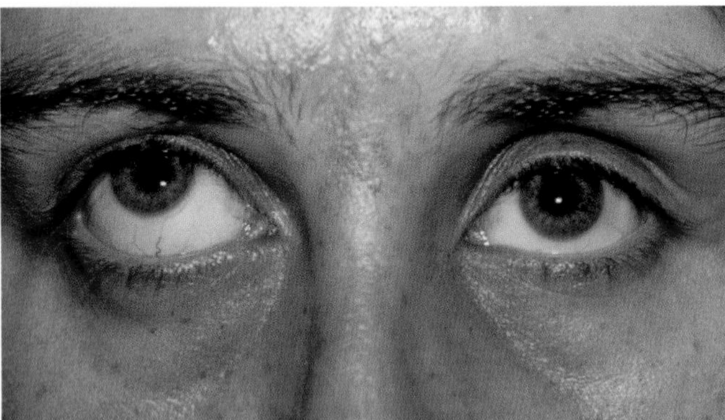

Fig. 16.13 Blow-out fracture of orbital floor
(a) This young man was punched in the left eye, causing a blow-out fracture of the orbital floor. **(b)** Note failure of upward gaze on the left due to trapping of the extraocular muscles in the fractured orbital floor

dental surgeon as the dental pulp may be exposed or endangered. Partially avulsed teeth need to be pushed back into position. This can usually be done with the fingers after local anaesthetic infiltration. Urgent dental referral for tooth splintage and root canal treatment is then required.

If a tooth is completely avulsed, it can often be successfully reimplanted by a dentist if it has been carefully cleaned and wrapped in a sterile, saline-soaked swab. Note that success with reimplantation diminishes proportionately to the time the tooth is out of the socket: under 30 minutes gives the best results. The discovery of missing or broken teeth in an unconscious patient should alert the examining doctor to the possibility of inhalation of tooth material into the bronchi or impaction in the lips or pharynx. Chest X-ray and examination of the perioral soft tissues should be performed in these cases.

COMMON ENT EMERGENCIES

The most common ear, nose and throat emergencies are illustrated in Figure 16.15.

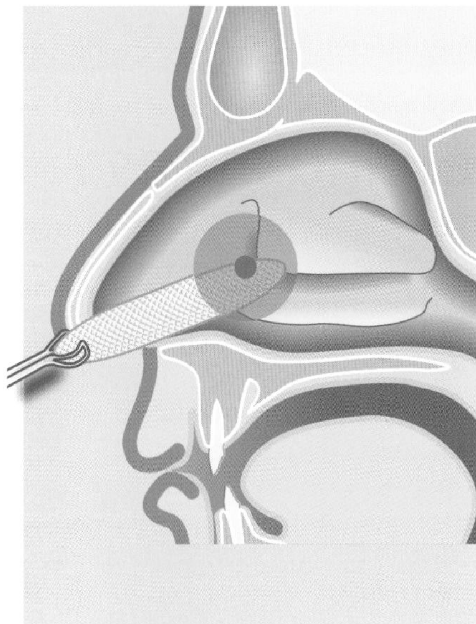

1. Active epistaxis

Management: apply topical local anaesthetic (e.g. Instagel). Pack gently with ribbon gauze or preformed sponge

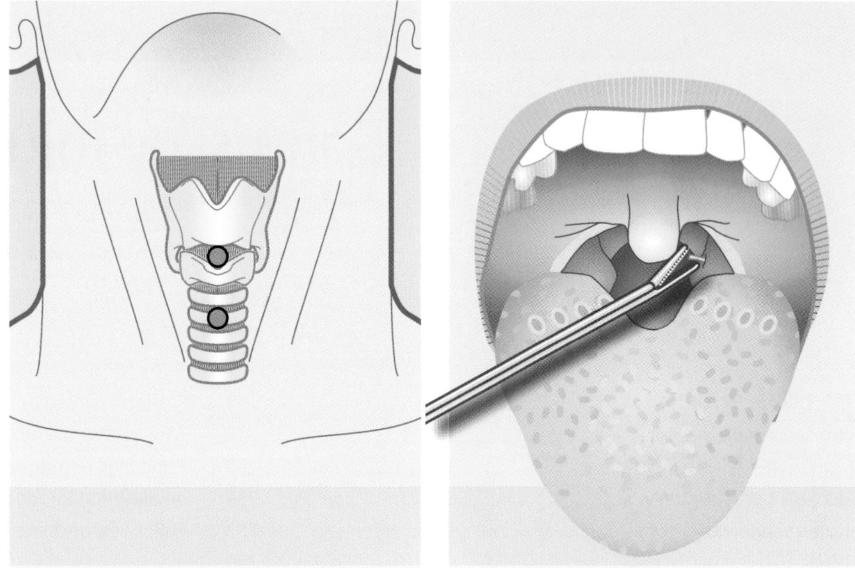

2. Acute upper airway obstruction

Management: sweep mouth with gloved finger for foreign body/denture; Heimlich manoeuvre to dislodge food inhaled into larynx. If these fail; stab laryngotomy (or rapid tracheostomy if trained and equipment to hand).
If in a restaurant, extend neck with rolled clothes under shoulders. Incise with steak knife and insert sheath from ball point pen

3. Fish bone in throat

Management: patient demonstrates position with finger tip, then apply lidocaine spray. Remove with forceps, using a headlight if available

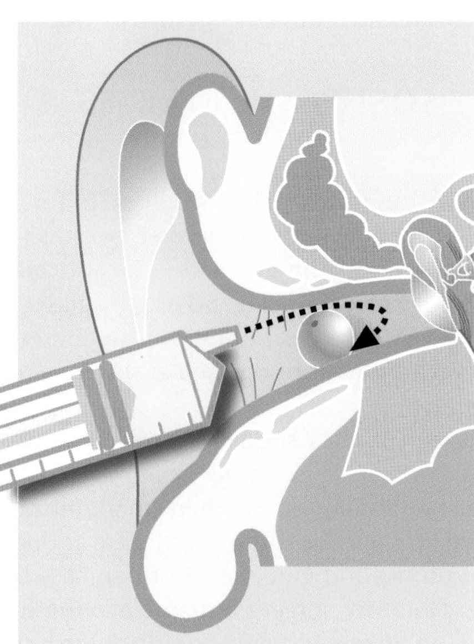

4. Foreign body in ear

Most commonly a bead in a child's ear.
Management: remove using special sucker tip or gently syringe using a 20 ml syringe and water at body temperature.
No forceps!

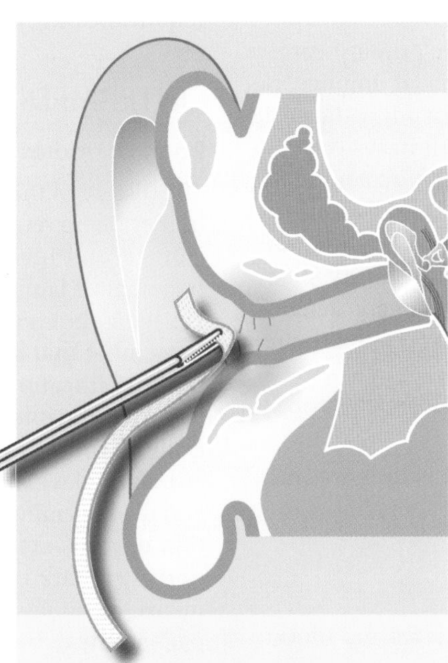

5. External otitis

Cause — usually *Staphylococcus* infecting hair follicles after swimming.
Management: Narrow ribbon gauze, soaked in antibiotic ointment + oral antibiotic against *Staphylococcus*, e.g. flucloxacillin

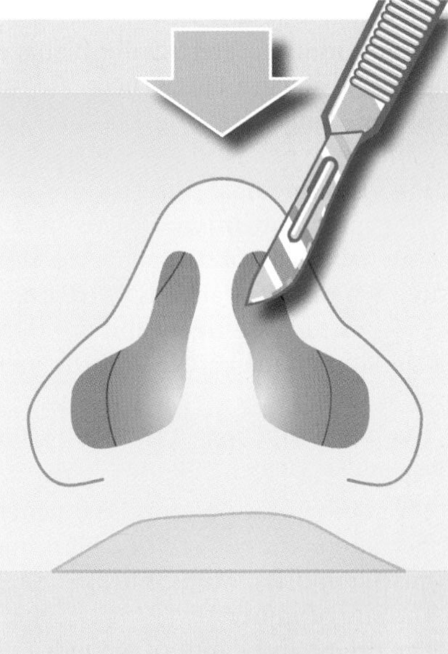

6. Septal haematoma following direct trauma

Note that the nose is blocked bilaterally.
Management: incise and drain under local anaesthetic. If untreated likely to become a septal abscess leading to collapse of cartilage

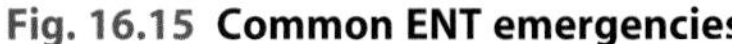

Fig. 16.15 Common ENT emergencies

17 Soft tissue injuries and burns

SOFT TISSUE INJURIES

Soft tissue injuries are defined here as cuts, lacerations, crushing injuries, missile injuries and impalements not involving bone or body cavities. The priority for treating soft tissue injuries depends on the primary survey determined by the ABCDE system (Ch. 15).

Minor injuries are usually managed in primary care or emergency departments. These are superficial injuries not involving 'danger areas' such as the eye or hand, without significant nerve or vascular injury and without heavy contamination. **Intermediate injuries** are not life-threatening but require special attention, usually in hospital. **Major injuries** require more complex management in hospital, often with more than one specialty involved, e.g. general surgery, plastic and reconstructive surgery and orthopaedic surgery. Penetrating and other major **eye injuries** need expert ophthalmic surgical care.

The management of a soft tissue injury depends upon the following factors:

- The mechanism of injury (e.g. penetrating knife wounds, lacerations in road crashes, blast injuries, gunshot and missile injuries, burns, bites)
- The site of injury
- The extent and depth of wounds
- The types of tissue involved including nerves and blood vessels
- The extent of tissue devitalisation
- Any contamination (e.g. with road dirt, soil or potential bacterial inoculation with animal or human bites)
- The possibility of retained foreign bodies

MINOR SOFT TISSUE INJURIES

Most minor wounds can be cleaned and sutured immediately or closed with tissue glue. Local anaesthesia is usually required. Tetanus must be considered in any wound more than purely superficial, and tetanus toxoid given if immunisation is inadequate. Deep, soil-contaminated wounds (however small) in a non-immunised patient also warrant prophylactic penicillin. **Grazes** may need cleaning of road dirt but generally just require dressing with non-adherent dressings such as Mepitel®.

INTERMEDIATE SOFT TISSUE INJURIES

Foreign bodies

The history of the injury can indicate the likelihood of foreign bodies being retained in the wound. The main types are agricultural and road dirt, wood splinters, and glass and metal fragments. Plain radiology reveals metal and usually glass (see Fig. 17.1) but a negative X-ray does not exclude its presence. Remember that a foreign body unrecognised at the time may result in litigation later.

As a principle, foreign bodies should be removed, especially if organic (e.g. wood) or likely to be contaminated. However, glass and metal fragments are often small, multiple and deeply embedded and may be difficult to locate at operation despite X-ray or ultrasound guidance. In these, it is best not to embark on exploratory surgery but to leave the fragments in situ where they rarely cause complications. The patient must be informed about what has been left and warned that fragments often work their way to the surface and are shed, and to return if problems occur. This must be recorded in the patient's notes in case of future legal action.

Flap lacerations

Relatively minor trauma to the tibia commonly produces a V-shaped **flap laceration** (Fig. 17.2) particularly in older patients or in patients on long-term corticosteroids. If untreated, this injury habitually fails to heal because of poor blood supply to flap and underlying tissue. Attempting to suture or tape a flap into place increases tension, causing

Fig. 17.1 Glass in soft tissue wounds

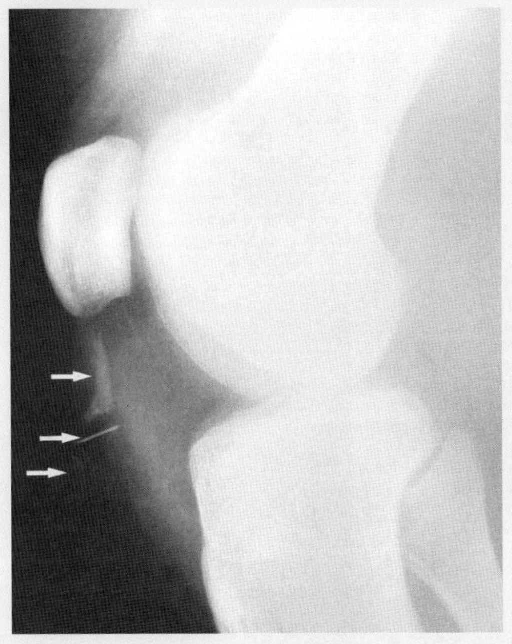

(a)

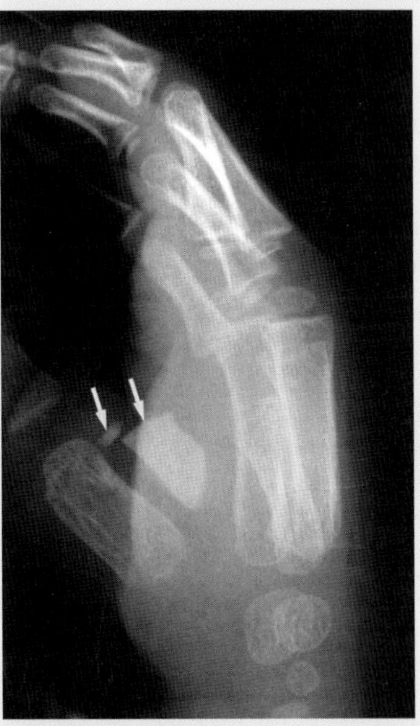

(b)

(**a**) A 19-year-old woman with lacerations near the knee after falling on to broken glass. Note several fragments of glass (arrowed) in the infrapatellar soft tissues. (**b**) Fragments of glass (arrowed) in the palm of a 12-year-old boy after he fell through a glass door. In both these cases, the fragments were missed by casualty officers because X-rays were not requested despite a history of glass injury

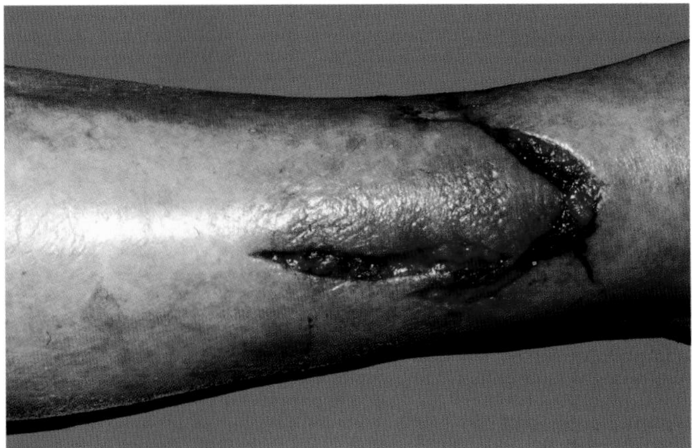

Fig. 17.2 Flap laceration
This wound was caused by a fall in which the patient's shin was scraped on a stone step. It is tempting to suture such a wound, but if this is done the flap will invariably undergo necrosis

ischaemia, tissue loss and ulceration. The most effective management is early excision and immediate split skin grafting. This can be performed under local anaesthesia and takes an average of 2 weeks to heal.

Facial lacerations

Minor facial lacerations heal well and can be primarily sutured in the accident department after careful cleaning. Infection is rare because of the excellent blood supply. Even ragged skin edges do not become devitalised and trimming is rarely necessary. The main consideration is the cosmetic outcome, so great care should be taken with technique, employing general anaesthesia if necessary. Complex lacerations, lacerations across the lip margin or eyelid and areas of substantial skin loss, especially on children and young people, should ideally be managed by plastic surgeons (see next section).

Scalp lacerations

With scalp lacerations, brain injury and skull fracture must be excluded and then determine whether the aponeurotic layer (galea) has been breached. Haemostasis must also be achieved; it is easy to underestimate blood loss from scalp lacerations, sometimes sufficient to cause hypovolaemic shock in the elderly. Assessment and thorough exploration is made easier by shaving the wound edges; large lacerations may need exploring under general anaesthesia. If the aponeurosis is breached, it should be repaired separately to prevent a subaponeurotic haematoma vulnerable to infection. Care should be paid to haemostasis from major scalp blood vessels lying in the superficial fascia between dermis and aponeurosis. Dense collagenous bands cross the area and can prevent torn vessels contracting, hindering the spontaneous arrest of bleeding. Torn vessels need to be individually ligated or sutured.

MAJOR SOFT TISSUE INJURIES

Major injuries of soft tissues alone requiring hospital treatment are uncommon and can be classified as in Box 17.1. A primary survey (Ch. 15) determines the order injuries are managed, with life-threatening injuries treated first. For other injuries, the urgency depends on the potential for deterioration (e.g. blood loss, ischaemia or loss of an eye), the risk of

Box 17.1 Classification of major soft tissue injuries

- Vital part of the body, e.g. eye, hand, extensive facial lacerations
- Vascular injuries involving blood loss or ischaemia
- Nerve and tendon injuries requiring meticulous surgical repair
- Animal or human bites
- Gunshot, missile and stab wounds
- Traumatic amputation of digits or limbs
- Injuries involving substantial skin loss likely to need skin grafting, e.g. degloving injuries to limbs
- Contamination with soil, road dirt—requiring debridement and/or prophylactic immune serum or antibiotics
- Crush injuries
- Chemical injuries, e.g. acid, bleach, fertiliser
- Burns of more than 5% of body area or involving inhalation

infection and the availability of the necessary specialists. Contused or contaminated wounds need early cleansing and excision of all devitalised tissue (debridement), usually under GA. If substantially contaminated, wounds are often left unsutured to prevent wound infection and are then sutured a few days later by **delayed primary closure**. Less commonly, wounds are left open and are allowed to heal by **secondary intention** (see Ch. 3, p. 36). Wounds involving skin loss may need early skin grafting.

INJURY TO A VITAL PART OF THE BODY

Eye

Injuries greater than 'sand in the eye' are best managed by ophthalmic specialists who require a slit lamp and other instruments to assess the injury. Typical injuries include abrasions to the cornea, penetrating injuries (dart or pellets) and firework injuries.

Neck

Penetrating injuries to the neck must be treated with respect. Vital structures are concentrated here and may be injured. These include major arteries and veins (carotid, jugular, subclavian, vertebral), the brachial plexus, some cranial nerves, the cervical sympathetic chain (see Fig. 17.3), and lung and pleura.

Lacerations to the limbs and hands

(for *Traumatic amputation*, see p. 236)

The main considerations with this type of injury are:

- **Possible nerve, tendon or vascular injury**—assessment includes testing sensation, movement, peripheral pulses and tissue perfusion (i.e. pulses, warmth, colour, capillary refilling after blanching). Tendon and nerve injuries are covered below
- **Tissue viability**—particularly important in crush injuries and flap lacerations such as in the pretibial area (see above)

CASE HISTORY

Fig. 17.3 Horner's syndrome caused by stab wound in the neck

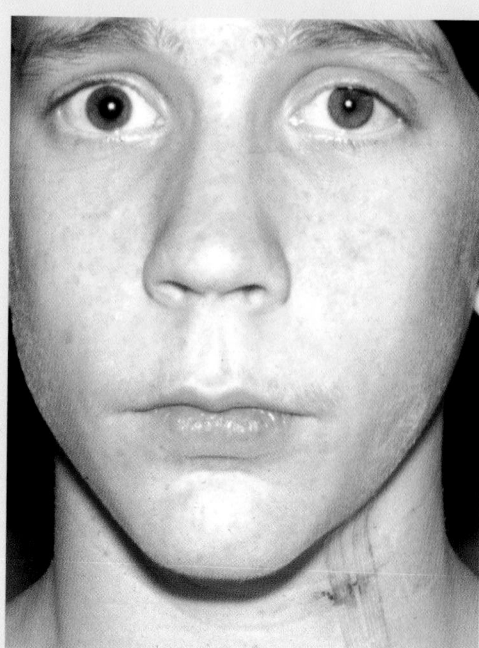

This 19-year-old was stabbed in the neck: the knife missed the great vessels but succeeded in damaging the cervical sympathetic chain, causing miosis (constriction) of the pupil as a result of unopposed parasympathetic activity

- **Risk of infection**—the fingers and hands are vulnerable to infection of pulp spaces and the deep palmar space. Wounds need antibiotic prophylaxis against staphylococci and streptococci (e.g. flucloxacillin plus amoxicillin). They also need meticulous cleansing and exploration, if possible by a specialist hand or plastic surgeon. Injuries from bites (especially by dogs or humans) and bones (usually in meat workers) almost invariably become infected (see below).

Extensive facial lacerations

Facial injuries should be thoroughly cleaned and examined under local or general anaesthesia to determine the extent of the damage before repair; ideally within 12 hours of injury. Facial wound edges need minimal trimming. Important anatomical boundaries should be aligned first; these include the vermilion border of the lip, the rim of the eyelid and the eyebrow. Tissue layers should then be approximated individually—mucosa, muscle, cartilage and skin. Parotid duct injury should be considered in deep lacerations of the cheek and the duct repaired if possible. Photographic documentation is useful to help the patient appreciate the extent of injury and to provide an accurate record of progress.

Facial nerve integrity should be determined before anaesthesia is given. Nerve branches should be repaired (usually by a plastic surgeon with microsurgical skills). Those caused by a laceration posterior to a vertical line from the lateral canthus of the eye do better than those anterior to this. Nerve repair should be performed no more than 72 hours after injury.

VASCULAR INJURIES INVOLVING BLOOD LOSS OR ISCHAEMIA

Where major **blood vessels** have been damaged, haemorrhage can usually be arrested, at least temporarily, by applying pressure on gauze swabs. If there is limb ischaemia, early vascular imaging and repair is needed. Vascular grafting is required if substantial lengths of vessel have been lost. If revascularisation is delayed, **reperfusion injury** is probable and **compartment syndrome** likely. Reperfusion injury occurs when blood flow is restored after a period of severe ischaemia. Much of the damage appears to be caused by free radicals formed in the inflammatory responses of damaged tissues and mediated by macrophages and inflammatory cytokines.

If a main artery and vein have both been severed, e.g. femoral artery and vein, the vein is always repaired first to allow venous drainage before repairing the artery. If nerves have also been cut, nerve repair is required using an operating microscope (microsurgery).

Compartment syndrome

The muscles of the leg below the knee and in the forearm lie within rigid fascial compartments. Delayed restoration of blood flow after ischaemia leads to reperfusion injury, which allows protein-rich fluid to leak from damaged capillaries. The intra-compartmental pressure rises (normally in the range of 0–10 mmHg) which compromises venous flow and later reduces capillary flow. This initiates a vicious circle that exacerbates the ischaemic insult and further increases the pressure. Arterial inflow is not usually impaired but compartment syndrome rapidly leads to irreversible nerve ischaemia and muscle necrosis.

If revascularisation follows a period of severe ischaemia and/or there have been signs of ischaemic anaesthesia or paralysis beforehand, the best management is pre-emptive **fasciotomy** at the same time. Fasciotomy involves incising the enclosing fascia of each compartment over a substantial length. The wound is left open and usually covered by split skin grafts a few days later. Fasciotomy can be performed later (but promptly) if early postoperative signs suggest a developing compartment syndrome. Signs include altered sensation or paralysis in the distribution of nerves passing through the compartment (e.g. foot drop caused by ischaemia of the common peroneal nerve), muscle tenderness and excessive pain on passive movement. Note that peripheral pulses may still be present. Treatment of established compartment syndrome is usually less satisfactory than pre-emptive treatment and may result in substantial disability.

ANIMAL-ASSOCIATED SOFT TISSUE INJURIES

Animals can cause human injury through bites, kicks, blunt trauma, goring with horns or lacerations from claws. Bite wounds in particular need prompt medical attention to reduce the risk of local infection. Tetanus is also a risk in puncture wounds or bites in a patient unprotected by tetanus immunisation.

Snakebite

Poisonous snakes are a hazard in many areas, although deaths from snakebite are rare. Snakebites are most common where dense human populations coexist with large snake populations (e.g. South-East Asia, sub-Saharan Africa, and tropical America). Highly dangerous snakes include the Australian brown snake; Russell's viper and cobras in southern Asia; carpet vipers in the Middle East; and coral snakes and rattlesnakes in the Americas. The venom of a small or immature snake can be even more concentrated than that of larger ones; therefore all snakes should be left well alone. Less than half of all snakebite wounds actually contain venom, but travellers are advised to seek immediate medical attention whenever a bite breaks the skin. First-aid measures should include immobilising the affected limb and applying a pressure bandage that does not restrict limb perfusion (not a tourniquet), then moving the victim quickly to a medical treatment centre. Incision of the bite is not recommended. Specific therapy varies and should be left to the judgement of experienced local emergency personnel.

Arthropod bites and stings

The bites and stings of some arthropods (which include insects) can cause unpleasant reactions. Travellers should seek medical attention if a spider or insect bite or sting causes excessive redness, swelling, bruising or persistent pain. Patients with a history of severe allergic reactions to bites or stings should consider carrying an adrenaline (epinephrine) autoinjector (EpiPen). Many insects and arthropods can transmit **communicable diseases**, even without the traveller being aware of a bite, particularly when camping or staying in rural accommodation. Travellers to many parts of the world should be advised to use insect repellents containing DEET, protective clothing, and mosquito netting around beds at night. Stings from **scorpions** can be painful but are seldom dangerous except in infants and children. Exposure to scorpion stings can be avoided by sleeping under mosquito nets and by shaking clothing and shoes before putting them on.

Animal bites

Domestic pets cause more bites than wild animals, with dogs more likely to bite than cats; however, cat bites are more likely to become infected. Their sharp pointed teeth cause puncture wounds and lacerations that may inoculate bacteria deeply. In Adelaide, about 6500 people are injured each year by dog attacks and 800 seek hospital treatment (7.3 per 10 000 population). Some 90% of children who were bitten suffered head and facial bites. In the USA, dog bites cause about 44 000 facial injuries requiring hospital treatment and 10–20 people are killed each year. This is about 1% of all emergency room visits. In the UK there was an average of 2.3 fatalities a year between 1999 and 2004. Unfortunately, most fatalities are in young children where bites to the face, neck or head are extremely hazardous. Children are often bitten in these areas because of their small stature.

Dogs typically cause a crushing wound because of their rounded teeth and strong jaws. An adult dog can exert 200–450 pounds per square inch (psi) of pressure, which can damage deep structures such as bones, vessels, tendons, muscle and nerves.

In general, the better the vascular supply and the easier the wound is to clean (i.e. laceration vs. puncture), the lower the risk of infection. Bites of the **hand** have a high risk for infection because of the relatively poor blood supply. The complex anatomical structure also makes adequate cleansing of the wound difficult.

The principles of treatment of bite wounds are inspection, debridement, irrigation and closure:

- Wounds should be **inspected** to identify deep injury and devitalised tissue. This nearly always requires a general or regional anaesthetic. Care should be taken to visualise the deepest part of the wound and to examine the wound through the range of motion
- **Debridement** is an effective means of minimising infection. Devitalised tissue, particulate matter and clots should be removed, as with any foreign body. Clean surgical wound edges result in smaller scars and promote faster healing
- **Irrigation** also helps prevent infection. A 19-gauge blunt needle and a 50 ml syringe provide enough pressure and volume to clean most wounds. In general, 100–200 ml of irrigation solution per cm^3 of wound is required. Large, dirty wounds need to be irrigated in the operating theatre. Saline solution is effective and inexpensive
- **Primary closure** can be considered in clean bite wounds or wounds that can be cleansed effectively. Others are best treated by **delayed primary closure**. Facial wounds are at low risk for infection, even if closed primarily. Bite wounds to the lower extremities, bites where there is a delayed presentation, or those in immunocompromised patients should generally be left open

Types of infection

Animal saliva is heavily contaminated with bacteria; over 130 disease-causing microorganisms have been isolated from dog and cat bites, thus nearly all infections are mixed. In rabies areas, bites from non-immunised domestic animals and wild animals carry the risk of rabies and the need for prophylaxis should be considered, in addition to tetanus prophylaxis. While local infection and cellulitis are the leading causes of morbidity, sepsis is a potential complication of bite wounds. Meningitis, osteomyelitis and septic arthritis are additional concerns in bite wounds. Rabies is a generally fatal complication. However, the three infections mentioned below are probably the most significant:

Pasteurellosis

Pasteurella multocida is a bacterium carried naturally by most mammals in their mouths, including healthy cats, dogs and rabbits, and by some birds and fish. The organism is responsible for the most common bite-associated infection. The first signs of pasteurellosis usually occur within 2–12 hours of the bite and include pain, reddening and swelling of the area around the bite. Pasteurellosis can progress quickly, spreading from the bitten area, and may cause flu-like symptoms such as fever, headaches, chills and swollen glands. If left untreated, it can cause pneumonia or systemic sepsis and, on rare occasions, death.

Streptococcal and staphylococcal infections

These bacteria can cause infections similar to those caused by *Pasteurella*. Redness and painful swelling occur at or near the site of the bite and progress proximally.

HUMAN BITES

Human bites can be as dangerous as animal bites because of the bacteria and viruses resident in the human mouth; the principles of contaminated wound management apply. In a closed-fist injury, an opponent's tooth often inoculates the extensor tendon and its sheath. The resulting contamination cannot be removed readily by normal cleansing and irrigation. Patients may need intravenous antibiotic therapy, and surgical drainage may also be necessary.

When fingers are bitten, tendons and their sheaths lying close to the skin can become infected. The wound may appear trivial, but careful inspection is needed to exclude deeper injury. When a person is bitten on the head, wounds may appear innocuous, but subgaleal bacterial contamination can be missed, especially in young children, who have thin soft skin over the scalp and forehead. Such wounds are best cleaned, left open and closed secondarily. Use of antibiotics is debatable and has not been shown to reduce infection rates.

HIV transmission has occurred very rarely after a human bite. Exposure to saliva alone is not generally considered a risk factor for HIV (or hepatitis) transmission.

GUNSHOT, MISSILE AND STAB WOUNDS

Gunshot wounds and missile injuries need special attention. High-energy missiles may cause a small entry wound but produce havoc within (see Ch. 15). X-rays need to be taken and wounds explored under general anaesthesia.

TRAUMATIC AMPUTATION OF DIGITS OR LIMBS

Principles of digit and limb replantation surgery

Complete amputation of digits is common, especially in industrial accidents, but sometimes whole limbs are severed. With clean-cut injuries, it is possible to reattach the amputated part using microsurgery to join the vessels and nerves. This cannot be done after crush or avulsion injuries or in grossly contaminated wounds. Even in ideal cases, recovery is slow and usually incomplete, necessitating many months away from work and much rehabilitation effort. Therefore, replantation should never be undertaken without carefully evaluating the likely benefits and ensuring the patient is fully involved in the decision. In digital amputation, the greatest disability results from loss of the thumb. Single digits are rarely replanted (except for example in a musician) because the remaining fingers rapidly adapt to the loss and rehabilitation is faster.

Replantation should only be considered if there has been no major crushing or degloving injury. Indications may include:

- Loss of whole upper limb or hand
- Loss of thumb alone
- Loss of all digits (replant thumb and one or two fingers)
- Loss of all fingers (replant one or possibly two fingers)

At the scene of the injury, the severed digit should be washed gently to remove obvious dirt and placed in a plastic bag which is then placed inside a second plastic bag containing ice or frozen peas. In this way it can be successfully preserved for up to 12 hours.

CONTAMINATION WITH SOIL AND ROAD DIRT

Superficial wounds such as grazes caused by motorcycle injuries and lack of protective clothing often become widely impregnated with road debris. These need to be scrubbed clean, often under general anaesthesia. In the case of large contaminated and contused wounds involving muscle, the potential for **gas gangrene** must be considered. Dead tissue must be thoroughly excised, benzylpenicillin given prophylactically, and primary closure avoided in favour of delayed primary closure. Note that **hydrogen peroxide** must **NOT** be used in any wounds other than purely superficial ones because of the dangers of oxygen embolism causing brain damage.

CRUSH INJURIES

Crush injuries occur most commonly in earthquakes and during wars after buildings have collapsed on people. Rhabdomyolysis follows prolonged heavy continuous pressure on muscle and **crush syndrome** is caused by reperfusion injury when the damaged muscle revascularises on removing compression. Damaged cells release potassium and potentially toxic substances such as myoglobin, phosphate and urate into the circulation. Water and extracellular electrolytes enter the damaged muscle. The net result is hypovolaemic shock with electrolyte disturbances leading to prerenal and toxic renal failure.

Following earthquakes, the incidence of crush syndrome is 2–5% of those buried under rubble. About half develop acute renal failure, and half of those need dialysis. Crush syndrome is also seen following industrial incidents, particularly in mining, and in road traffic collisions.

Diagnostic criteria for crush syndrome include:

- A crushing injury to a large mass of skeletal muscle
- Sensory and motor disturbances in the compressed limb
- Swelling and tenseness of the limb a few hours later
- Myoglobinuria and/or haematuria
- Elevated serum creatine kinase (CK) with a peak greater than 1000 U/L
- Renal insufficiency hours or days later. This may manifest with oliguria (urine output less than 400 ml in 24 hours), decreased plasma calcium concentration and elevated plasma urea, creatinine, uric acid, potassium and phosphate

Presentation

Crush syndrome presents with profound shock. A limb trapped will be pulseless on release; later it becomes red, swollen and blistered with loss of sensation and muscle power. Reperfusion injury causes **compartment syndrome** after release of compression. Once the compartment pressure exceeds capillary perfusion pressure (about 30 mmHg), tissues in the compartment become ischaemic.

Management

At the accident scene, after substantial crush injury, limb amputation on site will prevent crush syndrome. This takes fine judgement but a severely damaged limb may not be salvageable. Venous access should be obtained early, and saline infused at 1000–1500 ml/h during extrication.

Once urine flow is established, a mannitol-forced diuresis of up to 8 L/day should be maintained. Allopurinol can be given to reduce urate levels and protect the myocardium. If compartment syndrome seems likely, **fasciotomy** should be performed early.

Hyperkalaemia and infection are common complications and may lead to death. Intractable hyperkalaemia may benefit from dialysis. Disseminated intravascular coagulation can occur with massive tissue damage, and established acute renal failure requires appropriate management.

The earthquake in Marmara, northern Turkey, in 1999 was well documented and had a mortality rate for crush syndrome of 15%. Peak levels of CK give useful prognostic information: levels greater than 100 000 U/L virtually always signify that haemodialysis will be needed or that the patient is likely to die. Children with extensive injuries do very poorly.

PERIPHERAL NERVE INJURIES

Anatomy

In a peripheral nerve trunk, individual axons are sheathed in **endoneurium** and groups are bundled into **fascicles**. Each fascicle is covered in tough **perineurium** composed of collagen and elastin and may contain sensory and motor axons. A **peripheral nerve trunk** consists of a number of fascicles in a matrix of **epineurium** which also coats the nerve. Fascicles divide repeatedly along the course of a nerve, communicating with each other and intermixing rather than running neatly in parallel. This means the arrangement and type of axons and fascicles in one cross-section of the nerve may be very different from that in an adjoining cross-section. The difficulty of aligning the proximal with the distal arrangement is an important reason why functional recovery is poor if a segment of nerve is lost and has to be replaced with a nerve graft.

Types of injury

Nerve injuries were classified by Seddon in 1943:

- **Neuropraxia** is the mildest injury, where nerve continuity is preserved and only transient functional loss occurs. Recovery occurs within 6–8 weeks, without Wallerian axonal degeneration. The lesion is caused by compression, blunt impact or nearby low-velocity missile injuries and the injury is probably biochemical. Motor nerves are more sensitive to damage than sensory nerves and autonomic function is often retained
- **Axontmesis** occurs when there is interruption of axon and its myelin, but perineurium and epineurium are preserved. Axontmesis results from more severe crush injury or contusion; axonal continuity is lost and complete denervation occurs but supporting structures remain intact. Electromyography (EMG) confirms muscle denervation distal to the injury. Recovery eventually takes place by axon regeneration and is likely to be complete
- **Neurontmesis** involves complete functional disconnection and occurs with severe contusion,

stretching or laceration of a nerve. Axons and encapsulating connective tissues lose continuity and motor, sensory and autonomic functions are completely lost, and rarely recover without surgical intervention. The nerve is not usually completely severed but suffers internal structural disruption. In such cases, axonal regeneration causes fusiform swelling of the injured segment. If the nerve is divided, fibroblast proliferation produces dense fibrous scarring which inhibits sprouting axons from entering distal tubules; this seriously impairs nerve regeneration

Nerve regeneration

In **axontmesis**, calcium-mediated Wallerian (or antegrade) degeneration of the distal axon and myelin occurs early on. Within a few days, sprouting begins from the ends of proximal axons. Regenerating fibres eventually cross the injury site and then progress distally at 1–2 mm a day through undamaged tubules which provide a precise path for reinnervation of target organs.

In **neurontmesis**, nerve lesions close to the parent cell often lead to death of the cell body. If cell death does not occur, axons sprout (as in axontmesis) but the first barriers are the scar and any gap in the nerve. A neuroma forms on the proximal nerve end and no functional recovery occurs without operative repair. The most favourable injury for repair is a clean wound without segmental nerve loss.

Denervated muscle becomes irreversibly damaged after 18 months. Axons regenerate at about 2.5 cm per month provided they have an uninterrupted route, thus the distance between the injury and target muscle must be under 45 cm for any hope of functional recovery. As an example, if the ulnar nerve is injured in the brachial plexus, the wrist and finger flexors in the forearm may recover, but the intrinsic muscles of the hand may not. A further period is needed to achieve functional recovery because the new axon needs to mature, the synapse has to be reconstituted, the end-organ must recover from trophic changes, and a critical number of axons must reach the target end-organs to accomplish neural control.

Clinical types of nerve injury

Compression

Compression affects the largest myelinated fibres most. Motor control is lost first and discrete sensation follows. The underlying cause is probably ischaemia; large myelinated fibres are more susceptible to this than smaller unmyelinated ones. In partial injuries, smaller pain-bearing and sympathetic fibres are often preserved, causing pain and hyperaesthesia in the nerve distribution. Compression injuries include so-called **'Saturday night palsy'**, where the radial nerve becomes compressed over the back of a seat in a patient who passes out under the influence of alcohol. Total loss of motor and sensory function is likely to occur. Adverse effects are spontaneously reversible unless ischaemia persists for more than 8 hours.

Traction

Traction is the most common mechanism of nerve injury and is often associated with fracture or dislocation. Nerves have little elasticity and can only stretch 4% without injury. Luckily, most traction injuries are self-limiting and have a good prognosis; as many as 90% achieve good or fair recovery. The prognosis is worse when vascular trauma or open fractures are present, with only 65% recovering useful function.

Laceration

Lacerations such as those caused by a knife blade comprise up to 30% of serious nerve injuries. Exploration and repair is recommended in most cases.

Missile injury

Low-velocity gunshot missiles are less likely to sever nerves than sharp lacerations. However, about 70% of missile wounds that require exploration for other reasons demonstrate complete or partial transsection of a nerve. In high-velocity missile injuries, cavitation of soft tissues can produce nerve stretch injuries.

Repair of nerve injury

Direct repair

A clean sharp division of a nerve by a knife wound should be repaired by primary anastomosis within 24 hours of injury. Simple **epineural repair** involves re-approximation of the nerve ends using a circumferential line of sutures. This is technically easier than **fascicular repair** which involves microsurgical anastomosis of fascicles or groups of fascicles. Results of epineural repair are often good if the fascicular patterns at the cut ends are similar and where anatomic distortion is minimal. Even for proximal nerve trunk repair where a plexiform layout of fibres is more likely, the chances of the correct type of axons passing down the proper fascicles appear to be as good as in fascicular repair. Epineural repair is also stronger and resists tension better. With compression, stretching or contusion injuries, repair should be undertaken between 8 weeks, and 3 months of injury if there is no evidence of natural recovery.

Cable grafting

Autologous nerve grafting is needed if there is a large gap in a nerve. The most commonly used donor nerve is the **sural**, a large sensory nerve running down the posterior calf to the lateral dorsum of the foot. Several 'cables' are usually fashioned and attempts made to match proximal and distal fascicles. The plexiform and mixed nature of fascicles makes full recovery difficult to achieve.

Results of nerve repair

Assuming good technique, the following factors improve the prognosis for recovery after nerve repair:

- The repair involves purely sensory or motor nerves, e.g. the functional result of a severed peroneal nerve repair (motor) is likely to be better than an equivalent median nerve repair (mixed)
- The lesion is distal rather than proximal because distal trunks have a more linear arrangement
- The patient is younger; children have better results than adults, and younger adults better than older adults
- The repair is undertaken soon after injury

BURNS

INTRODUCTION

Burns affect everyone—young or old, rich or poor, in the developing or developed world—but the poor and underprivileged are more at risk and generally receive worse treatment. Burns cause devastating injuries. Initially there is severe pain and distress, but soon there is a massive assault on both physical and psychological aspects of those affected. There are visible physical scars and invisible psychological scars which together cause severe and long lasting disability.

EPIDEMIOLOGY

Thermal injury is common. Burns are the fourth most common trauma worldwide (after traffic collisions, falls and personal violence). Most burns are caused by flame injuries and many of the rest by scalds. Electrocution and chemical injuries are uncommon. In the UK, about 250 000 people are burnt each year; 112 000 attend accident departments and 13 000 are admitted to hospital. About 1000 have burns severe enough to need fluid resuscitation and, sadly, half of these are children under 12. In an average year, burns cause 250 deaths in the UK, although the incidence has decreased owing to prophylactic measures, e.g. curly cables on kettles; abandonment of open fires; and flameproof sofas and clothing. The incidence in the USA is higher, and is even more of a problem in the developing world, with 90% occurring in low to middle income countries. India alone has over 2 million burns a year. Mortality in the developing world is also much higher, e.g. Nepal has 1700 burn deaths annually in a population of 20 million, proportionately 17 times higher than in the UK.

Two-thirds of burns occur in the home and one third largely in industrial accidents. Around 60% of domestic burns are associated with cooking. Half of all deaths in domestic fires occur between 10 p.m. and 8 a.m. and excess alcohol often plays a role. Fireworks and bonfires are frequent causes of domestic burns. **Most burns are preventable.** Young children and the elderly are at greatest risk and also suffer disproportionate mortality. There is a male predominance except in the elderly; 10% of those burnt are over 65, often as a result of immobility, slowed reactions and decreased dexterity placing them at risk from scalds, contact burns and flame burns. Twenty per cent of all burns occur in children under the age of 4; 70% are scalds caused by spilling hot liquids or by exposure to hot bath water. Toddlers frequently pull containers or cups of hot liquid over themselves from cookers and tables which burn the outstretched arm, face, neck and front of the chest and can cover a large area (see Fig. 17.4).

Teenagers are often burnt as a result of illicit activities, e.g. with petrol, explosives or high tension electricity. Overall, 60% of burns occur between the ages of 15 and 64, of which half are flame burns, often with inhalational injury; burns tend to be deep dermal or full thickness (see Fig. 17.5).

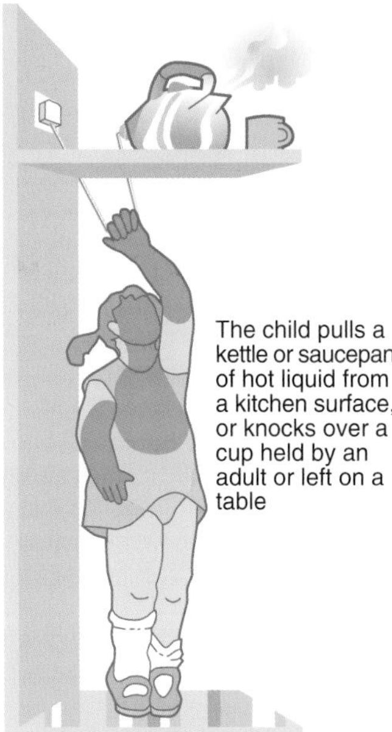
The child pulls a
kettle or saucepan
of hot liquid from
a kitchen surface,
or knocks over a
cup held by an
adult or left on a
table

Fig. 17.4 Typical pattern of burns in a young child The child pulls a teapot or cup of hot liquid from a table or when being held by a seated adult. The area shaded pink is typically burnt

PATHOPHYSIOLOGY OF BURNS

In thermal skin burns, the depth of destruction determines the local outcome. Skin burns are broadly divided into **partial** or **full thickness**. In partial thickness burns, epidermal elements are spared, eventually allowing spontaneous healing without skin grafting. In deep partial thickness burns, the only epithelial remnants may be hair follicles and sweat glands extending into the hypodermis, making regeneration slower. In full thickness burns, all the epidermis has been destroyed. Skin grafting is needed because epithelialisation from the margins is slow and prone to complications, in particular infection, fibrotic scarring and contractures.

The depth of damage is a function of the temperature and duration of exposure as well as the thickness of the skin (important in the very young and very old where the dermis is thinner). If applied for long enough, water at a temperature of only 45 °C will cause full thickness destruction and is often the mechanism of tragic burns in childhood. Note that the area of a major burn will not be uniformly deep.

Three zones of a major burn were described by Jackson in 1947. There is a central zone of **coagulation** where skin cells are irreversibly damaged. This is surrounded by a zone of **stasis** characterised by decreased tissue perfusion in which injured cells can survive or die according to the effectiveness of treatment. These zones extend deeply but the outer zone of **erythema** is superficial. Here the cells are minimally injured and recover in 7 days. This erythematous zone should not be included in calculating the burnt area.

SYSTEMIC EFFECTS (Box 17.2)

Extensive burns cause large fluid losses. Epidermal destruction removes the barrier that normally prevents evaporation of body water. In addition, inflammation causes exudation of protein-rich fluid into the extracellular space causing oedema

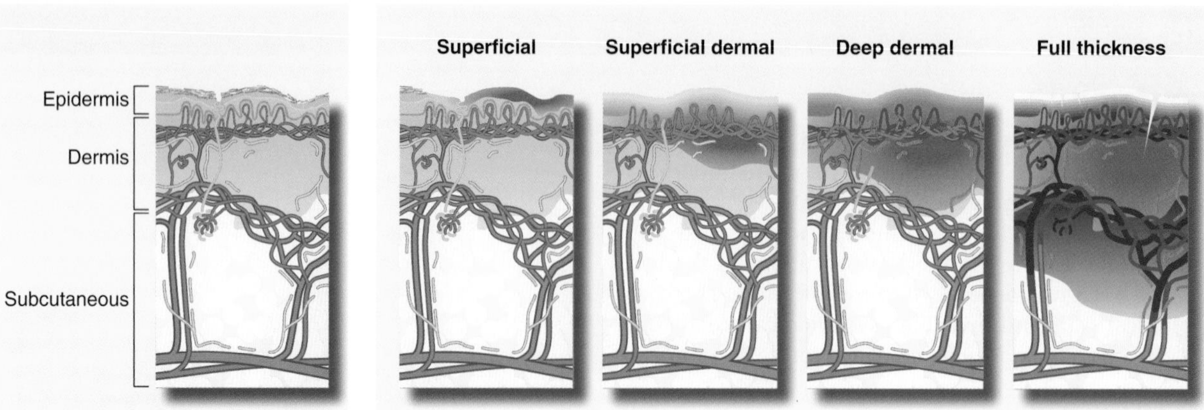

Fig. 17.5 Classification of depth of burns
Erythema—red, dry skin that easily blanches then rapidly refills (not illustrated here)
Superficial—red, moist wound that blanches and rapidly refills
Superficial dermal—pale, dry, blanching wound that regains colour slowly
Deep dermal—mottled cherry red and does not blanch (fixed capillary staining). The blood is thrombosed and fixed in damaged capillaries in the deep dermal plexus
Full thickness—dry, leathery or waxy, hard wound that does not blanch. In extensive burns, full thickness burns can be mistaken for unburnt skin

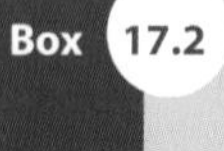
Box 17.2 Systemic changes occurring with large area burns (greater than 15% surface area in adults or 10% in children)

- Surface and third space fluid losses lead to hypovolaemia
- Systemic inflammatory response syndrome occurs once burns affect 30% of body surface area
- Myocardial contractility becomes depressed
- In smoke inhalation, bronchoconstriction and ARDS occur
- Basal metabolic rate (BMR) increases up to three-fold
- Function of the innate immune system becomes depressed
- General capillary permeability is increased
- Peripheral and splanchnic vasoconstriction occurs
- Red cells are destroyed by the burn
- Sepsis is likely if burns become infected, leading to organ failure and death

and blisters. The large volumes lost need to be replaced urgently (see Fig. 17.7, below), with the amount lost depending on burn area rather than depth. Once 30% of the body surface area is burnt, particularly if there is necrotic tissue, inflammatory mediators and cytokines spill into the circulation, causing a systemic inflammatory response. This provokes a generalised rise in capillary permeability, escalating the volume of plasma leaving the circulation into the 'third space'. Fluid losses are greatest in the first few hours but continue for at least 36 hours.

Epidermal loss and necrotic tissue place the patient at high risk of infection. The main organisms are *Streptococcus pyogenes* during the first week and *Pseudomonas aeruginosa* thereafter. If burns become infected, the risk of sepsis and organ failure increases and leads to substantial mortality, even in this antibiotic era.

ELECTROCUTION BURNS

Electrical burns result from the conversion of electrical energy into heat; electrocution is responsible for around 3% of admissions to burns units. The voltage is the key determinant of severity. Low domestic voltages just cause small but deep contact burns at exit and entry sites. High-tension injuries occur at voltages over 1000 V and cause large amounts of necrosis of bone and soft tissues and often limb loss. Muscle damage gives rise to rhabdomyolysis and renal failure. Contact with voltages greater than 70 000 V is invariably fatal.

The extent of burning is proportional to the electrical resistance of the tissue through which the current is transmitted. Bone offers the highest resistance; if current passes through a limb, the bones become heated and adjoining muscle is injured. Fasciotomy is likely to become necessary to decompress muscle compartments. Blood vessels also sustain intimal damage and thrombose. Deep tissue necrosis may not become clinically apparent until some days afterwards and the extent of damage is often much greater than suspected.

CHEMICAL BURNS

Chemical burns usually result from industrial accidents but may be caused by household chemicals. The severity depends on the agent, the concentration and quantity, and the duration of contact. Chemical burns tend to be deep because corrosives continue to act until fully removed. Alkalis such as cement tend to penetrate more deeply and cause worse burns than acids. **Hydrofluoric acid** is widely used in glass etching and circuit board construction and is a common cause of industrial chemical burns. It must be neutralised with topical or locally injected calcium gluconate to prevent the burning continuing. The initial management of chemical burns is similar for all agents, i.e. remove all contaminated clothing and dilute or wash away the chemical by thoroughly irrigating the area, often by showering the patient.

NON-ACCIDENTAL INJURY (NAI)

Between 3% and 10% of paediatric burns are due to non-accidental injury, i.e. deliberate harm to the child. Up to 30% of repeatedly abused children die. If non-accidental injury is suspected it is vital to follow the local NAI protocol.

ASSESSMENT OF THE BURNT PATIENT

HISTORY

The history should include information about the timing and source of the burn, the temperature and the duration of contact and whether there was any inhalation of noxious gases.

CALCULATING THE BURNT AREA

Early appraisal of the burnt area is important, not least because it helps determine the fluid volume required for resuscitation. Area estimation is often badly done even by experts and is complicated by the fact that erythema must be excluded to avoid overestimates. Preliminary evaluation can be done immediately but definitive assessment should be deferred for a few hours until erythema settles.

All of the burnt area needs to be exposed sequentially, ensuring the patient is kept warm. For adults, Wallace's rule of nines (Fig. 17.6) is fairly reliable for medium to large areas and is quick, but is inaccurate in children. Another method is to use the patient's palm and finger area to indicate 1% of body surface area. This is useful for small burns, and in very large burns where the **unburnt area** is measured. The most accurate method is to use **Lund and Browder charts** which compensate for variations in body shape with age; the charts are also accurate in children.

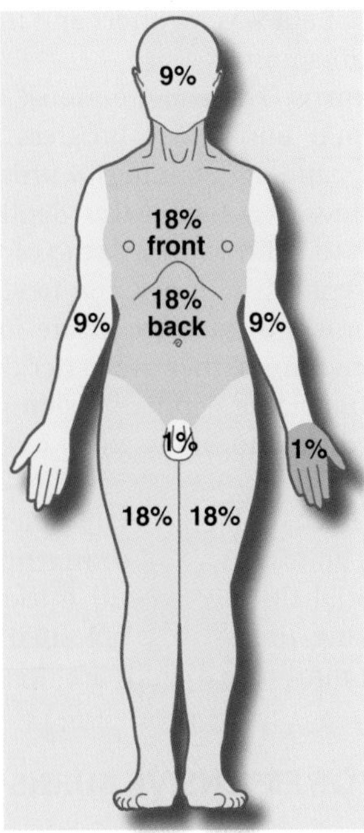

Fig. 17.6 Rule of nines Wallace's rule for estimating the percentage of the skin surface area burnt. A useful alternative estimate is that the area of the patient's own palm plus fingers is approximately 1% of the total skin area.

Early assessment of burn depth is difficult, not least because most large burns are a mixture of different depths. Burns are dynamic wounds where the eventual depth is influenced by the effectiveness of resuscitation and by inflammatory mediators, as well as external factors such as bacterial proliferation, dehydration and cooling. Thus it is essential to re-appraise the burn regularly until it heals.

Depth assessment is not relevant for calculating fluid resuscitation but is important for management of the burn. Figure 17.5 (p. 240) explains a widely used classification of depth, detailed below. In essence, partial thickness burns are capable of regenerating skin from preserved dermal adnexae whereas full thickness burns regenerate slowly from the edges and are likely to need skin grafting. By way of preliminary assessment, if the burnt area is erythematous, blanches on pressure and retains pinprick sensation, it is partial thickness; charred skin or thrombosed skin vessels invariably indicate a full thickness burn.

Partial thickness burns may be classified as follows:

- **Superficial** burns—affect the epidermis but not the dermis, e.g. sunburn
- **Superficial dermal** burns—destroy the epidermis and upper dermal layers; blistering usually occurs. The burn may be covered with soot or dirt, which needs removing, and blisters should be deroofed so that the base can be checked. Capillary refill can be tested by pressure from a sterile cotton bud. A 21 gauge needle is used to test sensation and bleeding; in superficial dermal burns, pain is felt normally and bleeding is brisk. Scalds tend to cause 'superficial' to 'superficial dermal' burns
- **Deep dermal** burns—these destroy all the epidermis and most of the dermis, leaving only the deepest skin adnexae, sweat glands and some hair follicles, all of which are scanty. Accurate depth estimation can be difficult. On needle testing, bleeding is delayed and only non-painful sensation is experienced
- **Full thickness** burns are insensate and do not bleed on needling

PRINCIPLES OF MANAGEMENT OF BURNS

Optimal treatment reduces the morbidity of burns as well as mortality in large burns. Effective treatment shortens the period of healing, speeds return of function and reduces the need for secondary reconstruction.

First aid

The first priority at the scene is to stop the burning process. The heat source must be removed and any flames doused. Clothing is removed unless stuck to the burn, and **active cooling** employed to remove heat and arrest progression. Ideally this is achieved by immersing the burnt area in tepid water (~15°C) for 15–20 minutes. This can cause hypothermia, especially in children.

Analgesia

Burns are very painful, with pain being greatest in superficial burns. Pain relief is best achieved by cooling and covering burns in addition to analgesic drugs. In larger burns, opioids are given initially and NSAIDs later.

Dressings

Cling film (PVC) is ideal as an initial burn dressing. It is essentially sterile and forms a pliable, non-adherent, impermeable barrier which is transparent to allow inspection. It should be laid on rather than wrapped around and covered with a blanket to keep the wound warm. Burnt hands are enclosed in plastic bags. Prepacked cooling hydrogels, e.g. Burnshield®, are available for applying at the scene of the burn.

Where should burns be managed?

Very small or erythema-only burns can be managed in primary care but all other patients should be assessed and resuscitated in an emergency unit. Initial assessment then determines whether treatment can continue as an outpatient in a general hospital, whether admission is required or whether transfer to a specialist burns unit is needed. Patients with extensive burns involving more than 30% of body surface should be transferred to a specialist burns unit right after initial treatment and resuscitation. Facial burns should also be referred after covering with bland paraffin ointment (repeated every 1–4 hours to minimise crust). Other referral criteria are summarised in Box 17.3.

OUTPATIENT MANAGEMENT OF MINOR BURNS

Patients appropriate for outpatient management are adults without inhalation injury or significant co-morbidity, with partial thickness burns affecting less than 10% of body surface area. Children with less than 5% burns are also suitably managed in this way. Patients with full thickness burns of up to 1% can also be managed as outpatients.

Immediate care involves analgesia and reassurance. Fluid resuscitation is not needed. The main objective of local treatment is to prevent dehydration and infection of the burn site; epithelialisation progresses faster in a moist environment. The burnt area is cleaned of soot and debris with soap and water or weak chlorhexidine if necessary. Larger blisters are de-roofed and covered with a non-stick impregnated gauze dressing. Tulle gras (paraffin gauze) has long been used but it soon dries out and adheres to the wound. A better, more expensive alternative is a soft silicone-coated net such as Mepitel. A generous layer of silver sulfadiazine cream (Flamazine) can be used instead; this antibacterial cream covers Gram-negative organisms including the common infecting organism, *Pseudomonas*. Either dressing is then covered by a thick absorbent layer of gauze and wool (Gamgee). Burns on the fingers and hands are best treated with a liberal coating of silver sulfadiazine cream and enclosing the hand in a plastic bag. Burnt areas should be checked at 24 hours and the dressing changed at 48 hours, by which time the depth should be evident and the treatment plan can be reviewed. Silver sulfadiazine cream can then be applied every 24–48 hours and skin slough excised as it separates. Partial thickness burns re-epithelialise within 14–21 days. If the burn has failed to heal within 3 weeks, the burn must be assumed to be full thickness and requires referral to a specialist unit.

Box 17.3 Criteria for referral to a burns centre

- Associated inhalational injury
- Partial thickness >5% in a child or >10% in an adult
- More than 1% full thickness burns
- Partial or full thickness burns to face, perineum, external genitalia, feet, hands and across joints
- Circumferential injury
- Chemical or electrical burns
- Extremes of age
- Non-accidental injury
- Co-morbidity
- Non-healed burn 3 weeks after injury

MANAGING BURNS OF SPECIFIC DEPTH

Superficial burns, typically sunburn, require only supportive therapy with regular analgesia and dressings for moist areas. Healing takes place within a week by regeneration from undamaged keratinocytes.

Superficial dermal burns. Blistering is common and exposed superficial nerves make these burns painful. Progression to a deeper burn is unlikely. Healing is expected within 2 weeks from keratinocytes within sweat glands and hair follicles. The rate depends on the density of adnexae, i.e. thin hairless skin on the inner arm or eyelid heals more slowly than thick or hairy skin of the back, scalp or face. Treatment is as above although Hypafix is a special dressing that preserves mobility and allows washing with the dressing in place. It is applied directly to hand burns, for example. This dressing needs changing at least weekly by soaking in oil. Awkward facial burns are left open but liberally coated with antimicrobial creams or ointment. If burns are still unhealed after 2 weeks, depth assessment was incorrect and the patient should be referred to a burns unit.

Deep dermal burns. These are the most difficult to assess as superficial dermal burns may progress to deep dermal burns (with fixed capillary staining) within 48 hours. The density of skin adnexae is less at this depth and healing is slower and subject to contractures. Some of these burns heal spontaneously if kept warm, moist and free of infection, but if deep dermal burns are extensive or are in functionally or cosmetically sensitive areas, they are better treated in a burns unit by excision to a viable depth and skin grafting within 5 days. This can reduce morbidity and accelerate return to normal function.

Full thickness burns. All regenerative elements have been destroyed; without grafting, wound contraction and distortion would be substantial. Ideally all full thickness burns need excision and grafting unless they are sited where function would not be compromised and are less than 1 cm in diameter.

MANAGEMENT OF EXTENSIVE BURNS

Major burns are those affecting more than 20% of the body surface area. Survival depends crucially on accurate assessment, prompt and effective resuscitation, also the premorbid condition of the patient and whether there has been smoke inhalation. The main early aspects of management are fluid replacement, assessment and treatment of inhalational respiratory problems and local management of the burns.

It is difficult to give an early prognosis. Clearly, aggressive treatment of someone who definitely will not survive is inhumane but victims of severe yet potentially survivable burns must be treated rapidly and effectively. The risk of dying is greater with increasing area, with inhalational injury and in children under 3 and adults over 60. Very high voltage electrical burns are particularly lethal. Other medical conditions also increase the risk, e.g. alcoholism, epilepsy, diabetes, atherosclerosis and drug abuse.

Resuscitation and fluid management

Adults with 15% and children with 10% body surface burns lose sufficient fluid to be at risk of hypovolaemic shock. Fluid replacement depends on the area of the burn and the patient's weight. Hypovolaemia in the presence of myoglobinaemia readily precipitates acute renal failure. Effective resuscitation maintains tissue perfusion in the zone of stasis, inhibiting depth progression. Most fluid is lost in the first 8–12 hours, during which there is a general shift of fluid from intravascular to interstitial. Substantial fluid losses continue for at least another 36 hours. Rapid boluses of fluid should not be given early on as raised intravascular hydrostatic pressure drives it rapidly out of the circulation.

Fluid requirements should be calculated from the time of injury, *not* the time of arrival in the emergency department. Colloids appear to offer no advantage over crystalloids and the volume required is estimated by referring to well-tried formulae such as that of Muir and Barclay shown in Figure 17.7, or the Parkland formula, Box 17.4. The Parkland formula has the advantage that it uses only crystalloids, it is easy to calculate and the rate can be adjusted by titrating against urine output.

These formulae are only a guide, however, and fluid balance must also be monitored according to pulse, blood pressure and urine output via a urinary catheter. Patients should also have 4–6-hourly estimations of packed cell volume, serum sodium, base excess and lactate. Note that patients with high-tension electrocution injuries need substantially more fluid than estimated by these formulae. In extensive full thickness burns, widespread red cell destruction occurs and blood transfusion may be needed.

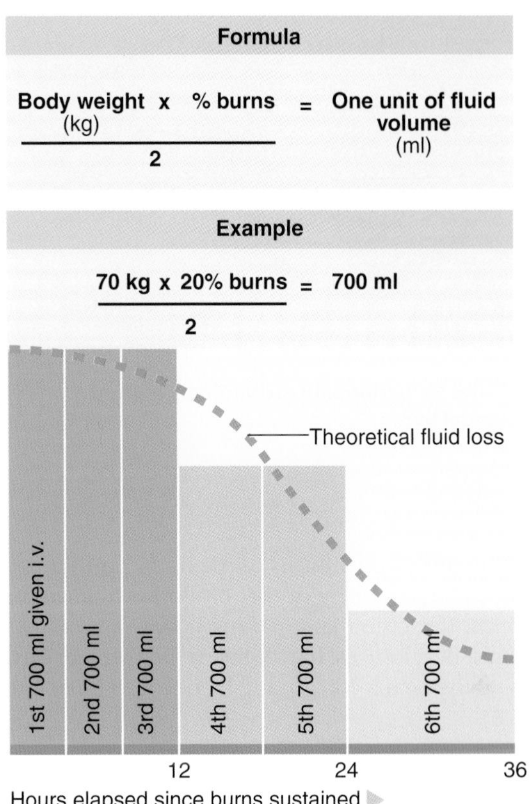

Fig. 17.7 Serious burns—a method for estimating fluid requirements over the first 36 hours (after Muir and Barclay)
The lower panel shows an example of a fluid replacement regimen for a 70 kg man with 20% burns. Each block represents one unit of fluid volume and is calculated as follows:

$$\text{Unit fluid volume} = \frac{70 \times 20}{2} = 700\,\text{ml}$$

Box 17.4 The Parkland formula for fluid resuscitation in the first 24 hours in major burns

- For adults, the total volume to be given over 24 hours is 3–4 ml Hartmann solution per kg body weight for each per cent surface area burnt
- For children, the calculation is the same as for adults plus normal maintenance fluids
- For all cases, half the estimated volume is given in the first 8 hours and the rest over the next 16 hours

Local management of the burns

All wounds should achieve epithelial cover within 3 weeks to minimise scarring. Partial thickness burns re-epithelialise spontaneously given proper care, but full thickness burns require excision and skin grafting. Fingers, eyelids, limb flexures and genitalia nearly always require primary grafting soon after injury. For optimal care, grafting should be performed within 5 days of injury and patients needing transfer to a burns unit should reach there within a maximum of 10 days.

The best covering for excised areas is autograft split skin from unburnt areas, ideally harvested near the recipient area to ensure best colour match. Sheets rather than postage stamp grafts should be used for hands and face. Wounds to be grafted must be free of infection; large areas of deep burns need excising and grafting early to prevent infection and systemic sepsis.

With extensive burns, skin grafting usually has to be performed in several stages because of a shortage of donor sites. Sites already used can be reused (**donor site rotation**) after 3 weeks or so; burnt areas can be primarily excised and covered with temporary covering until donor sites become mature. Temporary coverings include cadaveric allograft skin, xenograft skin (e.g. pigskin), specially developed synthetic products or cultured epithelial autografts (sheets can be available in 3 weeks, skin cell suspensions in 1 week).

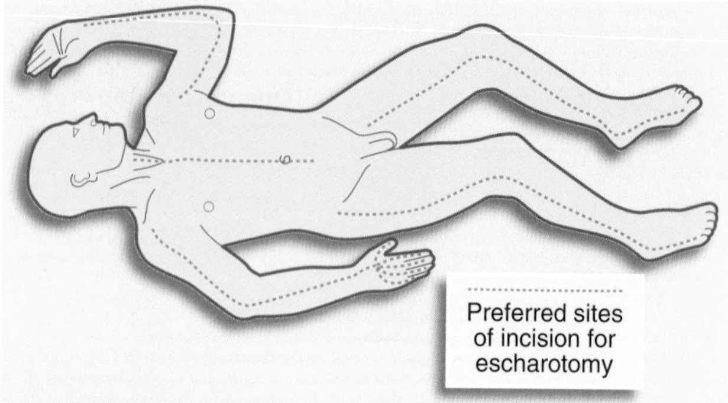

Fig. 17.8 Sites for performing escharotomy in deep circumferential burns

Box 17.5 Clinical indications of likely inhalational injury that may prompt endotracheal intubation and ventilation

- A history of flame burns or burns in an enclosed space
- Stridor, tachypnoea or dyspnoea
- Singed nasal hair
- Full thickness or deep dermal burns to face, neck or upper torso
- Changes in the voice with hoarseness or a harsh cough
- Carbonaceous sputum or carbon particles visible in oropharynx
- Erythema or swelling of the oropharynx on direct inspection

Deep circumferential burns of the limbs and thorax begin to contract early and may restrict blood flow and respiratory movements. If excision and grafting is not done early, and if these signs develop, **escharotomy** is performed, involving incision of the eschar longitudinally down to bleeding tissue (Fig. 17.8).

INHALATIONAL INJURIES

Respiratory and systemic damage from inhalation of hot air, smoke and toxic gases (e.g. carbon monoxide or cyanides from burning upholstery) is a major cause of death and complications even if skin burns are insignificant (Box 17.5). The heat of inhaled gases is often sufficient to cause inflammatory oedema of the oral, nasal and laryngeal mucosa or even serious burns. Blackening by smoke or burnt skin around the nasal or oral cavities warns of inhalation injury. In addition, noxious gases can injure the lung parenchyma, resulting in pulmonary oedema, atelectasis and secondary pneumonias a day or two later.

Investigations include chest X-ray, blood gas and carbon monoxide estimations and upper respiratory tract examination with flexible pharyngoscopy and bronchoscopy.

Initial treatment involves administration of humidified air by mask and antibiotics to prevent chest infection. More severe cases require oxygen by mask, progressing to endotracheal intubation and intermittent positive pressure ventilation if blood gases deteriorate or pulmonary oedema develops.

FOLLOW-UP AND LATE TREATMENT OF BURNS

Burnt areas should be protected from sun for 6–12 months by avoiding the sun or using sun block. Physiotherapy may be needed if mobility is impaired, and if deformity results from the burns or the treatment, prolonged psychological support is necessary, particularly if the face is involved.

Local symptoms of severe **itching** and **dryness** are likely to occur. These can be helped by topical lanolin and specially made pressure garments. These also minimise skin contractures. If limitation of functional movement at joints or around facial orifices is not helped adequately by physiotherapy, operations to release scars and skin grafting may be needed.

Full thickness burns across joint flexures (including around the neck) may undergo fibrotic contraction even after grafting, seriously limiting movement. This difficult problem is likely to require plastic reconstructive operations. Hypertrophic and keloid scars are also common and often require custom made pressure garments worn for a year or more, and sometimes surgical management.

Symptoms, diagnosis and management

4

Non-acute abdominal pain and other abdominal symptoms and signs

18

INTRODUCTION

The diagnosis of non-acute abdominal complaints is an important part of the general surgical clinic workload. Most patients with abdominal complaints can be managed as outpatients alone. Diagnoses made in a clinic are often quite different from those in emergency surgical admissions. Nevertheless, the surgeon in the clinic must remain alert to unfamiliar presentations which more usually present acutely, e.g. an appendix mass.

The principal presenting symptoms of non-acute abdominal disorders are shown in Box 18.1. In addition, patients are often referred to a surgeon after discovery of an **abdominal mass**, **obstructive jaundice** or an **iron deficiency anaemia** caused by chronic blood loss. As ever, the history can provide 70% or more of the clues to the diagnosis, and so must be taken thoughtfully, accurately and with great care.

PAIN

CHARACTER, TIMING AND SITE OF THE PAIN

Key points in taking a history of abdominal pain are summarised in Box 18.2. Pain is highly subjective and the description will be coloured by the patient's perception of it and its possible significance. Patients often use vague terms such as 'indigestion' and 'dyspepsia'; these terms are imprecise, so what the patient actually means should be clarified by further questioning. Time-related features of the pain are often highly significant in formulating a differential diagnosis but will only be elicited by diligent enquiry. It is important to establish when a pain first began. Sometimes, asking when the patient was last completely well helps pinpoint the real onset. When presenting a case history, say 'the pain began 6 days ago' rather than, say, 'it began last Thursday'.

Patients describe pain in many different ways, and as each entity tends to have its own pattern, recognisable patterns only come to light if all aspects of the pain history are enquired into.

The site of origin, distribution and radiation of the pain

These, and particularly the site it first manifested, suggest likely anatomical structures involved. These are shown in Figure 18.1 (p. 249).

DISEASES CAUSING NON-ACUTE ABDOMINAL PAIN—TYPICAL PATTERNS

- **Gallstones and gall bladder dysfunction**. Biliary colic presents with irregularly recurrent bouts of severe pain which, though described as colic, characteristically last continuously for 1–12 hours. Severe and prolonged episodes may bring the patient into hospital. Pain is usually located in the upper abdomen—most often on the right side—and may radiate around to the back. It is often precipitated by rich or fatty foods and may be associated with vomiting
- **Peptic ulcer disease**. Typically there is intermittent 'boring' epigastric pain which recurs several times a year and lasts for days or weeks at a time. It is not as severe as biliary colic unless there is perforation, which presents acutely. Retrosternal 'burning' occurs in peptic oesophagitis and tends to occur after large meals and on lying down. The relationship of pain with food varies according to the site of the ulcer disease: duodenal ulcer pain is relieved by bland food and recurs 3–4 hours afterwards, typically in the early morning, whereas the pain of gastric ulcer and oesophagitis tends to be aggravated by food, especially if acidic or spicy. Peptic pain is generally relieved by antacids and virtually always by H_2-blocking drugs (e.g. ranitidine) or proton pump inhibitors (e.g. omeprazole), this 'trial of treatment' providing evidence towards a diagnosis
- **Chronic pancreatitis and carcinoma of pancreas**. Either is typically associated with severe 'gnawing', persistent and poorly localised central pain which usually radiates

Box 18.1 Main presenting symptoms of non-acute abdominal disorders

- Abdominal pain
- Difficulty in swallowing (dysphagia)
- Weight loss
- Anorexia (loss of appetite)
- Nausea or intermittent vomiting
- Change in bowel habit, including rectal bleeding

Box 18.2 Assessing abdominal pain from the history

1. Onset and duration of pain
- How long ago did it start (hours, days, weeks)?
- Gradual or sudden onset? (sudden onset implies a mechanical cause)
- Any previous similar episodes or attacks?

2. Periodicity
- Does pain come in bouts recurring hourly, daily, weekly, monthly?
- Predominantly daytime or night-time?
- Any period free from pain?
- In females, any association with menstrual cycle? Possibility of pregnancy?

3. Location of the pain
- Where did the pain start and where is it now, e.g. central, epigastric, right or left subcostal (hypochondrial), in right or left iliac fossa, suprapubic, 'lower abdominal', or loin?
- Is pain well or poorly localised? (i.e. well localised if parietal peritoneum involved because of its somatic innervation)
- Is there any radiation of the pain? (i.e. spread to nearby areas)

4. Severity and character of the pain
- Discomfort only, moderate pain or severe pain?
- How much does it interfere with activities of normal living?
- What descriptive words does the patient use: 'sharp'; 'blunt'; 'burning'; 'crushing'; 'deep'; 'gnawing'; 'boring'; 'bloating'; 'knife-like'; 'stabbing'?
- Is the pain more likely to be physiological (e.g. pre-defaecation colic or dysmenorrhoea) or pathological?

5. Variation of pain severity with time
- Does the character of the pain vary during an attack, e.g. constant, intermittent or episodic, 'colicky' (i.e. coming in severe cramp-like waves), background pain with exacerbations?

6. Exacerbating and relieving factors
- e.g. improved or made worse by food, posture, exercise or drugs?

7. Associated symptoms
- e.g. vomiting, change in bowel habit, weight loss or nausea?

through to the back and is often associated with anorexia and weight loss. The pain may be relieved by leaning forwards ('the pancreatic position'). Early carcinoma of the pancreas, however, is usually painless

- **Irritable bowel syndrome and constipation**. These may cause a chronic symptom complex mimicking partial bowel obstruction and manifest by episodes of colicky pain. This is poorly localised, often 'bloating' pain, particularly post-prandially (after meals). Its intensity varies and it is often associated with transient disturbances of bowel function, particularly alternating diarrhoea and constipation. Passage of flatus or stool often temporarily relieves the symptoms
- **Diverticular disease and Crohn's disease**. Partial bowel obstruction can occur with sigmoid diverticular disease or with small bowel Crohn's disease. Symptoms are similar to those of complete bowel obstruction but more low-key. In incomplete bowel obstruction, there is often passage of some flatus or even faeces but the patient otherwise appears obstructed. The term subacute obstruction is meaningless and should be abandoned
- **Chronic renal outflow obstruction (hydronephrosis) caused by stone, tumour or fibrosis**. There may be a 'dull', poorly defined, fairly constant loin pain, which can radiate to the groin or genitalia and be accompanied by typical urinary tract symptoms, e.g. haematuria and dysuria. It is often aggravated acutely by high fluid intake
- **Gynaecological conditions**, particularly chronic pelvic inflammatory disease and ovarian tumours. These may reach the general surgeon because of poorly defined lower abdominal pain. A gynaecological history should be taken in female patients; pelvic examination may reveal the cause and ultrasound is usually diagnostic
- **Non-surgical (i.e. 'medical') disorders causing abdominal pain**. These include liver congestion in heart failure (common), splenic infarcts or diabetes (both uncommon but important), acute intermittent porphyria, sickle-cell anaemia or tertiary syphilis (very rare). Patients sometimes present with abdominal pain for which no organic cause can be found despite extensive investigation. In these, irritable bowel syndrome or sensitivity to certain foods, e.g. gluten or wheat protein, need to be considered. Only as a last resort should the pain be attributed to psychological disturbances

NON-ACUTE ABDOMINAL PAIN IN CHILDREN

This is common. The main organic causes are: 'infantile colic' (sometimes due to cow's milk allergy), irritable bowel syndrome in older children, chronic inflammatory bowel disease, recurrent streptococcal infections, and sometimes hydronephrosis caused by urinary tract obstruction. The so-called *'periodic syndrome'* is characterised by recurrent episodes of poorly defined and inconsistent abdominal pain and/or recurrent vomiting, sometimes sufficiently severe for the child to require admission and intravenous fluids. Abdominal migraine with or without nausea, pallor, photophobia and lasting for up to 3 days is most common in the years before puberty. Psychosomatic abdominal pain may be the explanation if organic causes have been excluded and thus psychological and

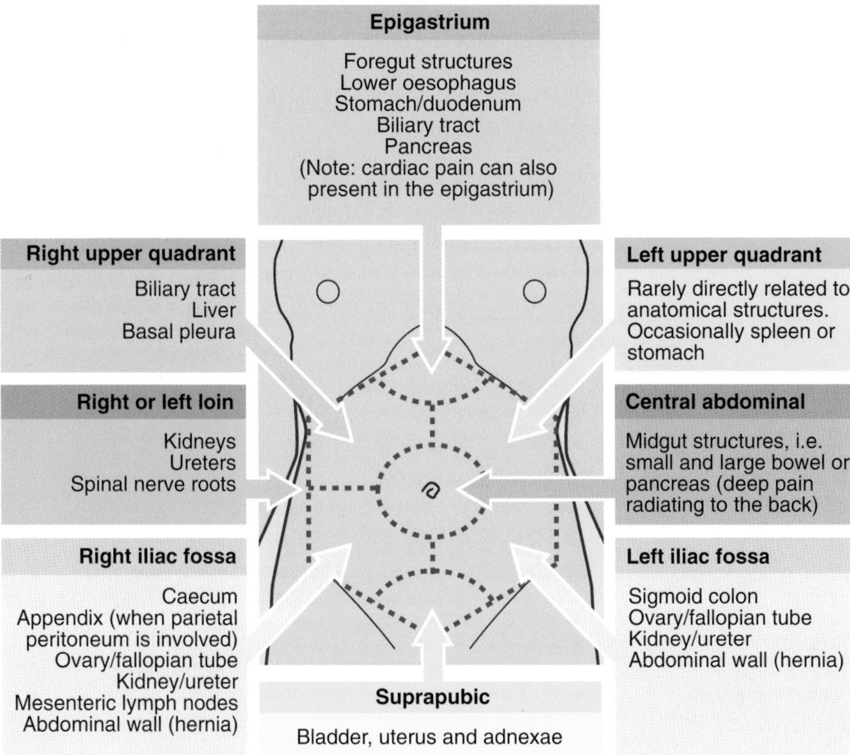

Fig. 18.1 Anatomical significance of the site of abdominal pain

environmental factors, including the possibility of child neglect and abuse, should be explored (see Table 51.2).

APPROACH TO INVESTIGATION OF NON-ACUTE ABDOMINAL PAIN

A differential diagnosis must first be made on clinical grounds (Box 18.3 and Fig. 18.1). The choice (and order) of investigations should be efficient and economical, after considering how each will support or help eliminate the most probable (and common) diagnoses and how it might influence management.

DYSPHAGIA AND ODYNOPHAGIA

CLINICAL PRESENTATION

Dysphagia is the term for difficulty in swallowing. The most common complaint is inability to swallow solids, which the patient describes as 'becoming stuck' or 'held up' before it passes into the stomach or is regurgitated. Fibrous foods such as chunks of meat, usually cause the most trouble. The patient can usually indicate a precise level for the perceived obstruction. The true level of obstruction is usually some distance below that point.

Dysphagia is almost always caused by disease in or near the oesophagus but occasionally the lesion is in the pharynx or stomach. Oesophageal narrowing usually causes symptoms only when the lumen is unable to expand beyond about 10 mm—the narrower the lumen, the more severe the symptoms. In many pathological conditions causing dysphagia, the lumen becomes progressively constricted and indistensible. Initially only fibrous solids cause difficulty but later this extends to all solids and later, even to fluids. Because narrowing is a gradual and insidious process, patients often compensate to a surprising degree (e.g. by liquidising all food) and may only present when they have difficulty swallowing fluids or even their own saliva. By this time there is usually marked weight loss.

The common causes of dysphagia are outlined in Box 18.4, p. 252. **Pain** on swallowing or **odynophagia** (usually provoked by both food and drink, particularly if hot) is a distinctive symptom highly suspicious of carcinoma.

Achalasia is an exception to the usual pattern of dysphagia, in that swallowing fluids causes more difficulty than solids. In achalasia, there is idiopathic destruction of the parasympathetic ganglia in Auerbach's (submucosal) plexus of the entire oesophagus, which results in functional narrowing of the lower oesophagus and peristaltic failure throughout its length. Thus the oesophagus becomes markedly distended and dilated, with solids settling towards the lower end and fluids spilling over into the airways causing **spluttering dysphagia**, particularly when the patient is lying flat. Achalasia often presents with chronic chest infection rather than dysphagia and the diagnosis is often reached late. Similar overspill symptoms can be caused by bulbar palsy, most commonly after a stroke.

Bolus obstruction is an acute form of dysphagia, where a lump of food sticks at a narrowed part, completely obstructing the oesophagus.

APPROACH TO INVESTIGATION OF DYSPHAGIA

Dysphagia, particularly of recent onset, must be regarded seriously and fully investigated. A plain chest X-ray should be

Box 18.3 Abdominal examination: 28 points to remember in examining a patient with abdominal symptoms

General examination

1. Well-looking or ill (thin, emaciated, weak)?
2. Alert and responding normally or obtunded and slumped in bed?
3. Dehydrated (poor skin tone, sunken cheeks)?
4. Abnormal skin colour (pale, jaundiced, grey)
5. Signs of surgical wounds or dressings
6. End-of-bed charts—fever, tachycardia, fluid balance, trauma chart, pain chart, drug chart (e.g. strength and frequency of analgesia), modified early warning scores (MEWS)
7. 'Medical accessories'—i.v. infusion, urinary catheter, parenteral nutrition, monitoring equipment, oxygen mask

Peripheral stigmata of abdominal disease

1. Fingernails for koilonychia (spoon-shaped nails in iron deficiency) and leuconychia (whiteness and opacity of nails, sometimes due to hypoalbuminaemia)
2. Hands for palmar erythema and Dupuytren's contracture (association with liver disease)
3. Eyes—yellow sclerae in jaundice, pale conjunctivae in anaemia
4. Mouth and tongue—for ulceration suggestive of Crohn's, angular stomatitis in anaemia, dehydration, telangiectasia in hereditary haemorrhagic telangiectasia
5. Supraclavicular fossa palpation for enlarged lymph nodes, particularly medial left-sided Virchow's node indicating upper GI malignancy (Troisier's sign)
6. Inspect abdominal skin for jaundice and scratch marks resulting from pruritus (itching), spider naevi (indicate likely liver disease)
7. Chest in males for gynaecomastia in liver disease

Abdominal inspection

1. Position the patient correctly (comfortable, near-flat, arms by sides) and expose the whole abdominal field ('nipples to knees', but not all at once)
2. Distended or scaphoid (sunken) abdominal shape?
3. Skin—wounds and scars, redness, purulent discharge or other signs of infection, erythema ab igne (see Fig. 18.2)
4. Bruising—umbilical or flank in acute pancreatitis; cloth printing (trauma cases)
5. Herniation (including usual primary sites and incisional hernias)
6. Caput medusae—enlarged veins radiating from umbilicus indicating portal venous obstruction
7. Visible peristalsis—usually indicating long-standing small bowel obstruction

Abdominal palpation (*do not hurt the patient; watch the face for signs of discomfort*)

1. Gentle overall palpation for obvious abnormalities
2. Overall firmer palpation at a deeper level provides detailed examination of abnormal masses—relationship to abdominal wall, size, shape, position, mobility, texture, hardness, fixation posteriorly or anteriorly, tenderness. Likely site or organ of origin?
3. Specific organ palpation—press in first, then ask the patient to breathe in deeply; gradually relax your pressure and seek the descending lower edge of the organ; repeat at 3 cm intervals moving upwards:
   - Liver—start as low as it might have reached, e.g. right iliac fossa, and work upwards as above. Map out palpable lower liver edge. If large, palpate surface for irregularities, e.g. metastases. The enlarging liver usually remains in contact with the anterior abdominal wall and is dull to percussion. Percuss also for upper border to gauge liver size; auscultate a large liver for vascular bruits
   - Spleen—tilt patient slightly towards right side, place left hand behind lower left ribs and gently lift. Start as low as enlargement might have reached, e.g. right iliac fossa, and palpate as for liver. Seek notch in lower edge. To be palpable, spleen needs to be enlarged 2–3 times normal. Percuss for overlying resonance due to gas in bowel superficial to it
   - Kidneys—as with the liver, a renal mass usually descends with inspiration since the kidneys lie just beneath the diaphragm. Bimanual palpation enables the posteriorly placed kidney to be felt by displacing it anteriorly (see Fig. 18.3). Place left hand in loin and attempt to push enlarged organ forwards on to examining hand
4. Examination for ascites (see Fig. 18.4)
5. Hernial orifices—inguinal and femoral for cough impulse; reducibility (see Ch. 32)
6. Rectal and/or vaginal examination if appropriate (see Table 18.1)
7. Percussion and auscultation if appropriate

taken to exclude bronchial carcinoma; occasionally an oesophageal fluid level behind the heart is seen, resulting from an oesophageal stricture, hiatus hernia or achalasia. In high dysphagia, flexible pharyngoscopy followed by a barium swallow and meal is the usual sequence of investigation. In lower dysphagia, flexible endoscopy (OGD) is usually performed, as this allows direct inspection and biopsy; however, contrast radiography can be helpful. In disorders of function, swallowing barium-soaked bread or a video record of a barium swallow may be diagnostic. Oesophageal physiology measurements using manometry and pH monitoring are helpful in reaching a diagnosis of achalasia, especially in its early stages.

WEIGHT LOSS, ANOREXIA AND ASSOCIATED SYMPTOMS

Marked weight loss (**cachexia**) and loss of appetite (**anorexia**) are frequently manifestations of serious, insidious, often malignant abdominal disorders. There may be other symptoms such as malaise, bloating, nausea, sporadic vomiting and regurgitation. These symptoms may have been unnoticed or dismissed as trivial by the patient and are only elicited by direct questioning.

The diseases which cause these symptoms may be grouped into four broad categories:

- **Intra-abdominal malignancies**, e.g. carcinoma of stomach or pancreas, metastatic disease in the liver or

Fig. 18.2 Erythema ab igne

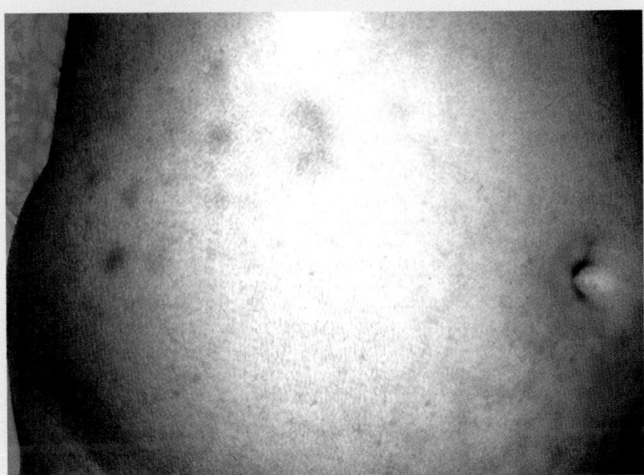

This woman of 45 suffered chronic pain in the right loin and had obtained some relief from regularly applying a hot water bottle to the area which resulted in typical skin damage. A staghorn calculus in the right kidney proved to be the cause

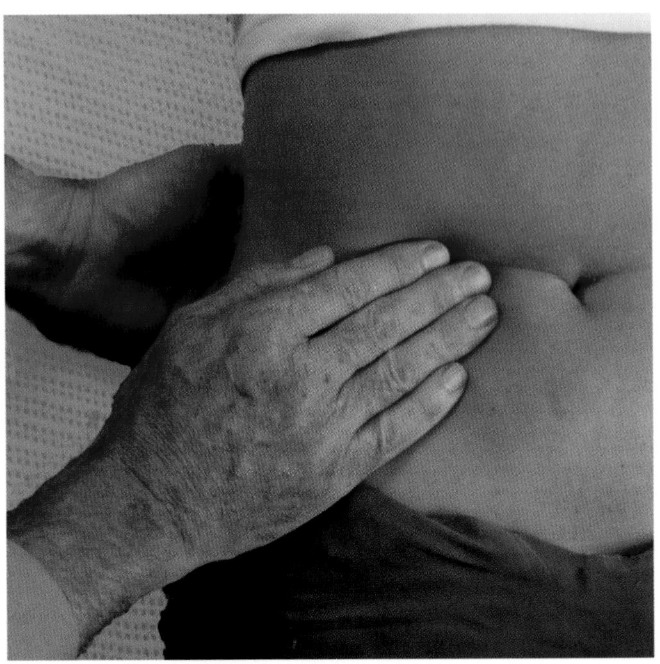

Fig. 18.3 Bimanual palpation of the abdomen
The posterior hand pushes forwards so that an enlarged viscus (usually retroperitoneal, e.g. kidney) or a mobile intra-abdominal mass is pushed onto the anterior examining hand. Note that this is not ballottement, which involves short, sharp palpation anteriorly, thus displacing ascites enabling a mass to bounce onto the examining hand

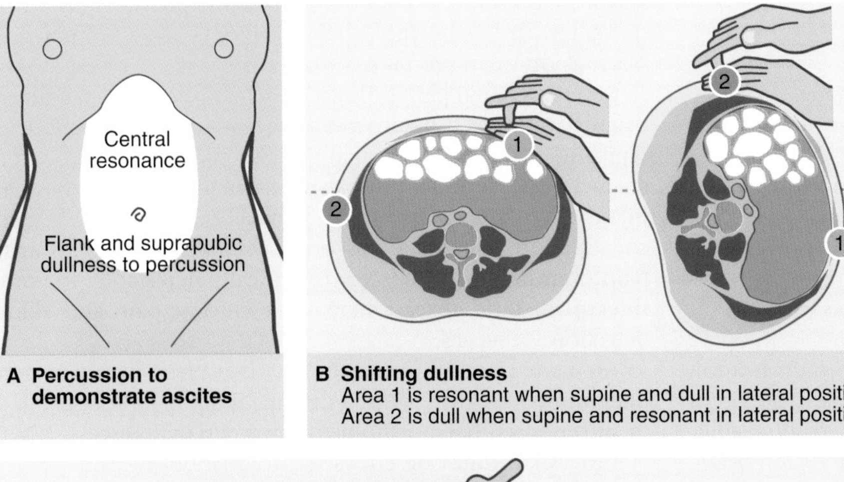

Fig. 18.4 Clinical signs of ascites

Box 18.4 Causes of dysphagia

Obstruction arising in the oesophageal wall

Common

- Peptic oesophagitis (often associated with hiatus hernia)—sometimes causes fibrous stricture
- Carcinoma of oesophagus or cardia (uppermost part) of the stomach

Uncommon

- Candida oesophagitis, particularly after major surgery

Extremely rare

- Pharyngeal pouch
- Oesophageal web (Plummer–Vinson/Paterson–Kelly syndrome)
- 'Oesophageal apoplexy' due to haematoma in the wall
- Leiomyoma of the oesophageal muscle

Disorders of neuromuscular function

- Achalasia—uncommon
- Bulbar or pseudobulbar palsy—rare
- Myasthenia gravis—rare

External compression of the oesophagus

- Subcarinal lymph node secondaries from carcinoma of the bronchus—fairly common
- Left atrial dilatation in mitral stenosis—rare
- Dysphagia lusoria (compression from abnormally placed great arteries)—very rare

widespread across the peritoneal cavity (arising particularly from stomach, large bowel, ovary, breast or bronchus), bowel lymphomas
- **'Medical' conditions**, e.g. alcoholism and cirrhosis, viral diseases (e.g. hepatitis or infectious mononucleosis), uncontrolled diabetes or thyrotoxicosis, malabsorption, renal failure, cardiac cachexia
- **Psychological disorders**, e.g. anxiety, depression, anorexia nervosa, bulimia
- **Chronic visceral ischaemia**, a very uncommon condition resulting from atherosclerotic narrowing of at least two of the three main visceral arteries—the coeliac axis and the superior mesenteric and the inferior mesenteric arteries—resulting in 'fear of food' and massive weight loss

APPROACH TO INVESTIGATION OF WEIGHT LOSS, ANOREXIA AND ASSOCIATED SYMPTOMS

There may be other clinical clues to the main diagnosis or to suggest a line of investigation, e.g. pain, signs of anaemia or jaundice, or a palpable abdominal or rectal mass. More difficult are cases where the symptoms occur alone. In that situation, basic screening investigations (full blood count and erythrocyte sedimentation rate, urea and electrolytes, liver function tests and urinalysis) begin to differentiate 'medical' conditions from 'surgical' ones. If these screening tests fail to produce a lead, abdominal imaging using ultrasound or CT scanning may be indicated to exclude liver metastases or occult intra-abdominal malignancy.

If investigations still reveal no cause, positive evidence of psychiatric disturbance should be sought. In practice, by this stage, previously concealed psychiatric features often become apparent, but except for anorexia nervosa or bulimia, these are rare.

ANAL AND PERIANAL SYMPTOMS

Anal bleeding

This is a very common symptom. It is well tolerated by patients who usually believe that 'piles' (haemorrhoids) are responsible. Patients often present when bleeding becomes excessive or when other symptoms develop. The characteristic feature of anal bleeding is fresh blood separate from stool which may only be seen 'on the paper'. Fresh bleeding, however, may arise from malignancy in the rectum, sigmoid colon or anal canal and must be treated seriously. In addition to digital examination and proctoscopy, all patients require at least sigmoidoscopy; patients over 40 require colonoscopy, barium enema or contrast CT examination to exclude large bowel cancer, whether or not a benign anal cause, such as haemorrhoids, has already been found.

Anal pain and discomfort

The principal causes of chronic anal pain and discomfort are haemorrhoids. Haemorrhoids usually cause intermittent bouts of discomfort and other anal symptoms rather than severe pain. Anal carcinoma is usually painless but may present with haemorrhoid-like symptoms. The difference is obvious on digital rectal examination.

Severe perianal pain following each episode of defaecation usually indicates a fissure-in-ano. This is a longitudinal tear typically in the posterior anal mucosa ending externally in a characteristic '**sentinel pile**', a small skin tag visible at the anal margin. A fissure is often initiated by a bout of unaccustomed constipation. A perianal abscess may be responsible for anal pain even before the abscess is clinically detectable; the rare **intersphincteric abscess** may cause chronic pain and elude detection for weeks.

An acute onset of anal pain may be caused by a **perianal haematoma**, clearly visible at the anal margin, by strangulated or thrombosed haemorrhoids or by a perianal abscess.

Proctalgia fugax describes recurrent shooting pains experienced in the anal area. Investigations should be performed to exclude local causes but usually no physical cause is found.

Perianal itching and irritation

The most common cause of these symptoms is inadequate hygiene resulting in local skin irritation. This is exacerbated by scratching or application of topical medications. The discharge associated with haemorrhoids, fistulae or tumours tends to cause itching and keep the perianal skin moist, predisposing to low-grade fungal and bacterial infections. The longer symptoms persist, the more difficult they are to eradicate and in fastidious patients a 'fixation' can develop. In children, threadworm infestation is a common cause of perianal itching, usually worse at night.

'Something coming down'

Haemorrhoids, skin tags ('memorials to past haemorrhoids') and occasionally mucosal or rectal prolapse cause this symptom. It is exacerbated by defaecation. Many patients tolerate the condition for some time before seeking medical advice and may have to push the lumps back manually after defaecation, presenting only when this becomes impossible. A pedunculated low rectal polyp may occasionally emerge through the anus and be confused with prolapsed haemorrhoids. Perianal warts are occasionally mistaken for lumps arising from within the anal canal.

Perianal discharge

This results from leakage of pus, inflammatory exudate or mucus from the anus or anal area. Pus may arise from a pilonidal sinus in the natal cleft or from an anal fistula. Inflammatory exudate or excess mucus may be produced by haemorrhoids, anorectal mucosal inflammation (proctitis), a villous adenoma or an ulcerating carcinoma.

APPROACH TO INVESTIGATION OF ANAL AND PERIANAL SYMPTOMS

Inspection of the anal area, careful digital rectal examination (DRE) and proctoscopy are mandatory (Table 18.1 and Fig. 18.5). Further examination follows the principles described earlier. If pain makes these examinations impossible, a young patient can usually be assumed to have a fissure. In an older person or those with specific risk factors (e.g. HIV positive), carcinoma of the anus must be excluded by examination under anaesthesia. Haemorrhoids appear as bulging bluish masses beneath the anal mucosa. They all arise above the squamo-columnar junction or dentate line ('internal piles') but may later extend beneath the perianal skin ('external piles') or prolapse through the anus ('intero-external piles').

A typical **anal fistula** appears as an inflammatory 'nipple' near the anal margin (see Fig. 18.6); it often exudes a discharge. In **proctitis**, the rectal mucosa is granular, erythematous and friable on proctoscopy. An anal or low rectal carcinoma is a discrete ulcerated lesion with an indurated (firm, woody) base and a thickened margin; diagnosis is confirmed by biopsy.

The lymphatic drainage of the anal canal below the dentate line is to inguinal lymph nodes and these should be examined when a suspicious anal lesion is found.

CHANGE IN BOWEL HABIT, RECTAL BLEEDING AND RELATED SYMPTOMS

Normal bowel habit varies widely between individuals in frequency and consistency of stool. Transient changes in habit are usually insignificant but persistent change definitely require investigation. The differential diagnosis of a change in bowel habit is summarised in Box 18.5.

FREQUENCY OF DEFAECATION AND STOOL CONSISTENCY

Chronic constipation or diarrhoea mark the extremes of change, although some patients develop an erratic bowel action. Any change may signify serious disease; the index of suspicion is further raised if there is rectal bleeding or tenesmus (for definition, see p. 256). Waking from sleep to

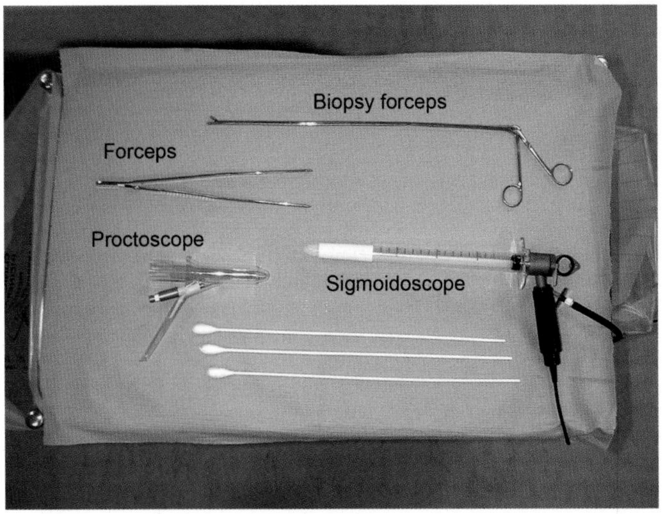

Fig. 18.5 Procto-sigmoidoscopy trolley
Typical layout of trolley prepared for proctoscopy and sigmoidoscopy in an outpatient clinic. Note the yellow waste bag on the left for contaminated swabs and waste and the paper bag on the right for waste wrapping from swabs, etc. Sigmoidoscopic biopsies are placed in a container of formol saline for fixation

Fig. 18.6 Anal fistula

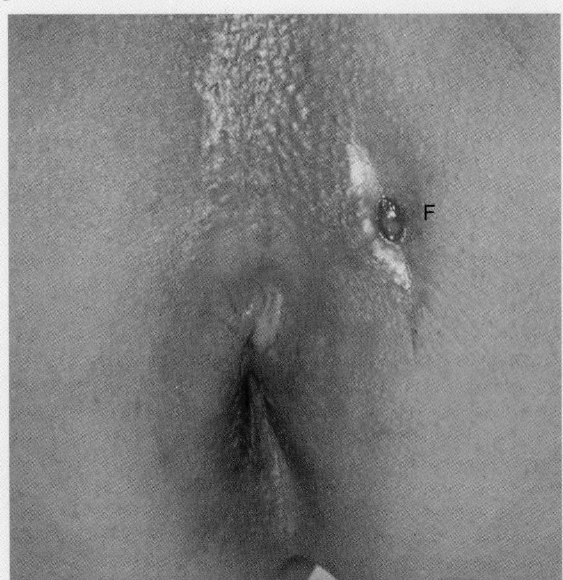

This man of 39 had presented with a perianal abscess 3 months previously that had been drained. He complained of persistent discharge which was found to be emanating from a fistulous opening **F** within the drainage scar. On further examination under anaesthesia this proved to be a low fistula

Table 18.1 Investigation of anal and colorectal symptoms

1. Digital rectal examination	
Purpose	Inspection of the anal and perianal area for skin changes and lesions Palpation of the anal canal and lower rectum and surrounding tissues. Normally the firm walls of the anal sphincter are felt over the first 5 cm or so. Above that level, the rectal walls are soft and mobile
Preparation	Chaperone if necessary 'Consent'—written or implied Patient position to maintain dignity—usually left lateral with knees drawn up Equipment—good light, surgical gloves, gel lubricant, tissues
Technique ● **Inspection**	 Sentinel pile; excoriation; ulceration, perianal haematoma; fistulous opening; scars; abscess; prolapsed mucosa or haemorrhoids; skin tags
● **Palpation** Always minimise pain and discomfort—if pain/spasm prevents examination a fissure or anal carcinoma may be present *Note*: in the female, the uterine cervix is often felt anteriorly as a firm but localised mass. In the male, the normal prostate gland is felt near the tip of the finger anteriorly as a smooth, firm swelling about 2 cm in diameter with a midline groove between the lateral lobes	*In lumen*—faeces/blood/foreign body *In wall*—ulceration, polyp, thrombosed piles, internal opening of tract or fistula; Crohn's thickening; anal carcinoma; lack of normal softness *Outside wall*—prostatic enlargement (usually benign) can be palpated, as can irregularity or nodularity which may represent carcinoma; cervix; frozen pelvis; mass in pouch of Douglas *Note*: glove should be checked for blood/mucus/colour of stool
2. Proctoscopy (Fig. 18.5; see also Ch. 30)	
Purpose	Direct visualisation of mucosa of anal canal Must be done even if rigid sigmoidoscopy/barium enema/MRI to be done Therapy, e.g. sclerotherapy/banding of haemorrhoids
Technique	The proctoscope with obturator in situ is lubricated and gently introduced into the anal canal to its greatest extent (10 cm). The obturator is removed and the instrument slowly withdrawn, ensuring that the mucosa of the entire anal canal is inspected
Findings in mucosa	Inflammation/granular surface Superficial ulceration Haemorrhoids—bleeding, degree of prolapse Anal carcinoma Solitary 'rectal' ulcer Pus Fistula Fibrous polyps Melanoma
3. Rigid Sigmoidoscopy (for flexible sigmoidoscopy see text)	
Purpose	**Visualisation** of the rectum up to rectosigmoid junction—18–20 cm **Biopsy** of suspicious lesions or abnormal mucosa
Technique	As for proctoscopy for 10 cm or so. Obturator removed and proximal end closed with lens. Gentle inflation whilst inspecting lumen, manipulating and advancing 'scope with least discomfort to patient Faecal loading may prevent visualisation; pain may limit examination to lower rectum only
Examples of pathology	Inflammation/granular surface Superficial ulceration Pus Polyps and adenomas Carcinoma Melanosis coli Strictures

Box 18.5 Differential diagnosis of change in bowel habit

- Carcinoma of colon, rectum or anus
- Diverticular disease
- Irritable bowel syndrome
- Crohn's disease of small or large bowel
- Ulcerative colitis
- Drug effects, e.g. codeine phosphate, iron, laxative abuse
- Reduction in fibre content of diet
- Parasitic infestations, e.g. giardiasis
- Following acute bacterial or parasitic colitis
- Changes in resident bacterial flora, e.g. antibiotic-associated diarrhoea
- Malabsorption syndromes
- Thyrotoxicosis

Note: in many cases, no cause is found

evacuate the bowels should be treated seriously, especially if it occurs persistently.

Stool consistency varies according to diet but the stool is usually 'formed'. Persistently unformed stools, i.e. 'looseness', is only abnormal if it represents a change from the patient's norm.

Constipation

Severe constipation arises for four main reasons:

- Incomplete bowel obstruction, e.g. faecal impaction, an obstructing carcinoma or stricture in the bowel wall, or occasionally an extrinsic lesion such as ovarian cancer
- Loss of peristalsis, e.g. acutely due to drugs such as narcotics, antidepressants or iron, chronic diverticular disease, chronic laxative abuse
- Inadequate fibre intake or poor fluid intake, which decrease faecal volume and prolong intestinal transit time
- In bed-bound patients, multiple factors including immobility, diet, inadequate fluid intake, drug effects

Diarrhoea

Chronic diarrhoea is most often caused by irritation or inflammation of small or large bowel. The inflammatory bowel diseases (ulcerative colitis and Crohn's disease) are important diagnoses. Chronic parasitic infestations of large bowel with amoebae or of small bowel with *Giardia lamblia* are easily overlooked. In areas where these diseases are not endemic, patients may give a history of foreign travel. Chronic diarrhoea may follow an acute attack of *Salmonella* or other coliform infection. Less commonly, a blind loop of small bowel remaining after bypass surgery becomes colonised with gut flora, causing changes in intraluminal metabolism (**blind loop syndrome**). The most common diagnosis in diarrhoea after intestinal infection is irritable bowel syndrome.

Bile salts irritate the bowel. Therefore if the enterohepatic circulation is disrupted, e.g. after distal small bowel resection, defective reabsorption of bile salts may cause diarrhoea. A less common cause is the increased volume of bowel contents in malabsorption syndromes. Finally, when no physical cause can be found, concealed laxative abuse or an anxiety state should be considered. Early morning diarrhoea on its own rarely indicates serious disease.

Erratic bowel habit

Some patients develop an erratic bowel habit with bouts of constipation interspersed with episodes of frequency and looseness of stool. The most common cause is **irritable bowel syndrome**, which can be attributed to a heightened pain response in conjunction with a possible over-production of enteric gas. Sometimes symptoms include a marked gastrocolic reflex, i.e. a call to stool immediately after eating. In **diverticular disease**, constipation and 'rabbit-pellet' faeces are the dominant characteristics (see Ch. 29). However, there may be episodic diarrhoea during periods of inflammation or following release of proximal liquefied stool past partially obstructed solid faeces (**spurious diarrhoea**). Incomplete bowel obstruction of this type may also occur in carcinoma of the left colon, Crohn's disease or faecal impaction.

Patients treated with broad-spectrum antibiotics, particularly the cephalosporins, may develop **antibiotic-associated diarrhoea**. If caused by *Clostridium difficile*, this is known as **pseudomembranous colitis** in its severe form; the symptoms are due to changes in colonic bacterial flora (see Ch. 12).

Changes in the nature of the stool

Stools are normally brown owing to the presence of urobilin, a breakdown product of bile. In biliary obstruction, bilirubin fails to reach the gut and stools become pale. In obvious jaundice, they are often described as 'putty-coloured' or 'clay-coloured'.

Stools may also be pale when they contain excess fat as in various malabsorption syndromes. In coeliac disease (gluten enteropathy) the stool is often loose and offensive. In fat malabsorption, the lipid rich stools tend to float and are difficult to flush away (**steatorrhoea**).

Undigested food in the stool indicates malabsorption or a 'short-circuit' in the bowel due to previous bowel resection or a fistula between bowel loops. Note that this can be normal when the diet is extremely high in fibre.

Presence of frank blood, altered blood or mucus in the stool

Note: acute gastrointestinal haemorrhage is covered in Chapter 19.

Frank rectal bleeding

When a patient has seen blood in the stool, it is important to know the colour, i.e. fresh or altered blood, and also the relationship of the blood to the stool. Bright red blood usually indicates a lesion in the rectum or anus. When blood is clearly separate from the stool it suggests an anal lesion (see above). If blood is on the surface of the stool it suggests a lesion such as an adenoma (see Fig. 18.7) or carcinoma in the rectum or descending colon. These observations have limited diagnostic reliability and all rectal bleeding should be assumed to be caused by a tumour until proven otherwise.

When older, darker blood is mixed with the stool, it usually indicates even more proximal disease, i.e. descending or

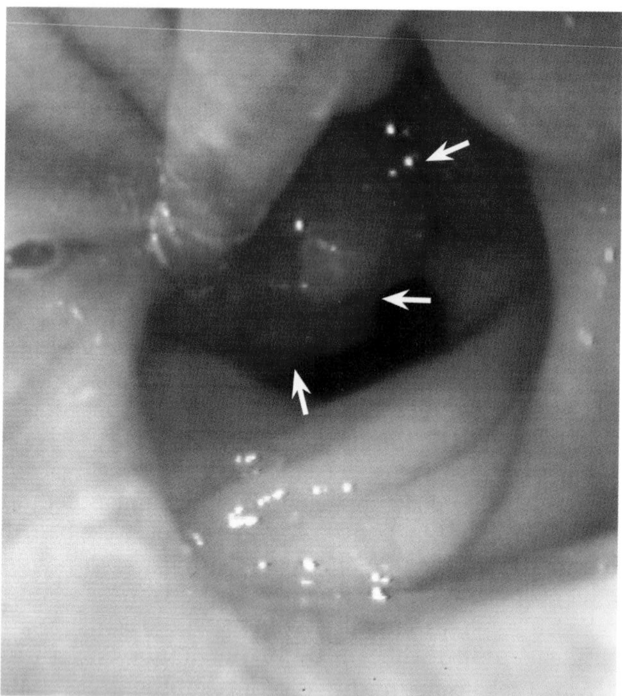

Fig. 18.7 Colonoscopic appearance of a polyp in the sigmoid colon
This 2 cm polyp (arrowed) was found to be the cause of rectal bleeding. It was easily removed with a colonoscopic snare soon after this photograph was taken

transverse colon. Carcinoma or inflammatory ulceration is often the cause. When the blood originates more proximally in the gastrointestinal tract, e.g. peptic ulcer, it is so altered by digestion that it may not be recognised as blood by the patient. The stool is typically shiny black or plum-coloured, has a characteristic odour, and with rapid bleeding, becomes fluid or 'tarry' (**melaena**). Patients on iron therapy have greenish-black, formed stools, not to be mistaken for altered blood; faecal occult blood testing should be negative.

Occult faecal blood loss
A persistent trickle of blood from the gastrointestinal tract may not alter the appearance of the stool but can cause serious iron deficiency anaemia. This 'occult' blood may be detectable only by chemical tests; these should be repeated three times to prevent false negatives.

Rectal passage of mucus or pus
Mucus ('slime') or pus may be passed alone or with the stool. The most common cause is irritable bowel syndrome. **Villous adenomas** typically secrete copious mucus, but this may also occur with rectal carcinoma. Mucus and pus may be noted in inflammatory bowel disorders and occasionally in diverticular disease. An anal leak of mucus may be a feature of haemorrhoids and causes itching (**pruritus ani**). A patient sometimes reports passing a mass of purulent material. This usually represents spontaneous discharge of a perianal or pararectal abscess, and will often be preceded by anal or perineal pain.

Tenesmus

Tenesmus is an unpleasant sensation of incomplete evacuation of the rectum. The sensation causes the patient to attempt defaecation (often with straining) at frequent intervals. The most common causes are irritable bowel syndrome or an abnormal mass in the rectum or anal canal (e.g. polyp; carcinoma). Occasionally a prostatic carcinoma invades around the lower rectum producing tenesmus. In some cases, despite extensive investigation, no organic cause is found.

APPROACH TO INVESTIGATION OF CHANGE IN BOWEL HABIT

In chronic diarrhoea, stool specimens should be examined for ova and parasites and cultured for *Shigella* and *Salmonella* species. After rectal palpation and proctoscopy, the next step is sigmoidoscopy. **Rigid sigmoidoscopy** (more accurately termed rectoscopy) permits visual examination up to the rectosigmoid junction and mucosal biopsy for histology and microbiology. **Flexible sigmoidoscopy** allows more precise examination as far as the splenic flexure, the area in which over 50% of large bowel cancers occur.

Further investigation is based on the differential diagnosis assembled during clinical examination. Barium enema X-ray, contrast CT scanning or colonoscopy is indicated in most cases. Low rectal lesions cannot reliably be demonstrated on barium enema, and so preliminary sigmoidoscopy is mandatory. Note that more than one colonic adenoma or carcinoma can occur at the same time (synchronous lesions), so a full colonic examination is needed if one lesion is found. If Crohn's disease is suspected, barium studies of small bowel may also be required.

IRON DEFICIENCY ANAEMIA

A common reason for surgical referral is persistent or severe anaemia believed to be caused by chronic intestinal blood loss. The patient may have presented with symptoms of chronic anaemia, namely lethargy, generalised weakness, breathlessness or even angina. Just as often, the anaemia has been recognised during general examination or on a blood count.

Chronic anaemia has many causes. Iron deficiency is the most common and the only one with a cause likely to need surgical treatment. In blood films, iron deficiency anaemia is characterised by hypochromic, microcytic red blood cells. Serum iron level is low and transferrin elevated. Iron deficiency anaemia can be caused by chronic low-grade blood loss (often occult), inadequate dietary iron intake or absorption, or a combination. The pattern of iron deficiency may be complicated by coexisting anaemia from another cause, particularly the 'anaemia of chronic illness'. For example, an elderly patient with rheumatoid arthritis may have a chronic normochromic, normocytic anaemia due to chronic disease, as well as an iron deficiency anaemia caused by gastric bleeding provoked by non-steroidal anti-inflammatory drugs. Pernicious anaemia or folate deficiency anaemia may also underlie iron deficiency anaemia.

APPROACH TO INVESTIGATION OF ANAEMIA

Investigation of a patient with suspected iron deficiency anaemia has five main components:

- History—seeking sources of blood loss from the various tracts (see Box 18.6) and excluding inadequate

Box 18.6 Conditions causing chronic occult blood loss

Lesions in the gastrointestinal tract

- Ulcerating tumours or polyps of the following (in order of frequency): caecum, stomach, the rest of the large bowel, and (rarely) stromal tumours of small bowel, e.g. leiomyosarcoma (GIST)
- Chronic peptic ulceration, i.e. hiatus hernia with reflux oesophagitis, gastric and duodenal ulcers or stomal ulceration following gastric surgery. All may be induced or aggravated by ingestion of aspirin and other non-steroidal anti-inflammatory drugs. These drugs can also cause chronic gastric haemorrhage from superficial erosions
- Other 'ulcerating' lesions of the bowel, e.g. haemorrhoids, angiodysplasias of colon or small bowel
- Chronic parasitic infestations, e.g. hookworm (extremely common in some developing countries)
- Angiodysplasias—small vascular malformations, single or multiple, occurring anywhere from stomach to rectum which bleed spontaneously

Lesions in the female genital tract

- Heavy menstrual loss (menorrhagia is an extremely common but easily overlooked cause)
- Carcinoma of uterus or cervix (usually presents as abnormal vaginal bleeding rather than anaemia)

Lesions in the urinary tract (rarely sufficient to cause anaemia)

- Transitional cell carcinoma of bladder, pelvicalyceal systems or ureters
- Renal cell carcinoma (may cause haematuria but rarely anaemia)
- Chronic parasitic infestations, e.g. schistosomiasis (common in some developing countries)

iron intake. Previous gastrectomy may cause vitamin B_{12} deficiency and also diminished acid output, which may diminish iron absorption. Drug history—aspirin, other NSAIDs and corticosteroids may be the cause of chronic gastroduodenal blood loss. A history of drug treatment for peptic ulcer or antacids for 'indigestion' may also indicate a source of blood loss

- Physical examination—seeking an abdominal mass, an enlarged Virchow's node in the left supraclavicular area (indicative of intra-abdominal malignancy), a rectal lesion or signs of a 'medical' cause
- Confirmation of iron deficiency anaemia and exclusion of common 'medical' causes of anaemia such as rheumatoid arthritis or chronic leukaemias—examine blood film, measure ESR, serum iron and transferrin, B_{12} and folate. When there is a 'mixed' anaemia, measuring iron stores in a bone marrow biopsy is the definitive method of diagnosing iron deficiency. Small bowel biopsies may demonstrate coeliac disease in a proportion of patients with simple anaemia without bowel symptoms
- Testing of specimens of stool for occult blood (at least three specimens)
- Pursuing clues that suggest the origin of bleeding with special investigations such as endoscopy and contrast radiology. When faecal occult blood is positive, colonoscopy is performed, looking for tumours, polyps, inflammatory bowel disease or angiodysplasias. If negative, this is followed by gastroscopy. Both can be performed in one session. If both are negative, it may be appropriate to proceed to small bowel contrast radiography, flexible small bowel enteroscopy or **capsule endoscopy** (see Ch. 5).

OBSTRUCTIVE JAUNDICE

THE NORMAL ENTEROHEPATIC CIRCULATION (Fig. 18.8)

The **haem** component of spent red cells is normally broken down to bilirubin (mainly in spleen and bone marrow), bound to albumin and transported to the liver. This relatively stable protein–pigment complex is insoluble in water and is not excreted in urine. In the liver, the complex is split and the bilirubin conjugated with glucuronic acid which makes it water-soluble, before being excreted into the bile canaliculi. The normal concentration of both conjugated and unconjugated bilirubin in the blood is very low. Bacterial action in the bowel converts conjugated bilirubin into colourless **urobilinogen** and pigmented **urobilin** which imparts the brown colour to normal faeces. Some urobilinogen is reabsorbed, passing to the liver in the portal blood, and is then re-excreted in the bile. The entire process is called an **enterohepatic circulation** (see Fig. 18.8). A small amount of urobilinogen escapes into the systemic circulation and is excreted in the urine, colouring it yellow.

Bile acids (salts) are synthesised in the liver from cholesterol-based precursors. These are excreted in bile to the duodenum and facilitate lipid digestion and absorption in the small intestine. About 95% of the bile acids are reabsorbed in the distal ileum and returned to the liver via the portal vein, only to be re-excreted in the bile. Thus both bilirubin and bile acids are involved in enterohepatic circulations.

PATHOPHYSIOLOGY OF OBSTRUCTIVE JAUNDICE

If biliary outflow becomes obstructed, conjugated bilirubin is dammed back in the liver from where it enters the bloodstream and causes a gradual rise in plasma bilirubin. Once the plasma bilirubin level exceeds about 30 μmol/L, jaundice should be clinically detectable. Conjugated bilirubin, being water-soluble, is excreted in the urine, turning it dark.

In obstructive jaundice there is diminished or absent excretion of bile into the bowel, causing changes in the faeces. There is less urobilin to darken the stool and fewer bile acids, resulting in defective fat absorption and characteristic 'putty' coloured stool.

A consequence of poor dietary fat absorption is malabsorption of fat soluble vitamins A, D, E and K. Lack of vitamin K

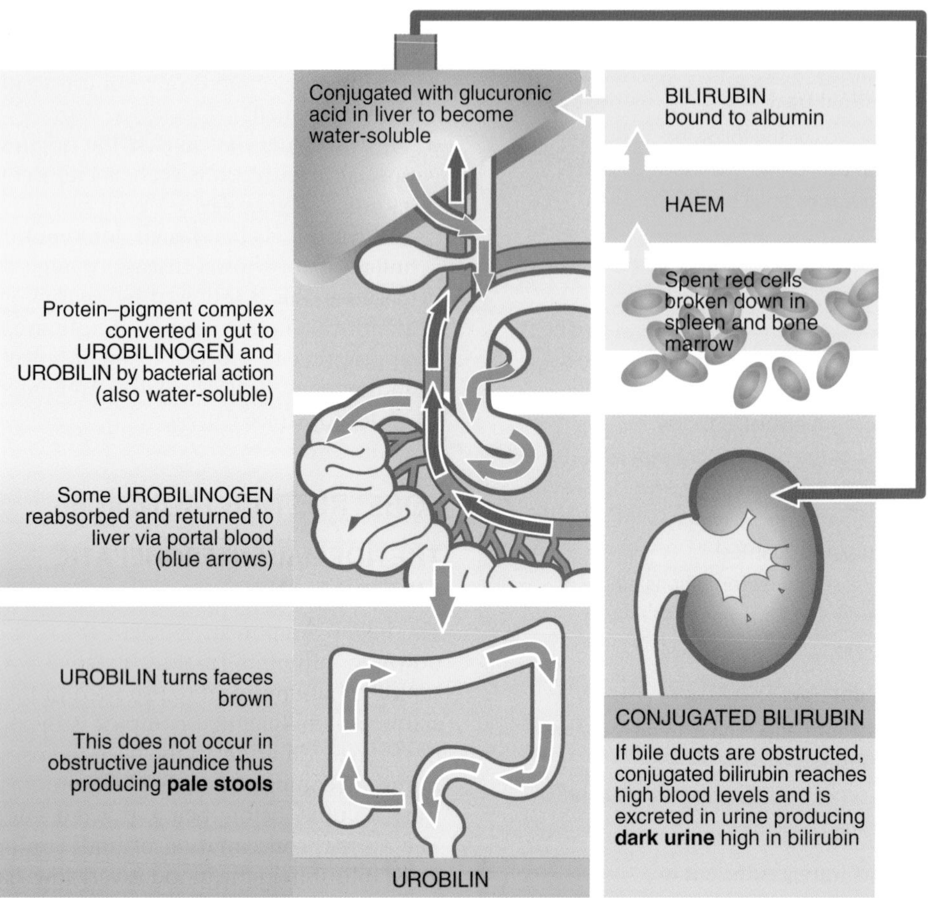

Fig. 18.8 Normal dynamics of bilirubin excretion and the effects of obstructive jaundice
Note that urobilinogen will appear in substantial quantities in the urine if large amounts are produced because of haemolytic anaemia, or if there is liver cell damage

leads to decreased hepatic synthesis of clotting factors, notably prothrombin (factor II), factors VII, IX, and X, and proteins C, S, and Z. Impaired blood clotting leads increases the risk of haemorrhage during invasive procedures, so a clotting screen must be checked beforehand. The coagulopathy is corrected with parenteral vitamin K or, in an urgent procedure, fresh frozen plasma. Biliary obstruction also dams back bile acids, which raises their blood concentration leading to deposition in the skin; this can cause intense itching.

HISTORY AND EXAMINATION OF PATIENTS WITH OBSTRUCTIVE JAUNDICE

History-taking

This should include enquiry about episodes of pain typical of gallstone disease, previous episodes of obstructive jaundice, biliary tract surgery or attacks of acute pancreatitis. Other important aspects of the history include:

- Change in colour of urine and stools, i.e. dark urine and pale stools
- Drug history, e.g. oral contraceptive pill—potential for intrahepatic cholestasis
- Risk factors for viral hepatitis—blood product transfusion, intravenous drug abuse, tattoos, shellfish ingestion, sexual exposure
- Alcohol intake—if excessive, predisposes to pancreatitis and cirrhosis
- Symptoms associated with malignancy—anorexia, weight loss and non-specific upper GI disturbance is common in carcinoma of the pancreas, a disease of later life
- A history of inflammatory bowel disease predisposes to **sclerosing cholangitis** although this is uncommon

Examination

Early jaundice is a subtle physical sign and can be missed unless the patient is examined in a good light, preferably daylight. Jaundice is first detectable in the sclera and soon afterwards in abdominal wall skin. In some cases of obstructive jaundice, the patient develops generalised itching (pruritus) and scratch marks may be evident. The general stigmata of liver disease, such as spider naevi and liver 'flap' of the wrists are found only when jaundice is caused by primary liver disease rather than extrinsic obstruction.

The abdomen should be examined, particularly for ascites, an enlarged liver or spleen, abnormal masses or a palpable gall bladder. An enlarged liver may be caused by primary or secondary malignancy, and in the tropics, schistosomiasis or malaria. In a jaundiced patient, splenomegaly with hepatomegaly is an important sign of chronic parenchymal liver disease (usually cirrhosis) and indicates portal hypertension. Ascites

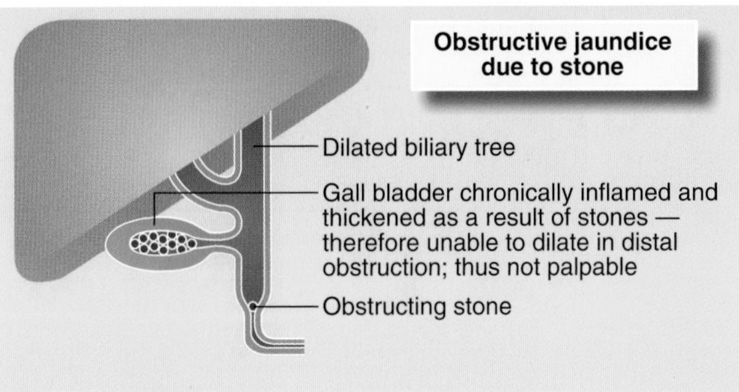

Fig. 18.9 Courvoisier's law

in a patient with obstructive jaundice is almost always due to disseminated intra-abdominal malignancy.

Courvoisier's 'law' (see Fig. 18.9) was formulated in 1890 and states that obstructive jaundice in the presence of a palpable gall bladder is not due to stone (and therefore likely to be caused by tumour). The argument is that gallstones cause chronic inflammation leading to gall bladder fibrosis or intermittent stone obstruction leads to hypertrophy of the gall bladder wall, either preventing its distension. In malignancy, progressive obstruction occurs over a short period and the non-thickened gall bladder distends easily.

Particular attention is paid to the colour of stool found on rectal examination, as a pale stool is characteristic of obstructive jaundice. The urine in obstructive jaundice is usually dark yellow or orange from the presence of conjugated bilirubin, and froths when shaken owing to the detergent effect of bile acids. Conditions causing obstructive jaundice are illustrated in Figure 18.10.

APPROACH TO INVESTIGATION OF JAUNDICE

Urine tests

The concentration of bilirubin in urine is easily established by dipstick tests. Substantial quantities usually mean biliary obstruction.

Blood tests

- Infective hepatitis should be excluded by serological screening for hepatitis B and C. A history of transfusion, intravenous drug abuse or travel to developing countries may increase the likelihood of an infection
- Confirm that the jaundice is obstructive by liver function tests, although these are not completely reliable. Obstructive jaundice is characterised by elevated plasma conjugated bilirubin and marked elevation of plasma alkaline phosphatase (liver isoenzyme). The transaminases, derived from hepatocytes, are usually only mildly elevated
- When biliary obstruction is intrahepatic (e.g. cholangiocarcinoma obstructing one duct) there may be a mixed biochemical picture with evidence of hepatocyte damage and duct obstruction. Liver function tests are an unreliable guide and liver ultrasonography is mandatory
- Mild jaundice is commonly found in patients with Gilbert's syndrome, caused by a mild congenital abnormality of haemoglobin metabolism without serious significance
- Coagulation studies should be performed because of likely defects in clotting
- Tumour markers should be tested for in patients with a previous history of GI malignancy

Imaging

Hepatobiliary ultrasonography

This is the simplest means of demonstrating dilated intrahepatic ducts (see Fig. 18.11), liver secondaries, a dilated extrahepatic biliary system or gall bladder abnormalities including stones. Ultrasound is unreliable for demonstrating pathology in the lower part of the biliary tree, and although it may show gallstones or lesions in the head of the pancreas, it is unreliable for excluding them.

CT scanning

This may be the next stage if ultrasound findings are equivocal. CT is particularly useful for demonstrating primary or secondary tumours but may miss a small carcinoma at the lower end of the common bile duct.

Endoscopic and magnetic resonance cholangio-pancreatography

If ultrasound demonstrates dilated ducts, endoscopic retrograde cholangio-pancreatography (ERCP) is often the next investigation (see Fig. 18.12). It is now usual practice to drain an obstructed bile duct at the same procedure if practicable, by sphincterotomy and stone removal or by placing an intraluminal **stent**. This may be the definitive treatment for duct stones or inoperable carcinomas; for patients requiring operation, stenting may be used to allow jaundice to settle and liver function to improve, but stents can interfere with endoscopic ultrasound staging of cancers. The role of diagnostic ERCP has been largely superseded by magnetic resonance cholangio-pancreatography (MRCP), described in Chapter 5.

Laparoscopy and liver biopsy

If bile ducts are not dilated, biopsy of liver or of demonstrated secondaries may be performed (with ultrasound or CT

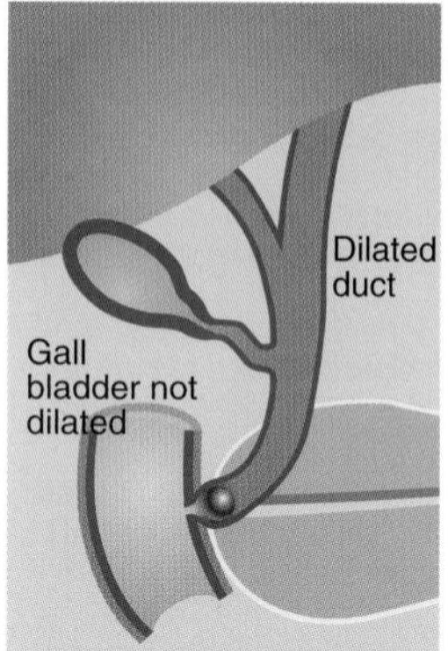

Stone impacted at lower end of CBD

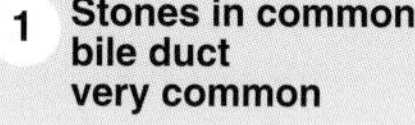

1 Stones in common bile duct very common

Suggested by a history of pain typical of biliary colic. Jaundice may be progressive (If stone is firmly impacted), fluctuant without ever disappearing altogether (if a stone alternately impacts and disimpacts), or intermittent (if multiple small stones successively impact then pass through the lower end of the common bile duct)

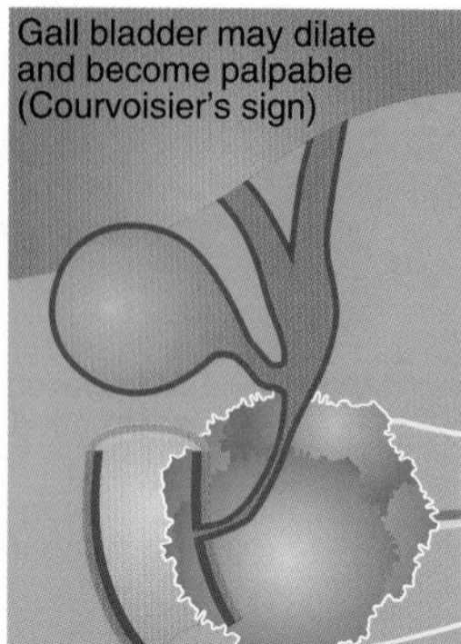

CBD compressed by carcinoma as it passes through the head of pancreas

May also invade or compress 2nd part of duodenum

2 Carcinoma of head of pancreas common

Typically causes painless jaundice which is persistent or progressive. The gall bladder may become palpable (Courvoisier's law, see Fig 18.9)

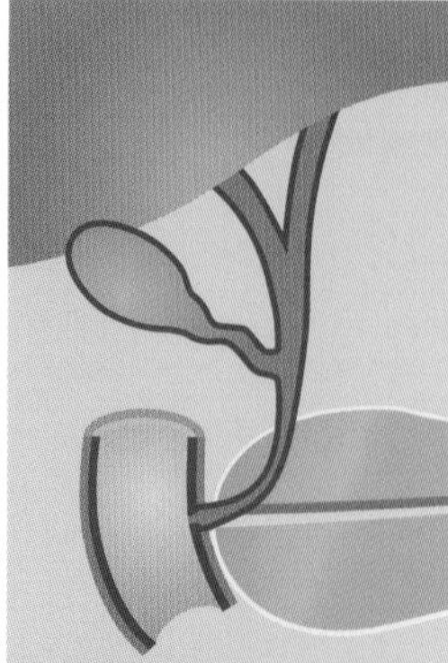

Acute or chronic pancreatitis may compress CBD in a similar way to pancreatic carcinoma in 2 by inflammation or scarring

3 Pancreatitis uncommon

Common bile duct is obstructed by inflammatory swelling in acute pancreatitis or by scarring in chronic pancreatitis

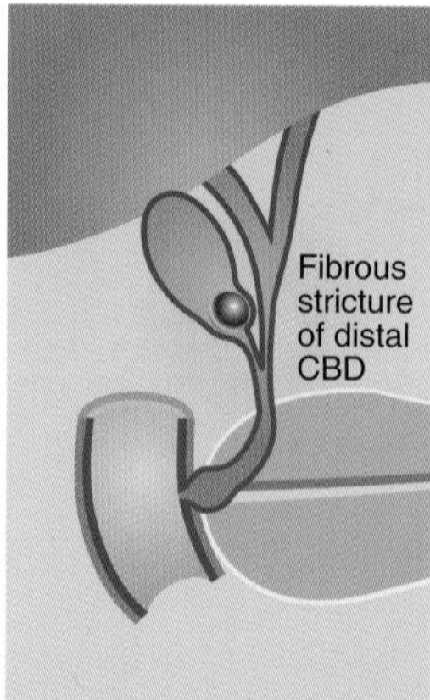

4 Mirizzi's syndrome rare

Found in about 1% of cholecystectomy patients. Gallstones impacted in Hartmann's pouch cause inflammation of the gall bladder which then fuses with the CHD causing secondary stenosis. Large impacted stones sometimes cause pressure necrosis of the adjoining duct walls leading to chole–choledochal fistula

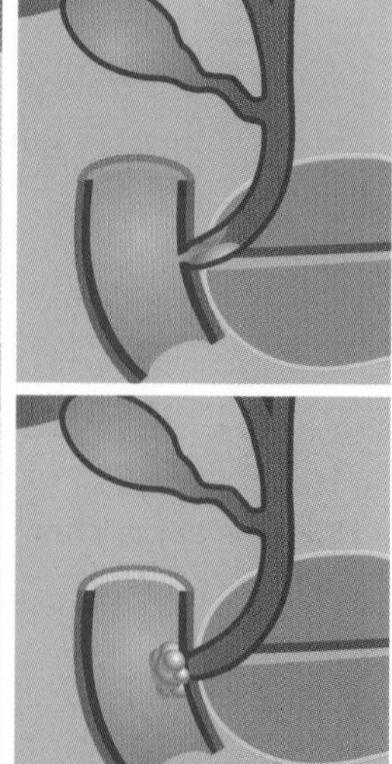

5 Periampullary malignant tumours uncommon

Include carcinomas of the ampulla, distal bile duct or duodenum (uncommon). Obstructive features are similar to carcinoma of head of pancreas

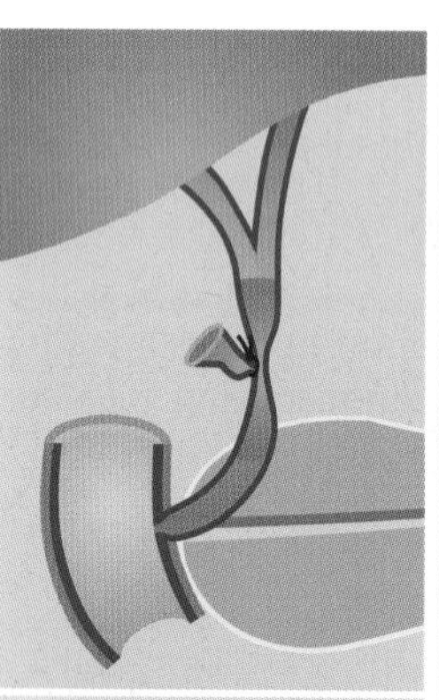

6 Benign strictures of the common bile duct uncommon

May be due to surgical damage (fairly common) or inflammation caused by previous stone. Obstructive features are similar to carcinoma of head of pancreas in 2

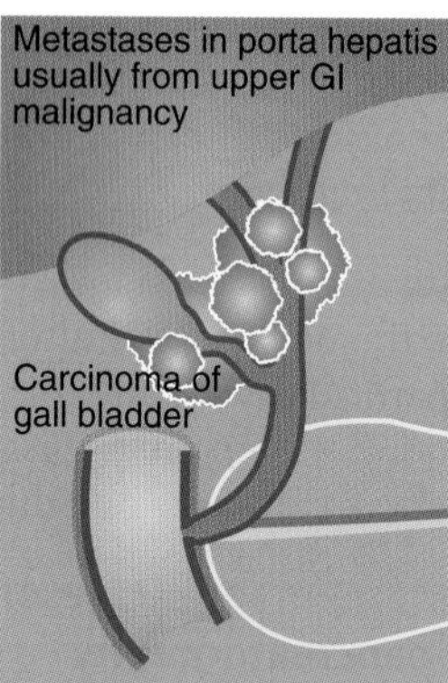

7 Other malignant tumours rare

May cause bile duct obstruction above the ampulla. Examples include lymph node metastases in the porta hepatis (fairly common), primary cholangiocarcinoma (uncommon) and carcinoma of the gall bladder

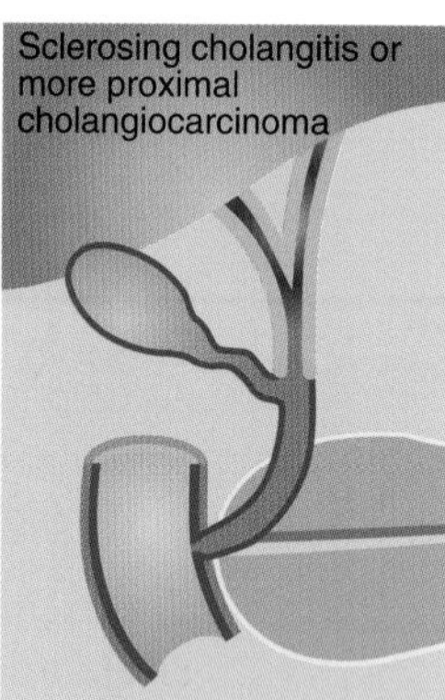

8 Intrahepatic or hilar bile duct obstruction rare

Primary cholangiocarcinoma; sclerosing cholangitis (rare)

Note: hepatic metastases rarely cause obstructive jaundice

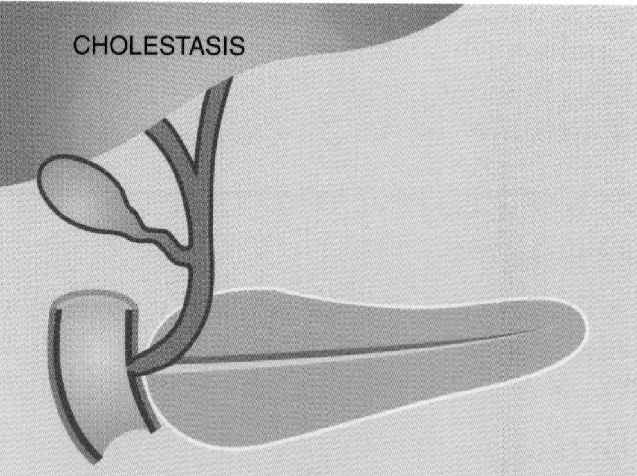

9 Intrahepatic cholestasis common

Viral hepatitis is a common cause.

Systemic sepsis often causes low grade jaundice (due to liver dysfunction).

Idiosyncrasy to certain drugs (including chlorpromazine, oral contraceptives and chlorpropamide) interferes with bile excretion from hepatocytes, presumably by affecting membrane transport.
Widespread hepatic lymphoma is a classical but rare cause

Fig. 18.10 Causes of obstructive jaundice

guidance), after correcting clotting abnormalities with vitamin K or fresh-frozen plasma.

In patients unsuitable for percutaneous biopsy, or those who require visualisation of other organs, laparoscopy can visualise the liver directly and obtain biopsy specimens from suspicious areas. Occasionally, a firm diagnosis cannot be made before a definitive operation; abdominal exploration and frozen section histology may provide the answer.

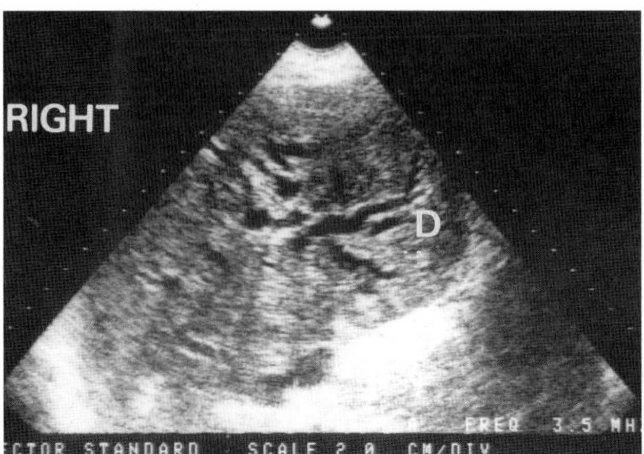

Fig. 18.11 Ultrasonogram showing dilated intrahepatic ducts
An ultrasound scan in an 80-year-old man with obstructive jaundice. This transverse section through the liver shows the characteristic 'double-barrel shotgun sign' **D**, with two parallel tubular structures representing major branches of the bile duct and portal vein. Normally, the portal vein is four times wider than the corresponding bile duct. Here they are the same diameter

PRINCIPLES OF MANAGEMENT OF OBSTRUCTIVE JAUNDICE

The primary aim of treatment is to relieve the biliary tract obstruction. Obstructed bile is often infected and a fulminant **acute cholangitis** can develop at any time. Back-pressure interferes with liver functions such as synthesis of albumin and clotting factors. Eventually structural liver damage ensues.

Three categories of obstruction can be defined according to treatment options:

- Potentially curable obstructions
- Obstruction due to incurable tumour
- Terminal disease

Potentially curable obstructions

These include bile duct stones and strictures as well as small tumours of the lower bile ducts, duodenum or ampullary region (*periampullary tumours*) (see Fig. 18.10, p. 260).

The number, size and position of **bile duct stones** may have been identified before operation by ERCP or MRCP. Stones can be removed at ERCP by dividing the ampullary sphincter using a 'bow-string' diathermy wire via the duodenal endoscope. Sometimes, if the stone is very large or impacted, obstructed bile may be drained by endoscopic placement of a stent (up to about 4 mm in diameter) alongside it within the bile duct without stone removal. Endoscopic procedures are treatments of choice for patients with common bile duct stones causing obstructive jaundice.

If cholecystectomy is the chosen treatment, bile duct stones can be identified by **perioperative cholangiography** and

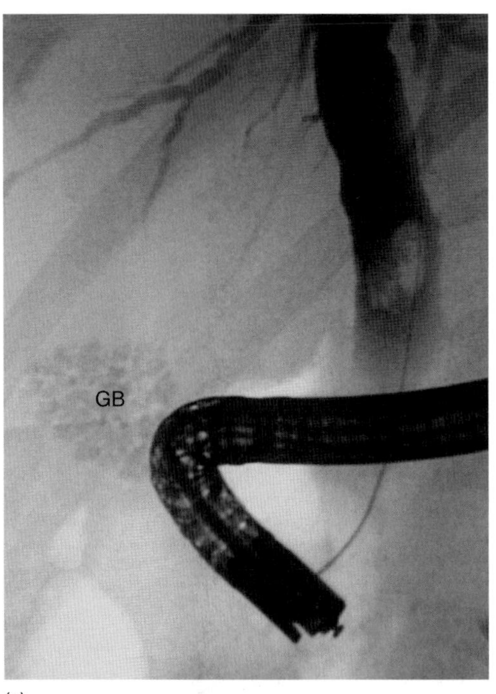

(a)

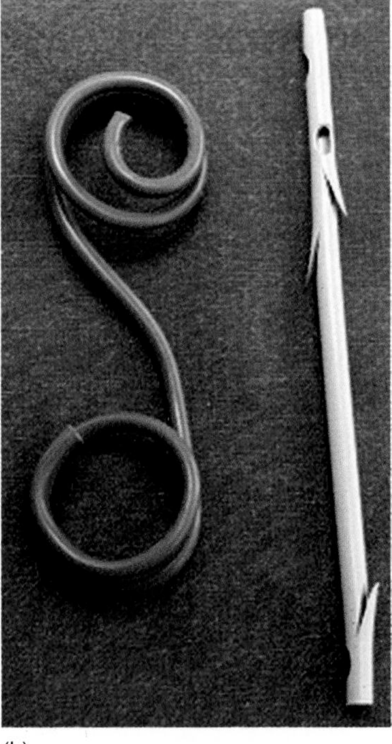

(b)

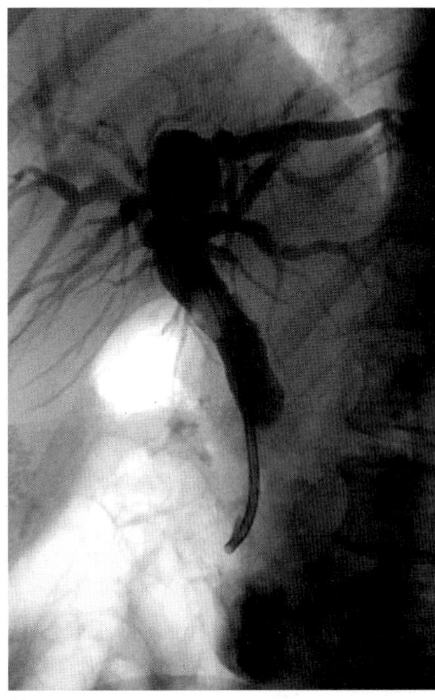

(c)

Fig. 18.12 Endoscopic stenting
(a) Diagnostic endoscopic retrograde cholangiogram (ERC) showing an enlarged common bile duct containing a single large stone. A collection of radiopaque gallstones is seen in the gall bladder (**GB**). **(b)** Two types of biliary stent: the pigtail type on the left and the notched variety on the right, as used in this patient. **(c)** Despite endoscopic sphincterotomy, the bile duct stone could not be retrieved so a tubular self-retaining stent has been placed to relieve the obstructive jaundice. The stone was successfully removed endoscopically on a later occasion

removed surgically using a **choledochoscope**, inserted via the divided cystic duct. Alternatively, an incision in the bile duct (choledochotomy) can be made, and closed primarily after stone extraction; however, this carries a risk of biliary stricturing and few surgeons perform this.

Many surgeons undertaking laparoscopic cholecystectomy routinely perform operative cholangiography but only a small proportion undertake laparoscopic exploration of the common bile duct as this is a difficult and time-consuming procedure.

Benign bile duct strictures can be treated by long-term stenting or surgical reconstruction, usually by anastomosing a loop of jejunum to the bile duct proximal to the obstruction (hepaticojejunostomy). Strictures are usually due to post-surgical fibrotic scarring (usually following iatrogenic injury) or from inflammatory scarring due to cholecystitis (**Mirizzi's syndrome**).

Small **periampullary tumours** may be amenable to complete excision, thereby relieving biliary obstruction and often achieving cure. **Adenocarcinoma of the pancreatic head** is a common cause of obstructive jaundice but the prognosis is poor even after successful radical pancreatico-duodenectomy. If an operation for potentially curable malignant disease is planned, the precautions in Table 18.2 should be employed.

Obstruction due to incurable tumour

Such obstructions are caused by carcinoma of the pancreatic head (common), lymph node metastases in the porta hepatis (uncommon) and from carcinoma of the gall bladder (rare). Stenting is the palliative treatment of choice for the bile duct and, if necessary, duodenum. The alternative is palliative triple bypass surgery to bypass both biliary and duodenal obstructions (see Fig 24.3, p. 328).

Terminal disease

By the time obstructive jaundice has appeared, some patients have reached a terminal stage of their cancer. In these cases, stenting may still be indicated but surgical interference may be difficult to justify; the aim should be to relieve distress and allow a dignified death with good palliative care. Some patients experiencing severe itching may be helped by drugs such as antihistamines or chlorpromazine. Oral colestyramine is not indicated because it only removes bile salts which are able to reach the bowel.

SPECIAL RISKS OF SURGERY IN THE JAUNDICED PATIENT

Despite the fact that most obstructive jaundice can now be relieved preoperatively by stone removal or stenting, surgery must still sometimes be performed in a jaundiced patient. This poses a greater risk from preoperative and postoperative surgical complications, as shown in Table 18.2.

ABDOMINAL MASS OR DISTENSION

An abdominal mass is sometimes discovered by the patient but more often by medical examination. An older patient with a palpable mass is likely to have a malignant tumour, but benign cysts, inflammatory masses, aneurysms or atypical hernias may be responsible. Occasionally masses have a

Table 18.2 Special precautions to be taken when operating on a patient with obstructive jaundice

Potential complication	Pathophysiology	Prophylaxis
Infection	Obstructed bile is usually infected with aerobic gut organisms, and is under pressure. Instrumentation may precipitate ascending cholangitis, leading to sepsis and multiple organ dysfunction Spillage of infected bile during operation causes peritoneal contamination and risks intraperitoneal or wound infection	Preoperative drainage of bile into the bowel by endoscopic sphincterotomy or stenting is sometimes used Prophylactic antibiotics against gut flora should be given
Endotoxaemia and renal failure	Endotoxins appear in the systemic circulation. These predispose to multiple organ dysfunction syndrome (MODS) by activating components of the inflammatory cascade and may precipitate a systemic inflammatory response. Renal function is particularly vulnerable if renal perfusion is already impaired Postoperative '*hepatorenal syndrome*' (i.e. acute renal failure) which manifests as oliguria and hyponatraemia	Prophylactic antibiotics Ensure adequate hydration during any period of restriction of oral fluid throughout—preoperative intravenous fluids and osmotic diuretics during operation Insert urinary catheter to monitor output
Hepatic impairment	Biliary back-pressure on the liver causes defective clotting factor synthesis (even if vitamin K given) and defective hepatic metabolism of certain drugs Patients with chronic parenchymal liver disease withstand the stresses of major abdominal surgery and anaesthesia poorly	Avoid drugs excreted by the liver. Give antibiotics to minimise endogenous endotoxin production
Fat malabsorption	Biliary obstruction causes diminished absorption of fats including fat-soluble vitamins such as vitamin K (a co-factor for prothrombin synthesis). This results in defective clotting	Monitor clotting Give parenteral vitamin K to improve prothrombin ratio, 24 hours preoperatively if possible; if necessary, fresh-frozen plasma perioperatively
Thromboembolism	Paradoxically, considering the clotting deficiency, postoperative deep vein thrombosis is common	Prophylactic subcutaneous low-dose heparin injections

'medical' cause, e.g. hepatosplenomegaly of chronic lymphocytic leukaemia. Commonly, one of the 'five Fs'—fetus, faeces, flatus, fat or fluid—may masquerade as a 'surgical' mass or distension. Patients with an abdominal mass usually have gastrointestinal symptoms, anaemia or jaundice in addition.

CLINICAL ASSESSMENT OF AN ABDOMINAL MASS

(see Table 18.3)

History

A thorough history often provides clues to the organ system involved. Important features include: how long has it been

Table 18.3 Causes of hepatosplenomegaly

Hepatomegaly	Splenomegaly	Hepatosplenomegaly
Physiological Riedel's lobe		
Malignant tumours Hepatocellular carcinoma Secondary carcinoma		
Infective **Viral** Hepatitis, Epstein–Barr virus, cytomegalovirus **Bacterial** Tuberculosis, leptospirosis, liver abscess **Protozoal** Malaria, schistosomiasis, amoebiasis, histoplasmosis, hydatid disease	Hepatitis, Epstein–Barr virus, cytomegalovirus Subacute bacterial endocarditis, typhoid, tuberculosis, leptospirosis Malaria, toxoplasmosis, brucellosis, schistosomiasis, leishmaniasis (kala-azar)	Hepatitis, cytomegalovirus Tuberculosis, leptospirosis Malaria, toxoplasmosis, brucellosis, schistosomiasis, leishmaniasis (kala-azar)
Alcoholic liver disease Fatty liver Early cirrhosis		
Systemic diseases Wilson's disease Haemochromatosis Cellular infiltration, e.g. amyloid, sarcoid	Sarcoidosis Amyloidosis Rheumatoid arthritis (Felty's syndrome) Storage diseases (e.g. Gaucher's)	Amyloidosis Storage diseases (e.g. Gaucher's)
Benign tumours Hepatic adenoma		
Congestive cardiac disease Right heart failure Tricuspid regurgitation (pulsatile liver) Budd–Chiari syndrome	**Congestive splenomegaly** Hepatic vein thrombosis Portal vein thrombosis Splenic vein thrombosis Cirrhosis with portal hypertension	**Congestive hepatosplenomegaly** Hepatic vein thrombosis Portal vein thrombosis Splenic vein thrombosis Cirrhosis with portal hypertension Budd–Chiari syndrome
Haematological disease **Lymphoproliferative disorders** Lymphoma Leukaemias	Lymphoma Leukaemias	Lymphoma Leukaemias
Myeloproliferative disorders	Chronic myeloid leukaemia Myelofibrosis Polycythaemia rubra vera Essential thrombocythaemia	Chronic myeloid leukaemia Myelofibrosis Polycythaemia rubra vera Essential thrombocythaemia
Anaemia	Haemolytic anaemia Megaloblastic anaemia	Megaloblastic anaemia
Miscellaneous Primary biliary cirrhosis Polycystic liver disease	Thyrotoxicosis	Infantile polycystic disease

there; how did the patient come to notice it; is it always present or does it sometimes disappear (e.g. a hernia may reduce); is it getting bigger or smaller? A history of intra-abdominal malignancy or malignant melanoma years before should be regarded with grave suspicion: the disease may have recurred, metastasised or a related new primary developed. This is especially common in colorectal cancer but uncommon once 7 years have elapsed since treatment.

General examination

General examination should seek systemic signs of disease (e.g. cachexia, anaemia and jaundice) or signs of malignant dissemination (e.g. supraclavicular lymphadenopathy in suspected stomach cancer). Abdominal and pelvic examination must be methodical and, if appropriate, proctoscopy and sigmoidoscopy performed.

EXAMINATION OF AN ABDOMINAL MASS

The location of the mass, its relations to other structures, its mobility and its physical characteristics, such as size, shape, consistency and pulsatility give valuable information about the organ of origin and the likely pathology. **Hernias**, e.g. incisional, umbilical and sometimes interstitial (Spigelian) hernias (see Ch. 32), may present as localised swellings but they usually shrink or reduce completely when the patient is supine or under anaesthesia unless they are incarcerated.

Examination of masses in specific regions of the abdomen (see Fig. 18.1)

Mass in the right hypochondrium (right upper quadrant or RUQ)

A right hypochondrial mass is usually of hepatobiliary origin. If so, it will be continuous with the main bulk of the liver to palpation and percussion. When the liver is diffusely enlarged, the inferior margin is regular and well defined and the consistency is usually normal. When infiltrated with primary or secondary cancer, it may be hard and irregular or the liver may appear diffusely enlarged. Carcinoma of the gall bladder is indistinguishable from hepatic cancer on palpation. Rarely, a Riedel's lobe—a congenitally enlarged part of the right lobe—is mistaken for a pathological mass but is soft and mobile. Less commonly, a right hypochondrial mass is a diseased gall bladder. A mass continuous with the liver above and having a typical pear-shaped rounded outline is likely to be a mucocoele of the gall bladder. A more diffuse, tender mass may be an empyema of the gall bladder.

Epigastric mass

A mass in the epigastrium is usually due to cancer of the stomach or transverse colon or sometimes omental secondaries from ovarian carcinoma. Cancer involving the left lobe of the liver may also present like this (Fig. 18.13). These masses are usually hard and irregular, and are mobile or fixed according to the degree of invasion. Occasionally an epigastric mass consists of massive para-aortic lymph nodes due to lymphoma or testicular secondaries. A pulsatile epigastric mass is likely to be an abdominal aortic aneurysm.

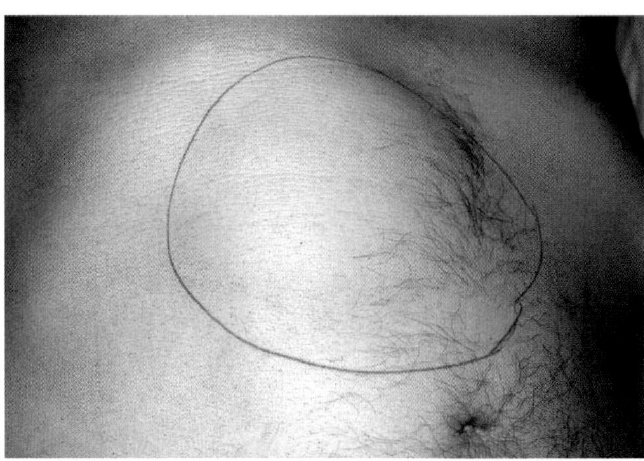

Fig. 18.13 Epigastric mass
This man of 44 presented having discovered an epigastric mass. It was asymptomatic. The margins of the mass are outlined on the skin. The mass moved downwards with respiration and proved to be a massive liver metastasis from a tiny pancreatic primary adenocarcinoma

Mass in the left hypochondrium (left upper quadrant or LUQ)

A cancer of the stomach or splenic flexure of the colon may present as a mass in the left hypochondrium. Tumour masses can usually be distinguished clinically from an enlarged spleen as the latter often has a discrete 'edge' and lies more posteriorly.

Mass in the loin or flank

A mass in the loin or flank is likely to be of renal origin and can best be felt on **bimanual palpation** (see Fig 18.3). Very rarely, a hernia occurs in the lumbar region; this reduces spontaneously as the patient rolls over.

Mass in the left iliac fossa

Masses here usually arise from the sigmoid colon. A hard faecal mass may be mistaken for cancer but it can often be indented like putty. A solid sigmoid mass is usually due to tumour or a complex diverticular inflammatory mass. Ovarian masses and sometimes eccentric bladder lesions may be palpable in either iliac fossa. These lesions, however, arise out of the pelvis and can often be pushed up on to the abdominal examining hand by digital pressure in the rectum or vagina (bimanual palpation—most effectively performed under general anaesthesia). Note that rectal examination is usually regarded as mandatory in a complete abdominal examination.

Hernias in the groin are common (see Ch. 32) and may be chronically irreducible (incarcerated). Occasionally, an interstitial (Spigelian) hernia develops above the groin in either iliac fossa. This presents a somewhat confusing picture on examination by virtue of its site and because the peritoneal sac herniates between the abdominal wall layers.

Suprapubic mass

Suprapubic masses usually arise from pelvic organs such as bladder or uterus and its adnexae. A palpable bladder is most commonly due to chronic urinary retention, easily confirmed on ultrasound. A distended bladder is dull to percussion and disappears on catheterisation. Bladder enlargement is usually symmetrical and may extend above the umbilicus. Only massive bladder tumours are palpable and these would be accompanied by urinary tract symptoms and urine abnormalities. Sometimes large bladder stones are palpable abdominally.

A uterus may be palpable abdominally when enlarged by pregnancy or fibroids. Bimanual examination involves vaginal and lower abdominal palpation. Ovarian tumours, particularly cysts, may become enormous and extend well up into the abdomen; again, bimanual examination (under general anaesthesia if necessary) helps distinguish the origin.

Mass in the right iliac fossa

The right iliac fossa is a common site for an asymptomatic mass. It may be due to unresolved inflammation of the appendix, surrounded by omentum and small bowel, forming an '**appendix mass**' (see Ch. 26, p. 342). There is usually a recent history of right iliac fossa pain and fever. Carcinoma of the caecum may become very large without causing obstruction because the caecum is large and distensible, and the faecal stream at this point is semi-liquid. Thus, caecal carcinoma often presents with an asymptomatic mass, and iron deficiency anaemia. Crohn's disease of the terminal ileum often presents with a tender mass, usually with typical symptoms of pain and diarrhoea.

Central abdominal mass

A central abdominal mass may originate in large or small bowel, be a result of malignant infiltration of the great omentum, or if they are large, from retroperitoneal structures such as lymph nodes, pancreas, connective tissues or the aorta. A common central abdominal mass is an abdominal aorta aneurysm. Aneurysms nearly all appear over 60 years of age and usually arise just above the aortic bifurcation (at umbilical level). A characteristic feature is **expansile pulsation**; other solid masses may transmit pulsation from large vessels nearby, but those masses are not expansile.

Several different types of hernia present near the centre of the abdomen. Most common is an **incisional hernia** protruding through part or all of an abdominal wall incision. This may occur any time after operation, from days to years later. It usually results from poor closure technique or postoperative infection. **Paraumbilical** or **umbilical hernias**, common in the obese, occur centrally and diagnosis is usually straightforward. **Divarication of the recti** (rectus abdominis muscles, not a true hernia) involves the recti being splayed apart, often as a result of pregnancy or obesity, leaving the central abdominal wall devoid of muscular support. This is easily recognised because of its typical 'keel' shape and its symptomless nature and the absence of an abdominal scar; treatment is rarely necessary. Divarication and midline hernias can best be demonstrated when abdominal muscles are contracted by asking a supine patient to raise both heels from the bed.

Rectal mass and findings on pelvic examination

An abdominal or pelvic mass may be palpable solely on rectal (or vaginal) examination. The mass may be a cancer of rectum or in the loop of sigmoid colon in the pelvic cavity; the latter is unlikely to be visible on sigmoidoscopy. Sometimes, secondary deposits from an impalpable tumour in the upper abdomen may seed the pelvic cavity. This may produce a hard anterior lump or even a solid mass filling the pelvic cavity (**frozen pelvis**). Frozen pelvis can also occur with endometriosis or local spread of a carcinoma of cervix or, rarely, prostate.

INTERPRETATION OF A FINDING OF ASCITES

Ascites is defined as a chronic accumulation of fluid within the abdominal cavity and has many causes, some malignant and some non-malignant. Ascites can usually only be recognised clinically when the volume exceeds 2 litres, but even then it is easily overlooked. Dullness to percussion in the flanks and suprapubic region with central resonance is suspicious of ascites and should be followed by an attempt to elicit a fluid thrill or 'shifting dullness' (see Fig. 18.4).

Malignant ascites

In intra-abdominal cancer, the peritoneum is sometimes seeded with tumour deposits that secrete a protein-rich fluid containing malignant cells (**malignant ascites**). The peritoneum may be peppered with thousands of minute seedlings or there may be several large masses hidden by ascitic fluid. Such widespread peritoneal involvement may cause abdominal distension but can be difficult to recognise on abdominal examination. It should be suspected if a patient with a past history of GI or ovarian cancer has other symptoms suggestive of malignancy such as anorexia or marked weight loss.

Lymphatic obstruction

A rare cause of ascites is major obstruction of abdominal lymphatic drainage. This is usually caused by malignant involvement of para-aortic lymph nodes with lymphoma or metastatic testicular malignancy. **Chylous ascites**, in which the ascitic fluid is milky-white, is rare and is caused by proximal lymphatic obstruction and the presence of chylomicrons in the fluid originating from mesenteric lymphatics.

Tuberculosis

Abdominal tuberculosis is an uncommon cause of abdominal swelling in developed countries but is common in the developing world. Tuberculosis can occasionally present as ascites; this form is characterised by multiple tiny peritoneal tubercles, only distinguishable from tumour secondaries by biopsy.

Non-surgical causes

Ascites is commonly caused by gross congestive cardiac failure, constrictive pericarditis, severe hypoalbuminaemia or portal venous obstruction, the last occurring in cirrhosis and occasionally with liver metastases.

Diffuse abdominal distension

In diffuse distension without a palpable abdominal mass, sinister causes must be excluded. Gas within bowel is a common cause for long-standing and often intermittent abdominal pain and distension. It usually occurs in healthy young adults, particularly women, in association with irritable bowel syndrome or air swallowing during hyperventilation. Chronic gaseous abdominal distension may also be found in elderly patients with partial volvulus of the sigmoid colon.

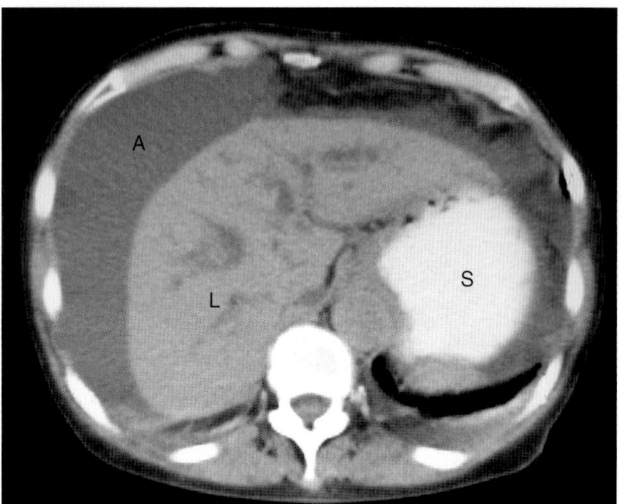

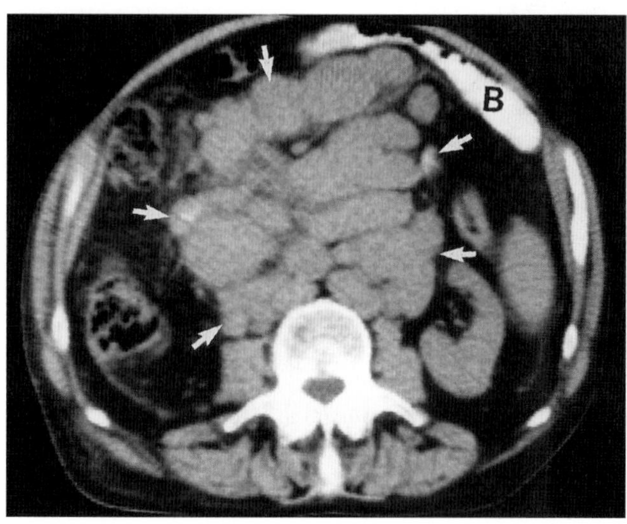

Fig. 18.14 CT scans showing gross ascites and enlarged lymph nodes
In **(a)** note the darker grey homogeneous shadow of fluid **A** around the liver **L** and the contrast in the stomach **S**. **(b)** Retroperitoneal mass of lymph nodes due to lymphoma. This CT scan was taken to assess the stage of spread of a known lymphoma. This 40-year-old woman presented with a large rubbery lymph node mass in her neck and was also found to have a large central abdominal mass. Abdominal CT scanning showed an enormous mass of lymph nodes (arrowed). Small bowel **B** is seen anteriorly, enhanced by orally administered contrast material

Clinical assessment usually diagnoses these problems and avoids unnecessary investigation.

Gross faecal loading may also be responsible for abdominal distension. This is often seen in children with abdominal pain and sometimes in young adults with irritable bowel syndrome. Asymptomatic chronic constipation is common in the elderly, and a faecal mass palpable through a thin abdominal wall can give the impression of a sinister mass.

APPROACH TO INVESTIGATION OF AN ABDOMINAL MASS OR DISTENSION

Laboratory tests

Blood, urine and stool investigations are performed as suggested by the history and examination, e.g. full blood count, function tests, dipstick urinalysis and faecal occult bloods.

Radiology

A chest X-ray should be performed if malignancy is suspected. Ultrasonography or CT scanning (see Fig. 18.14) is useful for demonstrating the size and origin of a mass. For pelvic masses, transvaginal or transrectal ultrasound is often the investigation of first choice although MRI is often helpful. CT scanning is most valuable for defining masses in the retroperitoneal area, e.g. pancreas, aorta or kidneys, but may be the preferred investigation for suspected large bowel cancer, particularly in frail patients. Ultrasound or CT scanning can be used to guide needle biopsy or aspiration cytology precisely. Contrast studies, e.g. barium meal, barium enema or intravenous urography, may be indicated by the clinical findings.

Endoscopy

Flexible endoscopic techniques such as gastroscopy, colonoscopy and ERCP enable direct examination and biopsy of many gastrointestinal lesions.

Other methods of tissue diagnosis

A tissue diagnosis should be obtained even if disseminated malignancy seems obvious. It can influence palliative and supportive treatment and, occasionally, an apparently hopeless case proves on histology to be treatable or even curable. Examples are tuberculosis, lymphomas or a germ cell tumour such as teratoma. Techniques of obtaining tissue for histology include needle or excision biopsy of enlarged cervical lymph nodes, and percutaneous biopsy of liver or an intra-abdominal mass. Paracentesis abdominis (i.e. needle aspiration of ascitic fluid) is a safe and simple way of obtaining a specimen for cytology and microbiology. Finally, when less invasive methods have failed to provide the necessary information, direct biopsy of tumour at diagnostic laparoscopy or open operation usually provides the definitive diagnosis.

Examination under anaesthesia, laparoscopy and exploratory laparotomy

Examination under anaesthesia (EUA) is sometimes necessary for estimating the mobility and spread of pelvic tumours. General anaesthesia with a muscle relaxant allows thorough abdominal palpation and bimanual examination of the pelvis via rectum and/or vagina and the taking of biopsies. This may not be possible without anaesthesia because of tenderness or abdominal wall muscle tone. EUA is often combined with cystoscopy or other rigid endoscopies.

Laparoscopy is now widely used as a diagnostic tool in general surgery. It allows direct inspection and biopsy of masses and visualisation of the extent of local spread governing resectability, as well as allowing a search for intra-abdominal metastases. Samples can be taken for cytology to demonstrate intraperitoneal spread. Special ultrasound probes may be applied directly to the liver and other organs where lesions are suspected.

The acute abdomen and acute gastrointestinal haemorrhage

19

INTRODUCTION

The term **acute abdomen** is widely understood but is difficult to define precisely. Typically, the symptoms are of acute onset and strongly suggest an abdominal cause; abdominal pain is almost always a prominent feature. The illness is of such severity that admission to hospital appears essential and operative surgery is a likely outcome. Many of the disorders causing an 'acute abdomen' are serious and potentially life-threatening unless treated promptly. On the other hand, simple and relatively trivial conditions such as constipation can produce acute and severe symptoms mimicking the early stages of an acute abdomen.

Major gastrointestinal haemorrhage is also a common reason for acute surgical referral, and is manifest by vomiting of blood (**haematemesis**) or profuse rectal bleeding or the passage of **melaena**. Many such patients are initially referred to a general (internal) physician or gastroenterologist, especially if the presumptive diagnosis is bleeding from a peptic ulcer or oesophageal varices.

Acute surgical emergencies constitute about 50% of all general surgical admissions. About half of these are for abdominal symptoms, predominantly pain, and half of those in this group resolve without operation.

BASIC PRINCIPLES OF MANAGING THE ACUTE ABDOMEN

The first goal is to resuscitate the patient with intravenous fluids and give analgesia. The next is to make a broad diagnosis on the history, examination, laboratory tests and imaging (Box 19.1). All help decide if an operation is necessary, and its urgency, and clarify any non-surgical treatment, e.g. antibiotics for diverticulitis or conservative measures for acute pancreatitis. The differential diagnosis encompasses the likely pathophysiological phenomena responsible.

DISORDERS AND DISEASES CAUSING THE ACUTE ABDOMEN

INTESTINAL OBSTRUCTION

PATHOPHYSIOLOGY OF INTESTINAL OBSTRUCTION

Any part of the gastrointestinal tract may become obstructed and present as an acute abdomen. Gastric outlet obstruction, however, presents differently and is described in Chapter 21. The causes of intestinal obstruction are many and varied, as outlined in Figure 19.1.

Obstruction leads to dilatation of bowel proximally and disrupts peristalsis. The manner of presentation depends on the level of obstruction in the GI tract (i.e. stomach, proximal or distal small bowel or large bowel) and on the completeness of obstruction. The most acute presentation is upper small bowel obstruction. This manifests within hours of onset because the large volume of gastric and pancreaticobiliary secretions is prevented from progressing, so it regurgitates into the stomach and is vomited. In contrast, distal large bowel obstruction is more chronic and may be present for days or a week before the patient seeks treatment.

SYMPTOMS OF INTESTINAL OBSTRUCTION

Symptoms and physical signs are summarised in Box 19.2.

Vomiting

Bowel obstruction eventually leads to vomiting; the more proximal, the earlier it develops. Vomiting can occur even if nothing is taken by mouth because saliva and other GI secretions continue to be produced and enter the stomach. At least

Box 19.1 Plain radiology in the acute abdomen—what to look for

Five main image densities are detectable on radiographs:

- White—metallic objects
- Off white—calcified structures
- Medium shades of grey—most soft tissues
- Dark grey—fat
- Black—gas

How to review an abdominal X-ray:

1. Check **name** is correct and **date** is current
2. Note **type of X-ray**, i.e. plain or contrast, erect or supine
3. Is the image of adequate **diagnostic quality**, i.e. appropriate density? Does it show the whole abdomen?
4. **Bowel gas and bowel wall**—note distribution and dilatation (small bowel diameter less than 3 cm, most large bowel less than 5 cm, caecum less than 9 cm). Absence of gas may indicate a displacing mass, ascites (central) or acute pancreatitis (ground glass appearance). Faeces appear mottled; 'faecal loading' may mean constipation or obstruction. Rigler's sign is strongly suggestive of bowel perforation
5. **Non-bowel gas**—free intraperitoneal gas, e.g. subphrenic gas in perforation of bowel, gas within bowel wall in necrosis, gas in biliary tree after sphincterotomy or fistula into bowel
6. **Calcification**—aortic wall in aneurysm, pancreas, renal and ureteric stones, gallstones, pelvic phleboliths (calcified old venous thrombi), teratomas, and fetus. Bones of spine and pelvis—osteoarthritis, metastases (lytic or sclerotic), Paget's disease, fractures
7. **Soft tissues**. Thickened bowel wall. Check outline of kidneys (are both present?; length equal to three or more vertebral bodies) and psoas muscles (obscured in retroperitoneal inflammation)
8. **Artefacts**—artificial objects placed by medical personnel—central venous line, nasogastric tube, metal vessel or Fallopian tube clips, biliary, vascular or bowel stents, inferior vena caval filter, intrauterine contraceptive device
   — foreign bodies—embedded bullets, glass fragments, objects inserted rectally
   — projection of buttons, safety pins, rings on hand, coins, body piercing

In patients with an acute abdomen, always review chest X-ray for the following:

- Hiatus hernia
- Heart size
- Lung fields
- Pneumothorax
- Diaphragms: relative height; gas under
- Bony changes
- CVP line position

WITHIN THE WALL

Tumours
benign or malignant, e.g. colonic carcinoma (especially left sided), gastric carcinomas near the pylorus and tumours of the small bowel (rare)

Inflammatory strictures
e.g. Crohn's disease or diverticular disease; certain tropical bowel disorders

Drug-induced strictures
e.g. NSAIDs

Lymphomas

Intussusception
a segment of bowel becomes telescoped into the segment distal to it. Usually initiated by a mass in the bowel wall (e.g. enlargement of lymphatic tissue or tumour) which is dragged along by peristalsis; rare in adults but common in children

OUTSIDE THE WALL

Adhesions
resulting from previous surgery or intra-peritoneal infection

Congenital bands
a rare cause of obstruction

Tumours
causing compression of the bowel

Hernias
internal and external (e.g. strangulated femoral or inguinal hernia)

WITHIN THE LUMEN

Impacted faeces
common

Solitary gallstones
rare

Phytobezoar
i.e. a mass of impacted vegetable matter such as orange pith (very rare except after partial gastrectomy)

Trichobezoar
rare, and found only in disturbed people who eat their own hair over a long period

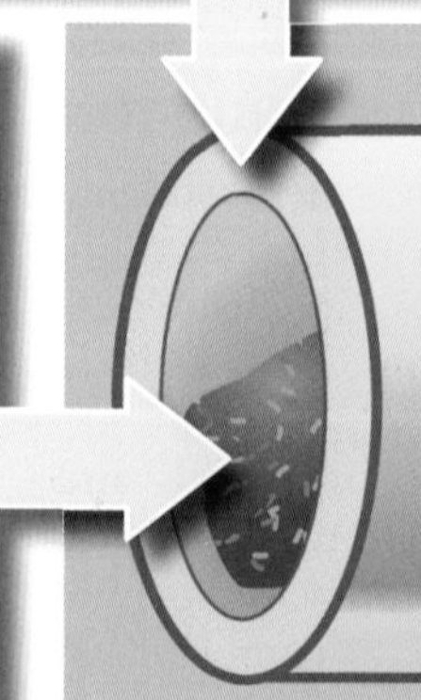

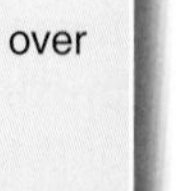

Fig. 19.1 Mechanical causes of bowel obstruction

Box 19.2 Clinical features of bowel obstruction and strangulation

Symptoms

- Vomiting—time of onset and nature of the vomitus suggest the level of obstruction
- Absolute constipation (i.e. no flatus or faeces passed rectally)—pathognomonic of complete obstruction (but not present in partial obstruction)
- Abdominal pain—usually colicky in character, often mild in uncomplicated obstruction and more severe in strangulation

Physical signs

- Dehydration—caused by vomiting, lack of fluid intake and fluid sequestration in obstructed bowel
- Abdominal distension—due to gas-filled loops of bowel. The more distal the obstruction, the greater the distension
- Visible peristalsis—uncommon finding; usually encountered in a very thin patient with prolonged but incomplete distal small bowel obstruction
- Abdominal tenderness—important feature distinguishing bowel strangulation from uncomplicated obstruction
- Central resonance to percussion with dullness in the flanks—gas within dilated bowel loops rising to the uppermost point in the abdomen
- Abnormal bowel sounds—exaggerated, lapping, sloshing, perhaps high-pitched or tinkling. Bowel sounds are absent or normal in adynamic obstruction

10 litres of fluid are secreted into the GI tract each day. The nature of the vomitus gives clues about the level of obstruction. For example, vomiting of semi-digested food eaten a day or two earlier suggests gastric outlet obstruction. Copious vomiting of **bile-stained fluid** suggests upper small bowel obstruction. If the vomitus becomes thicker and foul-smelling (**faeculent**), more distal obstruction is likely and this change is often an indication for urgent operation. The term faeculent is a misnomer as the vomitus contains altered small bowel contents rather than faeces.

Pain

Fluid and swallowed air proximal to an obstruction plus continuing peristalsis cause pain. The general area of the pain gives clues to the embryological origin of the affected bowel: upper, middle or lower abdominal pain originates in foregut, midgut or hindgut respectively. In obstruction, pain is not usually the most prominent symptom. It is usually colicky, occurring in short-lived bouts as peristalsis attempts to overcome the obstruction. In small bowel, the peristaltic action often increases for 24–48 hours after the onset of obstruction and then fades.

Constipation

Absolute constipation, i.e. no faeces or flatus passed rectally, is pathognomonic of obstruction. The longer the duration, the more noteworthy it becomes in the diagnosis of obstruction.

Effects of the competence of the ileocaecal valve

Symptoms develop more gradually in large bowel obstruction because of the large capacity of colon and caecum and their absorptive capability. However, if the ileocaecal valve remains competent, no retrograde flow of accumulating bowel contents occurs and the thin-walled caecum progressively distends and eventually ruptures; operation is clearly more urgent in these cases. The ileocaecal valve becomes incompetent in about half the cases of large bowel obstruction. This allows the small bowel to distend, delaying the onset of obstructive symptoms and perhaps their acuteness.

Incomplete obstruction

If bowel is partially obstructed, clinical features are less distinct. Vomiting may be intermittent and the bowel habit erratic. Chronic incomplete obstruction leads to gradual hypertrophy of bowel wall muscle proximally and strong peristaltic activity causes bouts of colicky pain, often more severe than in complete obstruction. In thin patients, the pain is often accompanied by **visible peristalsis**, the hallmark of incomplete obstruction. The most common cause is a slowly progressively obstructing colonic cancer. Incomplete obstruction should *not* be called subacute obstruction as the term is misleading.

PHYSICAL SIGNS OF INTESTINAL OBSTRUCTION

General examination

Vomiting, diminished fluid intake and sequestration of fluid in the small bowel lead to **dehydration**. Gas-filled loops of bowel proximal to the obstruction produce **abdominal distension**; the more distal the obstruction, the greater the distension. Examination may also reveal signs of anaemia or lymphadenopathy attributable to the primary disorder.

Groin examination

It is essential that the groins are examined for hernias as the resultant bowel obstruction will not settle with conservative treatment. An obstructed femoral hernia is usually very small and rarely causes local symptoms or signs, even when strangulated. Hence it is easily missed if not specifically sought. Instead it produces the symptoms and signs of small bowel obstruction. This is an important clinical point—an obstruction due to an irreducible hernia will not settle with the usual conservative treatment.

Abdominal examination

On **inspection**, scars of previous operations provide a map of previous surgical disease, and raise the possibility of adhesive obstruction. On **palpation**, the most striking feature is the lack of abdominal tenderness except when strangulation has occurred. Obstruction with tenderness *must* be diagnosed as strangulation or perforation, necessitating urgent operation after fluid resuscitation. Note that a large obstructing abdominal mass may be palpable.

On **percussion**, the centre of the abdomen tends to be resonant and the periphery dull because bowel gas rises to the most elevated point, mimicking ascites. On **auscultation**, obstructive bowel sounds are traditionally described as loud and frequent, high-pitched and tinkling; in practice, bowel sounds may or may not be increased but have an echoing, cavernous quality or else can sound like the lapping of water against a boat. A **succussion splash**, heard on gently shaking the patient's abdomen from side to side, may be heard in gastric outlet obstruction.

RADIOLOGICAL INVESTIGATION OF SUSPECTED BOWEL OBSTRUCTION

The most useful initial investigation is a plain supine abdominal X-ray (see Figs 19.2 to 19.4). The pattern and distribution of bowel gas often indicates the approximate site of obstruction. In small bowel obstruction, fluid levels may be visible on an erect or decubitus X-ray. Measuring the bowel diameter on X-ray gives the degree of distension. (See Box 19.1 for norms.)

Profound large bowel dilatation without small bowel distension is seen on X-ray in large bowel obstruction where the ileocaecal valve remains competent; this is a key determinant of the likely rate of deterioration of the patient. When the caecum reaches 10 cm, it is in imminent danger of rupture and an operation is needed urgently.

In large bowel obstruction of less acute onset, radiology helps demonstrate the site and nature of the obstruction (including sigmoid volvulus) and distinguish mechanical from pseudo-obstruction (see below). This may be a contrast enema but CT scanning is increasingly employed. CT scanning gives an indication of the level of obstruction but may not always give the precise diagnosis. Other useful information such as the presence of hepatic metastases may radically influence management, for example using a bowel stent to relieve the obstruction rather than operating.

THE ADYNAMIC BOWEL

This is covered in Chapter 12.

PSEUDO-OBSTRUCTION OF THE COLON

A form of adynamic bowel disorder peculiar to the large bowel is **pseudo-obstruction** although no mechanical obstruction is present. It can be caused by a range of apparently unrelated conditions that impair bowel peristalsis. These include retroperitoneal inflammation or haemorrhage, neurological conditions, biochemical abnormalities, certain drugs (e.g. anticholinergics), pregnancy and delivery, orthopaedic injuries or surgery (particularly in the elderly) and prolonged recumbency.

Physical signs are similar to those of mechanical obstruction except that bowel sounds are normal or inaudible. The diagnosis is based on the clinical findings and is confirmed if no mechanical obstruction is found on imaging.

Pseudo-obstruction usually eventually resolves with conservative measures, but it is important to identify and treat

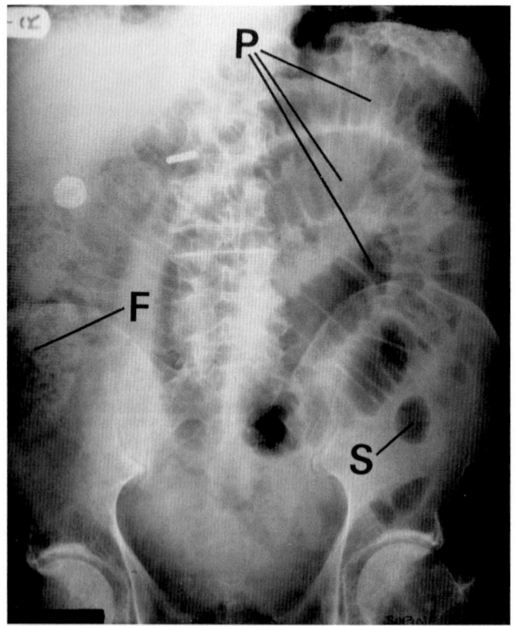

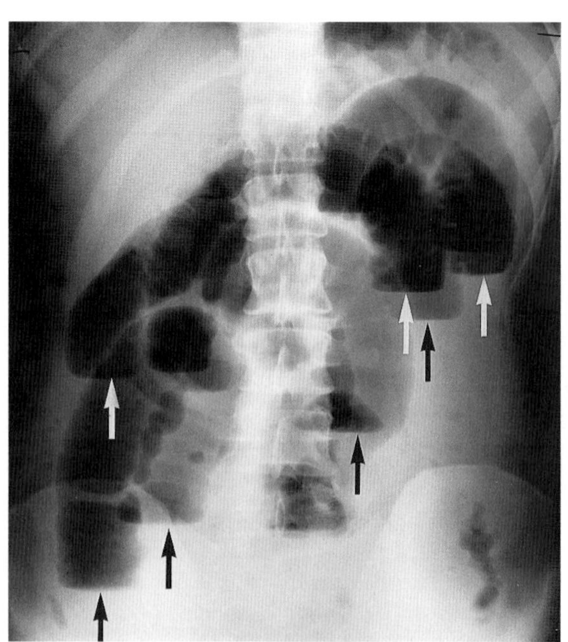

Fig. 19.2 Radiological appearances of obstructed bowel
(a) Supine abdominal film in a man of 67 presenting with vomiting and abdominal distension. The film shows mid small bowel obstruction. Dilated small bowel fills the upper left quadrant and centre of the abdomen, and can be identified by the valvulae conniventes (plicae circulares **P**) which extend across the whole width of the lumen. The small bowel distal to the obstruction is collapsed and is not visible on this film. The large bowel is also collapsed, with faecal loading of the ascending colon (**F**) and only a small amount of gas in the sigmoid colon (**S**). Note also the metallic tip of the nasogastric (NG) tube and the incidental radiopaque gallstone. **(b)** Erect film showing multiple loops of dilated small bowel and multiple fluid levels. The obstruction was caused by a small carcinoma of the medial wall of the caecum encroaching upon the ileal opening. *Note*: erect abdominal films are rarely taken nowadays

Fig. 19.3 Radiological appearances of obstructed bowel

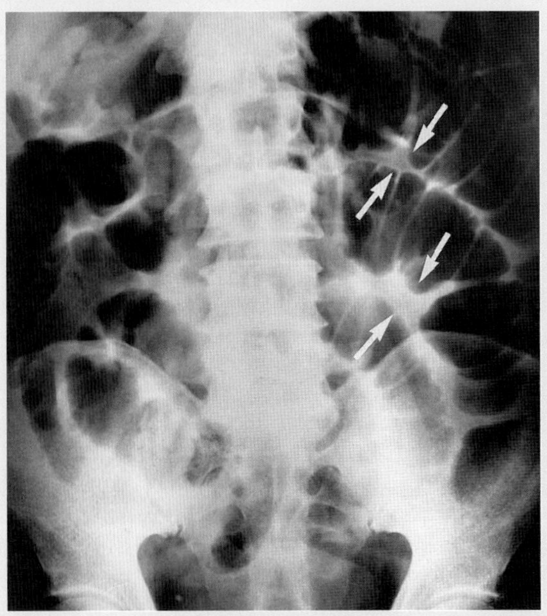

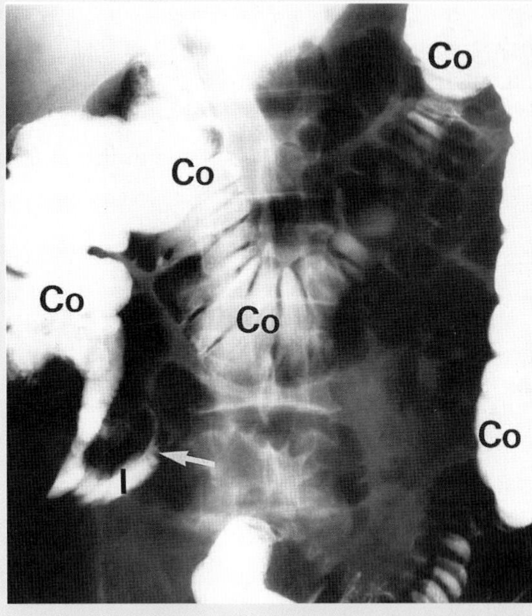

(a) Supine abdominal X-ray in a middle-aged man with several days of symptoms of small bowel obstruction. The abdomen is filled with grossly dilated small bowel loops. In addition, the small bowel wall is thickened, as shown by the apparent space between loops of bowel (arrowed); this is a characteristic feature of prolonged obstruction. **(b)** 'Instant' contrast enema showing contrast filling the normal colon **Co** and distal ileum **I** which abruptly terminates at the obstruction (arrow). The obstruction proved at laparotomy to be caused by a band adhesion resulting from an operation for appendicitis 25 years previously

any evident precipitating cause. Neostigmine is sometimes employed where conservative measures fail but needs close cardiac monitoring. Surgery is sometimes indicated if bowel perforates or if there is no recovery after prolonged conservative management.

PRINCIPLES OF MANAGEMENT OF INTESTINAL OBSTRUCTION

Once intestinal obstruction has been recognised and the approximate level of obstruction identified, management proceeds as follows:

- Resuscitation is an essential first step (see Ch. 4). Oral intake is discontinued and appropriate intravenous fluids given. After prolonged vomiting, patients may be seriously fluid and electrolyte depleted
- If the patient is vomiting and/or has marked small bowel dilatation, a nasogastric tube is passed and gastric contents aspirated. This controls nausea and vomiting, removes swallowed air and reduces gaseous distension. Most importantly, it minimises the risk of inhalation of gastric contents, particularly during induction of anaesthesia
- At least two-thirds of uncomplicated cases of obstruction are due to adhesions; these usually resolve with conservative measures employed for a maximum of 4 days
- Large bowel obstruction caused by faecal impaction can be relieved by enemas or manual removal of faeces
- Operation may be required to relieve the obstruction. Provided strangulation, obstructed hernia and caecal distension have been excluded, operation can safely be deferred for a day or two. This gives time for resuscitation and for any needed investigations. Nevertheless, few obstructions not beginning to settle within 48 hours resolve without intervention
- **Bowel stenting**—in some cases of left-sided colonic obstruction found to be due to cancer, the obstruction can be rapidly relieved with an endoscopically-placed expanding metal stent. Surgery can then be deferred until the patient's condition has been optimised. If incurable metastatic disease has been identified, resectional surgery may be avoided altogether
- At operation the cause of the obstruction is confirmed and dealt with appropriately (see Fig. 19.5)

BOWEL STRANGULATION

PATHOPHYSIOLOGY OF BOWEL STRANGULATION

Strangulation occurs when a segment of bowel becomes trapped so that its lumen becomes obstructed and its blood supply compromised. If unrelieved, this progresses to **infarction** and eventually perforation. Strangulation can occur when there is an external hernia, when loops of bowel become ensnared within the abdominal cavity or when there is mass rotation of bowel, twisting and compressing the mesentery (**volvulus**).

Fig. 19.4 Radiological appearances of obstructed bowel

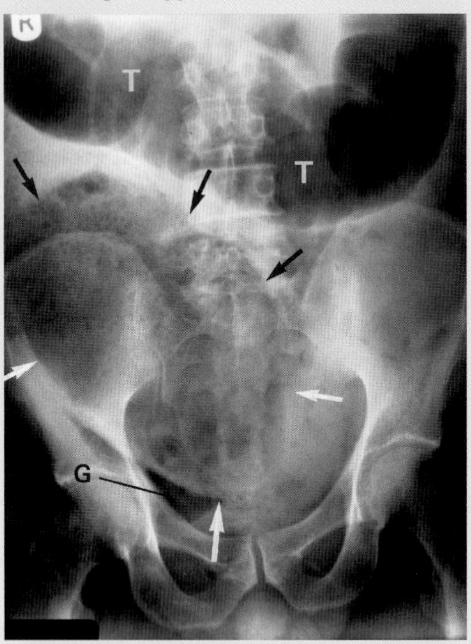

Supine film of an elderly man showing gross caecal dilatation with loss of haustration (surface folds). In large bowel obstruction, this typically occurs if the ileocaecal valve remains competent—a condition that carries a high risk of perforation. In this case, the transverse colon **T** is dilated with gas and there is complete absence of colonic gas on the left side of the abdomen where the descending and sigmoid colon lies. From this, it can be deduced that the colon is obstructed near the splenic flexure. In fact, this patient had an obstructing carcinoma at the splenic flexure and the caecum had perforated, as shown by the presence of gas **G** in the extra-peritoneal tissues

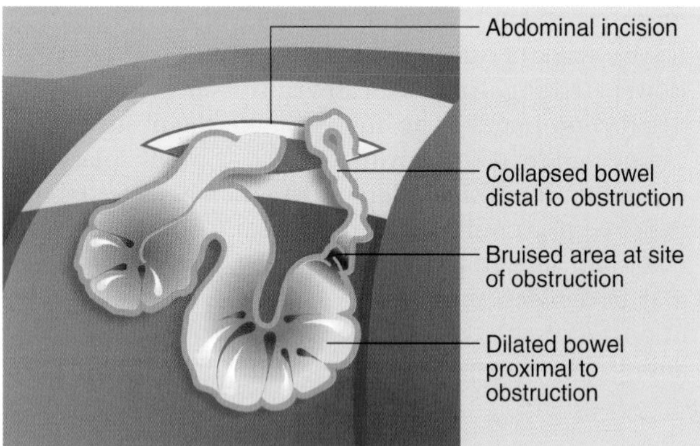

Fig. 19.5 Findings at operation for simple band obstruction of small bowel

Strangulation begins with partial obstruction of the bowel. Venous return is occluded causing bowel wall oedema which further aggravates the obstruction. The closed loop of bowel progressively dilates with gas from fermentation. The combination of gas pressure and venous back-pressure progressively inhibits arterial inflow, causing ischaemia and then infarction.

Strangulation most commonly occurs when small bowel is caught within an external hernia (inguinal, femoral, umbilical or incisional). The bowel undergoes necrosis and soon perforates within the hernial sac, after which generalised peritonitis usually ensues. Clinically, the patient first develops symptoms and signs of small bowel obstruction. A newly irreducible hernia can usually be found and is likely to be tender and inflamed. However, a strangulated femoral hernia is often deceptively small and non-tender and will be missed unless the groins are examined carefully.

Bowel may also become strangulated within the abdominal cavity if a loop becomes trapped by fibrous bands or adhesions (resulting from previous surgery or congenital) or passes through an omental or mesenteric defect. Similarly, strangulation occurs if a large loop of bowel becomes twisted on its mesentery, a condition known as **volvulus**. Small bowel volvulus is rare and occurs only when the mesentery has an unusually small base. Recognition is vital because the entire small bowel may be lost if treatment is delayed. The sigmoid colon (or occasionally the caecum) is particularly susceptible to volvulus if it becomes excessively distended; this is most commonly seen in elderly patients with chronic constipation and in countries where the staple diet is extremely high in fibre.

SYMPTOMS AND SIGNS OF BOWEL STRANGULATION

Intra-abdominal strangulation causes the usual symptoms and signs of bowel obstruction (see Box 19.2) but accompanied by **abdominal tenderness** which should be an alerting signal. When compared with uncomplicated obstruction, strangulation patients are systemically more unwell, with a rising tachycardia and a leucocytosis.

PRINCIPLES OF MANAGEMENT OF SUSPECTED BOWEL STRANGULATION

When strangulation is diagnosed or even suspected, operation must be performed urgently (after rapid fluid resuscitation) to try to prevent infarction and perforation (see Fig. 19.6). The patient is otherwise managed as for uncomplicated obstruction. Bowel strangulation is a clinical diagnosis best confirmed at laparotomy; there are no specific investigations to help.

PERITONITIS

PATHOPHYSIOLOGY AND CLINICAL FEATURES OF PERITONITIS

Peritonitis is defined as inflammation of the peritoneal cavity. At the outset, inflammation is often **localised** and the affected area contained by a wrapping of omentum, adjacent bowel and fibrinous adhesions. This may be insufficient to prevent spread, and **generalised peritonitis** results. Sudden perforation of any viscus almost invariably leads to life-threatening generalised peritonitis.

Localised peritonitis occurs near any primary intra-abdominal inflammatory process. Acute appendicitis is a typical example. When the parietal peritoneum becomes

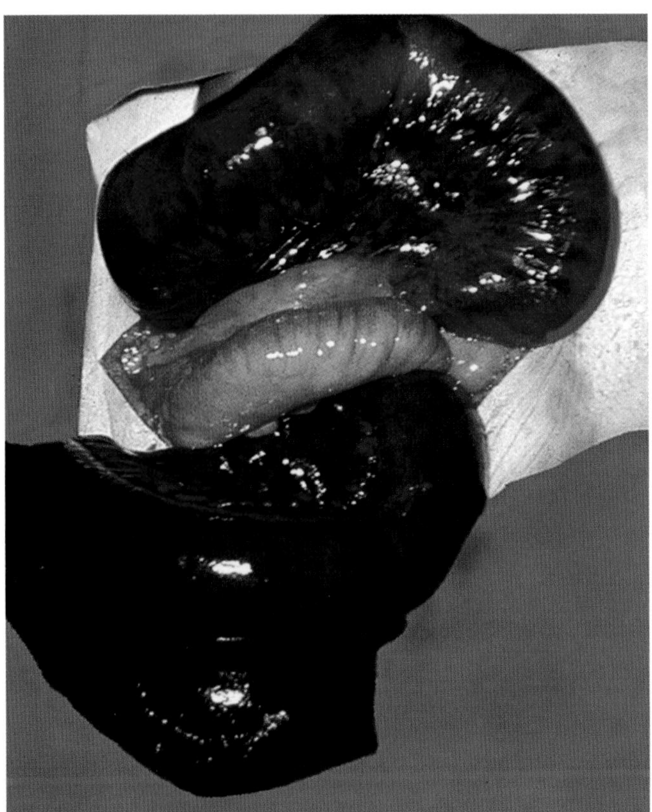

Fig. 19.6 Necrotic bowel after strangulation This photograph, taken at operation for bowel obstruction, shows a dilated necrotic loop of small bowel which has strangulated after passing through a congenital defect in the sigmoid mesocolon. The bowel was on the point of perforation

involved, pain then localises to the affected area and is exacerbated by abdominal muscle movement. The area is tender to palpation and overlying abdominal muscles contract when examination is attempted ('**guarding**'). If the palpating hand is quickly removed, the sudden peritoneal movement causes intense pain described as **rebound tenderness**. Rebound tenderness is better and more kindly elicited by gentle percussion. Rectal examination should be performed, as anterior peritoneal tenderness can be a sign of pelvic peritonitis. Localised peritonitis is usually accompanied by mild systemic 'toxicity', i.e. low-grade fever, malaise, tachycardia and leucocytosis.

With **generalised peritonitis**, the patient becomes seriously and rapidly ill. There is massive exudation of inflammatory fluid into the peritoneal cavity (causing hypovolaemia), toxaemia from absorbed products and if infection is present, systemic sepsis. The systemic illness is most severe when there is widespread contamination by faeces, pus or infected bile. Peritonitis is less severe when infection is absent (e.g. perforated duodenal ulcer in its early stages).

On examination in generalised peritonitis, the abdomen is rigid and tender (but may not be evident in the very elderly or mentally obtunded) and bowel sounds are absent because of peristaltic paralysis. CT scans are often performed but rarely change management and may delay definitive treatment. The causes of peritonitis are summarised in Box 19.3.

Box 19.3 Causes of peritonitis

Localised peritonitis

- Transmural inflammation of bowel, e.g. appendicitis, Crohn's disease, diverticulitis
- Transmural inflammation of other viscera, e.g. cholecystitis, salpingitis

Generalised peritonitis

- Chemical peritonitis: irritation of the peritoneum by noxious materials, e.g. bile, stomach or small bowel contents (due to perforation), enzyme-containing exudates of acute pancreatitis or blood
- Bacterial peritonitis: spreading intraperitoneal infection, e.g. rupture of intra-abdominal abscess or faecal contamination due to bowel perforation, trauma, surgical spillage or anastomotic leak after recent bowel surgery

INTRA-ABDOMINAL HAEMORRHAGE

Blood may come into the abdominal cavity from many sources including ruptured ectopic pregnancy, leaking aortic aneurysm or blunt trauma, especially to liver or spleen. Blood causes moderate peritoneal irritation and peritonitis-like symptoms, but often more muted. In an unstable patient with obvious intraperitoneal bleeding, this is best diagnosed and managed at laparotomy. If less urgent, bleeding may be confirmed by CT scan, which indicate the cause or help the difficult decision of whether to manage conservatively or by operation.

PRINCIPLES OF MANAGEMENT OF PERITONITIS

Local peritonitis is treated according to the diagnosis. For example, appendicitis requires appendicectomy whilst acute diverticulitis and salpingitis are usually managed with antibiotics.

With generalised peritonitis, the patient is at risk of dying from systemic sepsis. As soon as the diagnosis is made, high doses of antibiotics are given intravenously. With the exception of acute pancreatitis, generalised peritonitis requires urgent laparotomy to discover the cause, to clear the contaminating material (**peritoneal toilet**) and to undertake definitive treatment.

INTRA-ABDOMINAL ABSCESS

PATHOPHYSIOLOGY AND CLINICAL FEATURES OF INTRA-ABDOMINAL ABSCESS

There are two common causes of intra-abdominal abscess. The first occurs after bowel perforation, when omentum and adjacent bowel attempt to wall off the defect. The second is a complication of bowel surgery after localised faecal contamination during operation or an anastomotic leak later.

Appendiceal perforation may cause a local abscess or one which tracks into the pelvis. Diverticular disease often causes a **pericolic abscess** or **complex inflammatory mass** in the rectosigmoid area or pelvis. Less common examples include: perforated colonic carcinoma causing a pericolic abscess, gall bladder perforation resulting in a right-sided **subphrenic abscess** and posterior gastric ulcer perforation producing a **lesser sac abscess**.

Intra-abdominal abscesses tend to present with a worsening, continuous abdominal pain, diarrhoea or adynamic bowel disorder due to local bowel irritation and a swinging pyrexia. The last is an important sign of an abscess and there is usually marked leucocytosis. Patients are often relatively well, except with a postoperative abscess where a degree of systemic inflammatory response or multi-organ dysfunction is usual (see Ch. 3). There may be a palpable inflammatory mass, most commonly originating with acute appendicitis or acute diverticular disease. Rectal examination may reveal a hot, tender mass displacing the rectum backwards (a **pelvic abscess**)—a classic finding in the febrile post-appendicectomy patient. Patients usually complain of diarrhoea caused by inflammation near the rectum.

Ultrasound or CT of the abdomen and pelvis is most useful in demonstrating the site and size of an abscess, and drainage may be possible under imaging control (Fig. 19.7).

PRINCIPLES OF MANAGEMENT OF AN INTRA-ABDOMINAL ABSCESS

With a pelvic abscess in an otherwise well patient, there is usually no advantage in giving antibiotic treatment or attempting to drain the abscess because, given time, the abscess usually drains spontaneously and safely into the rectum. Discharge of the abscess is recognised when the patient passes pus and blood per rectum; this is followed by resolution of the fever and healing.

Small subphrenic abscesses may also resolve without intervention but larger ones can be drained percutaneously. Many intra-abdominal abscesses can be treated using percutaneous drainage under radiological control but this deals only with the abscess and not the underlying cause. Laparotomy may be required if the underlying cause needs treatment or if the abscess is unsuitable for percutaneous drainage.

PERFORATION OF AN ABDOMINAL VISCUS

PATHOPHYSIOLOGY AND CLINICAL FEATURES OF PERFORATION

Disease of any hollow viscus may be complicated by perforation into the peritoneal cavity. The common sites are stomach

CASE HISTORY

Fig. 19.7 Radiologically guided drainage of intra-abdominal abscess

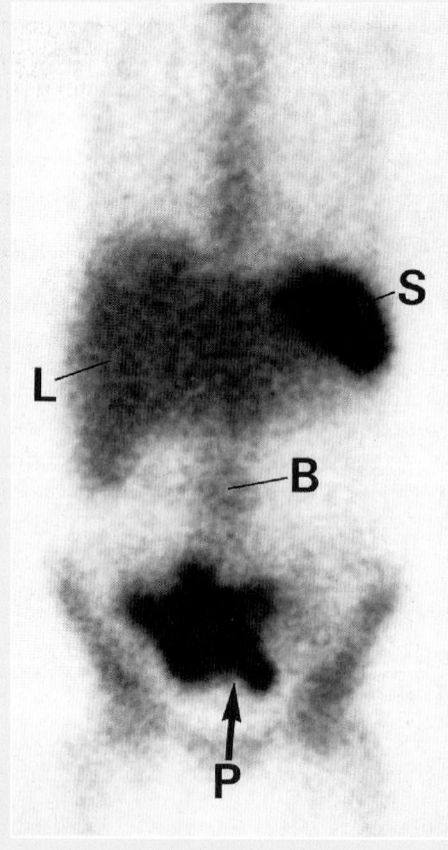

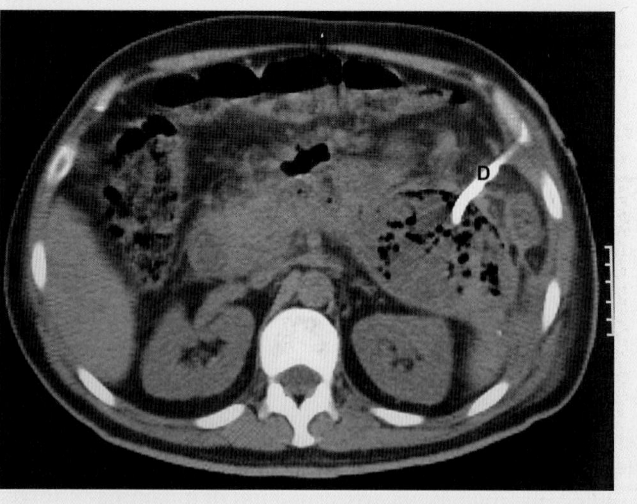

(a) Radionuclide scan of a 47-year-old woman who presented with lower abdominal tenderness and a swinging pyrexia. The patient's own leucocytes were labelled with a radionuclide. This image shows a large pelvic abscess (**P**), shown later to be due to diverticular perforation. Note also the radioisotope uptake by the spleen (**S**), liver (**L**) and bone marrow (**B**), which is a normal feature of such scans. **(b)** CT-guided percutaneous placement of a drain **D** into an abscess of the pancreatic tail following an attack of acute pancreatitis. *Note*: the pancreas remains generally swollen

and duodenum (from peptic ulcer), sigmoid colon (from diverticular disease or carcinoma) and the appendix (from acute appendicitis). The symptoms and signs of a perforated viscus depend on the nature of its contents, the volume of spillage and the effectiveness of local defences.

A small perforation may be immediately walled off by omentum and bowel but a local abscess then develops, giving symptoms of an intra-abdominal abscess. A common example is appendicitis in adults. A small diverticular perforation without faecal spillage may cause local peritonitis which may resolve spontaneously. At the opposite extreme, a large colonic perforation due to a stercoral tear from severe constipation causes sudden overwhelming faecal peritonitis, which is often fatal. A perforated peptic ulcer causes marked abdominal signs of peritonitis, typically 'board-like' rigidity, but little initial systemic upset because the fluid spilled is usually sterile. Acute cholecystitis occasionally perforates if inflammation is severe enough to cause necrosis.

Perforation is essentially a clinical diagnosis but can be confirmed by the presence of free gas in the peritoneal cavity on plain radiography (or CT scan). This is visible as a radiolucent line beneath the hemidiaphragms on an erect chest film (see Fig. 19.8) or a lateral decubitus abdominal film. Note that CT scanning is more sensitive than plain films for detecting small quantities of free gas. Free gas is rare in perforated appendicitis or perforated gall bladder. If imaging fails to support the clinical findings, action should be based on the clinical diagnosis.

PRINCIPLES OF MANAGEMENT OF PERFORATION

Perforation is a surgical emergency. Most cases require urgent operation to repair the defect or resect the segment of diseased bowel. Duodenal ulcer perforations can be plugged with omentum at open surgery or laparoscopically. In large bowel perforations, a Hartmann's procedure, which leaves a temporary colostomy (see Ch. 27), is frequently required because healing of an anastomosis may be impaired with gross peritoneal contamination, although there is a trend towards performing primary anastomosis even in these cases, together with a covering ileostomy. Very rarely, in perforation following colonoscopy, conservative management is appropriate if there are few clinical signs. This is because faecal contamination is minimal as the bowel is already clean. In the elderly or unfit, perforated duodenal ulcers may also be managed conservatively using restriction of oral fluids, nasogastric aspiration, acid suppression and antibiotics; however, the outcome is unpredictable and the approach should be reserved only for patients unsuitable for general anaesthesia or surgery.

ACUTE BOWEL ISCHAEMIA

PATHOPHYSIOLOGY AND CLINICAL FEATURES OF INTESTINAL ISCHAEMIA

Acute occlusion of the **superior mesenteric artery** (SMA) may lead to acute ischaemia of the primitive midgut-derived structures, i.e. jejunum, ileum and right colon (see Fig. 19.9). This causes massive infarction of the right side of the colon and most of the small bowel and later, fatal perforation. There are

CASE HISTORY

Fig. 19.8 Free perforation of abdominal viscus shown on plain chest X-ray

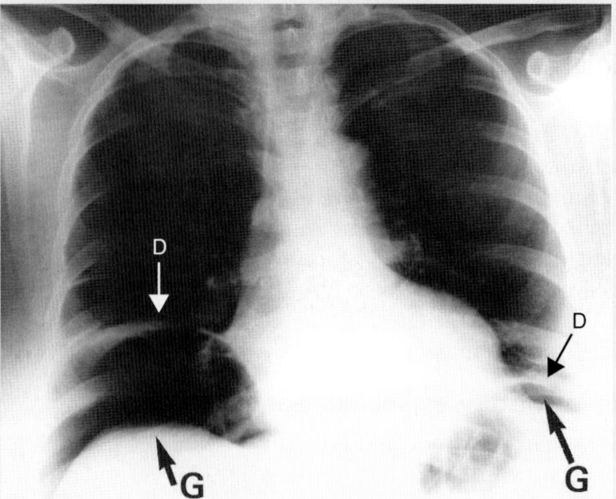

Erect chest X-ray from a man of 60 with a perforated sigmoid diverticulum who presented with a sudden onset of severe abdominal pain. The film shows large radiolucent gas shadows **G, G** under each hemidiaphragm **D, D**. Fortunately in this case, no faeces entered the peritoneum and the patient did not suffer shock or peritonitis

CASE HISTORY

Fig. 19.9 Intestinal ischaemia

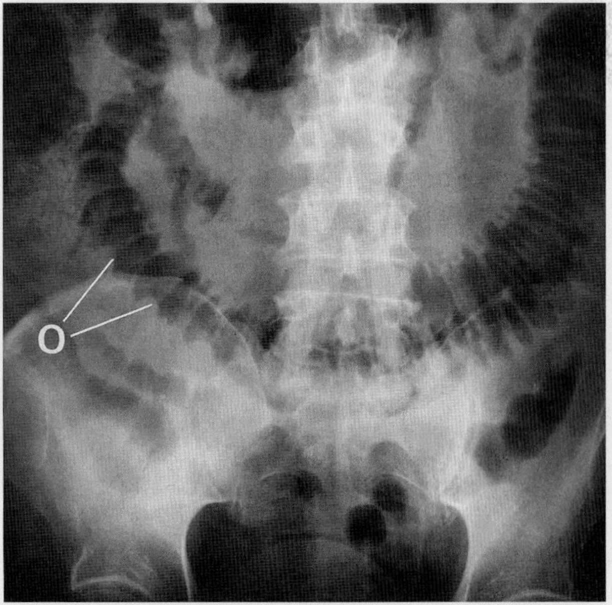

This 68-year-old woman with atrial fibrillation presented with collapse but only moderate abdominal pain. The patient had embolised her superior mesenteric artery (acute SMA occlusion) which supplies the embryological midgut-derived structures. The whole of her small bowel and the right half of her colon were necrotic but the left half of the colon was intact. This film shows the typical gross thickening of small bowel folds caused by swelling from oedema and intramural haemorrhage **O**

two types: **embolism** usually originates from left atrial thrombus in atrial fibrillation or from left ventricular wall thrombus after recent myocardial infarction; and **thrombosis** of the artery, usually a terminal event in gross low output cardiac failure or secondary to atherosclerotic stenosis. The vulnerability of the SMA territory is poorly understood, as is the sparing of the coeliac and inferior mesenteric territories, but it likely depends on the collateral blood supply.

Acute bowel ischaemia can be difficult to diagnose because of the lack of specific clinical features or diagnostic tests. In the early stages, pain is often very severe and out of proportion to the clinical signs. There may be mild diffuse tenderness but the abdomen is usually soft without guarding. As the process evolves, there is a disproportionate degree of cardiovascular collapse or shock. By this stage, arterial blood gas analysis will show a metabolic acidosis and the plasma lactate may be elevated. On plain abdominal X-ray, gas may be visible within the bowel wall. By this time, surgery is unlikely to succeed. Diagnosis therefore depends on clinical suspicion and rapid action, but for most cases the outlook is grim no matter how early the diagnosis is made.

Some cases of intestinal infarction are due to **mesenteric vein thrombosis**. The cause may be a prothrombotic disorder but is often idiopathic. In these patients, the infarction is often patchy and localised resections may allow some patients to survive.

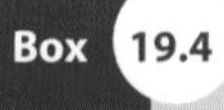

Box 19.4 Special points to note in examining a patient with an acute abdomen

General examination

See Box 18.3 (p. 250)

Abdominal examination

- Inspection
  - — distension, visible peristalsis, previous operation scars, obvious hernias, range of abdominal movement with respiration
  - — always inspect the loins and back
- Palpation and percussion
  - — tenderness, guarding, rigidity, rebound tenderness, pain on percussion
  - — free fluid, succussion splash
  - — groins for hernias and their reducibility, external genitalia
  - — abdominal masses (including a full bladder)
  - — abnormal pulsation (?aneurysm)
- Auscultation
  - — bowel sounds, mesenteric arterial bruits

PRINCIPLES OF MANAGEMENT OF INTESTINAL ISCHAEMIA

If intestinal ischaemia is suspected, laparotomy must be performed urgently unless it is clearly going to be fruitless. Very occasionally, it is possible to restore the mesenteric supply by embolectomy or bypass before the bowel necroses. If the infarcted segment is limited and the rest of the bowel looks healthy, resection gives a reasonable chance of recovery and an adequate amount of bowel to sustain nutrition. Even with short segments of residual small bowel, supplementary nutrition may allow prolonged survival but in nearly half the cases, the necrosis is so extensive that the patient should be allowed to die with minimal interference. In a few patients with arterial or venous infarction, massive resection and subsequent small bowel transplantation may be appropriate.

Examination and investigation of the acute abdomen are summarised in Boxes 19.4 and 19.5.

MAJOR GASTROINTESTINAL HAEMORRHAGE

PATHOPHYSIOLOGY AND CLINICAL FEATURES

Major gastrointestinal haemorrhage presents as vomiting of blood or passage of frank or altered blood rectally. Vomited blood (**haematemesis**) may be fresh or partly digested. In the latter case, it is dark and may have the typical appearance of 'coffee grounds'. Haematemesis usually indicates bleeding from the oesophagus, stomach or duodenum.

Blood loss beyond the duodenum is usually passed rectally. The extent to which it is altered by digestion and the degree of mixing with the stool are useful indicators of its level of origin and rate of bleeding. Upper gastrointestinal bleeding is often manifest by **melaena**. This is the passage of loose, reddish-black, tarry stools with a characteristic foul smell. With upper gastrointestinal bleeding proximal to the duodenojejunal (DJ) flexure, haematemesis or melaena or both can occur. Haematemesis is more likely if the bleeding is rapid. The main causes of major gastrointestinal haemorrhage are summarised in Figure 19.10.

MANAGEMENT OF UPPER GASTROINTESTINAL HAEMORRHAGE

Initial management and resuscitation

Any patient with severe upper gastrointestinal haemorrhage is at risk of dying from hypovolaemic shock. This may occur with the initial event or as a result of rebleeding. High-risk patients (see Fig. 19.11) have about a 50% risk of rebleeding during a hospital stay; a combined medical/surgical management policy can reduce mortality for all cases of upper GI haemorrhage from 10% to about 2%. Hospitals should have clearly written and agreed protocols for this so patients do not slip through the net and perish by default (Fig. 19.11).

Clinical history, examination and investigation

In Western countries, more than two-thirds of patients with upper gastrointestinal haemorrhage are over 60 and one-third of these have taken aspirin or other non-steroidal anti-inflammatory drugs. Alcohol consumption, previous peptic ulceration or gastric surgery, or a history of cirrhosis and variceal haemorrhage may also be important.

Abdominal examination is usually unremarkable but general examination may show signs of chronic liver disease suggesting possible gastro-oesophageal varices. Rectal

Box 19.5 Investigation of the acute abdomen

Blood tests

Haematology

- Haemoglobin
  - — may be normal immediately after an acute bleed
  - — low haemoglobin concentration may represent chronic anaemia due to occult blood loss rather than acute haemorrhage
- White blood count—leucocytosis is non-specific and rarely of much diagnostic value unless greater than about 14×10^3/L
- Blood group and ordering of blood for transfusion—for severely anaemic patients, in major haemorrhage or when major surgery is contemplated

Biochemistry

- C-reactive protein
  - — non-specific indicator of inflammatory activation
  - — confirms organic illness if substantially elevated
- Plasma amylase—whenever pancreatitis cannot be excluded
- Urea and electrolytes—indicated in vomiting and diarrhoea, dehydration, poor urine output, diuretic therapy, urinary tract disease, known or suspected renal failure, pancreatitis and sepsis
- Glucose—for diabetics or those with glycosuria (beware of hyperglycaemia due to acute stress or steroid therapy)
- Liver function tests and calcium estimation—for pancreatitis and acute biliary disease
- Clotting studies—for acute pancreatitis and septicaemia (disseminated intravascular coagulation), severe bleeding (consumption coagulopathy) or those with a history of bleeding disorders

Urine tests

- Ward ('stick') testing—for blood, protein, bile, glucose, nitrites and white cells
- Microscopy—for red and white blood cells, organisms
- Culture and sensitivity—in suspected urinary tract infections
- Strain urine for stones—in ureteric colic
- Pregnancy test in females if appropriate

Imaging (see Box 19.1)

Plain radiography

- Erect chest X-ray
  - — cardiovascular disease or abnormality, e.g. cardiomegaly, thoracic aneurysm, aortic dissection, cardiac failure
  - — respiratory disease
  - — suspected visceral perforation (gas under diaphragm)
- Supine abdominal X-ray (erect or decubitus if necessary)
  - — bowel (gas pattern and dilatation, fluid levels, gas in the wall, faeces and faecoliths)
  - — urinary tract ('KUB' = kidneys, ureters and bladder) shows kidney size and position, calculi
  - — biliary tract (gallstones, gas in biliary tree in gallstone ileus)
  - — aortic calcification (aneurysm)
  - — psoas shadows (obscured by retroperitoneal inflammation or haemorrhage)

Ultrasound

- Gallstones
- Pelvic abnormalities in obstetric and gynaecological practice
- 'Chronic' enlargement of the spleen
- Abdominal aortic aneurysm (AAA)
- Free abdominal fluid and gas indicating perforated bowel
- Other stones
- Dilated ducts; air in biliary tree
- Hydatid, teratomas and other cysts
- Intra-abdominal abscesses and masses

Contrast radiology

- 'Instant' barium enema in colonic obstruction or acute colitis
- Emergency intravenous urography in ureteric colic

CT scanning

CT can give rapid, cost-effective evaluation of acute abdominal pain but should not supplant clinical examination nor unreasonably delay surgical exploration in the deteriorating patient. Diagnostic value of CT is better if timing, contrast (i.v. and/or oral) and other variables are tailored to the working diagnosis.

- Assessment of abdominal trauma—severity and grading of solid organ injury, free intra-abdominal fluid and gas; retroperitoneal injuries including pancreatic and duodenal rupture and vascular injury
- Often first choice for ureteric colic, suspected aortic aneurysm or aortic dissection
- Useful where diagnosis remains in doubt, e.g. suspected bowel perforation (detects small amount of free gas), acute diverticulitis
- Investigation of postoperative complications—abscesses, fluid collections
- Severe acute pancreatitis, especially if necrosis suspected

examination may reveal melaena stool or altered blood and this can be helpful if the history of haematemesis has not been substantiated.

Estimating blood loss from the history is unreliable because a great deal of blood may remain in the bowel. It is essential to obtain good venous access early and then to perform a full blood count, urea and electrolytes and prothrombin ratio and liver function tests, to send blood for grouping and antibody screen (or cross-matching), and to order blood for transfusion in high-risk cases (see Fig. 19.11 and below). ECG and chest X-rays are useful in patients over 65 years or with cardiorespiratory disease. *Note*: the patient should be ready to go to the operating theatre at a moment's notice if he or she suddenly deteriorates!

COMMON CAUSES OF GASTROINTESTINAL BLEEDING

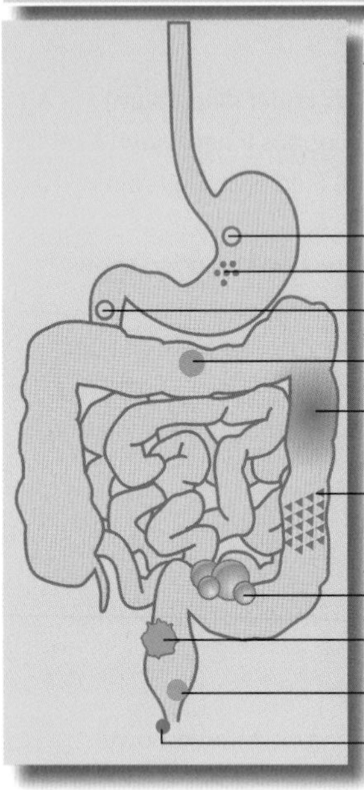

Pathology	Clinical features	Frequency
Acute and chronic gastric ulcers Gastric erosions Chronic duodenal ulcer	Haematemesis and/or melaena	Very common
Polyps or carcinoma of colon	Altered blood per rectum	Common
Ischaemic colitis	Abdominal pain then fairly fresh rectal bleeding	Fairly common
Angiodysplasias of colon	Pattern of bleeding depends on location within colon; increasingly recognised with the rise in colonoscopy	Fairly common
Diverticular disease	Fresh rectal bleeding	Common
Carcinoma of rectum Rectal polyps Haemorrhoids	Fresh rectal bleeding but rarely in large quantities	Common

UNCOMMON CAUSES OF GASTROINTESTINAL BLEEDING

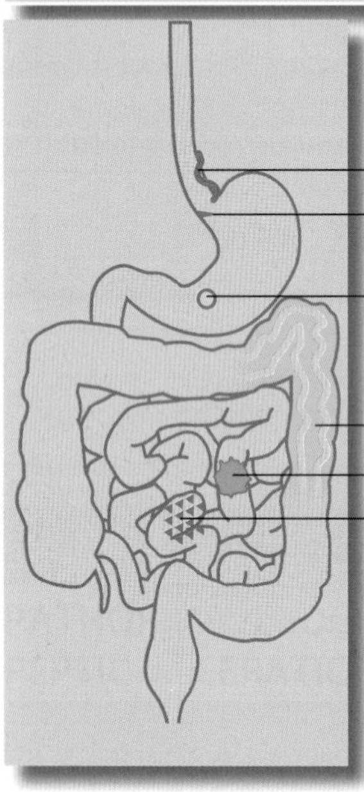

Pathology	Clinical features	Frequency
Oesophageal varices	Haematemesis and/or melaena	Uncommon
Mallory–Weiss oesophageal tears	Haematemesis or altered blood per rectum	Uncommon
Stress ulcers	Haematemesis and/or melaena	Uncommon
Acute or fulminant ulcerative colitis	Bloody diarrhoea	Uncommon
Malignant small bowel tumours	Altered blood per rectum	Rare
Angiodysplasias of small bowel	Altered blood per rectum	Rare

Fig. 19.10 Causes of gastrointestinal haemorrhage

Stratification of risk

Patients with acute upper GI haemorrhage should be stratified clinically into either a **low-risk group** (non life-threatening) or a **high-risk group** (where continued bleeding or likely rebleeding is potentially life-threatening) (see Fig. 19.11 and next section).

Patients with signs of shock must be monitored and resuscitated thoroughly; the rate and volume of i.v. fluid replacement (whether plasma expanders or blood) is adjusted against the responses of pulse rate, blood pressure, central venous pressure and hourly urine output.

Endoscopic management of acute upper gastrointestinal haemorrhage

Patients clinically at high risk should be assessed early by a surgical team, even if admitted under the care of a gastroenterologist or (internal) physician. Ideally, the same surgical team should remain responsible for that patient until recovery so that a prompt decision to operate can be made if conservative management fails.

Patients with upper gastrointestinal haemorrhage require endoscopy to determine the site and activity of bleeding, to diagnose oesophageal varices and to determine suitability for

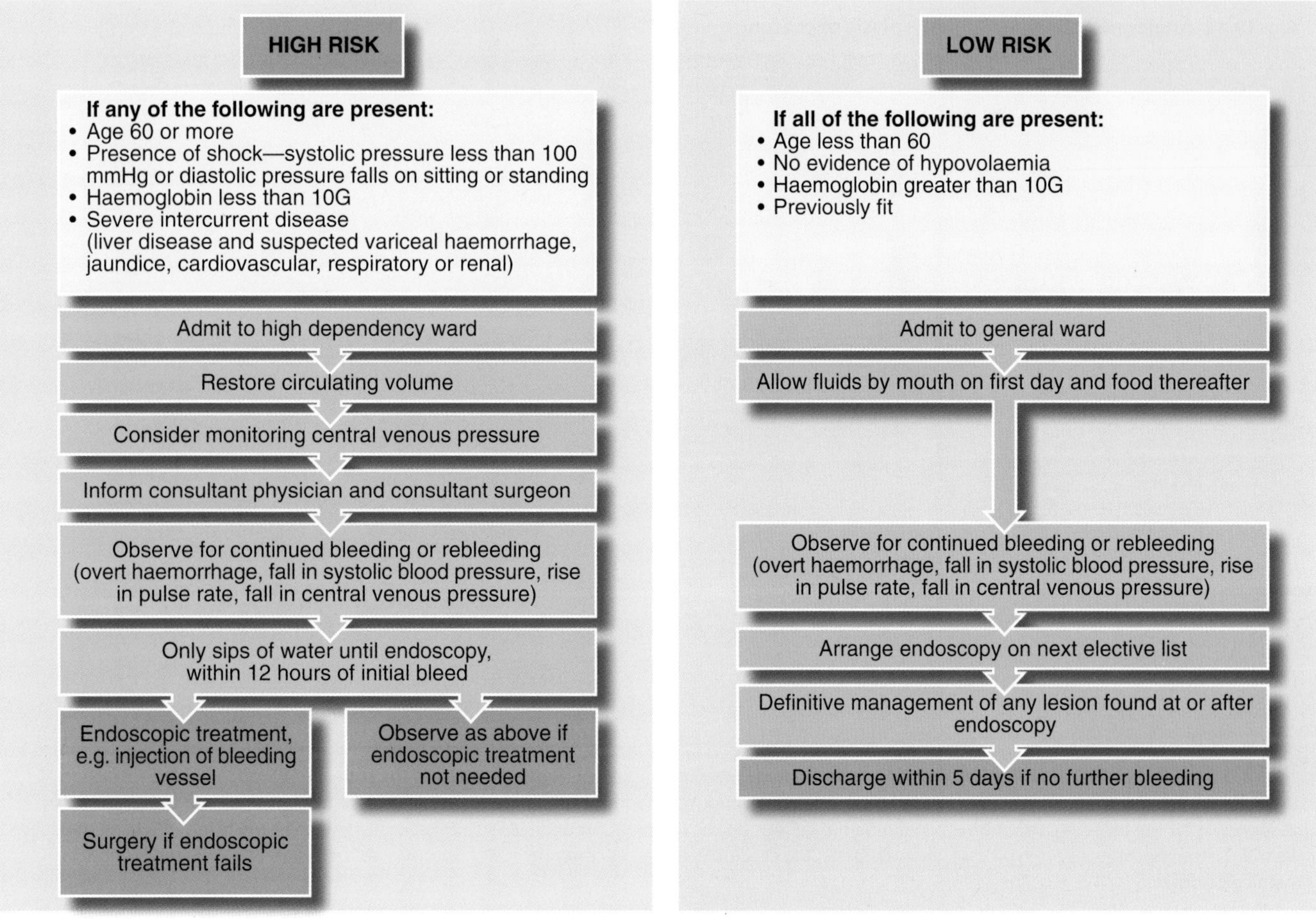

Fig. 19.11 Risk stratification in the management of acute upper gastrointestinal haemorrhage

endoscopic treatment. Endoscopy also assists in locating the source if surgery becomes necessary. Urgent endoscopy, within 12 hours of the first bleed, should be performed in high-risk patients; all others should be endoscoped on the next available list. Even in the most acute upper GI haemorrhage, gastroscopy can usually be performed on the operating table before operation. Duodenal or gastric ulceration should be easily identifiable, but its real value is the ability to diagnose unusual sources of bleeding (e.g. Mallory–Weiss tear; see Ch. 22) and to avoid operating on unsuspected variceal haemorrhage. Even in patients with known varices, endoscopy is essential, as in 50% of cases, blood loss will be from a completely different lesion, e.g. peptic ulcer or gastric erosions.

Certain endoscopic features may place apparently low-risk patients into a high-risk category. These are:

- **Active spurting from an artery in an ulcer bed**. Endotherapy by gastroscopic injection of adrenaline (epinephrine) or an adrenaline/sclerosant mixture should be attempted; there is a 25–40% rebleed rate even in expert hands and the patient must be closely monitored as these often need surgery
- **A visible elevated vessel or protruding adherent clot (Dieulafoy lesion)**. These lesions double the above risk of rebleeding to 50–80%. If the patient is hypotensive as a result of blood loss, the risk of rebleeding is 80%
- **Bleeding gastro-oesophageal varices**. Mortality is around 30%. Immediate treatment is required with endoluminal band ligation or injection sclerotherapy. Tamponade with special balloon catheters may also be necessary prior to endotherapy

High-risk patients should be commenced on a 72-hour intravenous infusion of high dose proton pump inhibitor. Low-risk patients usually stop bleeding with conservative management and are then unlikely to rebleed. They may be given sips of water, monitored for rebleeding, and endoscoped on the next available list.

Surgical management

A policy of early surgery for patients over 60 has been shown to reduce mortality. Urgent surgery is also required for patients defined clinically or endoscopically as at high risk, and who suffer one rebleed; or for any patient who suffers two rebleeds. Immediate surgery, including unguided laparotomy, is required for patients with exsanguinating haemorrhage or those unable to be stabilised during resuscitation.

Bleeding is arrested with under-running sutures after gastrotomy or duodenotomy and attempts are made to preserve

Fig. 19.12 Angiogram showing angiodysplasia of caecum

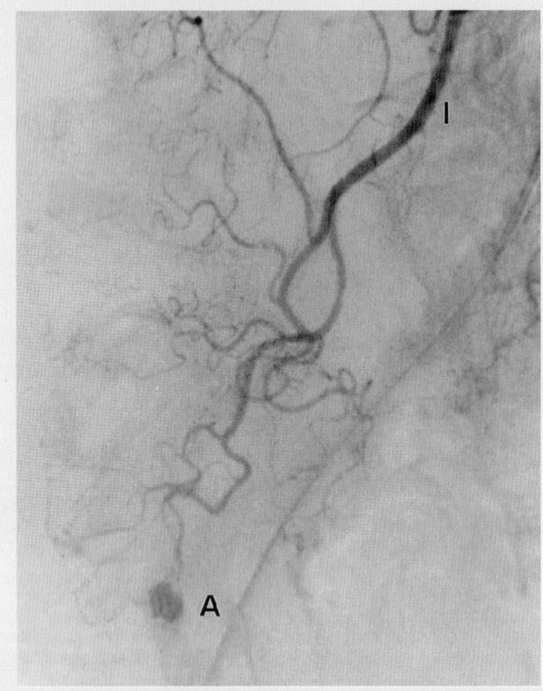

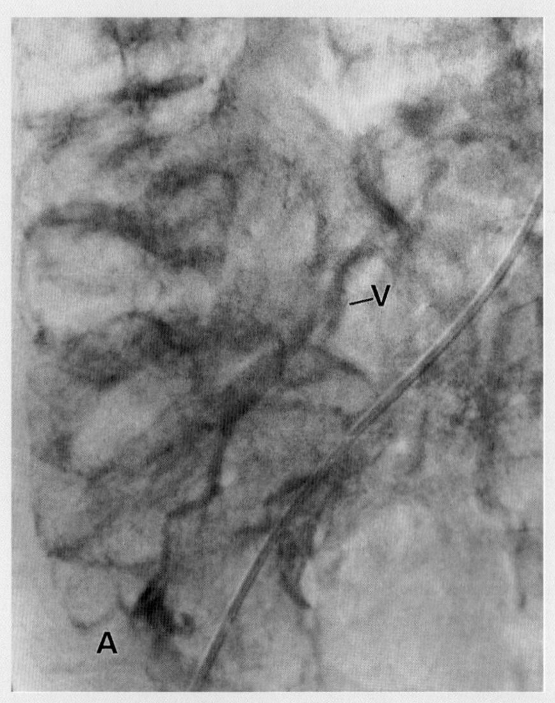

This man of 70 had been admitted to hospital on 12 occasions for rectal bleeding and chronic anaemia and had received 55 units of blood transfusion in all. On the last admission, this superior mesenteric arteriogram was performed, revealing the source of blood loss. **(a)** Subtraction film showing the arterial phase; the ileocolic artery **I** feeds a knot of abnormal blood vessels, an angiodysplasia **A**, at the lower pole of the caecum was responsible for the bleeding. **(b)** Subtraction film of the venous phase; the angiodysplasia **A** is still visible and there is early filling of a large draining vein **V**. These appearances are typical of angiodysplasia; the caecum is the most common site of occurrence. The lesion was resected by right hemicolectomy

the pyloric ring. Gastric and duodenal ulcers should be biopsied for *Helicobacter* testing, and for malignancy in gastric ulcers. Anti-*Helicobacter* therapy is given later if perioperative or postoperative testing is *H. pylori* positive.

MORE DISTAL GASTROINTESTINAL HAEMORRHAGE

More distal GI bleeding is not usually investigated immediately to find the site but is managed conservatively, anticipating spontaneous cessation. If bleeding continues, it is important that the source be localised by investigation so that treatment can be accurately targeted. 'Blind' laparotomy is often unsatisfactory because the source may be difficult or impossible to find or the cause may need non-surgical treatment.

Blood loss from diverticular disease (approximately 60% of cases) and ischaemic colitis is usually self-limiting. Several small bleeds may occur over a few days but the volume lost is usually small and hypovolaemia is rare. Typically patients present late and the bleeding has often stopped, with blood per rectum the only evidence.

Investigation involves **colonoscopy**, usually once the bleeding has stopped. Occasionally an unsuspected carcinoma or polyp is discovered. In ulcerative colitis, the diagnosis is evident from the other symptoms and signs, and management depends on the success of medical treatment (see Ch. 28). Persisting large bowel haemorrhage which is less rapid but recurrent is usually due to **angiodysplasias** (see Ch. 29). Colonoscopy can be both diagnostic and therapeutic for bleeding angiodysplasia. If colonoscopy is negative, impossible or unsatisfactory, radioisotope scanning using the patient's own labelled red cells can be used; this has the advantage of identifying bleeding at rates as low as 0.05 ml/min. Highly selective arteriography is increasingly used in diagnosis of gastrointestinal haemorrhage but relies on much more rapid bleeding (greater than 0.5 ml/min) (see Fig. 19.12). At the time of arteriography, bleeding can be controlled with localised delivery of vasopressors or by coil embolisation.

At laparotomy the whole bowel can be examined and any suspect area resected if appropriate. However, purely mucosal lesions are undetectable at operation so, as a last resort, a colonoscope inserted through an incision in the bowel wall can be used to examine the whole colon and small bowel for bleeding sites.

Gallstone diseases and related disorders

20

INTRODUCTION

Gallstones and related disorders account for all but a small proportion of biliary tract disease in most countries. Gallstone disease is also known as cholelithiasis and choledocholithiasis is when stones are present in the bile ducts.

Most gallstone-related disease presents with pain, typically located in the epigastrium or right hypochondrium (right upper quadrant or RUQ). The character of the pain varies but in most cases, it is acute and intermittent. Less commonly, gallstone disease presents as pain and jaundice caused by a stone passing into and obstructing the common bile duct.

STRUCTURE AND FUNCTION OF THE BILIARY SYSTEM

Bile collects in canaliculi between hepatocytes and drains via collecting ducts within the portal triads into a system of ducts within the liver. These progressively increase in diameter until they become the **right** and **left hepatic ducts** which fuse to form the **common hepatic duct**. This is joined further distally by the **cystic duct** to become the **common bile duct** (Fig. 20.1). The common bile duct is 4–5 cm long and passes down behind the duodenum then through the head of the pancreas to drain via the **ampulla of Vater** into the medial wall of the second part of the duodenum. In most cases, the **main pancreatic duct** joins the common bile duct at the ampulla although it may enter the duodenum independently. The **sphincter of Oddi** within the ampulla prevents reflux of duodenal contents into the common bile duct and pancreatic duct.

The **gall bladder** is a muscular sac lined by mucosa characterised by a single, highly folded layer of tall columnar epithelial cells. The lining epithelium is supported by loose connective tissue containing numerous blood vessels and lymphatics. Mucus-secreting glands are found at the neck of the gall bladder but are absent from the body and fundus. The proximal part of the duct is disposed into a spiral arrangement called the **spiral valve**, the function of which is not well understood. The gall bladder lies in a variable depression in the under-surface of the right hepatic lobe and is covered by the peritoneal envelope of the liver. The common bile duct is a fibrous tissue tube lined by a simple, tall columnar epithelium. Normally it is up to 0.6 cm in diameter and this can be measured on ultrasound scanning.

Bile is made continuously by the liver and passes along the biliary tract to the gall bladder where it is stored. Bile is concentrated there by as much as 10 times by a process of active mucosal reabsorption of water. Lipid-rich food passing from stomach to duodenum promotes secretion of the hormone **cholecystokinin-pancreozymin** (CCK) by endocrine cells of the duodenal mucosa. This hormone stimulates contraction of the gall bladder, squeezing bile into the duodenum. Bile salts (acids) act as emulsifying agents and facilitate hydrolysis of dietary lipids by pancreatic lipases. If biliary tract obstruction prevents bile from reaching the duodenum, lipids are neither digested nor absorbed, resulting in passage of loose, pale, foul-smelling fatty stools (**steatorrhoea**). Furthermore, the fat-soluble vitamins (A, D, E and K) are not absorbed. The lack of vitamin K soon leads to inadequate prothrombin synthesis and hence defective clotting. If surgery is necessary in a patient with obstructive jaundice, this may pose problems of haemostasis.

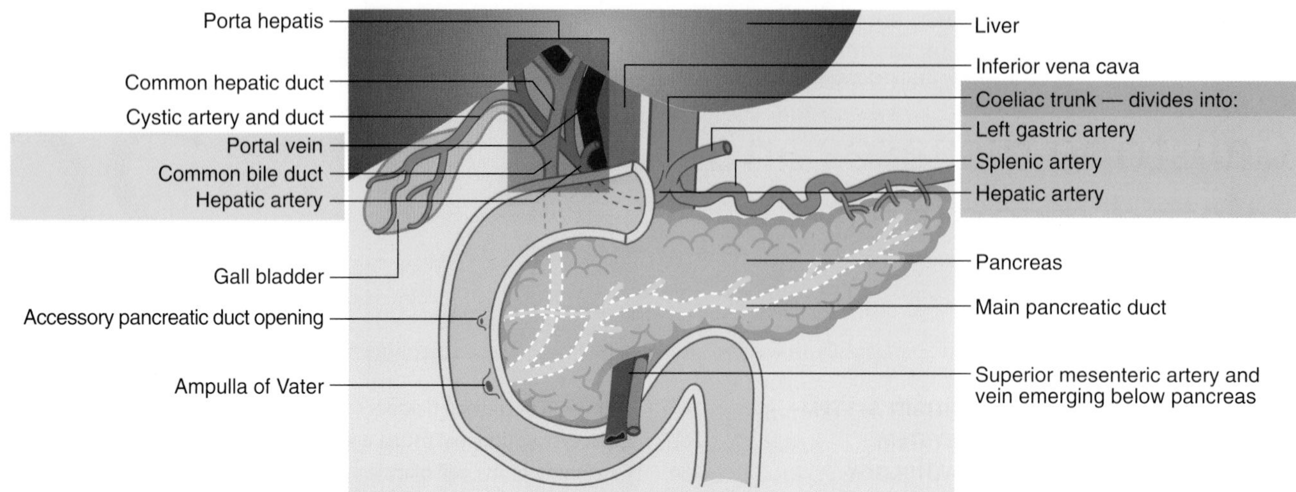

Fig. 20.1 Surgical anatomy of the gall bladder, biliary tract and pancreas
The coeliac trunk (the foregut artery) arises from the aorta and divides into the hepatic, splenic and left gastric arteries. The hepatic artery divides into right and left branches, mirrored by the extrahepatic right and left hepatic ducts. These join caudally to form the common hepatic duct; this in turn is joined by the cystic duct to form the common bile duct (CBD). The **porta hepatis** consists of the hepatic arteries, the extrahepatic bile ducts and the portal vein

PATHOPHYSIOLOGY OF THE BILIARY SYSTEM

GALLSTONE COMPOSITION

In developed countries, most gallstones are of **mixed** composition and contain a predominance of cholesterol; this is mixed with some **bile pigment** (calcium bilirubinate) and other **calcium salts**. A small proportion is virtually 'pure' cholesterol stones ('**cholesterol solitaire**'). In Asia, most gallstones are composed of bile pigment alone. The composition and pathogenesis of the various types of gallstone are summarised in Table 20.1 (and see Fig. 20.2), and some examples are illustrated in Figure 20.3.

The physical structure of mixed gallstones gives an insight into their sequence of formation. There is usually a small core of organic material, often containing bacteria. The main body of the stone is made up of concentric layers, demonstrating that stones form in a series of discrete precipitation events. Furthermore, in the same gall bladder, there are often several 'families' of gallstones, each of a different size. This suggests each generation began at a different time, presumably due to some transient change in local conditions. All families then build up at the same rate by lamination, leading to the range of different sizes. Radioisotope dating studies have shown that the average gallstone is 11 years old when removed!

The main factors in stone formation are: (a) changes in concentration of the different constituents of bile, (b) biliary stasis and (c) infection. It is likely that several subtle abnormalities combine synergistically to bring about precipitation of bile constituents.

Bile salts and lecithin are responsible for maintaining cholesterol in a stable **micelle** formation. The normal micellar structure of bile supports a greater concentration of cholesterol than could otherwise be held in solution and is therefore inherently unstable. An excess of cholesterol in proportion to bile salts and lecithin is probably one of the main factors in cholesterol stone formation. This is supported by the fact that patients in whom the terminal ileum has been resected or who have chronic distal ileal disease have a three-fold risk of developing cholesterol-rich stones. The mechanism is likely to be as follows: the terminal ileum is the main site for reabsorption of bile salts and when it is diseased or has been removed, reabsorption declines, leading to bile salt loss via the bowel and, eventually, a decline in the bile salt pool. The remaining bile salts are then insufficient to maintain the micellar structure of cholesterol in suspension.

Precipitation from bile is enhanced by **biliary stasis**. This occurs if the gall bladder becomes obstructed or contractility becomes defective. It is not known whether obstruction of the gall bladder outlet is a primary event in formation of stones but it probably plays a part in their continued accretion. Obstruction can be caused by dysfunction of the spiral valve in the cystic duct, by reflux of duodenal contents (which may be infected) or by small stones already formed. The muscular gall bladder wall is damaged by longstanding inflammation or infection which interferes with its ability to empty. Pregnancy is also a predisposing factor.

THE ROLE OF INFLAMMATION AND INFECTION

Inflammation and infection probably both play a part in gallstone formation. Abnormalities of bile composition may cause **chemical inflammation** of the gall bladder, resulting in inflammatory exudation and accumulation of inflammatory debris. **Bacteria** usually form the organic nidus upon which gallstones are built; they enter the gall bladder intermittently by reflux from the duodenum or via the bloodstream. This process is probably normal but becomes pathological if the bacteria are not flushed out, as occurs when the gall bladder does not adequately empty. In support of this is the fact that

Table 20.1 Composition and pathogenesis of gallstones

Chemical composition	Pathogenesis	Characteristics
Mixed stones (75–90% of all stones) Cholesterol is the predominant constituent Heterogeneous mixture of cholesterol, bile pigments and calcium salts in a laminated structure around a 'core' (Fig. 20.2)	Combination of: ● Abnormalities of bile constituents ● Bile stasis ● Infection	Multiple stones with several generations of different sizes often found together Stones may be hard and faceted (where they have developed in contact) or irregular, 'mulberry'-shaped, and softer Colours range from near-white through yellow and green to black Most are radiolucent but 10% are radiopaque
Cholesterol stones (up to 10% of all stones)	As for mixed stones	Large, smooth, egg- or barrel-shaped and usually solitary ('cholesterol solitaire') Yellowish. Up to 4 cm diameter and may fill the gall bladder. Radiolucent
Pigment stones Calcium bilirubinate (uncommon in developed countries, common in Asia)	Excess bilirubin excretion due to haemolytic disorders, e.g. haemolytic anaemias, infections, malaria, leukaemias	Multiple, jet-black, shiny 'jack' stones; 0.5–1 cm diameter. Usually of uniform size and often friable
Calcium carbonate stones (rare)	Excess calcium excretion in bile	Greyish faceted stones Radiopaque

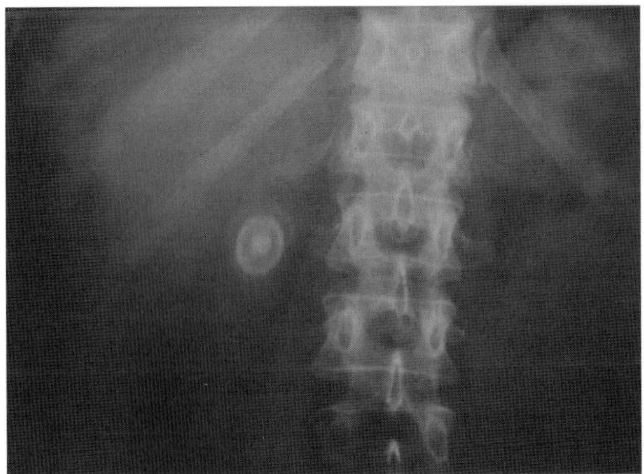

Fig. 20.2 X-ray of radiopaque gallstone
Plain abdominal X-ray showing large radiopaque gallstone in the right upper quadrant. Note that the stone is obviously laminated, having built up in layers over many years. Note also that only 10% of mixed stones are radiopaque

faecal organisms can be cultured from at least 25% of cholecystectomy specimens.

THE ROLE OF CHRONIC OBSTRUCTION

Most gall bladders removed for chronic pain show histological features more in keeping with a **chronic obstructive aetiology** than an infective one. These include atrophic mucosa, submucosal and subserosal fibrosis, hypertrophy of the muscular wall, and mucosal diverticula extending into the muscular layer (known as **Rokitansky–Aschoff sinuses**). Evidence of active or previous infection is uncommon. In some cases the gall bladder is so grossly scarred, distorted or contracted that its absorptive and contractile functions have been completely destroyed.

OTHER PATHOLOGICAL MECHANISMS

In about 10% of patients with typical symptoms of gall bladder disease, no stone can be found during investigation or at operation. In some of these, a stone may have passed out of the duct system into the bowel. In others, acute or chronic inflammation occurs independently of stones, called '**acalculous cholecystitis**'; once again, chronic obstruction may be the cause. Finally, the terms '**biliary dyskinesia**' and '**cystic duct syndrome**' may sometimes explain the condition where patients have typical symptoms of gall bladder disease but standard investigations are essentially normal. When biliary manometry is used, some patients have an abnormally high pressure in the sphincter of Oddi. Confirming this diagnosis is difficult but a fair proportion of patients suspected of this are cured by endoscopic sphincterotomy.

EPIDEMIOLOGY OF GALLSTONES

In developed countries, at least 10% of adults probably develop gallstones during their lifetime, although most remain asymptomatic. Gallstones are rare before adulthood and increase in prevalence with age. Women are affected four times more often and pregnancy appears to be an important predisposing factor; obesity and diabetes may also play a part. The typical patient is said to be a 'fair fat fertile female of forty', but many gallstone patients do not fit this description. Gallstone disease is rare in rural communities of developing countries but is increasing with urbanisation. Western-style processed foods, high in fats and refined carbohydrates but poor in fibre, may be responsible. Dietary contributions to gall bladder disease support the theory that changes in composition of bile are important in stone pathogenesis.

(a)
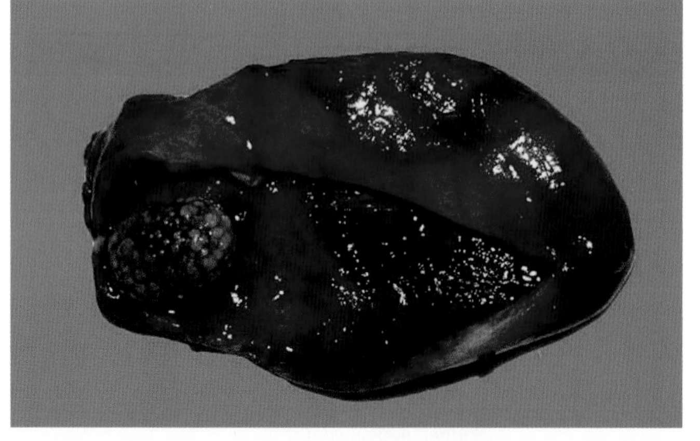

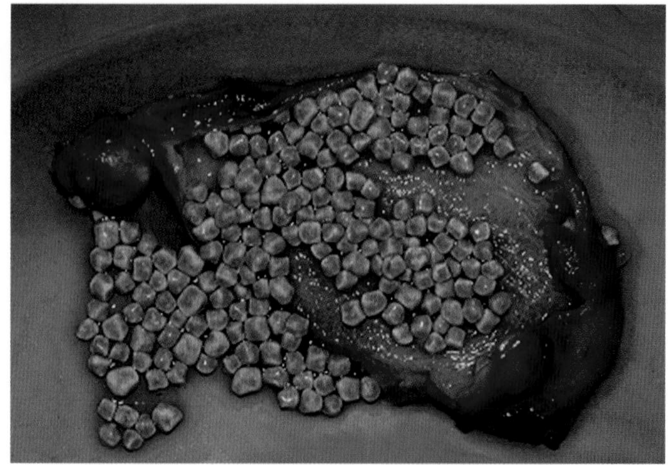
(b)

(c)
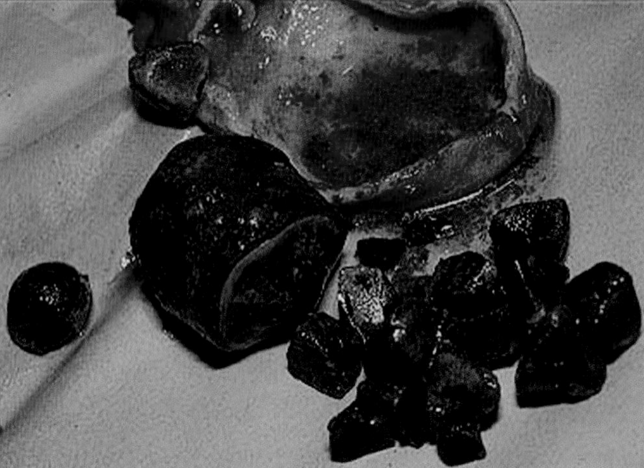

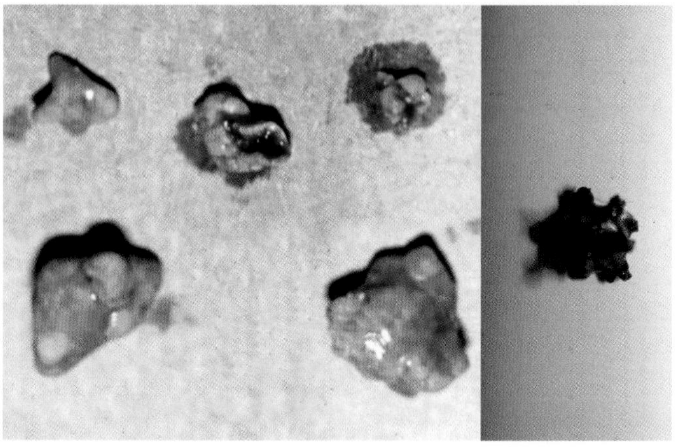
(d)

Fig. 20.3 Types of gallstone
(a) Thick-walled chronically inflamed gall bladder found to be obstructed at its neck by a single stone. Note the stone is an aggregate of many smaller stones **(b)** Multiple small gallstones in the gall bladder, all of much the same 'generation'. **(c)** Gall bladder containing one huge stone and multiple smaller stones. These stones all fitted together with adjoining facets. **(d)** Different types of gallstones—pale irregular stones of different ages on the left and a pigment 'jack' stone on the right

INVESTIGATION OF GALL BLADDER PATHOLOGY

When gallstone disease is suspected, investigation has the following objectives:

- Exclude haematological and liver abnormalities and other metabolic disorders
- Establish if gallstones are present in the gall bladder and/or common duct and whether the gall bladder wall is thickened
- Assess the integrity and patency of the bile duct system and the pancreatic duct (if there is any suggestion of obstruction)

Blood tests for haematological and liver abnormalities

Haemolytic disorders such as hereditary spherocytosis, thalassaemia and sickle-cell trait should be considered as they may predispose to pigment stones. Liver function tests (LFTs) are indicated to look for indications of common duct stone obstruction if there is any suggestion of jaundice and to exclude other liver abnormalities.

Imaging in investigating gall bladder pathology

Ultrasonography (see Fig. 20.4) can reliably identify stones in the gall bladder and any increase in thickness of the wall (caused by inflammation or fibrosis). Ultrasound also provides a simple and accurate means of demonstrating **dilatation of the common duct system**, often indicating distal duct obstruction. Unfortunately, it is unreliable for directly identifying bile duct stones, particularly at the lower end, because the image tends to be obscured by overlying duodenal gas. Ultrasound has the great advantage of being suitable for use in the seriously ill or jaundiced patient as it is non-invasive and can be performed at the bedside.

Investigating the biliary duct system

See Figure 20.5.

THE NON-JAUNDICED PATIENT

Patients with gallstones but no history of obstructive jaundice do not require preoperative investigation for duct stones apart from an ultrasound scan and LFTs. If cholecystectomy is needed, **intraoperative** (or perioperative) **cholangiography** may be carried out. A cannula is passed through the cystic duct into the common bile duct and radiopaque contrast material injected to fill the biliary tree. X-rays or fluoroscopic imaging are then used to demonstrate the duct morphology and abnormalities such as duct dilatation, filling defects caused by stone, or distortion of the tapering lower end of the common duct, as well as obstruction of flow into the duodenum. If cholangiography shows stones, the duct may be explored at the time or else dealt with later by endoscopic retrograde cholangio-pancreatography (ERCP).

Patients with a history of **transient jaundice** possibly attributable to stones will have either operative cholangiography at cholecystectomy or preoperative ERCP.

Fig. 20.4 Biliary ultrasound scans
Longitudinal scan of gall bladder in a 46-year-old woman who complained of intermittent attacks of right upper quadrant pain. The scan shows the outline of the gall bladder **GB** and a layer of gallstones (arrowed) along its posterior wall. The stones each cast a clear acoustic shadow **AS** beyond them. Note that these shadows can be projected back to the transducer **T**

THE JAUNDICED PATIENT

When obstructive jaundice has been diagnosed, it is important to distinguish between stone and tumour in order to plan appropriate management. **Ultrasonography** is usually the initial investigation. This shows the extent of dilatation of intrahepatic and extrahepatic ducts and may even show a stone lodged at the lower end of the duct. If stones are in the gall bladder, this suggests stones are blocking the duct rather than tumour, but the two can coexist. The ultrasound scan will usually demonstrate the presence of a carcinoma of the pancreatic head or enlarged lymph nodes in the porta hepatis; either may cause extrahepatic biliary obstruction.

Ultrasound may make the diagnosis, but if more information is required, biliary tract morphology can be outlined using **magnetic resonance cholangio-pancreatography (MRCP)** which produces images of the biliary tree and pancreatic ducts (see Ch 5, p. 65; Fig. 5.6). If MRCP does not yield the necessary information, the ducts can be visualised by direct introduction of contrast. There are two methods: ERCP and, more rarely, percutaneous transhepatic cholangiography. ERCP is the more useful investigation; it also allows the ampullary region to be inspected for tumour. If stones are found in the common bile duct, it is often possible to perform immediate **endoscopic sphincterotomy** to release the stones, thus diagnosing and relieving the jaundice in one procedure. This may be life-saving for the patient with ascending cholangitis and is the treatment of choice on its own for the patient who is a poor risk for laparotomy or laparoscopy.

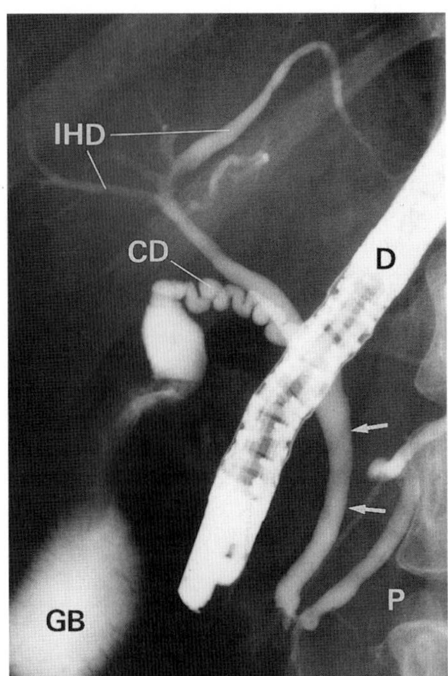

(a)

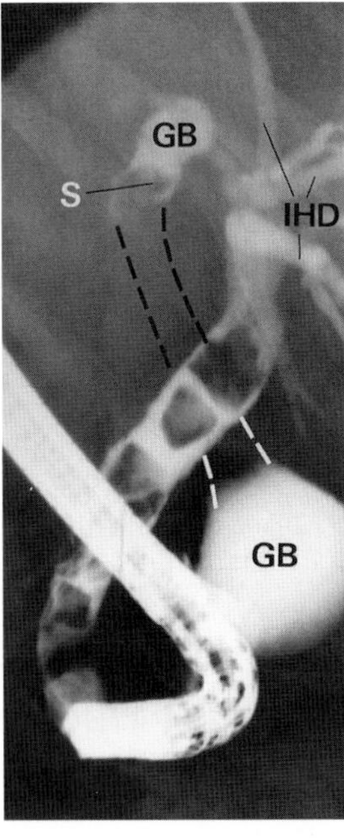

(b)

Fig. 20.5 Investigation of the biliary duct system
(a) Normal ERCP showing duodenoscope **D** in the second part of the duodenum. Contrast has been injected first into the pancreatic duct **P** and then into the common bile duct (arrowed). Note also the cystic duct **CD**, gall bladder **GB** and intrahepatic bile ducts **IHD**. **(b)** Endoscopic retrograde cholangiogram in a woman of 77 who presented with mild epigastric pain and obstructive jaundice. The film shows multiple large stones in the common bile duct, represented by filling defects. The common bile duct is moderately dilated, but the intrahepatic ducts **IHD** are not. The fundus and neck of the gall bladder **GB** are shown, but the body is empty of contrast (dotted lines). There is a stone **S** near the neck of the gall bladder

Percutaneous transhepatic cholangiography (Ch 5, p. 65; Fig. 5.6) is used in exceptional circumstances, for example if ERCP is unsuccessful because of previous gastric surgery. It involves inserting a long, fine (22 gauge) needle through the skin into one of the dilated intrahepatic ducts under radiological control. Contrast medium is then injected. An obstructing stone produces a characteristic rounded filling defect, contrasting with the tapering stricture typical of tumour.

Endoscopic ultrasound scanning (EUS), i.e. scanning via the endoscope, is a useful technique to show greater detail at the lower end of the common bile duct or to examine lesions in the ampulla or head of the pancreas with greater clarity.

CLINICAL PRESENTATIONS OF GALLSTONE DISEASE

Gallstones may cause chronic, low-grade symptoms, often labelled **chronic cholecystitis**. However, many of these symptoms may be due to irritable bowel syndrome or chronic aerophagia (air swallowing). Transient obstruction of the gall bladder by stone may cause episodes of acute pain (**biliary colic**). If the obstruction persists, the gall bladder becomes chemically inflamed causing **acute cholecystitis**. If obstruction does not resolve by itself and the contents do not become infected, the gall bladder becomes distended with mucus; this is known as a **mucocoele**, and is often palpable and tender. If the contents become infected, an abscess develops within the gall bladder and this is known as an **empyema of the gall bladder**.

Rarely, free **perforation** of the gall bladder may occur. Equally rarely, large stones in the common bile duct ulcerate directly into the duodenum causing **fistula** formation. If they pass down the small bowel and impact in the terminal ileum and cause obstruction, this is called **gallstone ileus**. Finally, gallstones probably predispose to **carcinoma** of the gall bladder in the very long term. The spectrum of clinical disorders associated with gallstones is summarised in Figure 20.6.

CHRONIC SYMPTOMS SUGGESTIVE OF GALL BLADDER DISEASE

Many patients are referred with a history of intermittent pain in the right upper quadrant or epigastrium often accompanied by nausea or even vomiting. The pain may be brought on by large or fatty meals and may radiate around towards the back. Symptoms are often vague and ill defined so patients often delay consulting a doctor. Examination rarely reveals more than vague upper abdominal tenderness. Many turn out not to have gallstones on ultrasonography and the pain may be due to irritable bowel syndrome but the differential diagnosis includes peptic ulcer disease, urinary tract infection and chronic constipation. Note that even if a patient has upper abdominal symptoms and demonstrable gallstones, this does not prove the pain is caused by stones. When symptoms are less specific, a more extensive diagnostic search is needed, perhaps including upper gastrointestinal endoscopy, plasma amylase and ECG as well as bowel investigations.

BILIARY COLIC

CLINICAL FEATURES

The most common reason for symptoms from gallstones is probably intermittent cystic duct obstruction by stone. The pain is severe; it typically rises to a plateau over a few minutes then continues unrelentingly. Note that this pain does not have the strikingly intermittent brief peaks of other forms of colic (e.g. ureteric). These patients may be in agony until the pain resolves spontaneously after several hours or after opiate analgesia. Vomiting is often associated with the attack and the patient feels exhausted and sore for the next day or so. There is commonly a history of previous similar episodes. There are few positive findings on examination: the patient is afebrile but there may be some local tenderness due to gall bladder distension. If the attack does not settle within 24 hours, acute cholecystitis is a more likely diagnosis (see below).

MANAGEMENT

Most cases of biliary colic can safely be managed at home if the diagnosis is recognised. Relief of pain usually requires only one injection of an opiate and the attack passes. Severe attacks of biliary colic usually prompt emergency hospital admission since the differential diagnosis includes other conditions that may require urgent operation, e.g. perforated peptic ulcer. Ultrasound examination should be performed early since early diagnosis may save several unnecessary days in hospital. In acute gallstone disease, cholecystectomy scheduled for the next available list is preferred by many surgeons and is generally safe, but others perform the operation electively at a later date. Early operation appears to be the better option, reducing the risk of the complications of gallstones.

If a mucocoele of the gall bladder is found on ultrasonography, the attack is likely to persist and there is a high risk of an **empyema of the gall bladder** developing. In this case, cholecystectomy often becomes obligatory during the current admission.

Cholecystectomy is the definitive treatment for attacks of biliary colic. Patients are frequently put on a low-fat diet initially or whilst awaiting operation and this often relieves symptoms, presumably by removing a stimulus to gall bladder contraction. In younger patients, cholecystectomy is typically straightforward. The gall bladder is usually found to contain stones or thick dark biliary sludge and its wall is often thin, although it may sometimes be inflamed. In some patients, the gall bladder is thickened and scarred and technically more difficult to remove. Techniques of cholecystectomy are discussed on pages 290 onwards.

ACUTE CHOLECYSTITIS

PATHOPHYSIOLOGY AND CLINICAL FEATURES

Several factors contribute to causing acute inflammation in an obstructed gall bladder. These include physical and chemical

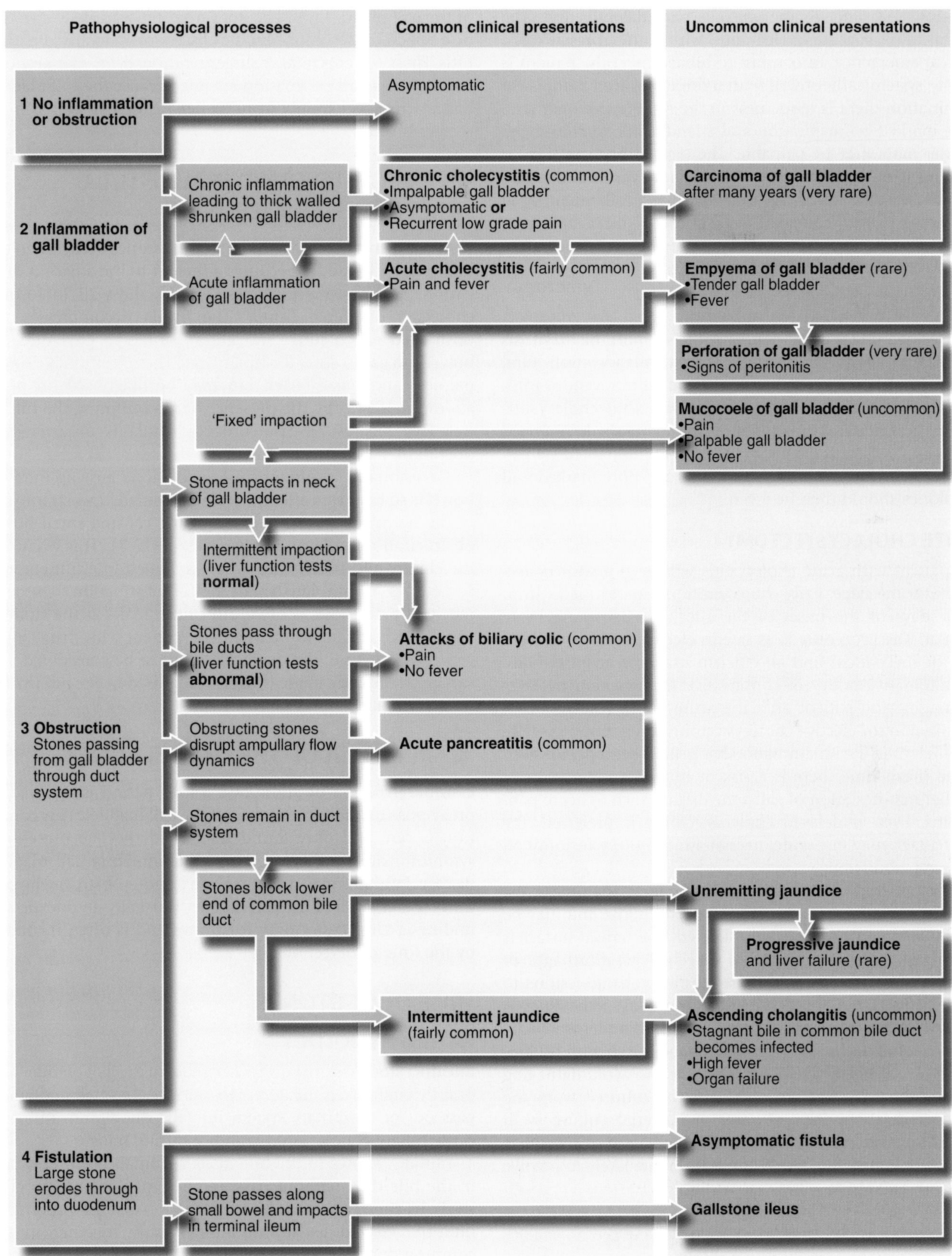

Fig. 20.6 Clinical consequences of gallstones

irritation and, later in the episode, bacterial infection. The clinical result is acute cholecystitis, which often presents as a surgical emergency. In contrast to biliary colic, the patient is usually systemically unwell with a fever and tachycardia. On examination there is tenderness in the right upper quadrant, more marked on inspiration and a tender inflammatory gall bladder mass may be palpable. The term '**Murphy's sign**' is often misused in this context; it was originally used to describe tenderness at the tip of the ninth rib. Being inflammatory in origin, the clinical course of acute cholecystitis is more prolonged than biliary colic, usually lasting several days before settling or else precipitating urgent surgery.

MANAGEMENT

Ultrasonography is usually sufficient to support the diagnosis by revealing stones and a thickened gall bladder wall. Oral intake should be restricted to fluids, and an intravenous infusion set up if necessary. Most patients with acute cholecystitis have only a chemical inflammation and therefore do not need antibiotics. When acute cholecystitis is accompanied by gall bladder infection, symptoms and signs are more marked and antibiotics should then be given.

ACUTE CHOLECYSTECTOMY

The patient with acute cholecystitis will need a cholecystectomy at some stage. Early cholecystectomy, performed within a few days of the onset of the attack, is becoming more popular. The procedure is as safe as elective surgery, convenient for the patient and an efficient usage of hospital beds. The alternative policy of conservative management involves discharging the patient after the acute attack resolves, with readmission for elective cholecystectomy after about 6 weeks, by which time the inflammation has usually settled. However, in the mean time there is a risk of further acute attacks or another manifestation of gallstone disease such as acute pancreatitis. Even if delayed cholecystectomy is preferred, the acute attack may not settle, necessitating cholecystectomy on the same admission.

When operation is performed during the acute illness, the gall bladder is found to be obstructed and tense and may be grossly inflamed, thickened and scarred. The serosal surface is oedematous and inflamed with petechial haemorrhages or even purulent exudate and there are fibrinous adhesions to nearby structures. The gall bladder neck or cystic duct is blocked by an impacted stone and the gall bladder is usually found to contain further stones or sludge mixed with inflammatory exudate. Great care must be taken to avoid damaging the bile ducts. Bowel organisms can be cultured from the contents in about 70% of cases. A bacterial culture swab should be taken from within the gall bladder at operation as any postoperative infective complications are likely to involve the same organisms.

EMPYEMA OF THE GALL BLADDER

In a more extreme clinical variant, the gall bladder becomes distended with pus. The condition, known as an empyema, represents an abscess of the gall bladder. As with abscesses elsewhere, a swinging pyrexia is often found. Sometimes part of the gall bladder wall becomes necrotic, leading to perforation which causes a subphrenic abscess or generalised peritonitis. These patients require surgery without delay. **Gangrenous cholecystitis** and perforation are rare because the gall bladder has a rich blood supply from its hepatic bed as well as from the cystic artery.

CHOLECYSTO-DUODENAL FISTULA AND GALLSTONE ILEUS

These uncommon complications of gallstones occur when the inflamed gall bladder becomes adherent to the adjacent duodenum and a stone ulcerates through the wall to form a cholecysto-duodenal fistula. The fistula decompresses the obstructed gall bladder and allows stones to pass into the bowel and gas to enter the biliary tree. The condition is usually painless and unsuspected but may be diagnosed on plain abdominal X-ray by the presence of gas outlining the biliary tree (see Fig. 20.7). Sometimes a fistula is discovered at operation.

Occasionally, a solitary cholesterol stone passing into the bowel is so large that after traversing the small bowel it impacts in the narrowest part, the distal ileum, causing small bowel obstruction or **gallstone ileus** (see Fig. 20.7). This occurs in the elderly and presents as an unexplained intermittent and sometimes incomplete small bowel obstruction. Unfortunately, the diagnosis is often difficult to make as the stone is usually radiolucent so in an elderly patient with distal small bowel obstruction, the diagnosis needs to be considered and can be confidently made if gas is recognised in the biliary tree on a plain abdominal X-ray.

CARCINOMA OF THE GALL BLADDER

Chronic irritation by stone over a long period is believed to predispose to adenocarcinoma of the gall bladder. This condition is rare and only found in the elderly. The presenting symptoms are similar to chronic inflammatory gall bladder disease. Jaundice may develop if the tumour obstructs the bile ducts. Carcinoma of the gall bladder is usually an unexpected finding at cholecystectomy for stones and is often incurable by the time of detection.

BILE DUCT STONES

PATHOPHYSIOLOGY

Bile duct stones nearly always originate in the gall bladder and pass through the cystic duct. Most stones are small enough to pass out of the biliary system into the duodenum but may cause biliary colic or mild jaundice during transit.

Initially, stones in the bile ducts are small but if they stay in the bile duct without passing, they may enlarge progressively in situ. This is evident from the occasional finding of multiple faceted gallstones fitting neatly together in the common duct and which could only have formed within the duct. The common bile duct is narrowest at its lower end and stones too large to pass out tend to lodge there. Such a stone becomes impacted, causing **progressive jaundice**, or acts as a ball-valve, causing **intermittent jaundice**. Obstruction results

CASE HISTORY

Fig. 20.7 Gallstone ileus

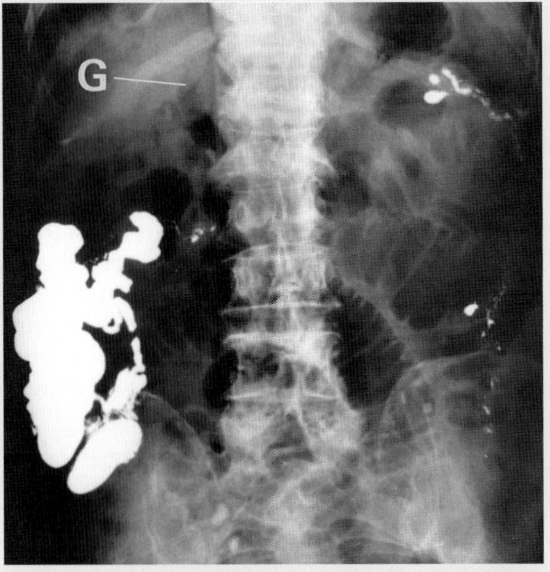

(a)

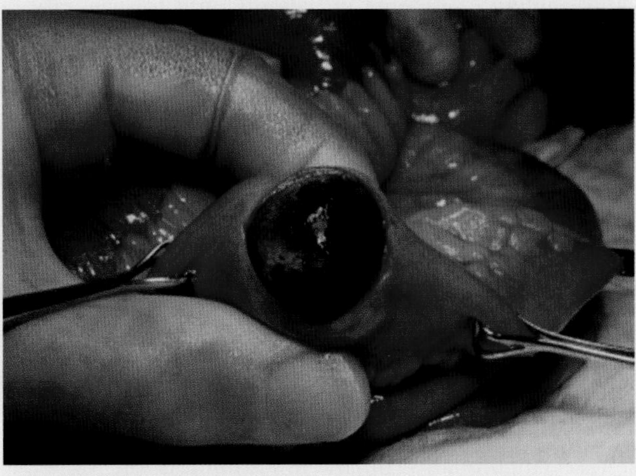

(b)

This 78-year-old woman presented with a gradual onset of small bowel obstruction. A large cholesterol solitaire stone had ulcerated from the gall bladder into the duodenum travelled down the small bowel and finally impacted in the distal ileum causing complete obstruction. **(a)** This plain supine abdominal X-ray shows widespread small bowel dilatation. The diagnostic feature is the presence of gas **G** in the biliary tree (in this case, the common bile duct and cystic duct). **(b)** Photograph showing 'cholesterol solitaire' stone being removed from the distal ileum at operation. This had caused gallstone ileus by obstructing the terminal ileum. The gall bladder and fistula did not require surgery

in gradual dilatation of the biliary tree; longstanding dilatation does not regress even after the obstruction is removed and may lead to stagnation of bile and further stone formation. Note that the gall bladder rarely distends in this condition even when the common bile duct is completely obstructed, because of the inflammatory fibrosis or mural hypertrophy caused by gallstones (Courvoisier's law—see Ch. 18, p. 259).

CLINICAL PRESENTATIONS OF STONES IN THE BILIARY TRACT

Obstructive jaundice

Stones in the common bile duct, as stated earlier, are a common cause of obstructive jaundice and must be considered in the differential diagnosis; details are given in Chapter 18.

Asymptomatic duct stones

Any patient with gallstones may have duct stones although asymptomatic duct stones are rare. Standard practice used to be to perform operative cholangiography at every operation. However, most surgeons now perform selective cholangiography in patients with signs, symptoms or investigations suggesting passage of stones.

Acute pancreatitis

Stones passing through or lying near the ampulla of Vater may interfere with drainage of pancreatic enzymes into the duodenum. Bile reflux into the main pancreatic duct may then cause acute pancreatitis (see Ch. 25).

Ascending cholangitis

Bile stasis in the common duct occurs with chronic obstruction and dilatation and predisposes to bacterial infection. The condition is known as ascending cholangitis and is a potent cause of systemic sepsis. It is characterised by intermittent attacks of pain, swinging pyrexia and jaundice. This triad is referred to as **Charcot's intermittent hepatic fever** and is often accompanied by marked weight loss. Ascending cholangitis is a serious condition and may culminate in life-threatening **acute suppurative cholangitis**. The bile duct must be drained urgently, either by surgical operation or preferably by endoscopic sphincterotomy.

MANAGEMENT OF GALLSTONE DISEASE

NON-SURGICAL TREATMENT OF GALLSTONES

Whatever the clinical manifestation of gallstone-related disease, most cases are treated surgically. A small proportion of patients is not fit for surgery and can be considered for oral drug therapy. **Chenodeoxycholic acid** (a bile acid) and related drugs increase the bile salt pool and inhibit hepatic cholesterol secretion. When administered over a long period, these drugs cause slow dissolution of cholesterol stones. Unfortunately, the drugs have several disadvantages:

- Very slow action
- Only small—less than 1 cm—cholesterol-predominant stones can be dissolved

- High rate of stone recurrence after successful treatment—up to 50% after 2 years
- Frequent drug-related side-effects, e.g. severe diarrhoea and hepatic damage

For these reasons, drug therapy has largely gone out of favour and should only be considered in patients unfit for general anaesthesia with small radiolucent stones in a gall bladder which concentrates contrast and contracts in response to a fatty meal.

SURGICAL MANAGEMENT OF GALLSTONES

INDICATIONS FOR SURGERY AND PREPARATION OF THE PATIENT

There are two main indications for cholecystectomy:

- Symptomatic gallstone disease
- Asymptomatic gallstones when there is a reasonable likelihood of future symptoms or complications

In most cases high-quality biliary ultrasound is the only imaging study required. This demonstrates gall bladder disease and gallstones and the diameter of the intrahepatic and extrahepatic bile ducts. Information from ultrasound about gall bladder wall thickness or the number and size of stones has not proved useful in predicting the feasibility of laparoscopic surgery. If there are stones in the duct system, common duct exploration is added to cholecystectomy or else stones are extracted at ERCP.

Any jaundiced patient is at particular risk during surgery because of infection, hepatic impairment, defective clotting, acute renal failure and venous thrombosis (see Table 18.2, p. 262). It is often preferable to relieve obstructive jaundice before surgery by endoscopic sphincterotomy and stone extraction or bile duct stenting to minimise some of these complications. In patients presenting with jaundice caused by operable carcinoma of the pancreas, however, the obstruction is often intentionally not relieved preoperatively because duct dilatation simplifies its anastomosis to bowel. It also minimises the risk of introducing infection into a stagnant biliary tree.

CHOLECYSTECTOMY—OPEN VERSUS LAPAROSCOPIC SURGERY

Laparoscopic cholecystectomy is now the gold standard treatment for gallstones. All surgeons performing this operation **must** also be able to competently perform the laparoscopic operation but also a potentially difficult open operation to cope with the occasional conversion to open operation brought about by unexpected difficulties or complications arising during a laparoscopic operation.

Laparoscopic management of gall bladder disease

Absolute contraindications to laparoscopic cholecystectomy include the late stages of pregnancy and uncorrected major bleeding disorders. Relative contraindications for less experienced surgical teams include morbid obesity, acute cholecystitis, untreated bile duct stones including obstructive jaundice, previous abdominal surgery (adhesions) and intra-abdominal malignancy.

In most centres, 1–5% of elective patients require conversion, so patients undergoing laparoscopic surgery should be prepared for and have consented to open surgery in case conversion proves necessary. If bile duct stones are suspected, preoperative ERCP (or equivalent magnetic resonance investigation) is advisable and stone extraction may be carried out. With experience, 95%+ of stones can be successfully extracted by endotherapy. Some surgeons favour operative cholangiography in every case to give a 'road map' of the duct anatomy, to exclude bile duct stones and to provide experience for when cholangiography becomes essential. However, other surgeons practice 'selective' cholangiography in only those patients who have had abnormal liver function tests at any time, have a dilated duct on ultrasound scanning, or with clinical evidence of earlier passage of stone (e.g. previous acute pancreatitis or jaundice).

Operative technique

The main steps in cholecystectomy are shown in Figure 20.8 and a common operating theatre set-up for laparoscopic cholecystectomy is shown in Figure 20.9. The patient is anaesthetised and a pneumoperitoneum established via an open Hassan procedure using an automatic gas insufflator. The open method is very safe and has largely superseded the blind Veress needle technique. A 10 mm cannula is then placed into the abdomen to accommodate a video laparoscope and the abdominal cavity inspected for other pathology. Three additional abdominal punctures are usually made to introduce operating instruments. The cystic duct and artery are identified and an operative cholangiogram performed (if desired) percutaneously across the abdominal wall. It is extremely important to be certain of the ductal anatomy before cutting anything because of the distortion introduced by retraction of the gall bladder and the limitations of two-dimensional imaging systems. If in doubt, perform a cholangiogram.

The cystic duct is doubly secured with metal or plastic clips, the gall bladder is dissected from the liver bed using diathermy or ultrasonic coagulation probes, and haemostasis is secured. The now free gall bladder is usually removed via the umbilical port. To achieve this, the laparoscope is moved to the upper midline port and forceps inserted through the umbilical cannula. The neck of the gall bladder is grasped and pulled into the cannula and the entire cannula and gall bladder neck withdrawn through the abdominal wall. If large stones prevent its passage, the incision is enlarged. The umbilical fascial defect should be sutured to prevent herniation but the upper midline puncture and the lateral punctures are usually left unsutured.

Results of laparoscopic cholecystectomy

Most patients are able to walk and tolerate food within 6 hours of operation and up to 80% can be discharged within 24 hours. The intervals before return to work and other normal activities are significantly reduced compared with open cholecystectomy.

Bile duct injuries occur in approximately 0.5% of patients. The risk of bile duct injuries is undoubtedly related to the experience of the operating team but has been reported to be twice as high in laparoscopic surgery as open surgery. The

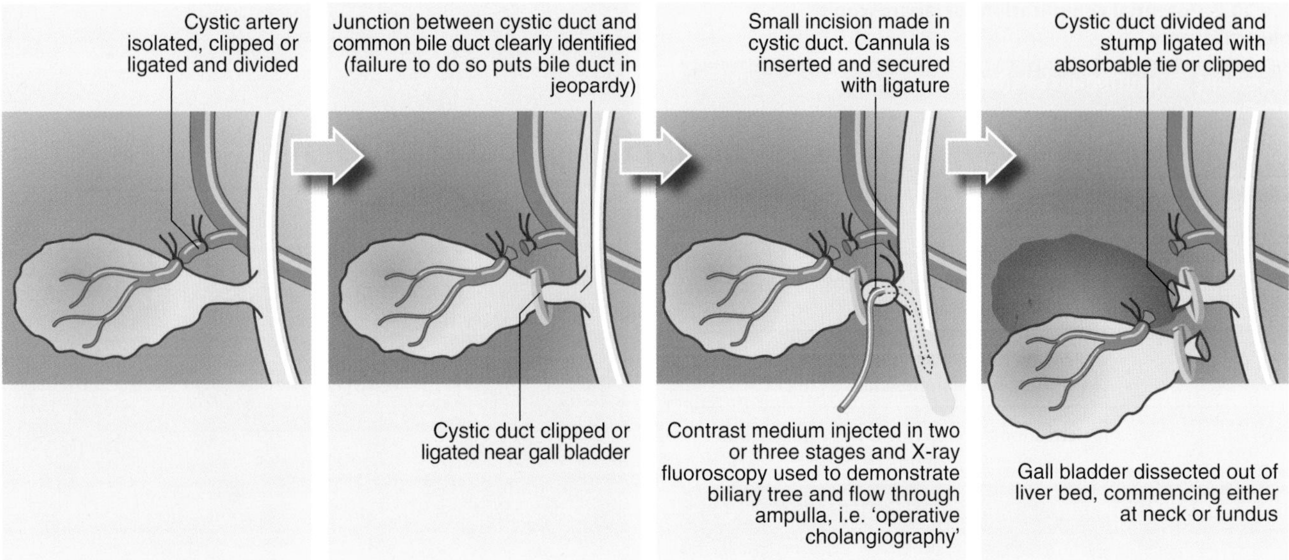

Fig. 20.8 Principal steps in cholecystectomy

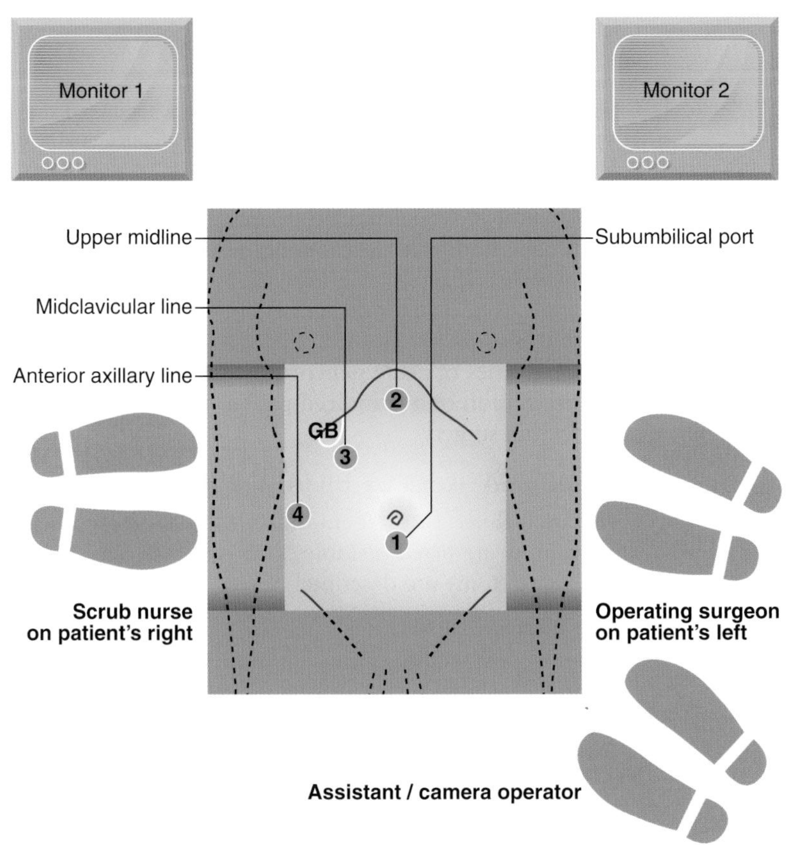

Fig. 20.9 Operating theatre arrangement for laparoscopic cholecystectomy
A common arrangement of the various operating ports (numbered **1–4**) is shown. The subumbilical port (**1**) is usually placed with the Hassan open technique to take a 10 mm video laparoscope. A Veress needle is still sometimes used for initial gas insufflation. At the upper midline port (**2**) a 10 mm trocar is placed 5 cm below the xiphoid under video vision to the right of the falciform ligament. This is used to introduce operating instrument—curved dissectors, clip applier, and suction and irrigation tubes. At the mid-clavicular (**3**) and anterior axillary (**4**) lines, 5 mm trocars give access for grasping forceps, which are used to retract the gall bladder, and liver retractors

consequences of bile duct injury can be catastrophic; patients have died with multi-organ failure resulting from unrecognised biliary peritonitis whilst others have required open operations to repair bile ducts and have risked the consequences of long-term bile duct strictures. Other potential complications are listed in Table 20.2.

OPERATIONS ON THE COMMON BILE DUCT

Exploration of the common bile duct

If stones are known to be present in the bile ducts, the common duct may be explored laparoscopically or at open surgery. The duct is opened through a longitudinal or transverse incision

Table 20.2 Potential complications of laparoscopic cholecystectomy

Stage of procedure	Complication
Placement of insufflation needle, trocar or other instruments	
During operation	Injuries to bowel Injuries to blood vessels, e.g. iliac artery Diaphragmatic injury with tension pneumothorax
Postoperative	Bleeding from trocar insertion sites Subcutaneous emphysema
Late	Herniation through trocar entry points and bowel strangulation
Trauma to biliary system	
During operation	Injuries to common bile ducts and hepatic ducts Bleeding from cystic or right hepatic artery Gall bladder perforation with spillage of bile and stones
Postoperative	Bleeding and bile leakage from liver bed Bile leakage from cystic duct remnant Retained bile duct stones
Other complications	Bowel damage by diathermy or laser

and stones retrieved by a combination of manipulation, irrigation, grasping with stone forceps or a Dormia basket or use of a balloon catheter. **Operative choledochoscopy** is often used to check for residual stones and to remove difficult stones. A flexible fibreoptic choledochoscope gives good visibility and manoeuvrability and can also be used in laparoscopic surgery. After exploration, a latex T-tube is usually inserted to drain bile to the exterior, with the transverse limb placed within the common bile duct. The main purpose of a T-tube is to provide access to the biliary tree for a further cholangiogram about 1 week after operation (**T-tube cholangiography**, see Fig. 20.10). This is to ensure that no stones remain and to allow any oedema at the ampulla to settle.

Endoscopic management of bile duct stones

With the widespread availability of ERCP and endoscopic sphincterotomy, stones in the common duct can often be retrieved without an operation. This technique represents a real advance in the management of duct stones over the earlier need for open surgery but does carry its own risks. **Endoscopic sphincterotomy** may be employed in the following circumstances:

- Urgent drainage of the bile duct in obstructive jaundice complicated by cholangitis. Definitive surgery can then be deferred until the risks of infection have been minimised

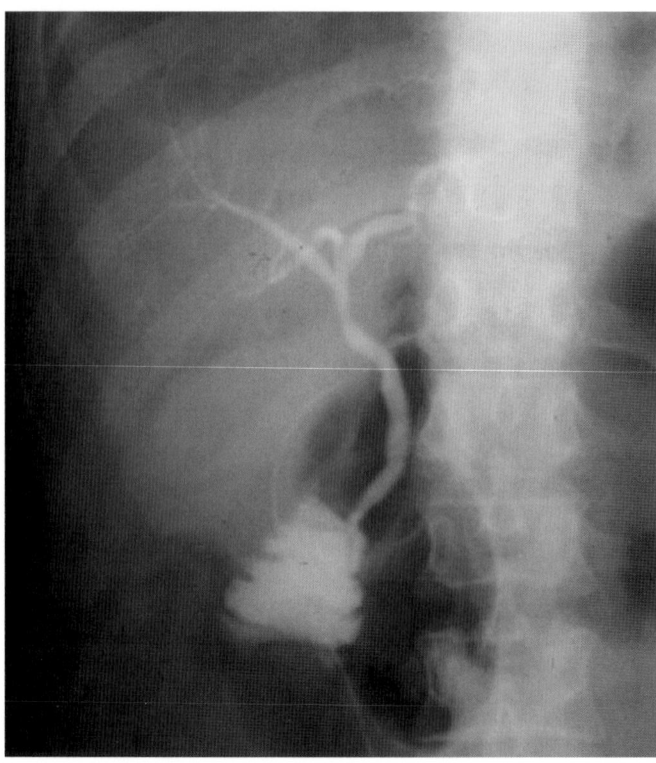

Fig. 20.10 Operative cholangiograms
Normal operative cholangiogram. The bile ducts are not dilated, the hepatic ducts fill, and contrast flows easily into the duodenum. There are no filling defects in the duct and the duct tapers normally at its lower end

- Retrieval of stones missed at operation. This avoids a difficult and hazardous operation to explore or re-explore the duct
- Removal of duct stones in patients unfit for operation (gall bladder left in situ)
- Some cases of acute pancreatitis due to gallstones
- Preparation of a jaundiced patient for elective gall bladder surgery

COMPLICATIONS OF BILIARY SURGERY

The procedure-specific complications of laparoscopic cholecystectomy are listed in Table 20.2. General complications of cholecystectomy are described below.

The retained stone

Despite considerable care at exploration of the common duct, stones occasionally remain in the duct system after operation and are revealed by postoperative T-tube cholangiography. Retained stones are usually retrieved by ERCP and sphincterotomy, although it is possible to retrieve retained stones percutaneously via a mature T-tube track using steerable grasping forceps or a Dormia basket.

Retained stones sometimes make themselves known many years later, when, having enlarged, they cause pain or obstructive jaundice. This possibility should be considered if a patient with previous biliary tract surgery develops typical pain or obstructive jaundice.

Biliary peritonitis

Bile leaking into the peritoneal cavity is an irritant and causes a chemical peritonitis. If the bile is infected, it causes generalised peritonitis and sepsis with a high risk of fatality. Bile tends to leak through suture lines because of its detergent action. Therefore, whenever the duct system has been opened, a drain should be left in the vicinity for at least 5 days. Small leaks after biliary operations usually settle spontaneously but if biliary peritonitis develops, the area must be urgently drained percutaneously or, more often, re-explored surgically and drained, with intravenous antibiotic cover.

Bile duct damage

The bile ducts can easily be damaged at cholecystectomy or common duct exploration unless their anatomy, which is commonly aberrant, is carefully displayed. The most serious error is unrecognised transection or ligation of the common duct. This presents as a major biliary leak or increasing jaundice in which case, urgent re-exploration and reconstruction is mandatory. Lesser degrees of bile duct damage from crushing, overuse of diathermy or a careless ligature will heal but eventually cause a fibrotic stricture which presents much later with obstruction. Regardless of how the bile ducts are damaged, complex reconstructive surgery is usually required, often at a tertiary referral centre, although endoscopic placement of a long-term stent allows rescue of some strictured ducts without operation. In the medium term, however, stents inevitably become blocked and have to be replaced every 3–6 months.

Haemorrhage

The cystic and hepatic arteries and the vascular liver bed are vulnerable to operative trauma and bleed profusely. Removing a grossly inflamed or fibrotic gall bladder is particularly hazardous. Manoeuvres to control haemorrhage may damage other structures, passing unnoticed at the time; this is a common cause of bile duct trauma.

Hazards of pre-existing jaundice

These are discussed under *Obstructive jaundice* in Chapter 18 (p. 262).

Ascending cholangitis and other infections

Ascending cholangitis can be a late complication of biliary surgery where an anastomosis has been formed between bile ducts and bowel. Reflux of intestinal contents and organisms takes place continually in such cases but active infection only occurs when bile stagnates in the duct system because of inadequate drainage. Usually the diameter of the anastomosis has shrunk to a point when it no longer drains adequately. Ascending cholangitis may also occur early after common duct exploration for jaundice, since bile in this situation is nearly always infected. Prophylactic antibiotics should always be used when operating on jaundiced patients with duct obstruction to minimise this complication.

An early complication of biliary surgery is a **subphrenic abscess**. This must be considered if the patient develops an unexplained swinging fever a few days after operation. Diagnosis may be elusive and is best made by ultrasound. Treatment is by percutaneous needle drainage under ultrasound guidance or occasionally by open operation.

21 Peptic ulceration and related disorders

INTRODUCTION

Peptic ulcer disease affects the oesophagus, stomach and duodenum. The conditions share the symptom of epigastric pain and the common aetiology of mucosal inflammation associated with gastric acid–pepsin secretions. The most important aetiological factor in gastric and duodenal ulcer disease is chronic mucosal infection with the bacterium *Helicobacter pylori*. Peptic disorders, together with gallstone disease, are the most common causes of organic upper abdominal pain.

With highly effective pharmacological agents to block acid secretion and more reliable diagnostic, treatment and monitoring techniques such as flexible endoscopy, surgery for peptic ulcer disease has declined by over 90% in developed countries in the last 30 years. Recent antibiotic and other treatments against *H. pylori* result in permanent cure for many peptic ulcer disorders. Most patients with suspected peptic ulcer disease are treated by family practitioners; the rest are largely managed by gastroenterologists. Only a minority present to surgeons because of failed medical treatment. Rates of emergency complications such as perforation and haemorrhage have remained relatively static but peptic pyloric stenosis has markedly declined as chronic ulceration has become less common. Nevertheless, because of the diagnostic difficulties posed by upper abdominal symptoms, surgeons still manage many patients who turn out to have peptic disorders.

PATHOPHYSIOLOGY AND EPIDEMIOLOGY OF PEPTIC DISORDERS

PATHOPHYSIOLOGY OF PEPTIC ULCERATION

Inflammation, probably initiated by *H. pylori* infection and sustained by the combined effect of gastric acid and pepsin on the mucosa, is probably the cause of all peptic disorders of the upper gastrointestinal tract other than reflux oesophagitis. *H. pylori* is a Gram-negative microaerophilic spiral bacterium which has the ability to colonise the gastric mucosa over a very long period. In many cases, infection appears to have been acquired in childhood, often with poor living conditions in early life. Normally, a dynamic balance is maintained between the inherent protective characteristics of the mucosa (the mucosal barrier) and the irritant effects of acid–pepsin secretions. The delicate balance between the two may be disrupted by diminution of mucosal resistance or excessive acid–pepsin secretion or a combination of both. The mucosal surface may become eroded by direct action of an external agent, e.g. alcohol. Whatever the aetiology, the range of pathological outcomes is similar and is summarised in Figure 21.1.

OUTCOMES OF BREACHES OF THE MUCOSAL BARRIER

When the protective mucosal barrier is breached, the delicate underlying connective tissue is exposed to acid–pepsin attack, exciting an acute inflammatory response. If the protective balance is restored at this early stage, inflammation resolves and epithelium regenerates. Little if any residual damage will result. If the healing balance is not restored, continued acid–pepsin attack on the unprotected submucosa leads to an **acute peptic ulcer**. This tends to become progressively larger and deeper.

Sometimes the ulcerative process continues virtually unchecked through the full thickness of the gut wall. The ulcer either erodes posterior tissues or perforates so that intestinal contents escape into the peritoneal cavity causing peritonitis. More often, the layer of necrotic slough and acutely inflamed underlying tissue in the ulcer base temporarily resist acid–pepsin attack. This allows granulation tissue to form which initiates the process of fibrous repair. If acid-reducing drugs are used, the ulcer may heal, leaving a small scar with normal

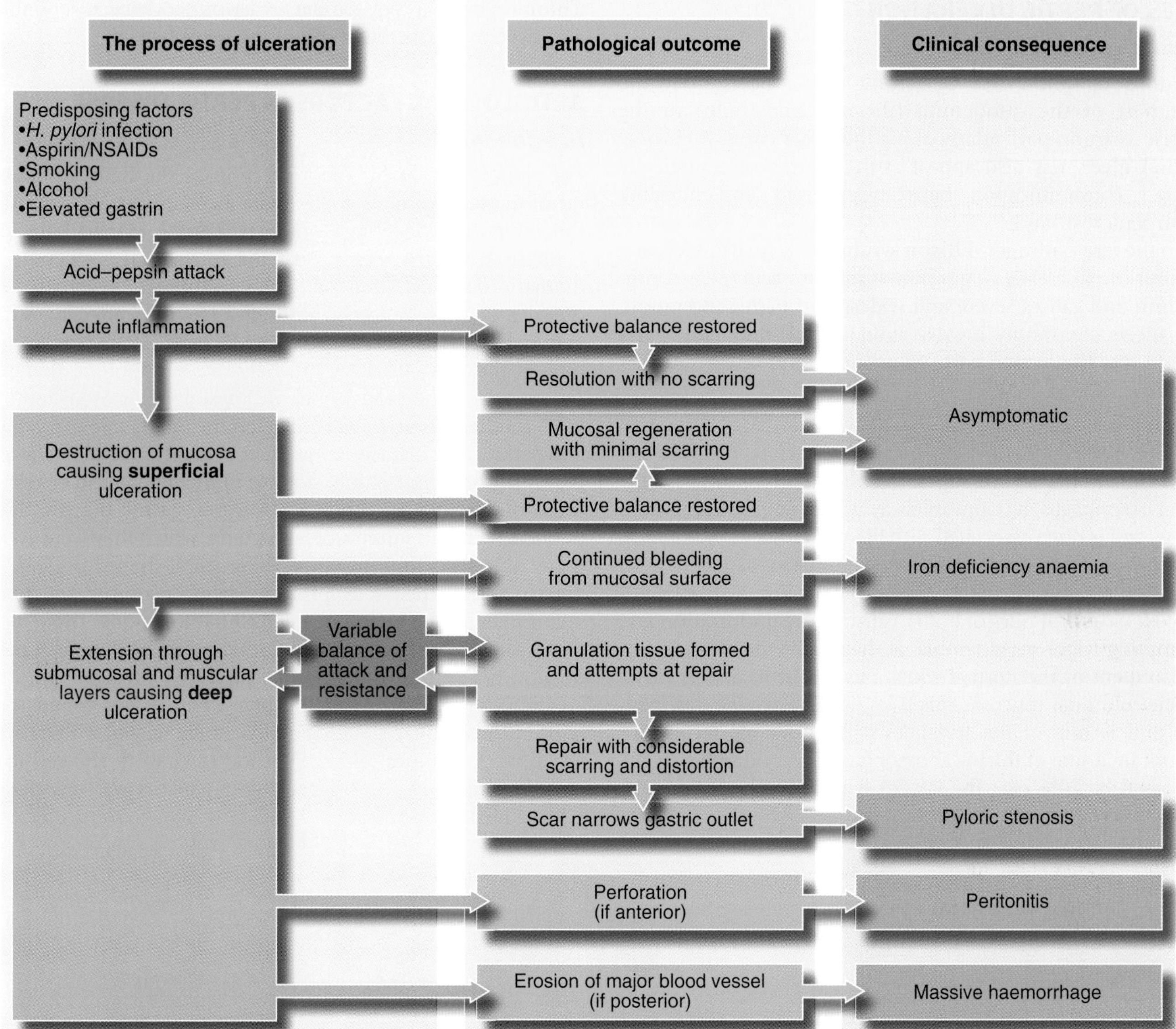

Fig. 21.1 Pathogenesis of peptic ulceration and its possible outcomes Note that pain is a common factor in any active ulceration

overlying mucosa. Usually, however, a tenuous balance is established between resistance and attack, matched by an unstable equilibrium between the rates of repair and tissue destruction. A chronic peptic ulcer then results which may persist for years, its size and symptoms varying as mucosal resistance and exacerbating factors fluctuate.

If local or systemic factors change and swing the balance in favour of repair, the lesion may heal completely. On the mucosal surface, the healed ulcer site is usually puckered by scar contraction in the muscular wall. If scarring occurs in a narrow part of the tract, e.g. the pyloric region, the lumen may stricture, and subsequent acute mucosal inflammation and swelling may precipitate **gastric outlet obstruction**. If healing does not occur, a chronic ulcer may slowly enlarge and deepen. Continual bleeding from the ulcer may cause **chronic anaemia**. Ulceration **posteriorly** may erode into the gastroduodenal artery causing acute major haemorrhage; if the ulcer lies on the anterior wall, it may perforate into the peritoneal cavity.

EPIDEMIOLOGY AND AETIOLOGY OF PEPTIC ULCER DISEASE

THE SIZE OF THE PROBLEM

Chronic peptic ulcer disease is very common in developed countries, affecting around 10% of the population at some time in their lives. The incidence of **duodenal ulcer** has been falling over the last 30 years, probably because of improved living conditions, reduced smoking and good medical therapy. The incidence of **gastric ulcer** is probably constant, although increasing numbers of cases are revealed as a result of NSAID-provoked haemorrhage.

Peptic ulceration is less common in developing rural communities, despite a high incidence of *H. pylori* gastroduodenal infection. This implies that environmental factors associated with Western life are additional aetiological factors in the disease.

SITES OF PEPTIC ULCERATION (see Fig. 21.2)

Stomach and duodenum

The most common sites for chronic peptic ulcers are in the **first part of the duodenum** (the duodenal bulb) or the **gastric antrum**, particularly along the lesser curve. A chronic **stomal ulcer** may also appear at the margin of a surgically created communication between stomach and intestine (gastroenterostomy).

In the rare **Zollinger–Ellison syndrome**, a gastrin-secreting tumour of pancreatic origin over-stimulates acid–pepsin production and causes severe and widespread peptic ulceration. The ulcers commonly involve stomach and duodenum and extend into the second part of the duodenum or even further distally.

Oesophagus

Peptic inflammation and superficial ulceration may involve the lower oesophagus. It is almost always secondary to acid–pepsin reflux, and is often associated with hiatus hernia. *H. pylori* infection (see below) is probably not an important factor here. Reflux causes intermittent destruction of the lower oesophageal mucosa by acid or bile (or both), causing **linear ulceration** and prompting vigorous attempts at healing. One outcome is replacement of the normal squamous epithelium with metaplastic columnar mucosa. This is known as **Barrett's oesophagus** and is one of the few known predisposing factors for adenocarcinoma of the lower oesophagus, a condition that has increased by 70% over the last 25 years (see Ch. 22, p. 311). Chronic peptic ulcers, similar to gastroduodenal ulcers, may also develop at the lower end of the oesophagus.

AETIOLOGICAL FACTORS IN PEPTIC DISEASE

H. pylori infection

The importance of *H. pylori* infection as the main initiating factor in peptic ulceration has finally been universally accepted following the pioneering work of Dr Barry J. Marshall and Dr J. Robin Warren in Perth, Australia in the early 1980s. In a dramatic demonstration of Koch's postulates, Marshall produced a duodenal ulcer in himself a few days after ingesting cultured *H. pylori*. The ulcer proved to be *H. pylori*-positive on biopsy and was cured by anti-*Helicobacter* antibiotic therapy. The pair won the Nobel Prize in Physiology or Medicine for 2005 for their discovery of the bacterium and its role in gastritis and peptic ulcer disease. Before their work, it had been believed that microorganisms could not live in the highly acid environment of the normal stomach. However, gastric biopsies had frequently shown intramucosal bacteria, which they were eventually able to culture in vitro. These spiral-shaped organisms appear able to penetrate protective surface mucus and then accumulate in the region of intercellular junctions. There they may excite inflammation, stimulating excess acid–pepsin production or compromising normal protective mechanisms.

The jigsaw began to fit together when it was found that peptic ulcers could regularly be successfully treated with a combination of bismuth and antibiotics. Later work showed that *H. pylori* infection in duodenal ulcer patients was associated

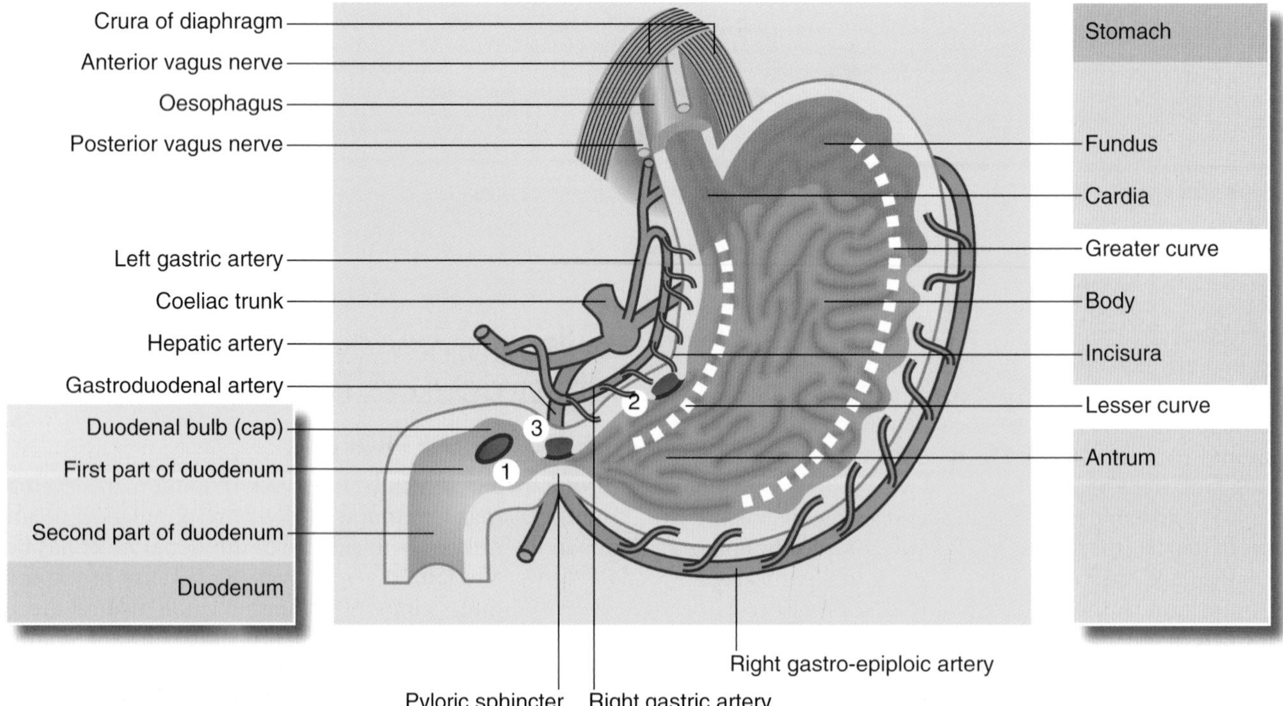

Fig. 21.2 Surgical anatomy of stomach and duodenum showing common sites of peptic ulceration
Acid secretion by the gastric mucosa is controlled by two mechanisms: **(a)** the vagus nerve stimulates acid secretion by the parietal cells (cholinergic stimulation) and **(b)** gastrin (produced by the APUD cells in the antrum) promotes secretion of acid and pepsin by the parietal and peptic cells of the fundus and body. The second is mediated via H_2-receptors. **(1)** Marks the common site for duodenal ulcers which may be anterior or posterior; **(2)** the common site of lesser curve gastric ulcers; and **(3)** the site of pyloric channel ulcers

with a six-fold increase in gastric acid production which remitted when the infection was eliminated. There is now evidence that *H. pylori* is sometimes carcinogenic, initiating certain types of gastric lymphoma and some cases of gastric cancer. The broad picture is now evident: *H. pylori* causes a chronic infection with complications that include gastric and duodenal ulcer, gastric mucosa-associated lymphoma and gastric cancer. Only a small percentage of patients with duodenal or gastric ulcers are *H. pylori* negative. Tests for *H. pylori* infection include stool antigen tests, serum anti-*H. pylori* IgG and hydrogen breath tests. However, the most reliable method of diagnosis is endoscopic biopsies with immediate testing for urease produced by the organism (see below, Fig. 21.7) and histological examination of biopsy specimens.

Further details of this fascinating story remain to be worked out; for example, why not all patients with *H. pylori* infection develop upper gastrointestinal lesions, and why not all patients with certain gastric cancers have been exposed to *H. pylori*. There is even speculation that elimination of *H. pylori* may predispose some patients to gastric cancer.

Acid–pepsin production

Parietal cells secrete acid in direct or indirect response to acetylcholine, gastrin and histamine. It is likely that the common mediator is histamine via H_2-receptors. The final common pathway for hydrogen ion secretion is via activation of a specific enzyme, H^+/K^+ ATPase, which exchanges hydrogen ions generated in the parietal cell for potassium ions in the gastric lumen using a mechanism known as the **proton pump**. In **duodenal ulceration**, the fundamental abnormality appears to be excessive production of acid–pepsin by the stomach, both basal (i.e. overnight) and stimulated. This may be a defensive response to *H. pylori* infection.

In patients with **gastric ulcers**, measured acid secretion is either normal or low, and the essential problem seems to be diminished resistance to acid–pepsin attack, probably related to the quantity or quality of mucus produced. Nevertheless, reduction of acid production by medical or surgical means is effective in healing gastric ulcers.

Mucosal resistance

There are several mechanisms which protect the upper gastrointestinal mucosa against autodigestion. Somatostatin and COX1 induced prostaglandins are inhibitors of parietal cell secretion and the latter have other cytoprotective properties. Two forms of mucus, soluble and insoluble, are secreted continuously by gastric and duodenal mucosa; they contain bicarbonate and together maintain the cell surface pH at neutrality.

Non-steroidal anti-inflammatory drugs (NSAIDs) prescribed for arthritic disorders are commonly identified as the causative factor for acute presentations of peptic ulceration. NSAIDs probably have their greatest effect systemically rather than locally, via their blocking effects on prostaglandin production. Indeed, in elderly patients presenting with upper gastrointestinal bleeding or perforation, ulceration may occur after only a few NSAID tablets have been taken or at any time during their use. This risk is not diminished by enteric-coated preparations, nor by administration by routes other than orally, e.g. as suppositories. The risk of NSAID-induced ulceration increases steeply in later life. All NSAIDs have been incriminated and their power to provoke peptic ulceration is in direct proportion to their effectiveness at relieving arthritic symptoms. A history of 'indigestion' in patients taking NSAIDs must be taken seriously.

Other mucosal irritants

Aspirin and other NSAIDs are known to induce acute mucosal inflammation directly (**acute gastritis**). In a susceptible individual, inflammation may persist, resulting in chronic ulceration. Prolonged heavy alcohol intake is also a recognised risk factor. The junction between parietal and antral cells on the lesser curvature of the stomach has been noted to be particularly vulnerable to gastric ulceration, although the reason is not understood. Cigarette smoking is twice as common in patients with chronic peptic ulcer disease as in the general population. Its pathogenic role is attributed to increased vagal activity, and its effect on producing relative gastric mucosal ischaemia. Ceasing smoking greatly assists in the healing of peptic ulcers.

INVESTIGATION AND CLINICAL FEATURES OF PEPTIC DISORDERS

INVESTIGATION OF SUSPECTED PEPTIC ULCER DISEASE

The diagnosis and management of peptic disorders relies mainly on flexible endoscopy, which revolutionised the process after its introduction in the late 1960s. Barium meal contrast radiography has largely been superseded by endoscopy.

ENDOSCOPY

Oesophago-gastro-duodenoscopy, also known as OGD or gastroscopy, involves visual examination of the mucosa using a steerable, flexible endoscope. Gastroscopy enables direct and comprehensive examination of the whole of the upper gastrointestinal tract prone to peptic ulcer disease.

In peptic ulcer disease, gastroscopy has definite advantages over contrast radiography, which by its nature can only demonstrate substantial structural abnormalities and then only as two-dimensional images. Benign gastric or oesophageal ulceration can be reliably distinguished from malignancy if endoscopic biopsies are taken from several places around the ulcer edge. In patients with peptic disorders, biopsies of distal gastric mucosa are now taken routinely to investigate *H. pylori* infection.

In acute upper gastrointestinal haemorrhage, gastroscopy is almost mandatory, as described in Chapter 19. Gastroscopy can identify the site of the bleeding and is particularly useful if gastro-oesophageal varices are suspected to be the source of bleeding but are found not to be. Gastroscopy also allows recognition of features which can help stratify patients into low or high risk of rebleeding and it provides an important means of treating bleeding sites by injection of vasoconstrictors or sclerosants.

CONTRAST RADIOLOGY

Contrast radiography of the upper gastrointestinal tract is used largely to determine swallowing function, to define anatomy, particularly with large hiatus hernias, and to give an idea of the effectiveness of gastric emptying. It involves the patient swallowing barium suspension (**barium meal**). During the investigation, the patient is tilted and rolled in various directions to demonstrate the whole region of interest. Effervescent tablets are given to produce gaseous distension of the stomach and duodenum and spread the contrast in a thin, even layer over the mucosal surface. This standard **double contrast technique** improves the imaging of mucosal detail.

PRESENTING FEATURES OF PEPTIC ULCER DISEASE

The various ways in which peptic inflammation affects the oesophagus, stomach and duodenum are summarised in Table 21.1.

Epigastric pain (usually described as 'boring', 'gnawing' or 'burning') is the principal presenting symptom and is common to peptic disorders whatever the site. Pain is often accompanied by other forms of discomfort, often described by the patient as 'indigestion' or 'dyspepsia'. A more specific description may suggest particular diagnostic entities. Retrosternal pain ('heartburn') and bitter regurgitation ('waterbrash') suggests reflux oesophagitis. Nausea or vomiting, anorexia (loss of appetite) and abdominal fullness or bloating are common in gastric ulcer and pyloric stenosis, but may also occur in a variety of other upper gastrointestinal disorders, e.g. gallstone disease and irritable bowel syndrome.

The relationship of symptoms to food intake may help to distinguish gastric from duodenal ulceration; gastric ulcer pain is typically exacerbated by food and duodenal ulcer pain relieved by it.

Peptic ulcers may be virtually asymptomatic, particularly those caused by NSAIDs. Diagnosis may then only occur on acute presentation with bleeding or perforation or on investigation of iron deficiency anaemia.

NON-ACUTE PRESENTATIONS OF PEPTIC ULCER DISEASE

PEPTIC DISORDERS OF THE OESOPHAGUS

All peptic disorders of the oesophagus are associated with reflux of gastric contents. These disorders range from mild reversible inflammation, through moderate acute inflammation with superficial ulceration (**reflux oesophagitis**), to severe persistent inflammation which may lead to **fibrotic scarring and stenosis** (see Fig. 21.3) and sometimes **chronic peptic ulceration**. In many patients, reflux is associated with hiatus hernia (see Ch. 22).

On gastroscopy, reflux oesophagitis is characterised by mucosal reddening and, in more severe cases, by typical linear superficial ulceration (see Fig. 21.4). Peptic strictures occur in the distal oesophagus and are usually located just above the oesophago-gastric junction, which itself often lies above the diaphragm because of inflammatory shortening of the oesophagus. The normal oesophago-gastric junction is about 40 cm from the incisor teeth when seen on endoscopy. Specialised intestinal metaplasia, dysplasia and carcinoma must be excluded by biopsies because the visual appearances may not be characteristic. Occasionally, a deep chronic ulcer occurs in the lower oesophagus; this looks and behaves like an often linear gastric or duodenal ulcer. When squamous oesophageal epithelium is repeatedly damaged by reflux, it may be replaced by metaplastic columnar epithelium. This is known as **Barrett's oesophagus** and there is strong evidence that it predisposes to malignant change. If found, it should be biopsied to exclude dysplasia. When dysplasia is severe, there is about a 1% annual risk of malignant change and endoscopic resection or surgery is necessary. Standard protocols are usually employed for surveillance of Barrett's oesophagus with repeated endoscopy every 2–3 years.

PEPTIC DISORDERS OF THE STOMACH

Peptic disorders of the stomach range from mild inflammation (**gastritis**) to **chronic gastric ulcers** and most often occur in the antral region and along the lesser curve beyond the incisura.

Chronic gastric ulcers must be distinguished from malignant ulcers. The site may aid recognition of a benign ulcer, but carcinoma may occur in any part of the stomach, with the region of the gastro-oesophageal junction now the most common. Malignancy can only be excluded by histological examination of multiple representative biopsies taken from around the ulcer circumference (not the base). In most cases, carcinoma probably arises de novo but occasionally a benign ulcer may undergo malignant transformation.

Gastritis

Gastritis appears as widespread reddening of the mucosa. If biliary reflux from the duodenum into the stomach is evident, the condition is sometimes referred to as '**biliary gastritis**' on the assumption that it is caused by the irritant effect of biliary and pancreatic secretions. Acute gastritis, often caused by alcohol (chronic alcoholism or single alcoholic binges) or aspirin/NSAID ingestion, can cause symptoms of sufficient severity to warrant gastroscopy. The mucosa often exhibits patchy shallow ulceration (**erosive gastritis**) and is friable and easily traumatised, causing bleeding.

Stress ulcers

Acute 'stress' ulcers are single or multiple small discrete superficial lesions that may develop rapidly in seriously ill patients, often in intensive care units. The condition may be a complication of extensive burns, systemic sepsis (possibly via visceral hypoperfusion), multiple trauma, major head injuries, uraemia or terminal illness. Stress ulcers typically present with haemorrhage (**haemorrhagic gastritis**), which is sometimes catastrophic, and occasionally with perforation. There is minimal mucosal inflammation around the ulcers and the

Table 21.1 Clinical consequences of peptic ulcer disease in different anatomical sites

Pathological process	Clinical lesion	Symptoms
Oesophagus		
Transient acid–pepsin reflux	Mild reversible acute inflammation, i.e. transient oesophagitis	Burning retrosternal pain (i.e. 'heartburn')
Recurrent acid–pepsin reflux or failure of oesophagus to expel acid by peristalsis (often found in hiatus hernia)	Episodes of acute inflammation, i.e. reflux oesophagitis—probably reversible with no scarring	Recurrent epigastric and retrosternal pain. Chronic iron deficiency anaemia may occur
Persistent severe reflux	Chronic low-grade blood loss Continuous severe inflammation with superficial ulceration. May lead to chronic ulceration and/or stricture	Severe retrosternal pain, dysphagia and sometimes recurrent small haematemeses
Stomach		
Acute gastric irritation, e.g. by NSAIDs or alcohol	Acute (reversible) mucosal inflammation, i.e. acute gastritis or erosive/ haemorrhagic gastritis	Epigastric pain, vomiting, acute upper gastrointestinal bleeding
Acute reduction in mucosal resistance provoked by visceral ischaemia or the systemic inflammatory response syndrome (usually in intensive therapy unit patients or after burns)	Widespread superficial gastric ulceration (gastric erosions)	May bleed uncontrollably or perforate
Chronic *H. pylori* infection, probably with longstanding diminished resistance to acid–pepsin attack, with or without extrinsic irritation	Chronic or recurrent gastric ulceration	Epigastric pain—characteristically exacerbated by food (especially if acid or spicy), anorexia and weight loss Symptoms of chronic anaemia
Duodenum		
Episodic acid–pepsin attack	Acute (reversible) mucosal inflammation, i.e. duodenitis	Episodic epigastric pain
Chronic *H. pylori* infection, probably with persistent acid–pepsin attack	Duodenal ulceration (may involve pyloric canal)	Epigastric pain—typically relieved by food and occurring several hours after food, especially at night
Pre-existing duodenal scarring causing pyloric stenosis with superadded acute inflammation and mucosal swelling	Complete pyloric obstruction	Symptoms of chronic anaemia Severe vomiting, dehydration, shock, gross electrolyte disturbance (hypochloraemic alkalosis)
Both stomach and duodenum		
Periodic loss of protective equilibrium	Recurrent ulceration	Intermittent symptomatic episodes
Erosion of a major vessel in ulcer floor	Severe haemorrhage	Massive haematemesis or melaena
Unchecked ulceration	Perforation and peritonitis	Acute severe abdominal pain and shock

aetiology may be primarily mucosal ischaemia rather than peptic. The risk of this life-threatening complication can be minimised in vulnerable patients by prophylactic treatment with proton pump inhibitors.

Chronic gastric ulceration

Chronic gastric ulcers vary greatly in size but the majority are small (less than 2 cm in diameter). **Giant ulcers** (up to 10 cm) are occasionally seen in the elderly; if posteriorly situated, they may erode through the stomach wall, obliterating the lesser sac and adhering to the surface of the pancreas. In these cases, the ulcer base or floor is composed of pancreatic tissue and erosion may cause catastrophic haemorrhage.

Benign gastric ulcers are typically regular in outline with a base consisting of white fibrinous slough. The ulcer gives the impression of having been punched out of the gastric wall, and there is no heaping-up of the mucosal margin as seen in malignant ulcers. The surrounding mucosa is surprisingly normal, although there may be radiating folds resulting

Fig. 21.3 Peptic stricture of the oesophagus

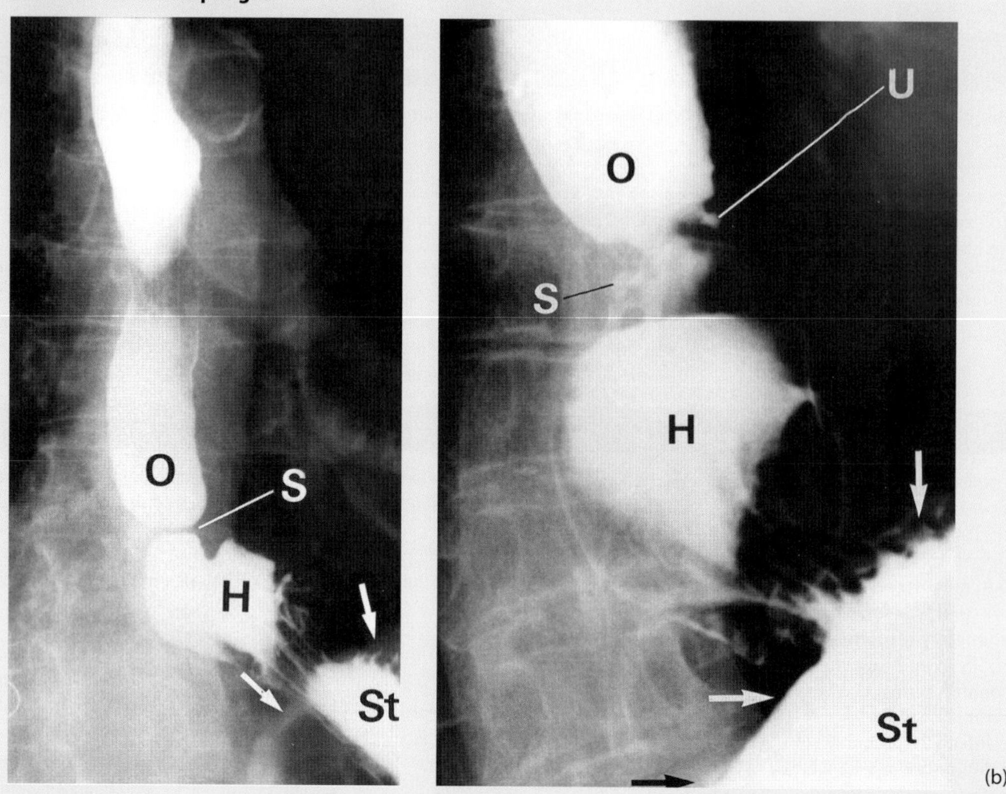

(a) A barium swallow in a 60-year-old woman who complained of burning retrosternal pain when lying flat (present for several years) and the recent onset of pain and difficulty when swallowing solid foods. The X-rays show the lower end of the oesophagus **O** and stomach **St**, part of which lies above the level of the diaphragm (position arrowed), forming a sliding hiatus hernia **H**. There is a tight stenosis in the last 2 cm of the oesophagus due to a peptic stricture **S**. **(b)** At greater magnification, barium can be seen filling the crater of a chronic peptic ulcer **U** immediately above the stricture

from chronic fibrotic contractures. The typical endoscopic appearance of a gastric ulcer is shown in Figure 21.5a.

Peptic disorders of the stomach typically cause severe, often disabling, epigastric pain which tends to be exacerbated by food, especially if acidic or spicy. The pain may be so severe that patients lose weight and develop a fear of food. Symptoms tend to persist for weeks or months, fluctuating in intensity and then disappearing completely, only to recur weeks or months later. Symptoms are a poor guide to disease activity or response to treatment. Indeed, major ulcers may be silent. Both can be monitored only by repeated gastroscopy until healing. A rare complication of peptic disease is perforation of a gastric ulcer into the transverse colon. The resulting gastro-colic fistula causes true faecal vomiting.

PEPTIC DISORDERS OF THE DUODENUM

Duodenitis

Duodenitis, a non-ulcerative form of duodenal inflammation, has a similar endoscopic appearance to gastritis. It is commonly discovered in patients suspected of having duodenal ulceration, and probably represents a mild form of peptic disease.

Fig. 21.4 Reflux oesophagitis

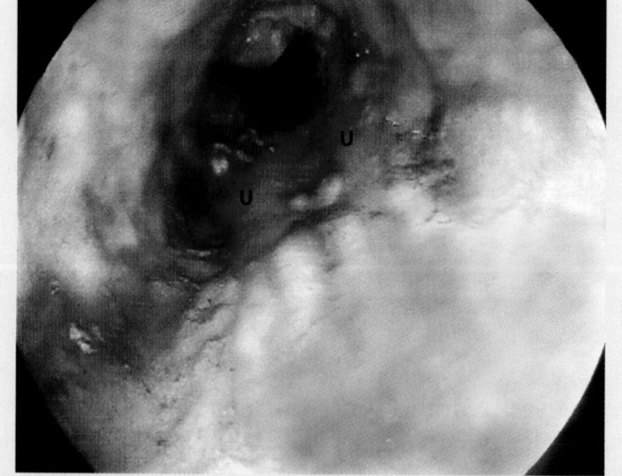

Gastroscopic view of the lower end of the oesophagus in a woman of 62 with a long history of reflux. Note the patchy ulceration **U** and the irregular fibrotic cardia caused by recurrent ulceration and attempts at healing. Further scarring may cause stricture formation

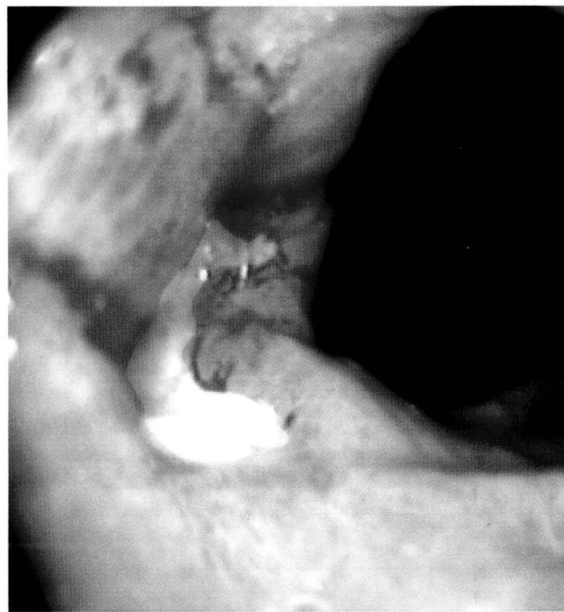

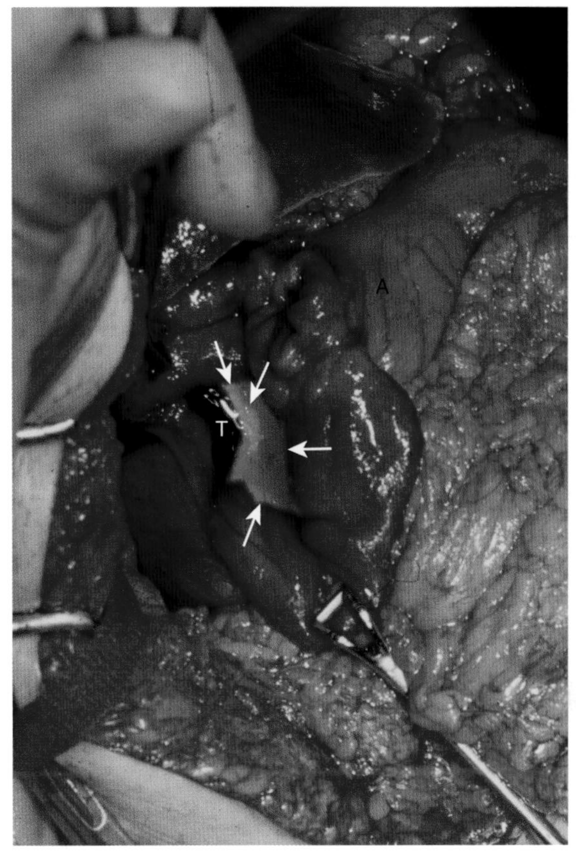

(a) (b)

Fig. 21.5 Peptic ulcers
(a) Lesser curve benign gastric ulcer as seen through a gastroscope. At the original examination, the ulcer could be viewed from several directions and biopsies taken of the edge to exclude malignancy. **(b)** Photograph taken at emergency laparotomy for bleeding duodenal ulcer. The pylorus has been opened longitudinally and a deep chronic posterior ulcer crater is identified (arrowed). Thrombus **T** overlying an eroded artery is visible. A bleeding artery in the ulcer crater was under-run with sutures to arrest the haemorrhage

Chronic duodenal ulceration

Chronic duodenal ulcers almost exclusively occur in the pyloric channel and the first part of the duodenum. The latter area is known endoscopically as the 'duodenal bulb' and radiologically as the 'duodenal cap'. On endoscopy, duodenal ulcers have a range of appearances similar to chronic gastric ulcers. There is usually a single ulcer but two or more ulcers at one time are common ('kissing ulcers' occur on opposing walls of the duodenum). Malignancy is very rare in the duodenal bulb, so biopsy of the ulcer for this purpose is seldom necessary; biopsy of the gastric antrum for confirmation of *H. pylori* infections is, however, indicated. The endoscopic characteristics of a duodenal ulcer are shown in Figure 21.6.

Duodenal ulcer symptoms follow the same general pattern as gastric ulcer but with important exceptions. The pain tends to appear several hours after a meal ('hunger pain') and is relieved by eating. A typical history includes episodic early morning waking (often around 2 a.m.) with epigastric pain; this pain is relieved by drinking milk and eating bland foods. Consequently, undiagnosed patients tend to gain weight from the increased intake of food and milk. This is in contrast to the weight loss often associated with gastric ulcer. Symptoms in duodenal ulcer are more useful as a guide to disease activity and response to treatment than in gastric ulcer.

MANAGEMENT OF CHRONIC PEPTIC ULCER DISEASE

Both the nature and the management of peptic ulcer disease have undergone extraordinary changes over the past four decades. Back then, medical management was relatively ineffective and was largely confined to simple antacid drugs, bland diets and bed rest. The only definitive treatment was major surgery and it was widely employed, often after a long period of chronic symptoms. Surgery was deferred as long as possible in the hope of spontaneous remission, and patients often had to 'earn' their operations by years of suffering! Partial gastrectomy offered the best cure rate and was thus the most common operation despite its mortality of 2–10% and its serious long-term complication rate. Later, various versions of surgical vagotomy were shown to be almost equally effective, but with fewer complications.

The principles of modern management of peptic disorders are summarised in Box 21.1.

Control of predisposing or aggravating causes

The patient's history may reveal adverse factors which can be easily eliminated. These are summarised at the start of Box 21.1. Radical dietary modification is unnecessary; patients should merely be advised to avoid food which they find

Fig. 21.6 Duodenal ulceration

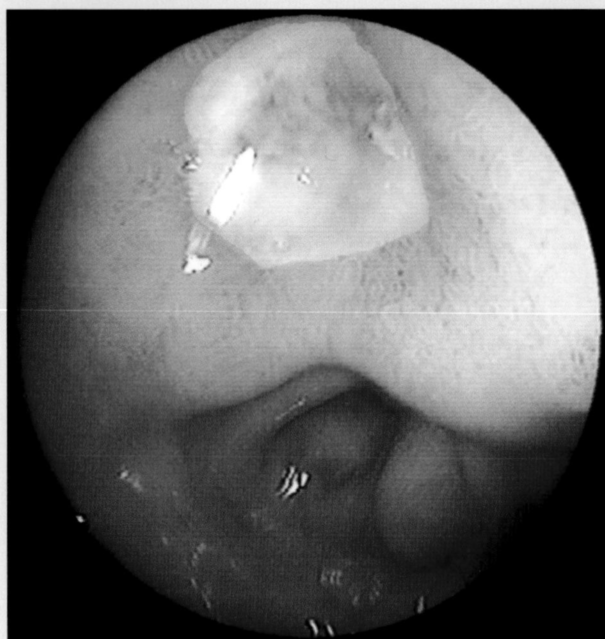

Endoscopic view of lesser curve gastric ulcer. This ulcer has probably only been present for about 4 months. It does not show surrounding scarring and distortion of the gastric wall that would be characteristic of longstanding ulcers

Box 21.1 Principles of management of peptic disorders

Control of predisposing or aggravating causes

- Modify diet, reduce alcohol intake, cease smoking, avoid irritant and ulcer-provoking drugs (aspirin and other NSAIDs), avoid stress, reduce oesophageal reflux by losing weight and attention to posture

Elimination of proven *H. pylori* infection

- Combined therapy with anti-acid and antibiotic combinations

Diminishing of irritant effects of acid–pepsin

- Simple antacid drugs, alginate preparations, liquorice derivatives, bismuth preparations

Administration of mucosal protective agents

- Sucralfate

Reduction of acid secretion

- H_2-receptor-blocking drugs (cimetidine, ranitidine), proton pump inhibitors (PPIs, e.g. omeprazole), surgical vagotomy (rarely employed nowadays)

Surgical removal of intractable ulcers and gastrin-secreting tissue

- Partial gastrectomy

Correction of secondary anatomical problems

- Dilatation of oesophageal strictures, operations for pyloric stenosis and hiatus hernia

aggravates the symptoms. Spicy or acidic foods are often blamed.

Aspirin and other NSAIDs should be avoided, although this is often difficult in patients with arthritic disorders. The ulcerogenic effect of these drugs is directly proportional to their effectiveness and relates largely to their systemic anti-cyclooxygenase (COX1) activity, an agent protective of gastroduodenal mucosa. There is therefore little to be gained from changing drugs within the group or by using them in enteric-coated or suppository form. If NSAIDs cannot be avoided in patients with a predisposition to peptic ulceration, concurrent use of cytoprotective drugs may be indicated.

Patients with oesophageal reflux, especially if associated with hiatus hernia, can minimise the damage by simple mechanical measures such as losing weight, elevating the head end of the bed and being aware of posture in daily activities.

Elimination of proven *H. pylori* infection

Once *H. pylori* has been confirmed, treatment involves a course of acid inhibition combined with antibiotic treatment. Eradication usually produces long-term ulcer remission, and *H. pylori* reinfection is rare. A triple regimen including a proton pump inhibitor (e.g. omeprazole) and two antibiotics (clarithromycin plus either amoxicillin or metronidazole) given for 1 week eliminates *Helicobacter* in over 90% of cases, although increasingly strains of *H. pylori* are demonstrating antibiotic resistance and local antibiotic protocols should be followed. Longer courses give potentially higher elimination rates but produce more side-effects and lower compliance. Confirmation of eradication can be achieved by re-endoscopy and rapid urease testing (Fig. 21.7), or by breath testing.

Diminishing of irritant effects of acid–pepsin

An array of proprietary antacid preparations is available over the counter and on prescription. When used assiduously, they promote ulcer healing almost as effectively as any other drug, although more slowly. They all utilise a few main active ingredients. **Sodium bicarbonate** offers rapid but temporary relief of symptoms, while **magnesium trisilicate** or **aluminium hydroxide** promotes ulcer healing. Some of these agents, however, interfere with proton pump inhibitors. **Colloidal bismuth compounds** have been in use for many years. They have an antacid action and have been found to be active against *H. pylori*.

Alginate preparations form a foamy layer on the surface of gastric contents, coating the upper stomach and lower oesophagus and protecting it from oesophageal reflux.

Administration of mucosal protective agents

Sucralfate is a complex of aluminium hydroxide and sulphated sucrose that is minimally absorbed from the gastrointestinal tract. It is believed to act by binding to denuded areas of mucosa and protecting them from acid–pepsin attack. It has been shown to be as effective as H_2-blockers in providing symptom relief and healing when given in the dose of 2 g twice daily. It does not interfere with other drugs and is safe in pregnancy. It is also effective for preventing stress ulcers in seriously ill patients.

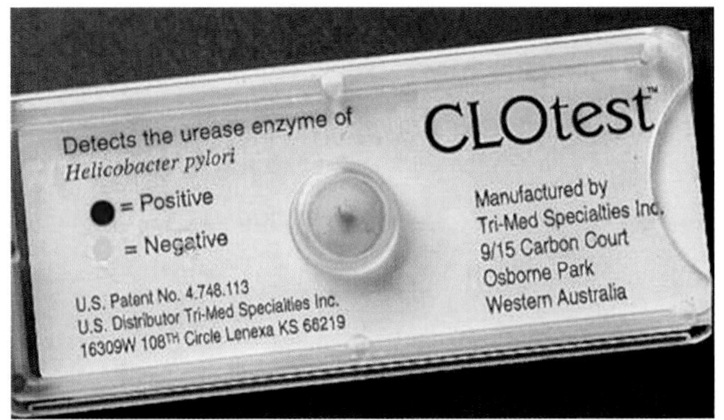

(a)

(b)

Fig. 21.7 Proprietary urease testing kit for *H. pylori*
Biopsies of gastric or duodenal mucosa are placed in the well and the result read after a set period. A positive result is indicated by the colour change seen here in **(b)**

Reduction of acid secretion

Acid secretion by the gastric mucosa is normally controlled by two mechanisms:

- Direct cholinergic stimulation of parietal cells mediated via the **vagus nerve**. This is under reflex control originating in the cerebral cortex triggered by the sight and taste of food
- Gastrin is secreted by APUD cells in the gastric antrum and promotes acid secretion via histamine released from mast cells in the vicinity of the parietal cells. The histamine receptors on the parietal cells are distinct from those elsewhere in the body and are designated as **type 2 (H_2) receptors**; these receptors are not blocked by standard 'antihistamine' drugs such as chlorphenamine. Gastrin secretion is partly controlled by the vagus and partly by local (vagally independent) reflexes initiated by gastric distension and the presence of food or alcohol in the stomach

From this, two practical methods have been found to reduce acid secretion: drugs which selectively block H_2-receptors or the proton pump mechanism (described earlier), and surgical division of the vagus nerve.

H_2-receptor blockade and proton pump antagonists

H_2-receptor blocking drugs were developed in the 1970s and were the first 'medical' revolution in the management of peptic disorders. **Cimetidine** was the first but was joined by **ranitidine**, which has a few minor advantages but is no more effective for healing ulcers. H_2-receptor antagonists are highly effective in reducing gastric acid secretion. Symptomatic response is rapid, usually within a day or two, and healing follows within a few weeks in 70–90% of cases. Recurrence rates, however, are high even with maintenance therapy, with 50–75% of patients developing further symptoms within 2 years.

A newer group of drugs, the substituted **benzimidazoles**, are extremely potent and reduce acid production to near zero by direct inhibition of the proton pump. **Omeprazole** and other variants are now often the first line treatment for most peptic ulcer disorders. In all cases where *H. pylori* infection is present, the use of these drugs must be combined with eradication antibiotic therapy.

Vagotomy

Vagotomy was first performed in the 1920s and popularised by Dragstedt from 1943. It gradually superseded classic partial gastrectomy as the surgical treatment of choice for chronic duodenal ulcer. The vagotomy operations illustrated in Figure 21.8 are now only of historical interest. The simplest involved dividing the anterior and posterior vagal trunks close to the abdominal oesophagus just below the diaphragm (**truncal vagotomy**). The operation is effective in promoting ulcer healing but paralyses gastric motility and slows pyloric emptying. A surgical **drainage procedure**, usually **pyloroplasty** ('V & P'), or less commonly **gastro-jejunostomy**, was therefore a necessary part of the operation.

Attempts to reduce the gastric emptying complications of truncal vagotomy led to operations designed to preserve the innervation of the distal antrum and pylorus whilst denervating the proximal acid-secreting portion of the stomach. **Highly selective vagotomy** preserved the nerves of Latarjet and avoided the need for a gastric drainage procedure. Early postoperative side-effects were fewer but ulcer recurrence rates were higher than for truncal vagotomy.

Surgical removal of intractable ulcers and gastrin-secreting tissue

Partial gastrectomy was occasionally used for patients where medical management had failed to heal a benign **gastric ulcer** or to treat repeated recurrences. The operation had the dual role of removing the ulcer and the gastrin-secreting mucosa. The classic gastrectomy for chronic gastric ulcer was known as the **Billroth I** type (Billroth, 1881) and involved removing the distal two-thirds of the stomach. The gastric remnant was then anastomosed to the first part of the duodenum (see Fig. 21.9).

The standard partial gastrectomy for **duodenal ulcers** was a **Polya-type gastrectomy** (Polya, 1911), also involving resection of the distal two-thirds of the stomach but anastomosing the cut end of the stomach to the side of a loop of proximal jejunum (gastro-jejunostomy). This is also known as a Billroth II operation. The cut end of the duodenum (duodenal stump) was closed and the ulcer left in situ to heal (see Fig. 21.9). Numerous variations on gastrectomy have been described over the years, but the essential difference is whether the gastric remnant is anastomosed to the duodenum (Billroth I-type) or to a jejunal loop (Polya-type).

In general, partial gastrectomy was highly effective in relieving symptoms and preventing recurrence of peptic disease, but long-term side-effects were a serious problem affecting 30–40% of patients.

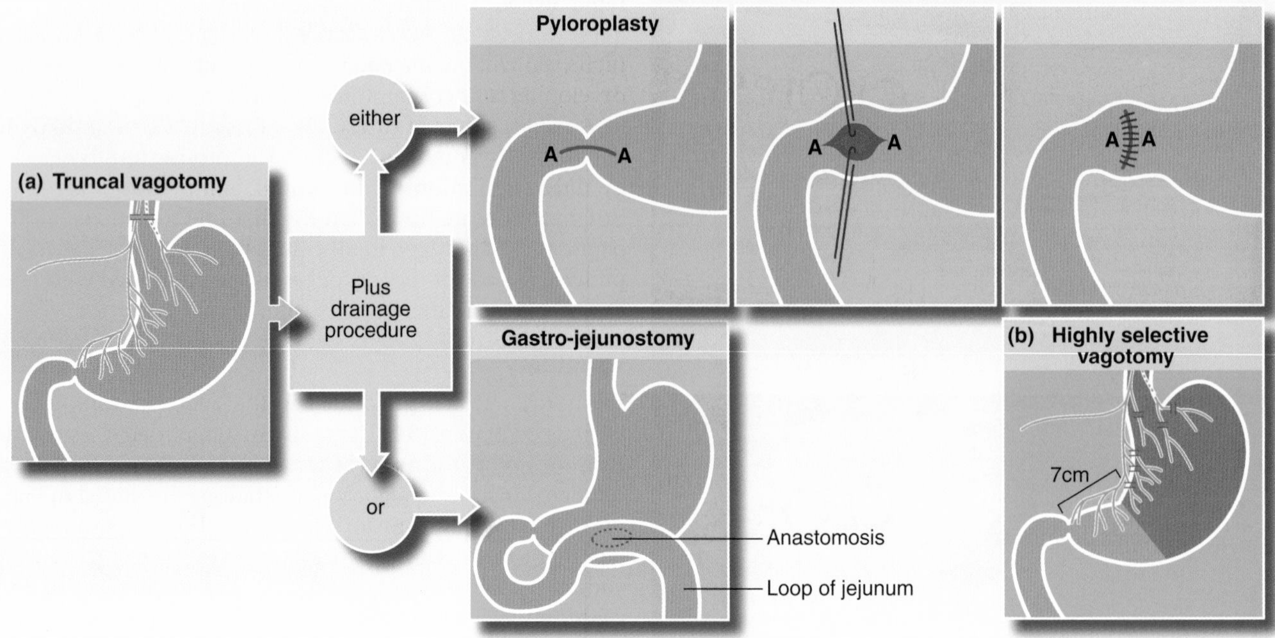

Fig. 21.8 The vagotomies and gastric drainage procedures (rarely performed nowadays but of historical interest)
(a) Truncal vagotomy is followed by a drainage procedure, either pyloroplasty (Heinecke–Mikulicz is illustrated) or gastro-jejunostomy. In gastro-jejunostomy an anastomosis is created to the most dependent part of the stomach; a short efferent loop of jejunum is brought up either in front of the transverse colon and sutured to the anterior wall of the stomach (antecolic), or behind the transverse colon via an incision in the mesocolon and sutured to the posterior wall of the stomach (retrocolic). **(b)** Highly selective vagotomy does not require a drainage procedure. Only the parietal cell mass is denervated, preserving the innervation of the pylorus and antrum plus the rest of the abdominal viscera

Complications and side-effects of partial gastrectomy

The main complications of partial gastrectomy occur in the long term and may not become manifest for years (see Box 21.2). Recurrent ulceration after partial gastrectomy was rare and occurred in the gastric remnant or at the stomal margin. The usual reason was that insufficient stomach had been removed, but occasionally malignant change was responsible (3% risk over 15 years). Abnormally high acid production was another cause, sometimes due to Zollinger–Ellison syndrome or hyperparathyroidism.

Correction of secondary anatomical problems

The main anatomical problems secondary to peptic disease are oesophageal stricture and pyloric stenosis.

Oesophageal strictures can usually be managed by periodic dilatation and medical or surgical treatment of the underlying cause. With the patient intravenously sedated, a guide-wire is inserted across the stricture endoscopically, and then metal, plastic or balloon dilators are inserted over it. Occasionally, reflux continues to cause damage and stricturing; it may then become necessary to perform anti-reflux surgery.

Box 21.2 Side-effects of partial gastrectomy

- Inability to eat normal-sized meals due to reduced gastric capacity
- 'Dumping' due to rapid emptying of stomach contents—common but most patients adapt with time
- Episodic bilious vomiting due to reflux of bile into stomach via the anastomosis
- Tendency to bolus obstruction of the gastric outlet stoma
- Weight loss due to a combination of above factors and malabsorption—especially common in women
- Vitamin B_{12} deficiency due to loss of gastric intrinsic factor; may present as macrocytic anaemia or subacute combined degeneration of the spinal cord—potentially catastrophic, occurring many years after operation and preventable by regular vitamin B_{12} (hydroxycobalamin) injections
- Iron deficiency anaemia due to reduced iron absorption—common but easily prevented by taking iron tablets, e.g. once weekly
- Malignant change in gastric remnant possibly due to bacterial production of carcinogens—rare

EMERGENCY PRESENTATIONS OF PEPTIC ULCER DISEASE

The emergency presentations of peptic ulcer disease are acute haemorrhage, perforation and, much less commonly, pyloric stenosis. Peptic ulcer disease was responsible for much major emergency abdominal surgery until the early 1970s. Since then there has been a remarkable reduction in emergency presentations of peptic ulcer, and emergency surgery is now uncommon. This change was well under way in the West before the introduction of effective modern drug therapy and can probably be attributed to the progressive improvement in living standards after the Second World War.

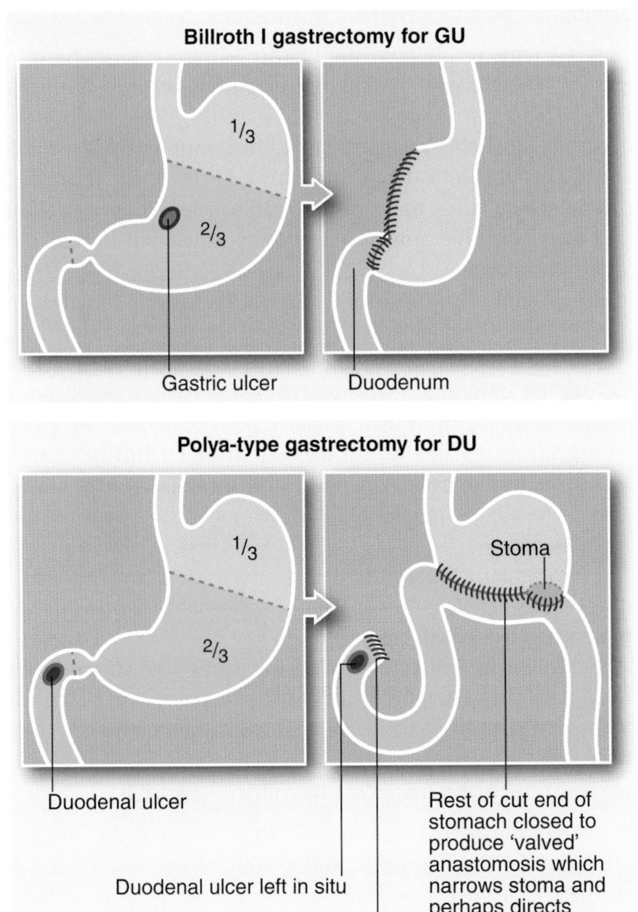

Fig. 21.9 Types of partial gastrectomy formerly performed for peptic ulcer disease

HAEMORRHAGE FROM A PEPTIC ULCER

Acute bleeding from a peptic ulcer presents with haematemesis or melaena or both. Management is discussed in detail in Chapter 19.

PERFORATION OF A PEPTIC ULCER

Perforation of a gastric or duodenal ulcer into the peritoneal cavity causes peritonitis. Perforations of peptic ulcers occur most commonly in elderly patients taking NSAIDs and in patients consuming excess alcohol.

Duodenal ulcer perforations are two or three times more common than gastric ulcer perforations. The perforation typically occurs on the anterior surface of the duodenal bulb just beyond the pylorus. About half the patients with a peptic ulcer perforation have had recent ulcer symptoms but the other half are asymptomatic.

Gastric ulcer perforations virtually always occur in the elderly. About a third of these are due to perforation of a gastric carcinoma. Thus standard surgical treatments for gastric perforation include excision or extensive biopsy of the ulcer.

Clinical presentation of perforated peptic ulcer

Perforation of a gastric or duodenal ulcer usually presents as a sudden onset of epigastric pain, rapidly spreading to the whole abdomen. The pain is continuous and is aggravated by moving about. Paradoxically, there may be vomiting of brownish or even blood-stained fluid. On examination, the patient is in obvious pain but is not shocked or toxic.

There is generalised involuntary abdominal guarding, which in younger patients is so tense as to be described as '**board-like rigidity**', although this may be absent in the elderly. There is also generalised abdominal tenderness but this may be difficult to detect because of guarding. After several hours, abdominal wall rigidity tends to relax although tenderness remains. Peptic ulcer perforation initially causes a chemical, as opposed to bacterial, peritonitis, unlike more distal bowel perforations. This explains the lack of general toxicity in the early stages. If untreated for more than 24 hours, secondary infection may take place and systemic signs appear.

If posterior wall gastric ulcers perforate, they leak gastric contents into the lesser sac, which tends to confine the peritonitis. These patients thus present with less marked symptoms.

Diagnosis of perforated peptic ulcer

Diagnosis of an upper gastrointestinal perforation can usually be made from the symptoms and signs alone. A plain erect radiograph of the chest often reveals gas under the diaphragm, confirming the perforation of a hollow viscus but not its origin. This radiographic evidence of perforation, however, is not always present. If perforation is suspected but the signs are equivocal, an abdominal radiograph may be taken after the patient has swallowed 25 ml of water-soluble contrast; this may confirm the leakage. Diagnostic gastroscopy is contraindicated because the stomach must be inflated during this examination and air and gastric contents would erupt into the peritoneal cavity. CT scanning is commonly used and reveals free gas within the abdomen together with free fluid, although again the origin may not be clear. Laparoscopy is increasingly used to diagnose perforated ulcers.

Surgical management of peptic perforation

Emergency surgery is indicated in nearly all cases of upper gastrointestinal perforation. The patient is first resuscitated and a nasogastric tube inserted. The operation is most commonly performed at laparotomy, but laparoscopic management of perforated duodenal ulcers is now well established with equally good results. The principles are similar in either case. At surgery, the abdomen is inspected and the diagnosis confirmed. 'Peritoneal toilet' is performed to remove fluid and food contaminating the peritoneal cavity. A perforated duodenal ulcer is usually obvious as a punched-out hole near the pylorus. An anterior gastric perforation is also obvious, but a posterior gastric ulcer is not visible unless the lesser sac is opened, usually along the greater curve.

In duodenal perforation, simple closure of the perforation by suturing a vascularised flap of omentum over the defect is the treatment of choice. This should be followed by *Helicobacter* eradication therapy as 90% of duodenal ulcers are associated with *H. pylori* infection.

In perforated gastric ulcer, the classic operation was Billroth I gastrectomy, including the whole ulcer in the resection. However, local excision of the ulcer and simple closure are safely employed, provided the ulcer is believed to be benign. In any case, the ulcer edge must be biopsied in several places to be certain.

Conservative management of perforated duodenal ulcer

If an elderly, unfit patient presents late with a perforated duodenal ulcer, many surgeons treat this conservatively. This involves nasogastric aspiration, intravenous fluids, gastric acid suppression and antibiotics. Many of these patients who might otherwise have succumbed with major surgery recover satisfactorily.

PYLORIC STENOSIS

The pyloric canal and the immediate pre-pyloric area are common sites of chronic ulceration. There may be typical symptoms of chronic duodenal ulcer or the presentation may be with pyloric stenosis and a minimal history of ulcer pain. Chronic ulceration near the pylorus causes fibrosis, which may progress to stricture formation. In the early stages, this leads to partial gastric outlet obstruction. An acute exacerbation of the ulcer leads to mucosal swelling and pyloric sphincter spasm, which then precipitates complete luminal obstruction.

CASE HISTORY

Fig. 21.10 Gastric outlet obstruction

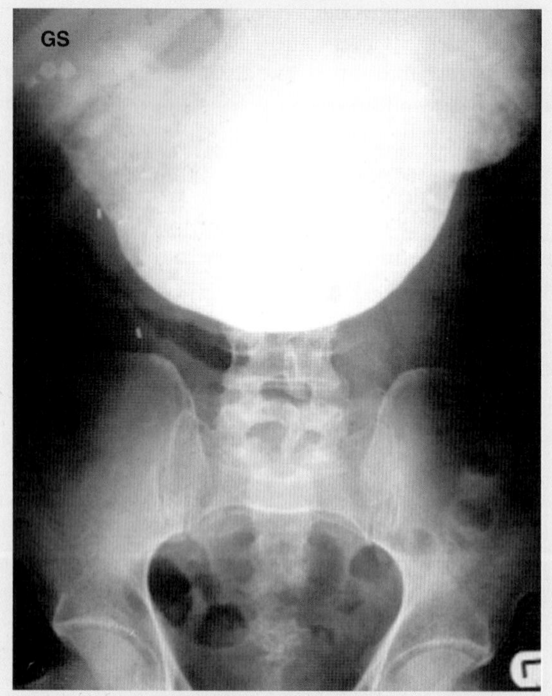

Barium meal examination in a woman of 78 who presented with a 2-week history of vomiting. She was grossly dehydrated with a hypochloraemic alkalosis. She was resuscitated and a nasogastric tube passed. This film shows huge gastric dilatation and no flow of barium beyond the pylorus. She also has incidental gallstones (**GS**). The obstruction proved to be due to chronic duodenal ulceration, but a diagnosis of carcinoma of the gastric antrum must be considered in such a patient

Clinical features of pyloric stenosis

These patients rarely give any history of peptic ulcer pain but tend to present with a short history (a few weeks at most) of episodic and sometimes projectile vomiting. This is unrelated to eating, and the vomitus typically contains foul-smelling semi-digested food eaten a day or more previously. It does not contain green bile. Often patients do not seek medical advice until they have become severely dehydrated with gross electrolyte disturbance.

On clinical examination, undernourishment, dehydration, constipation, weakness and weight loss may dominate the picture. Because the stomach is full of residual fluid and food, shaking the patient's abdomen from side to side produces an audible **succussion splash**. Gastric peristalsis may be visible in longstanding cases and a dilated stomach full of residual food may be palpable. On plain abdominal X-ray, it may be possible to see the grossly dilated stomach filled with mottled food material.

Several gastric washouts using a large-bore oral tube may be necessary to clear the gastric residue before endoscopy or barium meal is attempted.

The differential diagnosis of gastric outflow obstruction also includes carcinoma of the head of the pancreas (with or without obstructive jaundice) and, rarely, chronic pancreatitis.

Biochemical abnormalities in pyloric stenosis

The biochemical disturbances in these patients are complex and depend on the volume and composition of fluid lost by vomiting and on the body's compensatory mechanisms. Hydrogen and chloride are the principal ions lost in the vomitus. In response, the kidney conserves hydrogen ions by exchanging them for sodium ions (and some potassium ions), which are necessarily lost in the urine. The kidney also conserves chloride ions by exchanging them for bicarbonate ions. The net result may be a profound depletion of total body sodium (which is not accurately reflected in the plasma sodium level), profound hypochloraemia and profound metabolic alkalosis (**hypochloraemic alkalosis**). The plasma urea level is often high as a result of dehydration. Finally, the proportion of ionised calcium in the serum may fall as a result of the alkalosis, inducing tetany.

Management of pyloric stenosis

The first management priority in gastric outlet obstruction is resuscitation. Fluid and electrolyte deficiencies are corrected by infusion of physiological saline with added potassium chloride. The volume required often amounts to 10 litres or more. Rehydration will usually return the blood urea level to normal but may unmask anaemia serious enough to require blood transfusion.

Often the obstruction has a significant inflammatory element, and acid suppression and *Helicobacter* eradication will produce a significant clinical response. If these fail or malignancy is suspected, endoscopy should be repeated and careful balloon dilation of the stenosis may achieve the desired result. If the obstruction persists, operative treatment may then become necessary in the form of either a gastro-jejunostomy to bypass the obstruction, or more rarely a partial gastrectomy.

Disorders of the oesophagus

22

INTRODUCTION

Benign oesophageal diseases form a small but significant part of upper GI surgeons' workload. Most are managed by medical gastroenterologists except those likely to require surgery; then close collaboration is needed between medical and surgical specialists. Oesophageal cancer surgery is largely performed in specialised units.

Difficulty in swallowing, **dysphagia**, is the most common presenting symptom. **Reflux oesophagitis** and other peptic disorders of the lower oesophagus (often associated with hiatus hernia) and **oesophageal carcinomas** are the main conditions encountered. **Achalasia** and **pharyngeal pouch** are occasionally seen; **oesophageal web** (as in Plummer–Vinson syndrome) and **leiomyomas** (gastrointestinal stromal tumours, GIST) are extremely rare.

Oesophageal varices secondary to cirrhosis usually present as massive haematemesis and are usually managed with non-surgical therapy.

CARCINOMA OF THE OESOPHAGUS

PATHOLOGY AND CLINICAL FEATURES

The oesophagus is lined by stratified squamous epithelium. Historically the majority of oesophageal malignancies were **squamous carcinomas**. The rest were **adenocarcinomas** in the lower third, probably derived from metaplastic intestinal mucosa, i.e. Barrett's oesophageal changes. However, over the last few decades there has been a slow but steady reversal in these proportions; currently adenocarcinoma makes up 60–70% of new cases. Both forms tend to behave aggressively.

Tumours at the gastro-oesophageal junction originate from three areas: the distal oesophagus ('type 1'), the gastric cardia ('type 2') or the subcardial gastric wall ('type 3'). Oesophageal cancers may fungate into the lumen but more often infiltrate diffusely along and around the oesophageal wall. Once through the wall, the tumour invades adjoining mediastinal organs.

Difficulty in swallowing (dysphagia) is the classic symptom, but it tends to develop insidiously. Patients initially have trouble with solids but tend to compensate (liquidising their food, for example) before seeking medical advice. Later they have trouble swallowing liquids. By the time dysphagia manifests, the cancer is often incurable and lymphatic spread has already occurred to mediastinal nodes. Sometimes, involvement of other mediastinal organs, e.g. recurrent laryngeal nerve invasion or an oesophago-tracheal fistula, produces the first symptoms. Low oesophageal lesions tend to metastasise to upper abdominal nodes and the liver.

EPIDEMIOLOGY AND AETIOLOGY

The incidence of oesophageal cancer in Western countries is relatively low compared with cancer of the colon or stomach. It accounts for about 5% of all deaths from cancer, with men at two-fold greater risk than women. The disease is usually advanced by the time of presentation, hence the mortality rate is appalling, with 70% dying within a year and only 8% surviving 5 years (see Fig. 22.1).

Oesophageal carcinoma is uncommon before the age of 50 years. At least 50% occur in the lower third and only about 15% in the upper third. Heavy alcohol intake is associated with at least 20 times greater risk and smokers have five times the risk of non-smokers; however, these risk factors classically predispose only to squamous cell carcinoma.

Since 1980, adenocarcinomas have increased by 70% relative to squamous carcinomas in many Western countries. This may be connected with the widespread use of acid-suppressing medication and possibly with dietary changes. There is no familial predisposition but people with structural and functional disorders, such as peptic oesophagitis and stricture, achalasia, oesophageal web or pharyngeal pouch, are at considerably greater risk. Areas of exceptionally high incidence have been reported in China, elsewhere in the Far East, and around the Caspian Sea. There is some evidence that a fungus which grows on food grain may be responsible. These epidemiological patterns suggest that chronic tissue irritation is an important aetiological factor. One common finding in dietary studies is an association with low fruit and vegetable intake.

INVESTIGATION OF SUSPECTED OESOPHAGEAL CARCINOMA

Dysphagia or pain on swallowing (**odynophagia**) in a middle-aged or elderly patient demands urgent investigation

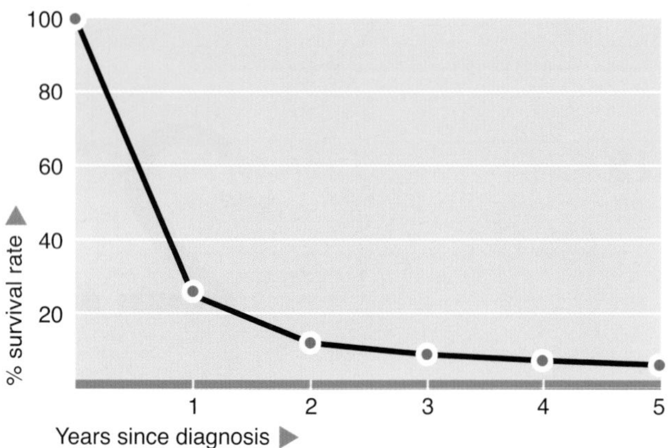

Fig. 22.1 Survival after diagnosis of oesophageal carcinoma

Box 22.1 Guidelines for recognising symptoms suspicious of upper gastrointestinal cancer*

Dyspepsia alone

- Patients over 55 with recent onset, unexplained and persistent dyspepsia

Dyspepsia plus any of the following 'alarm symptoms' at any age. *Note*: patients with symptoms marked ‡ should be referred even without dyspepsia

- Progressive unintentional weight loss‡
- Persistent vomiting‡
- Iron deficiency anaemia‡
- Epigastric mass‡
- Dysphagia
- Chronic gastrointestinal bleeding
- Suspicious barium meal result

Dyspepsia—unexplained worsening plus:

- Anaemia
- Known Barrett's oesophagus, dysplasia, atrophic gastritis or intestinal metaplasia
- Surgery for peptic ulcer over 20 years before

Unexplained upper abdominal pain and weight loss

- May need urgent ultrasound

Obstructive jaundice

- May need urgent ultrasound

*Based on recommendations of the National Institute for Health and Clinical Excellence (NICE), UK 2005. Patients referred with suspected cancer are expected to be seen by a specialist within 14 days

to exclude carcinoma (see Box 22.1). General physical examination is usually unrewarding except in advanced disease. In these cases, there may be signs of **wasting**, **hepatomegaly** due to metastases, a **Virchow's node** in the left supraclavicular fossa or sometimes **hoarseness** from recurrent laryngeal nerve involvement. Gastroscopy allows direct inspection of the oesophagus using a flexible endoscope and biopsies are taken of any suspicious areas (Fig. 22.2).

Staging the cancer

Once oesophageal carcinoma is diagnosed, it is important to establish the extent of local invasion and whether metastasis has occurred to thoracic or abdominal lymph nodes, liver or peritoneum; this will determine whether potentially curative treatment is appropriate. CT scanning of chest and abdomen is the principal investigation but it often understages the disease. **Staging laparoscopy** for lower third tumours can show peritoneal or visceral metastases not seen on CT scan; some units employ staging **thoracoscopy** to assess the pleural cavity for the same reasons. **Endoscopic ultrasound (EUS)** demonstrates very clearly the different layers of gut wall and thus helps to delineate the tumour more accurately in length and, more importantly, depth of invasion (T stage). It also has high sensitivity and specificity for involvement of local lymph nodes and can enable biopsy of suspicious nodes in otherwise inaccessible locations (**EUS-guided biopsy**), enhancing the staging process and in some cases preventing unnecessary surgery. The greater the number of involved nodes, the lower the chances of surgical cure. Increasingly patients are also undergoing fluorodeoxyglucose positron emission tomography (FDG-PET), known as PET scans, which localise any cancerous tissue more accurately than CT scanning alone.

MANAGEMENT OF CARCINOMA OF THE OESOPHAGUS

The ideal treatment would be to eliminate the cancer. In practice, this can rarely be achieved because of overt or occult spread. Even if cure is impossible, oesophageal obstruction must be relieved to allow the patient to eat and to prevent the appalling consequences of complete obstruction, namely inability to swallow even saliva.

The choice of treatment depends on the patient's fitness and the stage, but surgical resection of the tumour is only employed when the aim is cure. Co-morbidity such as chronic lung disease or cirrhosis (often from the adverse effects of alcohol and cigarettes) may influence the decision. Cardiac fitness is assessed clinically and by electrocardiography (ECG), echocardiography, and cardiopulmonary exercise testing (CPEX). In addition, spirometry and blood gases should be performed to assess fitness for thoracotomy. If the FEV_1 is less than 2 L, single lung ventilation used during thoracotomy is unlikely to be tolerated. Adjuvant therapy in addition to surgery has a role in some patients, although clinical trials are continuing to determine precise indications. Most often, chemotherapy is given alone or in combination with radiotherapy (chemoradiotherapy) before surgery (**neoadjuvant therapy**) in an attempt to shrink or downsize the tumour.

Historically, radiotherapy has been given as the sole form of treatment for squamous carcinoma. Intubation of the tumour was often needed before radiotherapy to prevent complete obstruction in the short term as a result of swelling. Results of this were often disappointing because of adverse local effects. Radiotherapy nowadays tends to be reserved for palliation.

Fig. 22.2 Barrett's oesophagus and oesophageal carcinoma

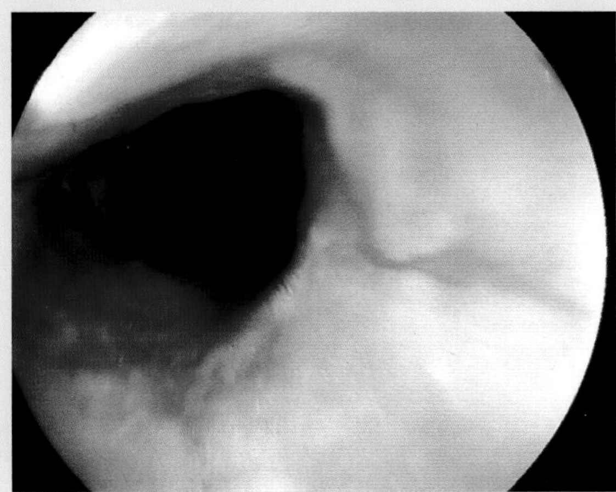

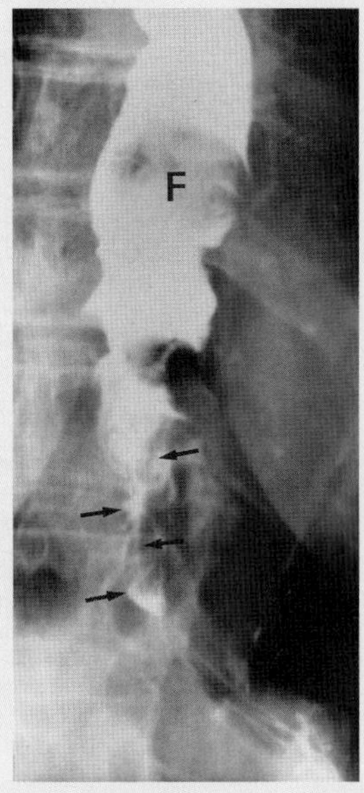

(a) (b)

(a) Endoscopic view of Barrett's oesophagus demonstrating linear ulceration and deeper red mucosa with chronic ulceration at the oesophago-gastric junction. Diagnosis is confirmed on biopsy. This condition is potentially premalignant. **(b)** Barium swallow in an elderly man who presented with almost complete dysphagia. The film shows the lower end of the oesophagus which has an irregular narrowing of the lumen (arrowed). This appearance did not alter in several views of the same area and is characteristic of malignancy. Nevertheless, endoscopy is usually performed to obtain histological confirmation by biopsies. The oesophagus above is moderately dilated and contains a bolus of food **F** which cannot pass onwards

For incurable patients with dysphagia, palliative procedures to restore swallowing, such as argon plasma tissue coagulation, laser treatment or stent insertion, can be effective and are preferable to major surgery, particularly if life expectancy is short.

Surgery

Once a decision has been made to operate, the choice of operation depends on the level of the lesion. In general, the aim is to remove the tumour with an appropriate safety margin, to perform a two-field lymphadenectomy (removing mediastinal and abdominal lymph nodes) and to achieve a leak-free anastomosis.

Lesions above the carina (tracheal bifurcation) are usually dealt with by a three-stage **oesophagectomy** known as the **McKeown operation**, with all stages performed at the same operation. The first stage is to mobilise the tumour and oesophagus via a right thoracotomy with the patient in the left lateral position. The second stage involves rolling the patient into a supine position and performing a laparotomy to allow the stomach to be mobilised and fashioned into a conduit. A third incision is then made in the neck through which oesophagus and tumour are delivered. The tumour is resected and the gastric conduit anastomosed to the cervical oesophagus. A cervical anastomosis is safer than an intrathoracic one, as the consequences of anastomotic leakage are less devastating.

If the tumour arises lower in the oesophagus, a two-stage **Ivor Lewis operation** is usually performed. The abdomen is opened first, and the stomach mobilised and fashioned into a conduit. The patient is then turned into a left lateral position and the right chest opened, the oesophagus mobilised and the tumour and lymph nodes excised. Finally the gastric conduit is drawn up into the chest and anastomosed to the proximal oesophageal remnant. If this is impossible, a loop of jejunum or a single end of jejunum (Roux-en-Y) is drawn up to make the connection (see Fig. 22.3). Controversy exists about whether extending lymphadenectomy into the neck, so-called 'three-field lymphadenectomy', is beneficial. The procedure increases operative risks and only appears to benefit a subgroup with proximal tumours and fewer than five involved nodes.

An operation that gained popularity is **transhiatal oesophagectomy**. A thoracotomy is avoided by mobilising the oesophagus and the cancer by blunt dissection from below via the diaphragmatic hiatus and from above via a neck incision, performing the anastomosis in the neck after resection. However, interest is waning because the safety margins of excision may be insufficient for potential cure and adequate lymphadenectomy is impossible in the chest. There is also a risk of damaging veins during dissection (particularly the azygos) and causing catastrophic haemorrhage.

There is increasing interest in laparoscopic approaches to these cancers, and many units are now regularly performing laparoscopic oesophagectomies and gastrectomies. Techniques involve combined laparoscopic and thoracoscopic approaches. Perioperative morbidity and mortality and cancer recurrence rates appear to be at least comparable with open surgery, and there are the additional benefits of minimal access surgery.

Oesophagectomy is always a major undertaking and carries the potentially fatal risk of anastomotic breakdown. This

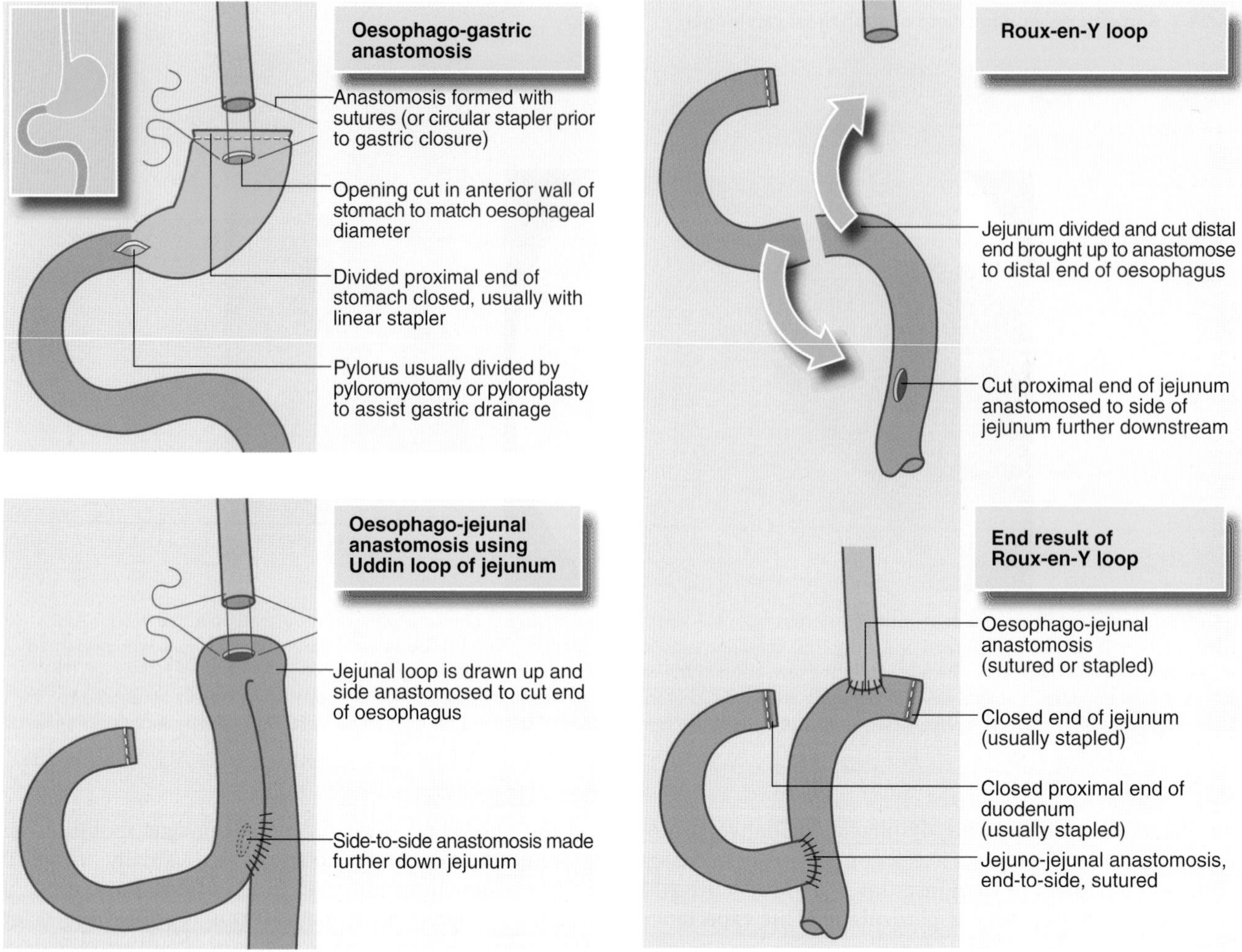

Fig. 22.3 Methods of reconstruction after distal oesophagectomy and partial or total gastrectomy

may lead to mediastinitis, lung abscess or oesophago-pleural fistula. Patients need to be made aware of the risks in relation to the benefits, as well as the likely prolonged convalescent period and the long-term morbidity. Postoperative problems include dysphagia, small capacity for food (early satiety), and reflux.

Inoperable lesions

If operation is inappropriate, oesophageal patency can often be restored by palliative ablation of the tumour with laser therapy or argon plasma coagulation via a gastroscope. These treatments can be repeated as the tumour regrows. Alternatively, the oesophagus can be intubated with an expanding metal stent (see Fig. 22.4) through the lesion. This is usually done under intravenous sedation, using the endoscopic technique of **pulsion intubation**. First the oesophageal lesion is dilated then the stent inserted using X-ray guidance. These tubes relieve symptoms, but food has to be liquidised and the tube kept 'clean' by taking fizzy drinks after eating. Patients are more susceptible to acid reflux, for which antacid medication may need to be prescribed. Chemotherapy, external beam radiotherapy and intraluminal brachytherapy (local radiotherapy) are increasingly used for palliation.

HIATUS HERNIA AND REFLUX OESOPHAGITIS

PATHOPHYSIOLOGY

The oesophagus is essentially a tube of smooth muscle conveying food to the stomach by peristalsis. At the lower end there is a tonically active sphincter mechanism. Its contraction coordinates with oesophageal peristalsis, relaxing to allow food to enter the stomach. The purpose of the sphincter mechanism is to prevent reflux of stomach contents into the oesophagus. After passing through the diaphragm, the oesophagus continues for about 2 cm within the abdomen before joining the stomach. The sphincter mechanism is not completely understood but it probably involves several components: a functional (but not anatomical) sphincter of the oesophageal wall immediately above the diaphragm and the smooth muscle at the gastric cardia. This mechanism is reinforced by diaphragmatic crural contraction, by the acute angle at which the oesophagus enters the stomach and by the '**flutter valve**' effect of intra-abdominal pressure on the abdominal oesophagus causing luminal collapse.

Hiatus hernia occurs when the proximal part of the stomach passes through the diaphragmatic hiatus up into the chest (see Fig. 22.5). Around 90% of hiatus hernias are of the **sliding type**, in which the gastro-oesophageal junction is drawn up into the chest and a segment of stomach becomes constricted at the diaphragmatic hiatus. The hernia tends to slide up into the chest with each peristaltic contraction. These hernias may become huge and, rarely, may contain the whole stomach including pylorus and first part of the duodenum, sometimes with part of the colon as well. In the 10% of non-sliding cases, the gastro-oesophageal junction remains below the diaphragm and a bulge of stomach herniates through the hiatus beside the oesophagus. These are described as **para-oesophageal** or **rolling hiatus hernias**.

In sliding hiatus hernia, the lower oesophageal sphincter mechanism often becomes defective, causing reflux of acid–peptic stomach contents. This is not a problem with rolling hiatus hernias which more usually present with pain or dysphagia.

Hiatus hernia in adults is commonly associated with smoking and obesity. The pressure of intra-abdominal fat may be contributory. Hiatus hernia can also be a congenital abnormality presenting in early infancy.

CASE HISTORY

Fig. 22.4 Intubation of oesophageal cancer: cloth-covered metal stent in situ

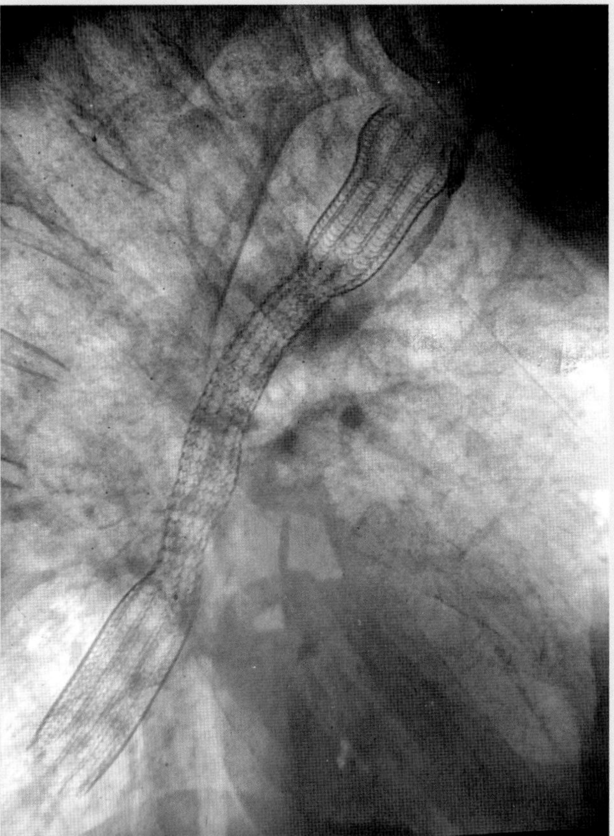

This 70-year-old man presented with inoperable carcinoma of the middle third of the oesophagus. The malignant stricture was dilated via a flexible gastroscope and a Dacron-covered metal stent inserted to keep the stricture open as a palliative measure. This lateral chest X-ray shows the stent in situ

CLINICAL FEATURES OF REFLUX OESOPHAGITIS

Hiatus hernia is common, especially in women, and becomes more common with advancing years. Only a small proportion of patients with hiatus hernia experience symptoms of **acid–peptic reflux**, i.e. 'heartburn'; moreover, reflux can occur without a hiatus hernia. Reflux causes acute inflammation (**oesophagitis**), experienced as burning retrosternal pain (**heartburn**), bitter-tasting regurgitation or other forms of 'indigestion'. Symptoms are typically worse at night when the patient lies flat or on bending forward during the day.

If reflux is severe and persistent, mucosal destruction is recurrent and inflammation becomes chronic. Progressive scarring leads to fibrosis of the wall and this may lead to luminal narrowing (stricture) and dysphagia. Longstanding oesophageal reflux predisposes to **Barrett's oesophagus**, with normal squamous oesophageal epithelium being replaced by metaplastic columnar mucosa. Barrett's oesophagus is the only known predisposing factor for adenocarcinoma of the lower oesophagus. Histological examination of biopsies may reveal **specialised intestinal metaplasia** (SIM) or **severe dysplasia**; both are markers for malignant change, supporting the metaplasia/dysplasia/carcinoma model for evolution of lower oesophageal cancer.

Occasionally, oesophageal reflux symptoms are severe and acute, causing chest pain which can easily be mistaken for

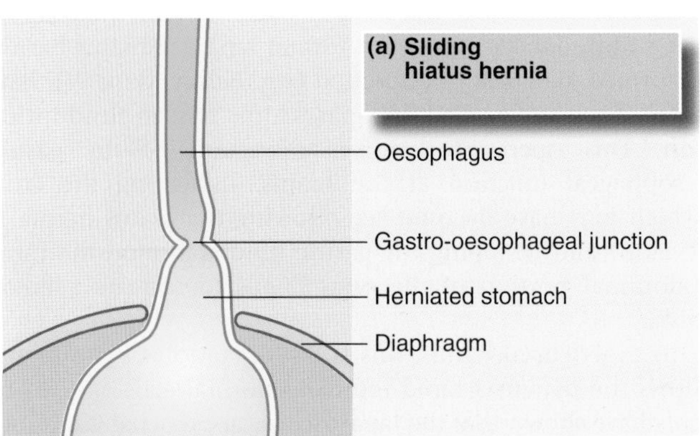

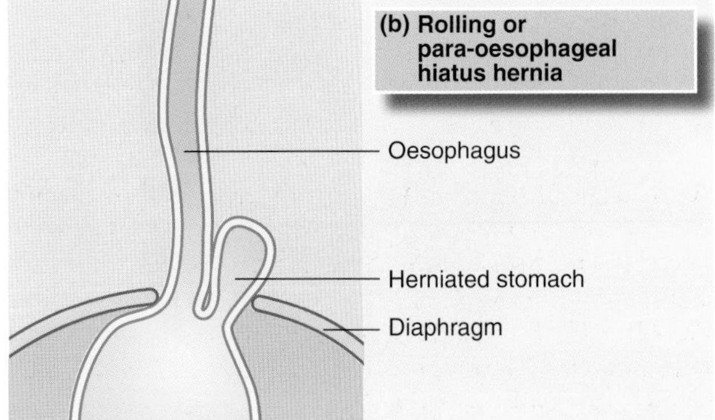

Fig. 22.5 Types of hiatus hernia
(a) Sliding hiatus hernia, which is common. This type disrupts the physiological anti-reflux mechanism. **(b)** Rolling or para-oesophageal hiatus hernia, which is rare. The anti-reflux mechanism is usually left intact

angina or even myocardial infarction. There is often an element of **oesophageal spasm** which, like angina, is relieved by glyceryl trinitrate and similar drugs, which may confuse the diagnosis.

In general, hiatus hernias are assessed at endoscopy, with biopsy if necessary. The latter is important to exclude carcinoma, especially in dysphagia. In specialised units, **oesophageal manometry studies** can assess the oesophageal muscular function and **oesophageal pH studies** assess the extent and severity of reflux. These studies help determine which patients are likely to benefit from surgery. Rarely barium swallow examination (see Figs 22.6 and 22.7) may be necessary to delineate complicated anatomy.

MANAGEMENT OF HIATUS HERNIA AND REFLUX OESOPHAGITIS

Most patients can be managed conservatively, with surgery reserved for intractable cases. Treatment is aimed at reducing acid–pepsin activity and preventing reflux.

Reducing reflux

Weight reduction, where appropriate, is the most effective long-term anti-reflux measure. Changes in diet often of themselves improve symptoms of reflux. For example, **alcohol** causes the sphincter to relax and many medical students can personally vouch for the combined effect of beer and spicy food! Other foods known to precipitate reflux are caffeine, high fat foods and chocolate. Reflux can be reduced substantially by taking smaller, more frequent and drier meals, by using blocks to elevate the head of the bed at night and by sleeping on more pillows in an upright position. **Smoking** induces sphincter relaxation, and quitting often reduces reflux dramatically. Patients should also be advised to wear loose-fitting clothing, and avoid bending or straining soon after meals. **Alginate drugs**, available in liquid or chewable tablet form, produce a foamy surface layer on the stomach contents and are said to coat the lower oesophagus, protecting it from reflux effects. These drugs are most effective if taken soon after food.

CASE HISTORY

Fig. 22.6 Sliding hiatus hernia

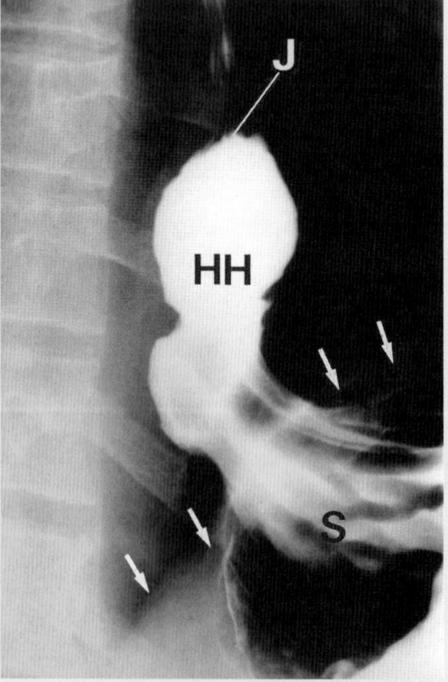

Sliding hiatus hernia in a 63-year-old woman. The hiatus hernia is marked **HH**, the stomach **S** and the oesophago-gastric junction **J**; the position of the diaphragm is arrowed

Prokinetic agents

Drugs that stimulate motility can have a useful effect in reflux. **Metoclopramide** and **domperidone** are dopamine antagonists that stimulate oesophageal clearance and gastric emptying and increase small bowel transit, as well as enhancing contraction of the oesophageal sphincter.

Reducing acid–pepsin production

This is probably the mainstay of treatment for reflux disease. Simple antacid drugs and H_2-receptor antagonists are sometimes effective but in most cases **omeprazole** or another proton pump inhibitor (PPI) is the drug of choice.

Management of strictures

Inflammatory fibrous strictures used to be regularly dilated with gum-elastic **bougies** of progressively increasing size under general anaesthesia via a rigid oesophagoscope. Nowadays, dilatation is usually performed under intravenous sedation using flexible gastroscopy under X-ray control, with a balloon to dilate the stricture. If the stricture recurs and causes dysphagia despite conservative treatment for reflux, an anti-reflux operation may be indicated. This usually allows healing of mucosal damage and may prevent further stricture formation.

Surgery for hiatus hernia and reflux oesophagitis

Surgery has historically been reserved for intractable symptoms, recurrent stricture and chronic oesophagitis which fail to respond to PPI therapy. This especially includes patients with Barrett's oesophagus (having excluded those with a high risk of malignancy by biopsy). Surgery may also be indicated for the young or middle-aged patient in whom PPIs produce a response but who do not wish to take long-term medication. The traditional operations for formal repair of hiatus hernia, performed via chest or abdomen (e.g. Belsey Mark IV), have largely been superseded by laparoscopic **Nissen fundoplication**. This operation involves dissection of the gastro-oesophageal junction at the hiatus, tightening the crura (which may have become lax, allowing the hiatus hernia to develop) and wrapping the gastric fundus around the intra-abdominal portion of the oesophagus to recreate a flutter valve.

In experienced hands, this is the operation of choice and allows the patient a rapid return to normal activity. Clinical trials have shown that the laparoscopic approach gives results comparable to open fundoplication. Typical side-effects of any Nissen operation include temporary dysphagia, gas-bloat syndrome (due to retained air and decreased ability to belch)

Fig. 22.7 Sliding hiatus hernia

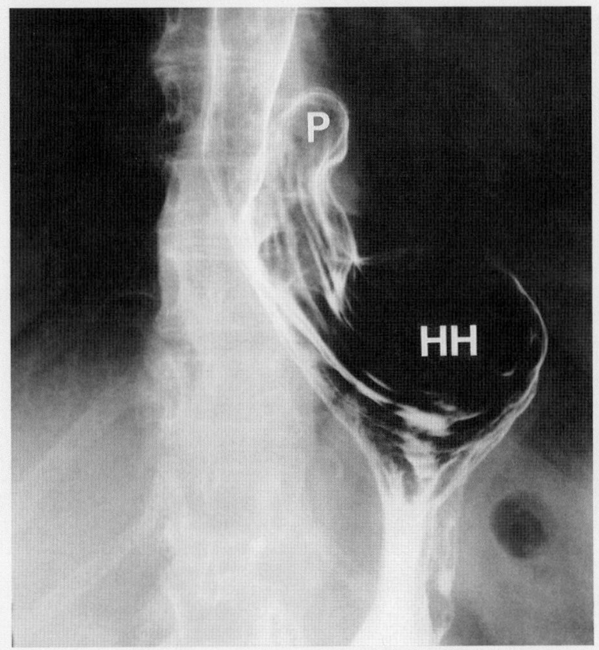

(a)

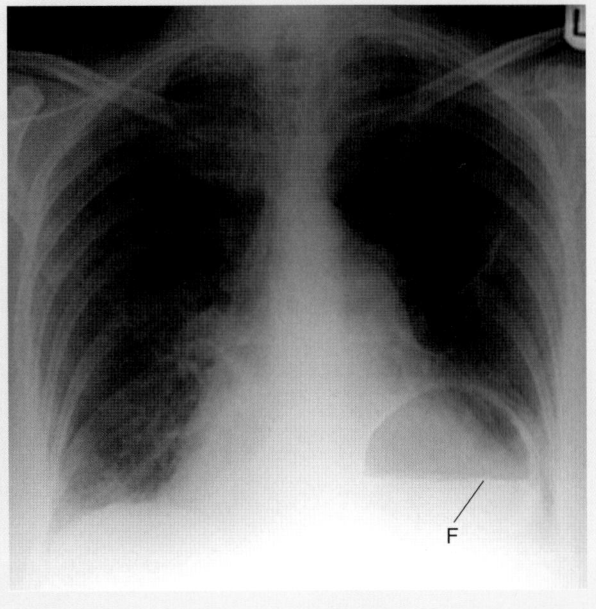

(b)

(a) Large incarcerated (irreducible) sliding hiatus hernia in an elderly woman with few symptoms. Note there is also a small para-oesophageal 'rolling' hiatus hernia **P**. **(b)** Plain chest X-ray of the same patient showing a fluid level **F** strongly suggestive of a hiatus hernia

and consequently increased flatus. These problems usually settle in time, but must be clearly explained to the patient before obtaining consent for operation. The most significant (but fortunately rare) postoperative complication is that of a **slipped wrap**. In this case, the fundal wrap slips down onto the stomach, or up through the hiatus into the chest (usually after a bout of excessive vomiting). In either case, the patient usually presents with acute onset chest and/or upper abdominal pain and dysphagia. This complication should be managed as a surgical emergency with diagnostic confirmation followed by early reoperation.

ACHALASIA

PATHOPHYSIOLOGY AND CLINICAL PRESENTATION

Achalasia is an uncommon disorder of oesophageal motility. In pathological terms, there is a poorly understood neurological defect involving Auerbach's myenteric (parasympathetic) plexus. Peristalsis is disrupted throughout the entire oesophagus, causing uncoordinated contractions and inadequate relaxation of the lower oesophageal sphincter.

The condition presents in two main age groups, young adults and the elderly. In the latter, the cause may be a central rather than a local neurological deficit. Achalasia, as with any structural oesophageal abnormality, predisposes to cancer with a 5% lifetime risk of developing squamous oesophageal carcinoma, usually 15–20 years after diagnosis of achalasia.

Clinically, the cardiac sphincter becomes constricted and the proximal oesophagus dilates with accumulated fluid and solids. Difficulty in swallowing is the usual presenting symptom, together with halitosis, weight loss, reflux of food into the back of the throat. Solids tend to sink to the lower end of the dilated oesophagus, whereas fluids spill over into the trachea causing **spluttering dysphagia** (see Ch. 18, p. 249) and coughing, particularly at night. Vomiting and retrosternal pain may occur in more severe cases.

INVESTIGATION OF SUSPECTED ACHALASIA

Chest X-ray may show the mediastinal shadow is widened by a dilated oesophagus; sometimes a fluid level in the oesophagus is visible behind the heart Fig. 22.7(b). At endoscopy the typical appearance is of a capacious distal oesophagus, usually with food and fluid residue, and a tight lower oesophageal sphincter that may or may not admit the tip of the gastroscope. It is important to see the oesophago-gastric junction to exclude an occult neoplasm masquerading as achalasia (**pseudoachalasia**). Barium swallow examination reveals gross dilatation of the oesophagus with a tapering constriction (often described as a 'bird's beak' or 'rat's tail') at the lower end. The constriction barely allows contrast to enter the stomach (see Fig. 22.8). Under fluoroscopic screening, uncoordinated purposeless peristaltic waves can often be seen; these are described as **tertiary contractions**, distinct from normal coordinated primary and secondary contractions. Oesophageal manometry is the cardinal test for achalasia, demonstrating excessive lower oesophageal sphincter pressure that fails to relax on swallowing, and abnormal peristalsis in patients with a more chronic history.

MANAGEMENT OF ACHALASIA

The condition is by its nature incurable, and treatment aims to relieve the distal obstruction. The standard operation is a laparoscopic abdominal procedure involving a longitudinal incision of the lower oesophageal and upper gastric muscle

CASE HISTORY

Fig. 22.8 Late-stage achalasia in a 60-year-old man

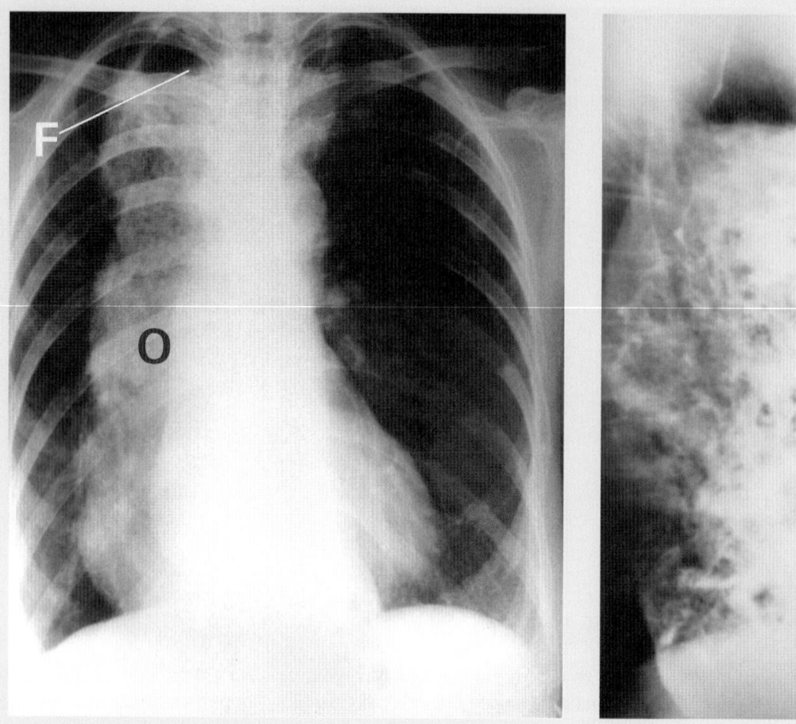

(a) The chest X-ray shows gross mediastinal widening caused by a massively dilated oesophagus **O** filled with food debris. Note the mottled appearance of the oesophagus and the fluid level **F** at its upper end. Note also the absence of a gastric air bubble below the diaphragm. This is characteristic of achalasia. **(b)** Barium swallow in the same patient. This confirms the findings on the chest X-ray

wall until the mucosa bulges through (**Heller's cardiomyotomy**); this is best combined with a partial fundoplication to overcome the almost inevitable reflux it will cause. Balloon dilatation is sometimes used as an alternative but often needs to be repeated. Botulinum toxin (Botox) is now often used to relax the lower oesophageal sphincter and is an excellent temporising measure, but needs to be repeated after 3–6 months as the effect wears off. Patients with achalasia should be followed up and periodically endoscoped to exclude developing squamous carcinoma (see Fig. 22.9).

PHARYNGEAL POUCH

Pharyngeal pouch is a rare cause of dysphagia. It arises at the junction of pharynx and oesophagus, and probably results from lack of coordination between the inferior constrictor muscle and cricopharyngeus during swallowing. At this point, there is an area of relative weakness known as **Killian's dehiscence**. The result is a progressive mucosal outpouching between the two muscles. The condition is best diagnosed by barium swallow (see Fig. 22.10). Pharyngeal pouch is easily perforated during endoscopy, and therefore in endoscopy to investigate 'high' dysphagia, the procedure should be performed by an experienced endoscopist. Treatment of pharyngeal pouch is by surgical excision from the side of the neck, or via a completely endoluminal approach using a stapler to join the pouch to the oesophagus.

OESOPHAGEAL WEB

Circumferential mucosal folds (or webs) in the oesophagus may produce annular narrowing and cause dysphagia. They also predispose to carcinoma in the long term. In the upper oesophagus, webs are associated with severe iron deficiency anaemia, particularly in women. The triad of dysphagia, anaemia and atrophic glossitis is known as **Plummer–Vinson** or **Paterson–Brown-Kelly syndrome**.

GASTRO-OESOPHAGEAL VARICES

PATHOPHYSIOLOGY

Gastro-oesophageal varices result from **portal venous hypertension**. The most common cause is cirrhosis of the liver, usually linked with alcohol abuse. Less common causes include portal vein thrombosis, hepatic vein thrombosis (**Budd–Chiari syndrome**) and schistosomiasis.

As resistance to flow and pressure rises in the portal venous system, abnormal communications develop between the peripheral portal system and the systemic venous circulation. This is known as **portal-systemic shunting**. Multiple large veins appear in the peritoneal cavity and retroperitoneal area, making any form of abdominal surgery hazardous. Large submucosal veins also appear at the lower end of the oesophagus and gastric fundus, and are known as **gastro-oesophageal varices** (see Fig. 22.11). These varices can cause

CASE HISTORY

Fig. 22.9 Oesophageal carcinoma secondary to achalasia

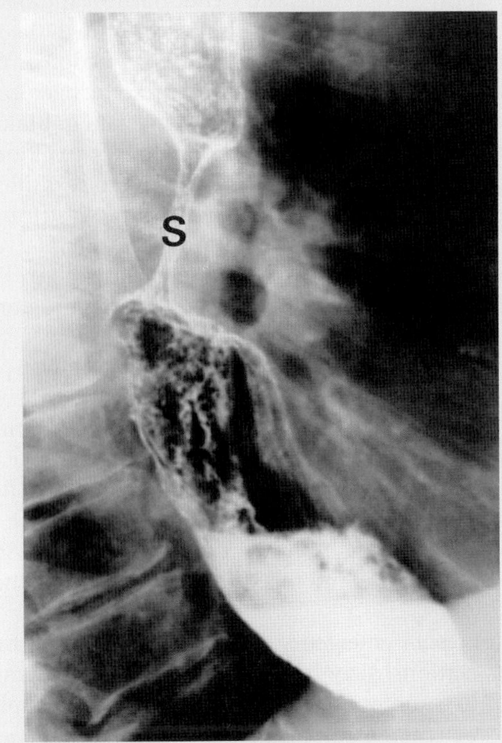

Malignant stricture **S** in the middle third of the oesophagus in a 60-year-old woman with achalasia of long standing. She had a Heller's myotomy at the age of 26. Note that this surgery does not reduce the inherent predisposition to carcinoma

CASE HISTORY

Fig. 22.10 Pharyngeal pouch

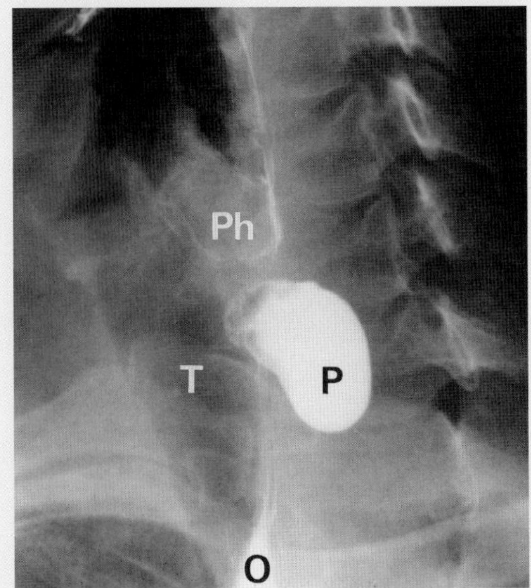

Lateral view during barium swallow examination in a 41-year-old man complaining of mild dysphagia; the X-ray shows a contrast-filled pouch **P** extending from the pharynx **Ph**. Note the gas-filled trachea **T** lying anteriorly. **O**=oesophagus

CASE HISTORY

Fig. 22.11 Endoscopic view of oesophageal varices

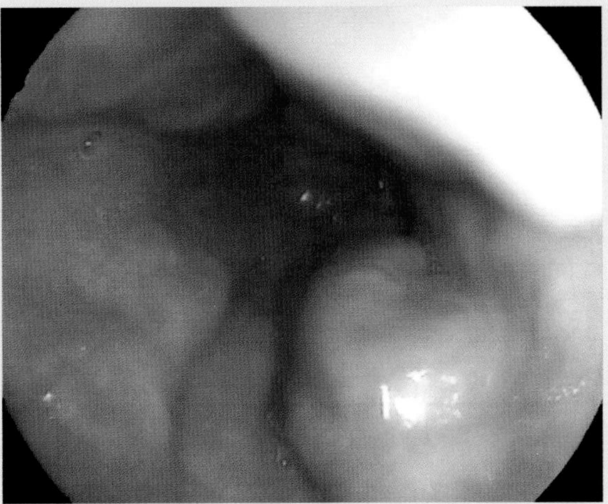

This man of 63 was known to have alcoholic cirrhosis and had suffered one acute gastrointestinal haemorrhage, treated successfully by injection of bleeding varices. The bulging blue masses can be seen protruding into the oesophageal lumen

massive gastrointestinal haemorrhage, possibly related to rises in intravariceal pressure. Up to 40% of cirrhotic patients suffer variceal haemorrhage at some stage.

ELECTIVE MANAGEMENT

Gastro-oesophageal varices are not usually treated unless they have bled. Occasionally, elective treatment is carried out in cases where haemorrhage is considered highly likely, with the improving efficacy of banding and sclerotherapy. After recovery from an acute bleed, varices should be treated at planned intervals by banding or injection sclerotherapy until they are eliminated.

MANAGEMENT OF BLEEDING GASTRO-OESOPHAGEAL VARICES

Diagnosis and resuscitation

When a patient with known cirrhosis or varices presents with massive upper gastrointestinal haemorrhage, the first priority is resuscitation. The source of haemorrhage is next sought by endoscopy. Only about half of these patients will be bleeding from oesophageal varices. The rest have bleeding gastric varices, gastric erosions, a peptic ulcer or Mallory–Weiss tears of the lower oesophagus. In this last condition, arterial bleeding is the cause and it does not respond to measures designed to treat bleeding varices, but is usually self-limiting. Whatever treatment is undertaken, it must be remembered that cirrhotic patients often have defective clotting, further exacerbated by massive haemorrhage. It is prudent to perform clotting studies and give specific corrective factors.

Treatment

If bleeding is from varices, an attempt may be made at endoscopy to band or inject them with a sclerosant (e.g. ethanolamine or sodium tetradecyl sulphate (STD)). The mainstay of initial treatment is an **infusion of vasopressin**

Table 22.1 Child's criteria for assessing operative risk in portal hypertension

Risk factor	Score points 1	2	3
Encephalopathy	None	Minimal	Marked
Ascites	None	Slight	Moderate
Bilirubin (μmol/L)	<35	36–50	<50
Albumin (g/L)	>35	28–35	>28
Prothrombin ratio	<1.4	1.4–2.0	>2.0

Each criterion is scored and the total added:
Child's grade A (good risk) scores 5–6
Grade B (moderate risk) scores 7–9
Grade C (bad risk) scores 10–15

or an analogue such as terlipressin. Octreotide has also been used successfully. More than 75% of patients initially respond to this therapy. Meanwhile, resuscitation continues with blood volume replacement, fresh-frozen plasma and platelets. Excess water and sodium should be avoided as this rapidly migrates into the peritoneal cavity as ascites. Hepatic encephalopathy should be anticipated as a result of the protein load of blood in the bowel and oral neomycin or lactulose administered. Delirium tremens may also require treatment if the patient is alcoholic.

In patients not responding to octreotide, an attempt is made to apply tamponade. After endotracheal intubation to protect the airway, a special tube is passed through the mouth into the stomach and a balloon inflated. Traction is exerted on the upper end for up to 4 hours to arrest the haemorrhage. Several varieties of tube are in use: the **Sengstaken–Blakemore tube** has separate intragastric and oesophageal balloons and depends for its action upon physiological arrest of bleeding. Most cases cease bleeding with inflation of the gastric balloon alone plus traction. The **Linton balloon** is an alternative comprising a single large intragastric balloon (300–600 ml) which allows simultaneous endoscopy and rubber banding or injection sclerotherapy of varices.

If variceal haemorrhage continues despite effective conservative therapy, transjugular intrahepatic portal-systemic stenting (**TIPS**) is sometimes used. This involves cannulating the internal jugular vein and placing an angiography catheter within the intrahepatic vena cava. Using combined fluoroscopy and ultrasound, the catheter is guided into the portal system within the liver. Then an expanding metal stent is placed to connect the intrahepatic portal system to the vena cava.

As a last resort, emergency surgical treatment is performed, but all operations carry high mortality in such seriously ill patients. The simplest operation is **transgastric oesophageal stapling**. A circular stapler is passed into the oesophagus via a gastrotomy, a ligature tied around the oesophagus between the staple cartridge and the anvil, and the gun fired. This places two rows of staples through the full thickness of the oesophageal wall, disconnecting the longitudinal veins. Operative risk in these patients has been calculated using **Child's criteria**, shown in Table 22.1.

Tumours of the stomach and small intestine

23

INTRODUCTION

Most gastric tumours are malignant: nearly all are adenocarcinomas, and the rest are lymphomas or else the occasional carcinoid tumour or sarcoma. True adenomatous **gastric polyps** are rare; most gastric polypoid lesions are small benign hyperplastic nodules.

Tumours of small bowel are rare. Of the malignant tumours, lymphomas and gastrointestinal stromal tumours (GIST) are much more common than adenocarcinomas. **Peutz–Jeghers syndrome** is a rare inherited disorder characterised by multiple benign polyps in the small bowel and perioral pigmentation plus increased risk of breast, colorectal and other cancers. Patients are fairly commonly encountered at student examinations (see Ch. 27, p. 353).

CARCINOMA OF STOMACH

PATHOLOGY OF GASTRIC CARCINOMA

Gastric carcinomas are almost exclusively adenocarcinomas. Two distinct histopathological groups are recognised, each with its own epidemiological associations. The **intestinal type** has histological features similar to intestinal epithelium. Cells grow in clumps and there is marked inflammatory infiltrate. The second variety is the **diffuse type**. Here the cells are singular, often arranged in single file and surrounded by a marked stromal reaction. Tumour cells have large intracellular **mucin** droplets which displace the nucleus to the cell periphery, giving the characteristic **signet ring appearance** (Fig. 23.1). Intestinal-type carcinomas have a better prognosis than mucin-producing signet ring carcinomas.

Gastric carcinomas develop in three morphological forms described below; the intestinal type largely produces fungating tumours and malignant ulcers, and the diffuse type causes infiltrating carcinomas:

- **Fungating tumours**—these polypoid lesions may grow to a huge size
- **Malignant ulcers**—these probably result from necrosis in broad-based solid tumours. Malignant ulcers are often larger than peptic ulcers (except for giant benign ulcers of the elderly) with a heaped-up indurated (hardened) margin
- **Infiltrating carcinomas**—this form spreads widely beneath the mucosa, and diffusely and extensively invades the muscle wall. This causes thickening and rigidity and the entire stomach contracts to a very small capacity. This is known as **linitis plastica** and its appearance likened to a 'leather bottle'. Linitis plastica affects a slightly younger age group than intestinal-type cancer and has a very poor prognosis. Diagnosis may be delayed because endoscopic changes are often subtle and standard biopsies of mucosa may not show malignancy

'**Early gastric cancer**' is defined as cancer limited to the mucosa and submucosa. This is found most often as a result of endoscopic screening or whilst investigating possible peptic ulcer. Results of surgery in this group are excellent, with a surgical cure rate of about 90%.

EPIDEMIOLOGY OF GASTRIC CARCINOMA

Gastric cancer is the fourth most common cancer in the world, causing 8% of cancers, but is the second most frequent cause of cancer deaths at 10%; its mortality is surpassed only by that of lung cancer (2008 figures). The disease is rare before the age of 50 and increases in frequency thereafter. Males have two to three times the risk of females, and the disease is more common in lower socio-economic groups. Korea has overtaken Japan in having the highest annual incidence—a crude rate of 70 per 100 000 per year in men and 27 in women (2002). In the UK, equivalent rates are 12.6 for men and 5.2 for women. The offspring of Japanese immigrants to America carry no greater risk than other Americans, evidence that environmental rather than racial factors are central in the aetiology. In much of the Western world, the incidence and death rates of gastric cancer have steadily decreased over recent years, and this is almost entirely due to a decline in the intestinal type. In Japan, the age standardised incidence for men has fallen from 80 per 100 000 per annum in 1975 to 50 in 2005.

The epidemiology gives enticing clues as to the causes of the disease. There are marked regional variations in incidence,

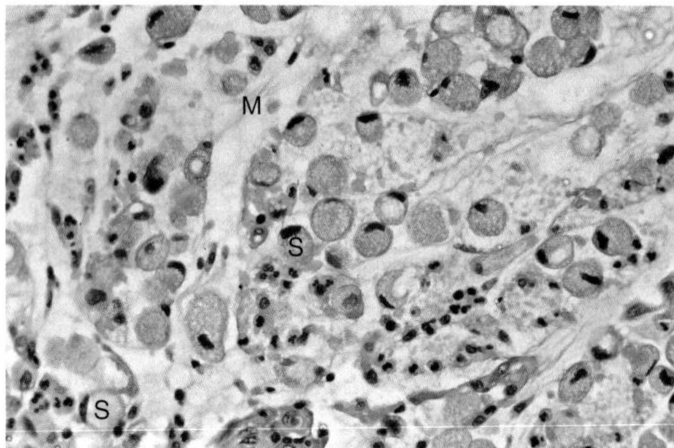

Fig. 23.1 Signet-ring carcinoma of the stomach—histopathology High-power view of typical infiltrating type of gastric carcinoma showing numerous signet ring cells **S**. This appearance is due to the presence of intracellular mucin **M**

largely explained by disparities in the rate of intestinal-type carcinomas. This, and the fact that this type is more prevalent in lower socio-economic groups, suggests that environmental factors are important in its genesis. There is probably no universal aetiological factor but rather a combination of co-factors that bring about malignant change. Japan, with its very high incidence of this disease, continues to play a leading role in research into early detection and management.

AETIOLOGY OF GASTRIC CARCINOMA AND PREMALIGNANT CONDITIONS

Atrophic gastritis

Multifocal atrophic gastritis (type B) is a condition that precedes intestinal-type gastric cancer. It probably represents one step of a sequence running from superficial gastritis, via atrophic gastritis, to intestinal and colonic metaplasia, dysplasia and eventually to cancer. Multifocal atrophic gastritis is the result of **chronic inflammation**. Risk factors for type B gastritis include *Helicobacter pylori* infection and certain items of diet. The **diffuse corporeal type of gastritis (type A)** of pernicious anaemia is a much weaker aetiological factor for cancer. Patients with this have a three- to six-fold increase in risk, but the absolute risk remains low.

Helicobacter pylori infection

H. pylori is known to initiate peptic ulceration, and chronic *H. pylori* infection has become a prime suspect for initiating intestinal-type gastric cancer. The organism can colonise gastric mucosa over long periods and cause chronic gastritis which may progress to type B multifocal atrophic gastritis. In one biopsy study of gastric cancers, *H. pylori* was found in 90% of intestinal-type cancers, whilst only 30% of the diffuse type were infected. The carcinogenic mechanism of *H. pylori* may involve alterations to the gastric acid–pepsin environment, with increased cell turnover and possibly enhanced mucosal susceptibility to ingested carcinogens. *H. pylori* eradication does not reverse gastric atrophy but does improve the enzymic and hormonal secretory capacity of the stomach. *H. pylori* also appears likely to be involved in **gastric lymphoma** of the **mucosa-associated lymphoid tissue (MALT)** type (see p. 322).

Box 23.1 Presenting features of gastric carcinoma

- Often asymptomatic until a late stage
- Non-specific epigastric pain and dyspepsia
- Iron deficiency anaemia
- Nausea and vomiting
- Anorexia and early satiety
- Feeling of abdominal fullness or discomfort
- Marked weight loss (cachexia)—late stage
- Epigastric mass (late stage)
- Left supraclavicular mass (metastasis in Virchow's node)
- Obstructive jaundice (metastases in the porta hepatis)
- Pelvic mass (metastases to ovaries)

Dietary factors

Dietary factors shown to increase the incidence of gastric cancer include excess intake of salt and nitroso compounds and a low intake of ascorbic acid. In this respect, diets high in dried and salted fish and salt-cured and smoke-cured meats appear to be a particular risk. Lettuce grown in temperate climates appears to offer some protective effect.

CLINICAL FEATURES OF GASTRIC CARCINOMA

Symptoms are often minimal until late in the course of the disease so that 70% of patients present with advanced local and/or metastatic disease. Lesions at the inlet or outlet of the stomach cause **obstructive symptoms** earlier than those elsewhere where the diameter allows for substantial growth before encroachment. Vomiting occurs if the gastric outlet becomes obstructed, typically by tumours of the antrum, and dysphagia occurs with gastro-oesophageal tumours.

In **advanced disease**, up to half the patients are asymptomatic and the rest have pain, nausea, vomiting, anorexia or a feeling of fullness after small meals (**early satiety**). Sometimes these symptoms are there months before the patient presents. **Anaemia** from chronic occult blood loss is common and one-third have positive stool tests for occult blood. One-third have **cachexia** (severe weight loss and wasting). This usually indicates metastatic disease and may be the only manifestation of cancer at the time. Of the 70% who present with advanced local disease (stage T_3), more than half have extensive abdominal nodal spread and half have distant metastases. The presenting features of gastric carcinoma are summarised in Box 23.1.

Spread of gastric cancer

Invasive gastric cancer progresses to involve submucosal lymphatics, and the depth of penetration through the gastric wall correlates closely with the likelihood of nodal metastases. The TNM system is now the standard staging structure agreed internationally, with additional Japanese nomenclature designating particular groups of lymph nodes draining the stomach as **stations**, numbered 1–16. Lymphatic metastatic spread initially involves nodes in the coeliac axis and periduodenal area; these are known as perigastric stations 1–6. Involvement of these is considered N_1 in the TNM system. Positive nodes in the para-aortic area, splenic hilum and porta hepatis indicate a more advanced stage, with porta hepatis nodes sometimes causing obstructive jaundice. Involvement of these 'secondary' stations signals N_2, N_3 or even M_1. Clearance of more distant lymph node stations is achieved by the radical R2 gastrectomy (pioneered in Japan). Node histology enhances the accuracy of TNM staging and improves the ability to predict long-term survival after surgery.

Direct spread and metastasis

- **Direct spread** into the transverse colon is not unusual in advanced cases and sometimes results in **gastro-colic fistula** formation, with true faecal vomiting
- **Transperitoneal (or transcoelomic) spread** may involve the surface of the ovaries (**Krukenberg tumour**) or form masses in the pouch of Douglas; a mass is often palpable on rectal examination
- **Remote lymph node spread**—the left supraclavicular (**Virchow's**) lymph node classically becomes invaded via the thoracic duct, giving a palpable mass (**Troisier's sign**) sometimes found at initial presentation
- **Haematogenous spread** to involve liver, lungs, brain and bone is common

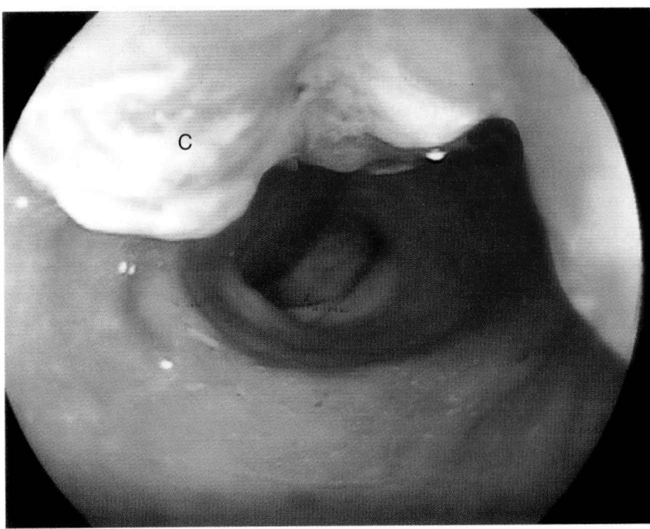

Fig. 23.2 Endoscopic view of carcinoma of the stomach
Gastroscopic view of large fungating intestinal-type carcinoma of stomach in the prepyloric region **C**. Diagnosis was confirmed by endoscopic biopsy

CASE HISTORY

Fig. 23.3 Barium meal showing linitis plastica

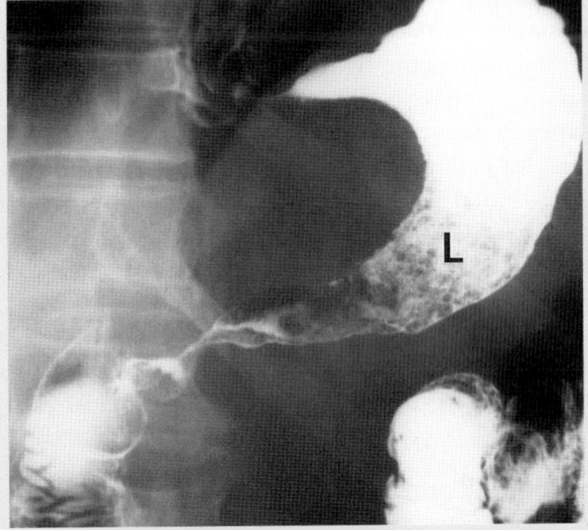

Linitis plastica-type infiltrating carcinoma of the stomach **L**. Note the shrunken appearance of the whole stomach caused by widespread submucosal invasion of the tumour. Endoscopic biopsy may not give the correct diagnosis because the mucosa is often intact. This 60-year-old woman presented with anorexia. She had a total gastrectomy but died 5 months later of widespread metastases

INVESTIGATION OF SUSPECTED GASTRIC CARCINOMA

Initial diagnosis

Early detection radically increases the chances of curing the condition. A high index of suspicion and early endoscopy for non-specific symptoms improve these chances. In one American series where early endoscopy was the rule, only 15% of gastric cancers were unsuitable for operation at initial diagnosis, and half the operations were performed with the aim of cure.

In areas with a high incidence of gastric cancer, **endoscopic screening** (Fig. 23.2) is an effective and popular method of detecting early disease. It is widely employed in Japan, with the result that over 40% of cancers operated upon after screening have been in a pre-symptomatic stage and can truly be defined histologically as 'early gastric cancer'. About 90% of these patients undergo potentially curative operations.

Barium meal used to be the standard investigation but it was difficult to differentiate between benign gastric ulcer and carcinoma. The radiological appearances of a typical gastric malignancy is shown in Figure 23.3 for historical reasons. **Endoscopy**, which allows visual inspection and biopsy, is now the standard investigation for suspected carcinoma of the stomach. The site of a lesion may be important as benign ulcers are usually found on the lesser curve or in the prepyloric area whereas carcinomas arise in any part of the stomach. The initial endoscopy in a patient found to have carcinoma gives an accurate diagnosis in 90% of those with **exophytic** lesions (where the tumour grows out into the lumen) but only 50% for **infiltrating** lesions. Multiple biopsies improve these rates, as do repeat endoscopy and re-biopsy of suspicious lesions.

Staging

Once cancer is diagnosed, knowing the stage helps determine the most appropriate treatment and whether surgery is likely to benefit the patient. **CT scanning of chest and abdomen** is often the first investigation, and many patients are found to already have local tumour invasion, lymph node involvement and hepatic metastases at this stage. If the CT scan is clear, **laparoscopy** improves the accuracy of staging, and is an important way to identify serosal involvement, omental disease and small liver metastases not seen on CT scanning. **Endoscopic ultrasonography** (EUS) via a flexible endoscope is highly accurate for determining the depth of penetration of small gastric cancers, and hence the 'T' (tumour) stage. Local spread (e.g. into pancreas), nodal involvement, left hepatic lobe metastases and ascites are also demonstrable by this method. Finally Fluorodeoxyglucose positron emission tomography (FDG-PET), known as **PET scanning**, is increasingly used to search for metastatic disease not identified by any other modality.

MANAGEMENT OF GASTRIC CARCINOMA

Like oesophageal cancer, gastric cancer is increasingly managed in specialist centres. This consolidates surgical, radiological and oncological expertise and ensures that other professionals such as anaesthetists, theatre staff, ITU/HDU staff, dieticians and physiotherapists become experienced in managing these cases and can all contribute to a multidisciplinary team (MDT).

Radical surgery

As described, metastasis from gastric cancer is often early, widespread and occult. For this reason, **radical surgery** offers the only prospect of cure even when the tumour appears small. Radical gastrectomies are very major operations and careful staging is needed to ensure that there is a realistic chance of cure, together with thorough assessment of general fitness.

Japanese surgeons have developed radical R1 and R2 gastrectomies for patients where cure is the intention. Both involve total or subtotal gastrectomy; R1 also removes local nodal stations whilst R2 removes local and secondary nodal stations. In Japan, if the cancer proves to be confined to mucosa and submucosa, 5-year survival approaches 90%; with local node involvement, survival is about 50%. With more distant spread, survival falls dramatically to 5%. Western results have not yet matched these, largely because of higher surgical complication rates.

Chemotherapy and radiotherapy

Gastric cancers respond to both chemotherapy and radiotherapy. The epirubicin–cisplatin–5-FU (ECF) regimen is effective against gastric cancer and the MAGIC trial published in 2006 improved 5-year survival from 23% for surgery alone to 36% for preoperative chemotherapy and surgery. Combined pre- and postoperative treatment is now the standard of care for resectable gastric cancer.

Radiotherapy has not been regularly used in gastric cancer but may have a place in palliation, particularly for local recurrence.

Palliative procedures

For patients with advanced cancer, it is wrong to perform heroic but ultimately ineffective surgery. Palliative surgical bypasses or local resections are rarely necessary with modern methods of palliation. If tumour bleeding, necrosis or encroachment on the gastric lumen results in distressing symptoms such as nausea, anorexia, vomiting or symptoms of anaemia, palliative chemotherapy or radiotherapy may be required. Gastric outlet obstruction may be relieved by placing a self-expanding intraluminal stent, but a laparoscopic bypass procedure may occasionally be required.

GASTRIC POLYPS

Most gastric polyps are benign **hyperplastic nodules** of gastric mucosa. They may be single or multiple and can occur anywhere in the stomach. They almost never become malignant.

Genuine **adenomatous polyps** are rare. These are true neoplasms, with histological and morphological forms similar to adenomatous polyps of the large intestine (see Ch. 27). Adenomas are usually single, large and asymptomatic. Most are found incidentally on endoscopic examination. Up to 40% show histological features of malignancy. Treatment is by endoscopic excision biopsy (**submucosal resection**).

GASTROINTESTINAL STROMAL TUMOURS (GIST)

Gastrointestinal stromal tumours are rare mesenchymal tumours that can arise anywhere in the GI tract. They were once thought to be leiomyomas because of the histological similarity but immunocytochemical markers can now distinguish mesenchymal tissue types and differentiate them from muscle and nerve tumours. GISTs have now been identified as originating from the **interstitial cells of Cajal**, the so-called 'pace-makers' of gut motility. GISTs are most frequently found in the stomach and can range from <1 cm to >20 cm. The risk of malignancy is determined partly by tumour location but mostly by size and histological mitotic index (see Table 23.1). Most gastric GISTs are small (<5 cm) and have a low mitotic index.

GISTs are often diagnosed incidentally at endoscopy. They can be sessile (domed) or pedunculated intramural lesions covered by normal mucosa (Fig. 23.4b). Small lesions may be asymptomatic; large lesions produce symptoms or signs of any abdominal mass. Gastric tumours are prone to

Table 23.1 Risk of aggressive behaviour of gastrointestinal stromal tumours (GIST)

Risk of aggressive behaviour (malignant potential)	Greatest dimension (cm)	Mitoses per 50 microscope high-power fields
Very low	<2	<5
Low	2–5	<5
Intermediate	<5	6–10
	5–10	<5
High	>5	>5
	>10	Any number
	Any size	>10

Fig. 23.4 Gastrointestinal stromal tumour

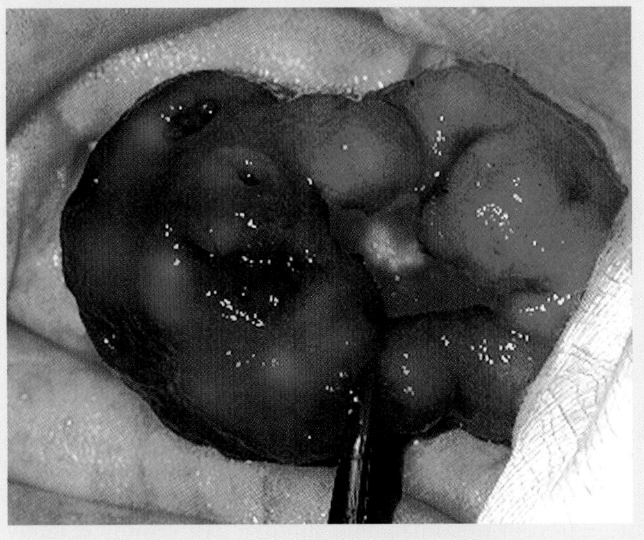

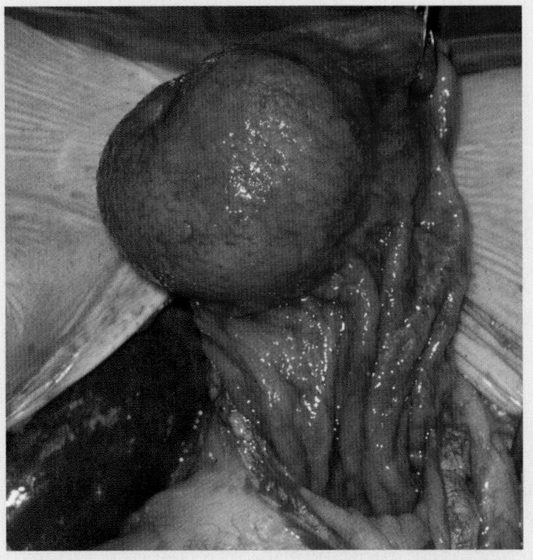

(a) This 64-year-old woman presented with recurrent iron deficiency anaemia. A large ulcerated polyp had been seen at endoscopy. Here, the stomach has been opened at laparotomy and the polyp is held up in the surgeon's hand. Deep peptic ulcers can be seen on its surface. Histologically, it proved to be a gastrointestinal stromal tumour (GIST). **(b)** Another gastrointestinal stromal tumour which had become impacted in the pylorus causing gastric outlet obstruction. It was delivered through the gastrotomy, excised and the defect closed with sutures

Fig. 23.5 Malignant gastrointestinal stromal tumour (leiomyosarcoma) of the jejunum

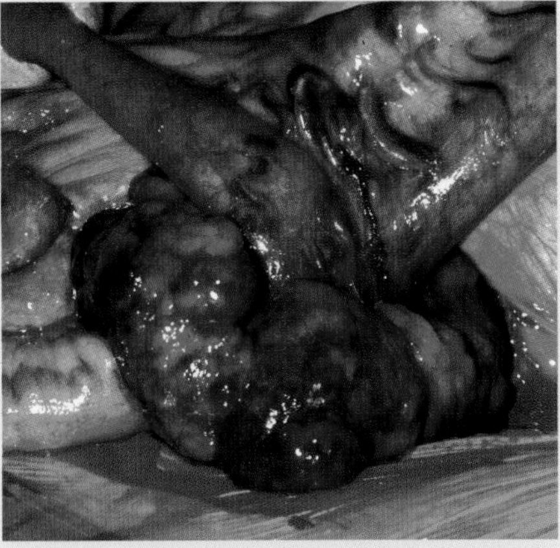

This operative specimen shows a large fleshy lesion on the outer surface of the upper jejunum. The patient was a 33-year-old woman who presented with iron deficiency anaemia refractory to oral iron. An abnormality was finally seen on a barium small bowel study after many fruitless investigations. This tumour was histologically well differentiated and amenable to resection; after 5 years, there was no recurrence

Fig. 23.6 Intussuscepting tumour of small bowel

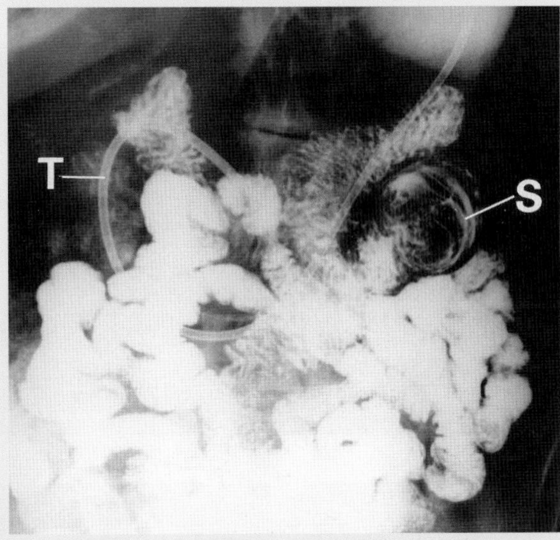

This 35-year-old woman suffered several self-limiting episodes of small bowel obstruction. During one of those episodes this small bowel barium enema was performed by placing the tip of a naso-jejunal tube **T** just distal to the duodeno-jejunal flexure and instilling barium. A small bowel intussusception is demonstrated by the 'coiled spring' sign **S**, due to the presence of barium between the telescoping layers of bowel. At surgery, a gastrointestinal stromal tumour was found to be responsible

haemorrhage via a central 'umbilicated' ulcer (Fig. 23.4a); these are typically found after an acute episode of haematemesis. Following diagnosis and before surgery, the patient may need to be staged by CT to confirm the size and exclude metastases (local, nodal or hepatic). Suitable biopsies allow immunocytochemical analysis, but it can be difficult to obtain sufficiently deep samples. Local resection is appropriate if the lesion has low malignant potential; malignant lesions require full oncological clearance as for other gastric cancers.

GIST tumours are highly resistant to traditional chemotherapy; however, the c-kit tyrosine kinase inhibitor imatinib (Glivec) is highly effective for advanced and metastatic disease and has improved 2-year survival rates to 75–80%.

Small bowel gastrointestinal stromal tumours

GISTs of small bowel are histologically similar to gastric tumours but may present by obstructing the lumen or growing out from the serosal surface of the bowel (Fig. 23.5). Primary resection and anastomosis is the usual treatment and survival is influenced by the size and mitotic counts.

GASTRIC AND SMALL BOWEL LYMPHOMAS

PATHOLOGY AND CLINICAL FEATURES OF LYMPHOMAS

Primary lymphomas sometimes arise in the stomach or small bowel. They constitute about 10% of gastric malignancies. As with peptic ulcer and intestinal-type gastric adenocarcinoma, *H. pylori* infection is an important initiating factor. In non-Hodgkin lymphoma, small bowel lymphoid tissue may become involved.

In the stomach, most lymphomas are non-Hodgkin lymphomas of B-cell origin. They may become extensive, diffusely infiltrating the stomach wall or, less often, projecting into the lumen as bulky ulcerating masses. The symptoms and endoscopic appearances closely resemble gastric adenocarcinoma but recognising lymphoma is important because the treatment is very different and the prognosis much better. Unlike gastric carcinoma, lymphomas tend to occur in children and young adults. Some cases of low-grade lymphoma involving the mucosa-associated lymphoid tissue or 'MALToma' have been reported to resolve following *Helicobacter* eradication, but this is only successful if the disease is detected early.

In the small intestine, lymphomas also produce bulky lesions which may obstruct, ulcerate, bleed or even perforate. Occasionally, a lymphoma provides the focus for an intussusception (see Figs 23.6 and 23.7 and also Fig. 50.12, p. 624). Small bowel lymphoma may be a complication of coeliac disease but the risk is only about six times higher than for the general population.

MANAGEMENT OF LYMPHOMAS

Gastric lymphomas are usually treated with primary chemotherapy using the CHOP regimen, sometimes with the addition of rituximab, and subtotal gastrectomy is rarely needed unless the tumour bleeds persistently or perforates. Primary **small bowel** lymphomas are often localised lesions, amenable to surgical excision. Postoperative radiotherapy or chemotherapy or both may be necessary. Treatment gives a 5-year survival rate of around 50%.

CASE HISTORY

Fig. 23.7 Intussuscepting tumour of small bowel

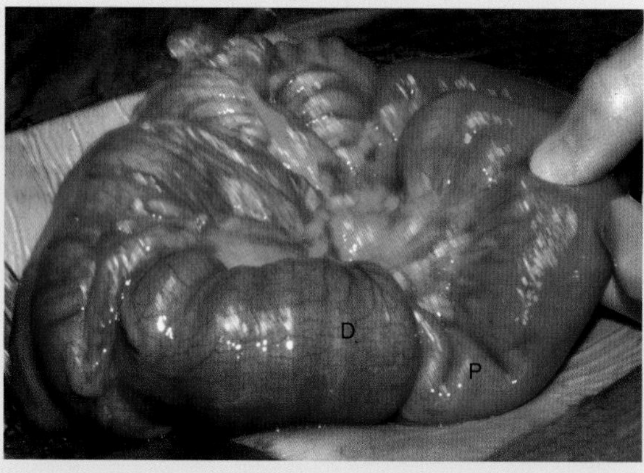

(a)

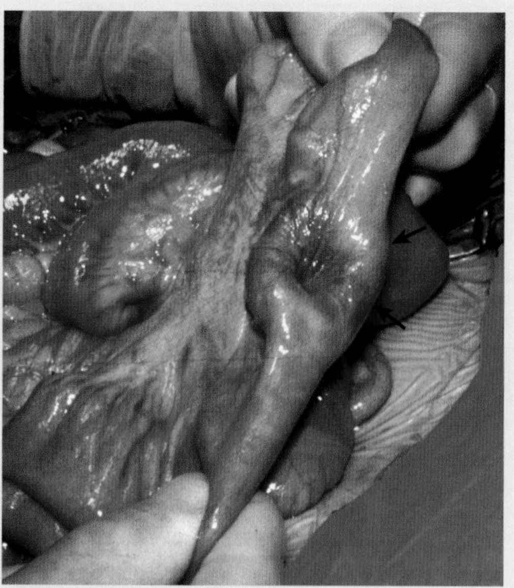

(b)

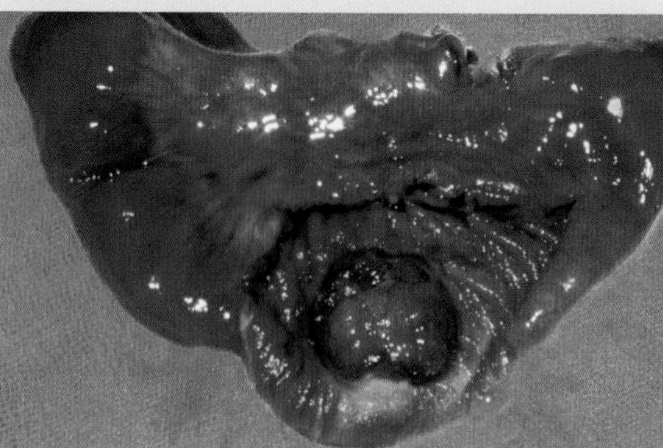

(c)

This 22-year-old man presented with small bowel obstruction. At laparotomy, the obstruction was found to be caused by an ileo-ileal intussusception. This set of operative photographs **(a)** shows how the proximal ileum **P** had intussuscepted into the distal ileum **D**. When this was reduced **(b)**, an abnormality of the bowel wall could be seen to have formed the apex of the intussuscipiens (arrowed). In **(c)**, a polypoid tumour **P** can be seen on the luminal surface, which proved histologically to be a lymphoma

CARCINOID TUMOURS

PATHOLOGY OF CARCINOID TUMOURS

Carcinoid tumours probably arise from APUD cells of the GI endocrine system. Thus, they can arise anywhere in the GI tract or in tissues embryologically derived from it including the pancreas and biliary system. More than 50% of carcinoid tumours are found in the appendix, and most of the rest occur in the small intestine.

CLINICAL PRESENTATION OF CARCINOID TUMOURS

Appendiceal carcinoid tumours are usually discovered incidentally in appendicectomy specimens and virtually always remain small and benign. In contrast, carcinoid tumours elsewhere spread locally in the bowel and mesentery, later becoming disseminated to the liver and other sites. The bowel lesions themselves usually present with symptoms of partial or complete obstruction.

Carcinoid tumours secrete a variety of catecholamines, including **serotonin**. When there is a large volume of tumour, usually in the form of liver metastases, enough catecholamines are secreted to cause the **carcinoid syndrome**. This is characterised by an array of clinical phenomena including transient 'hot flushes', hypotension, asthma and diarrhoea. A metabolite of serotonin, **5-hydroxy-indoleacetic acid** (5-HIAA), can be measured in the urine as a diagnostic marker.

MANAGEMENT OF CARCINOID TUMOURS

Treatment usually involves excising the primary lesion along with local lymph nodes. An appendiceal carcinoid present at the tip only and less than 2 cm in diameter can be treated by simple appendicectomy. In patients with metastatic disease, the condition progresses very slowly. It responds well to surgery, and in the typical young patient a more radical approach can be recommended than for other intra-abdominal malignancies. Metastatic carcinoid is not curable by radiotherapy or chemotherapy.

The full carcinoid syndrome is usually associated with large volume hepatic metastases. It is uncommon and symptoms can be controlled with the help of drugs such as **octreotide**, a somatostatin analogue. Radiotherapy is useful if pain is caused by massive liver enlargement as it may induce some shrinkage.

OTHER TUMOURS OF THE SMALL INTESTINE

Small bowel tumours include **solitary benign angiomas**. These are usually found incidentally at operation or autopsy but sometimes present with intussusception or chronic haemorrhage.

Adenocarcinomas do occur in the small intestine, especially in the duodenum, but are rare compared with stomach and large bowel. Small bowel adenocarcinomas present with bowel obstruction, biliary obstruction when in the periampullary region, bleeding or symptoms of metastases. Barium follow-through examination for chronic symptoms may demonstrate the lesion, but more commonly it is found and resected at a laparotomy for acute obstruction, only being recognised on histological examination. Unfortunately, metastasis to regional lymph nodes or the liver has already occurred in many patients by the time of presentation.

Peutz–Jeghers syndrome is described in Chapter 27 (p. 353).

24 Tumours of the pancreas and hepatobiliary system; the spleen

INTRODUCTION

More than 90% of pancreatic cancers are adenocarcinomas derived from exocrine ductal cells. These have the worst survival of all GI malignancies, with only about 12% surviving 1 year and 2% surviving 5 years. Much less commonly, neoplasia arises from **exocrine acinar (secretory) cells** (2%) or from **endocrine islet cells** (8%). Most endocrine tumours present with excess hormone secretion, e.g. insulin, glucagon or gastrin. Around 90% of insulinomas are benign but most others are malignant, although survival is often prolonged.

Ductal adenocarcinoma typically presents late, with intractable abdominal pain, weight loss and obstructive jaundice caused by common bile duct compression, also a frequent presentation of the uncommon **periampullary carcinomas**. These include biliary cholangiocarcinomas and adenocarcinomas of the ampulla of Vater and duodenum.

Primary sclerosing cholangitis (PSC) is a rare, non-malignant liver disease involving inflammatory fibrosis of bile ducts. It presents similarly to pancreatic cancer and is therefore included in this chapter. The uncommon **carcinoma of gall bladder** often presents with cholecystitis symptoms, with jaundice developing later.

Primary liver tumours are rare in developed countries but common in some developing countries, where hepatitis B and C are the main predisposing factors. **Secondary liver tumours** are common everywhere from haematogenous spread of many types of cancer. Surgical disorders of the spleen are covered at the end of this chapter.

CARCINOMA OF THE PANCREAS

PATHOLOGY

This is usually an adenocarcinoma arising from cells lining the ducts. About 80% arise in the head (the largest part) and 20% in the body or tail. Cancers often form a well-differentiated ductular pattern but despite this, it is a highly malignant tumour. It metastasises early to lymph nodes, to peritoneum, and to liver via the portal vein (see Fig. 24.1). At presentation, less than 20% are resectable and the overall prognosis is dire.

Pancreatic cancer presents at a mean age of 65 and is rare under 50. The incidence is similar in males and females, and in the Western world, ranks equal third with oesophageal cancer among GI cancers, after large bowel and stomach. In absolute numbers it is uncommon, being responsible for about 7000 deaths each year in the UK, although numbers in developed countries continue to rise. Risk factors include cigarette smoking (2–3 times the risk and presenting 15 years earlier), chronic pancreatitis (18 times risk, increasing to over 50 times in hereditary pancreatitis), obesity/type II diabetes (twice the risk), and positive family history.

CLINICAL FEATURES OF DUCTAL PANCREATIC CARCINOMA

There are no useful screening tests and so pancreatic cancer nearly always presents with symptoms and signs. The main features are substantial weight loss (80%), abdominal pain (60%) and obstructive jaundice (50%). Ascites and an abdominal mass are uncommon (Box 24.1).

Pain and other abdominal symptoms and signs

The **pain** of advanced pancreatic carcinoma is severe and continuous and typically described as 'deep' and 'gnawing'; it may drive patients to suicide. It is often nocturnal and poorly relieved by analgesics but sometimes alleviated by leaning forwards from sitting ('the pancreatic position'). Severe pain usually represents locally advanced disease with extrapancreatic invasion into retroperitoneal nerves around the coeliac axis. There are often ill-defined **dyspeptic symptoms** such as anorexia, nausea or sporadic vomiting and usually profound **weight loss**.

Obstructive jaundice

Jaundice, often without pain early on, develops over several weeks, and is associated with pale stools and dark urine. These clinical features are dramatic and never ignored. The jaundice is caused by common bile duct compression in its course through the pancreatic head. As a result, the proximal bile duct dilates and the gall bladder may become palpable (**Courvoisier's law**, see Ch. 18, p. 259). Bile duct obstruction may

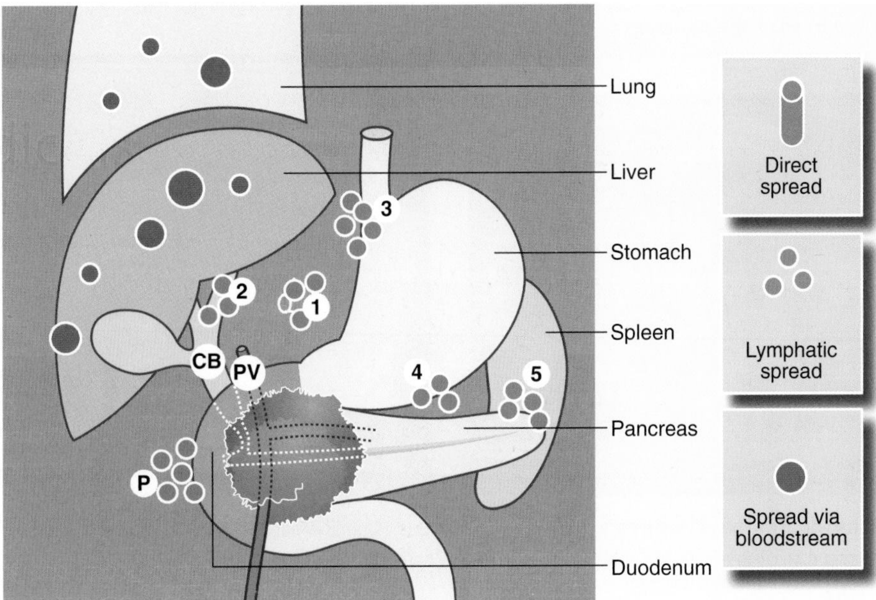

Fig. 24.1 Spread of carcinoma of the pancreas
Direct spread may involve the common bile duct **CB** where it traverses the pancreas, the duodenum and the portal vein **PV**. Lymphatic spread may reach the paraduodenal peritoneum **P** and the nodes of the coeliac axis **1**, the porta hepatis **2**, the lesser and greater curves of the stomach **3**, **4** and the hilum of the spleen **5**. Spread may also occur via the bloodstream to the liver, lungs, etc.

Box 24.1 Presenting features of pancreatic carcinoma

Common presenting features

- Substantial weight loss (about 80% of cases)
- Abdominal pain (about 60%)
- Obstructive jaundice, often without pain (about 50%)

Less common presenting features

- Acute pancreatitis (rare)
- Diabetes mellitus (preceding or following diagnosis)
- Gastric outlet obstruction (due to external compression)
- Thrombophlebitis migrans (recurrent superficial venous thromboses)
- Pancreatic steatorrhoea (due to pancreatic duct obstruction)

Box 24.2 Investigation of suspected pancreatic carcinoma

If patient jaundiced—suspect diagnosis from age, typical history, signs, liver function tests

If patient not jaundiced—suspect diagnosis on abnormal ultrasound or CT (differential diagnosis is often pancreatitis)

- **Primary imaging**—usually CT scan
- **Confirm histology**—CT-guided biopsy, endoscopic ultrasound-guided needle aspiration cytology
- **Assess primary tumour in detail**—site, size, local invasion especially of blood vessels using ultrasound, high-definition CT
- **Assess metastatic spread**—liver, nodes, peritoneum using CT, laparoscopy, ± laparoscopic ultrasound

also be caused by metastases in porta hepatis lymph nodes. Liver metastases alone rarely cause jaundice.

Note that pancreatic cancer and other obstructing biliary tumours typically produce a painless and progressive jaundice. In contrast, that of gallstone disease is less intense and fluctuates in intensity, and there is usually typical biliary pain.

APPROACH TO INVESTIGATION OF SUSPECTED PANCREATIC CARCINOMA (Box 24.2)

A patient with obstructive jaundice should be investigated as described in Chapter 18, p. 258. If pancreatic cancer is likely, optimum management is via a streamlined diagnostic pathway carried out in a specialised, high-volume pancreatic centre.

When investigations are complete, the multidisciplinary team considers whether curative treatment is feasible and how to plan and implement it, or if not appropriate, what palliative treatment is needed.

CT and ultrasound imaging

Ultrasound seeks masses in pancreas and liver, dilated bile ducts and stones in the gall bladder (abdominal ultrasound is unreliable for common bile duct stones). Additional detail about a mass comes from high-resolution CT scans, ideally before ERCP to ensure an artefact-free field. CT can show tumour extent and the presence and volume of liver metastases. It can demonstrate **vascular invasion** of superior mesenteric and portal veins, and superior mesenteric artery and coeliac axis, any of which lessen the feasibility of surgical resection. The extent of primary and/or metastatic disease on imaging may indicate the tumour is **inoperable** (i.e. not

Fig. 24.2 Carcinoma of the head of the pancreas

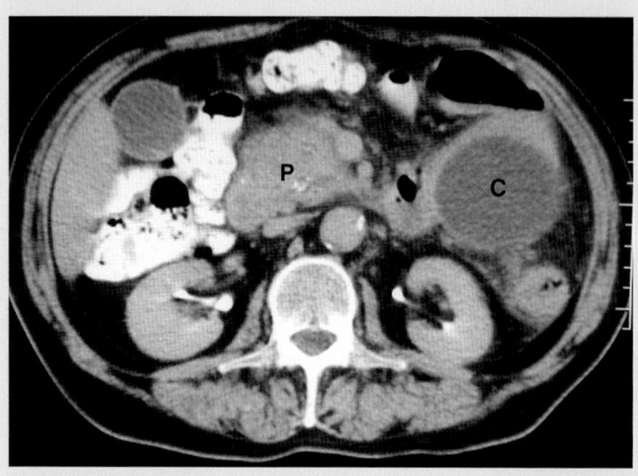

(a)

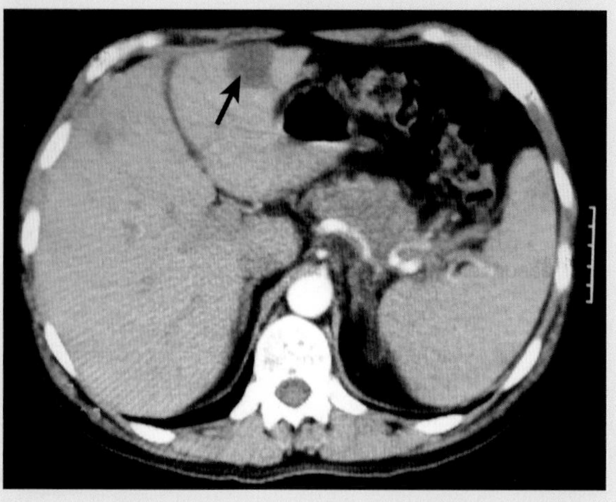

(b)

(a) CT scan showing enlargement of the head of the pancreas **P** most suspicious of carcinoma. The dark circular lesion within the tail of the pancreas is a secondary cyst or pseudocyst **C.** **(b)** CT scan further cephalad (towards the head) of the same patient showing one obvious low-attenuation lesion in the liver consistent with a metastasis (arrowed). The diagnosis of carcinoma of the pancreas was confirmed on percutaneous biopsy of the pancreatic lesion. Thus this 54-year-old man had inoperable disease. Unfortunately, this is all too common a presentation

resectable with intent to cure). Palliation can then be employed and the patient saved a fruitless attempt at resection.

Endoscopic ultrasound (EUS) and needle aspiration cytology

Where ultrasound and/or CT indicate a pancreatic head carcinoma may be resectable, **endoscopic ultrasound** can give added detail. In this, an ultrasound probe is positioned in the second part of the duodenum via a gastroscope. This allows precise examination of the pancreatic head and associated vessels as well as duodenum and ampullary region. Ultrasound-guided **needle aspiration** sampling of suspicious lesions can be performed via the gastric lumen for cytology, either before surgery or to guide oncological management. Endoscopic ultrasound is the gold standard for assessing tumour size, site and vascular involvement and thus potential operability. However, its accuracy is severely impaired if a stent has already been placed to relieve jaundice.

Magnetic resonance cholangio-pancreatography (MRCP)

In biliary obstruction, MRCP produces images similar to ERCP in diagnostic usefulness but is particularly useful for confirming choledocholithiasis (bile duct stones) or for obstructive lesions of the bile duct itself such as cholangiocarcinoma or primary sclerosing cholangitis.

Endoscopic retrograde cholangio-pancreatography (ERCP) and therapeutic intervention

ERCP is now largely employed for therapeutic intervention. For obstructive jaundice due to stone, ERCP is the main mechanism for removing duct stones. For inoperable carcinoma of the pancreatic head, placing a tubular stent across the obstruction allows palliation of jaundice by draining the biliary tree. Plastic stents eventually become encrusted and occluded so wider bore expanding metallic stents are more often employed.

Lesions in the body and tail of the pancreas

When pancreatic cancer is suspected in a non-jaundiced patient, abdominal CT can confirm the diagnosis more reliably than ultrasound, although small tumours may be missed (see Fig. 24.2a and b). CT scanning also indicates retroperitoneal and portal vein invasion; it shows metastases in liver and lymph nodes and CT-guided needle biopsy can obtain histopathology specimens, all of which can determine resectability. CT scanning can understage the disease, chiefly because it does not detect small-volume hepatic and peritoneal deposits.

Endoscopic ultrasound via the stomach can examine the pancreatic body and tail and allow aspiration cytology. Cancers here do not cause the early warning sign of jaundice and hence tend to present so late resectability is highly unlikely.

Staging laparoscopy may be included as a final evaluation before resection, allowing inspection and biopsy of peritoneum for small metastases; diagnostic laparoscopic ultrasound has largely been superseded by high-definition CT and endoscopic ultrasound. Accurate staging means resection can be offered to those most likely to benefit, whilst avoiding unnecessary surgery in the rest.

Cystic neoplasms of the pancreas

Cystic neoplasms are sometimes discovered incidentally on CT or ultrasonography, with the investigation prompted by non-specific upper abdominal symptoms. Cystic neoplasms can be difficult to differentiate from pancreatic pseudocysts but CT and endoluminal ultrasound (EUS) can define morphology and allow aspiration for cytology and biochemical analysis (e.g. CEA, CA19.9 and amylase). After excluding pseudocyst, the differential diagnosis includes **serous and mucinous cystadenomas** and **cystadenocarcinomas**. Radical resection is recommended for most since all cystic neoplasms may have malignant potential and are largely curable if treated early. If EUS-guided aspiration reveals a **serous lesion** without adverse radiological or biochemical features, observation by 'watchful waiting' may be an option, but the presence of mucus identifies a **mucinous pancreatic lesion** with greater malignant potential which should be resected.

MANAGEMENT OF PANCREATIC CARCINOMA

Surgical resection and adjuvant therapy

It is an unfortunate truth that most patients with pancreatic cancer present at an incurable stage. Only about 15–20% have apparently localised disease with a potential for surgical cure. **Whipple's operation** (pancreatico-duodenectomy, see Fig. 24.6, p. 330) is the standard type of operation where resection of the pancreatic head is indicated. It is a major undertaking with high operative morbidity and mortality; even in specialist centres, mortality is 1–2% with a 15–20% morbidity (pancreatic leaks, delayed gastric emptying, wound infections) and a 5-year survival of only 15–20%.

Postoperative chemotherapy with 5-fluorouracil (5FU) or gemcitabine confers a modest survival advantage. Clinical trials investigating the role of chemo-radiation, neoadjuvant therapy and immunotherapy are ongoing but prospects for cure remain poor.

Palliation of pancreatic cancer

When there is obvious widespread disease, the patient should be allowed to die with minimal surgical interference but with careful attention to symptom control. Good analgesia is fundamental; severe pain can often be relieved by permanent **coeliac ganglion blockade**, performed percutaneously. **Obstructive jaundice** can usually be relieved by inserting a biliary stent at ERCP. If unsuccessful, a percutaneous transhepatic cholangiogram (PTC) can help pass a guide-wire to the duodenum to facilitate ERCP or else place a stent from above; techniques are illustrated in Figure 24.3. Surgical bypass (usually a **'triple bypass'**, see Fig. 24.3) may provide longer-lasting relief from jaundice and duodenal obstruction than stenting. Duodenal obstruction alone can be bypassed by endoscopic stent placement or laparoscopic gastroenterostomy.

ENDOCRINE TUMOURS OF THE PANCREAS

Neuroendocrine cells of the islets of Langerhans give rise to several uncommon tumours. These often produce excess hormone secretions responsible for the presenting features. Islet cells make up 2% of the pancreatic mass and comprise cells of four types: **alpha cells** secrete glucagon, **beta cells** secrete insulin, **delta cells** secrete somatostatin and **F** or **PP cells** secrete pancreatic polypeptide.

INSULINOMAS (Fig. 24.4)

The most common endocrine tumours are **insulinomas** derived from beta cells, but they occur in only 1.7 per million people per year. The main symptoms are cerebral disturbances caused by hypoglycaemic attacks, often when fasting or exercising and relieved by oral or intravenous glucose. About 90% of insulinomas are single and 90% are benign and amenable to curative resection. They occur with equal frequency in the head, body and tail of the pancreas. Malignancy is only diagnosed if metastases appear.

The diagnosis is usually made late, often after hypoglycaemic attacks have caused accusations of alcoholism or referrals for psychiatric or neurological advice for abnormal behaviour or epilepsy. When inappropriate hyperinsulinaemia has been confirmed, CT scanning, MRI and endoscopic ultrasound usually identify the lesion. If unsuccessful, venous sampling may help and intraoperative ultrasound can usually locate otherwise invisible lesions. Insulinomas are usually small and can be treated by enucleation although larger or deep lesions may need pancreatic resection.

GLUCAGONOMAS

Alpha cells may give rise to **glucagonomas**; these are very rare and present with diabetes mellitus and a characteristic skin rash known as **migratory necrolytic erythema**.

GASTRINOMAS

Gastrin-secreting tumours (**gastrinomas**) occur once per million people per year. They arise in pancreatic islets or in ectopic cells in the duodenal wall. About 25% occur in patients with multiple endocrine neoplasia type 1 (MEN 1), described below. Gastrinomas cause severe and intractable peptic ulceration and diarrhoea known as **Zollinger–Ellison syndrome**.

The diagnosis is made by demonstrating persistently high serum gastrin. The tumour is localised by CT, MRI or endoscopic ultrasound, or in difficult cases using somatostatin receptor scintigraphy (SRS). Many lesions are too small to show on standard imaging and can only be located by intraoperative ultrasonography at laparotomy. About 60% are malignant but they grow slowly and metastasise late, so excision is often curative. If the primary tumour is inoperable, palliation with high-dose **proton pump inhibitors (PPIs)** often prevents peptic ulcer symptoms and complications.

MULTIPLE ENDOCRINE NEOPLASIA SYNDROMES (MEN)

Pancreatic neuroendocrine tumours sometimes occur in inherited autosomal dominant multiple endocrine neoplasia syndromes (MEN). Two main types are recognised, MEN 1 and MEN 2:

- MEN 1—islet cell tumours, pituitary adenomas and parathyroid hyperplasia
- MEN 2a—medullary thyroid carcinoma (often in childhood), phaeochromocytoma and parathyroid adenoma or hyperplasia
- MEN 2b—medullary thyroid carcinoma, phaeochromocytoma, mucosal and gastrointestinal neurofibromas and Marfanoid habitus

BILIARY AND PERIAMPULLARY TUMOURS

Adenocarcinomas originating from biliary duct epithelium are known as **cholangiocarcinomas**. They develop anywhere in the intra- or extrahepatic duct system but are more common near the confluence of right and left hepatic ducts ('Klatskin' tumour). The less common **intrahepatic**

Fig. 24.3 Palliative procedures for obstructive jaundice caused by carcinoma of the head of the pancreas or a periampullary tumour

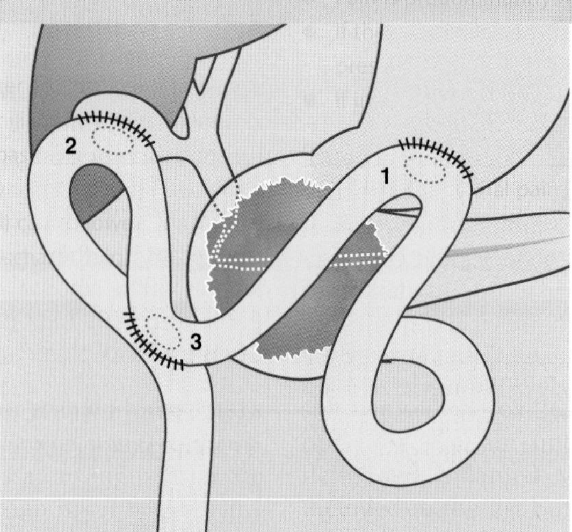

(a) Endoscopic stent placement. The sphincter of Oddi may require a preliminary endoscopic sphincterotomy prior to intubation. A self-retaining plastic stent, placed endoscopically or percutaneously, lies in situ across the biliary stricture. Note the 'pig-tail' ends of this type of stent which curl up when the wire is removed, retaining the stent in the correct position. **(b)** Triple bypass operation, less commonly performed nowadays because of the efficacy of endoscopic stenting and the short life expectancy of patients with pancreatic cancer

cholangiocarcinomas present like primary hepatocellular carcinomas but most of the biliary system remains patent so jaundice is rare. In contrast, **extrahepatic cholangiocarcinomas** usually obstruct bile drainage and present with painless progressive jaundice. Cholangiocarcinomas are more frequent in **primary sclerosing cholangitis**. Distinguishing cholangiocarcinoma from the hallmark multiple strictures of sclerosing cholangitis can be taxing.

Cholangiocarcinomas have a dense fibrous stroma and grow along ducts rather than producing focal proliferative lesions. The resulting smooth elongated stricture can be demonstrated by ERCP, MRCP or transhepatic cholangiography (see Fig. 24.5). Histological proof of malignancy may be elusive owing to the fibrous nature of the tumour. Unlike pancreatic cancer, cholangiocarcinomas are often slow-growing and metastasise late. Despite this, lymph node involvement at presentation is common, and extension along bile ducts and involvement of portal vein and hepatic arterial branches results in a low operability rate and an even lower long-term survival. Radical procedures combining partial hepatectomy with excision of the involved biliary tree and 'en bloc' portal vein resection and reconstruction may

CASE HISTORY

Fig. 24.4 Insulinoma as seen on a selective arteriogram (subtraction film)

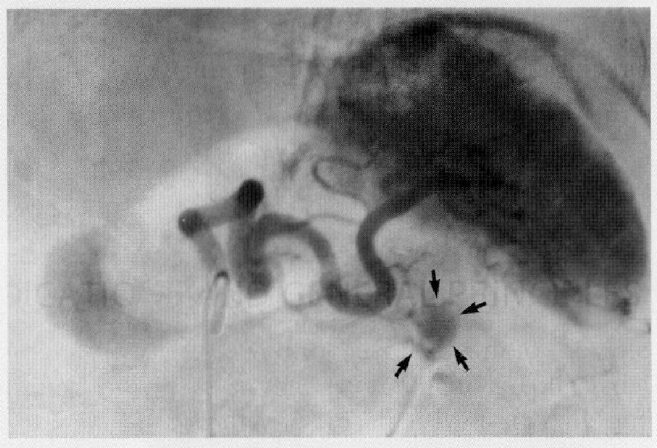

This 31-year-old woman suffered from bouts of faintness which proved to be caused by intermittent hypoglycaemia. Selective splenic arteriography demonstrated an abnormal mass of blood vessels about 1.5 cm in diameter (arrowed) in the tail of the pancreas representing an insulinoma. The tail of the pancreas was excised and the patient's symptoms disappeared

CASE HISTORY

Fig. 24.5 Cholangiocarcinoma

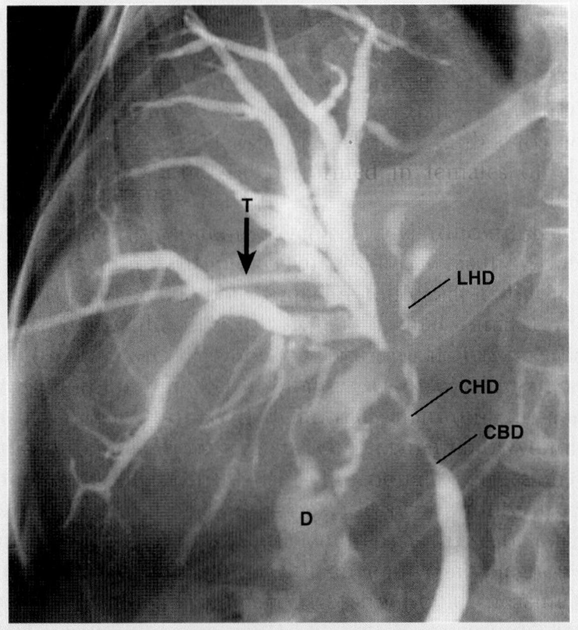

Percutaneous transhepatic cholangiogram in a 66-year-old man with painless progressive jaundice from an inoperable cholangiocarcinoma; this X-ray shows a long stricture of the common bile duct **CBD**, common hepatic duct **CHD** and left hepatic duct **LHD**. Some contrast has flowed through into the duodenum. The cystic duct is obliterated, preventing filling of the gall bladder. A percutaneous drainage tube **T** has been inserted into the right hepatic duct system prior to an attempt to place a stent across the stricture by the same route. Some contrast has flowed through into the duodenum **D**. Nowadays, most stents are placed endoscopically (see Fig. 24.3)

offer better clearance and improved survival for selected patients.

An unusual lesion is adenocarcinoma of the ampulla of Vater. Here it forms a polypoid lesion projecting into the duodenum and obstructing biliary drainage causing jaundice. Tumours are friable and bleed persistently, giving positive faecal occult bloods. An association with intestinal polyposis syndromes has been described. Diagnosis is made at endoscopy by inspection and biopsy. Very rarely, adenocarcinoma arises in the duodenal mucosa and causes obstructive jaundice if close to the ampulla. Again, the lesion is readily diagnosed at ERCP and biopsy.

MANAGEMENT OF EXTRAHEPATIC CHOLANGIOCARCINOMA AND PERIAMPULLARY CARCINOMA

Extrahepatic and periampullary cancers can often be successfully treated by Whipple's pancreatico-duodenectomy, Figure 24.6. Operative morbidity and mortality are similar to the operation for pancreatic cancer, but the prognosis is often better because the obstructing tumour is usually small, with less extensive spread.

CARCINOMA OF THE GALL BLADDER

Carcinoma of the gall bladder is a disease of old age and is nearly always associated with stones. Chronic inflammation is the likely carcinogenic factor. Early diagnosis is usually made incidentally at cholecystectomy and in this special case, wide excision of the gall bladder bed plus hilar lymphadenectomy may offer a chance of cure. In most, the diagnosis is late with advanced disease and jaundice. Direct invasion of liver plus lymphatic spread make resection impracticable and survival is usually short.

PRIMARY SCLEROSING CHOLANGITIS

Primary sclerosing cholangitis (PSC) is a rare condition, probably of autoimmune origin, causing progressive fibrosis and multiple biliary strictures. Luminal narrowing causes gradual and progressive obstructive jaundice and, later, secondary cirrhosis. It may arise sporadically but often occurs in long-standing ulcerative colitis. Bile duct stenosis is usually diffuse, with a characteristic ERCP appearance (see Fig. 24.7), but just occasionally it is localised to the extrahepatic biliary system. Here the radiological appearance is indistinguishable from cholangiocarcinoma, causing a diagnostic predicament. Management is by endoscopic dilatation of clinically significant strictures and prescribing choleretic drugs to improve bile flow. In advanced cases, liver transplantation is an option; interestingly, up to a third demonstrate cholangiocarcinoma in the excised liver.

LIVER TUMOURS AND ABSCESSES

Primary malignant liver tumours are uncommon in developed countries; most are **hepatocellular carcinomas** derived from hepatocytes. Even less commonly, other elements give rise to tumours such as **angiosarcoma**. Benign liver lesions

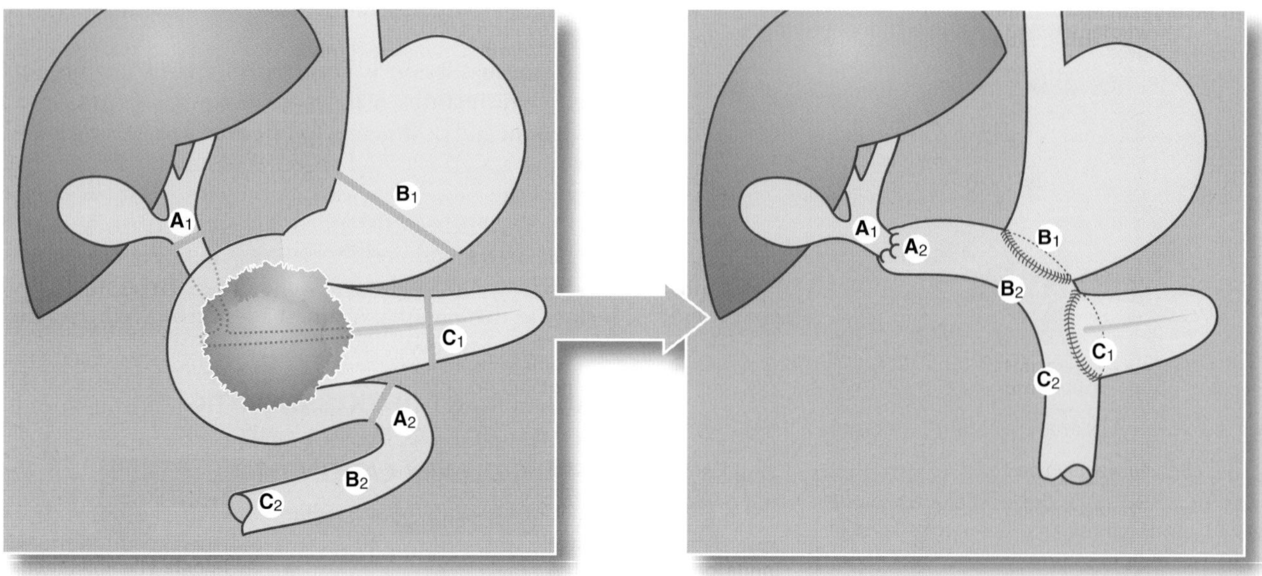

Fig. 24.6 Whipple's operation (pancreatico-duodenectomy)
(a) Structures are divided at the lines A_1, A_2, B_1, C_1. **(b)** The distal half of the stomach, the entire duodenal loop, the head and body of the pancreas and the lower end of the common bile duct are all removed, then reconstruction is performed with anastomoses between A_1 and A_2, B_1 and B_2 and C_1 and C_2

CASE HISTORY

Fig. 24.7 Primary sclerosing cholangitis (PSC)

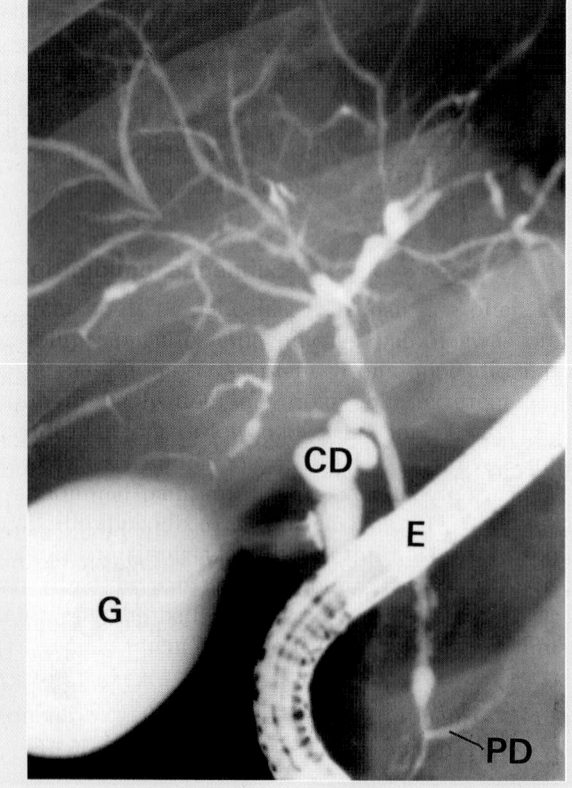

ERCP in a 52-year-old man with longstanding ulcerative colitis who developed painless jaundice. There is widespread irregular narrowing of both the intrahepatic and extrahepatic bile ducts typical of sclerosing cholangitis. Note the endoscope **E**, the normal gall bladder **G** and the cystic duct **CD** filling with contrast. The proximal part of the pancreatic duct **PD** also contains contrast

are increasingly found incidentally during ultrasound for gallstones. The most frequent are benign cysts and haemangiomas which need no treatment.

More rarely, benign solid areas of **focal nodular hyperplasia (FNH)** are discovered. These are more prevalent in women and often associated with the oral contraceptive pill. Other benign solid lesions include **hepatic adenomas**. Focal nodular hyperplasia is much more common than adenoma (ratio of 9 : 1) but adenoma may lead to hepatoma so most liver surgeons recommend resection whilst hyperplasia can safely be left. Both look similar on imaging, but focal nodular hyperplasia may have a characteristic central scar.

LIVER ABSCESSES

These usually present symptomatically with pyrexia, malaise and upper abdominal pain or tenderness. The most important cause worldwide is **amoebiasis**; about 10% of the world population is chronically infected with *Entamoeba histolytica*. Simple pyogenic abscesses can arise from biliary infection (e.g. ascending cholangitis), through the portal venous system (e.g. appendix or diverticular abscess) or generalised bacteraemia (e.g. endocarditis). Most liver abscesses are managed effectively with combined radiological drainage and long-course antimicrobial therapy. The key exception is **hydatid cysts** arising from *Echinococcus* infection, a zoonosis transmitted through contact with dogs or sheep. Draining hydatid cysts carries a serious risk of peritoneal dissemination and anaphylaxis, so complete surgical excision is undertaken with cover from an antihelminthic agent such as mebendazole.

HEPATOCELLULAR CARCINOMA

Hepatocellular carcinomas (also known as **hepatomas**) are malignant, slowly-growing tumours that often arise multicentrically and synchronously throughout the liver.

Hepatocellular carcinoma is the sixth most prevalent cancer worldwide and the third cause of cancer-related death. More than 700 000 cases were diagnosed in 2008 so it represents a substantial global burden. Unusually for malignancy, an aetiological factor can be identified in nearly all cases; factors include infection with hepatitis B and especially hepatitis C, alcoholic cirrhosis, haemochromatosis and chronic active hepatitis. Around 80–90% have some form of pre-existing cirrhosis. In developed countries, **alcoholic cirrhosis** and non-alcoholic fatty liver disease (associated with the metabolic syndrome) are the usual aetiological factors; indeed, hepatoma occurs in about 25% of patients with cirrhosis of more than 5 years' standing. The risk in patients with **haemochromatosis** and **chronic active hepatitis** is even higher.

Hepatocellular carcinoma is very common in parts of Africa and the Far East. Here the usual cause is hepatitis B-induced cirrhosis, but environmental carcinogens have also been implicated including **aflatoxin** from *Aspergillus* growing on stored grains and peanuts. Various **parasitic infestations**, e.g. schistosomiasis, *Echinococcus* (tapeworm) and *Clonorchis sinensis* (liver fluke), also predispose to it. In developed countries, the peak incidence is between the ages of 40 and 60, but in developing countries, most cases occur between 20 and 40.

Clinical features and management of hepatocellular carcinoma

The presenting features are anorexia, weight loss, abdominal pain and distension, often with jaundice and ascites, plus non-abdominal stigmata of cirrhosis. A liver mass may be palpable. Multiple modality imaging, combining ultrasound, CT or MRI scanning (along with markedly elevated α-fetoprotein) can establish the diagnosis and delineate the size and position of the liver mass or masses. Radiologically guided needle biopsy is used for indeterminate lesions but has a false negative rate of 30–40% and so a negative result should not rule out malignancy.

By the time of initial diagnosis, carcinoma is usually widespread in the liver, rendering curative resection impossible. However, in developed countries, asymptomatic tumours are often discovered incidentally, allowing potentially curative therapeutic intervention. Occasionally, small lesions are resectable but only in rare instances where coexisting cirrhosis is minimal. At one time, liver transplantation appeared to offer the necessary radical resection, but results with large tumours proved unsatisfactory and recurrence was the rule. Transplantation is more promising when there are fewer than three tumours, each smaller than 3 cm, or a single tumour smaller than 5 cm (the 'Milan' criteria). In these, outcomes are comparable to those for liver transplantation for cirrhosis alone, with 5-year survival around 70%.

Patients with known cirrhosis should ideally be in a 6-monthly ultrasound surveillance programme to identify developing hepatocellular carcinoma early. If tumours are discovered, the patient may be considered for transplantation or for palliation to curb tumour growth. Palliation may involve local cytotoxic drugs given by 'chemo-embolisation' via a hepatic intra-arterial cannula. Where resection or transplantation are not practicable (e.g. due to advanced age, co-morbidities or patient choice), radiofrequency ablation can manage neoplasms in cirrhotic livers, and in some centres, is the first-line treatment for small lesions. Chemo-embolisation and radiofrequency ablation can give many years of disease control.

SECONDARY LIVER TUMOURS

Secondary liver tumours are extremely common and arise from a wide variety of primary sources, especially stomach, pancreas, large bowel, breast and bronchus. Liver metastases are initially asymptomatic but the patient begins to feel ill with anorexia and weight loss as the parenchyma is progressively destroyed. Jaundice is unusual and appears only at a terminal stage when the biochemical picture tends to be a mixed hepatitic and obstructive pattern.

Many colorectal cancer patients can be cured by primary surgery, but those that eventually die almost all have metastatic liver disease. Whilst there is no benefit in resecting metastatic disease in most other sites, colorectal liver metastases are a special case, sometimes with a real chance of cure. Some 10–20% may be suitable for curative resection; recent optimistic outcome reports mean increasing numbers are considered for liver resection now better surgical techniques are available and surgeons more willing to undertake extensive or multiple resections.

The liver has a large reserve capacity and a remarkable regenerative capability. This means that up to 70% of liver tissue can be surgically resected, provided there is no other liver disease. Resection is sometimes combined with chemotherapy and/or radiofrequency ablation to 'downsize' the tumour in advance. This surgery is a major undertaking, best practised in specialised units with operative mortality of around 2% and 5-year survival of 30–40%. If further metastases appear in the hypertrophied regenerating liver, further resection can sometimes be done; even isolated lung metastases can be excised. In some series, this aggressive policy is extending 5-year survival close to 50%.

In other primary cancers such as breast and bronchus, liver metastases usually indicate surgically incurable disease, reflecting the systemic nature of the malignancy. Occasionally, however, metastases from renal cell carcinoma or neuroendocrine tumours have been successfully resected. If liver metastases are painful, palliation by systemic chemotherapy may retard growth and suppress symptoms. Multiple inoperable metastases can often be controlled by a range of physical methods including local cryotherapy, radiofrequency ablation, laser destruction and percutaneous alcohol injection. Such treatments are unlikely to extend survival and controlled clinical trials of benefit are notably lacking.

THE SPLEEN

The spleen plays a major role in defence against infections, particularly involving encapsulated organisms. It also filters and removes senescent or defective blood cells. Primary splenic diseases are uncommon but a range of haematological disorders may involve the organ and usually manifest as splenomegaly (see Ch. 18, p. 263). Historically, splenectomy was common in myeloproliferative disorders and often used for diagnosis, but is now rarely indicated except to treat hypersplenism, i.e. excessive consumption of cellular blood components or for symptom control in pain associated with massive splenomegaly. The surgeon is most frequently involved in repair, partial resection or removal of a normal spleen after trauma or iatrogenic injury (Ch. 15, p. 207).

ELECTIVE SPLENECTOMY

Patients undergoing elective (and emergency) splenectomy require immunisation against common encapsulated pathogens (*Pneumococcus, Haemophilus influenzae* type B and *Meningococcus*, ideally given at least 2 weeks before operation) and are advised to take lifelong antibiotic prophylaxis.

Laparoscopic splenectomy has become the standard technique for most elective cases and is outlined in Ch. 10, p. 145.

The most common elective indication for splenectomy is **immune thrombocytopenic purpura (ITP)** in which antiplatelet antibodies lead to platelet destruction and an increased risk of spontaneous haemorrhage. Splenectomy is curative in about 85% of cases.

When erythrocyte loss is severe or resistant to medical management, splenectomy is sometimes required for haemolytic anaemias, including hereditary spherocytosis, thalassaemia and autoimmune haemolytic anaemia. It is common to perform simultaneous cholecystectomy for secondary pigment gallstones. In addition, in sickle cell anaemia, splenic infarction or abscess formation may require splenectomy.

Rarely, primary lesions of the spleen may require partial or total splenectomy; these include haemangiomas, primary angiosarcoma and cysts.

Pancreatitis

25

INTRODUCTION

Pancreatitis is a common inflammatory disorder of the pancreas characterised by abdominal pain. Most cases present in an acute form known as **acute pancreatitis** and attacks range in severity from mild to severe. Severe attacks can be life-threatening, with a mortality of around 20%.

A small proportion of patients suffer a persistent form known as **chronic pancreatitis**; this is much more common in men and is often associated with high alcohol intake.

ACUTE PANCREATITIS

AETIOLOGY AND EPIDEMIOLOGY OF ACUTE PANCREATITIS

Gallstones and alcoholism together account for about 80% of acute pancreatitis worldwide. These and the other main causes of acute pancreatitis are listed in Table 25.1 (see also Boxes 25.1 and 25.2). **Opie** first pointed out the relationship between gallstones and pancreatitis in 1901 based on autopsy evidence. Small gallstones may cause transient obstruction as they pass through the ampulla via the bile ducts, or larger stones may impact at the lower end of the common bile duct, resulting in **pancreatic duct obstruction**. Beyond this, the precise mechanism of gallstone pancreatitis remains obscure.

The proportion of acute pancreatitis caused by alcoholism varies from country to country; for example, about two-thirds of patients in the UK have a gallstone aetiology whereas in parts of the USA and continental Europe about two-thirds have an alcohol aetiology. Longstanding high intake for at least 2 years is usually required to cause alcoholic pancreatitis; the mean daily intake of pure alcohol in subjects of one study was 140 g, compared with 40 g in controls. Occasionally acute pancreatitis can result from a single session of heavy drinking—students finishing exams beware! The mechanism of alcoholic pancreatitis is unknown but is probably the toxic effect of alcohol on the pancreas in genetically predisposed individuals.

In developed countries, the annual incidence of acute pancreatitis requiring hospital admission is about 1 : 2000 population and mortality is between 2% and 6%. About 15% fall into the category of **severe pancreatitis**. Women are affected more than men, but men are more likely to suffer recurrent attacks. The peak incidence is between 50 and 60 years. The reported incidence appears to have risen by a factor of 10 over the last 40 years, with only part of this attributable to improved diagnosis. Other factors are unknown.

PATHOPHYSIOLOGY OF ACUTE PANCREATITIS

Acute pancreatitis is characterised by the sudden onset of diffuse inflammation of the pancreas. A range of diverse factors initiate disturbances of cellular metabolism, chiefly concerned with membrane stability. This leads to inappropriate activation of zymogens (pre-enzymes) within the pancreas. Activation of **trypsin** is probably the key initiating event and this overwhelms intrinsic antitrypsin activity, leading to **interstitial oedematous pancreatitis**. Fortunately, the extent and severity of inflammation remain mild and self-limiting in most patients and systemic effects are mild. In the least severe cases, there is minimal peritoneal exudation and no pancreatic changes detectable on contrast-enhanced CT scanning. In more severe disease, the pancreas becomes swollen and oedematous but remains viable. If laparotomy is inadvertently performed at this stage, clear, non-infected peritoneal fluid is found, with whitish patches on great omentum and mesentery representing areas of **fat saponification** ('fat necrosis'). If it is extensive, calcium becomes sequestered in these areas and

Table 25.1 Aetiology of acute pancreatitis

Condition	Frequency
Obstruction	
Gallstones	30–70% of cases
Congenital abnormalities: pancreas divisum with accessory duct obstruction; choledochocoele; duodenal diverticula	5% of cases
Ampullary or pancreatic tumours	3% of cases
Abnormally high pressure in the sphincter of Oddi (over 40 mmHg)	1–2% of cases
Ascariasis (second most common cause in endemic areas, e.g. Kashmir)	Depends on locality
Drugs and toxins	
Alcohol excess	30–70% of cases
Drugs: ('**SAND**'—**S**teroids and sulphonamides, **A**zathioprine (and 6-mercaptopurine), **N**SAIDs, **D**iuretics such as furosemide and thiazides, and didanosine); also antibacterials such as metronidazole and tetracycline, H_2 blockers and many other classes of drug	1–2%
Scorpion venom	Very rare
Snake bites	Very rare
Iatrogenic and traumatic causes	
Following endoscopic retrograde cholangio-pancreatography (ERCP) or endoscopic sphincterotomy	2–6% of patients having the procedure
Following cardiopulmonary bypass	0.5–5% of patients having bypass
Blunt pancreatic trauma, usually due to motor vehicle accidents	Very rare
Repeated marathon running	Very rare
Metabolic causes	
Hypertriglyceridaemia (>11 mmol/L)	2% of cases
Hypercalcaemia	Rare
Hypothermia	Rare
Pregnancy	Rare
Infection	
AIDS: secondary infection with cytomegalovirus and others	About 10% in patients with AIDS
Other viruses: mumps, chickenpox, Coxsackie viruses, hepatitis A, B and C	Very rare
Idiopathic pancreatitis	
No definable cause after thorough diagnostic evaluation including ERCP; research studies show about two-thirds of 'idiopathic' cases have gallstone microlithiasis	10–12% of cases

this is incriminated in the drop in blood calcium characteristic of severe acute pancreatitis.

As severity increases, trypsin and other enzymes cause increasingly extensive local damage as well as activation of complement and cytokine systems leading on to systemic inflammatory response syndrome (SIRS) and organ failure. Manifestations include shock, acute respiratory distress syndrome (ARDS), renal failure and disseminated intravascular coagulation (see Ch. 2). At this stage, **acute peripancreatic fluid collections** become detectable on CT. The most severe pancreatitis is associated with **pancreatic necrosis**. Ischaemia within the gland plus reperfusion injury are likely mechanisms in transforming acute oedematous pancreatitis into this necrotising disease. Complications are common and mortality in this group (even without infection) is as high as 10%.

Box 25.1 Mnemonic for the causes of acute pancreatitis: 'I get smashed'

- I Idiopathic
- G Gallstones
- E Ethanol
- T Trauma
- S Steroids
- M Mumps
- A Autoimmune
- S Scorpion/snakes
- H Hyperlipidaemia/hypercalcaemia
- E ERCP
- D Drugs

Box 25.2 History and investigations helpful in determining the cause of acute pancreatitis*

History

- Previous gallstones
- Alcohol intake
- Family history
- Drug intake
- Exposure to known viral causes or prodromal symptoms

Initial investigations (acute phase)

- Pancreatic enzymes in plasma
- Liver function tests
- Ultrasound of gall bladder

Follow-up investigations (recovery phase)

- Fasting plasma lipids
- Fasting plasma calcium
- Viral antibody titres
- Repeat biliary ultrasound
- MRCP
- CT (helical or multislice with pancreas protocol)

*Adapted from UK guidelines for the management of acute pancreatitis. Gut 2005; 54: 1–9

A substantial proportion of these patients develop **infection** of the necrotic pancreas, usually with Gram-negative organisms translocated from bowel. This occurs within 2 weeks of the onset and greatly increases mortality. **Pancreatic abscess formation** is a different phenomenon, developing later and having a somewhat better prognosis.

In patients dying of acute necrotising pancreatitis, the peritoneal cavity becomes filled with dark, blood-stained inflammatory exudate containing fine lipid droplets. This is known as **acute haemorrhagic pancreatitis**. The peritoneal surface is grossly inflamed and semi-digested, and the pancreas is a necrotic mass.

Box 25.3 Clinical features of acute pancreatitis

Mild attack

- Acute abdominal pain
- Minimal or rapidly resolving abdominal signs, e.g. abdominal distension, some abdominal tenderness and guarding, absent bowel sounds
- Minimal systemic illness
- Moderate tachycardia

Severe attack

- Severe acute abdominal pain
- Severe toxaemia and shock
- Generalised peritonitis (diffuse abdominal tenderness, guarding, rigidity, absent bowel sounds)
- Acute respiratory distress syndrome (may develop during the first few days)

CLINICAL FEATURES OF ACUTE PANCREATITIS (see Box 25.3)

Acute pancreatitis presents as a patient with an acute abdomen who has severe abdominal pain coming on suddenly and continuously from the outset. Initially it is poorly localised in the central and upper abdomen and is often described by the patient as 'going through to the back'. Vomiting may be an early feature. In the early stages, the patient is restless and constantly changes posture in the search for a comfortable position. Pain is most often relieved by leaning forward in the '**pancreatic position**'. With the onset of chemical peritonitis, movement becomes increasingly painful and the patient lies very still. Clinical signs depend on the severity of the inflammatory process and the stage it has reached.

INVESTIGATION OF SUSPECTED PANCREATITIS

Acute pancreatitis must be excluded in any adult presenting with acute abdominal pain, and in any child with peritonitis not readily attributable to appendicitis. The British Society of Gastroenterology (BSG) and other organisations have produced comprehensive guidelines on the management of acute pancreatitis: (http://www.bsg.org.uk/pdf_word_docs/pancreatic.pdf).

Plasma amylase

Amylase is one of the enzymes released into the circulation in pancreatitis; measurement is a simple laboratory investigation and is generally a reliable diagnostic test. A level above 1000 i.u. /ml is usually regarded as diagnostic of acute pancreatitis but levels are often lower in alcoholic pancreatitis, particularly during recurrent attacks. Any inflammatory upper abdominal condition near the pancreas (e.g. cholecystitis, perforated peptic ulcer or strangulated bowel) can cause a moderate rise in amylase, although this rarely reaches 1000 i.u. /ml. Levels rise rapidly at the outset of an attack, and readings of

10 000 i.u./ml or more may be recorded on admission to hospital. However, levels fall as the patient recovers so a diagnosis of pancreatitis should not rely on an arbitrary threshold; rather the amylase level at any moment should be interpreted in relation to how much time has elapsed since the onset.

The peak amylase level is not an indicator of disease severity, but persistently raised levels over several days warn of developing complications. Note that false negative amylase results may occur in lipaemic serum. In this case, true results can be obtained on diluted specimens.

On rare occasions, plasma amylase may be normal in acute pancreatitis. This occurs where most of the gland has been destroyed by severe pancreatitis. It may also occur if a patient presents several days into an attack, by which time the amylase may have returned to normal. If pancreatitis is strongly suspected but the amylase is normal, the diagnosis may be confirmed by appropriate radiological imaging (see next section).

Plasma lipase estimation has been recommended for diagnosing acute pancreatitis as it is more sensitive than amylase and has a longer half-life, so it is easier to detect later in the course of the disease. It is not as widely used but is often useful in difficult or late-presenting cases. In addition, elevated alanine aminotransferase (ALT) levels are highly specific for gallstone pancreatitis.

Once the patient is in the recovery phase, fasting bloods should be taken for calcium levels and for plasma lipids, particularly triglycerides. Viral antibody titres may be useful in cases of idiopathic pancreatitis.

Imaging

Plain X-rays of chest (erect) to look for free gas under the diaphragm, and abdomen (supine) are usually performed during the initial investigation. The latter may show a featureless 'ground-glass' appearance. Bowel gas tends to be absent except perhaps for a '**sentinel loop**' of dilated adynamic small bowel in the centre. Note, however, that these signs are not specific for pancreatitis and are often absent. Rarely, radio-paque gallstones are visible.

An **ultrasound scan** of the biliary tree is essential but good images are not always obtained early; a delay of 48–72 hours may improve image quality. The goal is to look for small calculi in the gall bladder or bile ducts typically responsible for gallstone pancreatitis. If no definite cause for the pancreatitis is found, a repeat ultrasound should be performed following recovery.

CT scanning has a limited role in the diagnosis of acute pancreatitis. Initially, it is indicated only when clinical and biochemical findings are equivocal, particularly if amylase is normal and intra-abdominal pathology such as perforation or infarction needs to be excluded. CT scans performed too early cannot predict the final severity and are unlikely to influence management during the first week. In **severe pancreatitis**, contrast-enhanced CT is valuable for demonstrating necrosis, but this cannot be identified until at least 4 days after the onset of symptoms.

Endoscopy

In patients with severe acute gallstone pancreatitis, urgent ERCP and sphincterotomy should be carried out within 72 hours of the onset of pain. This is especially important in patients with cholangitis, jaundice or a dilated common bile duct. ERCP also has an important diagnostic role once the patient has fully recovered from the acute attack if a cause for pancreatitis is not evident from the history or initial imaging studies. In this group, a cause can be found in about 50%, e.g. small pancreatic or periampullary tumours, pancreatic duct stricture, gallstones, congenital pancreas divisum or a high-pressure sphincter of Oddi.

CLINICAL CLASSIFICATION

To provide **early warning** of severity, each patient with acute pancreatitis is sorted into one of two categories, **mild** or **severe**. This provides an indicator of prognosis within the first 48 hours, and is central to formulating a management strategy. Categorisation is based on thoroughly tested scoring systems originally developed by **Ranson** in USA (see Box 25.4) and modified by **Imrie** (Glasgow criteria—see Table 25.2). If three or more of the factors listed are present, the patient is diagnosed as having severe pancreatitis and should be admitted to an intensive care or high-dependency unit for careful monitoring. The more adverse factors present, the worse the prognosis. Even if a patient is initially placed in the mild group, continued observation is essential as deterioration to severe pancreatitis can occur at any time. The clinical features of acute pancreatitis are summarised in Box 25.3.

Mild acute pancreatitis

Mild attacks are common. The patient looks generally well with minimal systemic features. Nevertheless, there is often considerable pain. The abdomen is usually distended and

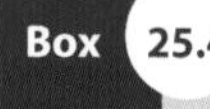

Box 25.4 Criteria for early identification of severe pancreatitis (after Ranson)

Severe pancreatitis, with a high risk of major complications or death, is defined by the presence of three or more of the following features:

On admission

- Age over 55 years (non-gallstone pancreatitis) or 70 years (gallstone pancreatitis)
- Leucocyte count greater than $16\,000 \times 10^9$/L
- Blood glucose greater than 10 mmol/L in a patient who is not diabetic
- Lactate dehydrogenase (LDH) greater than 350 i.u./L
- Serum glutamic oxaloacetic transaminase (SGOT) >100 u/L

During the next 48 hours

- Haematocrit increase of more than 10%
- Plasma urea increase of more than 10 mmol/L despite adequate i.v. therapy
- Hypocalcaemia (corrected serum Ca <2.0 mmol/L)
- Low arterial PO_2 (<8 kPa or 60 mmHg)
- Metabolic acidosis (base deficit more than 4 mEq/L)
- Estimated fluid sequestration more than 6 L

Table 25.2 A mnemonic ('PANCREAS') for remembering the modified Glasgow scoring system of severity prediction in acute pancreatitis (After E M Moore, with permission*)

Mnemonic letter	Criterion	Positive when
P	*PaO*$_2$	<8 kPA or 60 mmHg
A	Age	>55 years
N	Neutrophil count	$>15\times10^9$/L
C	Calcium (blood)	<2 mmol/L
R	Raised plasma urea	>16 mmol/L
E	Enzyme (plasma lactate dehydrogenase, LDH)	>600 i.u./L
A	Albumin (plasma)	<32 g/L
S	Sugar (plasma glucose)	>10 mmol/L

*E Moore A useful mnemonic for severity stratification in acute pancreatitis. Ann R Coll Surg Engl 2000; 82: 16–17

diffusely tender but with little guarding. Bowel sounds are absent as a result of inflammatory ileus. The patient may be mildly jaundiced from periampullary oedema. The differential diagnosis includes biliary colic, acute cholecystitis, an acute exacerbation of a peptic ulcer or even a perforation of a peptic ulcer. Lower lobe pneumonia or an inferior myocardial infarction may sometimes present like this. Sometimes the pancreatitis diagnosis is made after plasma amylase is unexpectedly found to be elevated.

Severe acute pancreatitis

In a severe attack the patient looks apathetic, grey and shocked and there are typical abdominal signs of generalised peritonitis, i.e. extreme tenderness, guarding and rigidity. In this case, the differential diagnosis includes other major abdominal catastrophes, especially faecal peritonitis from perforated large bowel and concealed haemorrhage from a leaking aortic aneurysm or ruptured ectopic pregnancy. Massive bowel infarction due to arterial occlusion may present like this but abdominal signs are less marked. An important early and dangerous complication of severe acute pancreatitis is acute respiratory distress syndrome (**ARDS**).

MANAGEMENT OF ACUTE PANCREATITIS

Mild attacks

The management of acute pancreatitis has been the subject of several international consensus conferences, the most important of which took place in Atlanta in 1992. This codified many definitions and circumstances within acute pancreatitis. Another important consensus meeting was in Washington in 2004. Numerous sets of guidelines are available; in the UK, the most used are published by BSG, updated in 2005.

Box 25.5 Recommended frequent investigations in severe acute pancreatitis

- Haemoglobin estimation and white cell count
- Arterial blood gas estimations
- Blood sugar
- Plasma electrolytes, creatinine and urea
- 'Liver function tests' (i.e. bilirubin, alkaline phosphatase, lactate dehydrogenase (LDH), transaminases, plasma proteins)
- Plasma calcium and phosphate
- C-reactive protein

Mild attacks require no further emergency investigation once diagnosed on plasma amylase, and are managed by fluid resuscitation and analgesia: recovery is usually rapid. These patients need no dietary restriction. Later management is aimed at treating predisposing factors. Gallstones should be sought by ultrasonography; if present, cholecystectomy is the definitive treatment and is ideally performed on the same admission or at worst 2–4 weeks after recovery. Ductal stones should be removed endoscopically before discharge from hospital. Alcohol abuse must be discouraged.

Severe attacks

A severe attack is defined by referring to a specified list of criteria which should be evaluated on admission and over the next 48 hours (see Table 25.2 and Box 25.4). Patients with severe pancreatitis may die early in the attack because of profound systemic toxaemia (SIRS), shock and multiple organ dysfunction syndrome (MODS); see Chapter 3, p. 51. ARDS develops rapidly with little warning but a deteriorating arterial *PO*$_2$ may herald its onset. This is an indication for urgent ventilatory support before the condition becomes established.

Even when pancreatitis is severe, supportive measures are still the mainstay of treatment. These include **oxygen** supplementation and carefully planned intravenous **fluid resuscitation**. A nasogastric tube is passed to aspirate the stomach only if gastroparesis causes troublesome vomiting. Enteral nasogastric or nasojejunal feeding has been reported to significantly decrease morbidity. If enteral feeding is not tolerated because of ileus, then total parenteral nutrition may be necessary.

Gross fluid and electrolyte disturbances as well as hypocalcaemia are also likely to occur. Fluid balance in the shocked patient is complicated by massive losses of protein-rich fluid into the peritoneal cavity and interstitially ('third space'). This sequestration of fluid needs to be countered by large amounts of intravenous fluids, carefully monitored by measuring central venous pressure and hourly urine output. Any patient with severe pancreatitis, or anyone with acute pancreatitis who develops signs of serious deterioration, should be admitted to an intensive care unit for close monitoring and vigorous treatment of cardiovascular, pulmonary, renal and septic complications. Box 25.5 lists recommended investigations to guide management.

There is probably little benefit in measuring plasma amylase again once the diagnosis is made. C-reactive protein (CRP) is more useful as it is a good indicator of systemic inflammation and hence developing necrosis and other complications. If the CRP is elevated >150 after 48 hours, complications are more likely. Biochemical estimations, particularly liver transaminases and bilirubin, are charted regularly, looking chiefly for evidence of biliary obstruction; renal function tests are performed for evidence of acute renal insufficiency.

Prophylactic parenteral antibiotics are no longer recommended as there is no evidence that they reduce either infective complications or mortality.

Endoscopy and surgery in severe acute pancreatitis

All patients suspected of having or proven to have a gallstone aetiology should undergo urgent therapeutic ERCP, which should take place within 72 hours of the onset of pain. This applies whether severe pancreatitis is predicted or confirmed. All of these patients require **sphincterotomy** of the sphincter of Oddi whether or not stones are found in the common bile duct. If stones are seen or if cholangitis or jaundice is present, biliary stenting is usually required.

There is no role for surgery during the acute attack but in patients with stones, laparoscopic cholecystectomy with operative cholangiography should be performed before discharge from hospital. This is because deferring cholecystectomy until months later increases the risk of another attack. In the small group of critically ill patients with infected necrotic tissue and infected peripancreatic fluid collections, surgical debridement with or without continuous peritoneal irrigation is unavoidable, but mortality remains high.

COMPLICATIONS OF ACUTE PANCREATITIS

Mortality

About 15% of patients admitted to hospital with acute pancreatitis have severe disease, which carries a high risk of potential complications. However, about a further 10% initially diagnosed with mild pancreatitis deteriorate markedly during admission and become severe. In severe pancreatitis, mortality is 10–30%, i.e. 2–5% of all cases, and obese patients have a higher mortality. About half of those that die, do so within the first week, usually of ARDS and pulmonary failure. Other early life-threatening complications are associated with **multiple organ dysfunction (MODS)**. Manifestations include cardiovascular collapse aggravated by fluid shifts, renal insufficiency made worse by hypotension, and disseminated intravascular coagulopathy. If death occurs after the first week, infective complications of pancreatic necrosis added to existing organ failure are the usual cause.

Pancreatic necrosis and infection

In severe pancreatitis, **pancreatic and peripancreatic necrosis** may manifest during the first 2 weeks of the attack (see Fig. 25.1). Necrosis is identified using intravenous contrast-enhanced CT scanning in which necrotic pancreas does not opacify, having lost its blood supply. Infection of devitalised pancreatic and peripancreatic tissues occurs in about one-third of patients with severe pancreatitis, and is often lethal. Infection may be suspected on CT by gas bubbles in pancreatic fluid collections but can only be confirmed by percutaneous aspiration (with microscopy and culture of the aspirate), usually performed under CT guidance. In proven infected cases, operative debridement, drainage and sometimes continuous peritoneal irrigation may be necessary, along with aggressive organ support.

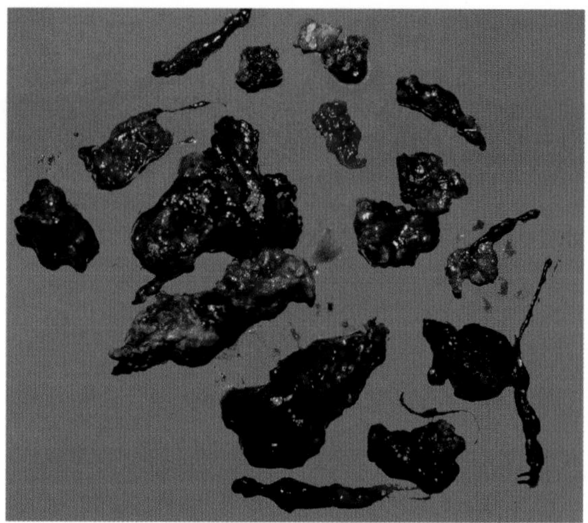

Fig. 25.1 Pancreatic necrosis
Necrotic pancreas removed 16 days after a severe attack of pancreatitis complicated by peripancreatic infection. The patient made a slow recovery but became diabetic in the convalescent period

Fluid collections around the pancreas

During the initial attack, **acute peripancreatic fluid collections** may develop. Most resolve spontaneously, but for those that do not, CT-guided percutaneous drainage is valuable. Fluid collections persisting for longer than 6 weeks are termed **pancreatic pseudocysts** (see below). Late in the course of the disease, a **pancreatic abscess** may appear. This is a well-localised collection of pus within the gland, and contrasts with **infected necrotising pancreatitis** which appears earlier and is not localised.

Pancreatic pseudocyst

A pancreatic pseudocyst is a collection of pancreatic enzymes, inflammatory fluid and necrotic debris, usually encapsulated within the lesser sac. Pseudocysts appear in 1–8% of cases of acute pancreatitis and are less likely to resolve spontaneously than the early acute fluid collections. A pseudocyst is not a true cyst (i.e. there is no epithelial lining) although the surrounding tissues become thickened by the inflammatory response. Pseudocysts may occur after even a moderate attack of pancreatitis and sometimes reach the size of a football! An upper abdominal mass may be palpable. If a pseudocyst is suspected, CT scanning is the investigation of choice (see Fig. 25.2).

Management varies according to the size of the cyst. Larger cysts, especially those larger than 10 cm, are unlikely to resolve. Those around 6 cm can be safely observed for up to 6 months, provided they have a typical appearance on CT scanning and are asymptomatic. If the cyst has failed to resolve

CASE HISTORY

Fig. 25.2 Pancreatic pseudocyst

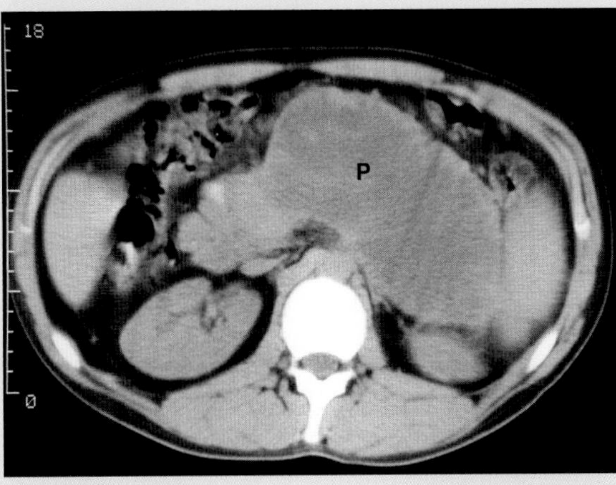

This 57-year-old man was admitted to hospital with an acute abdomen 3 weeks before this scan. He was found to have acute pancreatitis due to gallstones. The symptoms and signs of pancreatitis smouldered on and the CRP and plasma amylase failed to return to normal. This CT scan of his upper abdomen shows the cause of the persistent symptoms, a pseudocyst arising from the tail of the pancreas **P**

by then, operative intervention should be considered. Operation, either by laparoscopy or an open approach, involves 'marsupialising' the pseudocyst into the posterior wall of the stomach. This can be performed after about 6 weeks, when the wall of the pseudocyst has 'matured' enough to hold sutures.

Pancreatic abscess

Pancreatic abscesses occur in 1–4% of cases of acute pancreatitis. Certain patients remain systemically well despite pancreatic necrosis, with an illness that may grumble on for several weeks. There is a recurrent high swinging fever indicating the presence of an abscess. By that time, the necrotic pancreas is likely to have formed a discrete grey mass lying free within the pancreatic bed and bathed in pus. Pus may extend widely in retroperitoneal tissues. Surgery is then required to remove the necrotic tissue and drain the abscesses.

Complications of severe acute pancreatitis

Severe acute pancreatitis can cause wide-ranging complications in almost every body system:

- Multi-organ failure may lead to renal failure, respiratory failure, cardiac failure, and haematological and coagulation disorders
- Direct pressure effects, inflammation and hypotension may cause portal vein thrombosis
- Local pressure plus hypotension may cause bowel ischaemia—the transverse colon is commonly affected because of the position of the middle colic artery
- Pseudoaneurysms may form in vessels such as the splenic artery because of inflammatory damage to the arterial wall and fluid collections around them
- Internal pancreatic fistulae may form, particularly if necrosis causes disruption of the pancreatic duct or the wall of a pseudocyst. The result may be pancreatic ascites, mediastinal pseudocysts, enzymatic mediastinitis or pancreatic pleural effusions

Late complications of acute pancreatitis

Diabetes mellitus, and intestinal malabsorption due to loss of pancreatic secretions sometimes occur after severe attacks that have caused substantial pancreatic necrosis and loss of pancreatic tissue.

RECURRENT AND CHRONIC PANCREATITIS

RECURRENT ACUTE PANCREATITIS

Some patients suffer recurrent attacks, usually resulting from alcohol abuse or gallstone disease. The first and second attacks may be severe, but attacks after that almost never have lethal complications. The patient is entirely well between attacks. Attacks vary in severity in different patients but are rarely extreme.

CHRONIC PANCREATITIS

Some patients suffer persistent and severe upper abdominal pain, similar in character to a prolonged attack of acute pancreatitis. These patients do not develop the other features of acute pancreatitis and may not have elevated amylase levels. The pain is so severe and so persistent as to drive some patients to suicide. Carcinoma of the pancreas and chronic pancreatic inflammation should both be considered in patients with this pattern of pain. Inflammatory swelling of the pancreatic head occasionally causes obstructive jaundice but carcinoma in this position is a far more common cause of jaundice.

Despite the pain, there are usually no abnormal abdominal signs. Plasma amylase may be moderately elevated on occasions; the diagnosis of chronic pancreatitis may, however, be missed if raised amylase is not detected (because tests are not done at an appropriate time or the patient never has elevated levels). There is a danger these patients may be dismissed as suffering from psychosomatic pain.

In chronic pancreatitis, ultrasound or CT scans may show glandular swelling (sometimes difficult to differentiate from pancreatic carcinoma) and a dilated pancreatic duct. If ERCP is performed, the pancreatic duct system may look normal or else may be distorted and irregular in calibre, confirming chronic inflammation and fibrosis (see Fig. 25.3). Sometimes pancreatic duct stones are shown.

Chronic pancreatitis may cause years of misery, perhaps eventually 'burning out' as the gland atrophies completely. It is important to make the diagnosis early so pain can be relieved. In the long term, malabsorption or diabetes is more likely to develop than after acute pancreatitis.

Pancreatic calcification seen on abdominal X-rays is diagnostic of chronic pancreatitis but is a rare finding and is

CASE HISTORY

Fig. 25.3 Retrograde pancreatography

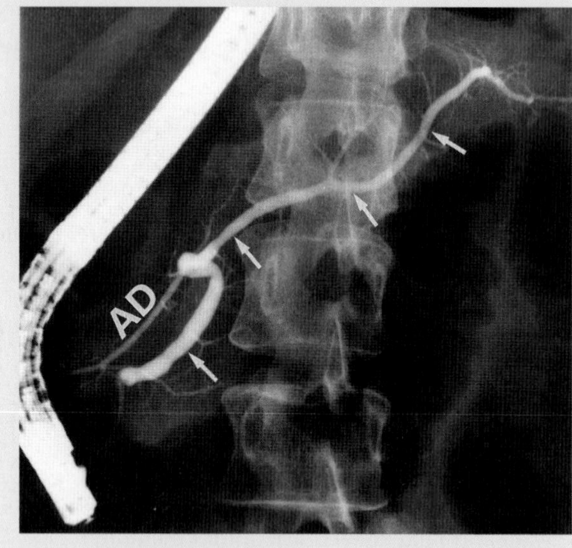

(a)

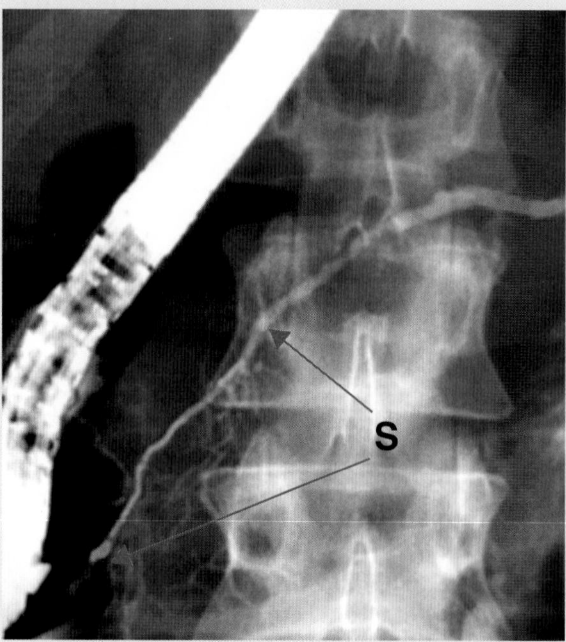

(b)

These films were both obtained by injecting contrast into the pancreatic duct using a flexible duodenoscope. **(a)** This pancreatogram is normal. The main duct (arrowed) narrows regularly towards the tail of the pancreas and there are no strictures or dilatations along its length. The accessory pancreatic duct **AD** also fills in this patient. **(b)** This pancreatogram is from a man of 26 with a history of severe upper abdominal pain. There is a long stricture of the main duct between the red arrows **S** of unknown origin. Typical changes of chronic pancreatitis, i.e. irregularity of the wall with dilatations and poor filling of small ducts, are seen in the duct distal to the stricture

CASE HISTORY

Fig. 25.4 Pancreatic calcification in chronic pancreatitis

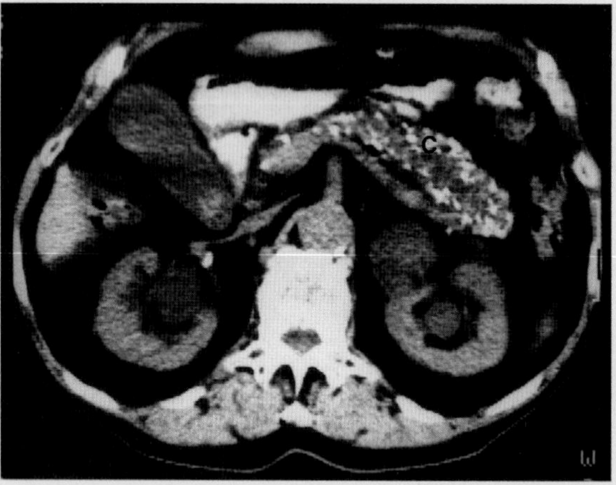

This obese 55-year-old man had a long history of severe abdominal pain and alcohol abuse. Pancreatic calcification was not visible on a plain abdominal X-ray but extensive calcification is clearly seen on this CT scan

sometimes found in asymptomatic patients (see Fig. 25.4). X-rays are therefore of little clinical value.

Treatment of chronic pancreatitis is far from satisfactory. Surgery is only useful if structural abnormalities can be found. Procedures include removal of pancreatic duct stones, partial pancreatectomy of body and tail for duct stenosis, sphincteroplasty of the pancreatic duct opening, or occasionally total pancreatectomy. Chemical coeliac ganglion blockade provides useful (and often permanent) pain relief, but does nothing to prevent inflammation. If there are multiple duct strictures, the pancreatic duct can be surgically split along its whole length and the side of a loop of jejunum sutured to it to allow unrestricted drainage. Interventional endoscopy can be employed for dilatation and stenting of isolated pancreatic duct strictures.

Appendicitis

26

INTRODUCTION

Acute appendicitis is the most common cause of intra-abdominal infection in developed countries and appendicectomy the most common emergency operation. In the UK, 1.9 females per 1000 have the operation each year compared with 1.5 males, and about 1 in 7 people eventually undergo the operation. Surprisingly, the incidence of appendicitis fell by about 30% between the 1960s and the 1980s, for reasons unknown.

Appendicitis can occur at any age but is most common below 40 years, especially between 10 and 20. It is rare below the age of 10 and very rare below 2 years. Appendicitis is rare in rural parts of developing countries, but the incidence approaches that of the West in the cities. Different susceptibility in similar people is probably related to reduced dietary fibre in city-dwellers.

Acute appendicitis should be considered in any patients presenting to hospital with acute abdominal pain. Even previous appendicectomy does not absolutely rule out the diagnosis. Despite lay impressions, a positive diagnosis is often difficult to make; this is partly because of the lack of specific tests to confirm or exclude appendicitis. At open operation a non-inflamed appendix is sometimes found but a small number of 'negative' operations may be unavoidable. Laparoscopy improves diagnostic accuracy, particularly in young women, and is used therapeutically to remove an inflamed appendix; it also has lower complication rates.

ANATOMY OF THE APPENDIX

The appendix is a blind-ending tube arising from the caecum at the meeting point of the three taeniae coli, just distal to the ileo-caecal junction. The appendix base thus lies in the right iliac fossa, close to **McBurney's point**. This is two-thirds of the way along a line from umbilicus to anterior superior iliac spine (see below, Fig. 26.6, p. 348). In most cases, the appendix is mobile within the peritoneal cavity, suspended by its mesentery (**meso-appendix**), with the appendicular artery in its free edge. This is effectively an end-artery, with anastomotic connections only proximally.

The appendix is described as lying in several 'classic' sites, but apart from the true retrocaecal appendix, the organ probably floats in a broad arc about its base (see Fig. 26.1). Only inflammation will fix it in a particular place. Its position then determines the clinical presentation. In about 30% of appendicectomies, it lies over the pelvic brim the ('**pelvic appendix**'). In some cases, the appendix lies retroperitoneally behind the caecum and often plastered to it by fibrous bands. Thus, an inflamed retrocaecal appendix may irritate the right ureter and psoas muscle, and may even lie high enough to simulate gall bladder pain.

Histologically, the appendix has the same basic structure as the colon. It is covered by serosa (visceral layer of peritoneum) becoming continuous with the meso-appendix serosa. A retroperitoneal appendix has no serosal covering. A prominent feature of the appendix is its collections of lymphoid tissue in the lamina propria. This often has germinal centres and is prominent in childhood but diminishes with increasing age.

The mucosa contains a large number of cells of the gastrointestinal endocrine amine precursor uptake and decarboxylation (APUD) system. These secrete mainly serotonin and were formerly known as **argentaffin cells**. Carcinoid tumours commonly occur in the appendix and arise from these cells.

PATHOPHYSIOLOGY OF APPENDICITIS

Appendicitis is probably initiated by luminal obstruction caused by impacted faeces or a faecolith. This explanation fits the epidemiological observation that appendicitis is more common with a low dietary fibre intake.

In the early stages of appendicitis, the mucosa becomes inflamed first. Inflammation eventually extends through the submucosa to involve the muscular and serosal (peritoneal) layers. A fibrinopurulent exudate on the serosal surface extends to any adjacent peritoneal surface, e.g. bowel or abdominal wall, causing localised peritonitis.

By this stage the necrotic glandular mucosa sloughs into the lumen, which becomes distended with pus. Finally, the end-arteries supplying the appendix thrombose and the infarcted appendix becomes necrotic or **gangrenous** at the distal end and the appendix begins to disintegrate. Perforation soon follows and faecally contaminated contents spread into the

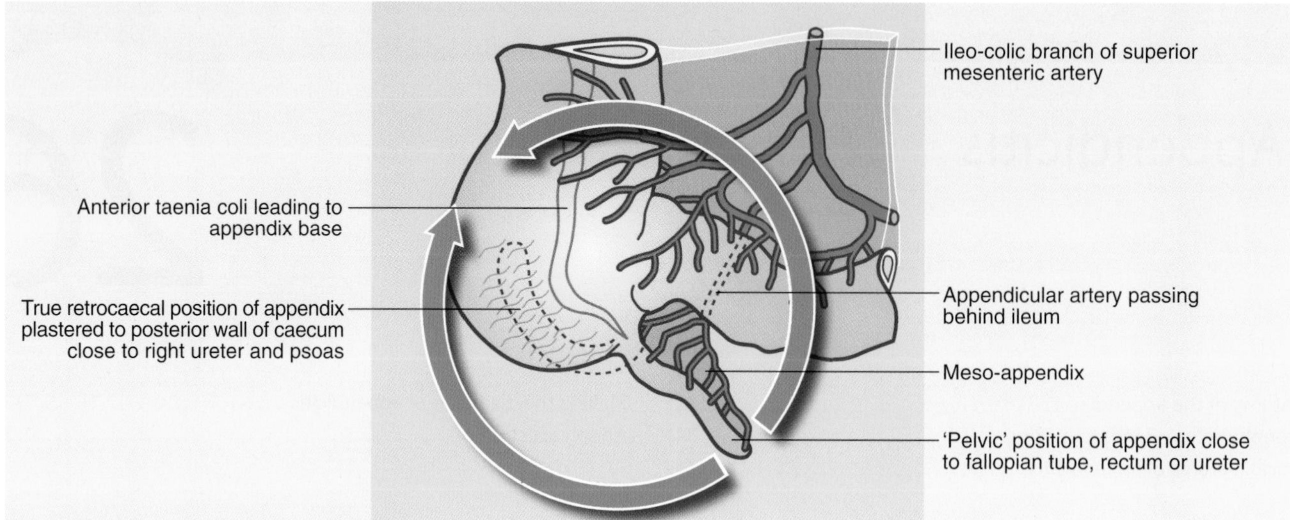

Fig. 26.1 Surgical anatomy of the appendix
The appendix can be positioned anywhere on the circumference shown by the arrowed arc

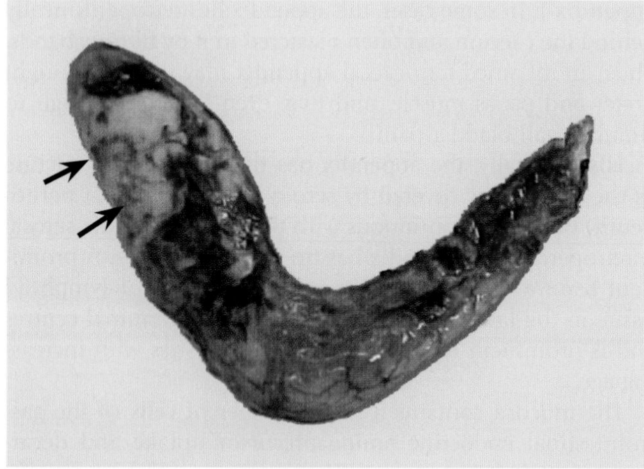

Fig. 26.2 Acute appendicitis
Macroscopic photograph showing acutely inflamed appendix. The distended tip shows a purulent exudate on the serosal surface (arrowed)

peritoneum. If the spilled contents are enveloped by omentum or adherent small bowel, a localised **abscess** results; otherwise spreading peritonitis develops. Acute appendicitis is illustrated histologically in Figure 26.2.

CLINICAL FEATURES OF APPENDICITIS

The pathophysiological evolution of appendicitis and corresponding symptoms and signs are illustrated in Figure 26.3.

CLASSIC APPENDICITIS

Acute appendicitis classically begins with poorly localised, colicky central abdominal **visceral pain**; this results from smooth muscle spasm as a reaction to appendiceal obstruction. Anorexia and vomiting often occur at this stage.

As inflammation advances over the ensuing 12–24 hours, it progresses through the appendiceal wall to involve the parietal peritoneum (innervated somatically). Then pain typically becomes **localised** to the right iliac fossa. Signs of local peritonitis can be elicited, i.e. tenderness, guarding and rebound tenderness. This classic picture is seen in less than half of all cases, largely because localising symptoms and signs vary with the anatomical relations of the inflamed appendix and the vigour of the body's defences.

OTHER PRESENTATIONS OF ACUTE APPENDICITIS

If the inflamed appendix lies in the pelvis near the rectum, it may cause local irritation and diarrhoea. If it lies near the bladder or ureter, inflammation may cause urinary frequency, dysuria and (microscopic) pyuria, i.e. leucocytes in the urine. These findings may be mistakenly interpreted as urinary tract infection. An inflamed retrocaecal appendix produces none of the usual localising symptoms or signs, but may irritate the psoas muscle, causing involuntary right hip flexion and pain on extension. A high retrocaecal appendix may cause pain and tenderness below the right costal margin. An inflamed appendix near the Fallopian tube causes pelvic pain suggestive of an acute gynaecological disorder such as salpingitis or torsion of an ovarian cyst.

The early phase of poorly localised pain typically lasts for a few hours until peritoneal inflammation produces localising signs. If untreated, the inflamed appendix may become gangrenous after 12–24 hours and perforate, causing peritonitis unless sealed off by omentum. The whole abdomen becomes rigid and tender and there is marked systemic toxicity. Perforation is common in young children. Sometimes, the pathological sequence is extremely rapid and the patient presents with sudden peritonitis.

In older patients, a gangrenous or perforated appendix is more likely to be contained by greater omentum or loops of small bowel. This results in a palpable **appendix mass**. This may contain free pus and is then known as an **appendiceal abscess**. As with any significant abscess, there is a tachycardia and swinging pyrexia. An appendix mass usually resolves spontaneously over 2–6 weeks. In the elderly, an appendix abscess is often walled off by loops of small bowel. There may

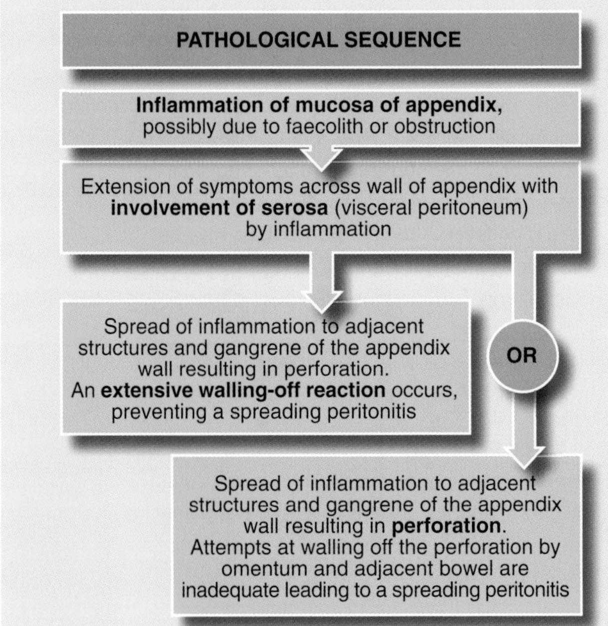

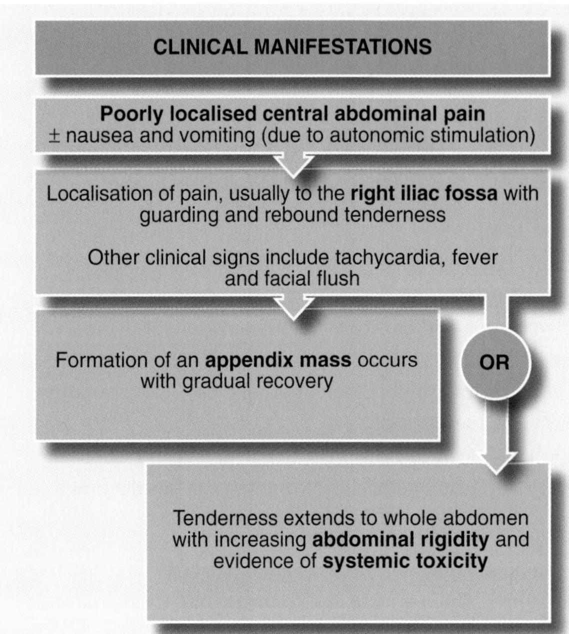

Fig. 26.3 Pathophysiology and clinical manifestations of acute appendicitis

Box 26.1 Cardinal features of acute appendicitis

- Abdominal pain for less than 72 hours
- Vomiting 1–3 times
- Facial flush
- Tenderness concentrated on the right iliac fossa
- Anterior tenderness on rectal examination
- Fever between 37.3 and 38.5°C
- No evidence of urinary tract infection on urine microscopy

be no palpable mass and the symptoms and signs may not suggest appendicitis. These include non-specific abdominal pain and features of small bowel obstruction due to localised paralytic ileus. Occasionally, appendicitis may present in a most unusual way. Examples include discharge of an appendix abscess into the Fallopian tube presenting as a purulent vaginal discharge, or appendicitis within an inguinal hernia presenting as a groin abscess.

MAKING THE DIAGNOSIS OF APPENDICITIS

Acute appendicitis is a clinical diagnosis, relying almost entirely on history and examination. Investigations are only useful in excluding differential diagnoses. Ideally, the diagnosis should be made and the appendix removed before it becomes gangrenous and perforates. This markedly reduces the risk of infective complications. However, unnecessary appendicectomies must be kept to a minimum.

Diagnosis of acute appendicitis poses little difficulty if the patient exhibits the classic symptoms and signs summarised in Box 26.1. However, the patient may present at a very early stage, or the signs may have some other pathological cause. At least two out of three children admitted to hospital with suspected appendicitis do not have the condition.

If evidence for acute appendicitis is insufficient and no other diagnosis can be made, the patient should be kept under observation, admitted to hospital if necessary and re-examined periodically. Eventually, the symptoms settle or the diagnosis becomes clear. Diagnostic laparoscopy may be needed in equivocal cases.

SPECIAL POINTS IN THE HISTORY AND EXAMINATION

Acute appendicitis typically runs a short course, between a few hours and about 3 days. If symptoms have been present for longer, appendicitis is unlikely unless an 'appendix mass' has developed. A recent or current sore throat or viral-type illness, particularly in children, favours a diagnosis of **mesenteric adenitis** (inflammation of mesenteric lymph nodes analogous to viral tonsillitis). Urinary symptoms suggest **urinary tract infection** but may also occur with pelvic appendicitis.

The patient with appendicitis is typically quiet, apathetic and flushed; the lively child doing jigsaw puzzles almost never has appendicitis! Oral foetor may be present but is not a reliable sign. Cervical lymphadenopathy may suggest a viral origin for the abdominal pain. Mild tachycardia and pyrexia are typical of appendicitis but a temperature much over 38 °C makes the diagnosis of acute viral illness or urinary tract infection more likely.

Signs of peritoneal inflammation in the right iliac fossa are often absent in the early stages. The patient should be asked to cough, blow the abdominal wall out and draw it in; these all cause pain if parietal peritoneum is inflamed. In children, it may be difficult to interpret apparent tenderness, especially if the child cries and refuses to cooperate. This can usually be overcome by distracting the child's attention whilst palpating

Box 26.2 Main differential diagnoses of acute appendicitis

Urinary tract infection (cystitis or pyelonephritis)

- Unlikely if nitrites are absent from dipstick testing of the urine and can be excluded if there are not significant numbers of white blood cells or bacteria on urine microscopy

Mesenteric adenitis

- Common in children and often associated with an upper respiratory infection or sore throat
- Inflammation and enlargement of the abdominal lymph nodes, probably viral in origin
- Fever is typically higher than in appendicitis (i.e. greater than 38.5°C) and settles rapidly
- A firm diagnosis can only be made at laparotomy or laparoscopy, but gradual resolution favours this diagnosis

Large bowel disorders

- Constipation may cause colicky abdominal pain and iliac fossa tenderness. There is no fever and the rectum is loaded with faeces
- Diverticulitis affecting the caecum or the sigmoid colon (when lying in the right iliac fossa) is usually diagnosed only at operation

Gynaecological disorders

- The pain of ovulation about 14 days after the last menstrual period (mittelschmerz) may cause right iliac fossa pain. There is often a history of similar pain in the past. There are no signs of infection and the pain settles quickly
- Salpingitis (most commonly chlamydial) causes lower abdominal pain, often with a vaginal discharge. Digital vaginal examination typically reveals adnexal tenderness, and moving the cervix from side to side induces pain ('cervical excitation')
- Torsion of, or haemorrhage into a right ovarian cyst may produce symptoms like appendicitis, but there is no fever. A tender mobile mass may be palpable in the right suprapubic region or on vaginal examination. This diagnosis can be confirmed with ultrasound
- Ectopic pregnancy. May present with anaemia and/or hypotension. A pregnancy test is mandatory

Small bowel pathology

- An inflamed or perforated Meckel's diverticulum (see Fig. 26.4) may present exactly like appendicitis
- Terminal ileitis due to Crohn's disease (or, more rarely, *Yersinia pseudotuberculosis*)
- Necrotic small bowel from strangulation usually presents with intestinal obstruction

Acute pancreatitis

- Pain is predominantly central
- If there is tenderness in the right iliac fossa, it will also be present in the epigastrium
- If in doubt, the serum amylase should be measured

Gastroenteritis

- Vague abdominal pain and tenderness which may be associated with vomiting and diarrhoea
- Usually improves steadily during a period of observation

the abdomen through the bedclothes or even with the child's own hand under the examiner's hand. Several signs (e.g. Rovsing's sign—pressure in the left iliac fossa causing pain in the right iliac fossa) are said to point to a diagnosis of appendicitis but all are unreliable. One useful test is to ask the child to stand, then to hop on the right leg. If this can be achieved, there is unlikely to be significant peritoneal inflammation.

Rebound tenderness was traditionally demonstrated by palpating deeply, then suddenly releasing the hand. However, this can cause excessive and unexpected pain. A kinder and more precise method is to perform gentle percussion in the right iliac fossa. This displaces and irritates inflamed peritoneum in a controlled way; if this is painful, then rebound is present. Anterior peritoneal tenderness on rectal examination (i.e. pelvic peritonitis) supports the diagnosis of appendicitis, provided other signs are consistent, but note the appendix itself cannot be palpated. In pelvic appendicitis, rectal tenderness may be the only abdominal sign. Lack of this sign does not, however, exclude appendicitis.

DIFFERENTIAL DIAGNOSIS

This theoretically includes all the causes of an acute abdomen. However, the conditions of practical importance are summarised in Box 26.2. These other conditions rarely need operation. Certain uncommon conditions such as *Yersinia* ileitis and inflamed Meckel's diverticulum (Fig. 26.4) are included in the list but they can only be distinguished from appendicitis at laparoscopy or operation.

THE EQUIVOCAL DIAGNOSIS

If acute appendicitis can be confidently diagnosed clinically, no further investigations are needed except for potential co-morbidity, anaemia or dehydration. It is worth emphasising there are no specific diagnostic tests; where the diagnosis is in doubt, the patient **must** be re-examined every few hours to detect clinical changes to ensure deterioration is detected early. Missing an evident clinical diagnosis and sending the patient home causes unnecessary problems and is likely to prompt a claim for medical negligence.

Certain investigations may be useful where the diagnosis is in doubt. The white blood count is usually unhelpful, as a modest rise occurs in many conditions. If there is a great rise (say to over 16×10^3), appendicitis is usually already clinically obvious, but a low WBC helps exclude non-suppurative gynaecological pathology. Urinalysis must be performed if urinary tract infection is possible. A

Fig. 26.4 Perforated Meckel's diverticulum

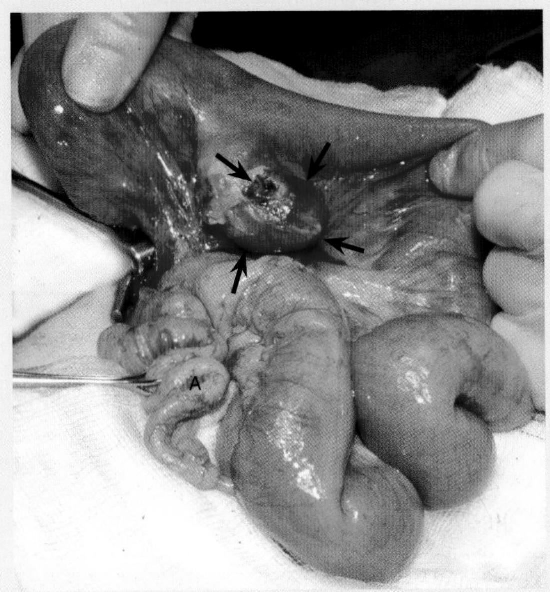

This man of 28 presented with a typical history and clinical findings of acute appendicitis. However, at operation he was found to have a normal appendix but a perforated Meckel's diverticulum (arrowed). The diverticulum was resected and the appendix also removed to prevent future confusion and the patient made a good recovery. On histological examination, the Meckel's was found to contain gastric mucosa

Table 26.1 Scoring system for the diagnosis of acute appendicitis based on the Alvarado score

Feature	Score
Migration of pain from central abdomen to right iliac fossa	1
Anorexia	1
Nausea or vomiting	1
Tenderness in right iliac fossa	2
Rebound tenderness	1
Raised temperature (≥37.5°C)	1
Raised leucocyte count ≥10×10^9/L	2
Neutrophilia of ≥75%	1
Total	**10**

The Alvarado scoring system is an objective, structured means of assessing patients with right iliac fossa pain, but has proved unreliable in diagnosing acute appendicitis. However, patients with an initial score of 4 or less are very unlikely to have appendicitis and do not need hospital admission unless symptoms worsen. In patients with appendicitis, 40% have rising scores, confirming this as a progressive disorder in which symptoms and signs evolve with time

pregnancy test should be performed in females of child-bearing age.

Various **scoring systems** have been devised to improve the accuracy of clinical diagnosis. The best known is the Alvarado score (see Table 26.1) but results are too variable for it to be of much clinical benefit.

Abdominal X-rays are not needed unless there is confusing evidence of abdominal pathology after a period of observation. A single right iliac fossa fluid level or even widespread small bowel dilatation suggests local adynamic bowel disorder due to appendicitis causing functional obstruction, but this is an uncommon finding. Even less commonly, a perforated appendix may allow sufficient free gas to escape to show on plain X-rays. In adults with an equivocal diagnosis of appendicitis, the plasma amylase should be measured to exclude acute pancreatitis. Abdominal ultrasound can be helpful to detect an abscess or mass, or non-appendiceal pathology, but cannot be relied upon to show uncomplicated appendicitis. CT scanning is claimed to be accurate but submits the patient to a high radiation dose and greatly increases the cost of investigation. Laparoscopy is increasingly used in women of menstruating age in whom gynaecological pathologies are common. However, this is an invasive investigation requiring a general anaesthetic and is best employed when an operation is clearly indicated but the diagnosis is still ambiguous.

PROBLEMS IN THE DIAGNOSIS OF APPENDICITIS

The very young

Appendicitis is rarely seen below 2 years of age, but when it does occur, the 'typical' abdominal symptoms and signs are obscure or absent. An infant or toddler may display signs of infection without revealing an abdominal origin. Abdominal X-rays may demonstrate dilated loops of bowel and fluid levels. Generalised peritonitis supervenes all too rapidly in this age group because abdominal defences are rudimentary, in particular the greater omentum 'wrapping' effect. Laparotomy is usually indicated in an ill infant with abdominal signs.

The elderly

Appendicitis usually develops more slowly in the elderly. The appendix wall becomes fibrotic with age and the area is more readily walled off by omentum and adherent small bowel. Indeed, many cases probably resolve spontaneously. In those who reach hospital, the history is often as long as 1 week. Features of obstruction may be present, including vomiting, colicky abdominal pain and obstructed bowel sounds. A mass may be palpable if the patient is relaxed and not too tender but often it can be palpated only under general anaesthesia. Abdominal X-rays may reveal fluid levels in the right iliac fossa.

Pregnancy

Appendicitis occurs at least as often during pregnancy as at other times but the diagnosis can be difficult. The appendix is displaced upwards by the enlarging uterus and abdominal pain and tenderness are in a higher position. The management of the pregnant patient must be shared with an obstetrician. Laparoscopy may be indicated but becomes technically

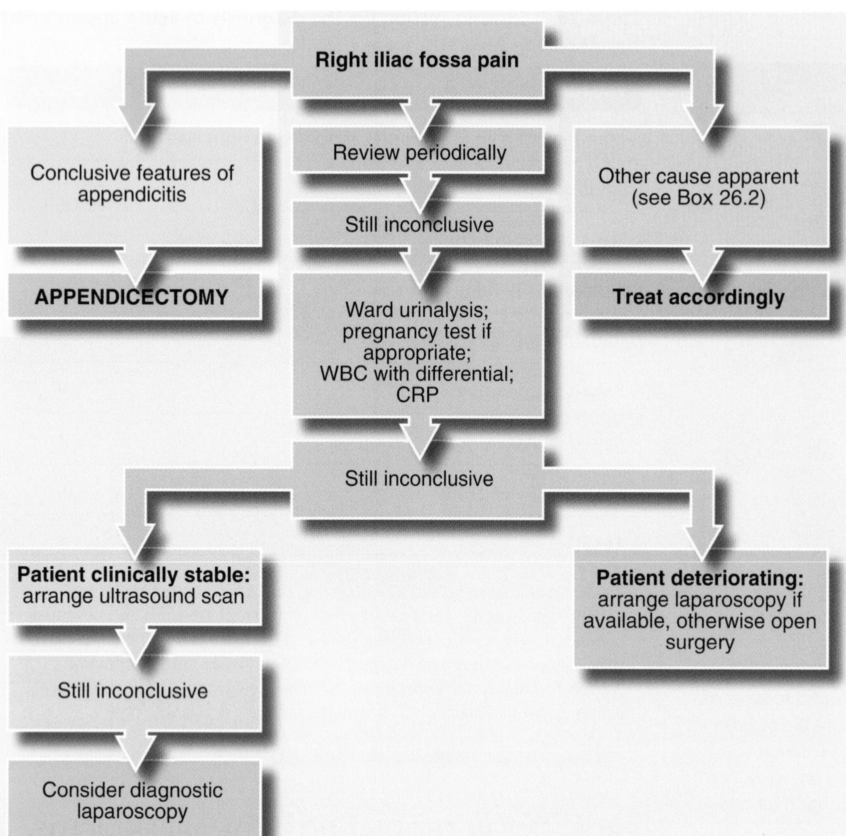

Fig. 26.5 Summary—management of suspected appendicitis

difficult beyond 26 weeks. Mortality from appendicitis for both mother and fetus rises as the pregnancy progresses and can be as high as 9% for the mother and 20% for the fetus in the third trimester.

The 'grumbling' appendix

Recurrent bouts of right iliac fossa pain are often labelled 'grumbling appendix'. Appendicular pathology is probably not the cause in most. Persistent chronic appendiceal inflammation probably does not occur, but recurrent bouts of appendicular colic or low-grade acute appendicitis undoubtedly do. These children may have several abortive admissions for abdominal pain and it may eventually be justifiable to remove the appendix to allay parental anxiety. A non-inflamed appendix containing a faecolith or threadworms (assumed to have caused the pain) is often found. The pain will be cured in no more than half.

The management of suspected appendicitis is summarised in Figure 26.5.

APPENDICECTOMY

The annual death rate from appendicitis has fallen dramatically since 1960. There were 3193 deaths in 1934 in the UK, whereas by 1982 this had fallen to 110. This results from better general nutrition, earlier presentation, better preoperative preparation and better anaesthesia. Deaths that now occur are usually due to dehydration and electrolyte changes unrecognised or ineffectively treated before surgery, often as a result of a late or missed diagnosis. Infective complications of appendicitis have fallen dramatically since the 1970s because of the widespread use of prophylactic antibiotics.

ANTIBIOTIC PROPHYLAXIS

In appendicitis, most intra-abdominal infective complications and wound infections occur in perforated or gangrenous appendicitis (see Box 26.3). Most infecting organisms are anaerobic and infections can largely be prevented by prophylactic metronidazole. Rectal suppositories are as effective as intravenous metronidazole and are cheaper but are best given 2 hours before operation. Aerobic organisms are involved in fewer cases and some surgeons advocate additional prophylaxis with an antibiotic such as a cephalosporin. In adults with moderate appendicitis, trials of antibiotic treatment alone compare favourably with appendicectomy but about a quarter present later with recurrent appendicitis.

TECHNIQUE OF APPENDICECTOMY

The principal steps are illustrated in Figure 26.6 and should be understood by any doctor assisting with the operation. Increasingly, laparotomy is being replaced by laparoscopic diagnosis and surgery, but the principles are similar. Surgeons performing appendicectomy need to be aware of possible appendiceal neoplasms, present in 0.5—0.9% of appendectomies. Most are innocent carcinoid-type tumours but others are mucinous adenocarcinomas.

Box 26.3 Complications of appendicitis (see also p. 346)

Intraperitoneal complications

Early

- Appendix stump blow-out—spillage of colonic contents into the peritoneal cavity
- Generalised peritonitis—perforated or gangrenous appendix, virulent organisms, late presentation or diagnosis
- Abscesses—local, pelvic, subhepatic, subphrenic
- Retained faecolith causing chronic local infection
- Haematoma due to slippage of a vascular ligature or a mesenteric or omental tear

Early or late (even many years later)

- Intestinal obstruction due to adhesions

Late

- Infertility due to tubal occlusion following pelvic infection

Abdominal wall complications

Early

- Superficial wound infection
- Deep wound infection
- Dehiscence

Late

- Incisional hernia

Notes:

1. Gangrenous or perforated appendix has much higher risk of infective complications
2. Undiagnosed appendicitis or a late diagnosis is likely to lead to a higher incidence of complications, particular infective ones such as generalised peritonitis and systemic sepsis

OPEN APPENDICECTOMY

A low skin-crease incision (**Lanz**) rather than a higher and more oblique one centred on McBurney's point is now favoured as it gives a better cosmetic result. The superficial (Scarpa's) fascia (well marked in children) is incised and the three musculo-aponeurotic abdominal wall layers split along the line of their fibres. This produces the '**gridiron**' **incision**, described as such because the fibres of external oblique and internal oblique run at right angles to each other. Peritoneum is then lifted and opened and may reveal pus or mucopurulent watery fluid; a swab is taken for microscopy and culture. The appendix is located with a finger and delivered into the wound; further exploration may be needed if it does not lie nearby. A retrocaecal appendix requires mobilisation of the caecum by dividing the peritoneum along its lateral side.

Once the appendix has been delivered, its blood supply in the meso-appendix is divided between clips and ligated. The appendix base is crushed with a haemostat which is then reapplied more distally. An absorbable ligature is tied around the crushed area. After this preparation, the appendix is then excised. A 'purse-string' suture may be placed in the caecum near the appendix base to invert the appendix, although this is not used in laparoscopic surgery and patients have not suffered from its omission. If the appendix is perforated or gangrenous, or if pus was found, thorough peritoneal toilet is performed. A sump sucker is guided down into the pelvis with a finger to aspirate fluid, and the area is gently swabbed with gauze to remove adherent infected material. Any pus or a faecolith left behind predisposes to a pelvic abscess.

The peritoneum, internal oblique and external oblique are each closed with two or three absorbable sutures. Drainage is not usually recommended unless there is a thick-walled abscess cavity which will not collapse. If the appendix is perforated or gangrenous, delayed primary closure of the skin is advisable as this reduces the high risk of wound infection. The superficial layers are left open initially and closed after 48 hours if the wound is clean.

After operation, oral fluids, followed by solids, are gradually increased unless vomiting or other complications occur, and most patients can be discharged on the second or third postoperative day.

LAPAROSCOPIC APPENDICECTOMY

Laparoscopy is a valuable technique that allows the appendix to be found wherever it lies. It also permits visual examination of the rest of the abdominal cavity and pelvis, improving diagnostic accuracy over open operation and minimising negative appendicectomies. It is strongly indicated in patients who are clearly unwell and in need of an operation but in whom the diagnosis is not clear. It is also useful in women of menstruating age and in any patient with pelvic symptoms. If the appendix is abnormal or if there is free fluid in the peritoneal cavity for which no other cause can be found, appendicectomy is performed. Laparoscopic appendicectomy is valuable in the obese, obviating the need for a large incision and a high risk of wound infection. Some surgeons use laparoscopy as a diagnostic tool and then convert to an open operation but laparoscopic appendicectomy may be performed if appropriate skills and instruments are available.

The principles and techniques are similar to open surgery but laparoscopy is more technically demanding. The meso-appendix may be clipped or divided by diathermy and the appendix base is ligated using pre-formed 'endo-loop' sutures. The appendix base is rarely buried and must never be diathermied. Superior visualisation and good access allow a thorough washout to be performed. Laparoscopic removal of the appendix has a lower wound infection rate and may allow an earlier return to normal activities.

THE 'LILY-WHITE' APPENDIX

If the appendix is found not to be inflamed at open operation (colloquially termed 'lily-white'), it should always be removed because an appendicectomy scar would lead future doctors to assume the appendix has been removed. The abdomen is explored as allowed by the incision to search for a cause for the symptoms:

- **Mesenteric lymph nodes** in children may be grossly enlarged by mesenteric adenitis—probably viral in origin

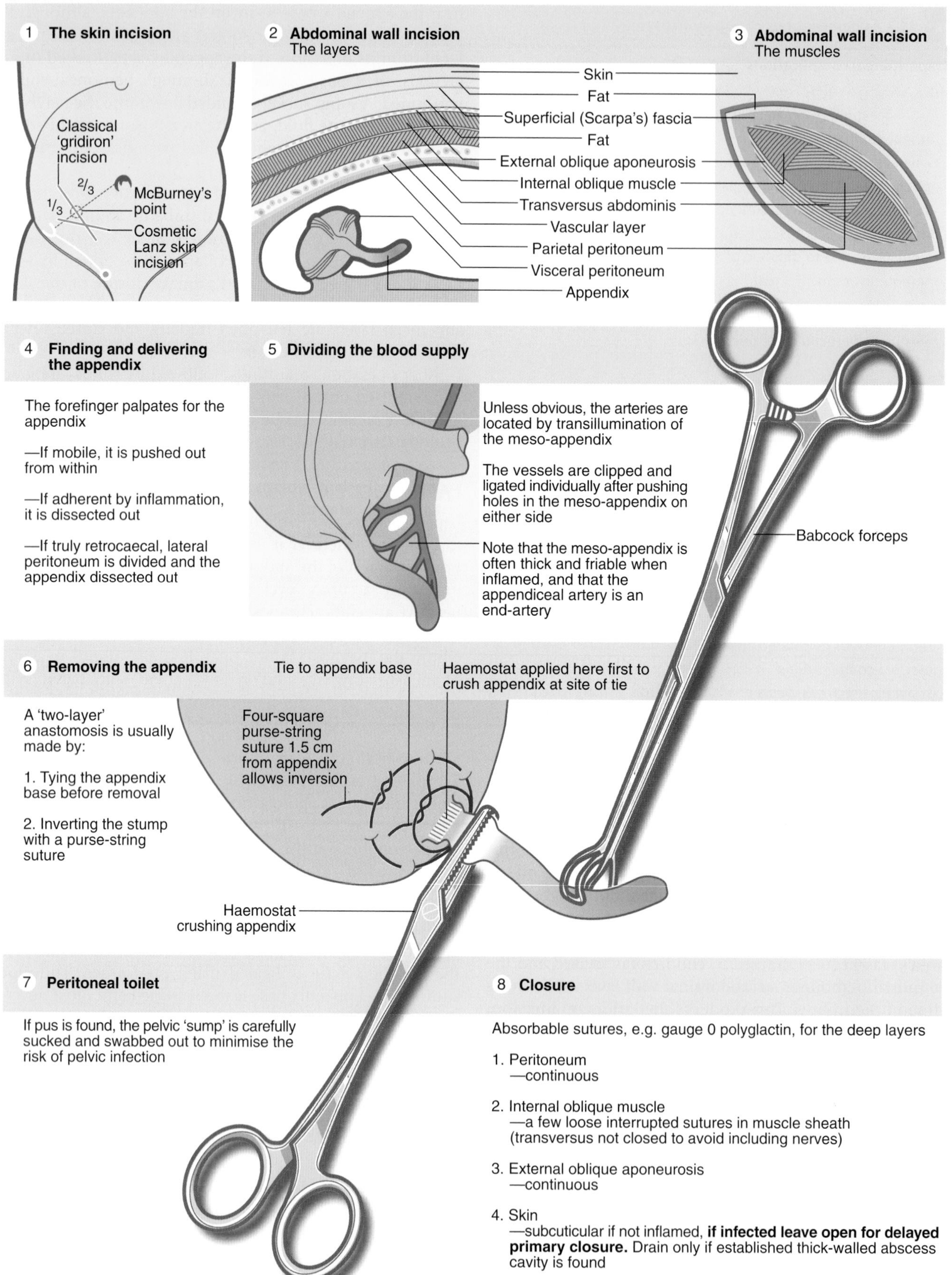

Fig. 26.6 Appendicectomy—operative technique

- **The terminal ileum** may be thickened and reddened by Crohn's disease or, more rarely, by *Yersinia* ileitis. The latter is a self-limiting condition caused by the organism *Yersinia pseudotuberculosis* and requires no specific treatment. The appendix is removed but the bowel left untouched. If possible, an enlarged mesenteric node is removed for histological examination
- **A Meckel's diverticulum** may be found within 60 cm of the ileocaecal valve—if inflamed, this is removed but a wide-mouthed non-inflamed diverticulum is usually left alone
- **Both ovaries can usually be palpated**—ovaries may be twisted, inflamed or enlarged or an inflamed Fallopian tube may be seen
- **Cholecystitis, sigmoid diverticulitis** (with the sigmoid displaced to the right), **inflammation of a caecal diverticulum, hydronephrosis** or a **leaking aneurysm** are rarely found

THE APPENDIX MASS

A vigorous response to appendicitis may result in a right iliac fossa mass, often with fever. Usually the patient has few systemic symptoms or signs of ill health. A conservative regimen followed by interval appendicectomy 6 weeks later (**Ochsner–Sherren regimen**) was advocated in pre-antibiotic days but is now less favoured. Early operation under antibiotic cover is now performed more frequently.

27 Colorectal polyps and carcinoma

INTRODUCTION

Carcinoma of the colon and rectum is the third most common malignancy in both men and women in Western countries. In the UK, the lifetime risk of colorectal cancer is 5%, although the condition is less common in the developing world. It is rare below the age of 50. Colorectal cancer is not only extremely common, it is also potentially preventable by screening the colon for premalignant lesions, namely **adenomatous polyps**, in people over 50. Surgery for large bowel cancer is generally rewarding, with high rates of cure achieved by timely resection.

Most cancers arise as a result of a complex interaction between genetic and environmental factors. The Western diet in particular has been incriminated in much of the geographical variation in incidence. About 5% of colorectal cancer is strongly genetically linked. It is important to recognise patients in this small group of **inherited colorectal cancer syndromes** as there are effective guidelines available for the screening and treatment of patients with these high-risk syndromes.

Most colorectal cancers originate in the glandular mucosa and are therefore histologically **adenocarcinomas**. Other forms of malignancy in the large bowel such as **carcinoid tumour** or **lymphoma** are rare. Squamous carcinomas occur at the anus or in anal canal skin, as do malignant melanomas, but these have an entirely different aetiology and different methods of management; they are discussed in Chapter 30.

Surgery is the mainstay of treatment for colorectal cancer. The common procedures and the complications of large bowel surgery are outlined in this chapter and the different types of intestinal stomas and their indications are described.

COLORECTAL POLYPS

The term **polyp** is simply a morphological description and describes any localised lesion protruding from the bowel mucosa into the lumen; it does *not* imply any specific pathology. This conforms to the use of the term elsewhere in the body, e.g. allergic nasal polyps. A simple pathological classification of large bowel polyps is shown in Box 27.1, emphasising the range of polyp types that can occur there.

Adenomatous polyps and adenomas

Polyps are common in the large bowel (Fig. 27.1). **The most significant** are **adenomas** (i.e. benign neoplasms) and all have potential for **malignant change**. In general, it takes 5–10 years to progress to invasive cancer. Early removal prevents progression from adenoma to adenocarcinoma. The process by which the epithelial cells acquire increasingly severe genetic mutations is termed the **adenoma–carcinoma sequence**. Thus, if adenomas are found at endoscopy, all of them should be meticulously removed (Fig. 27.1c) and subjected to histological examination.

Most adenomas are typically **pedunculated** or **sessile** (stalkless), allowing easy recognition and removal by diathermy snare. The much less common **flat adenomas** are particularly found in the Far East. These can be small and recognition at colonoscopy requires special dye-spray techniques. Flat adenomas can be removed by injecting saline into the submucosa to 'lift' the flat lesion before excising the abnormal mucosa with diathermy, sometimes in several pieces.

Adenomatous lesions examined histologically display a range of epithelial abnormalities from mild to severe dysplasia, to early invasive cancer. In invasive cancer, the cellular

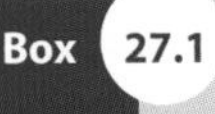

Box 27.1 Pathological classification of colorectal polyps and adenomas

Neoplasms

- Adenomas—very common, all potentially premalignant; these include villous, tubular and tubulo-villous types
- Early carcinomas—common
- Lymphomas—rare
- Leiomyomas and leiomyosarcomas—rare
- Lipomas and liposarcomas—rare
- Carcinoid tumours—rare

Hyperplasias

- Metaplastic mucosal polyps—very common
- Lymphoid aggregations—common in young children

Hamartomas

- Angiomas—uncommon
- 'Juvenile polyps'—uncommon; small malignant potential
- Peutz–Jeghers polyps—uncommon; small malignant potential

Inflammatory polyps

- 'Pseudopolyps' of severe ulcerative colitis

abnormality has breached the muscularis mucosae, from where extension progressively occurs into the submucosa. As a rule, the larger the lesion, the more likely it is to be malignant: only 1% of polyps smaller than 1 cm are malignant whereas about half of those larger than 2.5 cm are malignant.

Even in apparently benign lesions, there may be discrete areas of frank malignancy; so thorough histological examination is needed. When pedunculated lesions are removed by colonoscopic snaring, it is crucial to establish whether there is stalk invasion: if it is clear of cancer, further treatment is not usually required.

Classification of colonic adenomas

Three patterns of lesion are recognised histologically: tubular adenomas, villous adenomas and tubulo-villous adenomas.

Tubular adenomas are small pedunculated or sessile lesions in which the adenoma cells retain a tubular form similar to normal colonic mucosa. Tubular adenomas have the least potential for malignant transformation.

Villous adenomas are usually sessile (no stalk) and frond-like (papilliferous) lesions which tend to secrete mucus. The epithelial component of villous adenoma is more dysplastic than tubular adenoma and there is a correspondingly greater potential for malignancy; as with tubulo-villous adenomas, this potential is proportional to size.

Tubulo-villous adenomas are intermediate between tubular and villous adenomas and comprise the majority of colonic polyps (Fig. 27.1d). Most are pedunculated, and the stalk is covered with normal colonic epithelium. The stalk probably develops by peristalsis dragging the tumour mass distally and can range from about 0.5 to 10 cm long.

Distribution of colorectal adenomas

Although adenomatous polyps can occur in any part of the large bowel, three-quarters of them arise in rectum and sigmoid colon. This exactly parallels the distribution of carcinomas and provides verification that most cancers develop from polyps.

Adenomas often arise singly (particularly villous adenoma) but more than 20% of patients with colonic polyps have **multiple polyps**, most often tubulo-villous. Patients with proven carcinoma often have coexisting benign adenomas (**synchronous**), likely to become malignant later if not removed (see Fig. 27.2). This explains why the whole colon should ideally be examined before colectomy, preferably by colonoscopy, and why long-term follow-up after treatment of large bowel cancer should include regular colonoscopy.

Symptoms and signs of colorectal polyps

Many polyps cause no symptoms, and are found incidentally on colonoscopy, barium enema or CT colonography. Symptomatic polyps typically present with **rectal bleeding** and sometimes **iron deficiency anaemia** from occult blood loss. **Mucus production**, especially from villous adenomas, may be so copious as to be the main presenting complaint. Very occasionally, symptomatic **hypokalaemia** may develop because so much potassium-containing mucus is lost. Distal lesions occasionally produce **tenesmus** (a painful urge to defaecate) or may **prolapse** through the anus. Rarely, large polyps can cause obstructive symptoms or intussusception.

Diagnosis and management of colorectal polyps

For symptomatic patients, visualisation of the colon is needed. Most colorectal investigation is somewhat invasive and uncomfortable and the benefits have to be explained to patients, whilst their dignity and privacy is respected as far as possible. In the outpatient clinic, **rigid sigmoidoscopy** (which actually visualises the rectum) is often performed initially, as nearly half of all polyps lie within reach of the 25 cm instrument. **Flexible sigmoidoscopy**, usually performed without bowel preparation or after a phosphate enema, reaches past the sigmoid and descending colon to the splenic flexure, covering 75% of the area at risk, but to view the remainder of the bowel requires **colonoscopy**. Well performed colonoscopy is the 'gold standard' investigation: it allows visualisation of the entire large bowel mucosa, and polyps may be removed at the same time. For this reason, it is the first-line investigation in many centres. However, there are disadvantages: it requires a full day's bowel preparation and the procedure often requires sedation because of the discomfort. Furthermore, colonoscopy carries a 1 : 1000 risk of major haemorrhage or perforation. Sessile, small or flat adenomas in any location can be difficult to recognise even at colonoscopy and these potentially malignant lesions can be missed, especially if bowel preparation has been poor.

An alternative investigation growing in popularity and accuracy is **CT colonography**. Some studies have shown it to be virtually as sensitive for detecting polyps. It is less invasive and does not require sedation but bowel preparation is needed. Other alternative investigations include double contrast barium enema or unprepared CT scan.

Once an adenomatous polyp is found or a colorectal cancer has been treated, that patient is at risk of forming

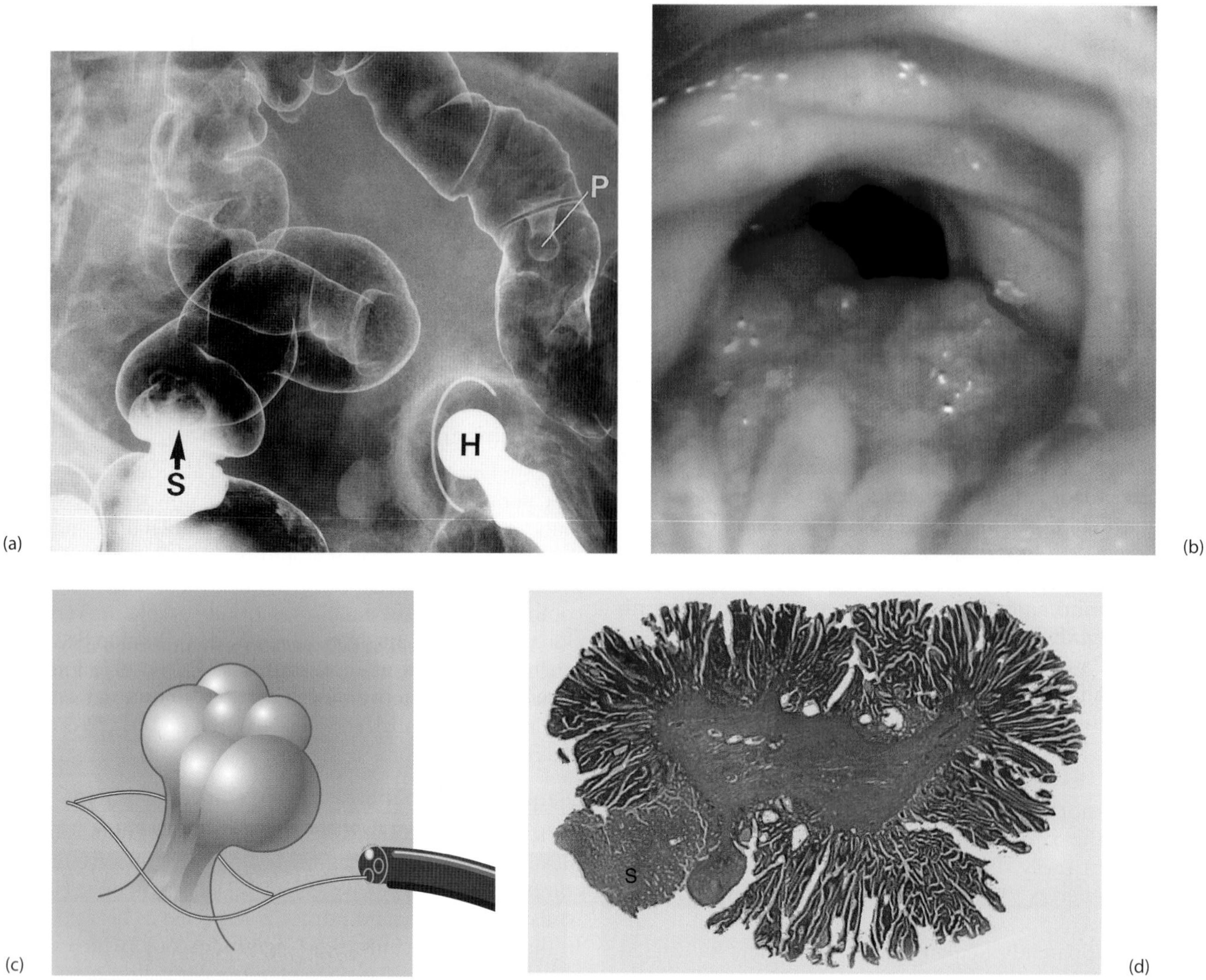

Fig. 27.1 Colorectal polyps
(a) This 65-year-old man was found to have positive faecal occult blood on colorectal cancer screening. This CT colography image shows a solitary polyp in the sigmoid colon, later removed by colonoscopic snaring. It proved to be a benign adenoma. **(b)** A 2 cm polyp on a long stalk in the sigmoid colon. **(c)** The snare loop is tightened around the stalk of the polyp before applying diathermy current to remove it and coagulate the blood vessels in the stalk. **(d)** Adenomatous polyp having mainly villous glandular architecture. The example shown has a well-defined stalk **S**, although this is more typical of tubular or tubulo-villous polyps, villous adenomas often having a broad base

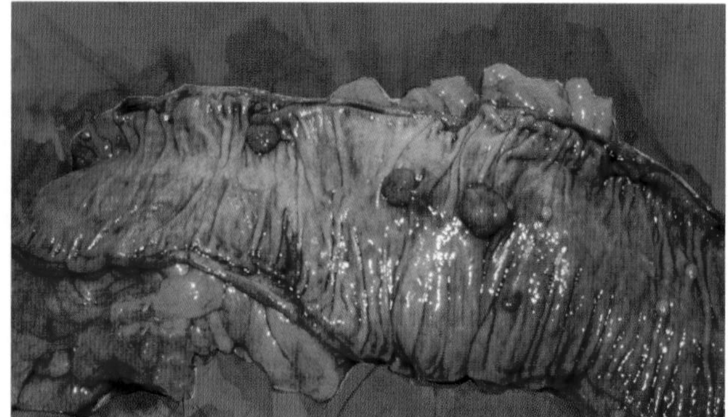

Fig. 27.2 Multiple colonic adenomatous polyps
This length of opened descending colon is from a 64-year-old man who presented with an invasive carcinoma of the rectum (not shown here). Several adenomatous polyps of various sizes can be seen in this part of the bowel; the larger polyps have greater malignant potential

further polyps elsewhere in the large bowel and needs follow-up colonoscopies. Intervals between colonoscopies are set according to guidelines determined by the number, size and pathology of polyps at each investigation and vary between 1 and 5 years.

Ideally, people at risk would undergo colonoscopic surveillance to detect asymptomatic polyps (as well as invasive cancers) so they can be removed before undergoing malignant change. The UK NHS national bowel cancer screening programme employs faecal occult blood testing every 2 years for people between 60 and 75 years of age. This test has been shown to aid detection of about 50% of asymptomatic cancers and is predicted to reduce mortality from colorectal cancer by at least 15%. Greater reductions could undoubtedly be achieved if patient compliance could be improved, and plans are under way to supplement this programme with a single flexible sigmoidoscopy offered to people aged 55–60.

ADENOCARCINOMA OF COLON AND RECTUM

EPIDEMIOLOGY OF COLORECTAL CARCINOMA

Table 27.1 shows that colorectal cancer is the third most common cause of death from cancer in the developed world; one in 20 people in the UK suffer from it at some point in their lives and almost a third arise in the rectum. The disease is rare before the age of 50 (except in inherited colorectal cancer syndromes, see later) but common after the age of 60. There is little difference in incidence between the sexes.

Apart from increasing age, **diet** seems to be an important factor. Since colorectal cancer is more common in developed countries, the Western low-fibre, high-fat diet may increase risk. High intake of meat, fats and ethanol may increase risk, whilst fish, fibre, antioxidants in fruit and vegetables may reduce it. Other protective agents may include **aspirin** and resistant dietary starch.

Ulcerative colitis, a chronic inflammatory condition of the large bowel (Ch. 28), carries an independent risk of bowel neoplasia. After 10 years of active disease, the cancer risk rises by 1% each year.

Finally, some **inherited genetic conditions** (discussed below) give rise to colorectal cancer. This explains the higher risk in first-degree relatives of patients with early-onset cancers and why it is important to ask about family history of bowel or other potentially inherited cancers in patients presenting with bowel symptoms.

INHERITED CONDITIONS CAUSING BOWEL CANCER

A small proportion of bowel cancers result from inherited conditions but they account for a disproportionate number of those presenting when young. Identifying these 'at risk' families allows counselling, surveillance and cancer prevention, best done through referral to specialist Familial Colorectal Cancer clinics. These inherited conditions may be divided into the **polyposis syndromes**, in which sufferers develop large numbers of polyps early in life, likely to undergo malignant change, and **hereditary non-polyposis colorectal cancer (HNPCC)**, in which sufferers have 'normal' or low numbers of adenomatous polyps which tend to progress to cancer. The latter is the most common inherited condition predisposing to bowel cancer.

Polyposis syndromes

The most important is **familial adenomatous polyposis (FAP)**, because it is reasonably common (1:30 000 people) and because large bowel cancer is inevitable if untreated. An autosomal dominant defect in the APC gene causes 100 or more adenomatous polyps to develop in the large bowel by the mid teens. Affected patients usually have one parent with the condition. Each affected individual is certain to develop colorectal cancer, at an average age of 40, unless preventative measures are taken. Ideally, prophylactic surgery to remove the area at risk should be performed in early adulthood. One option is subtotal colectomy and ileorectal anastomosis which removes nearly all the large bowel but has the retained rectum requires careful very long-term surveillance for malignancy. The alternative is to remove the rectum as well (**panproctocolectomy**) and perform an ileostomy or an **ileal pouch** restorative procedure.

Another polyposis syndrome is **Peutz–Jeghers** syndrome, which causes hamartomatous polyps throughout the gastrointestinal tract. Patients often have freckles around the mouth and on hands, feet and genitalia. Half of these patients are likely to die by the age of 50 because of polyp-related emergencies such as bowel intussusception or cancer. Patients are prone to develop cancers of small and large bowel, stomach, pancreas, testis and breast.

Hereditary non-polyposis colorectal cancer (HNPCC)

Hereditary non-polyposis colorectal cancer syndrome (also known as **Lynch syndrome**) results from defects in mismatch repair genes which repair damaged DNA. The condition carries a 70% lifetime risk of colorectal cancer, but also a substantially increased risk of one or more of other 'indicator' cancers such as those of endometrium, ovary, urothelium, small bowel and brain. Families can be difficult to identify because of the diversity of cancers and incomplete genetic penetrance (i.e. not everyone carrying the defect will develop cancer). When HNPCC is suggested by histological characteristics, young age of tumour onset, co-occurrence of tumours or family history, tumour tissue can be screened for markers. If abnormal, formal genetic tests are then undertaken. Those carrying a mutation are best offered colonoscopy every 2 years from the age of 25.

PATHOPHYSIOLOGY OF COLORECTAL CARCINOMA

Colorectal carcinomas exhibit a wide range of differentiation which broadly correlates with their clinical behaviour and prognosis (see Fig. 27.5). Most carcinomas are initially **exophytic** (i.e. protruding into the lumen) and later ulcerate and progressively invade the muscular bowel wall. Eventually, the tumour involves serosa and surrounding structures. Stromal fibrosis may cause luminal narrowing, responsible for the common acute presentation of **large bowel obstruction**.

Large bowel carcinomas metastasise via lymphatics and the bloodstream, and by the time of diagnosis as many as 25% of patients already have distant metastases (Fig. 27.4). Lymphatic spread is sequential, first to mesenteric nodes and then onward to para-aortic nodes. Occasionally lymph node involvement is directly responsible for the clinical presentation. For example, para-aortic nodes may present as a palpable mass or cause **duodenal obstruction**. Other enlarged nodes may compress bile ducts in the porta hepatis causing **jaundice**.

Haematogenous spread usually occurs later than lymphatic spread and is predominantly to the liver and less commonly to other sites such as lung or bone. Systemic manifestations may also occur.

Table 27.1 Death rates from colorectal cancer compared with other malignancies (UK 2004). Cancers are listed in order of frequency

Males (UK)	Number of deaths in 2010	Rate per million population	% of all male cancer deaths in 2010
1. Lung	19410	479	23.5
2. Prostate	10721	238	13
3. Colon and rectum	8574	209	10.4
4. Oesophagus	5105	130	6.2
5. Pancreas	3872	98	4.7
6. Bladder	3294	75	4
7. Stomach	3102	75	3.8
8. Leukaemia	2526	62	3.1
9. Kidney	2451	62	3
10. Non-Hodgkin lymphoma	2394	59	2.9
Other sites	21032		25.5
All male cancers	**82841**		
Females (UK)	**Number of deaths in 2010**	**Rate per million population**	**% of all female cancer deaths in 2010**
1. Lung	15449	313	20.7
2. Breast	11556	244	15.5
3. Colon and rectum	7134	127	9.5
4. Ovary	4295	91	5.7
5. Pancreas	4029	77	5.4
6. Oesophagus	2505	45	3.3
7. Non-Hodgkin Lymphoma	2042	38	2.7
8. Leukaemia	1978	36	2.6
9. Uterus	1937	39	2.6
10. Stomach	1858	33	2.5
Other sites	22011		29.4
All female cancers	**74794**		

Cancer mortality is decreasing in the UK, thanks to earlier diagnosis and improved treatments. For all cancers combined, mortality has fallen by approximately 26% and 20% in males and females respectively since 1990. The largest falls in mortality have occurred for stomach cancer (by 36% and 32% in males and females respectively), cervical cancer (by 28%) and breast cancer (by 19%). Mortality from lung cancer has fallen by 19% in males but increased by 6% in females, attributable to changes in patterns of smoking.

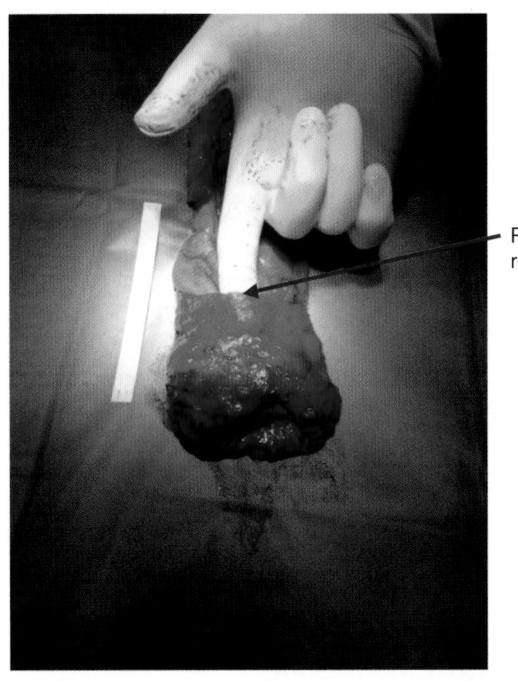

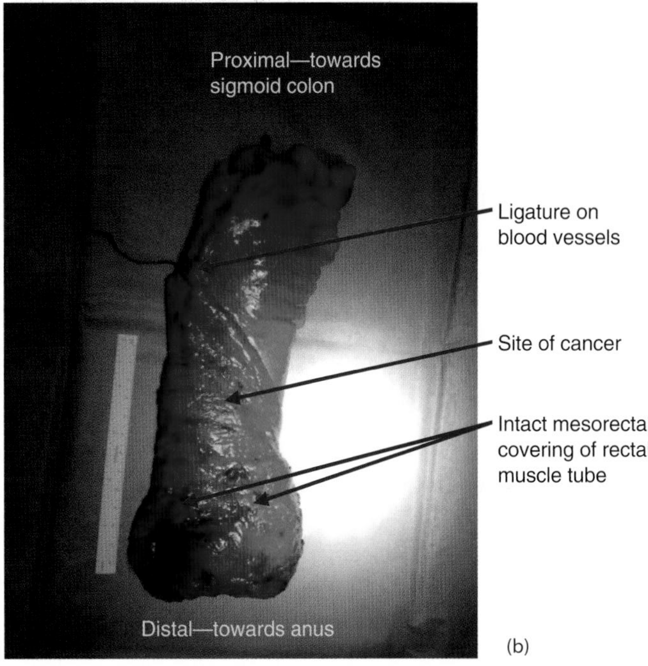

Fig. 27.3 Total mesorectal excision for low rectal carcinoma
Low carcinoma of rectum in a 70-year-old woman who presented with rectal bleeding and a change of bowel habit. A low anterior resection was performed with a covering loop ileostomy. The bowel was rejoined using the circular stapler. Two complete 'doughnuts' of tissue indicated successful firing of the stapler (see also Fig. 27.4)

CASE HISTORY

Fig. 27.4 Cancers of the colon and rectum

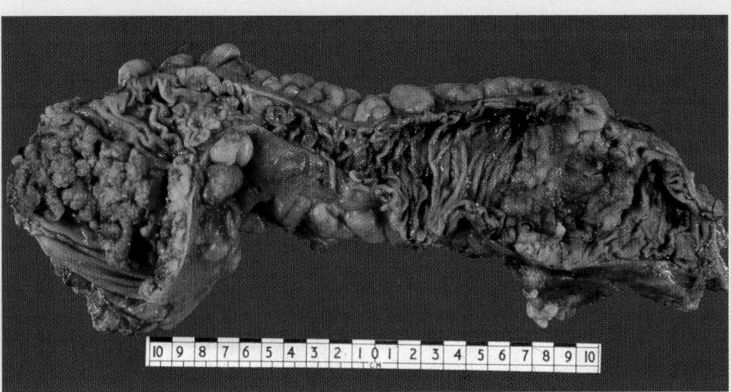

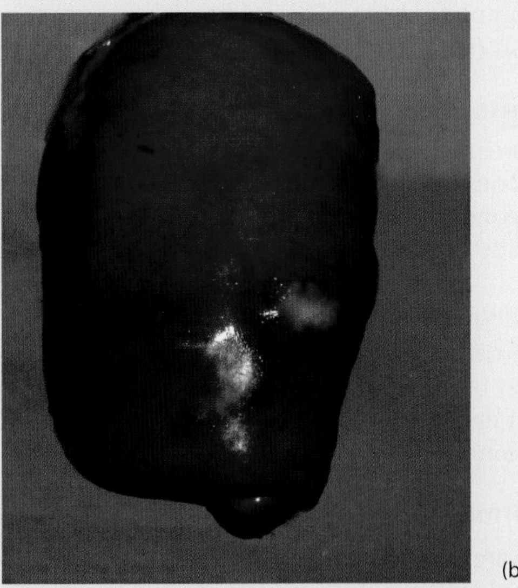

(a) Synchronous cancers of the transverse colon. This elderly man presented with a change in bowel habit, with constipation and overflow diarrhoea. Preoperative colonoscopy revealed two cancers that were biopsied and later resected at operation and the ends anastomosed. **(b)** This 49-year-old man presented with a 9-month history of rectal bleeding, found to be due to a sigmoid colon carcinoma which was resected. Two years later he was found on ultrasound screening to have a single metastasis in the right lobe of the liver. No other metastases were found so he underwent a resection of the right lobe of the liver; the resected specimen is seen here. Unfortunately, he returned 3 years later with a malignant paraduodenal mass and widespread peritoneal metastases, from which he died

PRESENTATION OF LARGE BOWEL CARCINOMA

Late presentations with metastases have been discussed. For local disease, the mode of growth and clinical presentation of large bowel cancer depend to some extent on the site.

Blood loss and anaemia

Carcinomas of caecum and ascending colon rarely obstruct unless the ileocaecal valve is involved. This is because the right colon has a larger diameter than the left and the faecal stream is more fluid. However, occult **bleeding** from the tumour surface commonly causes iron deficiency **anaemia**, and these patients typically present with anaemia and a palpable mass in the right iliac fossa.

Change of bowel habit and large bowel obstruction

Colorectal cancers usually secrete mucus and bleed into the lumen, which tends to change the bowel habit towards a looser stool. Thus a recent history of loose stool is more likely to predict cancer than increasing constipation, especially since constipation is so common in the elderly population. Faeces in the left colon are more solid and the intraluminal pressure is higher, thus distal cancers here are more likely to obstruct. Colonic cancers tend to progressively encircle the bowel wall, encroaching on the lumen and producing an **annular stenosis**, taking perhaps a year to involve each quarter of the circumference.

Large bowel obstruction may be partial or complete. **Partial obstruction** may present as a change in bowel habit, often noticed as constipation with intermittent 'overflow' diarrhoea. **Complete obstruction** precipitates emergency hospital admission (see Ch. 19).

Rectal bleeding

Carcinomas distal to the splenic flexure often cause visible blood to be passed per rectum. The character of the blood and the nature of its mixing with stool depend on how far proximally the lesion is from the anus.

Tenesmus

Carcinomas or polyps in the lower two-thirds of the rectum may be perceived as masses of faeces. This stimulates a persistent defaecation response, causing an unpleasant sensation of incomplete evacuation known as tenesmus.

Perforation

A cancer penetrating the bowel wall may stimulate a vigorous local inflammatory process resulting in a **pericolic abscess** which contains the perforation, at least for a while. This most often occurs in the rectosigmoid area and usually presents with left iliac fossa pain and tenderness and a swinging fever. The differential diagnosis is acute diverticulitis or a diverticular abscess.

A carcinoma anywhere in the colon (but rarely in the rectum) may perforate and present as an acute abdomen with **peritonitis**. Occasionally a carcinoma may erode into a nearby organ creating a malignant **fistula**. Fistulation can occur into stomach, bladder, uterus or vagina, or direct to the skin.

CLINICAL SIGNS IN SUSPECTED COLORECTAL CARCINOMA

These are illustrated in Figure 27.5. General examination may show features suggesting disseminated malignancy, e.g. obvious cachexia or supraclavicular node enlargement. Abdominal examination is usually normal but may reveal a mass in the colon, hepatomegaly due to metastases, or ascitic fluid. Unfortunately, all these signs represent late and often incurable disease.

Rectal examination is mandatory in all suspected cases as a high proportion of carcinomas occur in the lowest 12 cm and can be reached with an examining finger. In addition, intraperitoneal tumour spread into the pouch of Douglas may be palpable anteriorly through the rectal wall. The degree of **fixation** of a rectal tumour to surrounding structures can also be evaluated digitally to give some indication of operative difficulty. Finally, the glove should be inspected for stool colour and consistency as well as blood and mucus.

INVESTIGATION OF SUSPECTED COLORECTAL CARCINOMA

Proctoscopy and rigid or flexible sigmoidoscopy are usually performed at the initial consultation for anyone complaining of bowel symptoms. About 50% of colorectal cancers lie within reach of a rigid sigmoidoscope and 75% within reach of a flexible sigmoidoscope. Lesions can be biopsied through either instrument.

A history of rectal bleeding should be fully investigated in patients over about 45 years and in any patient if the symptoms or signs suggest malignancy. This applies even if a local cause such as haemorrhoids is found, since these are so common that they will often be found coincidentally. **Flexible sigmoidoscopy** is the initial investigation of choice for rectal bleeding because the causative lesion is probably in the left side of the colon. If a tumour is found, the rest of the bowel must still be examined for synchronous tumours or further polyps.

Where a change in bowel habit (particularly looser stools) or unexplained anaemia is present, any bowel lesion could be left or right sided, and thus the entire colon must be examined by colonoscopy or radiological imaging (Fig. 27.6).

Blood tests

Bowel neoplasms often cause anaemia but liver function tests remain normal until almost all parenchyma is replaced by tumour. Hypokalaemia rarely results from lesions producing excess mucin. Tumour markers are neither sensitive nor specific for a primary diagnosis of colorectal cancer but **carcino-embryonic antigen** (CEA) is used to monitor cancer recurrence.

Imaging for staging

When colorectal malignancy is diagnosed, surgery is likely to be necessary to relieve symptoms irrespective of distant spread. **Staging** is performed to guide oncological planning and counselling. Liver and lung metastases are sought, along with other evidence of spread within the abdomen or to bone. CT scanning is the most useful investigation for these but liver

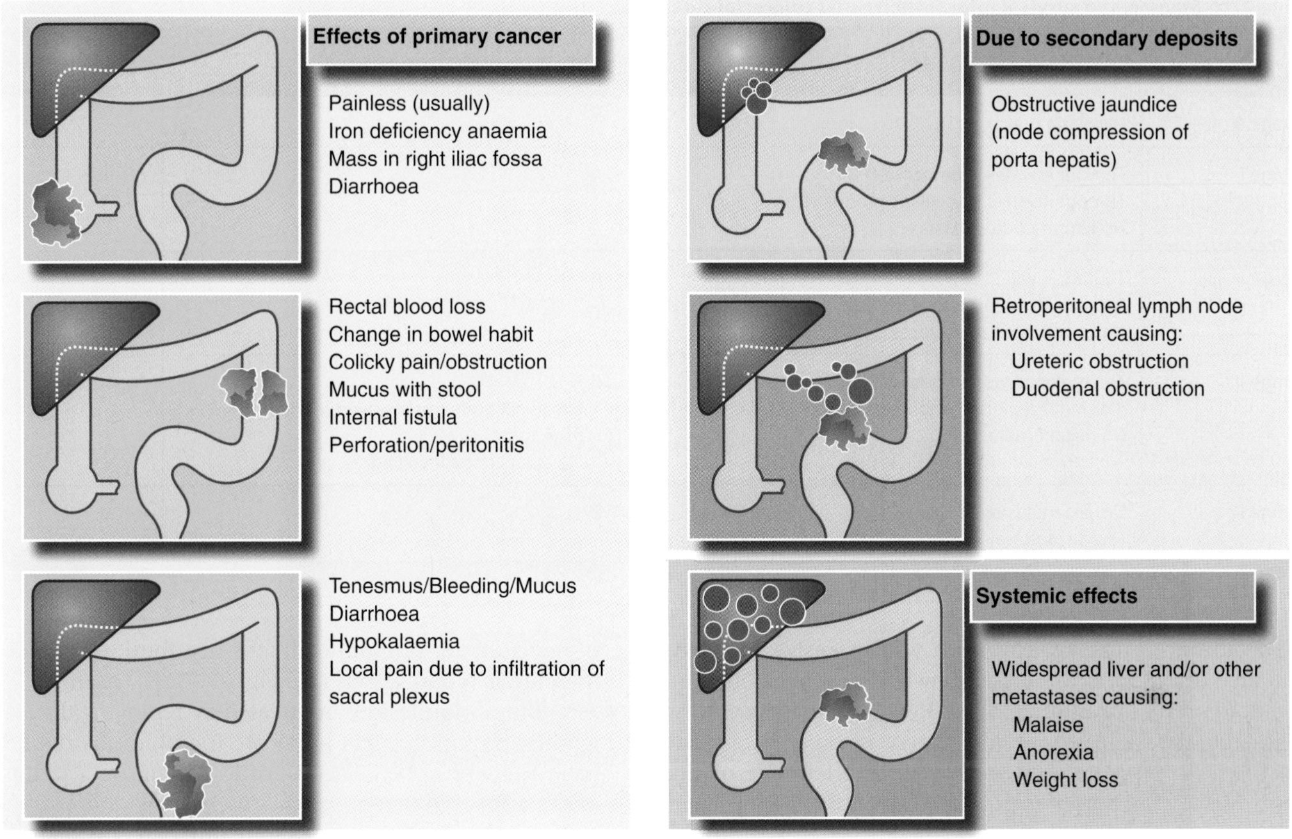

Effects of primary cancer

Painless (usually)
Iron deficiency anaemia
Mass in right iliac fossa
Diarrhoea

Rectal blood loss
Change in bowel habit
Colicky pain/obstruction
Mucus with stool
Internal fistula
Perforation/peritonitis

Tenesmus/Bleeding/Mucus
Diarrhoea
Hypokalaemia
Local pain due to infiltration of sacral plexus

Due to secondary deposits

Obstructive jaundice (node compression of porta hepatis)

Retroperitoneal lymph node involvement causing:
Ureteric obstruction
Duodenal obstruction

Systemic effects

Widespread liver and/or other metastases causing:
Malaise
Anorexia
Weight loss

Fig. 27.5 Symptoms and signs of colorectal cancer

ultrasound scanning may be more sensitive for detecting small liver metastases. MRI scanning can add important information about the precise extent of local spread of rectal cancer.

In a patient presenting as an emergency with complete large bowel obstruction, plain abdominal X-rays often show large bowel dilated by gas down to the level of obstruction and empty of gas beyond it. The level is often at the sigmoid colon or rectosigmoid junction. CT scan or sigmoidoscopy may confirm the likely diagnosis of carcinoma. Similarly, an 'instant' Gastrografin enema (i.e. without bowel preparation) can confirm the diagnosis and at the same time exclude **pseudo-obstruction**.

MANAGEMENT OF COLORECTAL CARCINOMA

Surgical excision is the main treatment. For tumours localised to the bowel wall, resection offers an excellent chance of complete cure; for tumours at a more advanced stage, chemotherapy and radiotherapy may increase the chance of cure. For rectal cancers, chemoradiotherapy may be given preoperatively (known as **neoadjuvant therapy**) to shrink the tumour to improve the chances of successful surgical removal. Management plans are ideally formulated by multidisciplinary team discussion, where surgeons, oncologists, radiologists, geneticists, palliative care physicians and colorectal specialist nurses discuss all aspects of the case.

CASE HISTORY

Fig. 27.6 Colonic carcinoma: barium enema examination

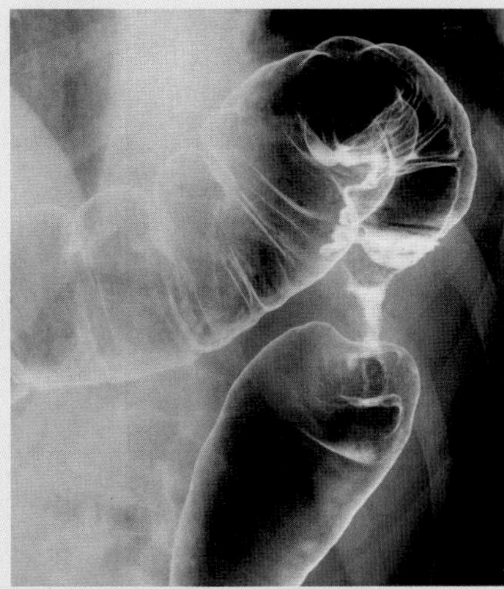

Typical 'apple-core' lesion just distal to the splenic flexure of a man of 39 who complained of rectal bleeding. With this degree of stenosis, it was surprising that he had had no change in bowel habit. Acute obstruction would probably soon have occurred if the tumour had not been recognised and resected. The patient is unusually young for colorectal carcinoma in the Western world

Table 27.2 Staging and survival rates from treated colorectal carcinoma

UICC stage	TNM stage	Modified Dukes' stage	Approximate 5-year survival
Stage 0	Dysplasia only		
Stage I	Tumour invades submucosa (T1) Tumour invades muscularis propria (T2) No lymph node metastases	**A**	85–95%
Stage II	Tumour invades beyond muscularis propria (T3) Tumour invades into other organs (T4) No lymph node metastases	**B**	60–80%
Stage III	1–3 regional lymph nodes involved—any T (N1) 4 or more regional lymph nodes involved—any T (N2) No distant metastases	**C** C1: apical node not involved (node furthest from tumour) C2: apical node involved	30–60%
Stage IV	Distant metastasis (M1) Any T stage, any N stage	**D**	<10%

For advanced disease, even with very extensive tumours, palliative resection is usually worthwhile to relieve obstruction or to prevent continuing blood loss. In frail patients with metastatic disease in whom any surgery is too risky, a **stent** can often be placed endoscopically on the left side of the colon to hold the bowel open and relieve obstruction.

STAGING OF COLORECTAL CARCINOMA

Staging of colorectal carcinoma influences the desirability of further treatment by chemotherapy or radiotherapy. It also gives an estimate of the statistical probability of surviving 5 years and the likelihood of cure. Final staging of colorectal cancer depends on information from several sources: the findings at laparotomy, histological examination of the resected specimen and the radiological and other imaging for distant organ spread. The two most widely used staging systems are the tumour/node/metastasis **(TNM)** and **Dukes' classification**, outlined in Table 27.2.

Approximately a quarter of all patients with colorectal cancer are incurable at presentation; all of these die within 5 years. Of those that undergo radical surgery with the aim of cure, 50% are alive and well 5 years later. Very few patients surviving 5 years die later of recurrent disease.

OPERATIONS FOR COLORECTAL CANCER

The principles of colorectal tumour resection are as follows:

- Before elective operations, the bowel may be prepared by giving a low residue diet and enemas. Oral purgatives are no longer given because of the potential dehydration
- Perioperative prophylactic antibiotics (e.g. gentamicin and metronidazole) are given
- Operative access is achieved laparoscopically, or by laparotomy, usually via a midline incision
- The affected segment of bowel is removed with a margin of normal bowel, usually 5 cm clear each side of the tumour. There must be a good blood supply to the cut ends of bowel to ensure healing so, in practice, lines of resection are determined by the distribution of mesenteric blood vessels (see Fig. 27.7). For example, ascending colon lesions are treated by removing the whole right colon (right hemicolectomy), as the right colic artery must be ligated in order to remove a section of the right colon
- A wedge-shaped section of colonic mesentery is removed with the bowel. This contains the primary field of lymph node drainage. If there are other obvious lymph node metastases, these are usually included in the resection specimen
- **Rectal cancers** are a special case and an outline of standard operations is given in Figure 27.8. The preferred operation is a sphincter-saving **anterior resection of rectum**; provided the lower edge of the tumour is 1–2 cm above the anal sphincters, the sphincter can usually be preserved. This operation involves excising the tumour with an appropriate length of bowel plus an intact envelope of fat around it (the **mesorectum** containing local lymph nodes). The proximal end of bowel is then anastomosed to the distal stump. Alternatively, a pelvic reservoir is created using a **J-pouch** technique (Fig. 27.8). This has been shown to reduce the frequency and urgency of defaecation without increasing surgical complications. A temporary defunctioning ileostomy or colostomy is sometimes used to aid healing of a low anastomosis. If the sphincter is involved, the entire rectum and anus has to be removed via an **abdomino-perineal excision (APE)**, with the proximal end of bowel brought out as a colostomy
- In most cases, the two cut ends of bowel can be anastomosed without the need for a temporary or permanent colostomy (the indications for stomas and their types and management are described on p. 361 onwards). The method used to rejoin the bowel depends on the site of the anastomosis, the preference of the surgeon and whether there is much disparity in diameter between the ends to be joined.

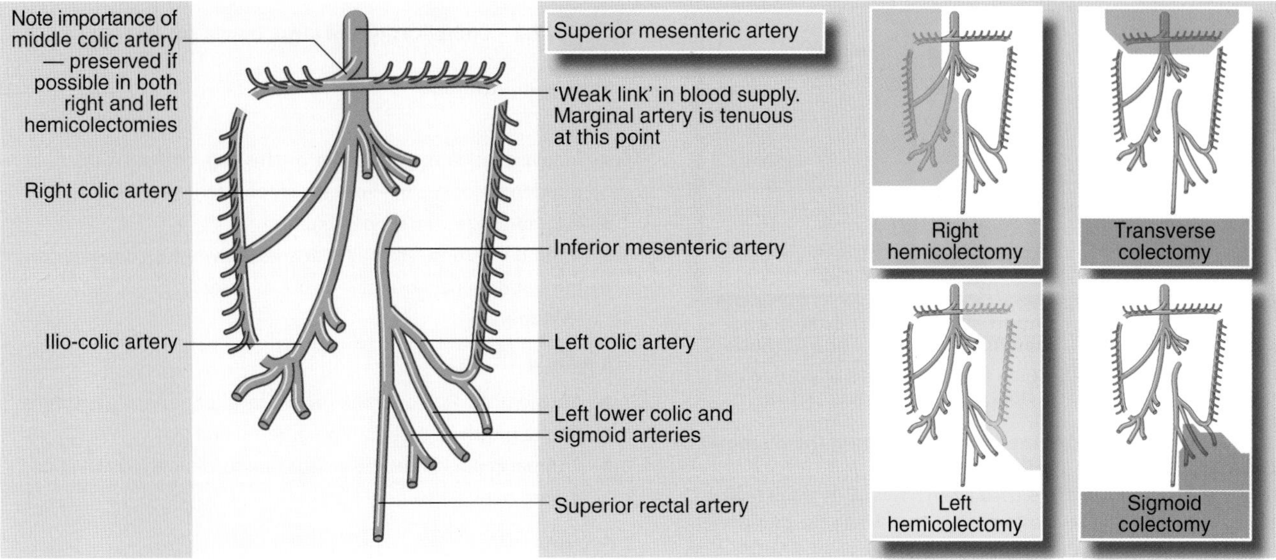

Fig. 27.7 Standard operations for colonic cancer

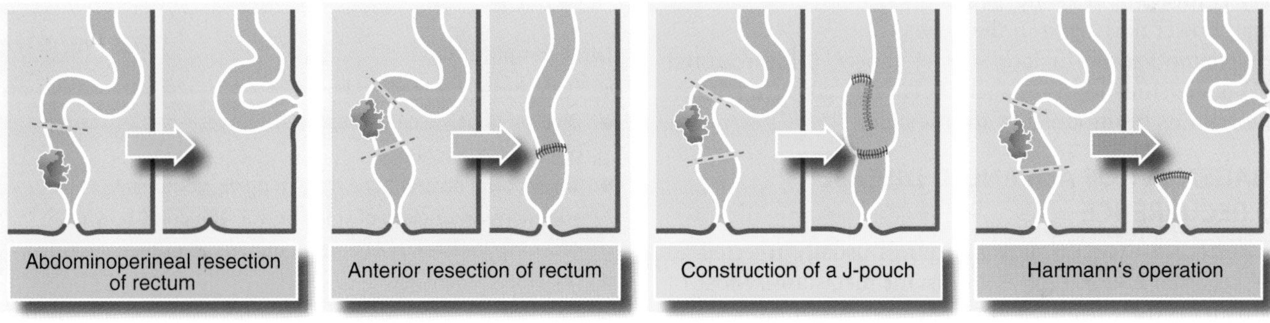

Fig. 27.8 Standard operations for rectal cancer
Hartmann's procedure is described on **page 363**

Methods of large bowel anastomosis are shown in Figures 27.9 and 27.10.

- Postoperatively, an 'enhanced recovery' program may be employed to encourage early eating and mobilisation (see Ch. 2, p. 26). These have been shown to lower complication rates and shorten hospital stays.

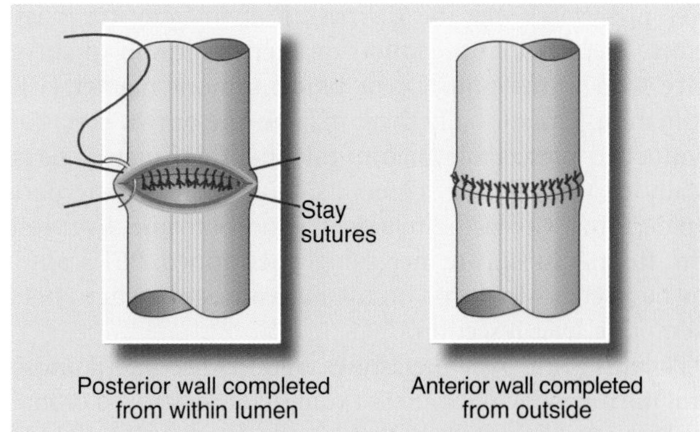

Fig. 27.9 Single-layer method of bowel anastomosis
A single-layer anastomosis using interrupted absorbable sutures is the safest and most commonly used method of anastomosis for nearly all types of bowel. If the bowel cannot be rotated, the posterior layer sutures are placed from inside the bowel and knotted within the lumen. Sutures usually incorporate the muscle wall and submucosa but not the mucosa

THE ROLE OF ADJUVANT RADIOTHERAPY AND CHEMOTHERAPY

Adjuvant radiotherapy and chemotherapy is usually offered to patients with Dukes' C cancers to increase the chance of prolonged survival. There is also a marginal benefit for those with Dukes' B but the potential advantages have to be weighed against the unpleasant side-effects of treatment. Neoadjuvant chemoradiotherapy is particularly relevant for rectal tumours tethered in the pelvis, where shrinking a large tumour can make it operable. Such therapy may enable the anal sphincter to be preserved by **downsizing** the tumour. Where rectal tumours extend through the bowel wall, particularly anteriorly, a course of radiotherapy directly before surgery has been shown to reduce local pelvic recurrence. Radiotherapy after

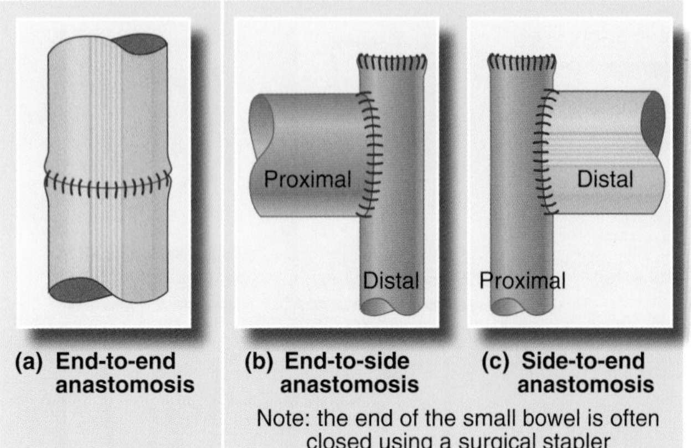

Fig. 27.10 Safe and reliable methods of matching the diameter of the bowel ends to effect a safe anastomosis
(a) An end-to-end anastomosis is used when bowel ends are of similar diameter. **(b)** An end-to-side anastomosis is used where the proximal end is greater in diameter than the distal end, e.g. in small bowel obstruction. **(c)** A side-to-end anastomosis is used where the distal end is greater in diameter than the proximal end, e.g. in right hemicolectomy

surgery is probably less effective and risks radiation damage to small bowel now lying in the pelvis.

For chemotherapy in large bowel cancer, **5-fluorouracil (5-FU)** is the chief adjuvant agent; it is often given in combination with its biomodulator, **folinic acid**.

MANAGEMENT OF ADVANCED DISEASE AND RECURRENCE

In advanced disease, primary tumour is usually resected to relieve its local effects even with distant metastases. Most of these patients die within 1 or 2 years and only about 1 in 10 survives 3 years. The exception is metastasis confined to the liver (see below), where partial liver resection is enabling prolonged survival in up to 40% of patients.

The **liver** is the most common site of distant metastasis. Liver metastases may be discovered at imaging for staging before operation, at operation or later as a result of surveillance with ultrasound, CT or blood tumour marker (CEA) estimation. Occasionally there may be one or two metastases confined to a resectable anatomical lobe. These may be excised locally or the affected segment of liver removed by partial hepatectomy. Given the relatively good outcome, liver resections for metastases are increasingly performed. PET scanning can be used to look for occult metastases elsewhere before attempting liver resection.

Patients with liver metastases seldom become jaundiced until the parenchyma is almost completely destroyed or major bile ducts are compressed at the porta hepatis. Specific treatment for this late event is rarely effective, although oral dexamethasone may temporarily reduce metastatic tissue oedema and relieve symptoms. Liver transplantation is fruitless. Colorectal tumours sometimes metastasise to **bone**, particularly the lumbar spine, and painful lesions may be palliated by radiotherapy.

Metastatic colorectal carcinomas are most often treated with 5-FU, with oxaliplatin as a second-line agent. This can substantially prolong survival and improve quality of life.

Box 27.2 Complications of large bowel surgery

Early complications

Local

- Inadvertent damage to other organs, e.g. ureter, bladder, duodenum or spleen—usually recognised at operation
- Haemorrhage, e.g. slipped ligature
- Wound infection—cellulitis, abscess or wound edge necrosis
- Intra-abdominal abscess—at site of surgery, pelvic or subphrenic

Regional

- Anastomotic leak or breakdown—local or general peritonitis
- Stoma problems—sloughing or retraction
- Compartment syndrome in legs due to prolonged elevation during perineal surgery (rare)

Systemic

- New onset atrial fibrillation or flutter—often indicates anastomotic breakdown
- Systemic sepsis leading to multi-organ dysfunction syndrome

Later complications

- Diarrhoea—due to short bowel
- Division of pelvic parasympathetic nerves—causes sexual/bladder dysfunction
- Small bowel obstruction—due to pelvic peritoneal adhesions or tangling of small bowel with colostomy or ileostomy, or later as a complication of radiotherapy causing small bowel damage

Colorectal carcinomas also respond to radiotherapy but its use is restricted because the radiation beam cannot avoid damaging nearby small bowel.

'Recurrences' within the colon usually represent new cancers arising metachronously from pre-existing or new adenomas. Careful examination of the entire colon before the first operation is likely to reduce such disease. Local recurrence in rectal cancer is now seen in 5–20% but this was more common before neoadjuvant radiotherapy and before the importance of mesorectal excision in anterior resection was realised (see Fig. 27.3). In abdomino-perineal excision, employing a prone patient position in theatre gives a clearer view of the anatomy and allows wider, more oncological margin clearance to be obtained. Recurrences often cause intractable perineal pain; occasionally a fungating mass grows in the anal region or buttocks. These very distressing complications may be palliated to a degree with radiotherapy.

COMPLICATIONS OF LARGE BOWEL SURGERY

The complications of large bowel surgery are summarised in Box 27.2. Infection arising from faecal contamination is the main early complication of large bowel surgery.

Contamination may result from perforation prior to operation, inadvertent faecal spillage during the operation or post-operative anastomotic leakage or breakdown.

Three main types of infection occur: wound infection and/or dehiscence, intraperitoneal abscesses and generalised peritonitis. Intra-abdominal infection carries a high risk of systemic sepsis and multi-organ dysfunction, particularly after emergency operations. All of these infective complications are radically reduced by appropriate use of prophylactic antibiotics.

STOMAS

INDICATIONS AND GENERAL PRINCIPLES

It is often necessary to divert the faecal stream to the anterior abdominal wall via a stoma. The effluent is collected in a removable plastic bag attached by adhesive to the abdominal skin. Stomas are named according to the part of the bowel opening on to the abdominal wall, i.e. **ileostomy** or **colostomy**. The term **urostomy** is used for the ileal conduit that connects ureters to the skin surface in patients whose bladder has been removed.

Stomas may be permanent or temporary. Wherever possible, the need for a stoma should be anticipated before operation and discussed with the patient. This is done to obtain informed consent and to prepare the patient for what is often perceived as a 'fate worse than death'. Specialised **stoma therapists** assist in planning and aftercare. Before the operation they counsel the patient, who is encouraged to try out a dummy appliance and talk to other stoma patients. The stoma therapist also identifies and marks the most suitable and comfortable site for the stoma appliance. This takes into account the patient's occupation and leisure activities, clothing and ability for self-care. Colostomies are usually fashioned in the left iliac fossa and ileostomies in the right iliac fossa.

Permanent stomas

These are necessary when there is no distal bowel segment remaining after resection or when for some reason the bowel is not to be rejoined. A **colostomy** is required after **abdomino-perineal excision** of a low rectal or anal canal tumour. An **ileostomy** (see Fig. 27.12) is employed after excision of the whole colon and rectum (pan-proctocolectomy) unless a pouch reconstruction is performed. Sometimes in patients with severe and permanent incontinence, a colostomy may make a better life possible.

Temporary stomas

Emergency procedures

A temporary stoma may be created (even by an inexperienced surgeon) as an emergency measure to relieve complete distal large bowel obstruction causing proximal bowel dilatation. If the ileocaecal valve remains competent in complete obstruction, the caecum can rupture and cause death by peritonitis. Thus if a patient with large bowel obstruction has a dilated caecum but no small bowel dilatation on plain abdominal X-ray, the ileocaecal valve is likely to be competent. If the patient develops right iliac fossa pain, perforation is imminent. Perforation can be prevented by a timely diverting stoma; the obstructing lesion may be removed at the same operation or later.

Defunctioning stomas

A 'defunctioning' stoma (ileostomy or colostomy) may be used to protect a more distal anastomosis at particular risk of leakage or breakdown by preventing intraluminal pressure rises and by diverting the faecal stream. Common examples are a technically difficult low rectal anastomosis (flatus and faeces may leak through the anastomosis), an anastomosis performed after resection of an obstructing lesion (distension may compromise the blood supply), or emergency resection involving unprepared bowel (solid faeces may remain impacted in the lumen). Reversing the temporary stoma to restore bowel continuity is often a relatively simple procedure, usually performed after 3–4 months. Some surgeons like to perform a limited contrast enema to demonstrate anastomotic integrity before closing the stoma.

Bowel rest

A temporary colostomy may be used to 'rest' a more distal segment of bowel or a perineum involved in an inflammatory process, by diverting the faecal stream. Examples include pericolic abscess, complex anorectal fistulae and major surgical perineal wounds.

TYPES OF STOMA

The way in which a stoma is fashioned depends on its purpose. The main types of stoma are described below and illustrated in Figure 27.11. Colonic stomas are designed with the bowel mucosa lying almost flush with the skin. Small bowel stomas are fashioned with a 'spout' of bowel protruding about 3 cm, to ensure that the irritant small bowel contents enter the ileostomy appliance directly rather than flowing on to the skin (Fig. 27.12).

Loop stoma

This type of stoma is designed so that both proximal and distal segments of bowel drain onto the skin surface (see Fig. 27.11a). This deflects proximal effluent to the skin surface and provides a 'blow-off' valve for the distal loop. Loop stomas are used mainly for temporary defunctioning to protect a distal anastomosis. It is straightforward to reanastomose the ends at reversal; the loop is then dropped back into the abdomen. The most common form of loop stoma is the **loop ileostomy**; occasionally a **loop transverse colostomy** is used.

Split or 'spectacle' stoma

This is the ultimate form of defunctioning stoma but has been largely superseded by the loop stoma. After resection, both

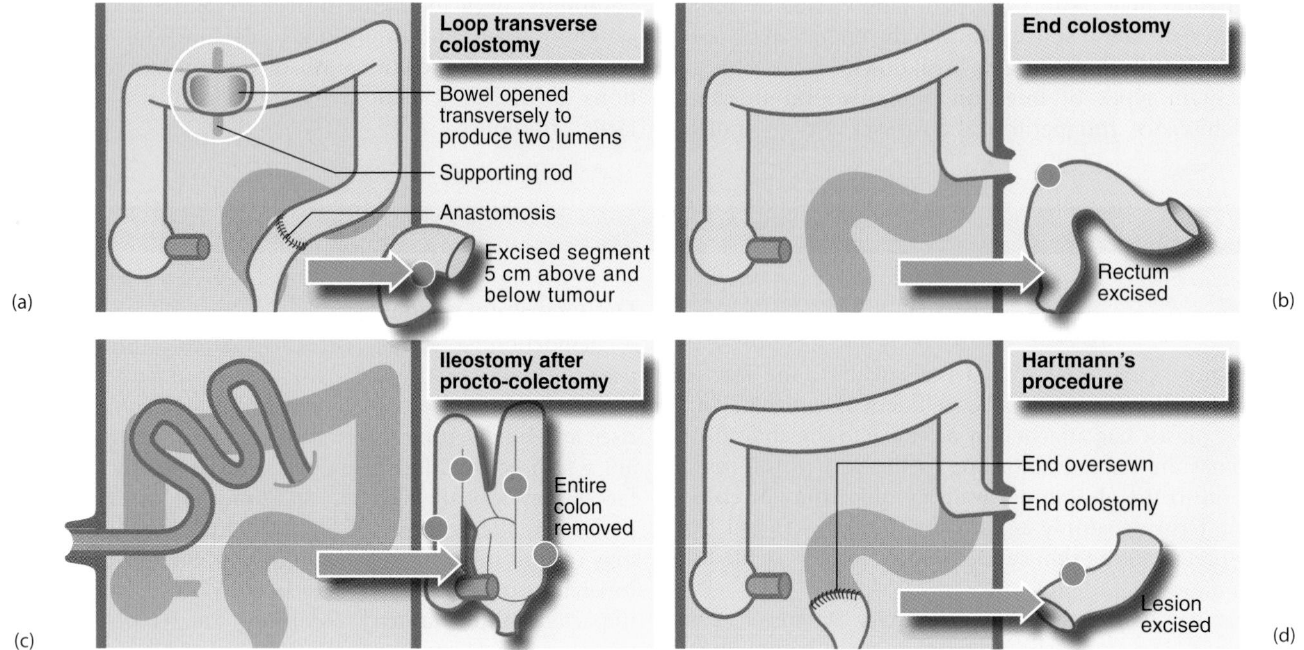

Fig. 27.11 Principal types of ileostomy and colostomy (a) Loop transverse colostomy is usually temporary, and is used to defunction the distal bowel. **(b)** End colostomy is usually permanent. **(c)** Ileostomy after procto-colectomy is permanent. Note the protruding 'spout' produced by everting the ileum. **(d)** End colostomy in Hartmann's procedure sometimes becomes permanent

CASE HISTORY

Fig. 27.12 End ileostomy

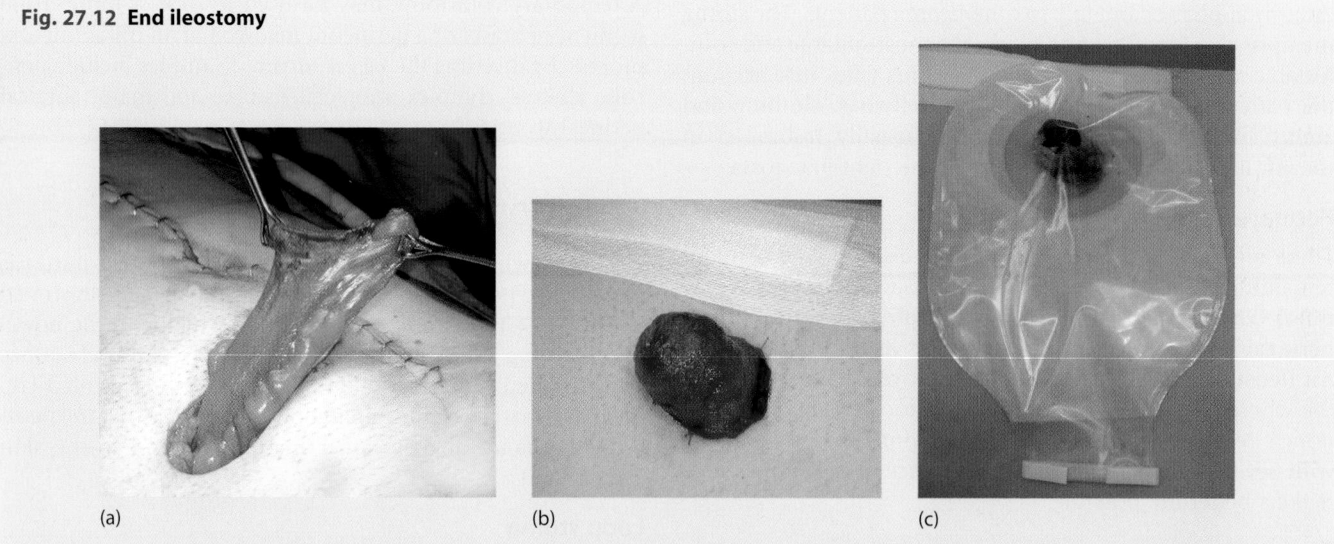

This man of 45 had suffered remittent ulcerative colitis for 12 years which could only be managed with high doses of steroids. He underwent subtotal colectomy and formation of this end ileostomy. Later, he will be considered for a pouch reconstruction. **(a)** Formation of ileostomy. The end of the ileum is brought to the surface via an opening made in the right iliac fossa at a point predetermined by the stoma therapist. **(b)** The end of the ileum has been turned back on itself like a cuff to form a spout or Brook ileostomy. **(c)** The stoma bag placed in the operating theatre

proximal and distal bowel ends are brought separately to the skin surface. The proximal end stoma passes stool into a stoma appliance; the distal stoma (or **mucous fistula**) defunctions the bowel beyond it and produces just a little mucus.

End stoma

This type of stoma is usually permanent. An end **colostomy** is most commonly used to 'resite the anus' on to the abdominal wall after removal of the rectum and anal sphincter (i.e. abdomino-perineal excision—Fig. 27.11b). An **ileostomy** may be employed after subtotal or pan-proctocolectomy, particularly in fulminant colitis (Fig. 27.11c). Later, some form of reconstruction may be considered, involving an ileal pouch or reservoir in the pelvis composed of loops of ileum sutured side-to-side connected to the anus. The anal sphincter mechanism is preserved so that the patient is usually continent and can control evacuation.

Table 27.3 Complications of ileostomy and colostomy

Complication	Treatment
Early complications	
Mucosal sloughing or necrosis of the terminal bowel due to ischaemia	Reoperation and refashioning of the stoma
Obstruction of stoma due to oedema or faecal impaction	Exploration with a gloved finger and sometimes glycerol suppositories or softening enemas
Persistent leakage between skin and appliance causing skin erosion and patient distress, often due to inappropriate location of stoma (e.g. over skin crease)	May respond to stoma nursing care or require a resiting operation
Late complications	
Parastomal hernia due to abdominal wall weakness	Resiting of stoma +/- mesh reinforcement of abdominal wall
Prolapse of bowel	Refashioning of stoma
Parastomal fistula	Refashioning of stoma, or local repair, possibly laparoscopic
Retraction of 'spout' ileostomy	Reoperation and refashioning of a new ileostomy
Stenosis of stomal orifice	Refashioning of stoma
Perforation after colonic irrigation	Emergency operation
Psychological and psychosexual dysfunction	May require counselling or measures to reverse stoma

Hartmann's procedure: end colostomy and rectal stump

Hartmann's procedure is a relatively safe technique, particularly for less experienced surgeons, and carries less overall risk than primary anastomosis. It is employed after emergency resection of rectosigmoid lesions where primary anastomosis is inadvisable because of obstruction, inflammation or faecal contamination or surgical inexperience. It may be the choice of treatment for frail or debilitated patients. At Hartmann's operation, the lesion is resected, the proximal bowel is made into an end colostomy (the same as that employed after an abdomino-perineal excision) and the cut end of the distal remnant is closed with sutures or staples (see Fig. 27.11d). Secretions from the residual rectum still pass through the anus. Several months later when local inflammation has resolved, a decision may be made to reconnect the bowel, depending on fitness and the preference of the patient. However, the colostomy is so well tolerated that some patients prefer to keep it permanently rather than undergo another major operation.

Irrigation technique for managing a colostomy

An ileostomy tends to work continuously during the day whereas a colostomy is intermittent. Some patients with a colostomy prefer to dispense with a stoma bag by using a technique of colonic irrigation. Once every few days the patient passes a litre or more of water into the colostomy via a special spout, then the water is allowed to drain out, with the aim of emptying the entire colon. After this, the stoma is covered with a dry dressing as a stoma bag is not needed until the next irrigation.

COMPLICATIONS OF COLOSTOMY AND ILEOSTOMY

These are summarised in Table 27.3.

28 Chronic inflammatory disorders of the bowel

INTRODUCTION

Substantial inflammation in any part of the small or large bowel usually presents with diarrhoea (i.e. frequent passage of loose stools). When inflammation affects the large bowel, the diarrhoea often contains blood. **Chronic diarrhoea** is defined as lasting for longer than 6 weeks, different from the acute diarrhoea of gastroenteritis which is usually of viral origin or related to food poisoning and is usually self-limiting, though often fatal in infants in the developing world.

A chronic change of bowel habit to looser and more frequent stools, whether containing blood or not, raises the possibility of three categories of diagnosis: **infective** (bacillary or amoebic), **inflammatory bowel diseases** (ulcerative colitis, Crohn's disease or rarer forms of non-infective colitis) and **neoplasms** (covered in the previous chapter).

The term **inflammatory bowel disease** usually means the two chronic bowel disorders, **ulcerative colitis** or **Crohn's disease**. They share many pathophysiological and clinical features. However, Crohn's disease can involve any part of the gastrointestinal tract, whilst ulcerative colitis is confined to the large bowel. When the large bowel alone is inflamed, it is important to differentiate between these conditions because management and the spectrum of complications differ substantially (see Table 28.1).

These diseases are chronic and relapsing by nature. They have variable responses to treatments, with a potential for complications after major surgery. The most effective management and best outcomes result from cooperation between medical and surgical gastroenterologists. Patients can mostly be managed on an outpatient basis but acute exacerbations or complications may require admission. Surgery is usually indicated when medical management has failed or when complications such as fulminant colitis, obstruction, toxic dilatation of the colon or perforation occur. In addition, ulcerative colitis is a long-term risk factor for **colorectal cancer**.

In developing countries, **infections** that cause chronic large bowel inflammation are more common and may also be contracted by travellers. **Amoebiasis** in particular may mimic ulcerative colitis, and **tuberculosis** may mimic Crohn's disease.

Pseudomembranous and other forms of **antibiotic-related colitis** are increasingly common in hospitalised patients after antibiotic treatment; they are discussed in Chapter 12. Whilst typical cases can be readily diagnosed and treated, severe forms may require emergency colectomy and may cause fatality in elderly patients. Symptoms may occur as long as 6 months after antibiotic use.

Infective causes must be excluded before inflammatory bowel disease is diagnosed because life-threatening complications can result from treating infective conditions with immunosuppressive drugs used for inflammatory bowel disease.

EPIDEMIOLOGY AND AETIOLOGY OF INFLAMMATORY BOWEL DISEASE

Ulcerative colitis and Crohn's disease are considered to be separate entities but in 10–15% of cases no clear distinction can be made; this is termed **indeterminate colitis**; it is possible that the diseases share aetiological factors or even represent different facets of the same disease.

Ulcerative colitis and Crohn's disease are relatively common in developed countries but the diseases seem rare in most of Africa, Asia and South America. In the West, the incidence of Crohn's disease appears to have increased over the past few decades (to 100 per 100 000 population per year), whilst ulcerative colitis (200 per 100 000) has remained static or may have even declined.

Most inflammatory bowel disease develops in the late teen years or twenties. Gender, social class and urban living seems to be irrelevant. In the USA, white people are three times more susceptible to ulcerative colitis than black people and five times more susceptible to Crohn's disease.

The aetiology of these diseases remains obscure. There is a familial incidence: 6–8% of patients with ulcerative colitis and about 20% of those with Crohn's disease have first-degree relatives with the same condition. It is likely that both conditions are genetically heterogeneous and polygenic. For Crohn's disease, implicated genes include *NOD2* and *CARD15*. For ulcerative colitis, genes *IBD1*, *IBD2* and *IBD3* have been identified. It is postulated that the presence of more than one of these genetic mutations may result in Crohn's disease.

Another similarity between the two diseases is the association with a range of non-gastrointestinal autoimmune disorders involving eyes, joints, skin and liver. The most

Table 28.1 Comparative features of ulcerative colitis and Crohn's disease

	Ulcerative colitis	Crohn's disease
Pathology		
Inflammation	Recurrent acute inflammation with intervening quiescent phases	Chronic relapsing inflammation
General distribution	Continuous involvement of affected part of colon	Skip lesions in any part of gastrointestinal tract
Rectal involvement	Always	About 25%
Ileal involvement	Backwash ileitis only	Involved in 80% of cases; exclusive to ileum in 50% of cases
Depth of wall involved	Mucosa only	Transmural, including serosa
Mucosal changes	Widespread irregular superficial ulceration with or without pseudopolyps	Fissured ulceration causing 'cobblestone' appearance
Granuloma formation	Absent	Characteristic but not always present
Mesenteric adenopathy	Reactive hyperplasia only	Lymph nodes often enlarged; granulomas may be present
Fibrosis of wall	Minimal	Marked
Main clinical features		
Diarrhoea	Severe during acute attacks, often causing incontinence	Less prominent
Rectal bleeding	Very common	Less common
Abdominal pain	Mild cramping 'pre-defaecation' pain with diarrhoeal attacks	Dominant feature—persistent or grumbling pain with severe acute attacks
Abdominal mass	No	Relatively common
General debility	Less marked	Characteristic
Complications		
Strictures	Rare	Common and often multiple
Fistulae	Rare	Common
Anal and perianal lesions	Uncommon	Common
Massive haemorrhage	Occurs in fulminant disease	Rare
Intestinal obstruction	Rare	Incomplete obstruction is common
Perforation	Complication of toxic megacolon	Free perforation rare but perforation causing local abscess formation or internal fistula common
Toxic megacolon	May occur in fulminant attacks	Rare
Malignant change	High risk with severe/longstanding disease	Low risk
Management		
Local 5-ASA/steroids	Left-sided active disease	Less effective
Systemic steroids	Severe exacerbations	Severe exacerbations
Oral 5-ASA	To treat mild attacks Long-term maintenance	Less effective
Immunosuppressives	In severe cases unresponsive to steroids As steroid-sparing agent	'Steroid sparing' in intractable cases
Surgery	Less common —in longstanding disease with evidence of dysplasia or malignancy —in fulminant colitis —in uncontrolled chronic disease	Commonly required

common for both ulcerative colitis and Crohn's disease is **ankylosing spondylitis**, which is usually associated with the lymphocyte surface antigen HLA-B27. In contrast, pericholangitis occurs often in ulcerative colitis but is rare in Crohn's disease, and occasionally progresses to **sclerosing cholangitis**.

Infection is believed to play a part in initiating some cases of both ulcerative colitis and Crohn's disease, as many cases follow an acute attack of gastroenteritis. Importantly, tobacco smoking is more common in patients with Crohn's disease, and smoking increases disease recurrence. Ulcerative colitis, by contrast, is more prevalent in non-smokers.

ULCERATIVE COLITIS

Ulcerative colitis is an inflammatory disorder of the mucosa and submucosa of the **large bowel** only. It is characterised by recurrent acute exacerbations and intervening periods of quiescence or chronic low-grade activity. The symptom severity corresponds to the level of disease activity. Extracolonic features affect a small proportion of patients and include anaemia, inflammation of joints (**arthropathy**) and inflammation of eyes, skin and biliary tract. The disease always

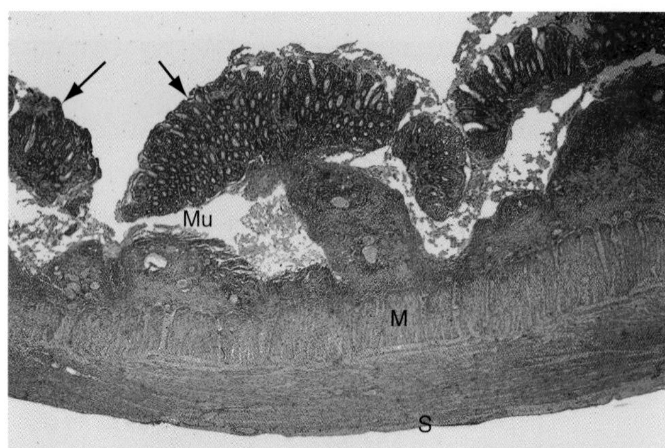

Fig. 28.1 Ulcerative colitis—histopathology
Erosion and undermining of the mucosa **Mu** by the inflammatory process has produced typical pseudopolyps (arrowed). Inflammation spares the muscle wall **M** and serosa **S**. Mucosal glands show reactive and regenerative changes

involves the rectum but often extends proximally in continuity to involve a variable length of colon. In nearly 20% of cases (but only those with pancolitis, i.e. colitis involving the whole large bowel), the distal end of the ileum becomes secondarily affected; this is described as **backwash ileitis**.

PATHOPHYSIOLOGY OF ULCERATIVE COLITIS

Initially, the colonic mucosa becomes acutely inflamed. Neutrophils accumulate in the lamina propria and within the tubular colonic glands to form small, highly characteristic **crypt abscesses**. Sloughing of the overlying mucosa produces small superficial ulcers. If the inflammatory process persists, the ulcers coalesce into extensive areas of irregular ulceration. Residual islands of intact but oedematous mucosa project into the bowel lumen; these inflammatory lesions are called **pseudopolyps** (see Fig. 28.1). The inflammation is usually confined to the mucosa and submucosa, only extending into the muscular wall and peritoneal surface in **fulminating colitis**.

Acute inflammatory episodes range from several days' to several months' duration. After subsiding, they can recur months or even years later. During quiescent periods, the acute inflammation resolves and the mucosa regenerates. The lamina propria, however, remains swollen by a chronic inflammatory infiltrate of lymphocytes and plasma cells. The colonic glands show a marked reduction in the number of mucin-secreting goblet cells, histologically termed '**goblet cell depletion**'.

After the disease has been present for some time, **dysplastic changes** can appear in the epithelium. Dysplasia (Latin for 'bad form') involves recognisable changes indicating early transformation to neoplasia. After prolonged or repeated episodes of inflammation, dysplasia may progress to **adenocarcinoma**. The risk of malignancy is greatest for those with early onset and extensive disease, and is approximately 5% after 10 years of colitis. Cancer diagnosis may be delayed if symptoms are mistaken for a relapse of colitis and are not investigated. Cancers in these patients are often particularly aggressive and occur on average 20 years earlier than in the general population.

Fig. 28.2 Radiological appearances (lateral decubitus) of ulcerative colitis

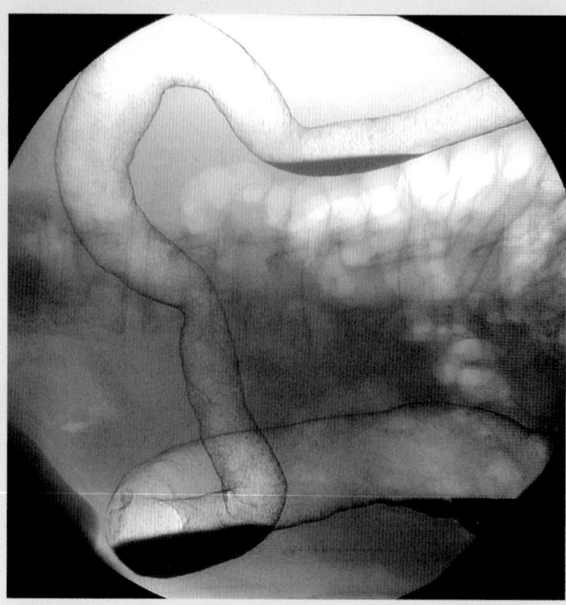

'End-stage' or 'burnt-out' ulcerative colitis in a 49-year-old office worker. He had suffered episodic, but not incapacitating, diarrhoea for 34 years, but presented on this occasion because of urgency and incontinence. Sigmoidoscopy showed only moderate rectal ulceration. This barium enema shows a typical smooth, shortened 'lead pipe' colon, with complete loss of haustration. Note that the film is orientated in the lateral decubitus position. He failed to respond to medical treatment and underwent proctocolectomy and ileostomy

In longstanding colitis, the mucosa and submucosa undergo fibrosis, resulting in smoothing out of haustrations and a shortened colon which has a characteristic radiological appearance, the so-called **lead pipe colon** (Fig. 28.2).

CLINICAL FEATURES OF ULCERATIVE COLITIS

Acute inflammatory attacks are marked by loose blood-stained stools streaked with mucus. This mucus results from inflammation of recto-sigmoid colonic mucosa. As the extent of inflammation increases, the diarrhoea may become severe. The patient may pass 20 or more loose stools a day, each time preceded by cramping abdominal pain. In many patients, the urge to defaecate is so precipitate that incontinence occurs unless a lavatory is immediately available.

Any attack of ulcerative colitis may progress to the severe form of **fulminant colitis**; the patient may become prostrated by dehydration, severe electrolyte disturbance and blood loss. Occasionally, the colon dilates massively and patchy necrosis eventually occurs. The patient is systemically ill with high fever, marked tachycardia and dehydration. This process, known as **toxic megacolon**, culminates in perforation and fatal peritonitis unless emergency colectomy is performed.

Ulcerative colitis should probably be regarded as a systemic disorder. It is sometimes accompanied by extra-gastrointestinal manifestations, summarised in Box 28.1. During active phases, inflammatory markers (erythrocyte sedimentation rate (ESR) and C-reactive protein (CRP)) are elevated and moderate

Box 28.1 Systemic manifestations of ulcerative colitis

Weight loss
- Frequent during exacerbations

Anaemia
- Typically chronic and non-specific (normochromic, normocytic)

Arthropathy
- Sacroiliitis/ankylosing spondylitis or rheumatoid-like arthritis, especially of large joints (approximately 20% of cases)

Uveitis and iritis
- Painful red eye or eyes (approximately 10%)

Skin lesions
- Erythema nodosum, i.e. tender red nodules on the shins (uncommon), pyoderma gangrenosum, i.e. purulent skin ulcers (rare)

Sclerosing cholangitis
- Progressive fibrosis of intrahepatic biliary system leading to cirrhosis, progressive liver failure, jaundice and eventually death (rare)

Fig. 28.3 Radiological appearances of ulcerative colitis

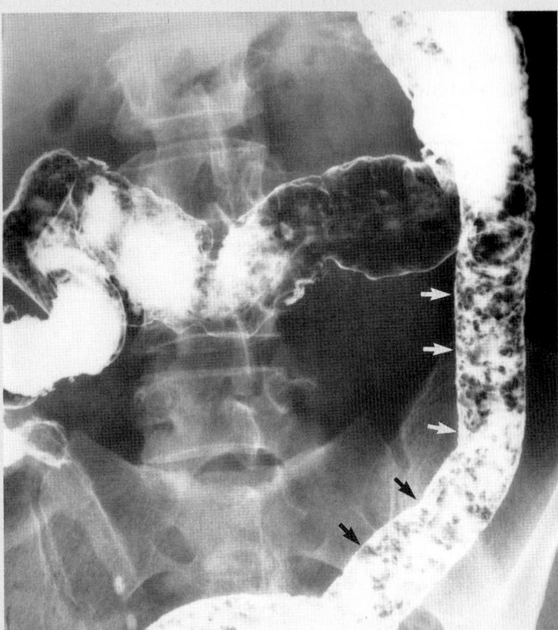

Severe and longstanding ulcerative colitis in a man of 50. The whole colon is affected (pancolitis) with loss of the normal haustral pattern. There is extensive pseudopolyp formation, particularly in the descending and sigmoid colon, manifest by multiple small filling defects (arrowed). Prolonged severe ulceration stimulates mitotic activity and is probably responsible for dysplastic changes and eventual malignant change in longstanding severe ulcerative colitis

anaemia and hypoalbuminaemia is common. Associated arthropathy, eye and skin disorders usually flare up in parallel with the colitis (although they may rarely precede the intestinal symptoms). However, the liver-related conditions—sclerosing cholangitis, chronic active hepatitis and bile duct carcinoma—are often independent of colitic activity and are therefore difficult to treat.

CLINICAL EXAMINATION AND INVESTIGATION OF SUSPECTED ULCERATIVE COLITIS

The typical patient referred for investigation of suspected ulcerative colitis is a young adult with a history of several weeks of frequent loose stools, later streaked with blood and mucus. The attack often starts with an attack of gastroenteritis or traveller's diarrhoea which fails to settle. There is sometimes a history of non-GI symptoms such as arthropathy or uveitis.

General examination often reveals anaemia but abdominal examination is usually unremarkable. Rectal examination, followed by proctoscopy and sigmoidoscopy, is mandatory to palpate, inspect and, if necessary, biopsy the rectal mucosa. The affected mucosa ranges in appearance from mildly hyperaemic and easily traumatised to extensive patchy ulceration.

At least three separate fresh stool samples should be analysed to exclude bacterial or parasitic causes or cytomegalovirus, as these conditions may closely simulate ulcerative colitis but require entirely different treatment.

Proctitis

Some patients with ulcerative colitis have inflammation confined to the lower rectum. The mucosa often has a granular appearance and the condition is described as **proctitis** or **granular proctitis**. Its cause is unknown and its course is self-limiting. It tends to recur at times of stress, often at protracted intervals. Proctitis usually responds to short courses of local 5-aminosalicylic acid suppositories (see later), but can occasionally progress into a distal or even a total colitis.

Contrast radiology

If the clinical picture and histological findings are consistent with inflammatory bowel disease, the extent and degree of colonic involvement can be assessed by barium enema examination. Radiological appearances are illustrated in Figures 28.2 and 28.3. Contrast radiology is not usually performed in acute disease.

Endoscopy

In an acute situation, an unprepared flexible sigmoidoscopy is usually performed. In non-acute situations, colonoscopy enables direct inspection of the entire colonic mucosa and the taking of multiple biopsies (see Fig. 28.4). Furthermore, in patients with longstanding total colitis, colonoscopy with narrow band imaging and multiple biopsies is used for annual surveillance for dysplastic change.

Fulminant ulcerative colitis

Fulminant attacks sometimes occur, with extremely frequent watery, blood-stained stools and severe systemic illness. An attack may progress to toxic dilatation and eventual colonic perforation. Urgent colectomy may be judged necessary to treat fulminant colitis resistant to medical therapy, or to treat toxic megacolon, once infective causes have been excluded.

Whatever the cause, patients with acute colitis require urgent hospital admission and resuscitation including fluid, electrolyte and blood replacement. Sigmoidoscopy and biopsy are performed to establish the diagnosis. Stool is sent for microscopy and culture. Plain abdominal radiography is performed to monitor for dilatation, which might indicate toxic megacolon (defined as a colonic diameter greater than 6 cm in the presence of pyrexia or tachycardia). In the absence of megacolon, plain radiography may demonstrate other features of acute ulcerative colitis as shown in Figure 28.5.

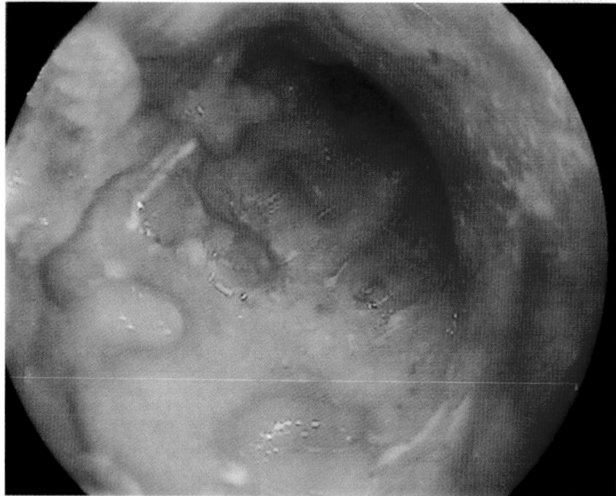
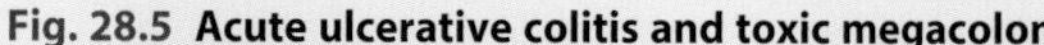

Fig. 28.4 Colonoscopic view of ulcerative colitis
This colon is quiescent with no evidence of current ulceration but inflammatory polyps are seen as memorials to past severe inflammation and ulceration

MANAGEMENT OF ULCERATIVE COLITIS

The choice of treatment depends on the severity of individual attacks, the amount of colon involved, the extent of chronic symptoms and the risk of long-term complications. The treatment options are summarised in Box 28.2.

Aminosalicylate preparations

Mild attacks of proctitis or procto-sigmoiditis are treated locally with 5-aminosalicylic acid (5-ASA) suppositories or enemas, which are more effective in acute proctitis than steroids. Mild attacks of pan-colitis are treated initially with oral 5-ASA preparations which are also employed as maintenance therapy in ulcerative colitis to prevent relapse. Although aspirin and other non-steroidal anti-inflammatories are chemically related to 5-ASA compounds,, these drugs should be avoided as they may worsen inflammatory bowel disease. The 5-ASA compounds are discussed later in this chapter as they are also used in the management of Crohn's disease.

CASE HISTORY

Fig. 28.5 Acute ulcerative colitis and toxic megacolon

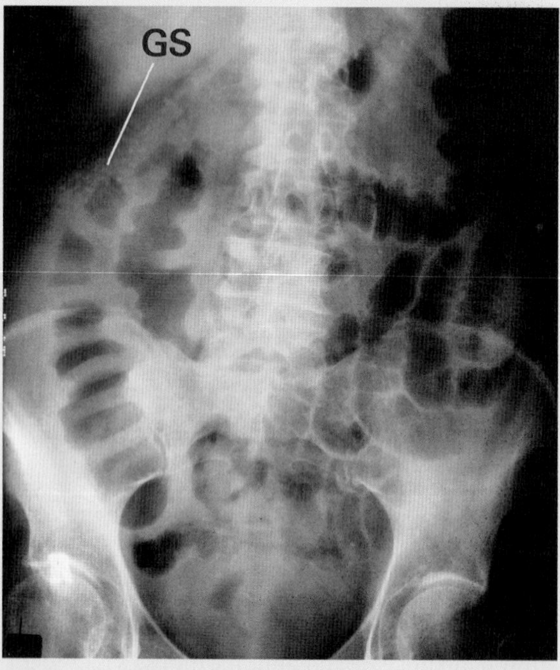

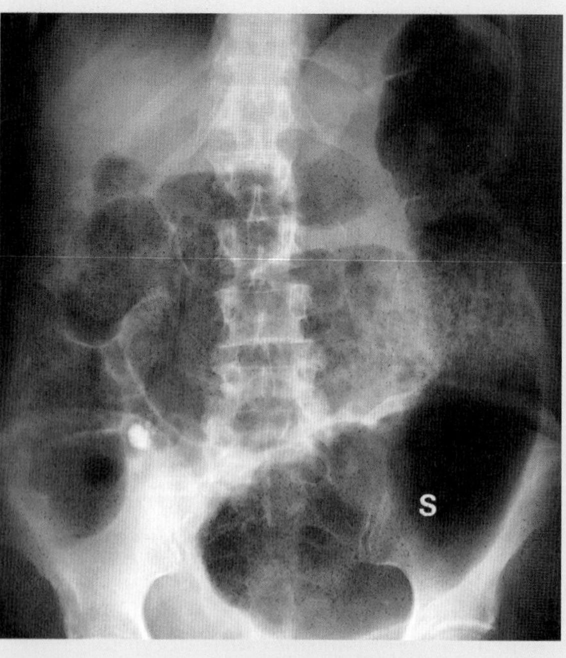

(a) This 44-year-old woman presented with fulminant ulcerative colitis. She was prostrated by frequent diarrhoea and consequent electrolyte abnormalities. This plain supine radiograph shows acute right-sided colitis. The caecum, ascending colon and proximal transverse colon are affected. In this area, there is absence of the normal 'convex outward' pattern and there are thick folds crossing the bowel lumen. This appearance is caused by oedema of the bowel wall; note the incidental finding of gallstones **GS**. **(b)** This patient presented in a similar way but became toxic while in hospital undergoing intensive medical treatment. There was an increasing tachycardia, fever and abdominal tenderness. Serial plain abdominal radiographs showed an increasing diameter of the left colon. This film shows the sigmoid colon **S** dilated to 10 cm and in imminent danger of perforation. This is known as toxic dilatation of the colon; it occurs most commonly in ulcerative colitis and usually affects the transverse colon

Box 28.2 Main treatment measures for ulcerative colitis

Local corticosteroid or 5-ASA preparations (suppositories, foam or liquid enema)

- Employed in cases of left-sided active disease

Systemic corticosteroids

- Suppress moderate or severe exacerbations (oral or intravenous administration according to severity of disease)

Oral (or sometimes rectal) aminosalicylate preparations, e.g. sulfasalazine, mesalazine (Asacol or Pentasa) or olsalazine

- Long-term maintenance therapy to minimise relapse

Surgical removal of the colon

- Emergency operation: incipient or actual perforation, serious haemorrhage, failure of fulminant colitis to improve on medical treatment
- Elective operation: failure of medical treatment, risk of malignancy

Corticosteroids

Steroid suppositories or enemas (foam or liquid) can be used for local treatment of rectal inflammation. Short courses of high-dose oral corticosteroids are used for more severe exacerbations (e.g. prednisolone 40 mg daily for 2 weeks then reducing the daily dose by 5 mg weekly). Intravenous administration is advisable in seriously ill patients. There is no evidence that 'bowel rest' (i.e. nil by mouth) and total parenteral nutrition (TPN) are of any value in ulcerative colitis. Immunosuppressive drugs, including **ciclosporin** and **azathioprine**, are often tried in patients who fail to respond to corticosteroids. Azathioprine is also used as a 'steroid-sparing' agent in patients whose disease settles on steroids but flares again as steroids are reduced.

Other supportive measures

In the acute case, anti-diarrhoeal agents such as codeine phosphate or loperamide should be avoided as they can precipitate toxic dilatation.

Patients with moderately severe chronic disease frequently become anaemic and lose weight, in part because of persistent stool loss of protein. These problems may be helped by medical treatment, a diet high in calories and protein, and oral iron supplements.

Surgery for ulcerative colitis

Surgery is required in only about 20% of patients with ulcerative colitis. Colectomy may be needed in the following:

- Urgent treatment of fulminant cases which fail to respond to intensive medical treatment. 'Failure to respond' has no precise definition but there should normally be symptomatic improvement after a week of intensive management
- Acute cases which progress to toxic megacolon, perforation or major haemorrhage
- Patients with chronic disabling symptoms of intractable diarrhoea with urgency, recurring anaemia and failure to maintain adequate weight and nutrition
- Children with failure to thrive and retardation of growth (both are exacerbated by corticosteroid therapy)
- Patients with longstanding colitis who develop dysplasia or malignancy

As a principle, surgery for ulcerative colitis requires removal of the entire large bowel and is curative. There are three main surgical options:

- **Subtotal colectomy with ileostomy** is the safest operation in the emergency situation when the patient is sick and on high-dose corticosteroids. Most of the diseased colon is removed, but the patient is left with an inflamed rectal stump. Months later, when the patient is well, this may be revised to one of the other surgical options. Alternatively the rectum may be retained and treated with local therapy plus endoscopic surveillance, although the cancer risk remains
- **Proctocolectomy with permanent ileostomy** (includes removal of rectum) is generally recommended for elderly patients in whom sphincter-preserving procedures are inadvisable
- **Restorative proctocolectomy (ileo-anal pouch, Parks' pouch)** is a sphincter-preserving operation which avoids a permanent ileostomy (see Fig. 27.8). The entire colon and rectal mucosa is excised and a **pouch** reservoir is fashioned from a loop of terminal ileum. The pouch is brought into the pelvis and anastomosed to the upper anal canal. A temporary ileostomy is usually retained for a few months to allow healing. Many patients have excellent continence and can evacuate their bowels in the normal way

CROHN'S DISEASE

Crohn's disease is a chronic relapsing inflammatory disorder of **any part** of the gastrointestinal tract (though nearly always small or large bowel) which predominantly affects younger people. About 60% of patients are under 25 years at the time of initial diagnosis, and on average, symptoms will have been present intermittently for 5 years. A useful website is http://www.crohns.org.uk/.

The disease often affects one or more discrete segments of bowel with intervening parts completely spared, unlike the continuous nature of ulcerative colitis. These discontinuous affected areas are known as '**skip lesions**' (see Fig. 28.11, p. 373).

The small bowel alone is affected in 50% of patients, the large bowel alone in 20% and both together in 30%. The terminal ileum is affected most commonly; in up to half of all cases, the disease is confined to the terminal ileum. In the original description of this disease it was named 'terminal ileitis'. Later, when it became clear that other segments of

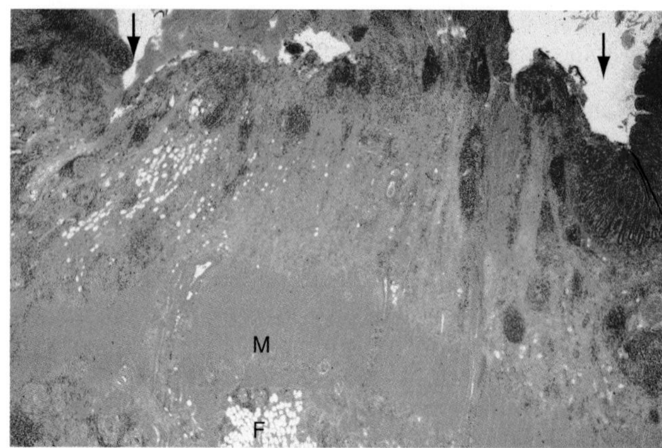

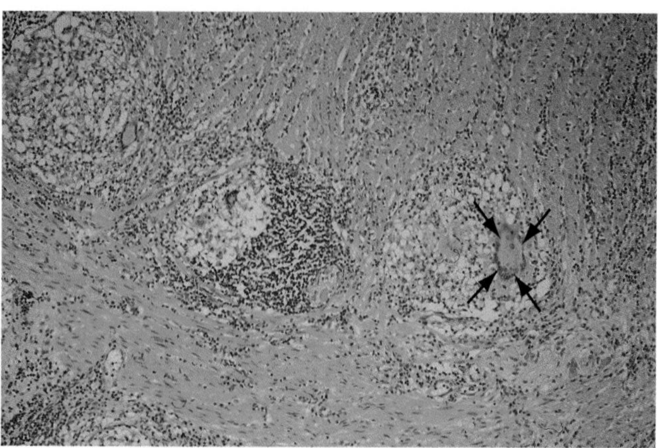

Fig. 28.6 Crohn's disease affecting the colon—histopathology (a) Inflammation has produced fissure ulcers (arrowed) which extend into the muscle wall **M**. Lymphoid aggregates are also present and the inflammatory process extends into serosal fat **F**. **(b)** High-power view showing well-formed granulomas with typical giant cells (arrowed), enabling a confident diagnosis of Crohn's disease to be made

bowel could be affected, the name was changed to **regional enteritis**, a term still used in the USA. Crohn's disease also commonly affects the perianal region, whether or not large bowel is involved. Occasionally, the disease involves the stomach, duodenum, oesophagus or mouth.

In contrast to ulcerative colitis, the inflammation involves the entire thickness of the bowel wall (**transmural inflammation**). Because of this, affected bowel may partially obstruct, fistulate or perforate, whereas this rarely occurs in ulcerative colitis. See Table 28.1 for comparisons between Crohn's disease and ulcerative colitis.

With each exacerbation, previously affected or new areas may become involved. The disease tends to run a protracted and unpredictable course.

PATHOPHYSIOLOGY AND CLINICAL CONSEQUENCES OF CROHN'S DISEASE

The essential pathological feature is chronic inflammation of bowel, with inflammation extending diffusely through the entire bowel wall. The wall becomes markedly thickened by inflammatory oedema, especially in the submucosa. The epithelium remains largely intact but is criss-crossed by deep **fissured ulcers**. These large serpiginous ulcers and the intervening areas of dome-shaped mucosa and submucosa give a typical 'cobblestone' surface appearance (Fig. 28.11).

Granulomas containing multinucleate giant cells (see Fig. 28.6) are usually scattered throughout the inflamed bowel wall as well as in local lymph nodes. (Although these non-caseating granulomas are typical of Crohn's disease, they are not always found, and ruptured crypt abscesses in ulcerative colitis may also cause them.) Longstanding inflammation leads to progressive **fibrosis** of the thickened bowel wall, which encroaches on the lumen, producing **elongated strictures**.

Effects of mucosal inflammation

Mucosal inflammation causes diarrhoea which, if the colon is involved, may be streaked with mucus and blood. Luminal narrowing in the small bowel results in partial obstruction that causes grumbling, colicky abdominal pain, sometimes with acute episodes. Pain is a prominent feature in Crohn's disease in contrast to ulcerative colitis, since inflamed large bowel does not obstruct in this way.

If small bowel is inflamed, diarrhoea occurs and digestive and absorptive functions may be compromised. Extensive disease results in general malabsorption causing protein-calorie malnutrition, iron and folate deficiency and anaemia. In children, Crohn's disease may cause marked growth retardation. Ileal inflammation disrupts **bile salt reabsorption**. Excess bile salts in the faeces cause colonic irritation (and more diarrhoea) while diminished recirculation of bile salts may result in gallstone formation. Involvement of the terminal ileum may reduce vitamin B_{12} absorption but serious deficiency usually occurs only after surgical resection.

Effects of transmural inflammation

Crohn's disease causes added problems if serosal inflammation extends to adjacent structures. If inflamed bowel impinges on **parietal peritoneum**, pain becomes localised and more severe and signs of local peritonitis develop. Indeed, Crohn's disease of the terminal ileum may mimic acute appendicitis. At appendicectomy, the terminal ileum is visibly inflamed and the bowel wall abnormally thick to palpation. In this case, the terminal ileum should not be excised as a firm diagnosis of Crohn's disease requires histological and microbacterial exclusion of *Yersinia* ileitis as well as tuberculosis. Both may simulate Crohn's, but are completely reversible with medical treatment.

Serosal inflammation may cause a diseased segment of bowel to adhere to adjacent abdominal structures. Several complications may occur if these become matted together by the inflammatory process:

- **Adhesions**. These tough, fibrotic post-inflammatory adhesions are rarely symptomatic but constitute a formidable obstacle if operation is needed later
- **Perforation**. Free perforation is rare but a contained perforation may occur which causes localised pericolic or pelvic abscess formation
- **Fistulae**. These may develop between diseased bowel and other hollow viscera causing unusual clinical phenomena.

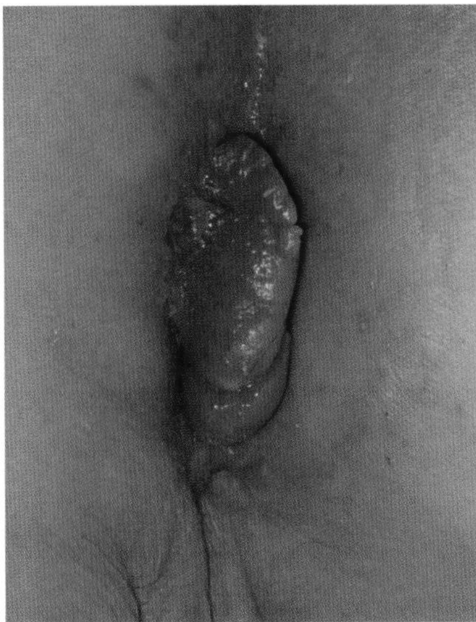

Fig. 28.7 Crohn's 'piles'
This appearance is typical of Crohn's 'piles'. They are pale and oedematous in contrast to ordinary haemorrhoids

Fig. 28.8 Multiple anal fistulae in Crohn's disease

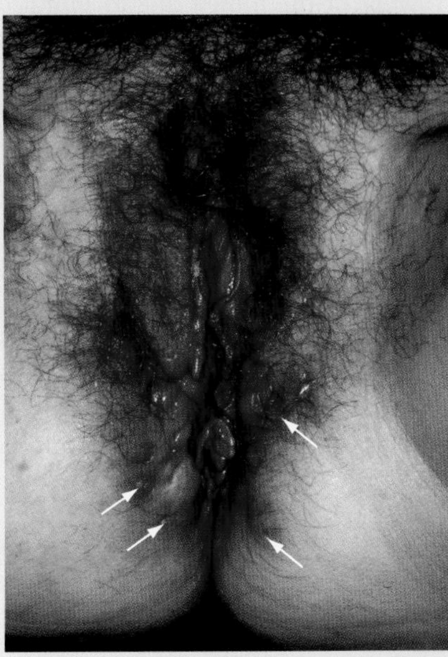

This 30-year-old woman had several 'skip lesions' of Crohn's disease in her small bowel and was troubled by recurrent perianal sepsis. This photograph shows a typical 'pepper-pot perineum', with several fistulous openings (arrowed) seen around the circumference of the anus. Anal skin tags are also visible

For example, a gastro-colic fistula may result in true faecal vomiting; an ileo-rectal fistula may aggravate diarrhoea. Entero-vesical fistulae cause severe urinary tract infections and pneumaturia (passage of urine containing air bubbles), and fistulae between bowel and uterus or vagina lead to vaginal passage of faeces. Entero-cutaneous fistulae between bowel and skin occasionally develop as a complication of bowel resection for Crohn's disease, or spontaneously

Perianal inflammation

Perianal inflammation occurs in 15% of patients with Crohn's disease. Symptoms include recurrent perianal abscesses, characteristic blueish, boggy 'piles' (see Fig. 28.7) and anterolateral anal fissures. The last two are quite distinct from ordinary haemorrhoids and posterior anal fissures. Multiple fistulae commonly develop between rectum and perianal skin and can extend into the labia or scrotum. Fistulae are sometimes so numerous as to cause a 'pepper-pot' or 'watering-can' perineum (see Fig. 28.8). Paradoxically, this is more often associated with small bowel disease than colorectal disease.

Systemic features

Like ulcerative colitis, Crohn's disease is a systemic disorder and has a similar range of non-GI manifestations (see Box 28.1, p. 367). In contrast with ulcerative colitis, it is usual for patients to feel generally ill during an acute attack. Specific systemic features affecting skin, joints or the eye are relatively uncommon and not necessarily related to bowel disease activity.

SYMPTOMS AND SIGNS IN CROHN'S DISEASE

Symptoms of Crohn's disease can be similar to those of ulcerative colitis, particularly when large bowel is involved (see Table 28.1, p. 365). Diarrhoea is usually less distressing and less likely to contain blood. Other characteristic symptoms include cramp-like abdominal pain, weight loss and general malaise. As an aide memoire, think of **pain, weight loss** and **diarrhoea** as symptomatic of Crohn's.

Physical examination may reveal generalised wasting and anaemia and sometimes other features like arthropathy. On abdominal examination, there may be areas of tenderness, an inflammatory mass in the right iliac fossa where omentum wraps around inflamed terminal ileum or the scars of previous surgery. The perianal skin should be examined for fissures, fistulae, Crohn's 'piles' or stenotic scarring from previous disease. Diseased rectal mucosa, with its typical firm surface nodularity, may be felt on digital examination. Sigmoidoscopic examination is usually normal but there may be mucosal oedema if the rectum is involved. In more severe cases, the typical 'cobblestone' appearance with fissured ulceration may be seen. Biopsies may be positive even when the mucosa is apparently normal.

APPROACH TO INVESTIGATION OF SUSPECTED CROHN'S DISEASE

Investigation of suspected Crohn's disease is similar to that for ulcerative colitis in respect of the large bowel, but follows a different pattern when there is suspected small bowel disease.

Colonoscopy enables a histological diagnosis to be obtained in colonic disease, and also allows biopsies of terminal ileum to be taken, which are often diagnostic. Barium 'follow-through' is the traditional method of examining small bowel but better images are sometimes obtained by controlled instillation of barium into the duodenum via a nasogastric tube. Typical radiological appearances of Crohn's disease include narrowing of the lumen due to mural oedema and fibrosis, nodularity and cobblestoning of the mucosal surface, deep fissured ulceration extending into the muscular wall, spiky 'rose thorn' ulcers and possibly evidence of fistula formation. Radiological changes in small and large bowel are shown in Figures 28.9 and 28.10. Note that large bowel abnormalities on barium enema may be difficult or impossible to distinguish from ulcerative colitis.

As in ulcerative colitis, full blood count, inflammatory markers (ESR and CRP) and liver function tests also give an indication of the disease activity; stool microscopy and culture is always undertaken to exclude an infective cause for diarrhoea.

Appearances of Crohn's colitis are shown in Fig. 28.10.

MANAGEMENT OF CROHN'S DISEASE

The aim of medical therapy in active Crohn's disease is to bring about and maintain remission. The treatments available may be broadly divided into three classes of medication:

Anti-inflammatory agents

- **5-ASA compounds**, as used in ulcerative colitis. These act locally, making it a challenge to deliver oral medication to inflamed small bowel without gastric inactivation. **Sulfasalazine** (a combination of 5-ASA and a carrier, sulfapyridine) is useful in ulcerative colitis and large bowel Crohn's disease because the active ingredient is released by colonic bacteria. However, some patients suffer side-effects related to the sulfapyridine. Mesalazine is useful for more proximal Crohn's disease as the active

CASE HISTORY

Fig. 28.9 Radiological appearances in Crohn's disease

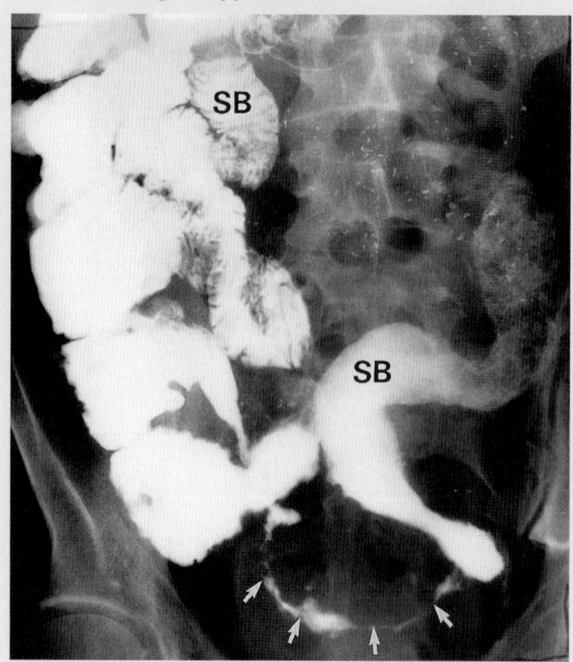

This man of 51 had recurrent attacks of colicky abdominal pain, with diarrhoea and loss of weight. This barium follow-through examination shows one of the characteristic radiological appearances of Crohn's disease. The terminal ileum is extremely narrowed by inflammation of the whole wall thickness (arrowed); this is known as the 'string sign of Kantor' and causes the symptoms and signs of partial obstruction. This film also shows dilatation of small bowel **SB** proximal to the stricture

CASE HISTORY

Fig. 28.10 Radiological appearances in Crohn's disease

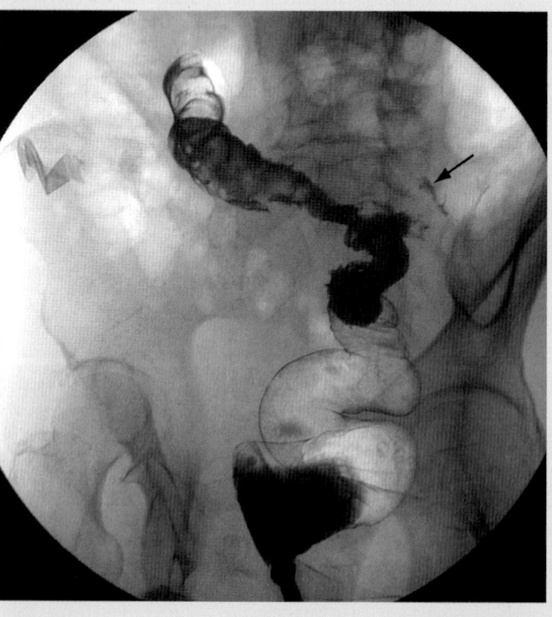

(a)

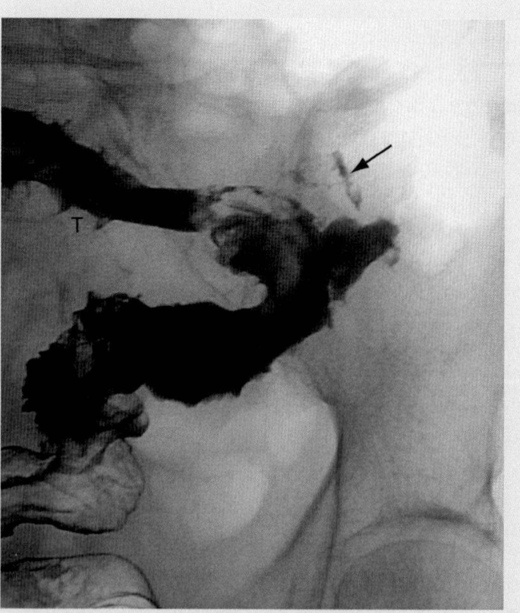

(b)

(a) Double contrast barium enema in a 28-year-old woman who complained of 8 months' history of recurrent abdominal pains and diarrhoea. She had not lost weight. This film shows a 'ragged' segment in the sigmoid colon with narrowing and 'rose thorn' ulcers **T**, better seen in the close-up view in **(b)**. In both views, contrast is visible outside the colon (arrowed). In fact, this is in small bowel because of a fistula between colon and small bowel

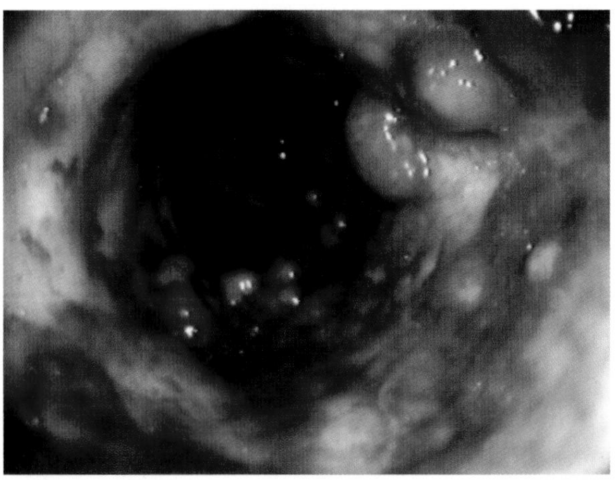
(a)

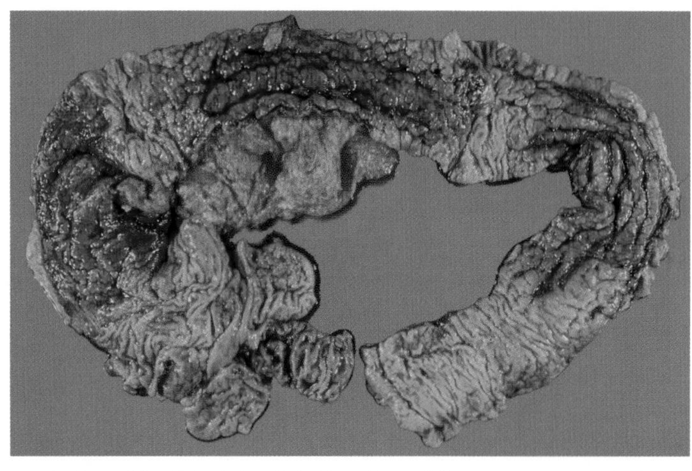
(b)

Fig. 28.11 Appearances of Crohn's colitis (a) This is a typical colonoscopic view of florid Crohn's colitis. Note the nodular appearance producing a 'cobblestone' surface with linear ulcers between the nodules. **(b)** This subtotal colectomy specimen was removed from a man of 54 with a long history of weight loss, diarrhoea and abdominal pain (see barium enema, **Fig. 28.10**). There are three 'skip lesions' typical of Crohn's disease, in the ascending colon, the transverse colon and the hepatic flexure showing thickening of the wall, cobblestone mucosal surface and narrowing of the lumen

compound is released earlier. Rectal Crohn's disease can be treated with 5-ASA suppositories or enemas, as in ulcerative colitis. 5-ASA compounds can be used as maintenance therapy in Crohn's disease but large doses are required
- **Corticosteroids** can act as systemic agents (e.g. prednisolone) or locally. Budesonide is a new oral steroid which is mostly released in the terminal ileum then rapidly inactivated by the liver after absorption, minimising systemic effects. Corticosteroids act rapidly to control flare-ups, but are rarely used for long-term maintenance

Immunomodulators

- **Azathioprine and 6-mercaptopurine** are immunosuppressants, sometimes used in more severe Crohn's disease. They can spare the need for damaging steroids, or they can help maintain remission in patients who relapse on 5-ASA compounds. About 10% of those treated are at risk of bone marrow suppression but those at risk can be predicted by pre-treatment testing
- **Methotrexate** acts both as an anti-inflammatory agent and an immunomodulator but has potentially serious side-effects upon liver and bone marrow
- **Infliximab** is a chimeric monoclonal antibody to TNFα, an inflammatory mediator. It is given by intravenous infusion for acute disease and is usually effective within 2 weeks. The drug can be given at 8-weekly intervals to maintain remission. Risks include developing antibodies to the drug. It should not be used where there is active infection or an abscess

Other supportive treatments

- Antidiarrhoeal drugs (e.g. loperamide) and antispasmodics are used in chronic symptoms
- Dietary modification: liquid/low-fibre diets for those with obstructive symptoms, and supplementary calories, iron and vitamins

THE ROLE OF SURGERY IN CROHN'S DISEASE

Surgery should not be considered curative in Crohn's disease, unlike ulcerative colitis. This is because operating on one section of bowel does not affect later recurrences elsewhere. Up to 70% of patients with Crohn's disease will eventually need surgery, of whom half will need further surgery within 5 years.

The main indications for surgery can be summarised as follows:

- Acute complications, e.g. abscess, perforation
- Persistent local ileal disease
- Intolerable long-term obstructive and other symptoms, e.g. abdominal pain, perianal disease, general ill-health
- Entero-cutaneous fistulae and symptomatic internal fistulae

The choice of operation depends on the site and extent of disease. The former belief that all disease must be resected has been abandoned. Given the diffuse nature of the disease and likelihood of further operations, as much bowel as possible should be preserved. Surgery for multiple small bowel strictures now involves **stricturoplasty** of each lesion, a technique of enlarging the lumen of diseased bowel without losing potential absorptive length. If disease is limited, resection of the diseased segment with a small margin of normal tissue may be performed, followed by wide side-to-side anastomosis. **Abscesses** are usually treated by simple drainage, with resection of the affected bowel at the same time or later.

Fistulae between abdominal viscera are treated by removing the diseased bowel. In contrast, entero-cutaneous fistulae, usually a complication of recent surgery, are a more formidable problem since they are often associated with complicating factors like intra-abdominal infection, gross fluid and electrolyte abnormalities and a hypercatabolic state. Patients with entero-cutaneous fistulae require intensive preparatory medical care and strategic surgical intervention before definitive treatment is possible.

For severe **large bowel disease**, the entire colon is generally removed (pan-proctocolectomy with ileostomy). This is because there are usually several colonic 'skip lesions' and recurrence is likely. Pouch procedures are not recommended because of the risk of recurrent disease in the small bowel reservoir.

Recurrent disease often necessitates further surgery. Careful medical treatment to reduce disease recurrence and hence increase intervals between re-operations is imperative: stopping smoking, 5-ASA preparations, and even azathioprine may be used, particularly if the patient has been left with a short bowel.

OTHER CHRONIC INFLAMMATIONS OF THE COLON

AMOEBIC COLITIS

Entamoeba histolytica is a protozoon parasite responsible for amoebic colitis. It is an endemic bowel commensal in many developing countries. Most of those infected have no symptoms but they are all carriers; less than 5% suffer amoebic colitis. In these, the organism invades the large bowel mucosa, causing chronic relapsing symptoms similar to ulcerative colitis. Encysted parasites are shed by carriers in faeces and infection is readily transmitted to new individuals via the faecal-oral route, contaminated hands or uncooked food.

The incidence of amoebiasis is likely to increase in the West as tourism expands into endemic areas. If sufferers are mistakenly treated with systemic steroids for inflammatory bowel disease, the result may be fatal. Occasionally, rampant invasion progresses to local perforation and a pericolic abscess or toxic megacolon.

In any case of amoebic colitis, amoebae passing to the liver in the portal veins sometimes produce **hepatic abscesses**, most frequently in the right lobe. These are usually solitary and are filled with reddish-brown necrotic material, said to resemble anchovy sauce.

Clinical features of amoebic colitis

The disease usually affects the proximal colon, causing colicky abdominal pain, erratic bowel habit with episodes of blood-stained loose stools and right iliac fossa tenderness. If the distal colon is involved, the patient suffers chronic watery diarrhoea with blood and mucus. When the entire colon is involved, there is generalised abdominal tenderness as well as systemic features, e.g. pyrexia and progressive weight loss. Large granulomatous colonic lesions known as **amoebomas** may be palpable and must be differentiated from carcinoma or diverticular disease.

If the patient develops an amoebic liver abscess, systemic features become more marked, with general ill-health and a swinging pyrexia with sweating attacks. There is pain in the liver area and an enlarged tender liver on palpation. The abscess may rupture spontaneously into the peritoneal cavity (causing peritonitis) or through the diaphragm into the chest. Secondary lung abscesses may then rupture into the bronchi and the patient coughs up 'anchovy sauce' sputum.

Diagnosis of amoebiasis

In developed countries, amoebic colitis should always be considered in the differential diagnosis of ulcerative colitis or Crohn's colitis. Amoebic colitis is best diagnosed by microscopic examination of fresh stool specimens; this may reveal trophozoites containing ingested red cells.

Liver abscesses cause serological tests for amoebiasis to become positive. The lesions are readily demonstrated by hepatic ultrasound and the diagnosis is confirmed by needle aspiration.

Treatment of amoebiasis

Metronidazole is the drug treatment of choice for amoebic dysentery and is given orally, 800 mg three times daily for 5 days, followed by diloxanide 500 mg three times daily for 10 days to eradicate cysts. Liver abscesses are treated with metronidazole 400 mg three times daily for 5–10 days followed again by diloxanide. Emergency surgery is occasionally necessary in fulminating amoebic colitis or less urgently for large liver abscesses.

MICROSCOPIC COLITIS

This recently described condition is so called because the histology is abnormal but the macroscopic appearance may be normal. It causes chronic watery diarrhoea and is thought to be the cause in up to 5% of patients complaining of this symptom. Its aetiology is still unknown, but a link with non-steroidal anti-inflammatory drugs has been noted. Specific histological findings (collagenous and lymphocytic types) are seen in biopsy specimens, although the colon may look macroscopically normal at colonoscopy. Treatment is not very effective: budesonide and bismuth may be tried for patients unable to control symptoms with antidiarrhoeal agents.

Disorders of large bowel motility, structure and perfusion

29

INTRODUCTION

Irritable bowel syndrome, chronic constipation and **diverticular disease** all arise from disordered peristaltic function and are at least partly attributable to the highly refined Western diet. These disorders could be regarded as endemic in developed societies.

Irritable bowel syndrome causes distressing abdominal discomfort in younger patients, whilst chronic constipation affects people of all age groups. Diverticular disease is probably caused by long-term dietary factors. These disorders make substantial demands on the time of family practitioners, physicians and surgeons, yet they are largely preventable. A hundred years ago, they were largely unknown in the West (apart from an obsession with constipation), as they still are in rural communities in many developing countries.

In addition to treating symptoms, the main surgical significance is that these conditions must be distinguished from inflammatory bowel diseases in the young and large bowel cancer in the older population. They have several symptoms in common:

- Intermittent attacks of abdominal pain, which can be severe
- Erratic bowel habit
- Abdominal bloating and passage of excessive flatus

Sigmoid volvulus is an acute condition resulting from chronic dilatation of the sigmoid colon plus an acute twisting of the sigmoid loop on a narrow mesentery, resulting in obstruction and massive dilatation (see below, Fig. 29.1, p. 378–379).

Angiodysplasia of the large bowel and **ischaemic colitis** are vascular conditions of the ageing gut, and both usually present with rectal bleeding and pain. Again, colorectal cancer has to be excluded as the cause of bleeding.

MODERN DIET AND DISEASE

EPIDEMIOLOGICAL OBSERVATIONS

Little scientific attention was paid to diet-related disease until the 1970s, although Gaylord Hauser had written about fibre in the diet in the 1930s. In the 1970s, the ideas of Surgeon Captain T. L. Cleeve, a Royal Navy physician, and later the remarkable epidemiological observations of Denis Burkitt, a long-time missionary surgeon in Africa, emerged. Now the subject of diet is respectable in surgical circles and has contributed to the understanding, prevention and management of many common diseases. Diseases such as irritable bowel syndrome, diverticular disease and appendicitis, common in Western society, are largely unknown in much of the developing world and this difference is almost certainly diet-related. Thus it follows that a dietary history is important in evaluating these patients, and dietary change is often a fundamental part of management.

Over millions of years as 'hunter-gatherers', humans subsisted on a staple diet of an extensive variety of vegetables and fruits, grains, legumes and nuts, supplemented by occasional meat or fish. The modern human gastrointestinal and metabolic systems are thus perfectly adapted to that diet. During the brief period (in evolutionary terms) of the last 100 years, the average Western diet has changed dramatically, due to affluence, fashion, convenience, food processing and advertising. Since the 1980s there have been similar dietary changes in the more prosperous parts of developing countries, particularly in the cities. The modern diet contains many more calories than the hunter-gatherer diet. These are largely in the form of refined carbohydrates and fats, especially saturated animal fats and 'trans' fats in artificially hydrogenated vegetable oils. Perhaps equally important, the modern diet contains far less non-absorbable fibre residue.

MECHANISMS OF DISEASE CAUSED BY MODERN DIET

Whilst the increase in calories and nutrients has brought benefits, it has also brought problems. The modern diet adversely affects both bowel function and metabolism, particularly of lipids. Box 29.1 outlines the important ways in which modern diet can induce disease and dysfunction. With regard to bowel diseases, the most important diet-related factors are likely to be faecal volume and consistency, together with

Box 29.1 Mechanisms by which refined diet may cause disease

Slowed gastrointestinal transit time

- Increases duration of contact between stool and bowel mucosa; this increases duration of contact of carcinogens, predisposing to colorectal cancer

Increased intra-abdominal pressure due to straining at stool

- Obstructs venous return making haemorrhoids and varicose veins more likely
- Predisposes to hiatus hernia, inguinal hernia and rectal prolapse

Reduced bulk and more solid consistency of faeces

- Make peristalsis less effective and constipation more likely
- Increase intraluminal pressure, perhaps predisposing to diverticular disease
- Hard stool increases friction, causing anal fissure and perhaps haemorrhoids
- Small stool bulk increases concentration of carcinogens
- May contribute to pathogenesis of appendicitis by obstructing appendiceal orifice

Decreased loss of bile salts in the faeces

- Increased bile salt pool predisposes to gallstone formation
- Increased bile salts in lumen may result in formation of carcinogens

Changes in bacterial flora of the bowel

- May result in formation of carcinogens
- May be implicated in appendicitis

Increased refined carbohydrate intake

- Predisposes to diabetes
- Contributes to excess calorie intake causing obesity

Increased dietary fat intake, particularly saturated animal fats

- Predisposes to atherosclerosis
- Predisposes to gallstone formation
- Contributes to excess calorie intake and obesity

Increased absorption of dietary fat because of reduced binding by fibre

- Increases fat absorption and blood lipid levels

Obesity

- Weakens abdominal wall muscles predisposing to hiatus hernia, abdominal wall hernias and vaginal prolapse
- Predisposes to thromboembolism
- Contributes to musculoskeletal and joint disorders

gastrointestinal transit time. The average Western adult passes between 80 and 120 g of firm stool each day with a transit time of about 3 days, although transit time can be as long as 2 weeks in the elderly. In contrast, rural dwellers in the developing world, with a diet similar to the hunter-gatherer, pass between 300 and 800 g of much softer stool each day, with an average transit time of less than a day and a half.

DIETARY FIBRE CONTENT

An essential part of managing many bowel conditions (other than irritable bowel syndrome) and preventing others is a substantial increase in dietary fibre intake. Box 29.2 lists foods with a high fibre content that can be eaten regularly with little effort or extra expense. Increasing the fibre content almost inevitably leads to reduced consumption of refined carbohydrates and saturated animal fats and lower total energy intake. Patients should introduce dietary fibre gradually because a sudden increase is likely to cause abdominal discomfort and distension and more flatus. Bulking agents (**ispaghula husk** preparations) can be taken in the early stages for a rapid result whilst avoiding unpleasant side-effects.

Box 29.2 Foods with a high fibre content

- Wholegrain and bran-enriched breakfast cereals, e.g. muesli, All-Bran, Weetabix (not cornflakes, puffed rice, etc.)
- Wholemeal bread (not white or 'brown')
- Other wholewheat products, e.g. wholewheat pasta, wholemeal pastry, digestive biscuits
- Other wholegrain, e.g. brown rice, cracked wheat
- Pulses of any kind, e.g. haricot beans (including canned baked beans), kidney beans, chick peas, other dried beans and lentils
- Potatoes (skins should be left on)
- Unpeeled fruit and vegetables (actually low in fibre compared with grains and pulses)

IRRITABLE BOWEL SYNDROME

Irritable bowel syndrome (IBS) has only been accepted as a pathological entity in recent years, although Osler coined the term *mucous colitis* in 1892 to describe mucorrhoea (excess mucus in the stool) and abdominal colic often found in patients with psychological problems. Another common name is '**spastic colon**'. The condition is widespread, particularly in young and middle-aged women.

CLINICAL FEATURES OF IRRITABLE BOWEL SYNDROME

Irritable bowel syndrome is a functional GI disorder characterised by abdominal pain and altered bowel habit without identifiable organic pathology. IBS can only be diagnosed clinically (after excluding organic causes) as there are no specific diagnostic tests. A group of experts formalised a diagnostic set of symptoms known as the **Rome II Criteria**. To fulfil a diagnosis of IBS, a patient must have the following symptoms continuously or recurrently for at least 3 months in a year: abdominal pain relieved by defaecation, and a change in stool frequency and consistency. Symptoms supporting the diagnosis include altered stool form, mucorrhoea and abdominal bloating.

The patient typically complains of episodic 'cramping' abdominal pain at any time of day and lasting from 15 minutes to several hours. The pain is unrelated to meals or other obvious provoking factors. It occurs anywhere in the abdomen but tends to arise peripherally, i.e. in either iliac fossa or epigastrium, and usually recurs in the same general area in any one patient.

Symptoms occur daily for weeks at a time and then resolve for weeks or months, only to return later. The patient may recognise that symptoms are worse at times of stress and are absent during weekends and holidays. The pain may provoke an urge to open the bowels, and evacuation may bring relief. An erratic bowel habit is characteristic of irritable bowel syndrome: passage of loose stools alternates with constipation, with small hard stools described as looking like rabbit pellets; but patients are divided into those for whom either diarrhoea or constipation is the predominant problem. Sufferers often complain of abdominal distension and excess flatus.

PATHOPHYSIOLOGY AND AETIOLOGY OF IRRITABLE BOWEL SYNDROME

The pathophysiology is poorly understood. Colonic motility studies show abnormal rises in intraluminal pressure and disordered peristalsis with segmenting, non-propulsive contractions. The small volume of faeces (because of little residual fibre) becomes excessively dehydrated and fragmented. However, some patients with irritable bowel syndrome appear to be hypersensitive to gut distension and their symptoms may be made worse by a high-fibre diet. These in particular may benefit from a low-fibre diet plus methylcellulose fibre substitutes that do not ferment, e.g. Celevac. Thus the patient avoids constipation without the fermentation and excess gas production of a high-fibre diet. There is growing support for the view that at least some IBS is due to specific food intolerance, particularly wheat protein, and it is worth excluding this in a trial of treatment.

MANAGEMENT OF IRRITABLE BOWEL SYNDROME

The diagnosis is made on the basis of a typical history and often after a trial of treatment. In the younger patient, where carcinoma is unlikely, abdominal and rectal examination (probably including flexible sigmoidoscopy) is all that is required. In IBS, these are normal except perhaps for mild tenderness in the area of pain. Other factors helping to exclude inflammatory bowel disease are a normal erythrocyte sedimentation rate (ESR) and C-reactive protein (CRP), and an absence of weight loss, ill-health and tiredness, troublesome diarrhoea or rectal bleeding. In cases of diagnostic difficulty, small bowel radiology and other investigations can exclude Crohn's disease.

Persistent upper gastrointestinal pain should be investigated, with gallstones or peptic ulcer disease in mind. In a patient over 50, irritable bowel syndrome is less likely, and cancer and diverticular disease must be excluded before IBS can be confirmed.

Treatment involves reassurance, adjusting the diet to test for wheat intolerance, treating the predominant symptom of constipation or diarrhoea, and antispasmodic drugs such as mebeverine and peppermint oil. Mebeverine plus codeine phosphate (as an analgesic) given immediately an attack comes on produces rapid relief and confirms the diagnosis. There is probably little benefit in giving continuous treatment. For selected patients, relaxation therapy or antidepressants such as amitriptyline may be beneficial.

CONSTIPATION

CLINICAL FEATURES OF CONSTIPATION

Whether or not they consider it a problem, many patients suffer from chronic constipation. Constipation is difficult to define but the essence is a subjective inability to evacuate the bowels with sufficient frequency, ease, completeness or satisfaction. Perception of normality varies greatly; some patients insist that daily evacuation is essential whilst others tolerate a bowel movement only once a week.

Constipation is often considered in two groups. The first is **slow transit** with a general failure of colonic propulsion. The second, much smaller group includes patients with an **evacuation disorder**. These patients often complain of incomplete evacuation and a sensation of obstructed defaecation: some disorders responsible (like rectal intussusception) can only be demonstrated on a dynamic X-ray study known as an **evacuation proctogram**. These patients also require specialised anorectal physiological assessment.

From a medical viewpoint, evacuation less than twice a week is abnormal. In the uncomplaining elderly, defaecation may occur much less frequently, causing vague discomfort and anorexia, and predisposing to urinary retention, incontinence and urinary tract infection. Severe constipation alone may lead to **faecal impaction** and **complete bowel obstruction** necessitating hospital admission. Faecal fluid may intermittently escape past the impacted faecal mass and cause soiling, overflow incontinence or apparent ('**spurious**') diarrhoea.

Abdominal pain may be the presenting symptom. The pain may be sufficiently severe to precipitate emergency admission with suspected appendicitis (usually children) or suspected intestinal obstruction (usually the elderly). As many as 25% of patients in these age groups admitted with abdominal pain are eventually diagnosed as suffering from constipation. There is no fever, tachycardia or vomiting, and signs of peritoneal inflammation are absent. There may be mild abdominal tenderness. The faecally loaded left side of the colon often forms a palpable column which indents on palpation with a putty-like consistency. Rectal examination usually reveals a palpable faecal mass, although in the elderly the faeces may be impacted higher up, so an empty rectum does not exclude constipation.

PATHOPHYSIOLOGY OF CHRONIC CONSTIPATION

For surgeons, chronic constipation is mainly a problem of children and the elderly. Patients present as emergencies and in the clinic. In most, the cause is a combination of low-fibre diet, poor fluid intake, obesity, inactivity and persistent failure to respond promptly to the urge to defaecate. Long-term use of **purgative drugs** such as senna may have an adverse effect on peristalsis. Some drugs, particularly **codeine** and **opiates**, slow large bowel motility, whilst yet other drugs such as **aluminium hydroxide mixtures** and **iron preparations** solidify the stool. Constipation is a characteristic feature of **hypothyroidism** and is also seen in **hypo-** and **hypercalcaemia**.

MANAGEMENT OF CONSTIPATION

Diagnosis of constipation in children is usually made on the history and examination; successful treatment confirms the diagnosis. If chronic severe constipation persists in infants despite treatment, a diagnosis of **ultra-short segment Hirschsprung's disease** (see Ch. 50) should be considered. In the elderly, a dietary and drug history should be obtained, and blood tests performed to exclude metabolic causes of constipation. It is vital to differentiate constipation from early large bowel obstruction in this group of patients. Carcinoma or the complications of diverticular disease should be excluded by sigmoidoscopy and barium enema, colonoscopy or CT pneumocolon.

In severe constipation, treatment involves a series of measures used progressively:

- Discontinue constipating medication
- Rectal measures: lubricant glycerine suppositories, small phosphate enemas, stool-softening arachis oil enemas, manual disimpaction (may require general anaesthesia)
- Oral agents (Box 29.3): senna, bisacodyl or osmotic laxatives containing macrogol (polyethylene glycol 3350). A more radical method is to use oral sodium picosulfate (as used in surgical bowel preparation), along with adequate oral or intravenous fluids to avoid dehydration. Note that if powerful oral laxatives are given to an obstructed patient, life-threatening perforation of the bowel can occur
- Oral 'maintenance' medications: sodium docusate as a stool softener, lactulose, Fybogel

In milder long-term constipation, dietary measures should be used. Many patients take a high-fibre diet but do not drink enough, failing to recognise that both are necessary to produce the benefits of fibre. Many women fail to gain from a high-fibre diet; clearly, increasing their fibre even more does not improve matters. If the condition is not severe, then eating more figs, apricots and prunes may solve the problem. Otherwise, a low dose of a stimulant laxative taken intermittently may be needed.

Box 29.3 Oral laxative agents

- Stimulant/irritant laxatives, e.g. dantron, bisacodyl, senna derivatives
- Faecal softeners and lubricants, e.g. Dioctyl, liquid paraffin
- Osmotic laxatives, e.g. lactulose, mixtures of magnesium hydroxide or magnesium sulphate
- Proprietary preparations, e.g. Milpar (liquid paraffin and magnesium hydroxide emulsion)
- Strong laxatives for single-dose use for bowel preparation or very stubborn constipation, e.g. sodium picosulfate (stimulant), mannitol solution (osmotic)

Note: bulking agents do not have a laxative effect in the short term

SIGMOID VOLVULUS (Fig. 29.1)

PATHOPHYSIOLOGY OF SIGMOID VOLVULUS

Patients with longstanding chronic constipation tend to develop a capacious, elongated and relatively atonic colon, especially in the sigmoid region. This is sometimes described as **acquired** or **idiopathic megacolon**.

Occasionally, a huge sigmoid loop, heavy with faeces and distended with gas, becomes twisted on its mesenteric pedicle (often abnormally narrow) to produce a closed-loop obstruction (see Fig. 29.1a–c). If this volvulus is not corrected, venous infarction ensues, followed by perforation and catastrophic faecal peritonitis. This full picture is uncommon, but there is often a history of transient episodes of abdominal pain diagnosed as constipation. Note that volvulus elsewhere, of the caecum, small bowel or stomach is unrelated to constipation.

CLINICAL FEATURES OF SIGMOID VOLVULUS

In Western countries, sigmoid volvulus is rare except in the elderly, those with severe learning difficulties, and long-stay patients in mental institutions; these groups all readily become faecally loaded. In contrast, it is very common in parts of the world where diet is extremely high in fibre, e.g. parts of Chile.

The patient with sigmoid volvulus is mildly unwell with abdominal distension and a variable degree of abdominal pain. There is absolute constipation (of both faeces and flatus) that has persisted for at least 24 hours. On digital examination, the rectum is empty but capacious. The abdomen is visibly distended and tympanitic to percussion but rarely tender. This is true even if the colon has reached the stage of venous infarction. Once perforation occurs, the full picture of faecal peritonitis will be evident.

MANAGEMENT OF SIGMOID VOLVULUS

Plain abdominal X-ray usually shows a single grossly dilated sigmoid loop, often reaching the xiphisternum (see Fig. 29.1). An erect film may reveal a characteristic 'inverted U' or 'coffee-bean sign' of bowel gas in the upper abdomen, with fluid

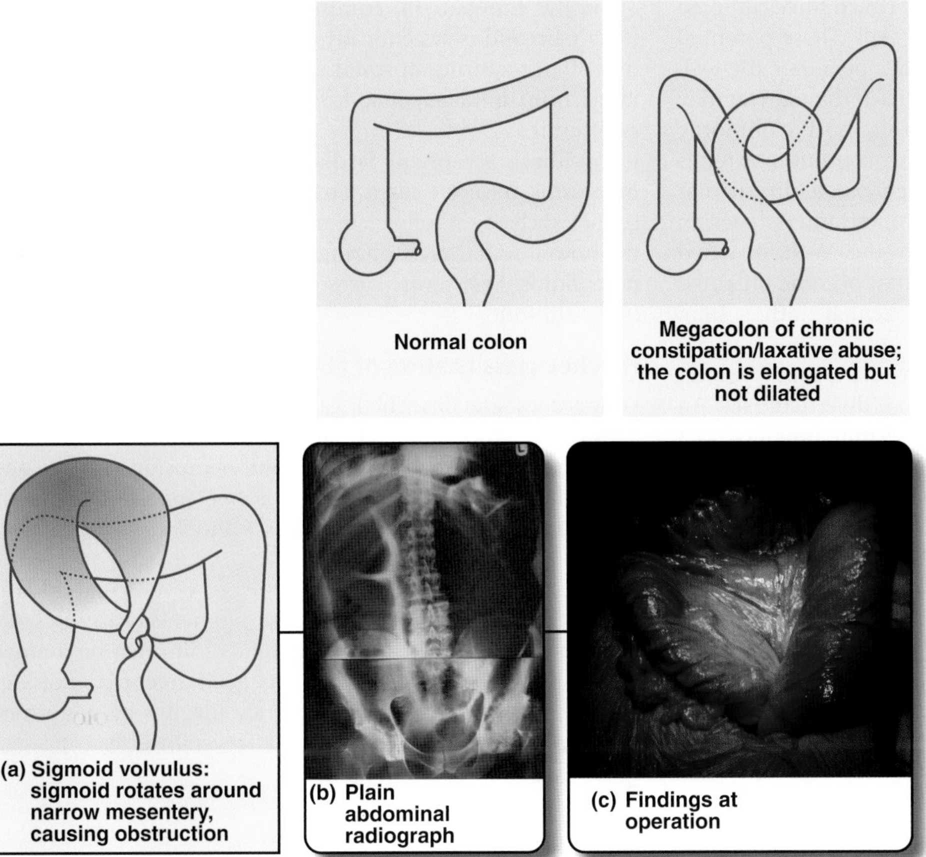

Fig. 29.1 Normal colon, megacolon and sigmoid volvulus
(a) Schematic diagram showing a grossly distended fluid-filled sigmoid colon twisted about its narrow neck, producing a 'closed-loop' obstruction; the loop is beginning to undergo necrosis. **(b)** and **(c)** This 35-year-old man with Down's syndrome presented with a massively swollen abdomen and total constipation. **(b)** Plain abdominal radiograph showing the abdomen filled with the dilated sigmoid loop, confirming the clinical diagnosis of sigmoid volvulus. Note the abdomen was so distended that two films were required to cover the area. The volvulus could not be relieved by gentle passage of a flatus tube. At operation **(c),** the hugely distended sigmoid emerged from the laparotomy wound. The loop had twisted three times around its narrow base and the colon was of doubtful viability. This sigmoid colon was resected without untwisting the volvulus

levels at the same height in the two bowel limbs in the lower abdomen; a lateral decubitus X-ray may reveal two parallel fluid levels running the length of the abdomen.

If sigmoid volvulus is diagnosed, a sigmoidoscope is gently passed as far as possible into the rectum and a flatus tube inserted through it. The end of the **flatus tube** is then gently manipulated through the twisted bowel into the obstructed loop. If this is successful, there is a gush of liquid faeces and flatus, relieving the obstruction. The flatus tube can be left in situ for 24 hours to maintain decompression, discourage re-twisting and allow recovery of the vascular supply of the bowel wall. Despite this, volvulus is likely to recur.

If plain X-ray and sigmoidoscopy do not confirm volvulus but large bowel obstruction is still suspected, an 'instant' **Gastrografin enema examination** is performed, without bowel preparation. This differentiates volvulus from other obstructions such as cancer and diverticular disease, and from pseudo-obstruction. In volvulus, pressure from the enema may cause the bowel to untwist, releasing a torrent of faeces and flatus.

If a volvulus cannot be released, operation is performed urgently. In most cases, the bowel is still viable but sigmoid colectomy is usually required to prevent recurrence. A safe alternative procedure is to excise the sigmoid and bring the divided ends of bowel out to form a **double-barrelled colostomy**, rather than risk a primary anastomosis in this dilated and unprepared colon. For recurrent volvulus, **sigmoid colectomy** or suturing the bowel to the abdominal wall to prevent twisting may be performed electively.

DIVERTICULAR DISEASE

Diverticular disease causes substantial morbidity in the older population, particularly in the West, and is a very common cause for hospital admission and operation. In developed countries, localised outpouchings or diverticula are present in the bowel wall in at least one-third of people over the age of 60. There is strong evidence that this can be caused or aggravated by a chronic lack of dietary fibre but there may also be a genetic element. Females are affected more often than males. (*Note*: the singular noun is *diverticulum* and the plural *diverticula*, not *diverticulae*; the adjectival form is *diverticular*.)

PATHOPHYSIOLOGY OF DIVERTICULAR DISEASE

In diverticular disease, the colonic circular muscle is thickened because of an excess of elastic tissue between muscle fibres rather than muscle hypertrophy. The likely mechanism for diverticular formation is functional **hypersegmentation**. In this, adjoining segments of colon contract at the same time, sending peristaltic waves towards each other. This causes very high luminal pressure in short segments which forces mucosa to herniate through weak points in the wall. These potential defects occur where mucosal blood vessels penetrate the wall from outside, between longitudinal muscle bands (**taeniae coli**). The sigmoid colon is the section most commonly affected by diverticular disease and the condition extends for a variable distance proximally. Right-sided diverticular disease is more common in Japanese, Chinese and Polynesian races and is common in Hawaii. In the West, isolated caecal diverticula sometimes occur and may become inflamed or perforate; these are probably congenital rather than acquired.

The presence of uncomplicated diverticula is unimportant; this asymptomatic condition is known as '**diverticulosis**'. An individual diverticulum may, however, become inflamed as a result of obstruction of its narrow outlet. This causes a **diverticular abscess**. The abscess lies outside the bowel wall and leads to complications described below.

COMPLICATIONS OF DIVERTICULAR DISEASE

Diverticular disease may lead to a range of complications:

- Spreading pericolic inflammation
- Pericolic abscess
- Intraperitoneal perforation
- Fistula formation into other abdominal or pelvic viscera
- Bowel-to-bowel adhesions
- Fibrous strictures of bowel
- Acute haemorrhage (which tends to occur without inflammation)

CLINICAL PRESENTATIONS OF DIVERTICULAR DISEASE AND THEIR MANAGEMENT

The consequences of diverticular inflammation are collectively described as **diverticulitis** and are summarised in Figure 29.3. Most people with diverticula are asymptomatic, and diverticula are a common incidental finding when the colon is investigated by barium enema or colonoscopy. Typical appearances are shown in Figures 29.2 and Fig. 29.4.

Chronic grumbling diverticular pain (see Fig. 29.3b)

This is probably the most common manifestation of diverticular disease and is usually managed in family practices. Peridiverticular inflammation is chronic, low-grade and recurrent. Local irritation provokes bowel wall spasm, causing pain and erratic bowel habit. There is chronic constipation with small pellet-like faeces and episodic diarrhoea. There are few abnormalities on clinical examination, except perhaps mild left iliac fossa tenderness and faecal loading. Endoscopy or radiological imaging is often performed to confirm the diagnosis and exclude malignancy.

In most patients, symptoms can be relieved by taking a high-fibre diet and bulking agents, although some patients find symptoms are better on a low-fibre intake.

Acute diverticulitis (i.e. spreading pericolic inflammation, see Fig. 29.3c)

This represents local extension of the inflammation described above. It involves pericolic tissues and parietal peritoneum. Typically, the patient complains of continuous left iliac fossa pain and is systemically ill with a pyrexia and tachycardia, often requiring hospital admission. Abdominal findings range from mild left iliac fossa tenderness to obvious local peritonitis.

Antibiotic treatment is directed against the usual faecal organisms. In severe cases, a combination of intravenous antibiotics such as ciprofloxacin and metronidazole is used, and the bowel 'rested' by stopping oral intake and giving intravenous fluids. Less severe cases can be managed at home with oral antibiotics.

Hinchey classification of abscesses and perforation

Four stages are described: stage 1 is a small pericolic or mesenteric abscess <4 cm; stage 2 is a large, often pelvic, abscess; stage 3 is a small perforation causing gaseous and purulent peritonitis; and stage 4 is free rupture with faecal peritonitis. Mortality rate for stages 1 and 2 is <5%, for stage 3, 13% and for stage 4, 43%.

In patients admitted with complicated diverticular disease, initial imaging is with CT scan. Stage 1 patients nearly all settle with antibiotics, stage 2 and 3 patients can often be drained percutaneously and stage 4 patients need urgent laparotomy. Endoscopy to exclude malignancy should not be performed until inflammation has settled, after several weeks.

Pericolic abscess (see Fig. 29.3d)

Pericolic abscess represents a further extension of the pathological process just described. The clinical presentation is

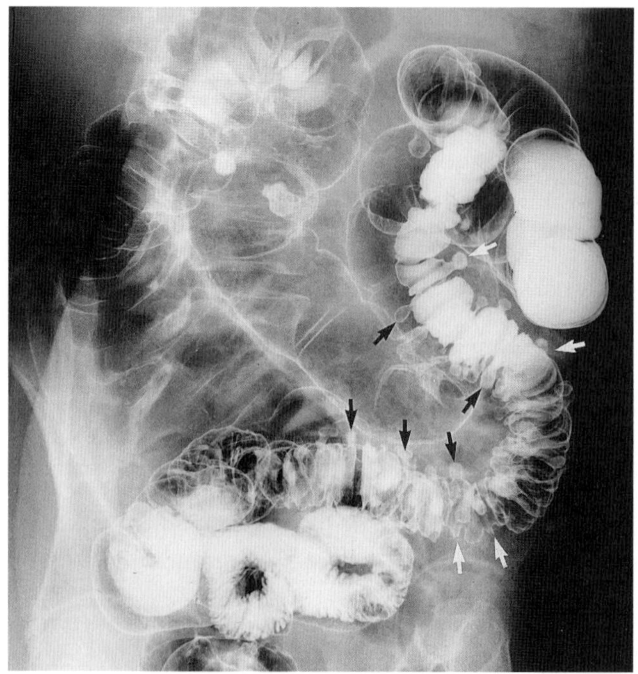

Fig. 29.2 Diverticular disease
Barium enema showing the typical appearance of multiple diverticula (arrowed) in the sigmoid and descending colon in a 77-year-old woman. A few diverticula are also present in the transverse colon

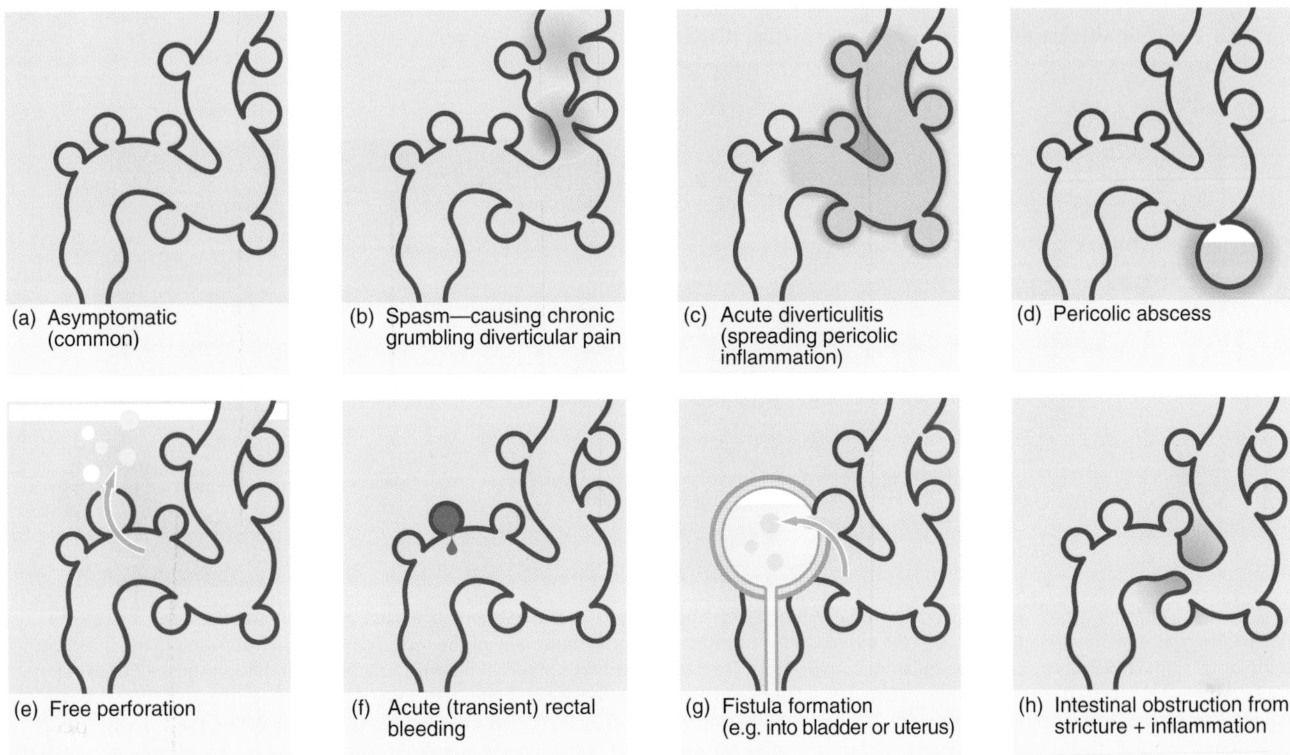

Fig. 29.3 Clinical presentations of diverticular disease

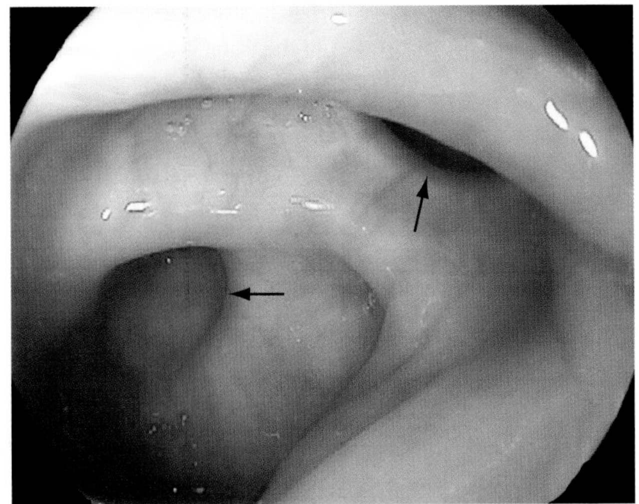

Fig. 29.4 Colonoscopic view of diverticula (arrowed)

similar at first but fails to resolve with antibiotics. The patient suffers persistent pain and tenderness, a swinging pyrexia and incomplete obstruction due to spasm of bowel wall muscle. Sometimes a pericolic abscess presents as 'pyrexia of unknown origin' or even systemic sepsis (septicaemia). A pericolic abscess may drain spontaneously into bowel, producing an attack of purulent diarrhoea; the condition then resolves. Diagnosis of a pericolic abscess is made on CT scan. A contrast enema may show leakage of contrast into the abscess cavity (see Fig. 29.5).

Antibiotic therapy is the first line of treatment for abscesses <4 cm. Ideally, this allows the abscess to be contained, and then resolve or drain spontaneously into bowel. Abscesses >4 cm can be drained percutaneously under radiological guidance. If this treatment fails, operation is required. This is a major procedure usually involving exploration and drainage of the abscess and diverting the faecal stream via a colostomy. The affected segment of bowel must be removed to prevent recurrence. Note that perforated carcinoma can present in a similar way and histological diagnosis is mandatory. The surgical options are to leave a rectal stump for later reanastomosis (Hartmann's operation, see Fig. 27.8, p. 359), a safe operation for non-specialists, or to primarily reanastomose the bowel ends. Reanastomosis is not attempted in faecal peritonitis or in a frail patient, as the chances of success are remote.

Diverticular perforation (Fig. 29.3e)

A small, asymptomatic diverticular abscess may rupture spontaneously, i.e. perforate, resulting in escape of gas and minimal bowel contents into the peritoneal cavity. The patient presents with an acute abdomen, the severity of clinical signs depending on the size of perforation and degree of peritoneal contamination. Perforations vary from pinhole size to a hole of 1 cm or more causing generalised faecal peritonitis and potentially fatal sepsis. With small perforations, symptoms and signs may be similar to acute diverticulitis; diagnosis of perforation is confirmed by finding free sub-diaphragmatic gas on CT or erect chest X-ray.

Conservative treatment employing percutaneous drain placement and bowel rest is appropriate for minimal

Fig. 29.5 Pericolic abscess due to perforated diverticular disease

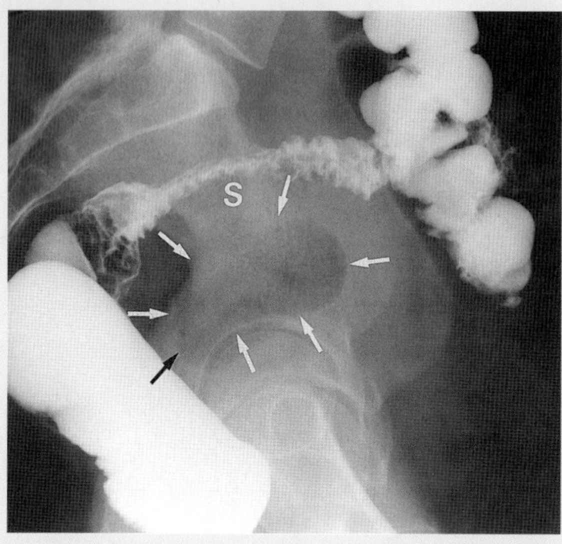

(a)

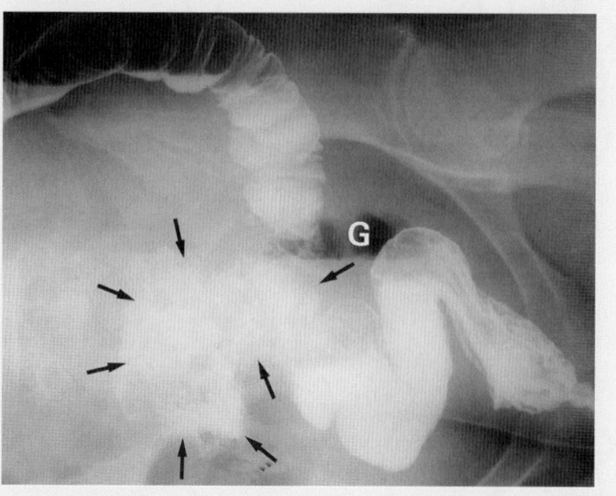

(b)

Barium enema films from a 49-year-old woman who presented with abdominal pain and tenderness, a mass in the left iliac fossa and a swinging pyrexia. She was treated with antibiotics but the pyrexia failed to settle. **(a)** Right lateral view of the rectosigmoid region showing marked narrowing of the distal sigmoid **S** due to spasm and inflammatory oedema. The radiolucent area antero-inferiorly (outline arrowed) represents a bubble of gas in a large pelvic abscess. **(b)** Lateral decubitus film (left side upwards) of the same patient taken later during the same examination. This shows barium which has leaked into the abscess cavity (outline arrowed). Note also a fluid level with a gas bubble **G** above it, within the abscess. At laparotomy, a large pericolic and pelvic abscess was found to be walled off. This was drained surgically, the sigmoid colon excised and the end of the descending colon brought out as a terminal colostomy in the left iliac fossa. The rectal stump was oversewn; 3 months later, the bowel was reconnected

perforations (Hinchey 3) but for Hinchey 4 perforations involves immediate parenteral antibiotics, followed by laparotomy for peritoneal toilet, diversion of the faecal stream and resection of diseased bowel.

Fistula formation into other abdominal or pelvic structures (Fig. 29.3g)

Fistula formation can occur when an inflamed diverticulum lies close to another hollow viscus. Inflammatory adhesions develop and the diverticulum then ruptures into the other viscus. A fistula between large bowel and small bowel (see Fig. 29.6) causes diarrhoea. A vesico-colic fistula causes **pneumaturia** and severe urinary tract infection. A fistula into the vagina after a previous hysterectomy causes a purulent vaginal discharge. Diverticular disease is the most common cause of these types of fistula but they may also be caused by Crohn's disease and sometimes colorectal cancers.

Fistulae rarely show up on barium enema examination. CT scanning may reveal a loss of normal tissue planes between bowel and viscus, and/or gas in the bladder. Diagnosis can also be made on the history, at operation or, in the case of bladder fistula, at cystoscopy. Surgery involves excision and histological examination of the affected segment of bowel and repair of the viscus.

Intestinal obstruction (Fig. 29.3h)

Diverticular disease occasionally presents with large bowel obstruction due to acute inflammatory thickening, muscle hypertrophy and spasm. **Incomplete obstruction** is more

Fig. 29.6 Diverticular fistula into the distal ileum

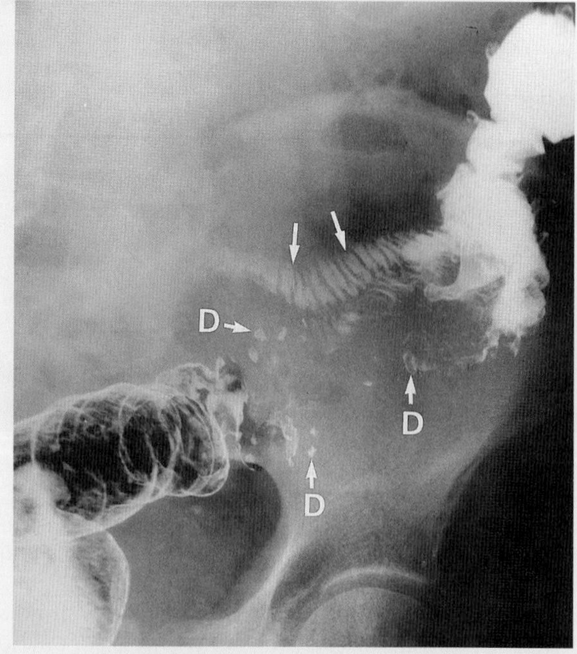

Barium enema of a 61-year-old man with a recently erratic bowel habit, who presented with pain and tenderness in the left iliac fossa. The X-ray shows the sigmoid colon, although part of it is poorly filled with barium which is only seen in the diverticula **D.** There is a loop of small bowel which contains contrast (arrowed), indicating the presence of a colo-ileal fistula caused by peridiverticulitis

common and presents as severe constipation. Chronic diverticular inflammation sometimes causes local fibrous strictures, particularly in the sigmoid, which cause intermittent bouts of constipation when the stool is dry. When detected radiologically or endoscopically, these strictures must be distinguished from malignancy or Crohn's disease by biopsy (Figs. 29.5 and 29.7).

When acute diverticular inflammation involves the pericolic tissues, small bowel may become involved. Thus, small bowel adynamic disorder may be the presenting feature, with obstruction-like symptoms.

Acute rectal haemorrhage (Fig. 29.3f)

Diverticular disease may present with acute rectal bleeding, which, unlike the other complications of diverticula, is not usually the result of inflammation. Blood loss is variable but the bleeding almost always stops spontaneously. The patient typically complains of having passed a mass of fairly fresh blood instead of the expected stool and is admitted to hospital urgently. The main differential diagnosis is **ischaemic colitis** but other causes of rectal bleeding such as carcinoma and haemorrhoids must be considered.

Management is rarely surgical but an angiogram and embolisation is sometimes performed by a specialist radiologist if the bleeding is severe. After necessary resuscitation, the patient is kept under observation for several days, after which it is safe to perform further investigations.

For further reading please see: http://www.nejm.org/doi/full/10.1056/NEJMcp073228

COLONIC ANGIODYSPLASIAS

Colonic angiodysplasias have been recognised as a common cause of acute or chronic rectal bleeding and iron deficiency anaemia since the mid-1970s. The lesions are tiny hamartomatous vascular lesions in the colonic wall, usually in the ascending colon, and produce bleeding out of proportion to their size (see Fig. 29.8). They may also occur in the stomach and small bowel. The origin of colonic angiodysplasias is unknown but since they occur later in life, they are probably acquired and degenerative.

If bleeding is acute and is occurring rapidly, selective mesenteric arteriography may demonstrate the source of bleeding. In chronic or recurrent haemorrhage, large bowel lesions can be visualised by colonoscopy. This underlines the importance of thorough colonoscopy in patients with unexplained GI blood loss. Lesions can often be treated by electrical coagulation via a colonoscope. If unsuccessful, the affected segment is excised. Similar lesions occur more rarely in small bowel and bleed in the same way.

ISCHAEMIC COLITIS

Ischaemic colitis is a condition of the elderly which usually presents with rectal bleeding. The history is characteristic; there is a bout of cramp-like abdominal pain lasting a few hours, followed by an attack of rectal bleeding. Usually the bleeding is dark red, often without faeces, and occurs one to

CASE HISTORY

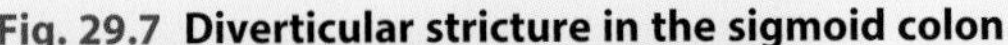

Fig. 29.7 Diverticular stricture in the sigmoid colon

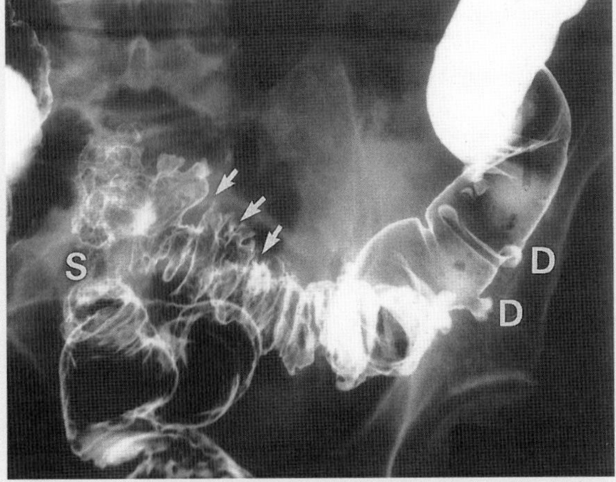

This 64-year-old man suffered several attacks of diverticulitis which settled with antibiotics. This frontal view of a barium enema shows diverticula **D** in the upper sigmoid colon and circular muscle hypertrophy in the distal sigmoid colon (arrowed) typical of diverticular disease. There is a stricture **S** near the rectosigmoid junction. This stricture does not show the typical 'shouldering' of a carcinoma, although carcinoma could not be excluded on barium enema. Colonoscopy confirmed that it was benign. This patient later had a severe attack of diverticulitis which required surgery and a Hartmann's operation was performed

CASE HISTORY

Fig. 29.8 Caecal angiodysplasia

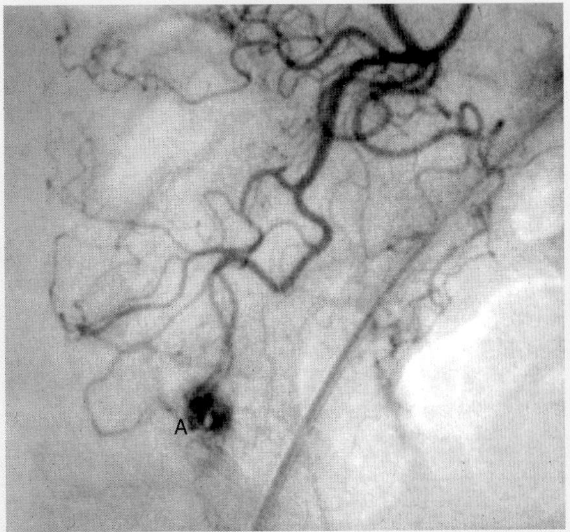

This 66-year-old man had been admitted to hospital on 12 occasions for rectal bleeding or anaemia and received a total of 77 units of blood by transfusion. This selective arteriogram was performed on the most recent admission and shows an abnormal mass of blood vessels **A** in the caecum typical of angiodysplasia. This part of the bowel was resected and the patient had not rebled 3 years later

CASE HISTORY

Fig. 29.9 Ischaemic colitis

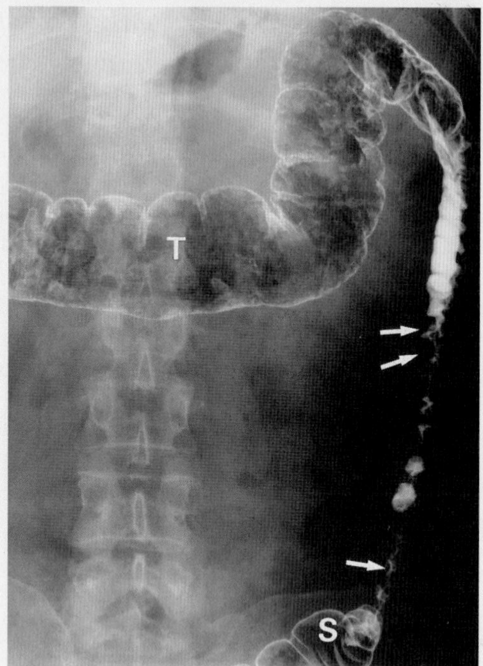

This 72-year-old man presented with a bout of severe abdominal pain 48 hours before this barium enema was performed. Soon after the pain, there was a single episode of fresh rectal bleeding. This film shows typical (though extensive) changes of acute ischaemic colitis, which characteristically involved the proximal descending colon. The transverse colon **T** and sigmoid colon **S** are normal. Note the extremely narrowed lumen of the ischaemic segment and the characteristic thumb-printing (arrowed) caused by mucosal oedema

three times over about 12 hours. The episode then ceases spontaneously. The differential diagnosis includes acute bleeding from diverticular disease. The cause is transient ischaemia of a segment of large bowel, followed by sloughing of the mucosa with the splenic flexure the most vulnerable. Further attacks occasionally occur but most patients have no further trouble. Investigation by barium enema in the acute stage may reveal colonic oedema in the affected segment (see Fig. 29.9). A rare late complication is fibrotic stricturing of the area affected by ischaemia.

Anal and perianal disorders

30

INTRODUCTION

Anal and perianal disorders make up about 20% of general surgical outpatient referrals. These conditions can be distressing or embarrassing and patients often tolerate symptoms for a long time before seeking medical advice. The common anal symptoms are summarised in Box 30.1 and interpretation is discussed in Chapter 18.

The range of anal and perianal disorders is illustrated in Figure 30.1. Haemorrhoids and other common benign conditions must be distinguished from rectal carcinoma and the rare anal carcinoma. Most anal and perianal conditions can be treated on an outpatient basis, although abscesses, and haemorrhoids that have become strangulated or thrombosed may present as surgical emergencies.

ANATOMY OF THE ANAL CANAL

At the anal verge outside the anal canal, there is normal skin composed of **stratified squamous epithelium** with skin appendages—sweat glands, hair follicles and sebaceous glands. The anal canal proper is about 4 cm long, extending from the lower to the upper border of the internal sphincter (see Fig. 30.2). There are three zones, each with different lining epithelium:

- The lowest or **distal zone** lies between the squamous–mucocutaneous junction and the level of the anal valves at the **dentate (pectinate) line**. This is lined by **non-keratinising** squamous epithelium without skin appendages or glands; the epithelium contains some melanocytes. This area is exquisitely sensitive, for example to injection
- The **anal transitional zone (ATZ)**. This lies between the zone of squamous epithelium below and the columnar mucosal zone above, and extends a distance varying between 0.3 and 2 cm. It consists of transitional epithelium resembling urothelium, 4–9 cell layers thick. Anal glands are present in the submucosa but there is minimal mucin production. A unique type of anal carcinoma develops from it with a viral aetiology
- The upper part of the anal canal is lined by rectal mucosa. On proctoscopic inspection, it is a dark reddish-blue where it overlies the submucosal venous plexus, becoming the typical pink of colorectal mucosa more proximally. This area of mucosa is relatively insensitive

The mucosa of the upper part of the anal canal is thrown into 6–10 longitudinal folds, the **columns of Morgagni**, each containing a terminal branch of the superior rectal artery and vein. The folds are most prominent in the left lateral, right posterior and right anterior sectors where the vessels form prominent **anal cushions**. These are important in fine control of continence. They may become pathologically enlarged to form **haemorrhoids**, which are complex collections of arterioles, arteries, venules, venous saccules and connective tissue. The anal columns are not readily visible on proctoscopy but the transition between glandular rectal mucosa and anal skin is clearly visible. The lymphatics of the upper anal canal drain to the pelvic and abdominal lymph node chain, whereas the lower part of the anal canal drains to inguinal lymph nodes.

The anal sphincter mechanism has three constituents: the **internal sphincter**, the **external sphincter** and the **puborectalis muscle**. The internal sphincter represents a downward but thickened continuation of the rectal wall musculature. The encircling external sphincter and the puborectalis sling (part of levator ani) arise from the pelvic floor. Continence is maintained principally by the anal sphincters squeezing the three anal cushions together to occlude the lumen. Continence is assisted by the rectum forming a compliant reservoir to accumulate faeces.

HAEMORRHOIDS

Haemorrhoids (piles) are extremely common, affecting nearly half of the population at some time. Men tend to suffer more often and for longer periods, whereas women are particularly susceptible in late pregnancy and the puerperium.

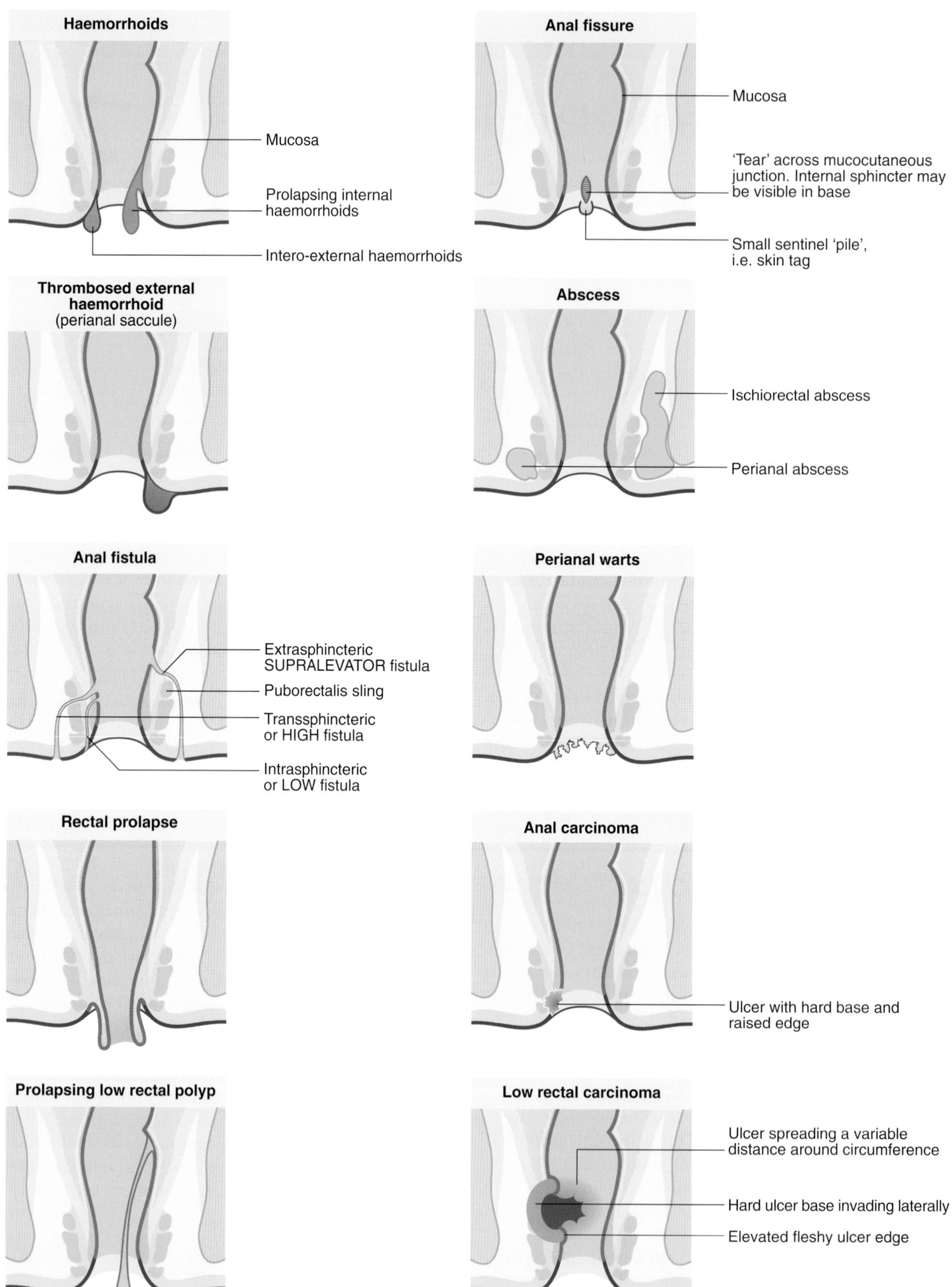

Fig. 30.1 Anal and perianal disorders

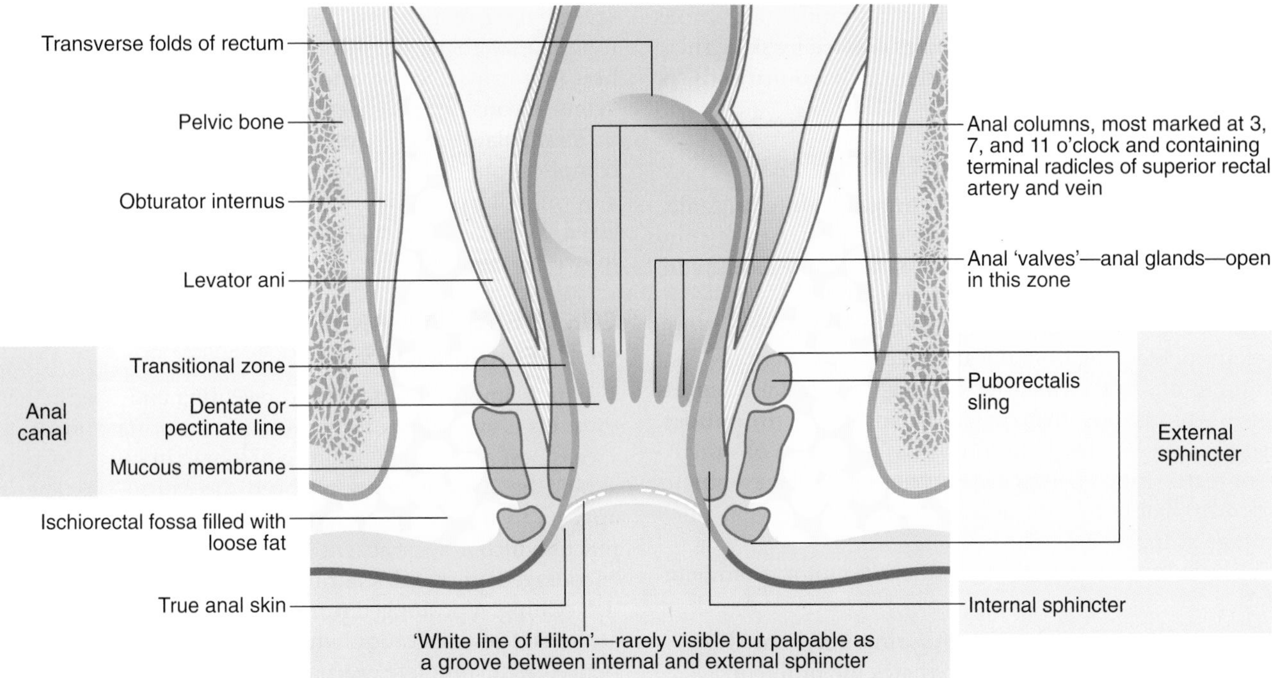

Fig. 30.2 Anatomy of the anal canal

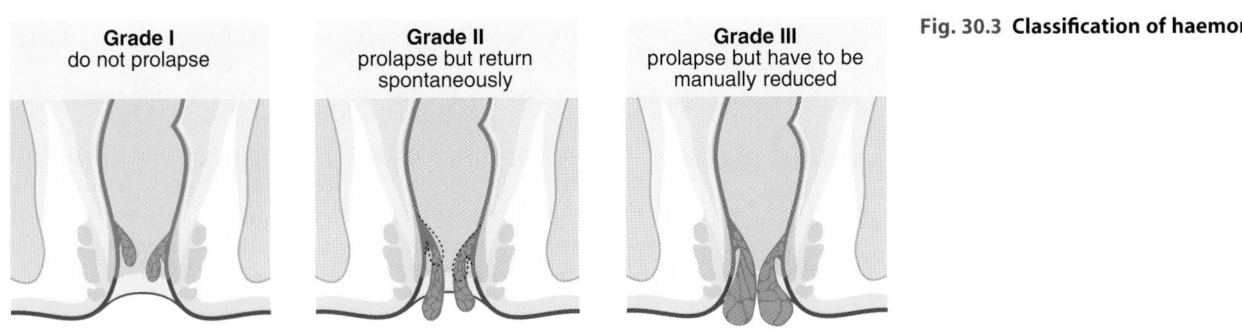

Fig. 30.3 Classification of haemorrhoids

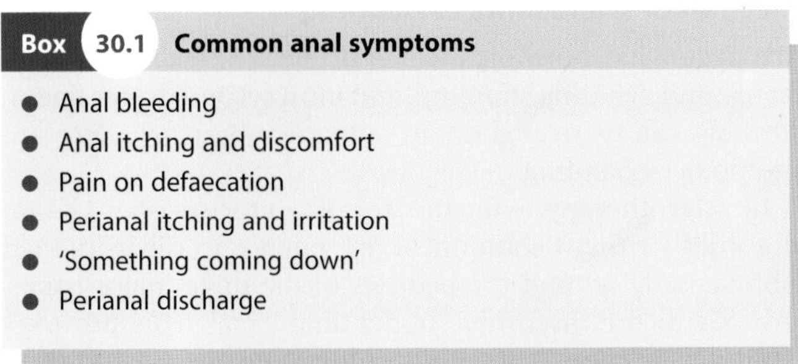

Box 30.1 Common anal symptoms

- Anal bleeding
- Anal itching and discomfort
- Pain on defaecation
- Perianal itching and irritation
- 'Something coming down'
- Perianal discharge

PATHOGENESIS OF HAEMORRHOIDS

Constipation and pregnancy are the most common triggers for development of haemorrhoids. Lack of fibre in the modern Western diet is a likely factor. Straining during constipation raises intra-abdominal pressure which obstructs venous return, causing the venous plexuses to engorge. The bulging mucosa is then dragged distally by the hard stool. Furthermore, persistent straining causes the pelvic floor to sag downwards, extruding the anal mucosa and causing a small degree of prolapse. Haemorrhoids are usually located in the 3, 7 and 11 o'clock positions when viewed with the patient in the supine lithotomy position. These correspond to the anatomical positions of the anal cushions. The venous component causes a problem only if it becomes thrombosed to form a **thrombosed external venous saccule** (sometimes inaccurately labelled a perianal haematoma).

In pregnancy-related haemorrhoids, venous engorgement and mucosal prolapse are probably the main mechanisms. Progesterone mediates venous dilatation, and the fetus obstructs pelvic venous return.

CLASSIFICATION OF HAEMORRHOIDS

Haemorrhoids (piles) are classified into first, second and third degrees according to the extent of prolapse through the anal canal. **First degree (or grade I) piles** never prolapse; **second degree (grade II) piles** prolapse during defaecation and then return spontaneously; **third degree (grade III) piles** remain outside the anal margin unless replaced digitally (Fig. 30.3). Most haemorrhoids can be described as 'internal' because they are covered by glandular mucosa. Large neglected haemorrhoids may extend beneath the stratified squamous epithelium so their lower part becomes covered by skin. These are correctly described as **'intero-external' haemorrhoids**, or more commonly 'external piles'.

SYMPTOMS AND SIGNS OF HAEMORRHOIDS

Haemorrhoids often produce symptoms intermittently. Attacks last from a few days to a few weeks, often with complete freedom from trouble between times. Episodes of constipation are often a precipitating factor.

Any haemorrhoid may **bleed** from stool trauma during defaecation. Bleeding from the arterial component of the anal cushion results in the characteristic bright red rectal bleeding. Large haemorrhoids may **prolapse** and then **thrombose**, causing acute severe pain if venous return is obstructed by sphincter tone. Longstanding haemorrhoids eventually atrophy, probably by thrombosis and fibrosis, leaving small **skin tags** at the anal margin.

The common chronic or intermittent symptoms of haemorrhoids are:

- Perianal irritation and itching (pruritus ani) caused by mucus leakage. Scratching exacerbates the problem
- Rectal bleeding (fresh blood, on the paper or separate from stool)
- Mucus leakage due to imperfect closure of the anal cushions
- Mild incontinence of flatus also due to imperfect closure of the anal cushions
- Haemorrhoidal prolapse

Most patients reaching the surgeon have tried various anaesthetic or soothing creams and suppositories, either self-administered or prescribed by the family practitioner. The usual reasons for referral are persistent symptoms or the need to exclude malignancy as a cause of bleeding.

On examination, external piles or skin tags may be visible in the anal area. Digital examination is essential to exclude carcinoma and provides a useful measure of anal tone. Haemorrhoids are not palpable unless they are large since the contained blood empties with finger pressure. **Proctoscopy** is needed to demonstrate internal piles, which are seen bulging into the lumen as the proctoscope is withdrawn. **Sigmoidoscopy**, rigid or ideally flexible, is important in patients over 40 years if there is a history of bleeding or any symptoms suspicious of malignancy; occasionally a rectal polyp will be diagnosed in this way. Since haemorrhoids are so common, they can mask an unrelated diagnosis of cancer.

ACUTE PRESENTATIONS OF HAEMORRHOIDS

Thrombosed or strangulated haemorrhoids present with acute severe pain and many patients are admitted to hospital as emergencies. These complications are common in the late stages of pregnancy and soon after delivery. The diagnosis of **thrombosed haemorrhoids** is usually obvious on inspection as an oedematous, congested purplish mass at the anal margin. Tight spasm of the anal sphincter makes digital rectal examination extremely painful. **Strangulated haemorrhoids** are even more painful, and the strangulated mass may become necrotic or even ulcerated. Symptomatic relief is provided by several days of bed rest and application of ice packs and topical anaesthetic gel; this conservative treatment may be the best that can safely be offered in late pregnancy. Some surgeons favour urgent haemorrhoidectomy for thrombosed or strangulated piles, accepting the slightly higher risk of complications in exchange for a more rapid recovery and a shorter hospital stay. Prophylactic antibiotics should be given to cover the operation because of the risk of infection in necrotic tissue.

CONSERVATIVE MANAGEMENT AND PREVENTION OF HAEMORRHOIDS

The most important means of preventing and treating haemorrhoids is avoiding constipation and ensuring a bulky stool. This is best achieved by taking a diet high in fibre. The patient should be advised to always heed the call to evacuate. This appears to be associated with a reflex release of lubricating mucus which may be absent later. Sufferers should be strongly encouraged to avoid straining and to spend minimal time defaecating. A prolonged ritual often leads to further straining at the end of defaecation when a mild prolapse can be experienced as incomplete evacuation of faeces. In many patients, these simple measures are enough to relieve symptoms. Note that repetitive straining occasionally leads to the formation of a '**solitary ulcer**' on the anterior wall of the proximal anal canal, which may be clinically indistinguishable from a malignant ulcer. With third degree haemorrhoids, symptoms can often be relieved by the patient replacing the prolapsing haemorrhoids digitally after defaecation.

Creams, suppositories and other topical preparations available with or without prescription are very widely used. Some contain local anaesthetic agents or steroids. They are useful for temporary symptomatic relief but do nothing to treat the underlying condition. Overuse may cause allergic reactions, maceration of the perianal skin and secondary infections.

SURGICAL TREATMENTS FOR HAEMORRHOIDS

Injection of sclerosants or banding

First degree haemorrhoids which do not regress with dietary change and avoiding straining, and most second degree haemorrhoids, can be treated on an outpatient basis by sclerosant injections or banding.

In **sclerotherapy**, with the aid of a proctoscope, 1–3 ml of a mildly irritant solution of 5% phenol in oil is injected submucosally around the pedicles of the three major haemorrhoids in the insensitive upper anal canal. This provokes a fibrotic reaction, effectively obliterating the haemorrhoidal vessels and causing atrophy of the haemorrhoids (see Fig 30.4). Injections are painless if the needle is placed correctly; direct injection into the haemorrhoid would be extremely painful. Sclerotherapy is usually repeated on 2–3 occasions at intervals of 4–6 weeks. *Note*: sclerotherapy is **not** suitable for patients with nut allergies because of the nut origin of the carrier oil.

An alternative treatment is **banding**. A cone of mucosa just above the haemorrhoidal neck is drawn into a banding instrument, often by suction, and tight elastic bands released around the base of the cone, constricting the haemorrhoidal vessels

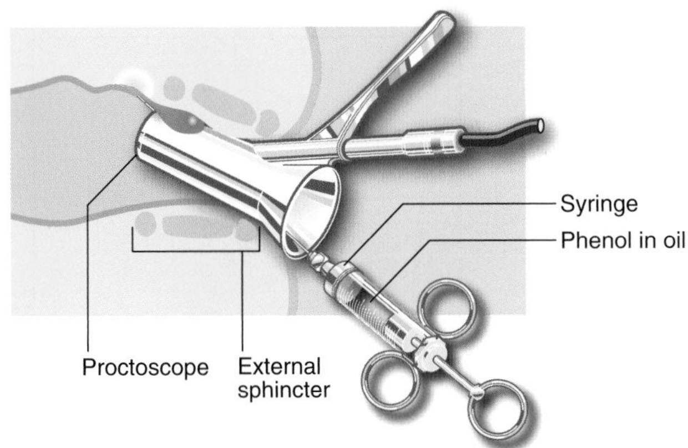

Fig. 30.4 Sclerotherapy or injection of heamorrhoids A mildly irritant solution of 5% phenol in oil is injected submucosally around the pedicle of the haemorrhoid

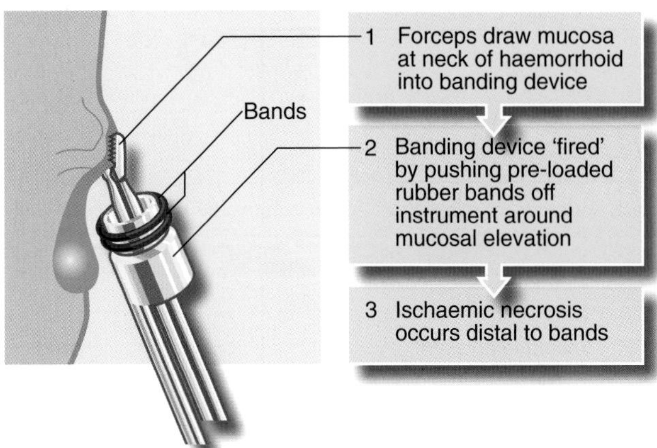

Fig. 30.5 Rubber banding technique for haemorrhoids Note that the haemorrhoid itself is not banded but the band is applied to the blood vessels at its base

(see Fig. 30.5). Importantly, the bands are not placed around the stalks of prolapsing haemorrhoids; this would be unbearably painful because of the somatic innervation of anal skin. The result of banding is that the haemorrhoid gradually shrinks. The bands separate with time and are passed.

Haemorrhoidectomy

Haemorrhoidal excision is indicated for third degree haemorrhoids and for lesser degrees when other treatments have failed. The most common operation is that described by **Milligan and Morgan** in which the haemorrhoidal masses are excised with overlying mucosa and some skin (Fig. 30.6). This leaves skin and mucosal defects which heal by secondary intention and wound contraction. A skin bridge **must** be preserved between each wound to prevent the serious late complication of anal stenosis. **Stapled haemorrhoidectomy** enjoyed some popularity for large haemorrhoids, particularly when mucosal prolapse is a feature. It aims to restore the anatomy of the anal cushions by excising a ring of low rectal mucosa, including the engorged necks of the piles. The metal staple line remains permanently in situ, palpable digitally and sometimes causing pain. This operation requires great skill and occasionally results in serious complications; this fact plus the residual staple line are contributing to a decline in interest in the operation.

Before haemorrhoidectomy, stool softeners such as bulking agents and gentle laxatives should be given to avoid constipation afterwards. The painful early postoperative period can be greatly eased by caudal analgesia given at operation.

Haemorrhoidal artery ligation operation (HALO)

This is a promising new procedure without an incision. It involves locating the artery supplying each haemorrhoid using ultrasound, then encircling it with a stitch via the insensitive lower rectal mucosa to cut off its blood supply. Over the following few days the haemorrhoids shrink, bleeding and local symptoms abate, although skin tags remain.

THROMBOSED EXTERNAL HAEMORRHOIDS

A thrombosed external haemorrhoid or **thrombosed external venous saccule** is an acutely painful anal condition (Fig. 30.7). The onset is sudden and, if untreated, there is persistent pain lasting 1–2 weeks, worse on defaecation. On examination, a blue-black hemispherical bulge is seen in the skin near the anal margin. This is sometimes called a perianal haematoma but this is inaccurate. The condition can occur in patients with haemorrhoids but is usually seen in isolation.

Most thrombosed external haemorrhoids subside over a few days and patients need only oral analgesia. If pain is severe or prolonged, the thrombosis may be incised and drained under local anaesthesia; some surgeons favour this as first line therapy.

ANAL FISSURE

An anal fissure is a longitudinal tear in the mucosa and skin of the anal canal, sometimes caused by passing a large, constipated stool. The tear is nearly always in the posterior midline of the anal margin. The fissure causes acute pain during defaecation and sphincter spasm, both of which persist for an hour or longer. There is often a small amount of fresh bleeding at defaecation. The result is fear of defaecation and this aggravates the constipation. This history alone is diagnostic of an anal fissure. On inspection, the fissure is concealed by the anal spasm but a small skin tag (sentinel pile) may be seen at the superficial end of the fissure (see Fig. 30.8). Rectal examination is extremely painful and rarely possible unless the fissure has become chronic.

Patients sometimes tolerate the pain of an acute fissure by using local anaesthetic creams and then present much later with a chronic anal fissure, prevented from healing by sphincter spasm and repeated tearing open of the fissure during passage of stools.

MANAGEMENT OF ANAL FISSURE

Anal fissure can be managed conservatively or operatively. Modern conservative treatment involves the use of topical glyceryl trinitrate (GTN) ointment 0.2–0.4%, applied three times a day for a month. This relaxes the sphincter spasm and increases blood supply to the fissure, allowing healing. Patients need to be warned that it may cause headaches. This treatment can cure most anal fissures. For the rest, diltiazem ointment,

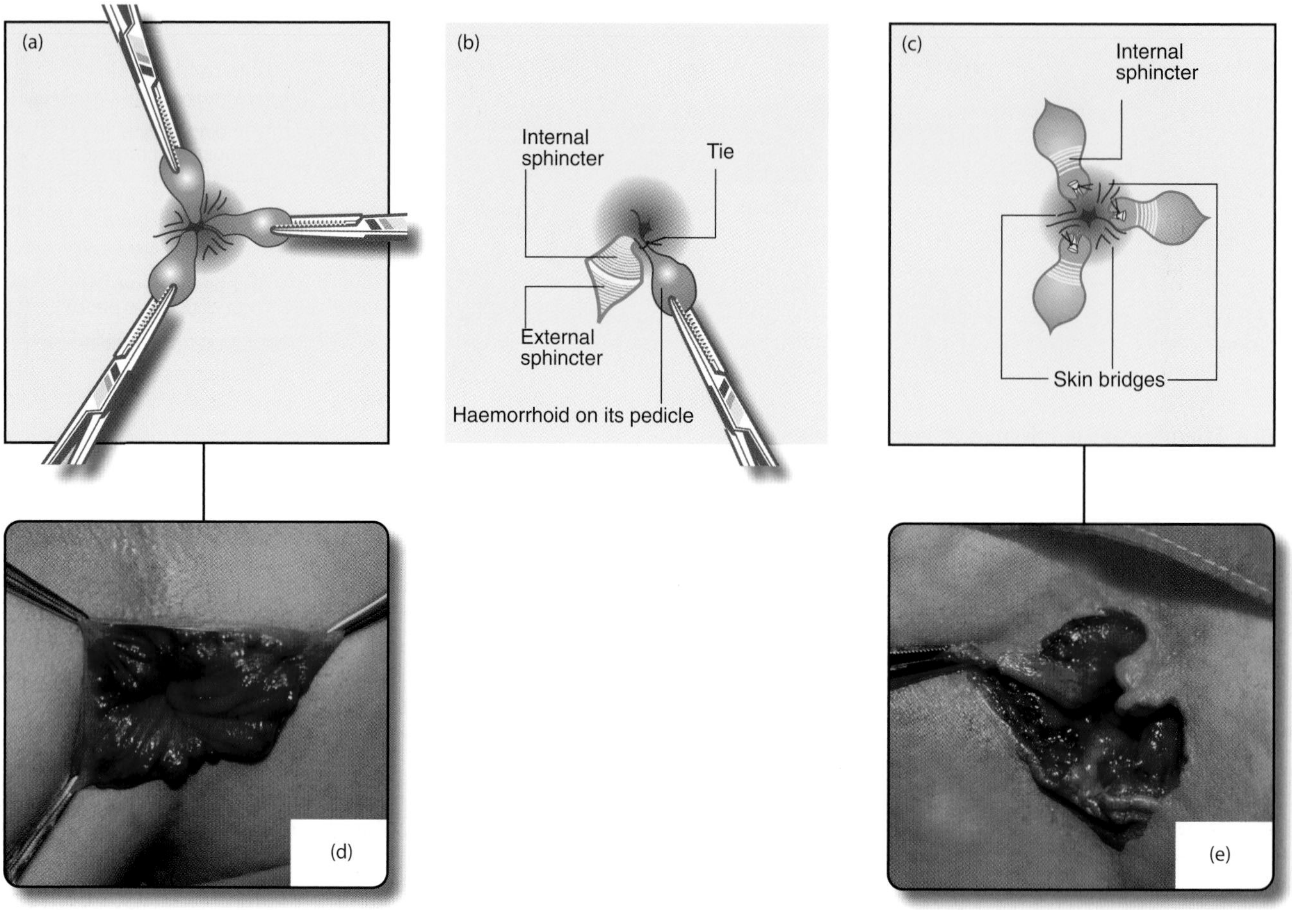

Fig. 30.6 Milligan–Morgan open haemorrhoidectomy
(a) and **(d)** Identification of the main haemorrhoids; the external part of each is clamped with a haemostat and retracted outwards. **(b)** Scissors are used to incise the skin around the external haemorrhoid, excess skin being excised at the same time. The haemorrhoid is then raised on its pedicle by dissecting it from the external and internal sphincters. The pedicle is transfixed and ligated at its base with an absorbable suture. The skin is not closed. **(c)** and **(e)** The process is repeated for the other primary haemorrhoids, ensuring that **skin bridges** are preserved at the anal margin between the areas resected or anal stenosis will occur as healing proceeds ('If it looks like a dahlia, it's a failure'). The completed haemorrhoidectomy has a 'cloverleaf' appearance ('if it looks like a clover, it's all over'). After haemostasis is ensured, wounds are dressed with a non-adherent dressing (e.g. Mepitel) and a surgical pad applied, held in place by elasticated net underpants

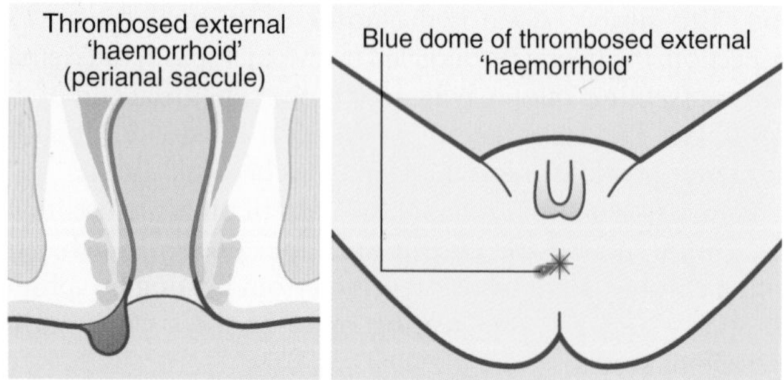

Fig. 30.7 Thrombosed external haemorrhoid

a calcium channel blocker, may be successful. Injection of botulinum toxin into the sphincter complex is another way to cause a temporary 'chemical sphincterotomy'.

Surgery in the form of **lateral submucous (internal) sphincterotomy** brings more immediate relief, but there is a 10–15% incidence of incontinence of flatus following this procedure. Surgeons tend to be reluctant to offer sphincterotomy to women because their sphincters are shorter and less robust, and because occult sphincter injury from childbirth may already have occurred. However, if conservative treatments fail and the patient is suitably informed of the risks, an internal anal sphincterotomy may be offered. This operation involves dividing about 1 cm of the lower rim of the internal sphincter via a small lateral incision. For chronic refractory fissures, anal advancement flap operations are sometimes performed; this avoids the sphincter muscle damage caused by sphincterotomy. **Lord's anal stretch**, which involved manual dilatation of the sphincter, led to unacceptable rates of incontinence due to sphincter damage and has long been abandoned.

ANORECTAL ABSCESSES

PATHOPHYSIOLOGY AND CLINICAL FEATURES

Abscesses in the anorectal area are common surgical emergencies. They present with constant and often severe perineal pain and local tenderness.

Anorectal abscesses begin as acute purulent infections of **anal glands**. These lie in the **intersphincteric space** between the internal and external sphincters and drain into tiny pits, the anal crypts near the dentate line. The ducts are very narrow and duct obstruction may be what initiates the infection. Rarely, an abscess remains confined between the sphincters and an **intersphincteric abscess** results. The only symptom may be chronic anal pain, and there is often little to find on clinical examination. The only clue may be localised tenderness on rectal palpation.

From the intersphincteric plane, infection tends to spread in one or more of three directions (see Fig. 30.9):

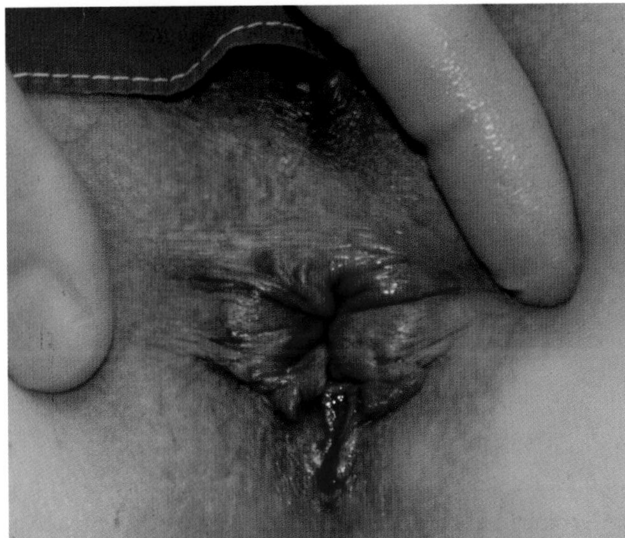

(a)

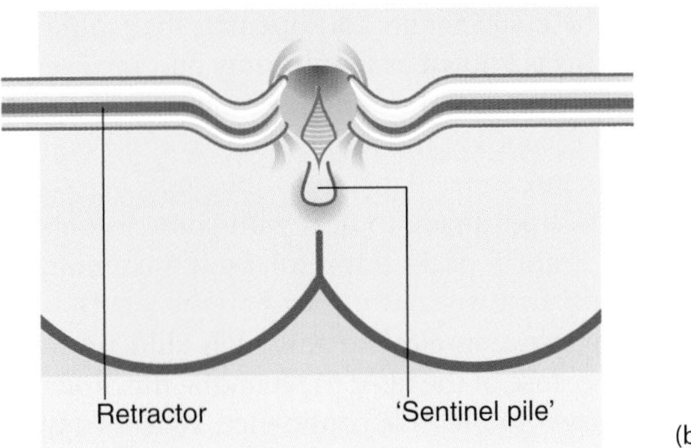

(b)

Fig. 30.8 Anal fissure (a) Chronic anal fissure with a 'sentinel pile'. Simple fissures are typically posteriorly located, as in this patient. **(b)** Explanatory diagram

- **Downwards** between the sphincters towards the anal verge, forming a **perianal abscess**. This is the most common presentation and accounts for 80% of anorectal abscesses. The patient presents acutely with a painful, tender, red swelling close to the anal verge
- **Outwards** through the external sphincter into the loose fibro-fatty tissue of the ischiorectal fossa, forming an **ischiorectal abscess**. There is little barrier to spread of infection once it has entered this space and a neglected or inadequately treated abscess may become enormous. Ischiorectal abscesses make up about 15% of anorectal abscesses. The patient presents with perineal pain and systemic signs of infection. There is tenderness over the ischiorectal fossa lateral to the anus but there may be no visible redness or swelling; rectal palpation reveals a tender mass lateral to the rectum
- **Upwards** between the sphincters to form a **supralevator abscess**, involving the pararectal tissues above the pelvic floor. These make up less than 5% of anorectal abscesses and present with systemic signs of infection, rectal pain and difficulty in micturition. On rectal examination, a tender mass is often palpable near the tip of the finger

TREATMENT OF ANORECTAL ABSCESSES

If perianal infection is seen very early, oral antibiotic treatment may abort it. Antibiotics used in this way by general practitioners, coupled with early referral, has reduced the number and severity of cases reaching the surgeon. However, once an abscess is diagnosed, **surgical drainage** is needed; antibiotics are only indicated in addition when there is spreading infection. Drainage is performed after careful examination (EUA) to determine the extent of the abscess under regional or general anaesthesia. **Perianal** and **ischiorectal abscesses** are drained via the perianal skin, ensuring all loculations are broken down. An **intersphincteric abscess** is drained via an internal sphincterotomy. A swab of the pus is sent for microbiological diagnosis to differentiate infection by skin pathogens (e.g. *Staphylococcus*) which occur spontaneously, from infections of bowel origin (e.g. *E. coli*) which suggest an underlying fistula. Large ischiorectal abscesses require packing or placement of a drain to keep the neck of the cavity open whilst granulation tissue gradually fills the space from its depths. Further examinations under anaesthesia after a few days are usually planned to ensure complete drainage and to inspect for fistulae. Supralevator abscesses are more complicated and require complex staged surgical procedures.

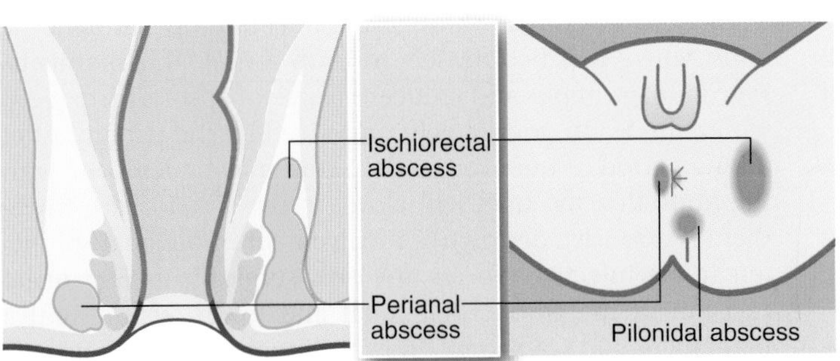

Fig. 30.9 Abscesses in the anorectal region

Incising a perianal abscess results in complete resolution in about 50% of cases; the other half develop an **anal fistula** (see below). The fistula is usually undetectable at the time of drainage but is recognised by a persistent discharge near the skin incision for several weeks afterwards (see Fig. 18.6).

Differential diagnosis of abscesses in the perianal area includes:

- **Crohn's disease**—may cause multiple abscesses and complex fistulae (see Ch. 28) and must be excluded
- **Hidradenitis suppurativa**—originates in perianal apocrine glands in the skin; it is easily distinguished from deeper perianal abscesses by careful inspection and palpation. There may be multiple infected glands in the natal cleft, groins and sometimes axillae
- **Pilonidal abscess**—occurs in the skin of the natal cleft (see Fig. 30.9) but may mimic a true perianal abscess if near the anal margin; careful examination shows no communication with the anal canal and often the presence of embedded hairs. Treatment is by incision and drainage but further procedures may be required to treat the associated pilonidal sinus (see p. 393)
- **Tuberculous abscess and fistula**—very rare

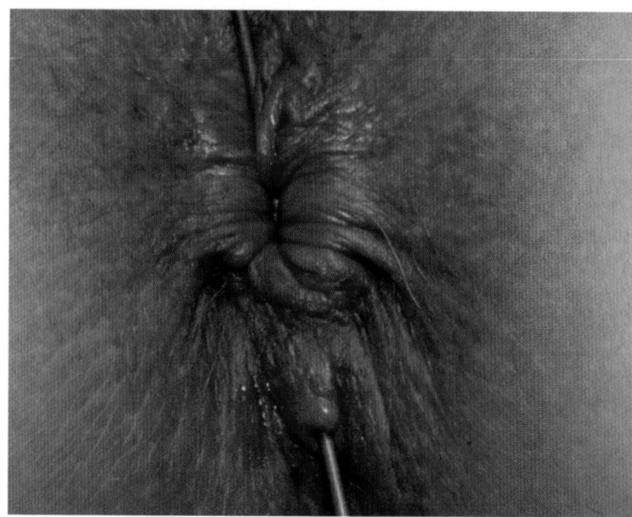

Fig. 30.10 Anal fistula A probe has been passed from the skin surface through a low anal fistula to emerge in the anal canal at the level of the dentate line. Treatment consisted simply of cutting down onto the probe, laying open the fistula along its length. The wound was left to heal by secondary intention

ANAL FISTULA

Anal fistulae usually develop as a complication of perianal, ischiorectal or supralevator abscesses. A fistula is an abnormal connection between two epithelial surfaces and consists of a chronically infected tract which may eventually become epithelialised. It extends from an **internal opening** at the level of the dentate line, and passes through the site of previous abscess to an external opening on the perianal skin near the old drainage scar. The communication between abscess cavity and bowel is established by spontaneous discharge of the enlarging abscess into the bowel before surgical drainage or after incomplete surgical drainage. To minimise the risk of fistula, any abscess in the anal region should be drained early and thoroughly.

The patient with a fistula typically complains of intermittent discharge of mucus or pus in the perianal region, often faecally stained. On examination, a small papilla of granulation tissue is seen on the skin within 2–3 cm of the anal margin (see Fig. 18.6). Pus may be expressed from it by compressing the underlying tract digitally between papilla and anus. This clinical picture is diagnostic of an anal fistula but this apparently trivial skin lesion is often dismissed as a pustule or an incompletely healed perianal abscess.

Most anal fistulae are simple and relatively superficial, with the internal opening located in a crypt at the level of the dentate line (well below puborectalis), most often in the posterior midline. These are known as **low anal fistulae** (Fig. 30.10). For successful treatment, it is essential to locate the internal opening so the entire tract can be dealt with.

Goodsall's rule helps to predict the course of a low fistula:

- If the external opening is **in front** of an imaginary transverse line across the anus, the fistula is likely to have a short **direct** tract to the anal canal
- If the external opening is **behind** the transverse line, the tract is likely to have a **curved** course towards an internal opening in the posterior midline

Assessment and treatment of fistulae requires general or regional anaesthesia. Examination under anaesthetic (EUA) is performed first. A malleable probe is gently manipulated through the fistula to try to demonstrate the internal orifice. If this is not found, hydrogen peroxide can be gently injected into the external opening. Provided the fistula is superficial and involves less than half of the sphincter bulk, treatment is by laying open the entire tract by cutting down on to the probe with diathermy, transecting the anal margin and opening the whole length of the fistula. This is known as **fistulotomy** and involves dividing some of the internal and external sphincter. The wound heals gradually by secondary intention. There should be no loss of faecal continence, but flatus may be less well controlled. Attempts have been made to deal with some fistulae by using tissue glues or fibrin packs but results so far are unimpressive.

If the fistula involves more than half the length of the anal sphincter complex, surgical treatment is difficult and highly specialised because of the need to retain the functional integrity of the sphincters to preserve continence. Where complex fistulae are suspected, the anatomy can be defined well by **magnetic resonance imaging (MRI)** so that careful staged surgery and/or appropriate conservative measures can be planned.

In many of the more severe cases, primary surgical cure is not attempted and infection is controlled long-term by placing a soft **Seton** or thread through the tract and out through the anus, where it is tied loosely to form a ring. This maintains free drainage of pus and reduces the risk of abscess formation, whilst the Seton goes largely unnoticed by the patient. After a long period of quiescence, the Seton may be removed with the hope that the tract will close. In the worst cases, where there is extensive destructive involvement of the anal sphincters in the infective process, the only surgical cure is perineal excision of the whole anal canal and lower rectum, and a permanent end colostomy. In exceptional cases, patients may choose this option to improve their quality of life.

Anal fistulae sometimes occur as a manifestation of **Crohn's disease**. Such fistulae tend to be multiple and in the most extreme cases form a 'pepper-pot' perineum (see Fig. 28.8, p. 371).

PILONIDAL SINUS AND ABSCESS

These conditions arise from the skin of the natal cleft rather than the anus. As the name implies, pilonidal sinuses, cysts and abscesses contain **'a nest of hairs'**. They are common in young adults, particularly hirsute men, and are found at the upper end of the natal cleft. Here, between the buttocks, there is often a congenital dimple or pit. Fragments of hair falling from the back or head accumulate in this nidus. The hairs slowly work their way into the dermis, with the cuticular scales on the hairs acting like barbs of an arrow. The process is encouraged by the massaging effect of sitting for long periods; pilonidal sinus is thus common in truck and tractor drivers. Sinuses also occur between the hairdresser's fingers from implantation of their clients' hair (see below).

Pilonidal sinuses tend to run a long indolent course with chronic or intermittent purulent discharge to the skin surface via one or more sinuses. Periodic acute exacerbations may progress to abscesses (Fig 30.11).

PILONIDAL ABSCESS

The mass of hairs and other skin debris in a pilonidal sinus excites a foreign-body inflammatory reaction, often resulting in a mildly or intermittently discharging sinus. If the cavity becomes secondarily infected, an abscess develops and causes acute pain and swelling. Pilonidal abscesses are often multilocular. They sometimes drain spontaneously but rarely heal completely. Many require surgical drainage because of pain.

TREATMENT OF PILONIDAL SINUS

Definitive treatment aims to eliminate the nidus of hairs and associated cystic cavities, chronic abscesses and sinuses. At operation, obvious plugs of hair are first removed and then the sinus network is explored with probes. In the past, surgical excision left large tissue defects extending to the sacral fascia which took months to heal. Currently the favoured surgical treatment is the **Bascom** 'cleft lift' procedure which may have the secondary advantage of flattening the cleft to minimise recurrence (see Fig. 30.12).

Despite surgery, pilonidal lesions commonly recur, although the Bascom procedure is promising in this respect. Recurrence may also be reduced by careful attention to

Fig. 30.11 Pilonidal sinus and abscess

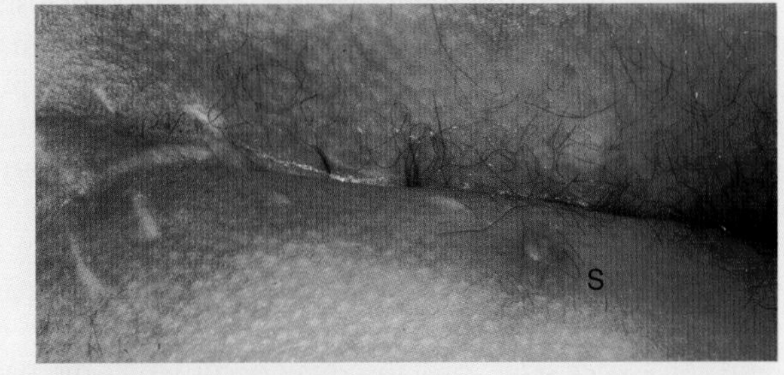

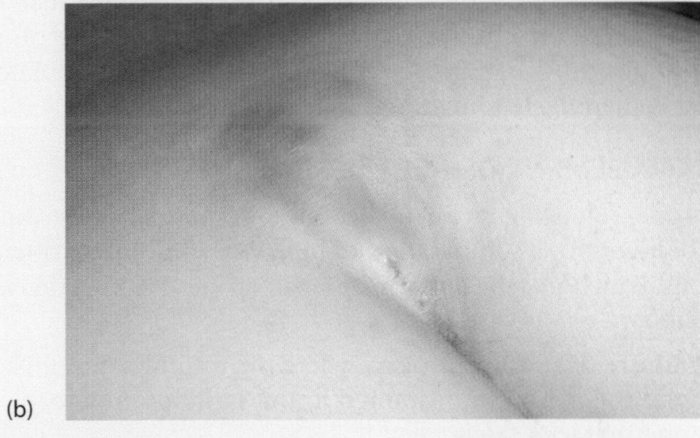

(a) Recurrent pilonidal sinuses. The scar from a previous operation for this condition is visible. There are several tufts of hair emerging from sinuses in the midline and a typical sinus opening **S** to one side.
(b) Pilonidal abscess in a different patient of 24. This is a common presentation and usually requires formal surgical drainage and curettage of the sinuses

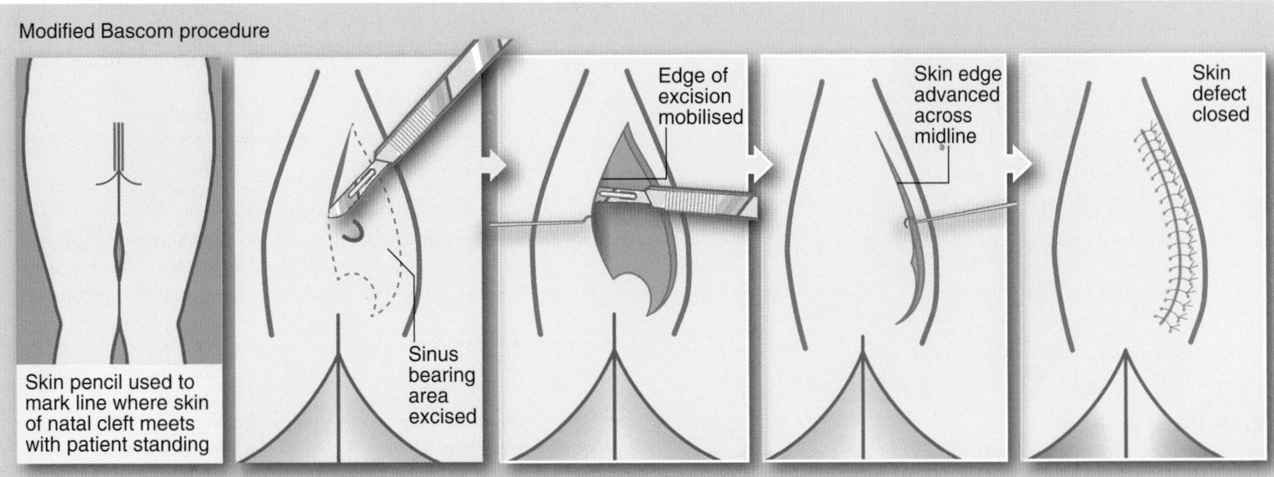

Fig. 30.12 Modified Bascom procedure

hygiene. Daily baths and regular shaving of the area are recommended.

RECTAL PROLAPSE

Rectal prolapse is a herniation of the rectum through the pelvic floor, so the mucosa and muscle wall effectively intussuscept through the anal canal (see Fig. 30.13). It is mainly seen in young children and the elderly.

In childhood, prolapse usually occurs around the age of 2 years. It tends to occur during toilet training and causes parental anxiety. Parents should be reassured that the prolapse will return spontaneously after defaecation or if not, gentle manipulation using water-soluble lubricant jelly may be required. These children should be given a high-fibre diet and taught not to strain during defaecation. More sophisticated treatment is rarely required.

In the elderly, rectal prolapse initially occurs only with defaecation and retracts spontaneously. Sometimes the patient has to reduce the prolapse manually, often with little complaint. At a later stage, prolapse may occur when the patient merely stands up. This can lead to incontinence because of dilatation of the internal anal sphincter. The patient becomes reluctant to leave home and often becomes socially isolated and is then likely to require surgical treatment.

MANAGEMENT OF RECTAL PROLAPSE

Rectal prolapse can be treated by abdominal or perineal procedures, or a combination of both. The **abdominal** operations, which may be performed laparoscopically, include two main types:

- **Suture fixation rectopexy**, where the rectum is mobilised and the mesorectum sutured to the sacral promontory and presacral fascia
- **Resection rectopexy**, where the rectum is mobilised and sutured in the same way, but a sigmoid colectomy is also performed to try to prevent the constipation that often accompanies suture fixation alone

The most popular **perineal** procedure is **Delorme's operation**, which is appropriate for most elderly patients because of its low morbidity and mortality. It involves excising redundant **rectal mucosa**, plicating the rectal wall and replacing the prolapsed rectum. More radical abdominal procedures or any procedure involving an anastomosis (e.g. Altemeier's perineal sigmoidectomy) is usually contraindicated because of greater risk.

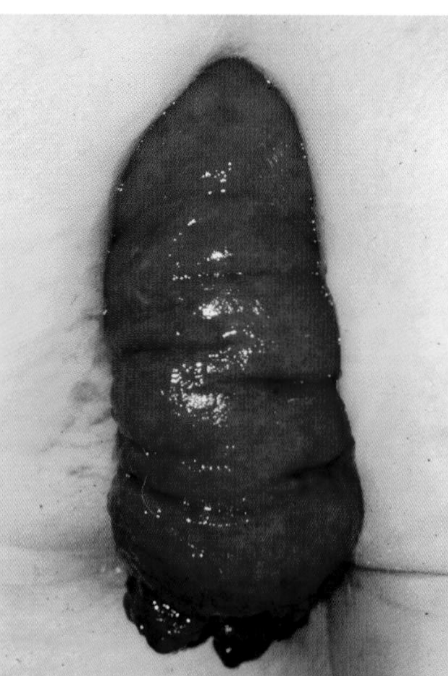

Fig. 30.13 Rectal prolapse
This complete rectal prolapse was in an 80-year-old woman. It emerged spontaneously whenever she stood, causing considerable discomfort and inconvenience, to say the least!

FAECAL INCONTINENCE (Table 30.1)

The process of maintaining continence is complex, involving higher behavioural control, sensory and motor pathways and the anal sphincter mechanisms. In addition, the rectal reservoir must function effectively. The continence mechanism has evolved to cope principally with semi-solid faeces and may fail if the stool is fluid. Incontinence presents in varying degrees: first for flatus, then for fluid and finally for solids as control is progressively lost. Declining mobility may also be a factor: mild incontinence that would otherwise be manageable may become a problem where debility and immobility impair the patient's ability to move to the toilet when required.

Table 30.1 Causes of faecal incontinence

Underlying problem	Disorders
Anorectal incontinence—pudendal neuropathy (previously known as 'idiopathic faecal incontinence'), anal sphincter and pelvic floor damage	Obstetric damage, operative damage, radiation damage, rectal prolapse, high anal fistula
Colorectal disease	Inflammatory bowel disease; polyps and tumours in rectum and anal canal
Faecal quality	Diarrhoea from any cause including infective; faecal impaction with overflow diarrhoea and incontinence
Rectal reservoir and sensation	Inflammatory bowel disease
Brain and higher cerebral functioning	Neurological disorders—dementias, psychological disturbances, impaired consciousness
Sensorimotor pathways	Spinal injury; neurological disorders
Mobility and access to toilet	Enforced bed rest or impaired mobility

Incontinence is socially debilitating. It is surprisingly common but often concealed. It particularly affects some younger parous women and many elderly people. Social embarrassment forces patients to alter their lifestyles so that they never stray far from a lavatory, using constipating agents like loperamide or simply staying at home all day. Assessment of the severity of incontinence should include enquiring about these coping strategies, as patients or carers may be too embarrassed to volunteer them. Standard rating scales can be used to assess incontinence and compare treatments, e.g. the Cleveland Clinic faecal incontinence scale.

Young faecally incontinent patients are mostly female and usually suffer from **anorectal incontinence**. In the elderly, the aetiology is usually multifactorial.

ANORECTAL INCONTINENCE

The main functional abnormality in anorectal incontinence is weakness of the external anal sphincter and pelvic floor muscles. This is sometimes due to direct injury from trauma or surgery but most cases were labelled idiopathic. It is now recognised that the most important cause of sphincter dysfunction in women is obstetric injury. Repeated childbirth, episiotomies or difficult forceps deliveries increase the risk. The mechanism is probably via traumatic **pudendal neuropathy** leading to atrophy of sphincteric and pelvic floor muscles. Even chronic straining at stool may cause pudendal neuropathy. In old age, degenerative changes in the spinal cord appear to be the principal cause of muscle atrophy.

If sphincters have been physically damaged, surgical sphincter repair may be undertaken but results are not always predictable or long-lasting. Continuous sacral nerve stimulation, where an implanted 'pacemaker' promotes increased sphincter tone, can be attempted. As a last resort, a colostomy may allow the patient a better quality of life.

ANAL WARTS (CONDYLOMATA ACCUMINATA)

Warts in the perianal region (see Fig. 30.14) have a viral aetiology (human papilloma-virus (HPV) types 6 and 11) and are generally transmitted by sexual activity. Just as cervical cancer is linked to specific strains of HPV infection, anal warts indicate an increased risk of anal canal carcinoma by virtue of their common aetiology. Immune suppression, for example in patients with organ transplants or with HIV infection, can lead to rapidly developing anal warts and progression to malignant change.

In small numbers, anal warts can be treated by topical applications of **podophyllin**. When large numbers are present, surgical excision under general anaesthetic is the only practical option. This involves meticulous excision of each individual wart by electrocautery. The normal skin between the warts is carefully preserved to avoid delayed healing or the disastrous complication of anal stenosis. Carefully mapped biopsies can also be undertaken to monitor for dysplastic change. In the future, prevention will come from human papilloma virus (HPV) vaccines in both sexes, shown to prevent papillomavirus-induced cervical cancer, genital warts, and some oral cancers.

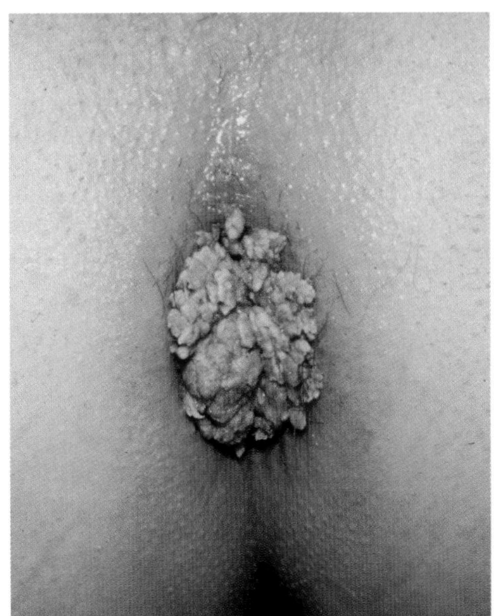

Fig. 30.14 Anal warts (condylomata acuminata)

SQUAMOUS CELL CARCINOMA OF THE ANUS

EPIDEMIOLOGY

The annual incidence of anal cancer in women and the general population is about 1 : 100 000; however, in men who have sex with men and who are HIV negative, the incidence markedly increases to 35 : 100 000 and it doubles if the men are HIV positive. The sharp increase of mainly non-keratinising cancers arising in the transitional zone in these groups is largely due to heightened rates of infection with HPV and the effects of immunosuppression fostering its progress. An effective vaccine has now been developed for HPV and, if administered in the early teens, should prevent infection and its consequences.

CLINICAL FEATURES

The symptoms of anal carcinoma are similar to those of haemorrhoids and other familiar benign anal conditions, namely fresh rectal bleeding, anal pain, discomfort and discharge. Later, incontinence can result from involvement of the anal sphincter. The patient may ignore the symptoms for a period and the doctor may initially overlook the diagnosis. On digital rectal examination, a localised firm or hard ulcer or a growth with an irregular surface and edge may be palpable and there may be surrounding woody induration. The lesion is usually visible on proctoscopy and the diagnosis confirmed by biopsy. Palpation of the groins may reveal hard, matted involved inguinal nodes. Anal canal carcinoma also metastasises to intra-abdominal superior rectal nodes, reflecting the mixed drainage of the anal canal.

Chemoradiotherapy has now largely superseded abdomino-perineal excision because of demonstrably better cure rates for non-surgical therapy.

Other rare anal neoplasms

The anal canal is the third most common site for **malignant melanomas** after skin and the eye. These cause non-specific anal symptoms of discomfort and bleeding and diagnosis may thus be delayed. These melanomas are usually non-pigmented and biopsy evidence is needed to make a firm diagnosis. Treatment outcomes are poor. **Adenocarcinoma** of the rectum may extend distally into the anal region, and rarely **basal cell carcinomas** may occur here.

PROCTALGIA FUGAX

Proctalgia fugax is a neuropathic type of pain which often manifests as brief episodes of severe lancinating pain in the perineum with sphincter spasms. It occurs at unpredictable times but often at night. It usually occurs independently of conditions such as anal fissure, complicated piles and anal or rectal neoplasms; the patient may be convinced that cancer is the cause and may suspect that the doctor thinks it is 'all in the mind'. The cause is unknown but is believed not to be psychological. Whilst it is difficult to cure, reassurance and recommending ice packs or warm baths may help. If this fails, therapy with amitriptyline or gabapentin may control symptoms.

PRURITUS ANI

Anal itching can be distressing. It is generally caused by mucus leakage and may occur without significant haemorrhoids; even a minute quantity of leaking mucus or faecal material causes profound irritation. Patients generally try to self-medicate with various creams but these tend to increase skin maceration and worsen the problem. Pruritus can be helped greatly if all topical creams are stopped and the perineum is washed and dabbed dry after defaecation using plain water. Even soap can aggravate the symptoms.

Thoracic surgery

31

INTRODUCTION

In its broadest sense non-cardiac thoracic surgery covers the diagnosis and management of all non-cardiac disease within the chest. However, the practice varies between countries. For example, in the UK, unlike North America, most oesophageal disease is no longer managed by thoracic surgeons but by gastroenterologists and upper GI surgeons. This chapter will review the management of benign and malignant conditions of the chest and mediastinal disorders that are commonly managed by UK thoracic surgeons. The principles of oesophageal surgery are covered in Chapter 22 and chest trauma in Chapter 15.

INVESTIGATIVE TECHNIQUES

Imaging

Chest X-ray, computerised tomography (CT), magnetic resonance imaging, ultrasound (US) and synchronized CT-positron emission tomography are the most commonly used modalities. Chest X-ray is useful as a 'baseline' and also for early post-procedure follow-up. CT provides the best anatomical information and is used for preoperative planning and for follow-up. low radiation-dose protocols protocols are being explored for lung cancer screening. Early evidence suggests that screening certain groups may lead to longer survival and this may become common practice. MRI is most useful to study soft tissues, and in particular in malignancy, to determine the extent of chest wall invasion, diaphragm invasion and for spread of cancers to the liver or brain.

US is useful to guide drainage of collections, siting of chest-drains and for biopsy of superficial or pleural-based lesions. Most modern thoracic surgeons can undertake basic bedside ultrasound to evaluate pleural effusions.

Ideally, before placing a non-emergency chest drain, US or preferably CT scanning should be performed to reduce the risk of complications.

Lung function tests

Lung function tests give a detailed portrait of the physiological effects of individual chest diseases and can track changes over time or as a result of treatment. When surgery is contemplated, lung function tests help assess the patient's capacity to withstand chest wall incision or lung resection. They include:

- Measurement of **air flow** into and out of the alveoli, i.e. FEV_1, FVC, peak air flow, total lung capacity, alveolar ventilation
- Measurement of **gas diffusion** across the alveolar–capillary interface, usually involving measuring rates of carbon monoxide diffusion
- Assessing the amount of dead space by calculating the **residual volume** and **total lung capacity**
- Assessing exercise capacity, e.g. by the 6 minute walk test or by formal cardiopulmonary exercise testing
- Baseline arterial or capillary blood gases

Bronchoscopy

Flexible bronchoscopy can be performed with minimal or no sedation and topical local anaesthesia. It is possible to examine as far as segmental bronchi, obtain small biopsies and clear secretions.

For cancer staging, transbronchial ultrasound (endobronchial US, EBUS) allows biopsy of lymph nodes close to the airway. This can be combined with transoesophageal ultrasound (EUS) to allow more lymph node stations and the left adrenal gland to be biopsied. Rigid bronchoscopy is

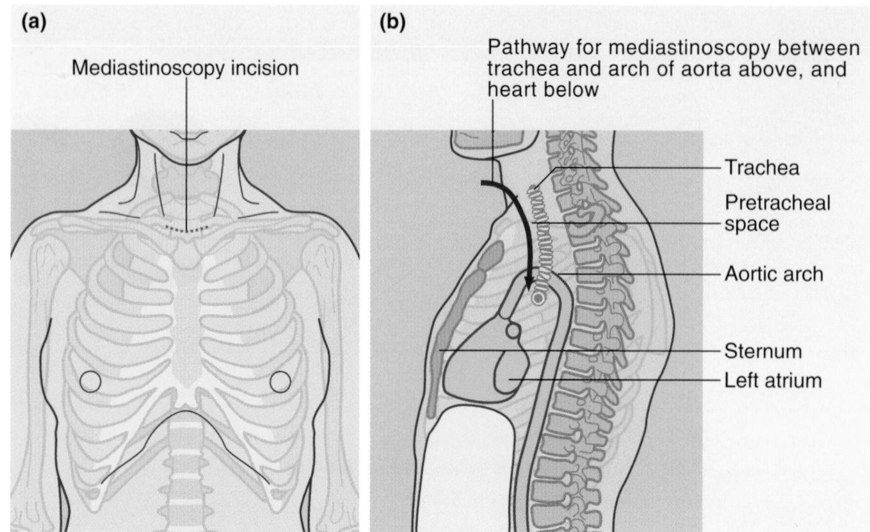

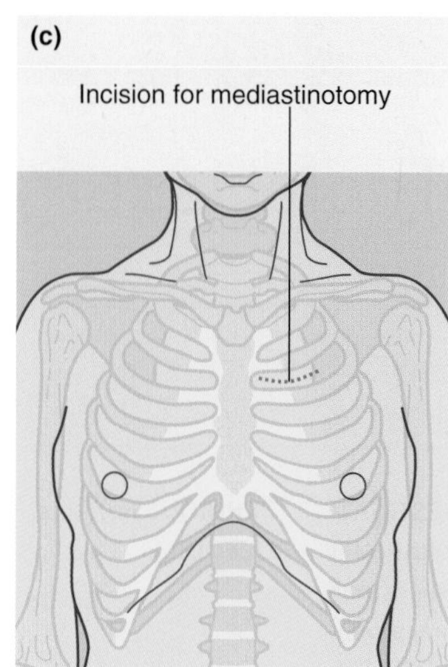

Fig. 31.1 Mediastinoscopy and mediastinotomy
(a) and **(b)** Mediastinoscopy for investigation of the posterior mediastinum. **(c)** Mediastinotomy

performed under general anaesthesia and allows passage of larger instruments, including a flexible bronchoscope, for removal of foreign bodies, obtaining large biopsies and control of bleeding.

Pleural aspiration and percutaneous biopsy

Aspiration of pleural effusions for cytological examination can be performed using a standard wide-bore needle and syringe. Blind pleural biopsy is now discouraged because of its relatively low yield rate and high complication rate. Many thoracic masses are amenable to percutaneous biopsy under US or CT guidance, although thoracoscopy or direct surgical cut-down to the lesion has the best yield.

Video-mediastinoscopy

A mediastinoscope is used to biopsy paratracheal and subcarinal lymph nodes. The instrument is a rigid tube incorporating fibreoptic light guides; it is inserted via a skin incision above the suprasternal notch and passed caudally along the plane of the pretracheal fascia (see Fig. 31.1a and b). The route passes close to the azygos vein, superior vena cava, innominate artery, arch of the aorta, pulmonary artery and the recurrent laryngeal nerves posterolaterally on each side. These structures and the oesophagus are at risk of damage and, although rare, this must be explained to the patient. Mediastinoscopy gives access to the mediastinum except for the subaortic fossa (below the aortic arch and often containing lymph nodes). Access to this area is obtained by anterior mediastinotomy or video-assisted thoracic surgery.

Thoracoscopy

This is the thoracic equivalent of laparoscopy and is sometimes known as **video-assisted thoracoscopic surgery** or **VATS**. It is usually performed under general anaesthesia but basic procedures use local anaesthesia with sedation. Instruments for viewing and operating are inserted through small incisions in the chest wall.

Thoracoscopy is the preferred technique for pleural biopsy, pneumothorax treatment and evacuation of early empyema and is also used to sample mediastinal lymph nodes and perform cervical (thoraco-dorsal) sympathectomy.

The range of procedures is becoming increasingly complex, e.g. extensive pleurectomy for mesothelioma or lobectomy. VAT lobectomy usually involves a non rib-spreading 'utility' incision of 5–10 cm and two or three further 'port' incisions to pass a video-telescope and surgical instruments. The resected specimen is placed in an extraction bag so it can be removed intact. The ports can be used to place drains.

Anterior mediastinotomy

Anterior mediastinotomy (see Fig. 31.1c), a form of mini-thoracotomy, may be used to obtain biopsies from anterior mediastinal lesions, e.g. thymic tumours. The approach can be left or right of the sternum, either intercostally or with costal cartilage resection. Left anterior mediastinotomy affords good access for biopsy of subaortic fossa masses. Increasingly, VATS is the preferred method of accessing these sites.

Thoracotomy

Thoracotomy, described on page 400, gives full access to the paratracheal, subcarinal and hilar lymph node groups, the great vessels, oesophagus, lung and pericardium and is used when less invasive procedures are inappropriate or have failed.

THERAPEUTIC PROCEDURES

TRACHEOSTOMY

Principles of tracheostomy

A tracheostomy (see Figs 31.2, 31.3) is an artificial opening into the trachea to provide a secure airway when the pharyngeal airway or larynx needs to be bypassed. With time, an epithelialised fistula develops between the skin and trachea which allows tracheostomy tubes to be changed and the airways cleaned with ease. In many units 'percutaneous tracheostomy' is performed using a 'Seldinger-type' technique. However, the technique of 'open' tracheostomy should be understood by most surgeons.

Indications for tracheostomy include:

- Permanent functional obstruction of the upper airway, e.g. carcinoma of larynx
- Temporary or potential upper airway obstruction, e.g. facial fractures, major head and neck operations or injuries
- Long-term ventilatory support, where prolonged endotracheal intubation would otherwise be likely to cause permanent laryngeal damage and prevent swallowing and speech. Tracheostomy also provides continuous access to the lower airways for bronchial aspiration and toilet

Tracheostomy should be a planned procedure performed in the operating room under general anaesthesia. It is *not* an emergency procedure for patients with upper airway obstruction. For these, endotracheal intubation or cricothyroidotomy (see Fig. 31.4) should be used.

Complications of tracheostomy

- **Haemorrhage** caused by erosion of the innominate (brachiocephalic) artery or vein
- **Tracheo-oesophageal fistula**, particularly where a nasogastric tube is in place
- **Displacement of the tracheostomy tube** may occur before the desired 'fistula' becomes established, making it difficult to reintubate the trachea
- **Tracheal stenosis**, usually the result of prolonged use of a high-pressure cuff (now rare due to the introduction of low-pressure cuffs)

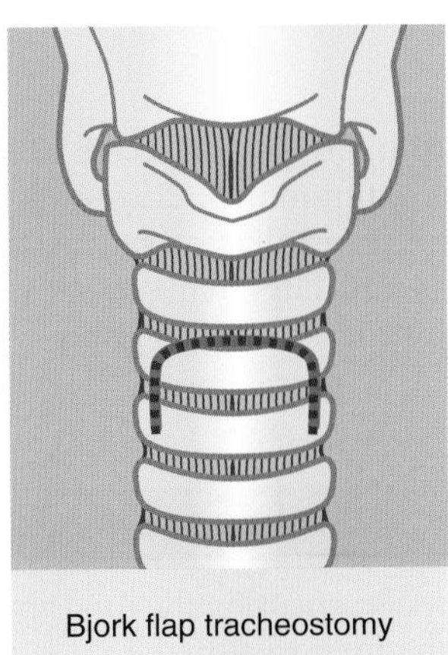

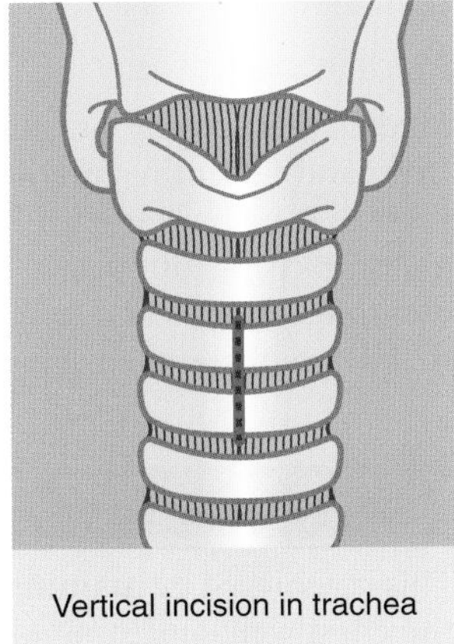

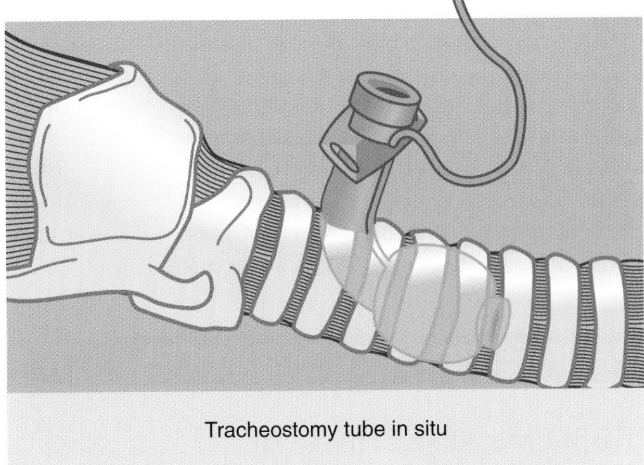

Fig. 31.2 Tracheostomy placement

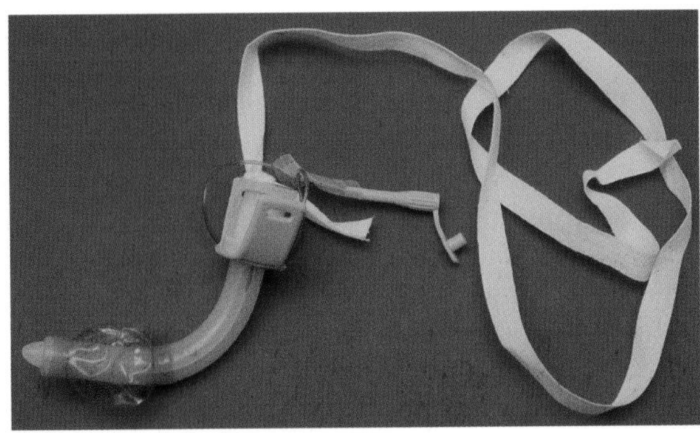
(a)

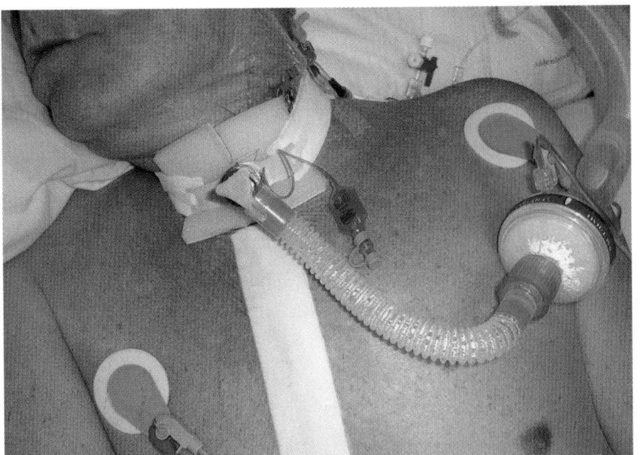
(b)

Fig. 31.3 Tracheostomy
(a) Disposable tracheostomy tube. Note the distal balloon which is inflated via the small tube to provide a snug fit inside the trachea. **(b)** Patient being ventilated via an elective tracheostomy after cardiac surgery

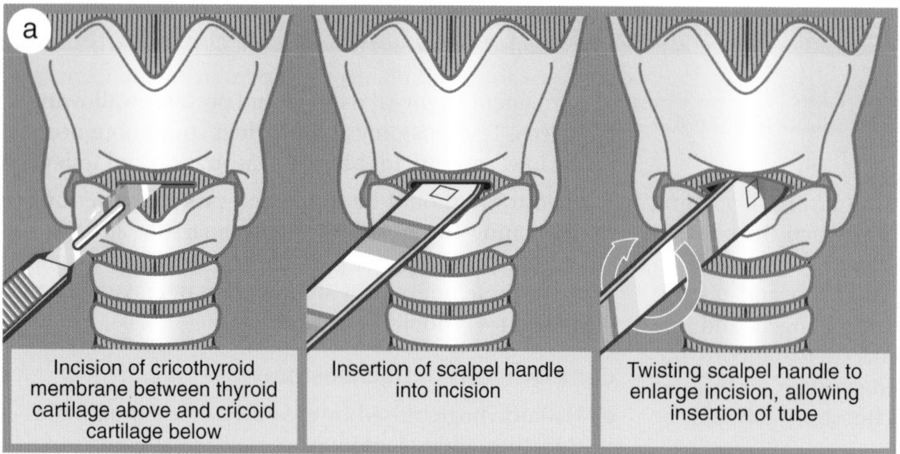

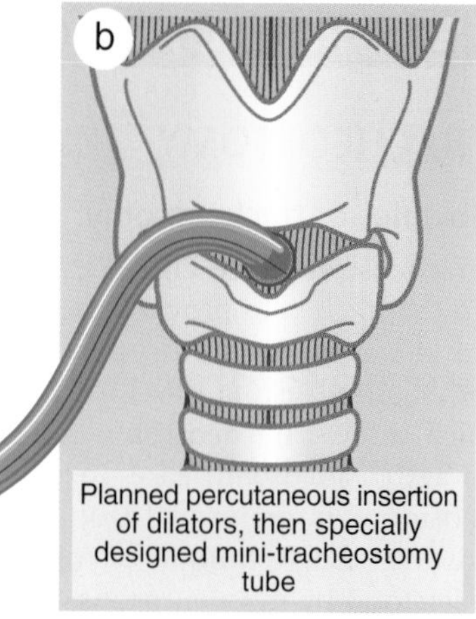

Fig. 31.4 Cricothyroidotomy
(a) In a dire emergency, this life-saving procedure can be rapidly employed to gain time. **(b)** Modern mini-cricothyroidotomy can be performed percutaneously by making a small incision through the cricothyroid membrane and progressively dilating it with graduated dilators before insertion of a specially constructed small-diameter tube, e.g. Minitrach or Quicktrach. These are used in accident victims and often in intensive care units

THORACOTOMY

All thoracotomies are now devised to spare at least some muscles from being divided.

Posterolateral thoracotomy

Posterolateral thoracotomy is the standard approach for lung and oesophageal resections as well as for surgery of the descending aorta. Generally a curved incision passes below the inferior angle of the scapula, latissimus dorsi is divided and the chest is entered through the bed of the (unresected) fifth or sixth rib. If necessary, the incision can be extended into the abdomen (thoraco-abdominal incision), e.g. for oesophago-gastrectomy or thoraco-abdominal aortic aneurysm.

Lateral thoracotomy

Lateral thoracotomy involves an incision extending between anterior and posterior axillary lines.

Anterior thoracotomy

This is used for diagnostic biopsy or pericardial window.

Median sternotomy

Median sternotomy or 'sternal split' gives wide access to the heart and the entire anterior mediastinum including the great vessels. It is the standard incision for cardiac surgery as well as for excision of thymic lesions and large retrosternal parathyroid tumours and, occasionally, resection of a goitre with massive retrosternal extension.

SPECIFIC THORACIC DISORDERS

PROBLEMS AFFECTING THE PLEURAL SPACE

INTRODUCTION

The pleural cavity is a potential space between the chest wall and lung, lined by a continuous sheet of mesothelium. That lining the chest wall is **parietal pleura** and that covering the lung is **visceral pleura**. The pleural space normally contains a minute amount of serous fluid to lubricate movement of opposed pleural surfaces and it causes them to adhere by surface tension. This, and the negative pressure arising from the tendency of the chest wall to expand, keeps the lungs expanded. Disease or injury may result in accumulation of air (**pneumothorax**) or fluid (**pleural effusion**) in the pleural cavity. Pleural effusions are classified as transudates or exudates. Fluid collections can be subdivided into pus (**empyema**), blood (**haemothorax**), chyle (chylothorax) and, rarely, lymph (lymphothorax).

The pleural space is not essential to life, and the principle of managing pleural problems is often to eliminate this space. This is achieved by draining the space, ensuring the lung abuts the chest wall, and stimulating the lung to adhere to it. Such pleural adhesions are known as pleuradhesis (or pleurodesis). Pleural adhesions may occur spontaneously.

PNEUMOTHORAX

Pneumothorax is classified as primary or secondary. Primary refers to 'spontaneous' pneumothorax, occurring without obvious lung disease. It is most common in people between the ages of 15 and 30, and is characteristically (but not exclusively) seen in tall, thin males. Secondary pneumothorax occurs in patients with other lung disease, most often COPD. It is most common after 50 years in patients with a smoking history but can occur in a range of conditions including *Pneumocystis* pneumonia and collagen disorders.

Primary or 'spontaneous' pneumothorax most often results from rupture of a 'bleb' on the pleural surface of the lung, usually a small air-filled cavity that communicates with lung parenchyma. Rupture allows air to escape into the pleural space and the lung collapses. **Traumatic pneumothorax** usually results from blunt chest injury, often from rib fractures

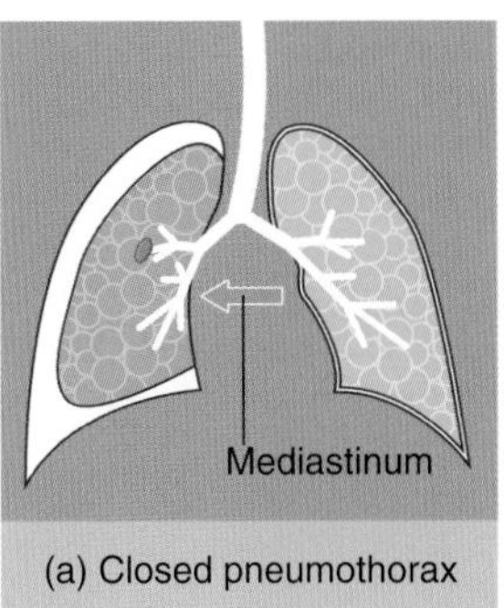

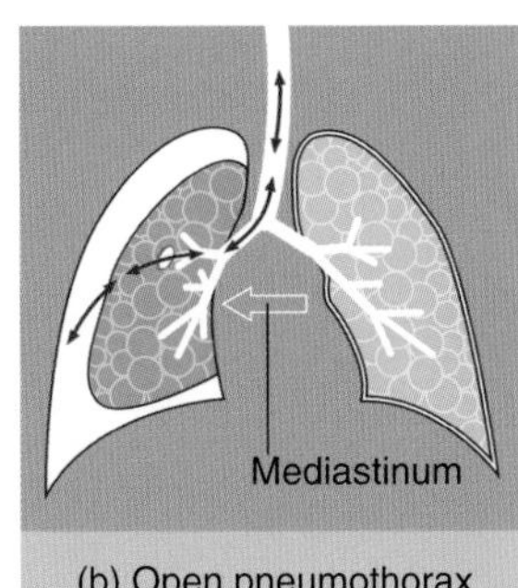

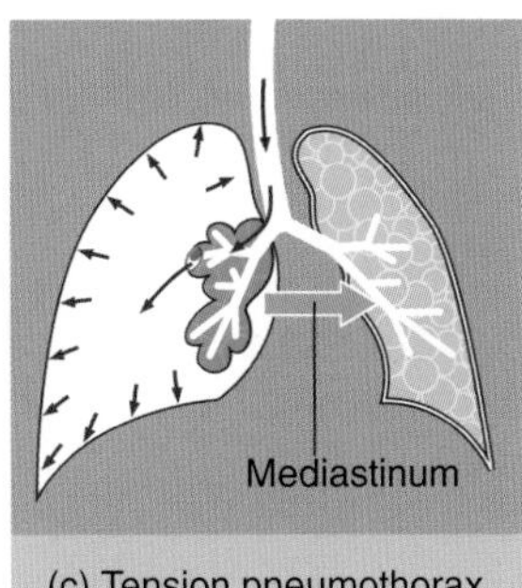

Fig. 31.5 Classification of pneumothorax
(a) In closed pneumothorax the pleural defect closes spontaneously, leaving a fixed amount of air in the pleural space. **(b)** In open pneumothorax there is free passage of air via an open defect in the visceral pleura. **(c)** In tension pneumothorax the pleural defect acts as a flap valve allowing progressive entry of air into the pleural space, collapsing the lung and pushing the mediastinum to the opposite side

penetrating visceral pleura. Penetrating chest injury, e.g. stab wounds, may also be responsible. Different types of pneumothorax are illustrated in Figure 31.5.

Sometimes, after trauma, if the site of air leakage acts as a one-way valve, a **tension pneumothorax** is created. The valve effect allows air to escape into the pleural space but not to return to the airway, causing lung collapse on the affected side. Rising intrapleural pressure reduces venous return and in extreme cases can push the mediastinum towards the opposite side. Reduced venous return leads to low-output cardiac failure which in turn worsens the venous return. The physiological upset is extreme, can progress rapidly, poses an immediate threat to life and must be treated urgently.

Treatment of a pneumothorax is required under the following circumstances:

- Where there is a tension pneumothorax
- When the lung volume is compromised by more than about 25% as calculated on a PA chest X-ray
- If the pneumothorax is increasing
- When a small pneumothorax is having a disproportionate effect on lung function because of pre-existing lung disease

Treatment of pneumothorax

Aspiration

An uncomplicated pneumothorax in an otherwise fit patient can be treated by aspiration. A 50 ml syringe is connected to a three-way tap or one-way valve and a needle. The needle is inserted intercostally into the pneumothorax and air aspirated or allowed to blow out. Progress is later monitored by chest X-ray. The process can be repeated, but formal tube drainage may be needed if the pneumothorax recurs.

In **tension pneumothorax**, rapid emergency relief can be obtained by passing a large needle into the pleural space. A relatively safe point is just lateral to the mid-clavicular line in the 2nd intercostal space. A formal chest drain must be inserted soon afterwards.

Intercostal tube drainage

The technique of intercostal chest drainage is described in Figure 31.6; see also Figure 31.7. If a pneumothorax needs a drain, a single small apical drain is used, e.g. 16F gauge. Smaller drains are used by non-surgeons but these have a high failure rate due to kinking and blockage.

Any intercostal tube drain must be connected to an apparatus to prevent lung collapse from air being drawn into the chest by negative intrapleural pressure. The usual arrangement is to connect the chest drain to a rigid tube secured below the water level in a bottle to form an underwater seal. This allows air and fluid to leave the chest cavity but not return. The bottle is kept below patient level so gravity assists. As the patient breathes, excess pleural air and fluid are gradually expelled into the bottle, and air bubbles from the exhaust tube. If there is a lung air leak via a breach in the visceral pleura, this is manifest by continued bubbling in the bottle and failure of the lung to expand. Continuous suction should then be applied to the underwater seal outlet for a few days; this usually helps the lung to expand and adhere to the chest wall, thereby remaining inflated and blocking the air leak.

Patients with intercostal drains must be transported with care to ensure the drainage bottle does not tip over and always remains below patient level to prevent fluid reflux into the chest. It is no longer recommended that chest tubes be clamped when patients are moved as this is dangerous (one exception to this is after pneumonectomy).

Intercostal drains are removed when the lung is fully expanded. For pneumothorax, cessation of bubbling in the bottle for 24 hours is an indication for removal; for fluid drainage, the duration varies with the underlying problem.

Treatment of persistent or recurrent pneumothorax

More extensive surgical intervention may be required for persistent or recurrent pneumothorax. The general rule is that surgery is offered for an unresolving pneumothorax, two pneumothoraces on the same side or one on each side. Patients in high-risk occupations, such as pilots, may be offered surgery after a single pneumothorax. Approaches include stapling of bullae to prevent air leakage and pleural abrasion or pleurectomy. In patients with fragile lungs, as in secondary pneumothorax, lung resection is sometimes avoided by insufflating talc to encourage a chemical pleurodesis (see Fig. 31.8). Most of this surgery is now performed by VATS.

EXCESS PLEURAL FLUID

Excess pleural fluid may be a watery transudate (e.g. in heart failure) or an exudate of variable viscosity (e.g. due to pleural infection).

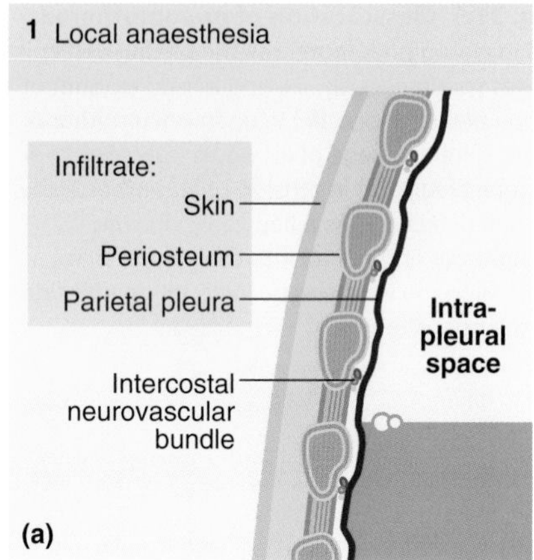

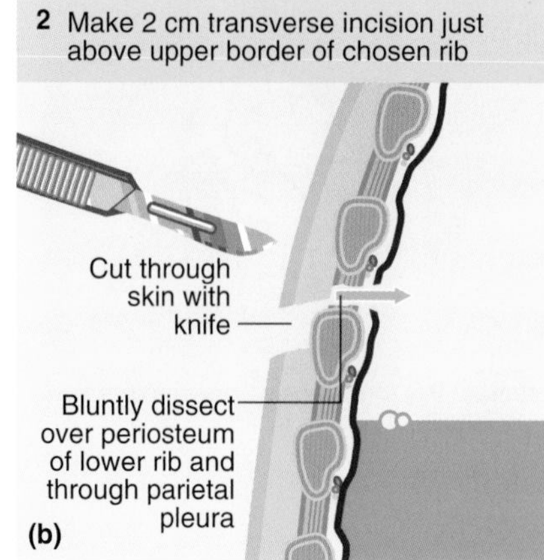

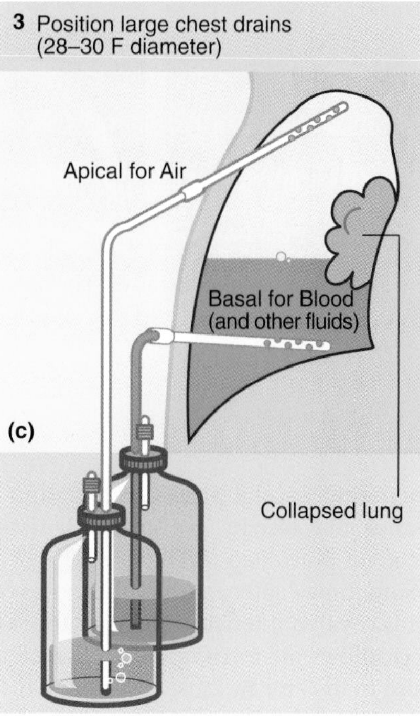

Fig. 31.6 Technique of intercostal tube drainage of chest (tube thoracostomy)

- Inject local anaesthetics to block sensitive structures and intercostal nerve and give time for this to take effect
- Make 2 cm incision near upper border of rib and parallel to it
- Bluntly dissect intercostal muscles down to parietal pleura with artery forceps. Stay near upper border of rib to avoid intercostal vessels
- Palpate lung with gloved index finger to free adhesions and ensure free entry for the drain
- Remove trocar from large-bore chest drain tube (at least 28 F gauge); 16 F can be used for pneumothorax alone. Grasp distal end with artery forceps and guide drain into chest in an apical or a basal direction according to purpose. Never insert a chest drain with the trocar in position as this is highly dangerous
- Attach drain to an underwater seal and suture drain to chest wall. Snug the skin around the drain with a purse string suture. Apply airtight dressing around the tube and tape tube to chest wall. Sit patient up to 45°
- Take a chest X-ray to confirm position of tube

Indications for draining a pleural effusion include:

- **Diagnostic**
  - empyema
  - suspected malignancy
  - traumatic haemothorax
- **Therapeutic**
  - removing the compressive effects of a large pleural fluid collection on the lung
  - draining pus from an empyema
  - arresting haemorrhage from damaged intercostal vessels causing haemothorax

Uncomplicated pleural effusions are usually drained via a large-bore tube (28 F gauge or larger) inserted towards the base of the pleural cavity in the most practicable dependent position. More than one drain may be required if fluid collections are loculated.

Malignant effusions

Malignant effusions (e.g. from breast cancer) usually recur after simple drainage and need to be treated in other ways. Methods include:

- Stimulating **adhesion formation** between visceral and parietal pleura (**pleurodesis**). This can be achieved by aspirating the fluid, injecting an irritant such as sterile talc and maintaining tube drainage until permanent adhesions develop. An alternative is to perform **pleural abrasion**. Via a small thoracotomy, the parietal pleura is widely abraded using a surgical swab. Again, chest drainage allows adhesions to form between the layers of pleura with permanent prevention of effusion
- **Parietal pleurectomy**. Traditionally performed by thoracotomy but now usually by VATS, this involves stripping the parietal pleura to cause diffuse adhesion of the lung surface to the chest wall (see Fig. 31.8b)
- **Pleuro-peritoneal shunting** using a tubular device connecting the two cavities. This is implanted beneath the skin and incorporates a one-way valve. Excess pleural fluid is manually 'pumped' from the pleura into the peritoneum by the patient several times a day where it is resorbed. Unfortunately the manual pumping can be uncomfortable and devices can become blocked
- **Tunnelled intrapleural catheter**. A small catheter is tunnelled a few centimetres from the skin to the pleural space and can be opened to intermittently drain the pleural space. The catheter can be inserted under local anaesthesia. Tunnelling reduces the infection risk

Empyema

When pleural fluid becomes infected, pus accumulates in the pleural cavity and is known as an **empyema**. Early on, an

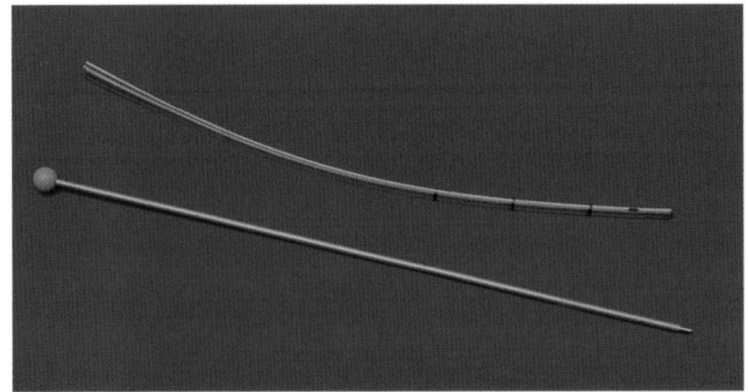

(a)

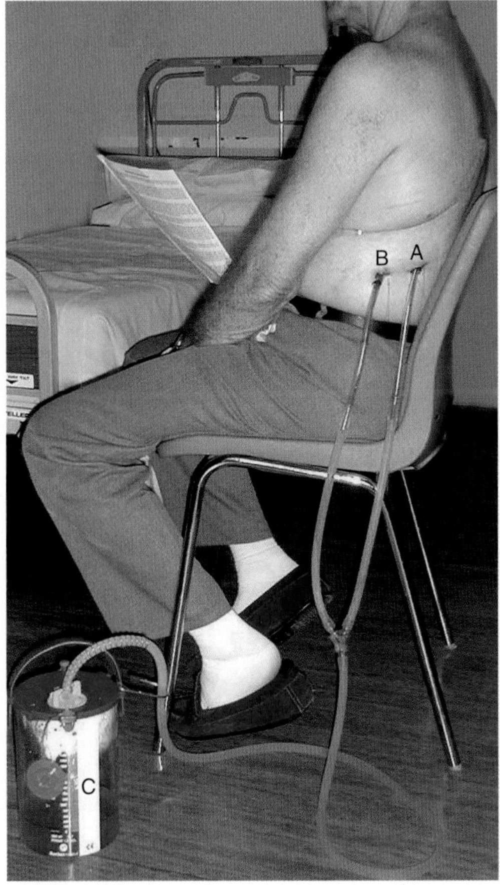

(b)

Fig. 31.7 Chest drain
(a) 30 F gauge tube (10 mm) with stylet removed (and thrown away!). Note the radiopaque line and the side holes near the tip. **(b)** Post thoracotomy and lobar resection of lung for cancer. This patient has two chest drains in situ, an **A**pical drain for Air and a **B**asal drain for Blood. Both are connected to an underwater seal, **C,** to prevent inflow of air that would cause a pneumothorax

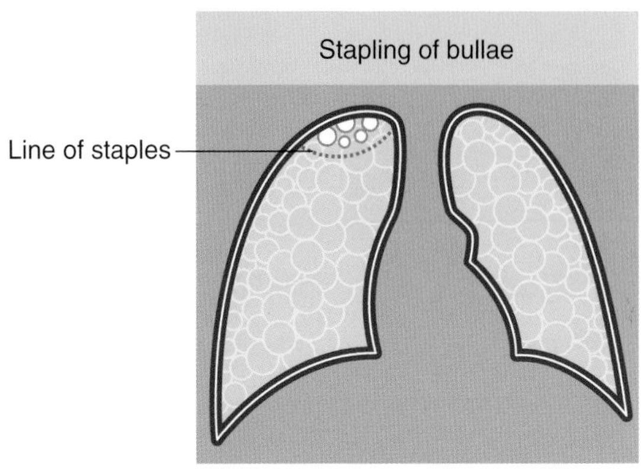

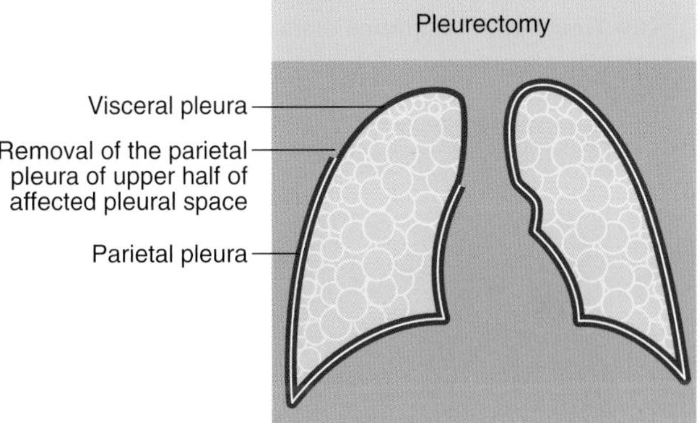

Fig. 31.8 Surgical approaches for treatment of persistent pneumothorax

empyema can be treated by dependent intercostal tube drainage with irrigation if necessary; some empyemas respond to treatment with fibrinolytics. In chronic cases, a thick fibrous wall or **cortex** gradually forms around the pus-filled space. Treatment options then include prolonged closed tube drainage, open tube drainage (sometimes involving removing a segment of rib), and surgical 'decortication' (see Figs 31.9 and 31.10), which releases entrapped lung and tethered chest wall and diaphragm, allowing the lung to re-expand.

Haemothorax

Following chest trauma, blood can accumulate in the pleural space. This usually needs draining via two large drains, one apically and one basally. A similar strategy is employed after open chest surgery. Clotted blood does not drain well and usually needs evacuation by VATS or thoracotomy. Removing blood allows the lung to expand against the chest wall and helps to arrest continuing haemorrhage from intercostal vessels. Persistent or increasing drainage of blood indicates continuing intrathoracic bleeding and requires intervention. Continued bleeding is usually from the systemic circulation (e.g. internal mammary, intercostal or great vessels) rather than from lung parenchyma.

LUNG ABSCESS

Lung abscesses have become much less common with effective antibiotic treatment of pulmonary infections. Onset of symptoms may be insidious, with clinical features including a swinging pyrexia, foul-smelling sputum and a cavitating shadow on chest X-ray. Primary lung abscess may follow bacterial lung infection, most commonly with *Staphylococcus aureus*, *Streptococci*, *Pseudomonas* or *Klebsiella*.

Secondary lung abscess may follow aspiration of gastric contents or occur in lung segments distal to bronchial obstruction by a centrally placed neoplasm or inhaled foreign body.

Lung abscesses are usually treated with antibiotics alone but occasionally a cavity requires drainage. Drains are usually placed percutaneously under ultrasound or CT guidance.

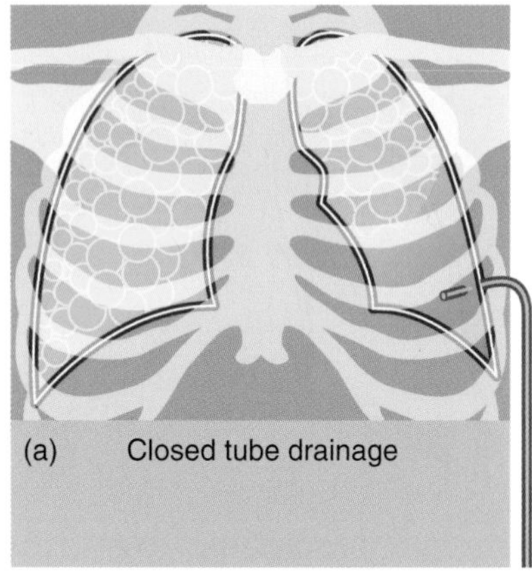

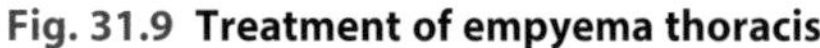
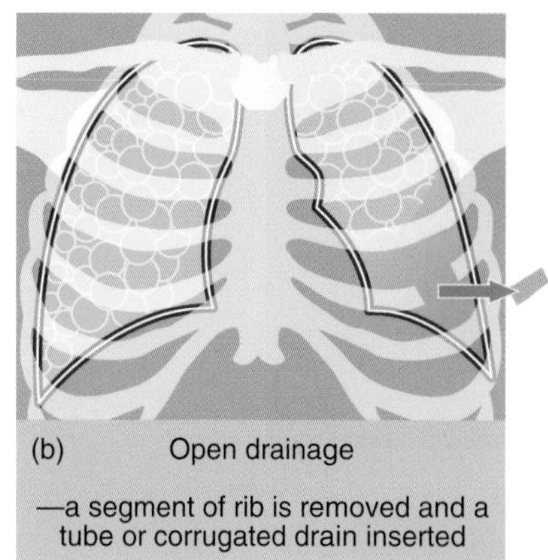

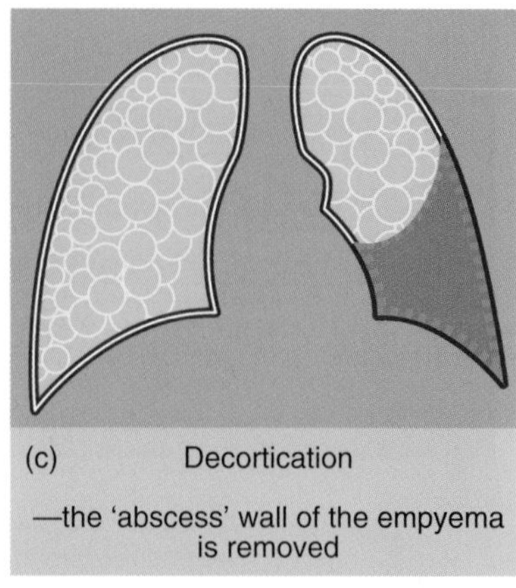

Fig. 31.9 Treatment of empyema thoracis

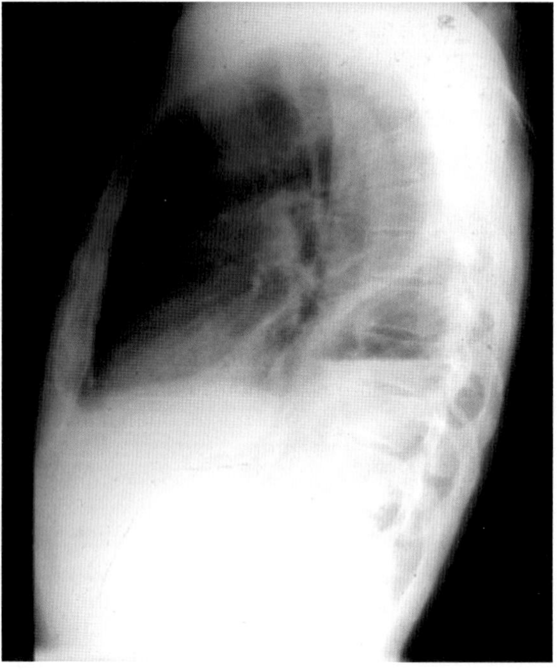
(a)

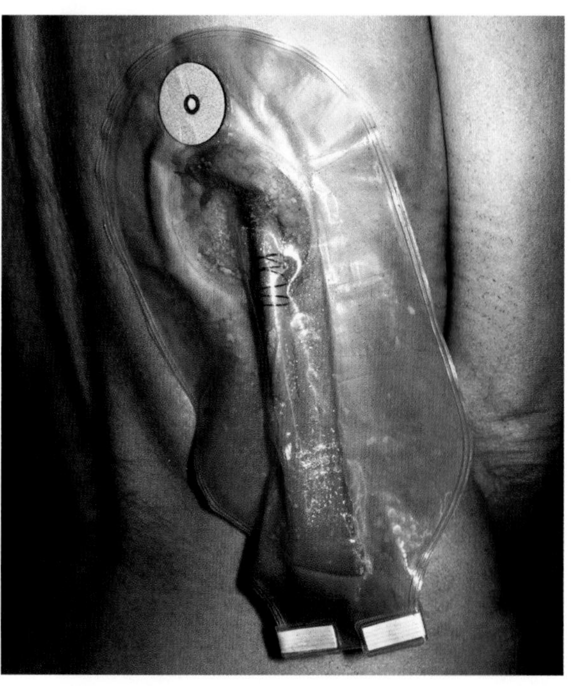
(b)

Fig. 31.10 Empyema thoracis
This 51-year-old man underwent a thoraco-abdominal oesophagogastrectomy for proximal gastric cancer. He suffered a small intrathoracic anastomotic leak and developed an intrapleural empyema, shown by the fluid level in **(a)**. **(b)** Drainage of empyema. A section of rib overlying the cavity was resected and a large red rubber tube was inserted to give dependent drainage into a bag. The drain was gradually shortened as the cavity closed. This patient was alive and well 15 years later

Surgery by deroofing ('marsupialisation') or resection of the abscess may be required. Good chest drainage is vital after the procedure.

CANCER OF THE LUNG

Lung cancers are either primary tumours or metastatic deposits from elsewhere. Smoking is the commonest cause of primary lung cancer. Due to smoking control, rates of lung cancer are starting to plateau and even fall in developed countries but continue to increase elsewhere. Of primary tumours, about 80% will have metastasised by the time of presentation. Lymph nodes in the hilar area are usually involved first, followed by other mediastinal nodes. The liver, adrenal glands, bone and brain are common sites of metastatic spread.

Primary lung cancers are classified into **small cell tumours** (10–15%) and **non-small cell lung cancers** (NSCLC). Small cell cancers are usually treated non-surgically as they have a very high risk of metastases and are more responsive to chemoradiotherapy than NSCLC. Non-small cell cancers are further classified as squamous cell carcinoma, adenocarcinoma, large cell carcinoma, undifferentiated carcinoma, and broncho-alveolar cell tumours. Many lung cancers grow rapidly and assessment must not be delayed if curative treatment with surgery or chemo-/radiotherapy is contemplated. A much less aggressive form of lung cancer is **typical carcinoid** tumours of the lung. They are still usually removed by surgery.

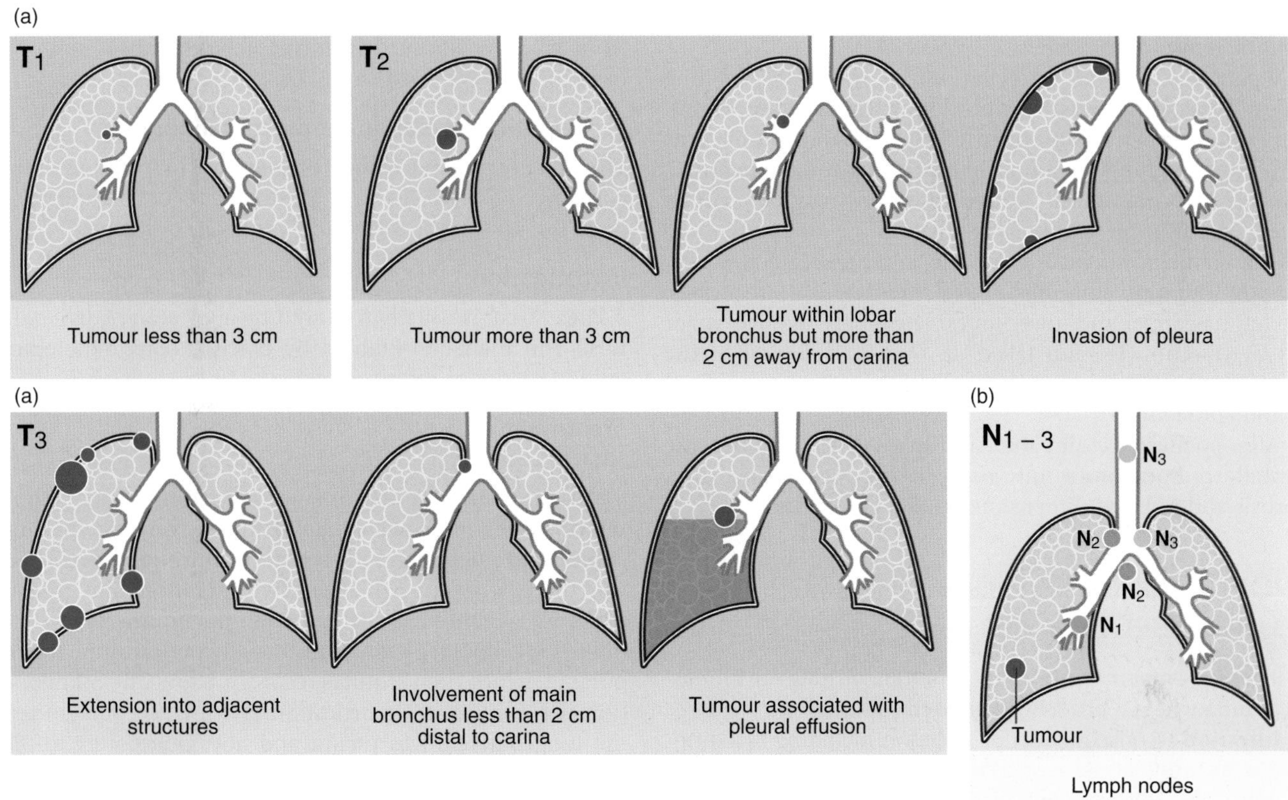

Fig. 31.11 Tumour staging using the TNM classification
(a) Tumour size and extent. **(b)** Lymph node involvement

STAGING OF LUNG CANCER AND ITS IMPLICATIONS

TNM staging of lung cancer is fundamental to planning appropriate treatment. This is periodically reviewed and the most recent classification (the seventh version) is shown in Figure 31.11. In staging, contrast-enhanced CT scanning of chest and upper abdomen is the first step. The likelihood of enlarged lymph nodes being malignant increases with size. The order of further tests varies with local practice but generally includes a CT-PET scan, brain imaging with CT or MRI and evaluation of enlarged or PET-positive sites by biopsy. If histological confirmation has not been achieved by biopsy of a suspicious node, the primary site may need biopsy.

If the lung cancer is confirmed to be 'early', i.e. stage I or II and selected patients with IIIa disease, fit patients are offered surgery. Stage 1a NSCLC can have a 5-year survival of >70% but very few patients present this early.

If preoperative staging of mediastinal lymph nodes is negative but N_2 disease is discovered at surgery (i.e. occult N_2 disease), around 50% can undergo a histologically complete resection; this subgroup would expect a 5-year survival of 30%.

Some patients with more advanced disease are also offered surgery, including patients with limited mediastinal node involvement, and very occasionally patients with a removable isolated distant metastasis.

Palliative treatment

For patients whose disease is too extensive for surgery, yet the tumour and lymph nodes can be encompassed within a radiotherapy 'field' with acceptable toxicity, they can be offered radiotherapy with curative intent, usually accompanied by chemotherapy. For advanced disease, radiotherapy can increase life expectancy as well as provide effective palliation for troublesome complications such as lobar collapse, haemoptysis, superior vena caval obstruction or symptomatic metastases in brain or bone. Advanced radiotherapy techniques such as stereotactic radiotherapy are under evaluation and may allow higher doses to be given with acceptable toxicity.

Chemotherapy adds around 5% on average to 5-year survivals and is offered to appropriate patients. New targeted therapies have been introduced and can have benefits. For example, patients with certain epidermal growth factor receptor mutations respond very well to modulator drugs of those pathways.

SURGICAL TREATMENT OF LUNG CANCER

The role of surgery varies according to cell-type, known responsiveness to other therapies, respiratory function, age and fitness of the patient for major surgery. Surgery is usually reserved for potentially curable patients. Surgical treatment of operable lung cancer involves wide resection of the primary with sampling of loco-regional (mediastinal) lymph nodes to establish accurate pathological TNM staging which influences any decision to employ adjuvant chemotherapy or radiotherapy.

Operation involves removing one or more affected lung lobes (**lobectomy**) or the whole lung (**pneumonectomy**), sometimes with resection of involved chest wall. In patients with impaired lung function, sublobar resection (**segmentectomy** or non-anatomical '**wedge**' resection) may be justified with the aim of preserving lung function.

The standard surgical approach is postero-lateral thoracotomy. The right lung has upper, middle and lower lobes, the left has upper and lower lobes. The empty thoracic space left by resection is soon taken up by hyperinflation of the remaining lung tissue, mediastinal shift and elevation of the hemidiaphragm.

After pneumonectomy there is a space which may become partially or sometimes fully occupied by mediastinal shift, fibrosis and reduced dimensions of that side of the chest.

NON-MALIGNANT INDICATIONS FOR LUNG RESECTION

- **Trauma**—major sharp injury to a lobe or lung, or blunt trauma where a bronchus has been ruptured
- **Infection**—consequences of infection including bleeding due to bronchiectasis or secondary fungal infection of a persistent, antibiotic 'sterilised' abscess cavity
- **Benign tumours**—if curative excision via bronchotomy is impracticable
- **Lung transplantation**—transplantation of a single lung is sometimes performed for non-malignant disease when there is minimal respiratory reserve and one lung is substantially more affected than the other. Bilateral lung transplantation is performed in patients with lung diseases involving infection, e.g. cystic fibrosis or bronchiectasis. Heart–lung transplantation is offered when both lungs and heart are irreparably damaged, e.g. Eisenmenger's syndrome (see Ch. 14)

MALIGNANT MESOTHELIOMA

This is a malignant proliferation of mesothelial cells and can arise in pleura (or rarely in peritoneum). There is usually extensive local spread, restriction of the lung and pleural effusion. Spread is usually late and can be to local lymph nodes and eventually more distantly. There are three main histological forms somewhat correlated with disease behaviour: **epithelioid** is the least aggressive, **biphasic** or mixed (histologically a mixture of epithelioid and sarcomatoid types), and **sarcomatoid** which is the most aggressive.

Malignant mesothelioma is strongly associated with asbestos exposure, either direct, as in a building industry worker, or indirect, such as in a family member. There is generally a long interval between exposure and development of the disease (20–40+ years). The carcinogenic agent is the asbestos fibre that provokes chronic inflammation that may eventually become malignant. Asbestos exposure is also associated with increased rates of lung cancer. Mesothelioma is likely to peak between 2010 and 2020 in developed countries, but is still rising in other parts of the world. This is due to the time lag from asbestos exposure. Unfortunately asbestos is still widely used in less developed countries.

Presentation of malignant mesothelioma

This usually presents with chest pain due to irritation of intercostal nerves, or shortness of breath due to loss of lung volume from the tumour or the pleural effusion, or both.

Investigation

A chest X-ray is usually followed by a CT scan. A tissue diagnosis can then be obtained by percutaneous radiologically guided biopsy or thoracoscopy.

Treatment

Unfortunately mesothelioma is rarely curable. Occasionally a localised malignant mesothelioma can undergo complete resection with hope of cure, but the more usual aim of surgery is maximum debulking ('cytoreduction') in advance of adjuvant therapy, or pure palliation. Two operations aim to achieve maximum debulking. Extrapleural pneumonectomy (EPP) involves removing pleura, lung, usually pericardium, and diaphragm, which then requires reconstruction. The other operation is pleurectomy-decortication (PD) which aims to retain the lung but removes pleura and any lung cortex to allow reinflation. Sometimes this also involves resection of diaphragm and/or pericardium. In specialist centres, approximately 30% 5-year overall survival can be expected.

Palliative procedures include thoracoscopic pleurectomy, simple talc pleurodesis, pleuro-peritoneal shunts and insertion of tunnelled intrapleural catheters.

Overall, chemotherapy has been shown to extend survival in mesothelioma by only about 3 months. The place of radiotherapy is also controversial. 'Port-site' radiotherapy has been used to reduce the growth of mesothelioma through previous incisions and high-dose hemithoracic radiotherapy to the operated side can be used after pneumonectomy with the aim of reducing recurrence.

BENIGN ASBESTOS DISEASES OF THE CHEST

Asbestos exposure may be associated with pleural effusions, pleural plaques, 'infolded lung' and lung fibrosis. These are not of themselves premalignant, but are markers of exposure. They may cause major problems, culminating in respiratory failure.

In some countries such as the UK, mesothelioma is considered an occupational disease and financial support is available from the government or other bodies.

DISORDERS OF THE MEDIASTINUM

Disorders of the mediastinum of surgical importance are summarised in Figure 31.12.

ANTERIOR MEDIASTINUM

Retrosternal thyroid

Rarely, the thyroid gland is ectopically located in the anterior mediastinum where it can become enlarged by any of the

Anterior mediastinum (between sternum and pericardium)	Middle mediastinum (pericardium and its contents and lymph nodes)	Posterior mediastinum (posterior to pericardium)
• Retrosternal thyroid • Parathyroid hypertrophy or tumour • Thymoma • Lymph node enlargement • Aneurysm of ascending aorta • Hernia through foramen of Morgagni • Germ cell tumour (seminoma/teratoma)	• Lymph node enlargement • Mediastinal cysts	• Neurogenic tumours • Aneurysm of descending aorta • Hiatus hernia • Congenital hernia through foramen of Bochdalek

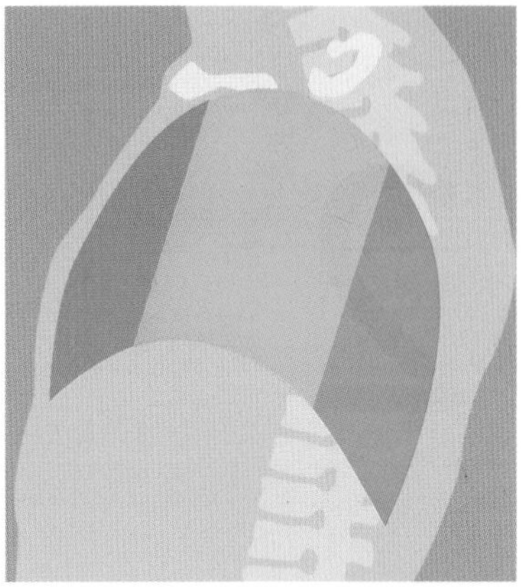

Fig. 31.12 Disorders of the mediastinum

processes discussed in Chapter 49. Alternatively, an inferior extension of a normally located thyroid gland may spread retrosternally into the anterior mediastinum. The adverse effects of retrosternal thyroid enlargement are usually related to progressive displacement of the trachea. Sudden enlargement of retrosternal thyroid tissue caused by haemorrhage can threaten the airway. Most retrosternal thyroids can be removed through a standard thyroidectomy collar incision and only rarely is a median sternotomy required.

Thymus

The thymus causes few pathological problems except for uncommon benign or malignant tumours. For benign thymomas or low-grade cancers, surgery alone may be sufficient and 5-year survival can be as good as 70% or better following complete resection. Thymic cancers are also often sensitive to chemotherapy and radiotherapy, and large, aggressive or invasive thymic cancers may benefit from neoadjuvant or adjuvant treatment.

Myasthenia gravis is an unusual clinical condition associated with certain thymic tumours or thymic hyperplasia. After thymectomy, some patients with myasthenia gravis improve but this is unpredictable.

Parathyroid

Benign and malignant parathyroid tumours usually occur in the neck but sometimes occur anywhere between the retrothyroid area and the aortic arch. If retrosternal lesions are suspected, exploration of the anterior mediastinum accompanied by thymectomy usually enables the abnormal parathyroid tissue to be removed.

Lymph node enlargement

Lymphoma can occur here and good biopsies are needed for diagnosis. The usual treatment is chemotherapy with or without radiotherapy.

Germ cell tumours

The anterior mediastinum is a relatively common site for these uncommon tumours. Generally these tumours are approached surgically by sternotomy, a collar incision or VATS.

MIDDLE MEDIASTINUM

This contains the pericardium and hila of both lungs. Disorders requiring surgical intervention include:

- Lymph node enlargement—lung cancer or lymphoma are the most common causes. Tumour type may be defined by biopsy, and the extent by CT scanning. Non-malignant granulomatous diseases can also manifest here (e.g. sarcoid)
- Aneurysms—those of the ascending aorta or the arch of the aorta are usually degenerative but may also appear as a late complication of aortic trauma or dissection. Syphilitic aneurysm is now rare
- Developmental cysts—these include pericardial, bronchogenic, enterogenous and cysts of uncertain origin. Mediastinal cysts occasionally become infected and even more rarely undergo malignant change
- Germ cell tumours—primary or secondary teratoma or seminoma occasionally occur. These are diagnosed by histology or raised serum markers and can usually be treated successfully with chemotherapy

POSTERIOR MEDIASTINUM

The posterior mediastinum lies behind the pericardium. Surgery may be required for the following conditions:

- Aneurysms of the descending aorta
- Tumours of neurological origin—these may be bilobed and extend into the spinal canal. These are usually benign
- Diaphragmatic hernia—hiatus hernia is common but is not always associated with gastric reflux. Most sliding hernias can now be treated with acid-reducing drugs, weight loss and other simple advice (see Ch. 22). The more unusual para-oesophageal or rolling hiatus hernia may lead to gastric infarction and many believe its presence is an indication for surgery. Congenital herniation into the posterior mediastinum (hernia of Bochdalek) is very rare. Thoracic or abdominal approaches for hiatus hernia are performed. The commonest operation for hiatus hernia with reflux is a laparoscopic fundoplication

32 Hernias and other groin problems

INTRODUCTION

This chapter describes the clinical presentation and diagnosis of lumps and swellings in the groin along with specific conditions causing these problems. Other hernias of the anterior abdominal wall (ventral hernias) are considered at the end of the chapter.

Groin lumps and swellings account for about 10% of general surgical outpatient referrals. In both sexes, the most common lumps in the groin are **hernias**, mainly inguinal but also femoral. Both are caused by abdominal contents protruding through an abdominal wall defect. The normal testicular descent is from the abdomen to the scrotum via the inguinal canal, and this area remains vulnerable throughout life; inguinal hernias are much more common in males. If large, an **inguinal hernia** may present as a scrotal rather than a groin lump, but it is obvious that it arises in the groin. In the female, the uterine round ligament pursues a similar course; this explains inguinal hernias in females. The femoral canal, below the inguinal ligament, is another potential weakness and may give rise to a **femoral hernia**, particularly in women.

Enlarged lymph nodes due to infection or malignancy also cause groin lumps or swellings. Less common are vascular abnormalities such as a **saphena varix** or a **femoral artery aneurysm**. Very rarely nowadays, a **psoas abscess** may track down beneath the inguinal ligament to present in the groin. This used to be a common complication of spinal tuberculosis but is now more often a result of infection tracking down from a perforation in the left colon.

The anatomy of the groin provides a good starting point for understanding surgical problems in this area and is explained in Figure 32.1.

LUMPS IN THE GROIN

CLINICAL EXAMINATION

Groin and scrotum must be examined to discover the anatomical origin of the swelling. Lumps in the groin are examined as lumps elsewhere but there are some special points to note:

- Examine the patient both standing and lying
- Examine for the presence of a cough impulse and test the reducibility of the lump
- Demonstrate the relationship of the origin of the lump to the inguinal ligament and the pubic tubercle

Position for examination

The patient must first be examined whilst standing, which increases intra-abdominal pressure, making any hernia more visible. Ask the patient to cough while palpating the lump: intra-abdominal pressure is thus transmitted through the abdominal wall and an expansile **cough impulse** is felt in a hernia. Small inguinal hernias may reduce on lying down, and a scrotal varicocoele (see Ch. 33) will empty.

Consistency and reducibility

Hernias are usually soft and 'squishy' but the most reliable diagnostic sign is if the lump reduces when the patient lies flat or can be reduced by gentle manipulation by patient or clinician. Most inguinal hernias are at least partly reducible, although longstanding hernias gradually become irreducible because of adhesions within the sac. These are said to be **incarcerated**, i.e. chronically irreducible. In contrast, femoral hernias are nearly always **irreducible** and have no cough impulse as the femoral canal is so narrow (see Table 32.1).

A **strangulated** inguinal hernia can be readily diagnosed by finding an irreducible hernia in the correct anatomical position; the lump is tender and often red. Conversely, strangulated femoral hernias are usually very small and unimpressive, often no more than the size of a grape, yet have serious consequences. Strangulated hernias, particularly femoral hernias, sometimes present with abdominal pain or signs of obstruction but without localised pain in the groin. This emphasises the importance of examining the hernial orifices in every patient with an acute abdomen.

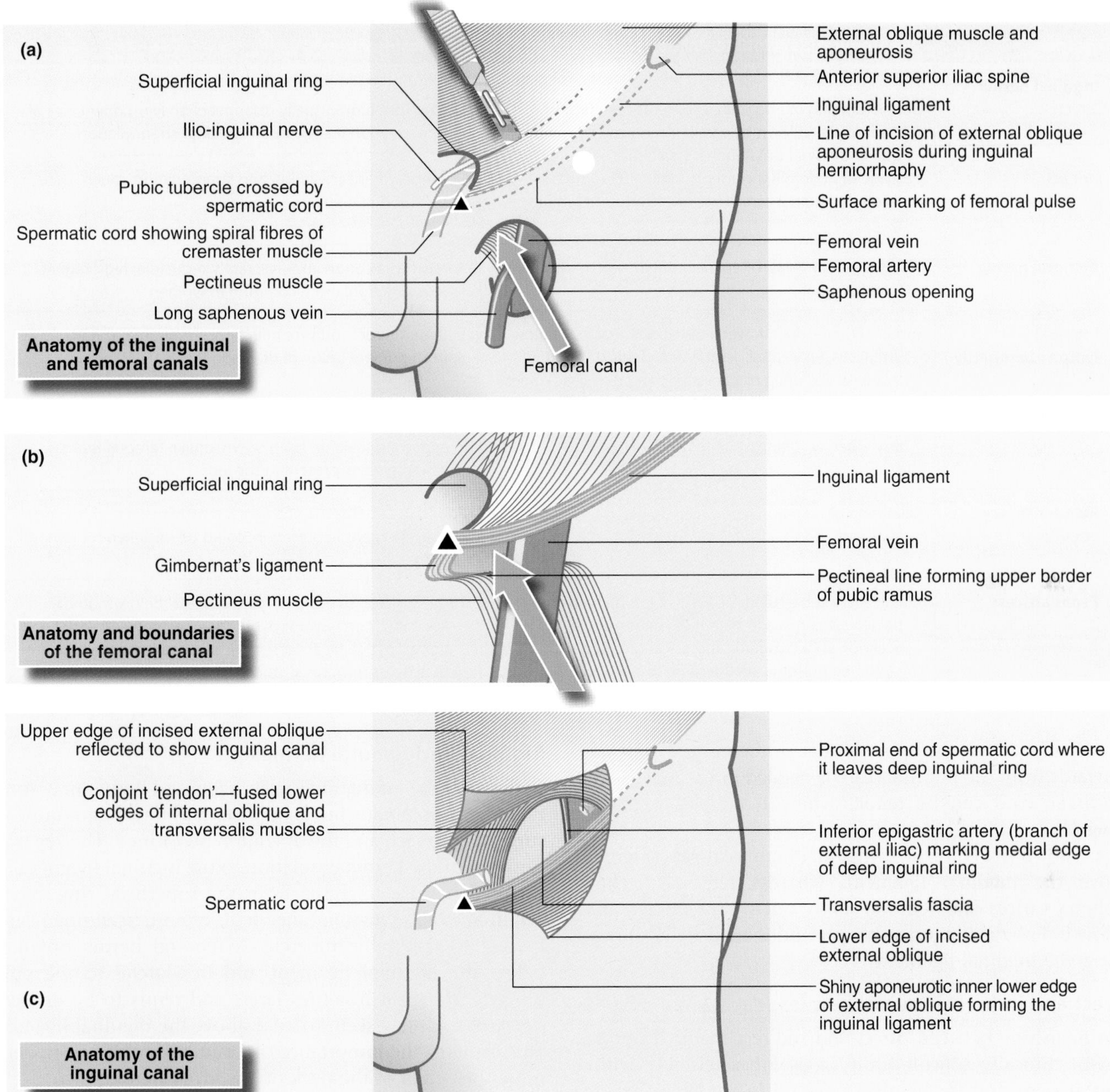

Fig. 32.1 Structure of the inguinal and femoral canals
(a) The entire groin area. The surface marking of the femoral pulse is shown, midway between the pubic symphysis and the anterior superior iliac spine; the deep ring lies 2.5 cm above it. **(b) Structure of the femoral canal**—the abdominal opening seen from below. **(c) Structure of the inguinal canal**. The inguinal canal displayed by incising the anterior wall (external oblique aponeurosis) as in the first stage of open repair; the spermatic cord has been removed for clarity

Enlarged inguinal lymph nodes vary in consistency, number and size depending on the pathological cause; they are of course not reducible. A **saphena varix** is very soft and disappears completely on palpation or if the patient lies down, refilling when pressure is released or if the patient stands. The leg on that side nearly always has obvious varicose veins. A saphena varix also exhibits a cough impulse. **Femoral artery aneurysms**, however, are firm but pulsatile. These vascular conditions must be diagnosed correctly as injudicious operation could be catastrophic!

Relationship to the inguinal ligament

The site of the lump in relation to the inguinal ligament needs to be identified. The ligament is not visible but stretches between two palpable bony prominences, the **anterior superior iliac spine** laterally and the **pubic tubercle** medially (see Fig. 32.1a). The pubic tubercle is higher than might be imagined from the skin contour, lying 2–3 cm above the groin crease. The iliac spine is easy to locate but the pubic tubercle can be difficult, especially in obese patients. It is best found

Table 32.1 Summary of groin lumps and swellings and their clinical features

Disorder	Anatomical/developmental basis	Clinical features
a. **Inguinal hernia**		
Direct	Simple bulging of abdominal contents resulting from inadequate support by weak or ruptured posterior wall of inguinal canal (transversalis fascia)	Discomfort; lump usually disappears on lying down; risk of incarceration if large but low risk of strangulation
Indirect	Passage of abdominal contents, often including bowel, through inguinal canal towards scrotum or labium majus	Potential for incarceration and strangulation; much more common in men
b. **Femoral hernia**	Abdominal contents, often including bowel, migrate into femoral canal	Rarely has a cough impulse; rarely reducible; high rate of strangulation; more common in women
c. **Inguinal lymphadenopathy**	Inguinal nodes drain lower limb, abdominal wall below umbilicus, anal canal, scrotal skin, penis (but not testes, which drain to para-aortic and para-iliac nodes)	Enlarged nodes indicate infection, lymphoma or metastases from primary lesion in drainage area
d. **Saphena varix**	Dilatation of long saphenous vein superficial to deep fascia before it enters the femoral vein	Can be mistaken for femoral hernia but empties on pressure and disappears on lying down, unlike femoral hernia; varicose veins present in the leg
e. **Femoral artery aneurysm**	Dilatation of common femoral artery just below inguinal ligament	Found in patients over 65 years, mostly male; classic clinical sign is expansile pulsation; could be mistaken for femoral hernia
f. **Psoas abscess**	Classically, a tuberculous abscess of lumbar vertebra tracking down inside sheath of psoas muscle; occasionally a pyogenic abscess originating within the abdomen presents via the same route	TB presents as swelling or 'cold abscess' below inguinal ligament; rare nowadays but may be confused with lymph nodes; pyogenic abscess typically 'hot'; rarely may be due to abscess from renal stones

by palpating along the upper border of the pubic symphysis, outwards from the midline (care is needed in the male as the spermatic cord can be tender where it crosses the pubic tubercle).

As shown in Figure 32.2, inguinal hernias always originate **above** the inguinal ligament, whereas femoral hernias, saphena varices and femoral artery aneurysms always arise **below** it. Enlarged inguinal **lymph nodes** are usually situated below the inguinal ligament.

Direct and indirect inguinal hernias (Fig. 32.3)

Distinguishing between direct and indirect inguinal hernias may be clinically difficult but it is a useful exercise in eliciting clinical signs and frequently comes up in student examinations! By definition, an **indirect inguinal hernia** is one in which the hernial sac lies within the spermatic cord, leaving the abdomen via the deep (internal) inguinal ring to pass along the inguinal canal, exiting through the superficial (external) ring. Thus, if the hernia can be completely reduced, finger pressure over the deep ring will prevent it reappearing on coughing (the deep ring is midway between the pubic symphysis and the pubic tubercle, 2.5 cm above the femoral pulse; see Fig. 32.1a). In contrast, a **direct inguinal hernia** leaves the abdomen through a weakness or split in the **transversalis fascia**, the posterior wall of the inguinal canal, emerging directly through the superficial ring and cannot be controlled by digital pressure over the deep ring. In practice, this test is often unreliable. The patient's age is perhaps the most useful indicator of the likely type of inguinal hernia, with indirect hernias most frequent under the age of 50 and direct hernias more common after that age.

Inguinal and femoral hernias

Differentiating an inguinal from a femoral hernia may sometimes be problematic but is important as it will determine the surgical approach and the operation performed. The key is the position of the hernia in relation to the inguinal ligament. An inguinal hernia, emerging from the superficial ring, has its origin above the inguinal ligament, often descending over or medial to the pubic tubercle. A femoral hernia originates below the inguinal ligament and lies lateral to the pubic tubercle. Rarely it becomes large, and tends to be deflected upwards and may seem to arise above the inguinal ligament. This explains the importance of careful examination to determine the origin of the neck of any groin hernia.

INGUINAL HERNIA

Inguinal hernia is one of the most common conditions seen in general surgical clinics. In a typical district general hospital, inguinal hernias account for about 7% of surgical outpatient consultations and about 12% of operating theatre time.

As shown in Figure 32.4, inguinal hernias in males are by far the most common type of groin hernia. Inguinal hernias occur eight times more often in males because of the abdominal wall deficiency caused by testicular descent. Femoral hernias are rare in males, comprising only 2.5% of groin hernias. Even in females, inguinal hernias are the most frequent (twice as common as femorals). Femoral hernias are twice as common in females as in males.

Inguinal hernias occur at any age. In childhood they always have a developmental origin and are common in premature

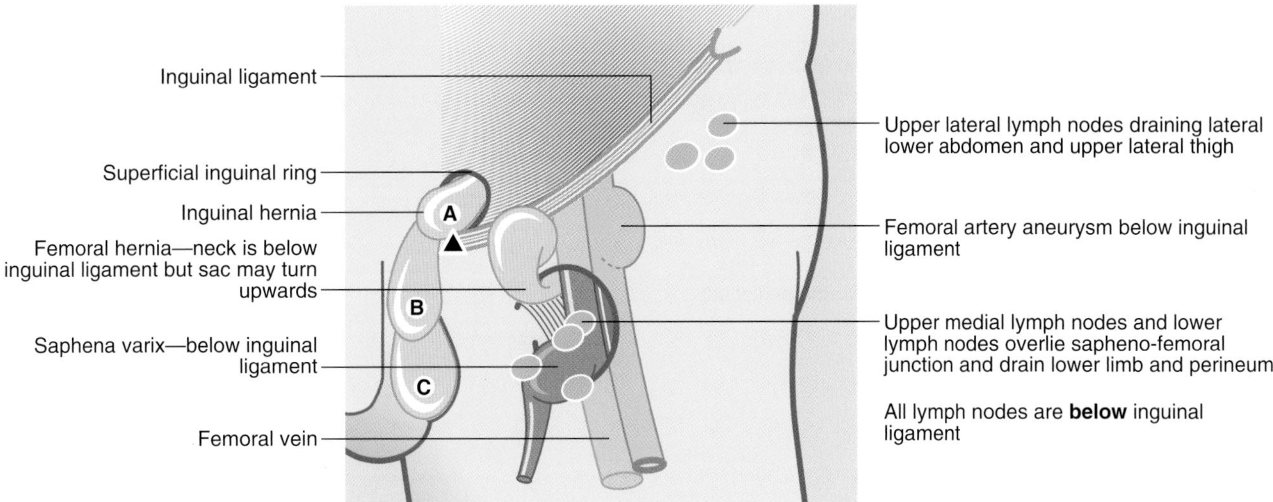

Fig. 32.2 Significance of the relationship of groin lumps to the inguinal ligament
A, B and **C** are stages in the enlargement of an indirect inguinal hernia. Note that the neck is above the inguinal ligament. A direct inguinal hernia enlarges forwards in position **A**, but occasionally extends into the scrotum

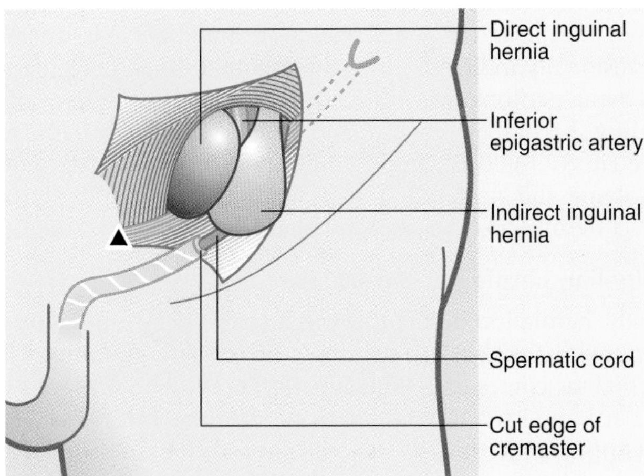

Fig. 32.3 Direct and indirect inguinal hernias
A direct inguinal hernia bulges medially to the inferior epigastric artery and is not usually attached to the spermatic cord. An indirect inguinal hernia leaves the deep inguinal ring lateral to the artery and lies within the cremaster muscle covering the cord

infants. In males, hernias appear most often before the age of 5 or after middle age. A smaller peak occurs in the late teens and early twenties. Hernias in these young men probably result from a congenital predisposition, exacerbated by work or sport. Most inguinal hernias should be repaired early to reduce the long-term risk of strangulation and the need for emergency operation. The exception is small, easily reducible painless direct hernias in elderly men or those with substantial co-morbidity.

ANATOMICAL CONSIDERATIONS

The surgical anatomy of the inguinal canal is shown in Figure 32.1c. The external oblique aponeurosis (or fascia) forms the anterior wall of the inguinal canal. In the diagram, it has been split obliquely from the external ring along the line of its fibres for about 5 cm laterally and the cut edges

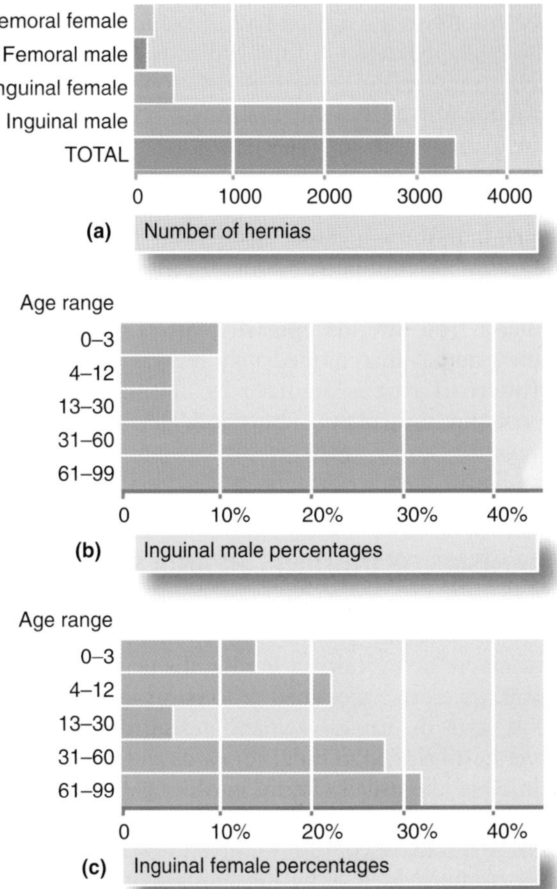

Fig. 32.4 Relative annual incidence of inguinal and femoral hernias in East Anglia (UK)
(a) Number of hernias by type and **(b)** Incidence of inguinal hernias in males by age. **(c)** Incidence of inguinal hernias in females by age

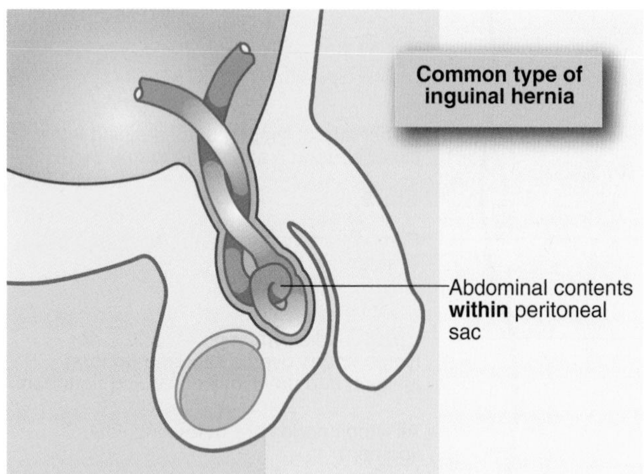

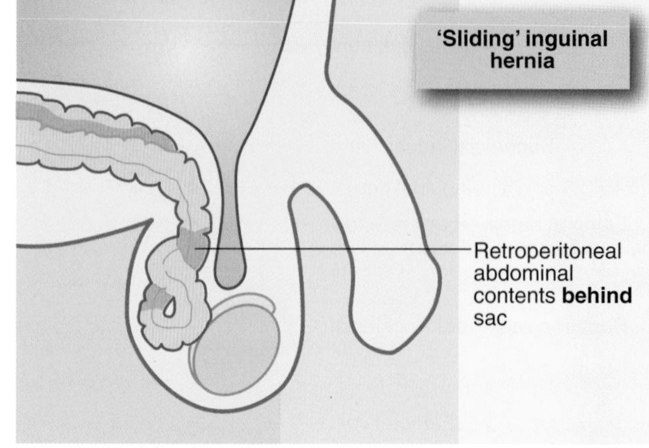

Fig. 32.5 Common and sliding inguinal hernias

reflected upwards and downwards to expose the inguinal canal. This is how it would appear after the first stage of an inguinal hernia repair operation.

The internal oblique and transversus abdominis muscles are deficient above the medial half of the inguinal ligament, with the D-shaped defect normally filled with the **transversalis fascia**. Transversalis is particularly strong here and forms the posterior wall of the inguinal canal, providing the only restraint to herniation of the abdominal contents. Arching over this, the inferior borders of the two muscles fuse to form the conjoint musculature and 'tendon' which extends from the lateral half of the inguinal ligament to the pubic crest.

The spermatic cord passes through the deep ring, a defect in the transversalis fascia at the most lateral part of the muscular defect. The **inferior epigastric artery** passes upwards from the external iliac immediately medial to it. Thus, the **deep (internal) ring** is bounded by the inguinal ligament below, conjoint musculature above and laterally, and the inferior epigastric artery medially. At operation, whether an inguinal hernia is direct or indirect is defined by its relationship to the inferior epigastric artery.

MECHANISMS OF INGUINAL HERNIA FORMATION

Inguinal herniation may be direct or indirect. In either case, the herniated abdominal contents are contained within a sac of peritoneum. In an **indirect hernia**, the peritoneal sac may represent a patent or reopened processus vaginalis and may extend as far as the tunica vaginalis and surround the testis.

Direct hernias tend to bulge forwards and rarely enter the scrotum. They are usually found in older patients with deficient muscles and weak transversalis fascia. The neck of a direct sac is broad, in contrast to the narrow neck of an indirect sac, confined as it is by the borders of the deep ring. Consequently, indirect inguinal hernias are more liable to strangulate. A direct hernia may occur suddenly after physical strain. In this case, the transversalis fascia has split, causing the appearance of a 'rupture'.

An indirect and a direct hernia can occur together on the same side—a **pantaloon hernia**. A hernia may consist merely of peritoneum and associated extraperitoneal fat, but if larger, the sac usually contains omentum or small bowel, or less commonly large bowel or appendix. Occasionally, the contents of the sac are diseased, e.g. large bowel carcinoma, an inflamed appendix (acute appendicitis) or peritoneal tumour metastases. Sometimes a retroperitoneal viscus 'slides' down the posterior abdominal wall and herniates directly (occasionally indirectly) into the inguinal canal, dragging its overlying peritoneum with it. Thus, the visceral contents of a **sliding hernia** lie behind and outside the peritoneal sac (see Fig. 32.5). This most commonly occurs in the left groin involving the descending and sigmoid colon or in larger direct hernias, may involve the bladder.

Spigelian hernia

Rarely, herniation occurs through a fascial defect in the linea semilunaris at the lateral border of rectus abdominis. The hernial sac comes to lie interstitially, i.e. between the layers of internal and external oblique or transversus abdominis. This is a **Spigelian hernia**. It has some clinical characteristics of an inguinal hernia but the bulge lies higher than an inguinal hernia and may be difficult to palpate because it is covered by one or more layers of the abdominal wall (see Fig. 32.6).

NATURAL HISTORY OF INGUINAL HERNIA

Inguinal hernias usually develop slowly, although exacerbated by any condition which persistently raises intra-abdominal pressure, e.g. obesity, constipation, straining at micturition or chronic coughing; continued heavy lifting probably has a similar effect. In infants, a period of severe coughing or crying may precipitate an acute indirect hernia which may become irreducible.

A chronically irreducible hernia that is not strangulated is described as **incarcerated**. However, the term is often used inaccurately when a clinician is uncertain if an acutely irreducible hernia is strangulated. In patients presenting as emergencies, it is safer to assume such a hernia is strangulated until proved otherwise.

Hernial strangulation

Inguinal hernias that are difficult to reduce or which intermittently cause pain are at particular risk of strangulation. Strangulation occurs if the hernial contents become constricted

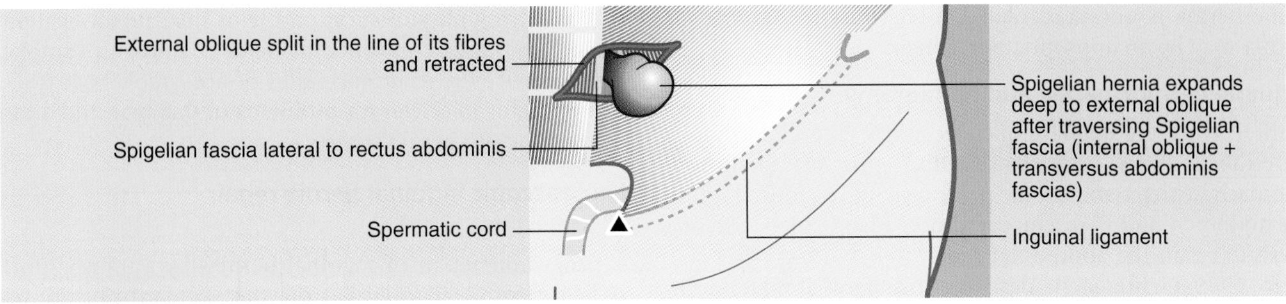

External oblique split in the line of its fibres and retracted
Spigelian fascia lateral to rectus abdominis
Spermatic cord
Spigelian hernia expands deep to external oblique after traversing Spigelian fascia (internal oblique + transversus abdominis fascias)
Inguinal ligament

Fig. 32.6 Spigelian hernia

CASE HISTORY

Fig. 32.7 Strangulated inguinal hernia

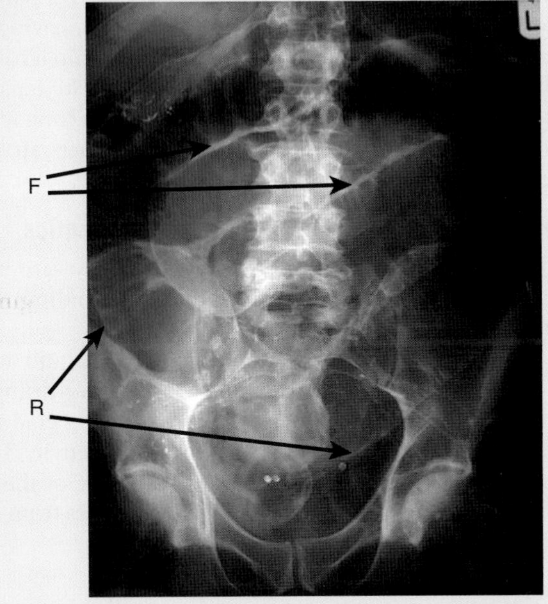

This 40-year-old man presented with symptoms and signs of distal small bowel obstruction evidently due to a strangulated inguinal hernia. At first, the abdomen, though distended and tympanitic, was not tender. However, during resuscitation, the abdomen became tender. This X-ray shows a clear outline of the outside of parts of the small bowel **R**, representing Rigler's sign. A false Rigler's sign is seen in other parts **F**; this is where two loops of thickened small bowel lie in contact

CASE HISTORY

Fig. 32.8 Inguino-scrotal hernia

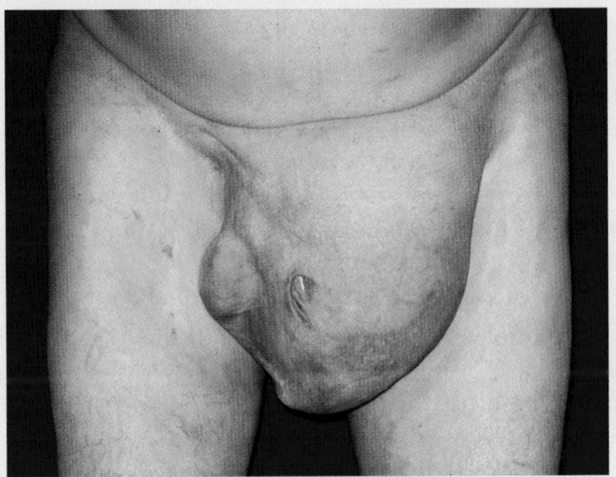

This man of 76 lived alone and only presented to a doctor when he had increasing difficulty controlling the direction of his micturition. His penis had disappeared altogether as the hernia had enlarged. The right testis is visible in the scrotum but the left side of the scrotum is filled with a large hernia. At operation, the abdominal wall defect was surprisingly small and was easily repaired by a standard method

by the neck of the sac or by twisting. Obstruction of venous return then leads to swelling and later to arterial obstruction. If strangulation is not relieved by manual or operative reduction, **infarction** follows. A strangulated inguinal hernia first becomes irreducible and then tender and later red. Symptoms and signs of bowel obstruction develop over the next few hours, followed by peritonitis if the bowel perforates (Fig. 32.7). Strangulation is a surgical emergency.

MANAGEMENT OF INGUINAL HERNIAS

Inguinal hernias in adults should ideally be repaired by **herniorrhaphy**, although there is evidence that small, reducible direct hernias in older men can safely be left alone.

Hernia operations are usually performed under general anaesthesia, although epidural or spinal or local anaesthesia may be used in patients with poor cardiovascular or respiratory function. Many surgeons favour an open repair under local anaesthesia for most cases; certainly if age or infirmity makes anaesthesia hazardous, this is a safe option.

Some hernias become intermittently irreducible, often with local pain and tenderness or even symptoms of bowel obstruction (vomiting, colicky abdominal pain, distension and absolute constipation). Such warning episodes are an indication for early operation. More severe and prolonged symptoms of this nature precipitate emergency admission to hospital, in which case strangulation must be assumed and operation performed urgently, preferably within 4 hours to maximise the chance of saving ischaemic bowel. In any patient with an obstructed or strangulated hernia, the first step is to ensure that the patient is fully resuscitated; more patients die of fluid and electrolyte problems than of delaying an operation by a few hours.

Very large 'wheelbarrow' hernias are invariably of long standing and are found mainly in elderly men (see Fig. 32.8). They only present when size becomes a handicap, if bowel strangulates within the hernia or if the anatomical distortion interferes with micturition. Bowel adhesions may make operation difficult and postoperative wound infections are common.

If the hernia is not strangulated, a bag truss to support the hernia may be an appropriate treatment.

Inguinal herniorrhaphy and herniotomy

Until recently, the standard open techniques of herniorrhaphy were mostly based on Bassini's 19th century extraperitoneal approach, which removed the peritoneal sac or reduced it into the abdomen and then employed non-absorbable sutures or mesh to repair the abdominal wall.

In 1989 **Lichtenstein** described his mesh implant technique which rapidly became the standard operation. This employs a 'tension-free' technique, using a patch of non-absorbable open-weave mesh to repair and reinforce the defect rather than pulling together muscle and fascial layers together under tension. Figure 32.9 shows the principles of the Lichtenstein type of inguinal hernia repair.

The mesh technique has several distinct advantages:

- The technique is easily learned and trainee surgeons can reliably produce good results
- Postoperative pain is substantially less, allowing increased mobility and early return to normal activities such as work and driving
- Recurrence rates appear to be exceptionally low

Having a foreign body implanted might be expected to increase the risk of infection but in practice it is exceptionally rare. The mesh used does not have to be expensive—studies are being published of successful hernia repairs in developing countries using sterilised mosquito netting!

In infants, the patent processus vaginalis is merely ligated and excised (**herniotomy**); formal repair of the abdominal wall defect is usually unnecessary. If the defect is enormous, a single stitch should be used on the medial side to narrow the deep ring.

Complications of hernia repair

Early complications of herniorrhaphy include scrotal haematoma or wound infection. Most surgeons employ prophylactic antibiotics for mesh repairs but there is little evidence of benefit. Late complications include recurrence (see below), chronic **groin pain** due to inadvertent trapping of the ilio-inguinal or another nerve in the repair, and **testicular atrophy** caused by inadvertent damage to the testicular artery, usually with diathermy, or over-tightening of the deep ring.

Recurrence

Inguinal hernias recur in 2–25% of cases over a lifetime. The rate is greatly increased when inadequate attention has been given to operative principles.

The causes of inguinal hernia recurrence include:

- Inappropriate technique—Bassini type repairs have a 25% recurrence rate
- Operator inexperience—Shouldice and laparoscopic repairs have a long learning curve
- Technical failure—failure to recognise and remove an indirect sac at operation; insufficient coverage of the defect; suture or mesh failure
- Missed diagnosis of a concomitant femoral hernia
- Inherently poor musculature, chronic cough, urinary obstruction, constipation or resumption of heavy work too soon after repair
- Underlying physiological problems that impair healing such as poorly controlled diabetes or smoking—smokers have twice the recurrence rates of non-smokers. It is important to screen for problems of this type and address them before hernia surgery

Laparoscopic inguinal hernia repair

(described in Ch. 10)

Laparoscopic repair of inguinal hernias by a transperitoneal or retroperitoneal route is now the standard operation for hernia repair in many centres. It offers less postoperative pain and a slightly quicker return to normal activities but has a slightly higher risk of major complications compared to open techniques for primary hernia repair. The method is particularly recommended for repair of recurrent hernias, having the advantage of allowing the mesh to be placed in virgin territory, and also for bilateral repair, when both sides can be repaired through the same three small incisions. There is a long learning curve for laparoscopic repair and the recurrence rate may be slightly higher than the Lichtenstein technique.

Postoperative care and return to normal activities

Most inguinal hernias are now repaired on a day case basis although some patients with significant co-morbidities may need to stay in hospital overnight.

During the first postoperative week, patients should avoid activities likely to strain the repair, such as heavy lifting or driving a car. Over the next 2 or 3 weeks, they should gradually return to normal activity, including usual sexual activity. Time to return to work depends on the physical nature of the job and whether activities cause pain, but usually varies from 2 to 4 weeks.

Trusses

A **truss** made of padded webbing may control certain types of hernia when surgery is inappropriate or unacceptable to the patient. They can safely be used only if the hernia is easily reducible and can be kept reduced and free of symptoms. For very large irreducible hernias, a 'bag truss' can support the hernia. Most trusses are ill-fitting and ineffective and are better avoided if possible. There is some evidence that trusses increase fibrosis and inflammation and may make repair more difficult—early repair is the best option if practicable.

FEMORAL HERNIA

A femoral hernia is formed by a protrusion of peritoneum into the potential space of the femoral canal. The sac may contain abdominal viscera (usually small bowel) or omentum. Around 40% of femoral hernias present with strangulation. The incidence is higher in women and increases with age (Figs 32.4 and 32.10). Increased intra-abdominal pressure and other factors related to pregnancy may be important in females since the incidence of femoral hernia is higher in parous than nulliparous women.

CLINICAL FEATURES OF FEMORAL HERNIA

The anatomy of the femoral canal is shown in Figure 32.1b, page 409. A femoral hernia is usually small, appearing as a

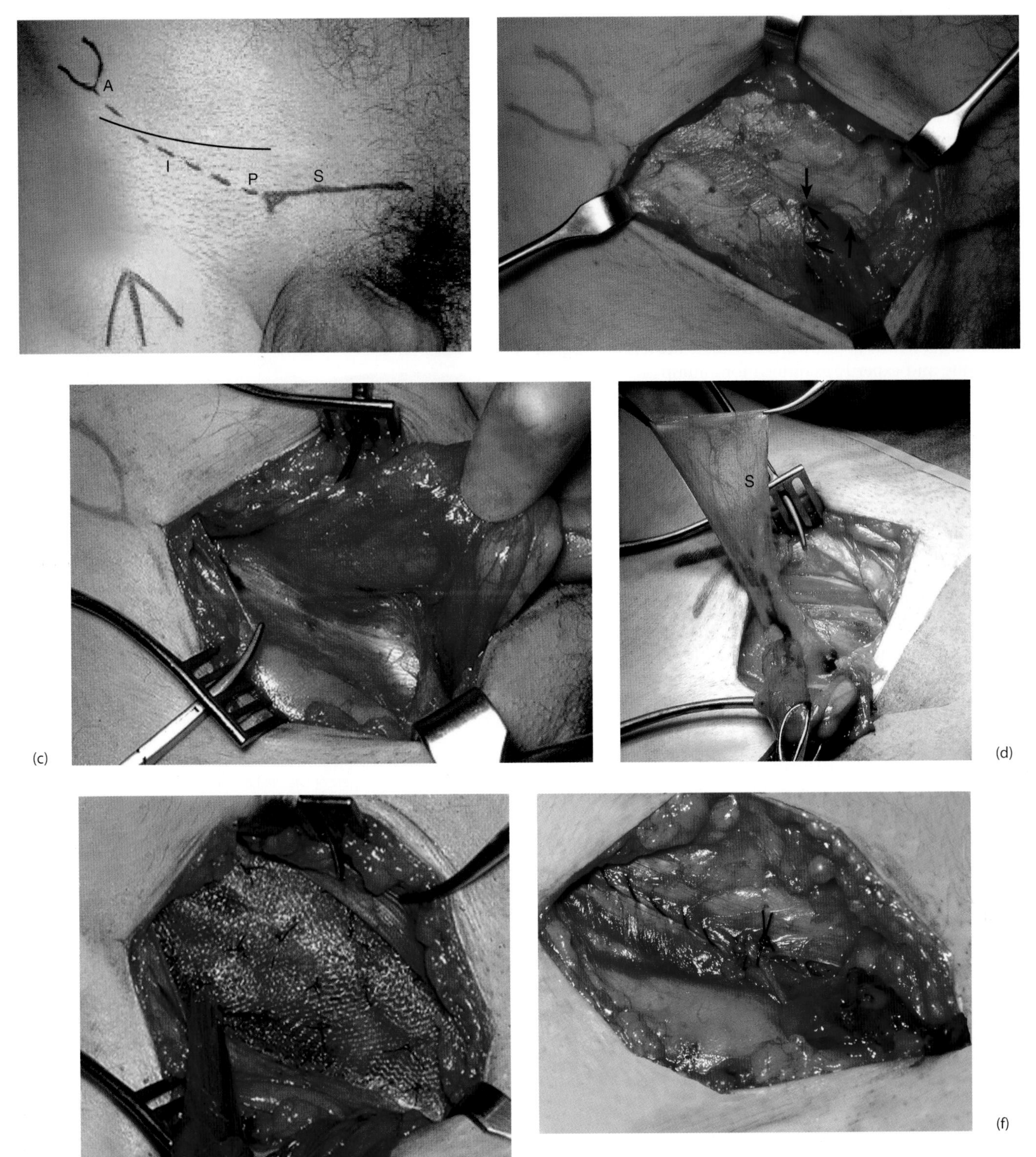

Fig. 32.9 Technique of mesh hernia repair
(a) Skin markings demonstrating the upper border of the pubic arch **S**, the anterior superior iliac spine **A**, the pubic tubercle **P** and the inguinal ligament **I**. Note the side of the planned operation has been marked with an arrow on the thigh to ensure the correct side is operated upon. The line of incision is shown as a solid line. **(b)** The dissection down to the external oblique aponeurosis. The external (superficial) ring is arrowed. **(c)** External oblique aponeurosis opened, demonstrating the shiny inguinal ligament, which is its inturned lower edge. **(d)** The indirect hernia sac **S** dissected out from the spermatic cord and held upwards before ligation and excision. The inferior epigastric artery and vein lie at the medial border of the deep inguinal ring. **(e)** Polypropylene mesh is cut to shape before insertion and sutured in place along the inguinal ligament and, in this case, tacked to the surface of the internal oblique with 'starry sky' sutures. **(f)** External oblique closed to recreate the inguinal canal before skin closure

lump immediately below the inguinal ligament and just lateral to its medial attachment to the pubic tubercle. Since the femoral canal is narrow, a cough impulse can rarely be detected, and the hernia is usually irreducible. Thus, small femoral hernias may be difficult to distinguish from other lumps arising in the femoral canal such as a lipoma or enlarged Cloquet's lymph node. However, a hernia is deeply fixed whereas the others tend to be more mobile.

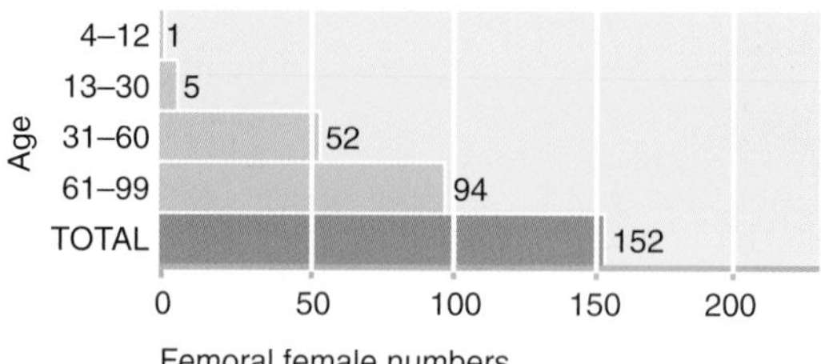

Fig. 32.10 Annual incidence of femoral hernias in females by age in East Anglia (UK)

Strangulated femoral hernia

In contrast to strangulated inguinal hernia, there are often no obvious localising symptoms and signs in strangulated femoral hernia, and the classic presenting features are those of distal small bowel obstruction. The diagnosis of strangulated femoral hernia is easily missed unless the femoral region is carefully and expertly examined for a lump.

In nearly 30% of strangulated femoral hernias, only a portion of the bowel circumference is trapped in the hernial sac. Although the bowel lumen remains patent and the patient continues to pass flatus, peristalsis is sufficiently disrupted for other signs of obstruction to occur, notably vomiting. This is known as **Richter's hernia** (see Fig. 32.11). Resuscitation and urgent operation are required as for completely strangulated hernias.

Fig. 32.11 Richter's hernia

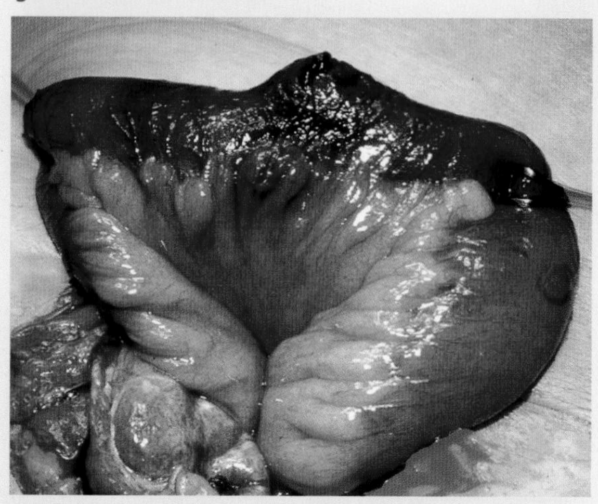

This 71-year-old woman presented with symptoms and signs of incomplete small bowel obstruction; these included vomiting, abdominal distension and colicky abdominal pain, but she continued to pass flatus. She had a 2 cm femoral hernia which was not tender. At operation, only a part of the wall of the ileum was trapped in the hernia. The photograph shows bruising around the area trapped in the hernia. Luckily, the bowel was viable and did not need resection. The hernia was repaired before closure

CASE HISTORY

MANAGEMENT OF FEMORAL HERNIA

The abdominal orifice of the femoral canal is small and indistensible so abdominal contents finding their way into the canal strangulate much more readily than in inguinal hernias. Thus, all femoral hernias, even if asymptomatic, should be repaired without delay.

Elective repair is performed by first isolating, emptying and excising the peritoneal sac (see Fig. 32.12). The femoral canal is then closed with non-absorbable sutures or a plug placed between pectineus fascia and inguinal ligament. The canal can be exposed by several different methods. The most common

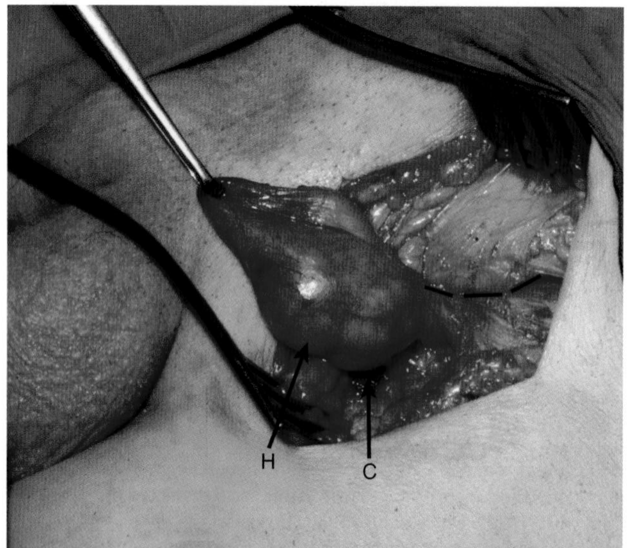

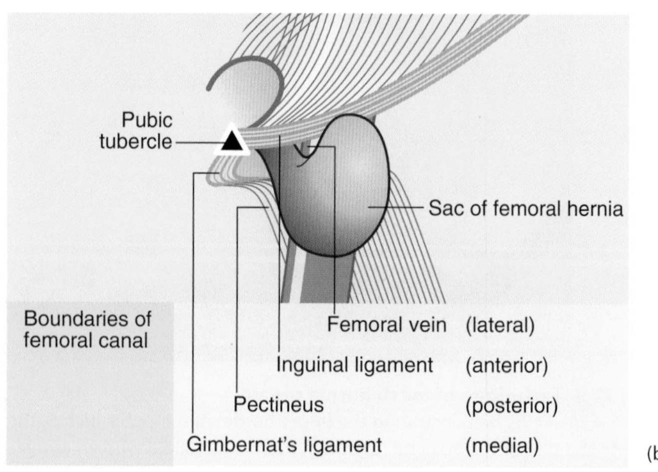

Fig. 32.12 Femoral hernia
(a) An average-sized femoral hernia **H** at operation. The patient's genitalia are to the left of the photograph. The line of the inguinal ligament is marked with an interrupted line and the opening of the femoral canal is seen at **C**. **(b)** The four margins of the femoral canal

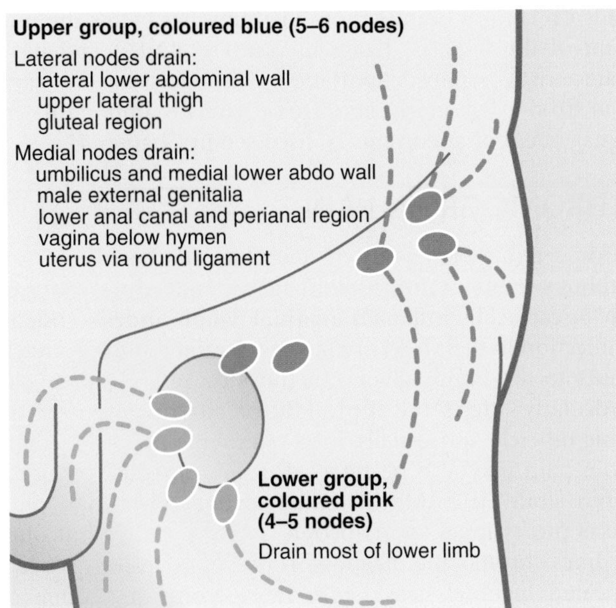

Fig. 32.13 Superficial inguinal lymph nodes of the groin
The lower group lie around the termination of the long saphenous vein. Both upper and lower groups drain to the external iliac nodes

are a) the **femoral** or low approach, b) the **Lotheissen** or high approach, via the posterior wall of the inguinal canal, and c) the **McEvedy** or pararectus extraperitoneal approach. The last is virtually a laparotomy and is rarely employed. Occasionally a femoral hernia containing bowel cannot be safely reduced via a local approach, or bowel of doubtful viability escapes back into the abdominal cavity. In either case, a laparotomy incision is required to safely complete the operation.

ENLARGED INGUINAL LYMPH NODES

The lymph nodes of the inguinal region are clustered into the three anatomical groups shown in Figure 32.13. These drain the lower abdominal wall and lower back, perineum (including vulva and vagina), anal canal, penis and scrotal skin and the whole lower limb. The testes are derived from the retroperitoneal area and hence drain to the upper para-aortic nodes within the abdomen rather than inguinal nodes.

Inguinal lymph nodes may become secondarily enlarged as a result of local disease in their field of drainage. Examples include infections of the foot, skin diseases, sexually transmitted infection or tumours. Inguinal node enlargement may also be part of a generalised lymphadenopathy in lymphoma or a systemic infection such as glandular fever or AIDS. Inguinal nodes may also become involved in tuberculosis. Multiple small firm ('shotty') nodes are commonly found and are accepted as normal if less than 1 cm in diameter. These nodes probably result from minor infections of the lower limb.

CLINICAL FEATURES OF ENLARGED INGUINAL LYMPH NODES

Enlarged inguinal lymph nodes present with pain or a lump in the groin but are often discovered incidentally. Enlarged lymph nodes are recognised by their anatomical position and by excluding hernias or vascular abnormalities. Enlarged nodes are usually mobile but become fixed to the surrounding tissues when infiltrated by tumour. If doubt exists as to whether nodes are enlarged, ultrasound scanning usually gives a definitive answer and can guide percutaneous needle biopsy. In general, nodes smaller than 1 cm are unlikely to be malignant.

The history may need to be reviewed for clues as to the origin of any nodes. A history of systemic manifestations of lymphoma, TB or acquired immunodeficiency syndrome (AIDS) should be sought. These include malaise, periodic fevers and weight loss. There may be a history of a 'mole' or 'wart' having been removed, even many years before. If this was a malignant melanoma or squamous carcinoma, it could now have metastasised. Other symptoms of tumours that metastasise to inguinal lymph nodes should be sought; for example, anal pain or bleeding might indicate an anal carcinoma, and an unretractable foreskin may hide a penile carcinoma.

Examination should include palpating lymph nodes in the neck and axillae, and palpating the liver and spleen. The skin of the whole drainage field should be examined closely, paying particular attention to the back, perineum and feet, including between the toes and beneath the toenails, and beneath the foreskin. The examination may reveal infection, squamous cell carcinoma or malignant melanoma. Rectal examination is mandatory to exclude anal carcinoma. A blood test for human immunodeficiency virus (HIV) may be indicated.

If enlarged lymph nodes cannot be explained by simple local factors or a systemic illness, nodes should be sampled for histology. If metastatic malignancy is suspected, fine needle aspiration or needle core biopsy is appropriate, but if lymphoma is likely, a node should be surgically removed or be subject to an open biopsy to obtain substantial tissue for histological typing.

SAPHENA VARIX

A saphena varix is a dilatation of the long saphenous vein in the groin, just proximal to its junction with the femoral vein (see Fig. 32.14). The varix is caused by valvular incompetence at this point; there are usually substantial varicose veins elsewhere in the long saphenous system.

The varix can reach the size of a golf ball or even larger. On examination, the swelling is soft and diffuse. The diagnostic feature is that it empties with minimal pressure and refills on release ('the sign of emptying'). A cough impulse is invariably present and a fluid thrill can be felt if varicosities further down the thigh are tapped lightly. Treatment is high saphenous ligation, as for sapheno-femoral reflux associated with varicose veins (see Ch. 43).

FEMORAL ARTERY ANEURYSM

Femoral aneurysms are uncommon as a cause of lumps in the groin. They may occur as part of a generalised aneurysmal disease involving the abdominal aorta, iliac and lower limb arterial system but can also occur in isolation. Diagnosis is

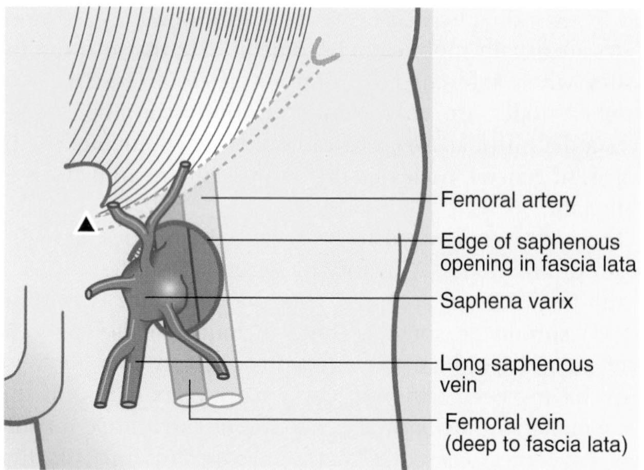

Fig. 32.14 Saphena varix

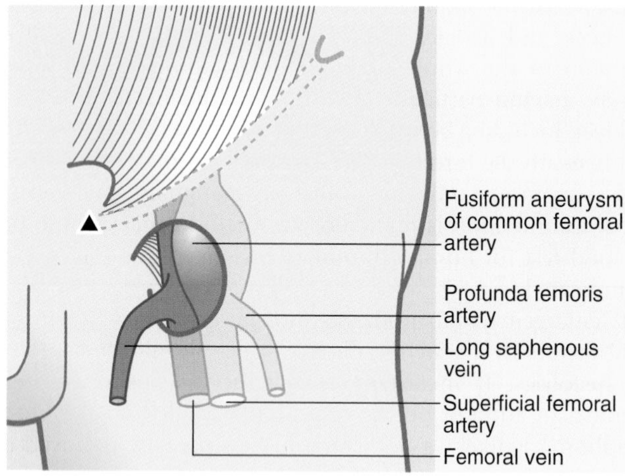

Fig. 32.15 Femoral artery aneurysm

made on clinical examination; the lump lies below the mid-point of the inguinal ligament (see Fig. 32.15) and has a characteristic expansile pulsation. Distinguishing an aneurysm from a femoral hernia is clearly vitally important. The management of aneurysms is discussed in Chapter 42.

CHRONIC GROIN PAIN

Chronic groin pain without any clues in the history and without swelling is difficult to diagnose and treat. Groin pain may be caused by **inflamed inguinal lymph nodes** secondary to infection in their field of drainage. **Strained muscle attachments** to the bony pelvis sometimes cause groin pain; this particularly affects the hip adductor attachments near the pubic tubercle and usually follows extreme physical activity. Groin pain may also be **referred** from a diseased hip joint. 'Groin strain' is a difficult entity to understand and often affects professional sports people. It starts acutely but often becomes chronic; the diagnosis is one of exclusion. A newly appeared inguinal hernia may cause groin pain, often on sitting, yet be too small to detect clinically. Unfortunately, there is no dependable test for an early hernia other than laparoscopy, although ultrasound in experienced hands is fairly reliable.

VENTRAL HERNIAS

Ventral hernias include epigastric, umbilical and paraumbilical hernias. Ventral incisional hernias occurring through previous surgical or traumatic wounds are considered in Chapter 12.

EPIGASTRIC HERNIAS (see Fig. 32.16)

These are midline herniations through defects in the linea alba, anywhere between xiphoid process and umbilicus. They are four times more common in males and are often tiny, with

CASE HISTORY

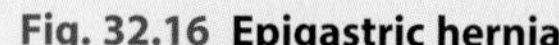

Fig. 32.16 Epigastric hernia

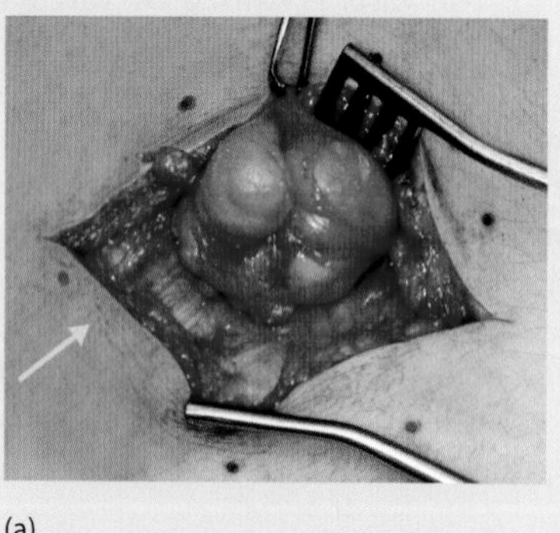

(a)

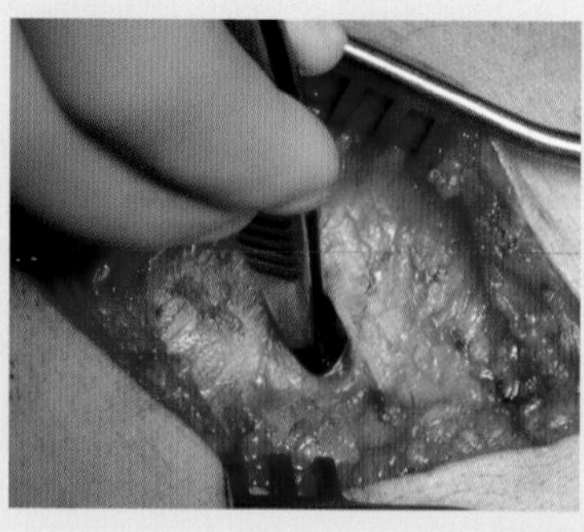

(b)

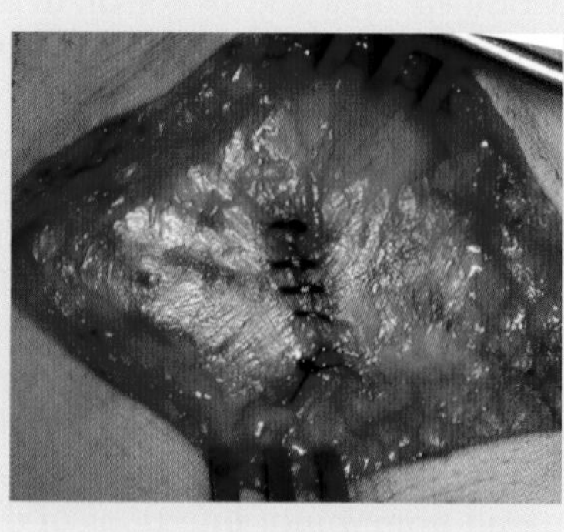

(c)

This man of 28 had an unusually large epigastric hernia that caused pain on exercise. It was situated in the midline, midway between the xiphisternum and the umbilicus.

(a) 'Mushroom-like' epigastric hernia mass protruding through the linea alba (fibres indicated by arrow)
(b) Relatively small defect in linea alba after mobilising and reducing the hernia
(c) After edge-to-edge repair of defect using continuous non-absorbable nylon suture

a defect less than 0.5 cm. Most are symptomless and the presence of a lump and sometimes episodic sharp pain on exertion are the usual presenting complaints. Treatment is by direct suture repair if the hernial defect is smaller than 1 cm. Larger hernias may require a tension-free mesh repair.

UMBILICAL AND PARAUMBILICAL HERNIAS

Umbilical hernias in children are discussed in Chapter 51. **Paraumbilical hernias** are acquired rather than congenital. They occur in all age groups but are five times more common in females. The abdominal wall defect is in the linea alba, generally above or below the umbilical cicatrix. The swelling lies adjacent to the umbilicus, with the umbilicus itself pushed to the side to produce the characteristic 'smile' of a paraumbilical hernia.

True umbilical hernias are the third most common abdominal hernia in adults and appear directly through the umbilical cicatrix. They also occur more commonly in females, and obesity and poor muscle tone are predisposing factors. Hernias range from asymptomatic small protrusions, through larger and occasionally painful lumps, to very large, irreducible and intermittently painful swellings. Both paraumbilical and umbilical hernias become progressively larger and surgical repair is the treatment of choice. This is by direct suture for the smallest defects or the use of mesh for larger defects.

33 Disorders of the male genitalia

DISORDERS OF THE SCROTAL CONTENTS

INTRODUCTION

Abnormalities of the scrotal contents include disorders of the testis or its coverings, the spermatic cord and inguino-scrotal hernias (see Ch. 32). Distinguishing between them usually requires only clinical examination. Diagnoses that must not be missed are testicular tumours and testicular torsion. Other problems include inflammation, hydrocoeles and cysts, maldescent and testicular trauma, as well as varicocoele. Male sterilisation and disorders of the penis are also covered in this chapter.

CLINICAL EXAMINATION OF SCROTAL LUMPS AND SWELLINGS

A lump or swelling in the scrotum may be:

- A solid or cystic mass arising from a component of scrotal contents or spermatic cord. These include testis, epididymis, epididymal appendage, vas deferens and pampiniform venous plexus
- A collection of fluid in the tunica or processus vaginalis (**hydrocoele**)
- An indirect inguinal hernia extending along the embryological path of testicular descent into the scrotum

The important disorders of the scrotum and contents are summarised in Table 33.1, with their anatomical and clinical significance.

The origin of a scrotal lump

The first objective is to determine if the swelling arises in the groin, the spermatic cord or the scrotum and is achieved by palpating the cord at the scrotal neck. In a hernia, the cord is broader than normal and the hernia can be shown to communicate with the abdominal cavity by a cough impulse or by reducing the hernia. Spermatic cord swellings (varicocoele or cyst) are usually easily recognised. In purely scrotal lumps, the spermatic cord is a normal diameter.

Testicular and epididymal lumps

With a scrotal abnormality, an attempt should be made to palpate testis and epididymis separately, and to determine their relationship to the lump. If the testis is enlarged or has a lump within it, this is a tumour until proven otherwise. Testicular swellings due to lymphoma, leukaemia or granulomatous infections (e.g. tuberculosis or syphilitic gumma) may be softer but this is unreliable. Any testicular pathology may cause a little fluid to accumulate in the tunica vaginalis producing a small **secondary hydrocoele** but this rarely interferes with testicular palpation.

Lumps in the epididymis (cysts, chronic epididymitis or, rarely, tuberculous granulomata) are discrete from, but attached to, an otherwise normal testis. Tiny focal lumps in the epididymis are rarely clinically important. Infective lesions cause diffuse and usually painful thickening of the epididymis, whereas epididymal cysts are almost always located at the upper pole. Epididymal cysts are filled with clear fluid and therefore transilluminate. **Transillumination** (Fig. 33.1) is demonstrated by shining a strong beam of light through the scrotum in a partly darkened room. If the lesion is fluid-filled, it will glow (except in the case of blood). About 10% of cysts in the epididymis, and most in the cord, are filled with an opalescent fluid containing spermatozoa (**spermatocoeles**) which can also transilluminate.

SCROTAL PAIN

ACUTE PAIN (Box 33.1)

In acute scrotal pain, **testicular torsion** *must* be excluded since the torted testis can be saved if operation is performed

Table 33.1 Summary of disorders of the scrotum and its contents and their clinical features

Disorder	Anatomical/developmental basis	Clinical features
1. Testicular disorders		
a. Incompletely descended testis (see also Ch. 51)	Failure of complete descent from retroperitoneal site into scrotum; testis may be arrested at any point of descent or in an ectopic site	Mainly a problem of infancy and childhood and requiring orchidopexy; possible cause of lump in groin; slightly increased predisposition to malignancy; fertility may be impaired
b. Torsion of testis	Rotation of testis in scrotum; twisting of the spermatic cord results in venous obstruction which may culminate in infarction; recurrent incomplete torsion may occur	Complete torsion causes severe acute scrotal pain (and sometimes abdominal pain); partial torsion may cause episodic pain
c. Inflammation of epididymis or testis	'Epididymitis, usually caused by common urinary tract pathogens or sexually transmitted organisms Acute orchitis is often viral (mumps) Chronic orchitis may be caused by tuberculosis or syphilitic gumma	Acute epididymitis is painful; must be distinguished from testicular torsion; usually associated with UTI Testicular pain and swelling Usually presents as painless testicular enlargement
d. Malignant testicular tumours	Derived from germ cells of testis; metastasise via lymphatics to para-iliac and para-aortic nodes or via bloodstream, commonly to lung	Present as painless swelling of testis usually with small secondary hydrocoele
2. Disorders of other scrotal contents		
a. Hydrocoele	Abnormal collection of fluid in space around testis; in children may still be in communication with peritoneal cavity (communicating hydrocoele)	Presents as a painless scrotal swelling which transilluminates; testis may be difficult to palpate within it until fluid is drained
b. Haematocoele	Collection of blood around testis; usually early result of trauma or surgery	Presents like a hydrocoele after trauma but does not transilluminate
c. Varicocoele	Dilatation of pampiniform venous plexus of spermatic cord	Presents as a scrotal swelling separate from testis and epididymis; feels like a 'bag of worms'; disappears on lying down, thus patient must be examined standing
d. Epididymal cyst and spermatocoele	Cysts derived from epididymal tissue	Epididymal cyst presents as a scrotal swelling which transilluminates; separate from the testis, often multiloculated Spermatocoele is unilocular, sometimes bilateral, in cord or epididymis and may be transilluminable
e. Torsion of hydatid of Morgagni	Torsion of epididymal appendage	Occurs in children; may present late as a small hydrocoele; in the acute phase, presents as scrotal pain and oedema and may simulate testicular torsion
f. Indirect inguinal hernia	Herniation of abdominal contents along the embryological path of testicular descent	Presents as a scrotal swelling, often with a cough impulse, that can be reduced back into the abdomen

promptly; an exploratory operation is mandatory if torsion cannot be confidently excluded. Torsion occurs mainly in adolescents but occasionally in young adults. Recurrent, incomplete torsion may cause transient episodes of severe pain or poorly defined lower abdominal pain. In these cases, the anatomical relationship of the testis to the tunica vaginalis is often abnormal so the testes lie horizontally rather than vertically when standing. These 'bell-clapper' testes are susceptible to torsion. The main differential diagnosis at all ages is acute epididymitis. Torsion of an epididymal appendage (hydatid of Morgagni) produces symptoms similar to testicular torsion in children but less severe; surgical exploration is usually still required to exclude it. A traumatic haematocoele also causes acute pain but the trauma or surgery that preceded it points to the likely diagnosis.

CHRONIC PAIN

Chronic scrotal pain is most often due to **inflammation**. It can often be traced to a vasectomy, although the cause is usually obscure and treatment often ineffective. Patients present weeks or months after the operation, complaining of localised tenderness at the operation site or a general ache in one side of the scrotum. If there is a small tender lump due to a stitch granuloma, this is usually cured by excision. Sperm leakage (**sperm granuloma**) following vasectomy may also

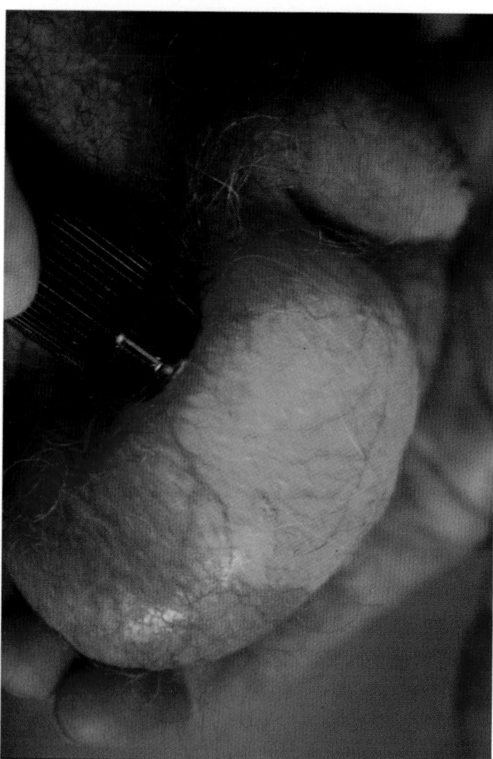

Fig. 33.1 Transillumination of a scrotal cyst
This 30-year-old man complained of a swelling in the right scrotum. On clinical examination there is a 3 cm soft rounded swelling at the upper pole of the epididymis. A confident diagnosis of epididymal cyst can thus be made

Box 33.1 Common causes of acute pain in the scrotum

Torsion of the testis
- Sudden onset of unilateral scrotal pain with or without poorly localised abdominal pain
- In early cases, the testis is high in the scrotum and exquisitely tender, and the cord is thickened; later these signs are often obscured by oedema
- The opposite testis may lie horizontally (bell-clapper testis)

Torsion of the epididymal appendage (hydatid of Morgagni)
- Nearly always in children
- Sudden onset of unilateral scrotal pain; the testis hangs normally. There is a tenderness only at its upper pole and minimal overlying oedema

Acute epididymitis
- Moderate or severe scrotal pain and tenderness with marked redness and oedema
- Often preceded by symptoms of urinary tract infection; urine usually contains white cells, nitrites and organisms

Haematocoele following trauma or scrotal surgery (e.g. vasectomy)
- History may be diagnostic although torsion is sometimes precipitated by trauma

cause chronic pain, Pain is a feature of chronic bacterial epididymitis, which usually follows an acute episode.

INFLAMMATION OF THE EPIDIDYMIS AND TESTIS

EPIDIDYMITIS

Bacterial epididymitis is the most common inflammatory disorder of scrotal contents. It is usually secondary to urethral infection that has ascended via the vas deferens. The source is a urinary tract infection with coliforms (in the 50–65 age group) or a sexually transmitted infection with *Chlamydia* or *Neisseria gonorrhoeae* (common in the 15–30 age group). Epididymitis is often incorrectly called orchitis or epididymo-orchitis. The testis is rarely infected, although the inflammation surrounding epididymitis may cause testicular tenderness.

In epididymitis, pain usually begins acutely. It may present as a surgical emergency and be clinically indistinguishable from testicular torsion. On examination, the affected side of the scrotum and its contents are swollen, oedematous and tender, and the scrotal skin can be red and warm. It may be difficult to palpate testis and epididymis separately once infection is established. In a boy under 15, epididymitis must never be diagnosed in the absence of urinary symptoms, a proven urinary infection or urethritis. Such an 'acute scrotum' must be explored to exclude torsion (see p. 428).

Treatment of acute epididymitis is initially with bed rest for pain relief and at least a month of an appropriate broad-spectrum antibiotic. The infecting organism is often not identified but attempts should be made to do so using urine cultures, blood cultures or culture of urethral discharge after prostatic massage. Ofloxacin is often favoured on a 'best-guess' basis as it covers *Chlamydia* and Gram-negative organisms. Persistent or chronic epididymitis may cause the patient to suffer chronic scrotal tenderness. Chronic epididymitis may also result from inadequate antibiotic treatment of an acute episode.

Tuberculous epididymitis

Tuberculosis may involve the epididymis via bloodstream spread from a pulmonary or other focus. A tuberculous urinary tract infection can spread to the epididymis, with swelling as the presenting complaint. Typically, the whole length of the epididymis is thickened, non-tender and 'cold'. In contrast to bacterial epididymitis, the epididymis can be readily distinguished from the testis on palpation. If untreated, the testis may also become involved.

Diagnosis requires analysis of serial early morning urine specimens (EMUs) for mycobacteria or, more reliably, histological examination of percutaneous needle biopsies. If tuberculosis is confirmed, a search must be made for pulmonary and urinary tract disease (see Ch. 38).

ORCHITIS

Primary bacterial orchitis is rare and may result from pyogenic infection in the genital tract or elsewhere. **Tertiary gummatous syphilis** may involve the testis, producing diffuse non-tender enlargement. This is now rare and there is usually a history of primary and secondary lesions. Sometimes a gumma is found unexpectedly during investigation of a suspected testicular tumour.

Viral orchitis is most often caused by **mumps**. In post-pubertal males, bilateral mumps orchitis produces infertility in 50%; elevated follicle-stimulating hormone (FSH) blood levels following orchitis usually indicate the patient is infertile. Mumps orchitis manifests 4–6 days after the onset of parotitis with extreme testicular tenderness and an inflammatory hydrocoele. Treatment is directed at symptomatic relief. Mumps has reappeared since the spurious MMR vaccine scare. Other viruses affecting the testis include Coxsackie, human immunodeficiency virus (HIV), Epstein–Barr, varicella and, in earlier times, smallpox.

HYDROCOELE

PRIMARY HYDROCOELE

A hydrocoele is an excessive collection of fluid within the tunica vaginalis, i.e. in the serous space surrounding the testis. Like the peritoneal cavity, the tunica normally contains a little serous fluid which is produced and reabsorbed at the same rate (Fig. 33.2).

In infants and children, a hydrocoele is usually an expression of a patent processus vaginalis (PPV). In some, the scrotal swelling disappears overnight, and is known as a **communicating hydrocoele**. Provided there is no hernia, hydrocoeles below the age of 1 year usually resolve spontaneously. For older children, ligation of the PPV is required.

Primary hydrocoeles may develop in adulthood, particularly in the elderly, by slow accumulation of serous fluid, presumably by impaired reabsorption. These can reach a huge size, containing several hundred millilitres of fluid but the lesions are otherwise asymptomatic. The swelling is soft and non-tender and the testis cannot usually be palpated. The presence of fluid is confirmed by transillumination.

CASE HISTORY

Fig. 33.2 Testicular hydrocoele

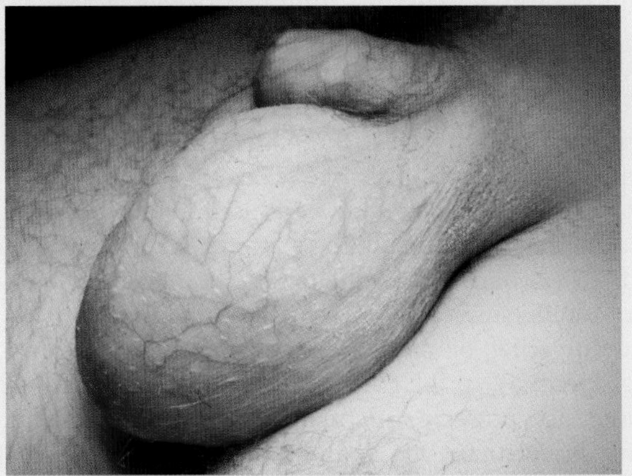

This man of 67 had a painless swelling of the left side of the scrotum for several years that was slowly enlarging. On examination, the swelling was confined to the scrotum and did not involve widening of the cord at the scrotal neck which might indicate a hernia. The testis was not palpable separately from the swelling, and the swelling transilluminated, confirming the diagnosis

Note that a secondary hydrocoele may develop in response to testicular tumour or inflammation. In most, the hydrocoele is small and the testis can easily be palpated to reveal the primary abnormality.

Management

For symptomatic patients, a hydrocoele operation can be performed by everting the sac and oversewing the edges (Jaboulay procedure) or plicating the sac (Lord's method). If the sac is thick, it is best excised. Alternatives include observation alone or periodic aspiration (rarely performed) if the patient is unsuitable for surgery. If a testicular tumour is a possibility, a hydrocoele must not be aspirated as malignant cells can be disseminated via scrotal skin to its lymphatic field.

HYDROCOELE OF THE CORD

Rarely, a hydrocoele develops in a remnant of the processus vaginalis somewhere along the course of the spermatic cord. This hydrocoele also transilluminates, and is known as an **encysted hydrocoele of the cord** (see Fig. 33.3). In females, a multicystic **hydrocoele of the canal of Nuck** sometimes presents as a swelling in the groin. It probably results from cystic degeneration of the round ligament.

FOURNIER'S SCROTAL GANGRENE

Fournier's scrotal gangrene is a form of **necrotising fasciitis** of genitalia and perineum and does not involve the testes. There is often consequent systemic sepsis. The underlying causes are varied and include pre-existing primary hydrocoele, genitourinary trauma, either accidental or iatrogenic, perirectal abscess and urethral stricture. Predisposing factors include diabetes mellitus, corticosteroids, chemotherapy and alcohol abuse. The infecting organism is principally an anaerobe but there is often synergistic aerobic infection. Treatment is urgent and includes intravenous antibiotics and surgical excision of all necrotic tissue, with the wound left open to heal by secondary intention.

EPIDIDYMAL CYST AND SPERMATOCOELE

Multiple cysts can develop in the upper pole of the epididymis and present as a painless scrotal swelling (see Fig. 33.3). Epididymal cysts affect a slightly younger age group than hydrocoeles. The testis can be palpated separately from the cysts, which transilluminate.

Less common is a **spermatocoele**, a single cyst containing spermatozoa. Spermatocoeles usually occur in the head of the epididymis and may present like a third testis. They are clinically similar to epididymal cysts but may or may not transilluminate. Occasionally they occur in the spermatic cord and surgical excision may cause obstruction to passage of sperm. If a patient wishes to remain fertile and the cysts are bilateral, excision may be contraindicated.

VARICOCOELE

A varicocoele (see Figs 33.3 and 33.4) represents dilatation and tortuosity of the pampiniform plexus of the spermatic vein in the cord. The condition is much more common on

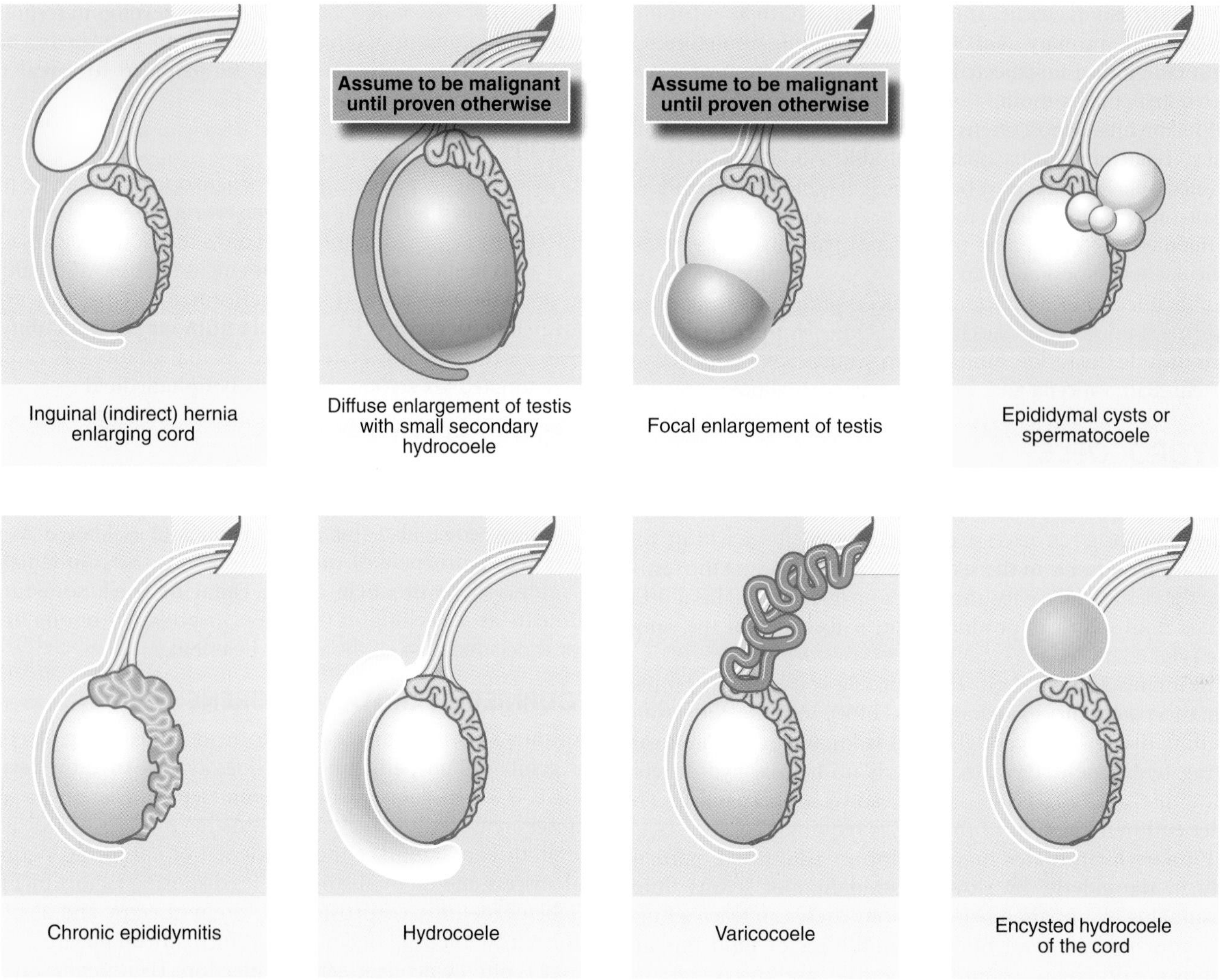

Inguinal (indirect) hernia enlarging cord

Assume to be malignant until proven otherwise

Diffuse enlargement of testis with small secondary hydrocoele

Assume to be malignant until proven otherwise

Focal enlargement of testis

Epididymal cysts or spermatocoele

Chronic epididymitis

Hydrocoele

Varicocoele

Encysted hydrocoele of the cord

Fig. 33.3 Causes of a lump or swelling in the scrotum

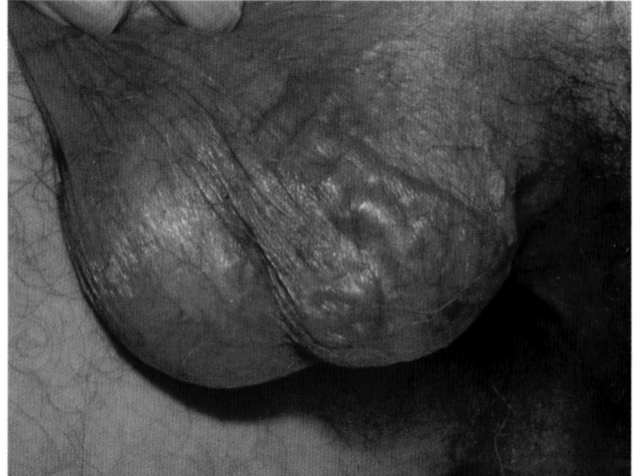

Fig. 33.4 Varicocoele
Note the 'bag of worms' appearance

the left (90%), so it may result from the different venous drainage of the two sides: on the left, the testicular vein drains into the high-pressure renal vein, whereas the right testicular vein drains directly into the inferior vena cava.

Varicocoele is common, affecting about 10% of young adult males. It is usually asymptomatic but is often discovered during examination for infertility. Varicocoele increases scrotal temperature, which may inhibit sperm function and cause possible loss of testicular volume. When lying flat, the distended veins often collapse and become impalpable. Varicocoele is best diagnosed if the patient is examined standing, when the varicocoele feels like 'a bag of worms'.

Rarely, a varicocoele may be caused by an invading renal cell carcinoma obstructing the left renal vein. Such varicocoeles do not collapse when the patient lies flat.

In adults, surgical treatment of varicocoele is only indicated for relief of pain or treatment of low sperm count (oligospermia). In the child or adolescent, treatment may be advised to preserve spermatogenesis. The treatment of choice is percutaneous embolisation. Alternatively, surgical ligation can be performed laparoscopically or via an open approach.

TESTICULAR TUMOURS

Testicular tumours are relatively uncommon, making up about 1.5% of male cancers, but they are the most common

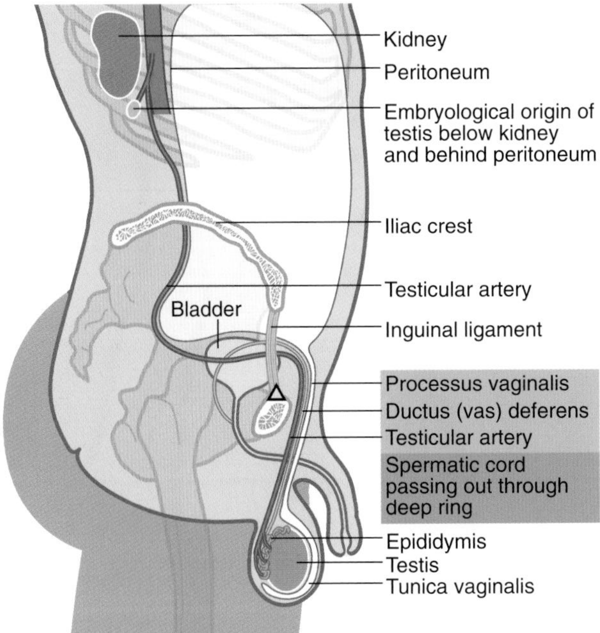

Fig. 33.5 Embryological descent of the testis
The testicular artery marks the line of descent of testis towards the scrotum. In the embryo, the arterial supply is direct from the aorta and this persists even when the testis has reached the scrotum

cancer in men in their third and fourth decades. They are important because curative treatment is now available for most of them. Testicular lymphatic drainage and the route of lymphatic metastases is towards intra-abdominal nodes and is determined by the embryology of testicular descent (see Fig. 33.5). Note that this is different from scrotal skin, which drains towards inguinal nodes.

There is roughly one new case of testicular malignancy in 20 000 males per annum, and half have already metastasised by the time of presentation. Undescended testes are at least 30 times more likely to turn malignant, although the individual risk is still low. These tumours are usually seminomas.

More than 90% of primary testicular tumours are derived from **germ cells**, the rest being classified by the World Health Organization as **sex cord/gonadal stromal tumours**. A detailed classification of malignant testicular tumours is shown in Box 33.2 and the WHO histopathological classification is shown in Box 33.3. Germ cell testicular tumours are generally fast-growing, aggressive tumours that metastasise to intra-abdominal lymph nodes and later via the bloodstream to the lungs.

Non-germ cell **Leydig cell tumours**, derived from the gonadal stroma, often present with excess hormone secretion rather than a testicular lump. This causes precocious puberty in a child and testicular feminisation in an adult.

Testes may be secondarily involved in more widespread malignancy such as lymphoma, chronic lymphocytic leukaemia or, in children, acute lymphoblastic leukaemia. These rarely present as lumps but the surgeon may be asked to perform testicular biopsy as part of monitoring.

Box 33.2 Classification of malignant testicular tumours*

- Seminoma
- Differentiated teratoma (TD)
- Malignant teratoma intermediate (MTI)
- Malignant teratoma undifferentiated (MTU)—also known as embryonal tumour
- Subvariant: malignant teratoma trophoblastic (MTT), also known as choriocarcinoma
- Yolk sac tumour

*Testicular Tumour Panel and Registry of the Pathological Society of Great Britain and Ireland. Unlike the WHO classification, this groups all non-seminomatous tumours under the heading of teratoma

Box 33.3 WHO histopathological classification of testicular tumours

1. Germ cell tumours (90%)
   — Seminoma (48%)
   — Non-seminomatous GCT (42%)
   — Teratoma (most common)
   — Embryonal carcinoma
   — Yolk sac tumour
   — Choriocarcinoma
   — Mixed NSGCT
   — Mixed GCT
2. Sex cord/gonadal stromal tumours
   — Leydig cell tumour
   — Sertoli cell tumour
   — Mixed
3. Miscellaneous non-specific stromal tumours
   — Ovarian epithelial tumours
   — Tumours of the collecting ducts and rete testis
   — Lymphoma, leukaemia, secondary metastases

PATHOLOGY OF TESTICULAR TUMOURS

Seminomas

More than half of malignant testicular tumours are seminomas, derived from spermatocytes (Fig. 33.6). They occur predominantly between the ages of 20 and 45 with a peak incidence at 35 years. The cut surface of a seminoma is typically pale, creamy-white and **homogeneous**. Histologically, tumour cells are uniform and tightly packed. A distinct but rare form of seminoma, **spermatocytic seminoma**, occurs between the ages of 50 and 70 years and almost never metastasises.

Teratomas

Teratomas are slightly less common than seminomas and their peak incidence is a decade earlier. Since they are

CASE HISTORY

Fig. 33.6 Seminoma

Testis: upper and lower poles are indicated by the thin arrows

The tumour is the hypoechoic area indicated by the thick arrow

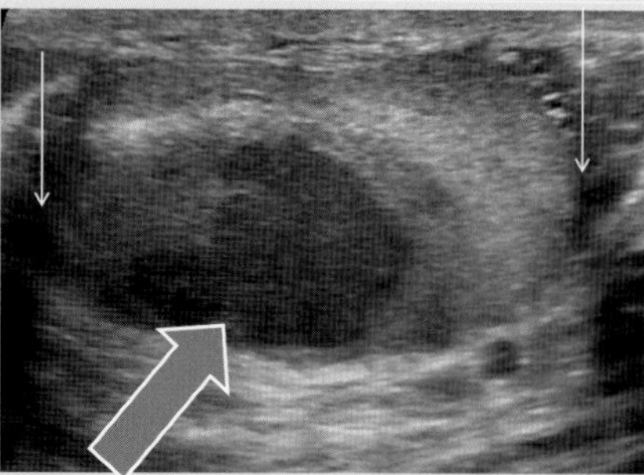

This ultrasound scan was performed on a 23-year-old man with a short history of an enlarged testis. There was no clinical sign of a hydrocoele. The scan shows a solid mass involving the whole testis with no evidence of fluid. The scan is fairly homogeneous, suggesting seminoma. Teratomas tend to be more variegated but making a definitive diagnosis requires surgical exploration

derived from multipotent cells, teratomas may contain tissue from all germ cell layers: ectoderm, mesoderm and endoderm. Teratomas exhibit a wide range of differentiation. Differentiated and intermediate tumours contain a collection of tissues resembling mature adult tissues: in particular, squamous epithelium (ectodermal), cartilage and smooth muscle (mesodermal), and respiratory epithelium (endodermal). Consequently, the cut surface often appears **variegated**, with cystic areas and patches of necrosis and haemorrhage; this is easily distinguished from seminoma with the naked eye.

CLINICAL FEATURES OF TESTICULAR TUMOURS

A malignant testicular tumour usually presents as a painless, progressively enlarging testicular lump. If the testicular capsule becomes involved, a **secondary hydrocoele** may appear but this is usually small and does not hinder palpation.

Seminoma and teratoma both spread via lymphatics to para-aortic nodes at about the level of L1/2. Spread is then proximally along the lymphatic chain then thoracic duct to supraclavicular nodes and the systemic circulation. Lung secondaries are particularly common in teratomas. Poorly differentiated testicular tumours metastasise early and may present as enlarged abdominal or cervical lymph nodes, or with symptoms of lung metastases. The primary testicular lesion may be very small or even impalpable.

A solid testicular lump **must** be assumed to be a tumour until proven otherwise. The history is rarely helpful but may include an episode of trauma which merely drew attention to the lump. On examination, the testis is either diffusely enlarged or contains a discrete lump which is firm and non-tender. Systemic examination may reveal evidence of metastases. Malignant cervical nodes may be palpable but inguinal nodes are not involved unless the tumour has spread to scrotal skin, which is rare except when biopsy or orchidectomy has been performed through a scrotal incision. Orchidectomy for suspected tumour should always be carried out via an inguinal approach.

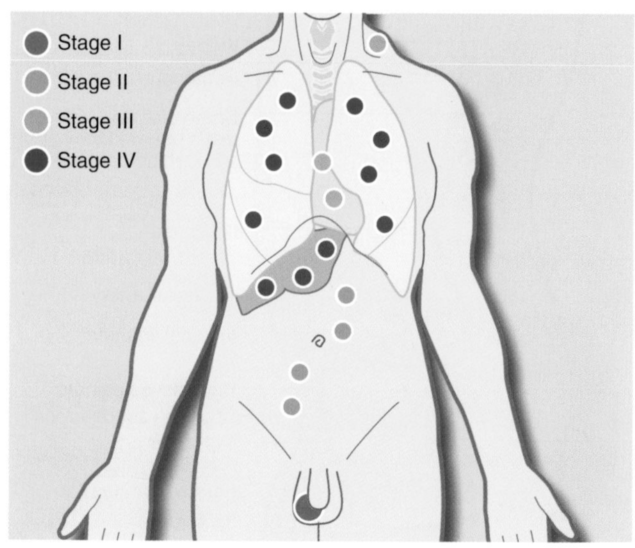

Fig. 33.7 Stages of spread of testicular tumours

Box 33.4 Stages of spread of testicular tumours

Stage I

- Tumour confined to testis

Stage II

- Retroperitoneal lymph node involvement
  - — IIa nodes <2 cm
  - — IIb nodes 2–5 cm
  - — IIc nodes >5 cm

Stage III

- Metastasis above the diaphragm confined to lymph nodes

Stage IV

- Extralymphatic metastases (usually lungs and liver)

INVESTIGATION AND TREATMENT OF TESTICULAR TUMOURS

The outlook for treated testicular tumours, even with metastases, is often good. Cure rates have improved dramatically over the past 35 years with the evolution of scientifically based treatment protocols and availability of CT scanning and tumour markers for staging and monitoring the disease. Investigation and treatment usually take place in parallel. The aims are to confirm the diagnosis, detect any metastases and stage the disease, then to treat according to the stage.

The first investigation is scrotal **ultrasonography**. If this confirms a solid testicular mass, surgical exploration is required. Preliminary staging investigations are usually performed next, including chest X-ray or CT (to look for hilar node involvement and lung secondaries), CT abdomen and pelvis to assess retroperitoneal nodes and blood levels of **tumour markers** (which must be measured before treatment). A standard method of staging testicular tumours is shown in Figure 33.7 and Box 33.4. Tumour markers contribute to diagnosis and staging and are useful for tracking residual or recurrent metastases because blood levels correlate with tumour bulk. Serial postoperative measurements help monitor disease progress and the impact of therapy.

Tumour markers

Human chorionic gonadotrophin (beta-hCG) is secreted by syncytiotrophoblastic cells and levels may rise in any tumour type, particularly poorly differentiated germ cell tumours. **Alpha-fetoprotein** (AFP) is produced by yolk sac elements. About 75% of patients with metastatic teratoma have elevated AFP levels but this marker is not expressed in seminoma. **Lactic dehydrogenase** (LDH) is elevated in more than half the patients with metastatic seminoma.

Surgical exploration

Orchidectomy is the only appropriate treatment for the primary tumour and is usually performed as part of the diagnostic process. The surgical approach is via an inguinal incision to avoid involving scrotal skin. The spermatic cord is temporarily clamped to prevent venous spread of tumour cells and the testis is brought out for inspection and palpation. If the testis is obviously malignant, orchidectomy is performed, dividing the cord at the internal inguinal ring. If there is diagnostic doubt, a testicular biopsy is taken and examined immediately by frozen section before proceeding. The other testis is usually unaffected and can be preserved. Further treatment is planned according to tumour type and stage.

Management of seminoma

For stage 1 seminoma, i.e. disease confined to the testis, some oncologists advise no further treatment after orchidectomy, although carboplatin-based chemotherapy is occasionally recommended. Seminoma is very radiosensitive and radiotherapy can also play a role for the primary, although it is not usually recommended by the European Association of Urologists in view of the high cure rate from standard treatment. For stages IIa and b (i.e. abdominal lymphadenopathy up to 5 cm diameter), radical radiotherapy to the ipsilateral (same side) para-aortic and iliac nodes gives a cure rate of about 95%. Oligospermia of the contralateral testis may occur even if it is lead-shielded but is usually transient. In stage IIb, chemotherapy is an alternative to radiotherapy using etoposide and cisplatin (EP), or cisplatin, eposide, bleomycin (PEB).

Management of teratomas and other non-seminomatous germ cell tumours

Up to 25% of patients with stage I disease would relapse within a year of orchidectomy without further treatment. Radiotherapy has no curative role in these types of tumour. There are three options for further treatment for stage I disease:

- Immediate chemotherapy
- Retroperitoneal lymph node dissection
- Surveillance and treatment if metastases occur

In the USA, lymph node dissection is often employed and provides a good cure rate but risks ejaculatory failure from autonomic nerve damage. In the UK, meticulous surveillance is the preferred option. Chemotherapy for relapse is virtually always successful and thus the 75% of patients that do not relapse are spared additional treatment.

Box 33.5 Treatment of testicular tumours

1. Removal of the affected testis—usually performed as part of the diagnostic process
2. No further treatment usually given if stage I disease (i.e. no metastases) but careful surveillance with tumour markers and CT scans required
3. Radiotherapy—local irradiation alone for moderate abdominal lymph node metastases in seminoma (stages IIa and IIb)
4. Chemotherapy with EP (etoposide and cisplatin) or BEP (bleomycin, etoposide and cisplatin)—for all cases of metastatic teratoma, and metastatic seminoma beyond stage IIb
5. Debulking surgery for lymph nodes treated by chemotherapy—sometimes necessary

Chemotherapy is indicated for all patients with known metastatic disease, including those in whom the only evidence of metastatic disease is elevated tumour markers. Results of chemotherapy for metastatic disease were transformed in the 1970s by the use of **cisplatin**. The Einhorn regimen, originating from Indiana, combined this with **vinblastine** and **bleomycin** and gave even better cure rates of 70%. Later, **etoposide** replaced vinblastine (bleomycin, etoposide, cisplatin—**'BEP'**) increasing cure rates to 85%. Three-quarters of patients with teratomas and other non-seminomatous germ cell tumours have **low-volume disease**, and in these, cure can be expected in 95%.

Long-term surveillance

After chemotherapy, surgical debulking ('salvage') of residual lymph node masses is occasionally indicated. In the long term, tumour markers and sequential CT scans are used to monitor the success of treatment. Recurrent disease can nearly always be successfully treated by radiotherapy, chemotherapy or surgery.

Fertility

Many patients with testicular tumours are already subfertile at presentation, and chemotherapy is likely to further adversely affect fertility. Patients need to be counselled carefully and, if required, semen can be collected and stored before treatment so that artificial insemination or in vitro fertilisation may be performed later. However, the success rate is poor.

Treatment of testicular tumours is summarised in Box 33.5.

ABSENT SCROTAL TESTIS (CRYPTORCHIDISM)

Failure of testicular descent or cryptorchidism occurs in 3–4% of male infants at birth and this falls to about 1% by 12 months. It can be classified as:

- **Retractile**—intermittent active cremasteric reflex draws the testis out of scrotum. It can be gently 'milked' back into the scrotum

- **Incomplete descent**—testis lies along the normal line of descent; intra-abdominal, inguinal or pre-scrotal (Fig. 33.5)
- **Ectopic**—abnormal line of testicular descent outside the external ring; testis may be palpable in the perineum, femoral region or base of penis
- **Atrophic**—secondary to trauma, iatrogenic (hernia operation or scrotal surgery) or androgen deprivation as part of prostate cancer treatment. Occasionally, an adult testis may become displaced upwards towards the inguinal canal following trauma or hernia surgery; this is known as a **trapped testis**. The testis is normal sized but is fixed in position by adhesions. If trauma was the cause and there were other major injuries, the scrotal injury may have been overlooked
- **Absent**—antenatal intra-abdominal torsion, orchidectomy after delayed diagnosis of torsion or bilateral orchidectomy for treatment of prostate cancer

MANAGEMENT OF MALDESCENT OF THE TESTIS

In developed countries, maldescent is usually identified at screening during early childhood and surgically corrected by orchidopexy at a young age (see Ch. 51); to best preserve spermatogenesis, the testis should be surgically placed in the scrotum between 6 months and 1 year. There is some evidence that orchidopexy before the age of 10 decreases the risk of testicular cancer.

CASE HISTORY

Fig. 33.8 Torsion of the testis

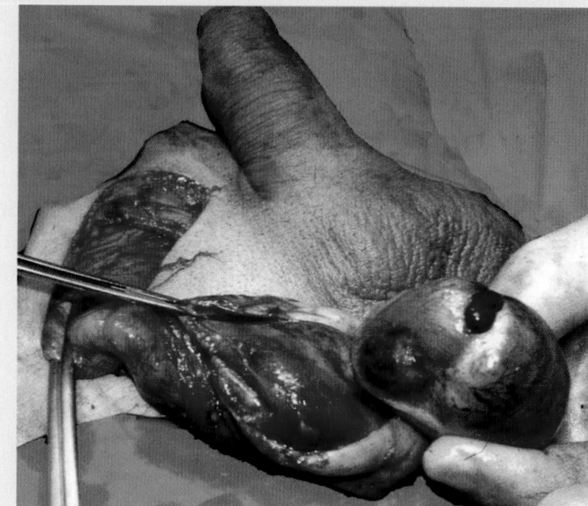

This 15-year-old boy experienced sudden severe lower abdominal pain extending to the scrotum during a football match. A provisional diagnosis of torsion was made and the scrotum explored within 2 hours of the onset of pain. At operation, the testis was twisted 2½ times around on its cord (arrowed) and was near infarction. On untwisting, however, it soon regained normal colour. Both testes were fixed to prevent future torsion

TORSION OF THE TESTIS OR EPIDIDYMAL APPENDAGE

TESTICULAR TORSION (Figs. 33.8 and 33.9)

In infants, the newly descended testis and its investing tunica vaginalis are mobile within the scrotum. These testes may undergo **extravaginal torsion** which presents as a hard, swollen testis. Later in childhood, the testis becomes suspended in a near vertical position, anchored by the spermatic cord and by attachments to the posterior scrotal wall. This attachment prevents rotation. Minor anatomical variations can produce a narrow-based pedicle with a horizontal ('bell-clapper') testicular lie, that allows the testis to twist about its axis within the tunica (**intravaginal torsion**). When this occurs, pampiniform plexus veins become compressed causing venous congestion. After a few hours, venous infarction occurs unless torsion is corrected. Trauma during sport may sometimes initiate the process, and there have been reports of successful manual untwisting on the sports field. In general, however, torsion is an emergency requiring prompt diagnosis and urgent surgical treatment to save the testis.

Torsion presents with a sudden onset of severe testicular pain often with poorly localised central abdominal pain (because the testis retains its embryological nerve supply) and sometimes vomiting. In the early stages, the affected testis is tender, slightly swollen and drawn up into the neck of the scrotum where the cord may be palpably thickened. With these features, the diagnosis is seldom in doubt. At a later stage, the scrotal skin becomes red and oedematous, making accurate palpation difficult. At this point, torsion may be difficult to distinguish from acute epididymitis and the scrotum must be explored surgically.

TORSION OF THE EPIDIDYMAL APPENDAGE (HYDATID OF MORGAGNI)

The hydatid of Morgagni is a small embryological remnant at the upper pole of the testis (see Fig. 33.9). This may undergo torsion and produce symptoms similar to testicular torsion, out of proportion to the small size of the infarcted tissue. Infarction of the hydatid is of no consequence except that it must be distinguished from testicular torsion.

MANAGEMENT OF SUSPECTED TESTICULAR TORSION

Differentiating between acute epididymitis and torsion can be difficult. If a firm diagnosis cannot be reached, surgical exploration is mandatory. Investigations are of little value: radionuclide studies and Doppler ultrasound examination may be employed to show testicular blood flow but results can be misleading.

Urgent operation is usually imperative as delay leads to testicular necrosis after about 8 hours. A scrotal incision is made and the testis is examined and untwisted. If the testis is black and fails to recover its colour, it is necrotic and should be removed to prevent it inducing a sympathetic contralateral orchiopathy. If some colour is restored, the testis is best left, although it may later atrophy. After untwisting, the testis is sutured to the tunica vaginalis or placed in a surgically created dartos pouch to prevent recurrence. Both testes should be secured as predisposition to torsion is usually bilateral.

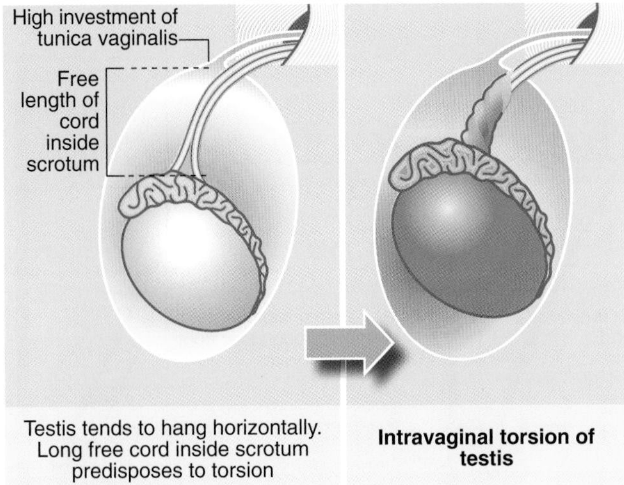

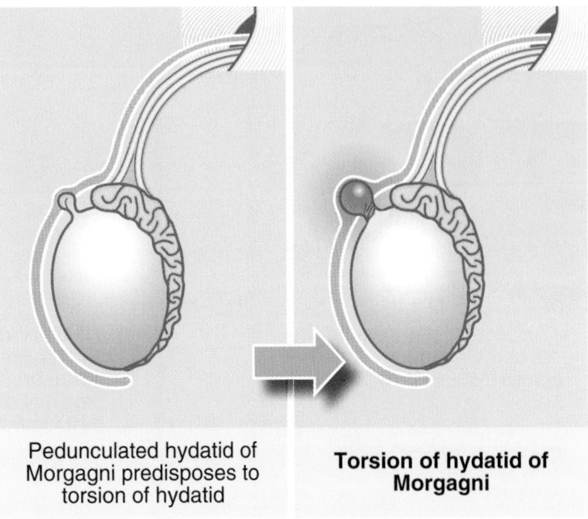

Fig. 33.9 Torsion of the testis and hydatid of Morgagni

TRAUMA TO THE TESTIS

The testes may be injured during contact sports or fights. The dense fibrous capsule investing the testis (tunica albuginea) may remain intact or it may split, but the testis is extremely painful in either case. If the tunica remains intact, a **testicular haematoma** results; if it splits, the testicular parenchyma bursts and bleeds into the tunica vaginalis cavity, resulting in a **haematocoele**.

If pain is severe and persistent, the scrotum can be explored surgically. Pain from a haematoma can be relieved by incising the tunica albuginea. Evacuating a haematocoele, however, may be impossible because blood infiltrates the tissues. If a haematocoele can be evacuated, the tunica albuginea rupture is best repaired.

MALE STERILISATION

Male sterilisation by vasectomy is a simple, effective method of birth control. It can be performed under local anaesthesia at little cost and requires no special equipment. The essential prerequisite is that the couple involved should have completed their family, since reversal is technically difficult and unreliable. A technique of vasectomy is illustrated in Figure 33.10.

Most procedures involve removing a section of the vas (ductus) deferens and ligating or cauterising the cut ends. For medicolegal reasons, the nature of the excised portion can be confirmed histologically. Spermatozoa remain in the proximal duct system for several months after vasectomy, so the operation cannot be considered a success until at least two successive sperm counts are negative. These need to be performed about 1 month apart, after 20–25 ejaculations. Despite correct operative technique and negative sperm counts, there is still a late failure rate of about 1 case in every 500. Failure suspected of resulting from spontaneous vas reconnection can be proved by a positive sperm count. This is because of the problem of determining paternity in the case of unexpected pregnancy!

Early complications of vasectomy include postoperative scrotal haematoma (usually operator error) and wound infection. Later, failure of sterilisation may become apparent, or a **sperm granuloma** may present as a tender scrotal swelling near the cut end of the vas for which further excision is usually required. Chronic debilitating pain can occur in the testis and the patient must be warned of this possibility at the time of consent. The patient must also be warned of the possibility of spontaneous reversal.

DISORDERS OF THE PENIS

Problems with the foreskin (prepuce) are common and form most penile surgical disorders. Other disorders are uncommon in adults but the most serious is **carcinoma of the penis**. In children, penile disorders are either developmental or minor inflammatory conditions, discussed in Chapter 51. Disorders of the foreskin include **balano-posthitis** (inflammation of the glans and foreskin), **phimosis** (stricture of the preputial meatus), **paraphimosis** (acute constriction of the glans by a tight retracted foreskin) and **balanitis xerotica obliterans** (idiopathic sclerosis of the foreskin). **Peyronie's disease** (idiopathic fibrosis of the corpora cavernosa) is now a frequent presentation in urological clinics (see below). Exclusion of cancer is usually the first step.

FORESKIN PROBLEMS IN ADULTS

PHIMOSIS

A common complaint is that the foreskin will not fully retract, causing pain on intercourse. Such phimosis is usually caused by fibrosis of the foreskin and may be due to chronic or recurrent low-grade *Candida* infection. Phimosis is aggravated by attempts at retraction which cause minor tears of the inner

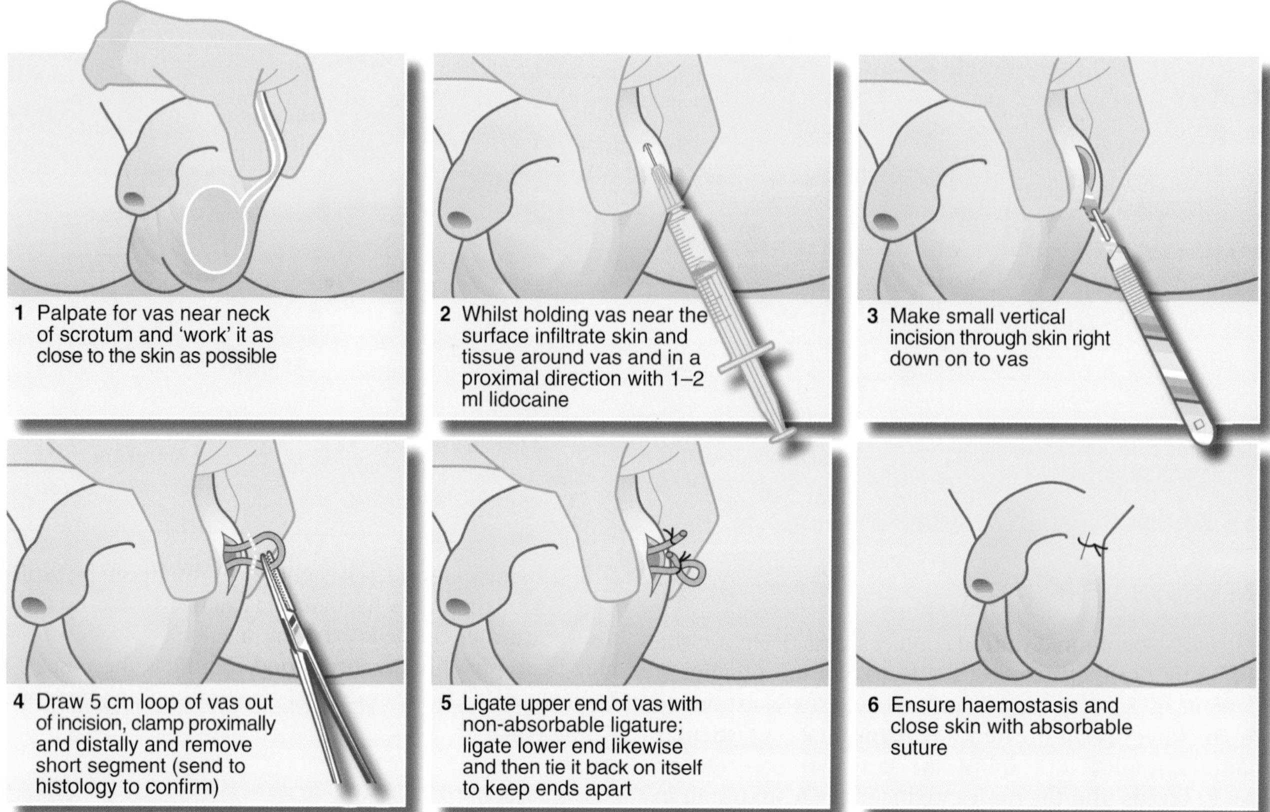

Fig. 33.10 Technique of vasectomy
Note that each side is dealt with separately

epithelial lining, inducing further inflammation and fibrosis. The condition may be accompanied by stenosis of the urethral meatus, also due to recurrent inflammation and fibrosis. Treatment usually involves circumcision but a preputioplasty or reshaping operation is sometimes successful.

BALANO-POSTHITIS (BALANITIS)

The term balano-posthitis refers to overt inflammation of the glans penis and foreskin (Greek: *balanos* gland, *posthe* foreskin); it is the correct term but the short form 'balanitis' has passed into common usage. The condition occurs most commonly in children. Inflammation alone is most often caused by *Candida* or faecal bacteria, but this problem rarely reaches the surgeon.

Balanitis xerotica obliterans is a fibrotic condition of the foreskin of unknown aetiology and is probably analogous to lichen sclerosus of the vulva in females. It produces a thickened, stenosed, often depigmented foreskin which is often adherent to the glans. Circumcision is usually curative. As many as 25% of children with phimosis have this condition. The process can involve the urethral meatus and may cause stenosis, sometimes requiring meatotomy or meatoplasty at the same time. More rarely it results in a urethral stricture likely to require urethroplasty.

PARAPHIMOSIS

If a phimotic foreskin is forcibly retracted, the tight meatal band may lodge in the coronal sulcus making reduction impossible. This is known as paraphimosis. Progressive oedema of the glans penis and foreskin then exacerbates the difficulty of reduction. It may occur at any age, but is particularly common in elderly men in whom the foreskin is not correctly pulled forwards after retraction for catheterisation or washing the glans (nurses and junior doctors are the main culprits). Paraphimosis also occurs in children and adolescents experimenting with foreskin retraction or cleaning beneath it. In most cases, the foreskin can be reduced by firm manual compression of the glans and foreskin. Local anaesthetic jelly is applied first for lubrication and pain relief. Sometimes, incising the tight ring may be necessary under local or general anaesthesia to effect reduction. **Preputioplasty**, in which the band is incised longitudinally and the skin sutured transversely, can often be performed at the same time to solve the problem in the long term. If not, circumcision or preputioplasty is usually performed at a later date when the oedema and inflammation have resolved.

CIRCUMCISION

Circumcision is or has been a widespread practice in many communities for religious or cultural reasons. From a strictly scientific or medical standpoint, however, it is difficult to support as a general health measure, although there is evidence that circumcision can reduce the risk of recurrent urinary tract infections, and definitely reduces the risk of transferring HIV. It also reduces the frequency of carcinoma of the penis. Routine circumcision for recurrent balanitis, phimosis and even paraphimosis in children has largely gone out of favour as most cases respond to local treatments or to

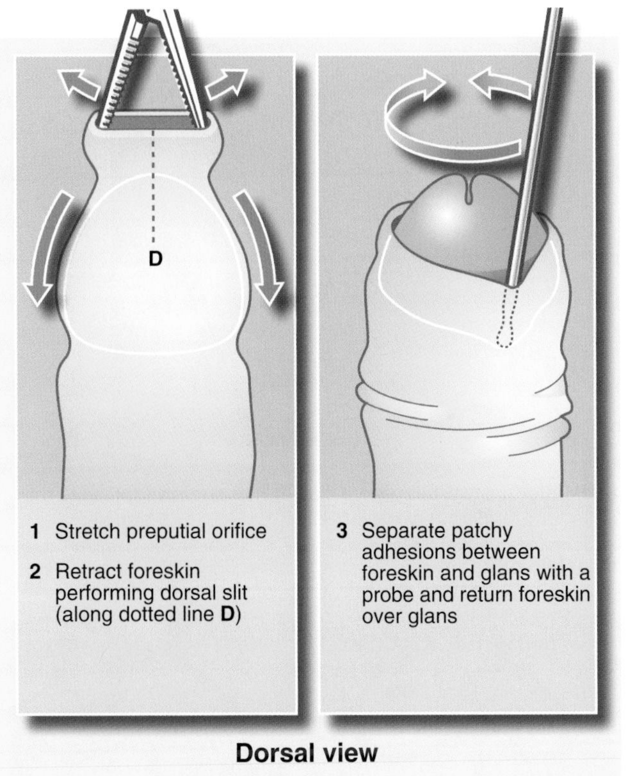

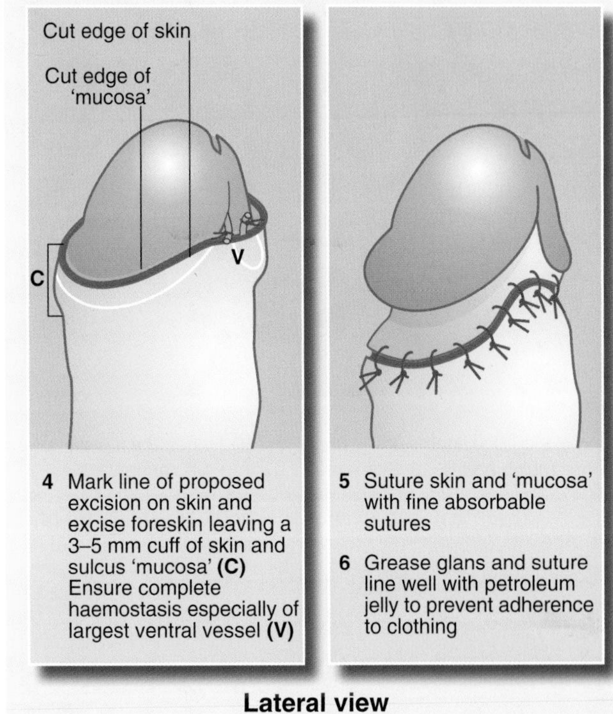

Fig. 33.11 Technique of circumcision

preputioplasty. Misguided circumcision in babies may predispose to ammoniacal nappy rash and meatal stenosis.

Circumcision should be reserved for unresolved phimosis, recurrent balanitis and sclerosis from balanitis xerotica obliterans. A surgical technique is shown in Figure 33.11. During the operation, the urethral meatus should be checked for stenosis. If present, a meatotomy may be required. An occasional early postoperative complication is haemorrhage which usually requires surgical re-exploration. Postoperative bleeding can best be prevented by meticulous haemostasis at operation.

PEYRONIE'S DISEASE

This disease of unknown aetiology occurs in young to middle-aged adults. Some cases are thought to result from penile trauma during sexual activity and others are associated with Dupuytren's contracture of the palmar fascia. Slowly progressive asymmetrical fibrotic plaques develop in the fascia surrounding the corpora cavernosa. The corpus spongiosum, including the glans, is spared. The plaques may become calcified and visible on X-ray. The condition causes the penis to bend towards the affected side on erection, making intercourse difficult and painful. There may be spontaneous partial resolution with time.

Severe cases require surgery. **Nesbit's operation** involves creating pleats in the corpus on the contralateral side. Another approach involves excision of the plaques, which are replaced by a patch of tunica vaginalis. Either procedure may restore symmetrical erection, although Nesbit's procedure results in a shorter penis. Penile prosthetic implants may be required if erection is inadequate for satisfactory sexual intercourse. 'Medical treatments' of Peyronie's disease, i.e. steroid injections or radiation, are of no benefit.

CARCINOMA OF THE PENIS

Carcinoma of the penis is rare in developed countries and almost unknown in circumcised males. Poor hygiene and accumulation of smegma are suspected aetiological factors but there is growing evidence of a viral aetiology linked to that of carcinoma of the uterine cervix in females (human papilloma virus).

Histologically, the tumours are squamous cell carcinomas, usually well differentiated, which arise from the inner surface of the foreskin or the glans penis near the coronal sulcus. The tumour invades locally and tends to penetrate the distal urethra (Fig. 33.12a). Metastatic spread is to inguinal lymph nodes (see Fig. 33.12b). **Erythroplasia of Queyrat** is the term given to severe dysplasia and carcinoma-in-situ of the glans that may represent a precursor of invasive carcinoma.

Most cases of carcinoma of the penis are found in the elderly. The disease is usually well advanced before an irregular lump, bleeding or discharge is noticed. In uncircumcised males, the lesion may be hidden by the foreskin. Figure 33.13 illustrates staging of the disease.

Local surgical excision or 'glansectomy' is often performed, with reconstructive surgery if feasible. In advanced cases, 'penectomy', and block dissection of inguinal lymph nodes if they are involved, may be required. Radiotherapy can be used in stage I disease if the urethra is not involved and for palliation in stage IV disease.

CASE HISTORY

Fig. 33.12 **Carcinoma of the penis**

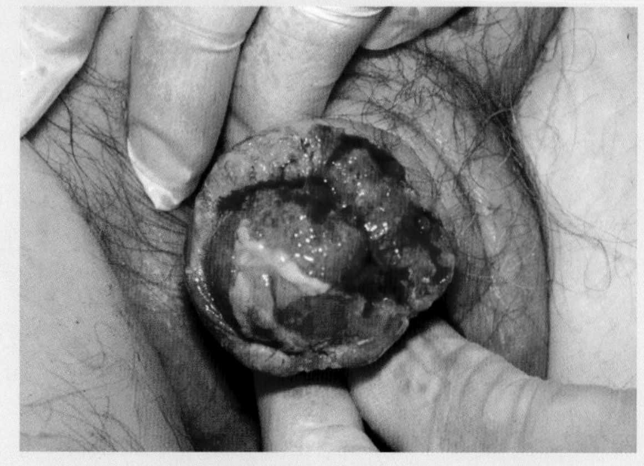

(a)

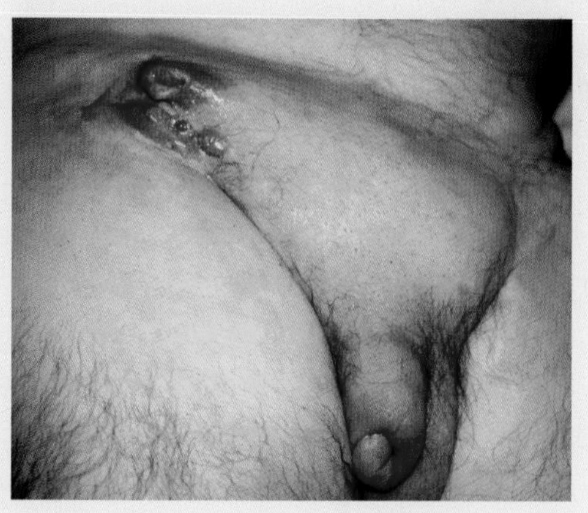

(b)

(a) An obvious carcinoma of the penis, revealed when the foreskin is retracted. **(b)** Unfortunately, this patient already had extensive spread to the inguinal lymph nodes

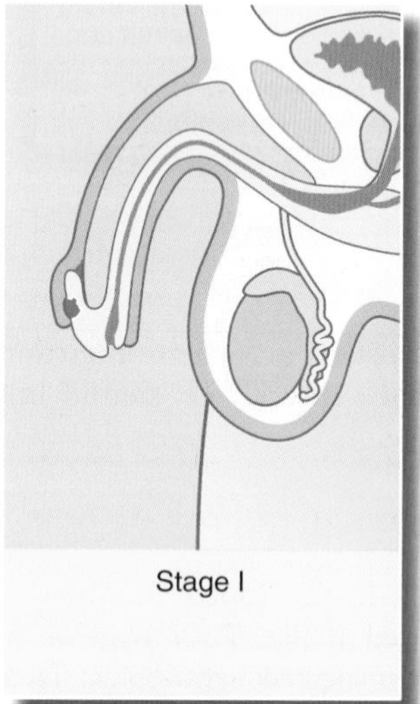

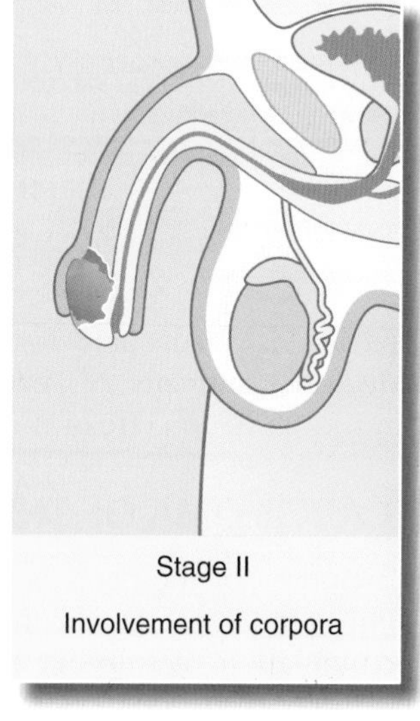

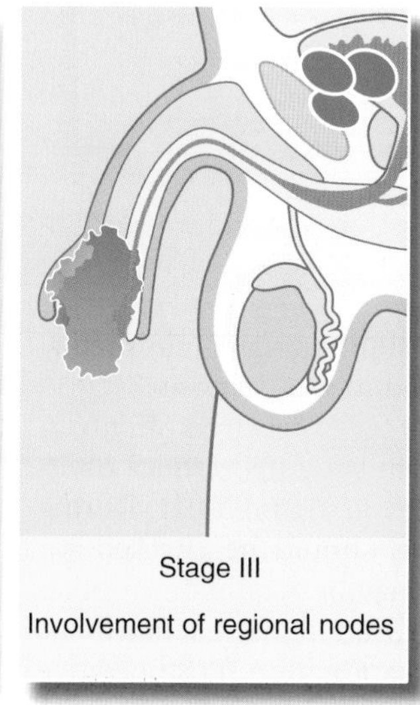

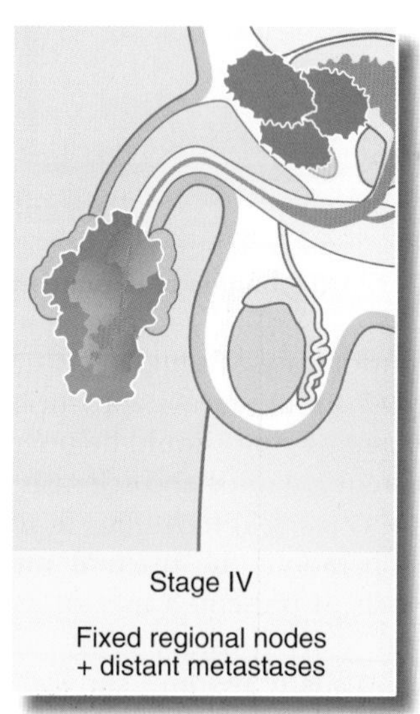

Fig. 33.13 **Stages in the spread of carcinoma of the penis**

PRIAPISM

Priapism is an abnormally prolonged penile erection lasting 4 hours or more. It is usually painful and can occur without sexual stimulation, and does not resolve after ejaculation. The abnormality affects only the **corpora cavernosa** and is caused by a disturbance of mechanisms that control penile detumescence. The corpus spongiosum surrounding the urethra and forming the glans penis is not affected and the glans remains flaccid.

There are two main types of priapism. **High-flow (arterial) priapism** occurs when an artery ruptures into the lacunar spaces of the corpora cavernosa. This is often associated with trauma and is relatively uncommon and painless. Compared with venous priapism, there is less tumescence and it is less painful. **Low-flow (venous) priapism** is due to prolonged corporeal venous stasis caused by occlusion of the venous outlet mechanism (veno-occlusive priapism). This eventually results in penile ischaemia. It is very painful and, unless treated, results in long-term fibrosis and impotence (loss of the ability to achieve an erection). In veno-occlusive priapism, tissue changes that will lead to fibrosis are already evident within 24 hours, whereas there is no such change in arterial priapism.

The most common cause of priapism is a side-effect of injected intracavernosal drugs used to treat erectile dysfunction.

Treatment of veno-occlusive priapism must be prompt to avoid long-term erectile problems. Ice packs and external compression are a useful temporising measure but usually will not give long-term relief. Aspiration of blood from the cavernosa using a butterfly needle is the next step. Intracavernous injection of an alpha-adrenergic agonist (phenylephrine) or oral terbutaline, a beta-2-adrenergic receptor agonist, usually produces detumescence. If these measures are unsuccessful, operative management by means of a surgical shunt may be necessary but results are sometimes disappointing.

UROLOGY

Symptoms, signs and investigation of urinary tract disorders

34

INTRODUCTION

Urinary tract disorders are common and comprise a significant part of the workload of GPs, general physicians, paediatricians and surgeons. Many general surgeons deal with urological problems, which make up about 25% of their workload. Prostate disorders account for at least half of the work in urological surgery. The main conditions are benign prostatic hyperplasia, affecting about 10% of ageing males in Western countries, and prostatic carcinoma, now the second most common cancer in men worldwide and the commonest cancer diagnosed in men in developed countries. The remaining surgical disorders of kidney and urinary tract can be divided into five broad groups: tumours, stone disease (**urolithiasis**), infections, congenital abnormalities and finally, local and systemic disorders secondarily involving the urinary tract.

This chapter deals with the symptoms, signs, approach to investigation and diagnosis of urinary tract disease. The various disease entities are then discussed in the following five chapters.

SYMPTOMS OF URINARY TRACT DISEASE

Urinary symptoms may be caused by intrinsic disease of the urinary tract or by disease of other structures.

SYMPTOMS CAUSED BY INTRINSIC DISEASE OF THE URINARY TRACT

Outflow of urine from the kidney may become impeded by urinary tract obstruction, which may secondarily interfere with renal function. Chronic obstruction to bladder outflow or bilateral upper tract obstruction may lead to renal failure, often without any localising symptoms.

Benign prostatic hyperplasia is the most common prostatic disorder, and usually presents with symptoms of bladder outflow obstruction (i.e. micturition disorders or urinary retention or both) and sometimes with haematuria. Prostatic obstruction predisposes to bladder infections or stones and the patient may present with the consequent symptoms.

Prostate cancer may present with bladder outflow obstruction similar to benign hyperplasia or it may be discovered at an asymptomatic stage at a medical check-up, by digital rectal examination (DRE) or by a blood test (prostate specific antigen, PSA). Some cases are first diagnosed because of symptoms of metastases, such as bone pain.

Chronic prostatitis may be bacterial or abacterial and usually presents with a chronic perineal ache. In the acute form, bacterial prostatitis can present as a systemic illness (or even Gram-negative sepsis) with urinary symptoms and an exquisitely tender prostate. Occasionally, a prostatic abscess develops.

The important urinary tract tumours, stone diseases and infections are outlined in Table 34.1. Any of these may present with haematuria. Disorders which cause urinary stasis also predispose to urinary tract infection.

Congenital abnormalities may involve the kidneys, ureters, bladder, urethra and genitalia, either alone or in combination. Most of the serious abnormalities are recognised antenatally by ultrasound, at birth or in early childhood. The exceptions are **polycystic disease** and **medullary sponge kidney**, which usually present in adulthood. Less serious congenital abnormalities such as duplex systems may predispose to urinary tract infections because of abnormal flow dynamics. These abnormalities may be discovered at any age during investigation of recurrent urinary infections. Congenital disorders which present mainly in adulthood are discussed in Chapter 39 and those presenting mainly in childhood in Chapter 51.

Table 34.1 Pathophysiology and clinical features of urinary tract tumours, stones and infections

Disease	Pathophysiology	Clinical features
Tumours		
Renal cell carcinoma (also known as renal adenocarcinoma and formerly as 'hypernephroma')—fairly common	Occurs in adults. Derived from renal tubular cells	Presents either incidentally (e.g. on CT scan) or with symptoms of haematuria, a mass or constitutional signs such as pyrexia or polycythaemia or is asymptomatic
Nephroblastoma (Wilms' tumour; see Ch. 51)—rare	Developmental origin; usually diagnosed before age 5	Presents as an abnormal mass with or without pain and haematuria
Urothelial carcinoma (transitional cell carcinoma or TCC)—common	May arise in transitional epithelium anywhere in urinary tract from pelvicalyceal system to urethra, but most common in bladder	Usually presents with haematuria. Predisposes to urinary tract infections. May cause ureteric obstruction
Squamous cell carcinoma—very rare	Arises in metaplastic squamous epithelium. Secondary to chronic stone or schistosomal irritation, especially in bladder. Also arises de novo in squamous epithelium of distal urethra	As for transitional cell carcinoma
Adenocarcinoma of bladder—very rare	Arises from columnar epithelium of urachal remnant	As for transitional cell carcinoma
Stone disease		
In general	Stones in situ may cause irritation of urinary tract epithelium	Present as pain or haematuria or recurrent infection
Stones may develop in pelvicalyceal system or bladder. Pelvicalyceal stones can pass into the ureter—very common	Chronic—renal stones may cause chronic pelviureteric or ureteric obstruction either directly or by causing fibrotic strictures Acute—renal stones may cause ureteric obstruction as they pass down the tract	Present with chronic pain (due to back pressure) or recurrent infection Present as acute colicky pain often with renal tenderness (renal or ureteric colic). Infection may supervene, destroying the kidney if untreated
Infections		
'Common' infections due to bowel organisms	Infection develops either via bloodstream (haematogenous) or lower urinary tract stasis predisposes to infection	Typically present with dysuria and frequency with or without haematuria. Any urinary tract abnormality or stasis predisposes to infection Ascending infection may cause pyelonephritis, i.e. infection of kidney and renal pelvis
Tuberculosis—uncommon	Kidney involvement via bloodstream from pulmonary or other primary disease. May spread via urine to ureters and bladder	May present as haematuria, persistent sterile pyuria, or as an incidental finding in pulmonary tuberculosis
Urinary schistosomiasis (also known as bilharzia)—very common in some developing countries; probably the world's most common cause of haematuria	Induces chronic inflammation and fibrosis in bladder wall leading to gross bladder distortion, stones and sometimes squamous cell carcinoma	Presents with haematuria and various symptoms of infection and bladder fibrosis
Urethritis	Usually caused by sexually transmitted infections, e.g. gonococcus or *Chlamydia*	Presents with urethral discharge and dysuria

URINARY SYMPTOMS CAUSED BY NON-URINARY DISEASE

The urinary tract sometimes becomes secondarily involved in local inflammatory conditions such as Crohn's disease or diverticular disease. Fistulae may form, resulting in passage of flatus and/or faeces in the urine (pneumaturia and faecuria). Retroperitoneal fibrosis, diverticulitis, tumours of the prostate, cervix or colon, and sometimes aortic or iliac aneurysms may secondarily involve the ureters and cause upper urinary tract obstruction.

THE COMMON SYMPTOMS OF URINARY TRACT DISEASE

These fall into eight categories:

- Abdominal pain
- Passage of blood in the urine (**haematuria**)

- Pain associated with micturition (**dysuria**)
- Disorders of micturition such as frequency or hesitancy
- Retention of urine (acute or chronic)
- Urinary incontinence
- Passage of bowel gas in the urine (**pneumaturia**)
- Passage of blood in the semen (**haemospermia**)

ABDOMINAL PAIN

Urinary tract disorders may cause abdominal pain with or without urinary symptoms.

Pain arising from the kidneys and upper tract

Both renal inflammation and stretching of the renal capsule cause pain in the renal angle, the posterior gap between the lowest rib and iliac crest. This area may also become tender to palpation or percussion. Renal stones, tumours or polycystic disease may cause dull and persistent loin pain even without obstruction.

In acute infections such as pyelonephritis (affecting renal pelvis and kidney) or bladder infection, the pain is severe and is usually associated with systemic features and urinary tract symptoms.

Acute upper ureteric obstruction and distension of the pelvicalyceal system produce excruciating loin pain. The pain is colicky (resulting from powerful ureteric peristalsis) and often radiates to the hypochondrium (right or left upper quadrant of the abdomen) or groin (see Fig. 34.1). This pain is known as **renal** or **ureteric colic**. When obstruction is low in the ureter, the pain may radiate to the genitalia.

Pain arising from the bladder and lower tract

Pain originating in the bladder (e.g. in cystitis) is experienced in the suprapubic area. Pain may be referred to the penis or vulva if the bladder trigone is involved. In adults, urinary symptoms such as dysuria and frequency are usually present as well, but children may have no localising symptoms or complain only of pain, making the diagnosis less obvious. Dysuria is usually the predominant symptom of urethral disorders, but pain arising in the male urethra (e.g. in sexually transmitted infections) is usually referred to the tip of the penis. Finally, the pain of prostatic inflammation (prostatitis) is usually felt deep in the perineum. The prostate is tender on rectal examination in the acute but not the chronic form.

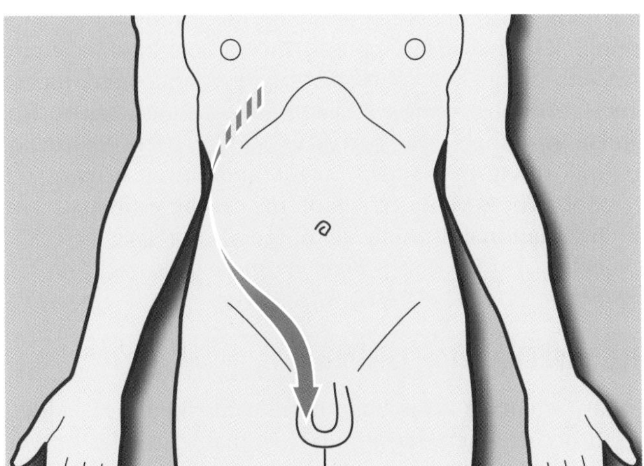

Fig. 34.1 Renal pain and its referral

Pain simulating urinary tract disease

Pain from other abdominal pathology may sometimes mimic pain arising from the urinary tract. Acute appendicitis may present with suprapubic pain, and biliary tract pain may be referred to the right thoracolumbar region, while posterior duodenal ulcers and pancreatic disease may cause pain in the central lumbar region. An expanding or leaking abdominal aortic aneurysm may sometimes mimic urinary tract disease, particularly if a ureter is compressed. Diseases of the thoracolumbar spine, such as metastatic cancer, tuberculosis, spondylosis and disc lesions, may also simulate upper urinary tract disorders. Suspected renal colic with a local rash is usually due to shingles (herpes zoster); the rash may not appear for several days after the onset of pain; perineal zoster may cause retention of urine. In women, pain arising from the ovaries or genital tract (e.g. pelvic inflammatory disease) may be confused with bladder pain.

HAEMATURIA

Patients may notice blood or even clots in the urine (**frank haematuria**) and this needs to be distinguished from urethral bleeding. More often, blood is discovered on 'dipstick' testing or microscopy of a midstream urine specimen (**microscopic haematuria**). Haematuria is often episodic rather than persistent, whatever the cause. 'Dipstick' testing for haematuria is extremely sensitive and yields many false positive results.

CAUSES OF HAEMATURIA

(see Fig. 34.2 for renal causes)

Tumours are a common cause of frank or microscopic haematuria and must be suspected even if another possible cause is found. Haematuria from tumours is typically painless. However, carcinoma-in-situ of the bladder, a dysplastic condition with a high probability of progression to invasive carcinoma, usually presents with irritative voiding, dysuria and haematuria. Irritation from infection or stones may also cause bleeding, but is usually accompanied by pain or dysuria. If the urethra is obstructed by prostatic enlargement, straining at micturition may cause bleeding from dilated veins at the bladder neck.

Trauma to a normal kidney may cause frank haematuria if substantial force has been applied, but microscopic haematuria is common after minor trauma in contact sports and rarely indicates significant injury. Enlarged kidneys are more susceptible to trauma, whatever the primary pathology. In hydronephrosis or polycystic kidneys, minor blunt trauma may cause gross haematuria.

Sometimes urine becomes red with haemoglobin rather than blood. In young people this may be induced by vigorous exercise such as jogging (**exercise haemoglobinuria** and **haematuria**). These patients are believed to have defective

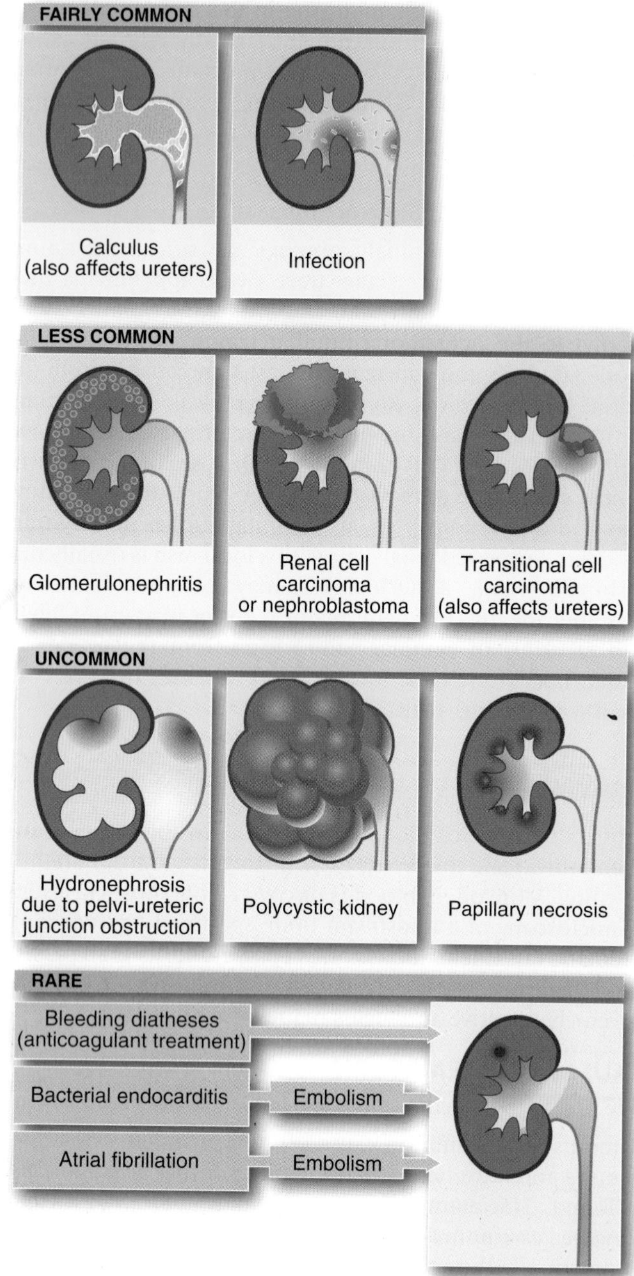

Fig. 34.2 Renal causes of haematuria

red cell membranes which makes them more vulnerable to trauma. Exercise haemoglobinuria is self-limiting and requires no treatment.

Haematuria also occurs in renal parenchymal inflammation such as glomerulonephritis or arteritis. Haematuria may also be caused by microemboli impacting in the kidneys, as in atrial fibrillation or infective endocarditis. Any urinary tract disorder with a potential for haematuria is more likely to be revealed when a patient is on anticoagulant therapy or develops a bleeding diathesis.

DIAGNOSTIC FEATURES OF HAEMATURIA

The stage of micturition at which blood appears is sometimes diagnostically useful. Blood from the kidneys, ureters or bladder wall will completely mix with the urine, and be present throughout the urinary stream. Urethral bleeding may leak out independently of micturition, or be seen only at the beginning or end of the urinary stream. Blood arising from the bladder neck or posterior urethra may sometimes present as terminal haematuria. Gross bleeding may result in the passage of clots.

Haematuria on dipstick testing should be confirmed by urine microscopy for red blood cells, and checked for infection by culture and sensitivity. Microscopic haematuria may represent a noteworthy lesion anywhere in the urinary tract and must be taken seriously; however, a significant cause is found in only 5–25% of patients.

DYSURIA

Dysuria describes pain or discomfort on micturition, often accompanied by difficulty in voiding. The pain is often described as 'burning' or 'scalding'. Any irritation of the urethra may cause dysuria. The most common cause is urinary tract infection, but recent urethral instrumentation or catheterisation can also cause dysuria.

DISORDERS OF MICTURITION

The normal bladder has a capacity of 350–500 ml. When this is reached, the detrusor muscle undergoes reflex contraction, initiating the desire to void. Micturition is normally initiated by conscious sphincter relaxation; detrusor contraction then empties the bladder completely. There are six common symptoms of disorders of micturition:

- Urinary frequency
- Nocturia
- Urgency
- Hesitancy
- Poor urinary stream
- Post-micturition dribbling

Features and common causes of these symptoms are summarized in Table 34.2.

LOWER URINARY TRACT SYMPTOMS (LUTS)

This term encompasses the symptoms of hesitancy, poor stream, terminal dribbling and incomplete bladder emptying with frequency, nocturia, urgency and urge incontinence. Although these occur in prostatic obstruction, similar symptoms also occur in bladder neck obstruction, urethral stricture, bladder calculi and lower urinary tract infection. The severity of symptoms can be estimated using the International Prostate Symptom Score (see Box 35.1, p. 446).

RETENTION OF URINE

Urinary retention is the inability to void when the bladder is full. It occurs when the sphincter is unable to relax or when there is proximal urethral obstruction, and the two causes may coexist.

Table 34.2 Symptoms of disorders of micturition

Symptom	Description	Causes
Urinary frequency	Frequent passage of small quantities of urine but with normal daily urine volume (unlike in polyuria)	**Bladder irritation** — infection (common), carcinoma-in-situ of bladder **Incomplete bladder emptying** — bladder outflow obstruction (prostatic hyperplasia), neurological (e.g. multiple sclerosis) **Overactive bladder** (detrusor instability) — sensitive voiding reflex **Small or indistensible bladder** — surgery, fibrosis (e.g., tuberculosis, schistosomiasis, radiotherapy) **Psychosomatic** (daytime only)
Nocturia	The need to pass urine at night, usually accompanied by frequency or polyuria	**Cardiac failure** — peripheral oedema returning to systemic circulation when supine **Old age** — enhanced renal blood flow when recumbent **Drugs** — e.g. some calcium channel blockers
Urgency	Sudden desire to void, may result in incontinence	**Cystitis** — bladder neck irritation **Prostatic hyperplasia** — abnormal entry of urine into proximal urethra, high detrusor pressure due to bladder outflow obstruction
Hesitancy	Difficulty in initiating micturition	**Prostatic hyperplasia** — insufficient urine entry into proximal urethra to cause sphincter relaxation **Psychosomatic** — often situational (e.g., in a urinal) in young males
Poor urinary stream	Slow or interrupted urine stream	**Urethral compression** — prostatic hyperplasia, bladder neck hypertrophy **Urethral stricture** — due to inflammation and scarring
Post-micturition dribbling	Continued flow of urine drops at the end of micturition, may amount to incontinence	**Weak bulbospongiosus muscle** — incomplete emptying of urethra **Abnormal sphincter function** **Pelvic floor weakness (women)**

ACUTE RETENTION

Acute urinary retention is often very painful and occasionally occurs in normal individuals, usually males, particularly postoperatively, when fluid overload, drugs, pain, the supine posture, anxiety or embarrassment are responsible. Similar factors may precipitate an episode in men with asymptomatic prostatic enlargement. Occasionally acute retention is caused by an obstructing blood clot (**clot retention**) or stone.

In females, acute urinary retention may also occur in pregnancy if the enlarging uterus becomes wedged in the pelvis at about 14 weeks' gestation. Large ovarian cysts or uterine fibroids may cause similar obstruction. Other possible causes include neurological disorders such as sacral nerve injury, herpes zoster and multiple sclerosis.

CHRONIC RETENTION

Chronic retention is often painless and occurs with structural or functional abnormalities of bladder muscle or the sphincter mechanism. Less commonly, it is caused by persistent urethral obstruction. In chronic retention, voiding of urine is often incomplete. The problem progresses until the residual volume approaches maximum bladder capacity. Voiding then usually occurs by 'overflow' and the bladder usually becomes abnormally distended. When obstruction is prolonged and severe, the bladder muscle hypertrophies, bladder diverticula may develop, and back pressure on the kidneys can cause uraemia and renal failure. At any stage, complete cessation of flow, i.e. **acute-on-chronic retention**, may be precipitated by overfilling (often alcohol-induced), urinary tract infection or constipation. The most common cause of chronic retention is bladder outflow obstruction caused by a hypertrophied bladder neck or prostatic enlargement. It may also be caused by lower spinal neurological problems, e.g. central protrusion of lumbar intervertebral discs damaging the S2, 3, 4 detrusor muscle innervation.

URINARY INCONTINENCE

Involuntary passage of urine is a distressing and socially debilitating symptom. The normal bladder has a capacity of approximately 350–500 ml. During filling, the detrusor muscle relaxes so the intravesical pressure does not rise until bladder capacity is approached. Once the bladder is filled, voiding occurs by detrusor contraction and sphincter relaxation. Both are mediated via a spinal reflex at the level of S2, 3, 4. Superimposed on this system is an inhibitory mechanism under cortical (conscious) control, to delay voiding if it is socially inappropriate. Conscious control, including nocturnal control, develops during early childhood. Nocturnal incontinence is known as **enuresis**.

The pathophysiology of incontinence can be divided into three categories based on disorders of structure and function which are described below and summed up in Box 34.1. Some disease processes may produce incontinence by more than one mechanism.

LOSS OF CORTICAL CONTROL

Loss of inhibitory control over reflex voiding may occur in disease of the cortex, such as the dementias, or in spinal cord disease above the sacral reflex level, such as multiple sclerosis. Traumatic paraplegia is a common cause of complete loss of cortical control. The resulting incontinence may be described as a **suprasacral neurogenic bladder**. The bladder fills to normal capacity and then empties spontaneously, more or less completely, leaving little residual urine.

DISORDERS OF SACRAL REFLEX CONTROL OF DETRUSOR AND SPHINCTER FUNCTION

If the sacral reflex arc is damaged on either afferent or efferent sides, reflex contraction of the detrusor and relaxation of the sphincter are lost. This may occur in low spinal trauma or systemic or local disease such as myelomeningocoele, diabetic neuropathy or invasive pelvic tumours. The bladder becomes grossly distended and urine passively overflows causing constant **dribbling incontinence**. This can be improved by regular manual emptying of the bladder by abdominal pressure, or more effectively by intermittent self-catheterisation (ISC). This form of incontinence is described as **sacral neurogenic bladder**. The large residual urine volume predisposes to infection and should be emptied regularly if possible.

In some patients, typically middle-aged women, reflex control of detrusor activity becomes hypersensitive so the voiding reflex is initiated when bladder filling is well below full capacity. This hypersensitivity results in small volumes of urine being passed frequently and precipitously to produce **urge incontinence**. The condition is known as **overactive bladder** or **detrusor overactivity** and can lead to a minor but upsetting form of incontinence.

Bladder infection produces excessive sensory irritation and activation of the voiding reflex. In young children and the elderly, this may be responsible for incontinence with none of the usual symptoms of infection.

Persistent bladder outflow obstruction due to prostatic enlargement causes progressive stretching of the bladder and damages the voiding reflex. The result can be a hugely distended, flaccid, **hypotonic bladder**. Dribbling overflow incontinence may persist even when the obstruction has been removed.

Box 34.1 Causes of incontinence of urine

Loss of cortical control

- Cortical disease
- Spinal cord disease, i.e. supra-sacral neurogenic bladder

Abnormalities of the sacral reflex mechanism

- Sacral neurogenic bladder
- Overactive bladder
- Infection producing bladder hyperactivity
- Hypotonic bladder

Detrusor or sphincter abnormalities

- Stress incontinence
- Post-prostatectomy
- Tumour invasion
- Urethral trauma
- Contracted bladder
- Rare congenital abnormalities

STRUCTURAL ABNORMALITIES OF THE BLADDER OR SPHINCTER

The most common condition in this category is **stress incontinence**, in which the sphincter is weak. Any sudden increase in pressure on the bladder (such as coughing, sneezing or laughing) causes small quantities of urine to leak out. Stress incontinence is usually seen in parous women and results from pelvic floor damage during childbirth. There is often a degree of uterine prolapse and cystocoele. Various operations can alleviate this.

Prostatectomy (transurethral or open) may damage the sphincter, as may locally invasive tumours or pelvic fractures involving the proximal urethra. Tuberculosis, radiotherapy and **interstitial cystitis** in its severest form may cause severe bladder contraction and frequency to the point of incontinence.

Incontinence is a feature of several rare congenital abnormalities such as epispadias or an ectopic ureter opening below the sphincter mechanism. These should be excluded in a child who fails to develop continence.

PNEUMATURIA

Pneumaturia is the passage of gas mixed with urine. It is caused by abnormal communication between bowel and urinary tract resulting in fistula formation. The commonest causes are diverticular disease and Crohn's disease, although it can also occur in carcinoma of the colon or bladder (see Box 34.2). Gross urinary tract infection is inevitable. The patient typically complains of symptoms of urinary infection (dysuria and frequency) and may also describe bubbles or even faeces in the urine.

Box 34.2 Causes of vesicocolic fistula and pneumaturia

- Diverticular disease and pericolic abscess bursting into bladder (most common cause)
- Carcinoma of bladder invading colon
- Colonic carcinoma invading bladder
- Crohn's disease inflammation fistulating into bladder

HAEMOSPERMIA

Haemospermia describes the presence of blood in semen. It is usually innocent but can be caused by prostatitis or a stone in an ejaculatory duct. In the older male patient it is a rare presenting symptom of prostatic carcinoma.

APPROACH TO THE DIAGNOSIS OF URINARY SYMPTOMS

SPECIAL POINTS IN THE HISTORY

A detailed history of the urinary tract symptoms should be taken, together with a general history to elucidate any systemic causes or contributing factors, e.g. diabetes or multiple sclerosis. A full history of medication, past and present, should be recorded.

In patients with haematuria, the occupational history may be important. Exposure to aniline dyes and other industrial chemicals that were once widely used in the rubber and cable industries greatly increase the risk of urothelial carcinoma (transitional cell carcinoma) of the urinary tract. Tobacco smoking is estimated to cause 50% of bladder cancers.

Haematuria can also be caused by infestation with *Schistosoma*, which is endemic in parts of the Middle East and Africa and is transmitted by water snails. A history of residence or travel in affected regions should therefore be sought. Similarly, tuberculosis is common in developing countries and can easily be overlooked in immigrants.

PHYSICAL EXAMINATION

GENERAL EXAMINATION

A full general examination should pay special attention to a sallow complexion and signs of weight loss which could indicate uraemia, particularly if accompanied by a uriniferous smell and scratch marks indicating itching. Blood pressure must be measured in every case as hypertension may be a feature of pyelonephritis, renal artery stenosis, polycystic kidneys or glomerulonephritis.

ABDOMINAL EXAMINATION

Abdominal inspection may reveal asymmetry due to a large renal mass; this may be a nephroblastoma in a child or polycystic kidneys in an adult. In chronic retention, a large, sometimes asymmetrical bladder may be visible. The loins should be carefully inspected from the back; a subtle fullness may indicate a renal mass or a perinephric abscess.

A bimanual technique is used when examining the abdomen for kidney enlargement. One hand palpates the subcostal region anteriorly while the other hand is placed posteriorly in the renal angle to push the kidney forward on to the palpating hand. The kidneys are impalpable unless they are enlarged or displaced, except in a very thin patient. A renal mass may move with respiration and, because it is retroperitoneal with bowel anteriorly, should also have an area of resonance on percussion overlying it. The main causes of an enlarged kidney are hydronephrosis, polycystic disease, renal cell carcinoma and nephroblastoma (Wilms' tumour) in children. Loin tenderness is uncommon in non-acute renal disorders except in chronic perinephric abscess. Tenderness is usually found in acute conditions, such as pyelonephritis or acute obstruction. Renal tenderness can be distinguished from vertebral tenderness by gently tapping the spinous processes. This will cause pain if the tenderness is vertebral.

The lower abdomen is palpated for an enlarged or distended bladder, which is felt as a soft mass arising from the pelvis, sometimes asymmetrically. It is dull to percussion and pressure on it may induce an urge to void; bladder distension is easily confirmed on ultrasound examination. A suprapubic mass in the male usually indicates urinary retention, but occasionally it is a colonic carcinoma or a large bladder tumour or stone (all firm to palpation). In the female, ovarian masses, pregnancy or uterine fibroids are more common causes of a suprapubic mass than urinary retention. Finally, auscultation along the 12th rib posteriorly may reveal the bruit of renal artery stenosis.

RECTAL EXAMINATION

Rectal examination should be performed in both sexes. In females, a vaginal examination may also be indicated. In the male, the prostate is palpated per rectum for size, shape and consistency (Fig. 34.3). The normal prostate is about 3 cm in diameter and weighs 10–15 g; it can be massively enlarged and weigh over several hundred grams, so that its upper edge may be out of reach of the examining finger. Most prostatectomy operations leave a capsular remnant so that the prostate appears palpable after prostatectomy and may be of a firmer consistency.

The severity of prostatic obstructive symptoms depends not on the prostatic diameter but on the extent of encroachment upon the urethra. In some cases, an enlarged median lobe lying posteriorly above the bladder outlet may act as a flap valve, intermittently obstructing urine outflow.

On palpation, the normal prostate has a smooth surface and a firm consistency and is divided into two lateral lobes by a midline groove. In prostatic hyperplasia, enlargement is usually symmetrical, and the midline groove is maintained. Consistency remains normal. In contrast, a prostate infiltrated with carcinoma is irregular and asymmetrical. There are often hard nodules, and the median groove may be lost. In advanced cases, the tumour may be felt invading laterally into the pelvis or posteriorly around the rectum (see Fig. 34.4). Digital examination can help distinguish benign from malignant prostatic enlargement in gross cases, but if carcinoma is suspected, **transrectal ultrasound scanning (TRUS)** using a rectal probe is performed, together with multiple needle biopsies under ultrasound guidance. Note, however, that there is a 2% risk of systemic sepsis and the procedure needs to be covered with a short course of antibiotics, e.g. ciprofloxacin. The symptom of prostatic tenderness is uncommon and may indicate prostatitis.

INVESTIGATION OF SUSPECTED URINARY TRACT DISEASE

In common conditions like prostatic hyperplasia or urinary tract infection, the diagnosis is usually evident from the history and examination. Symptoms such as haematuria, however, suggest several diagnostic possibilities and other diagnoses must be excluded.

A simple approach to investigation of urinary tract disease is to consider the following questions:

- Are any blood tests likely to be helpful in diagnosis?
- What urine tests are indicated?
- Where is the lesion?

ARE ANY BLOOD TESTS LIKELY TO BE HELPFUL IN DIAGNOSIS?

Blood tests that can be useful are summarised in Box 34.3.

When prostate cancer is suspected, **prostate specific antigen (PSA)** levels should be estimated and fractionated into **free PSA**, **total PSA** and their **ratio**. The free PSA is more likely to be raised in carcinoma and is a reliable indicator if the level is markedly elevated, although the higher the level, the greater the volume of cancer. In biopsy-proven prostatic cancer, persistently raised PSA levels above 20 are likely to indicate metastatic disease. However, the level may be normal in the presence of a small-volume cancer.

Total PSA rises with age and, in benign hyperplasia, tends to rise in proportion to prostate mass. Acute retention, urinary tract infection, any urethral instrumentation or biopsy of the prostate causes elevation of the PSA for up to 6 weeks; standard digital rectal examination does not affect PSA level.

WHAT URINE TESTS ARE INDICATED?

Any urinary symptoms should prompt collection of a clean **midstream urine (MSU) specimen** for microscopy and bacteriology. Microscopy will show the presence or absence of significant numbers of red blood cells (**microscopic haematuria**), white cells (**pyuria**) and bacteria (**bacteriuria**). However, the cells can lyse if the specimen is kept overnight at room temperature.

Bacteriuria of more than 5×10^5 per cubic millimetre is considered to indicate significant infection. The urine is cultured to identify the organisms, and organisms are tested for antibiotic sensitivity. Culture-negative urine (**sterile pyuria**) is characteristic of urinary tract tuberculosis, urinary stone, bladder tumour, prostatitis or (most commonly) a partly treated urinary tract infection. In sterile pyuria, three early morning urine specimens should be examined for acid-fast

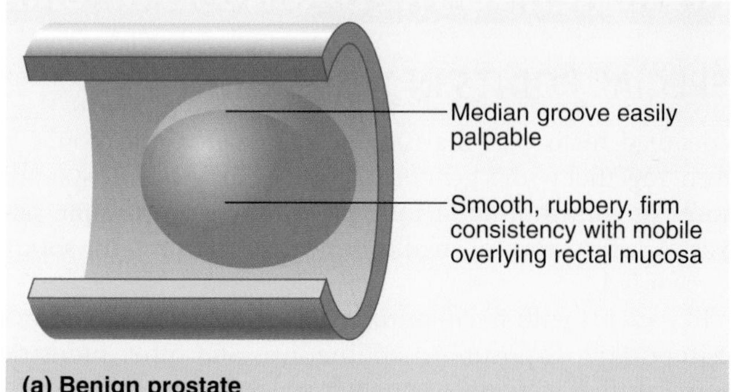

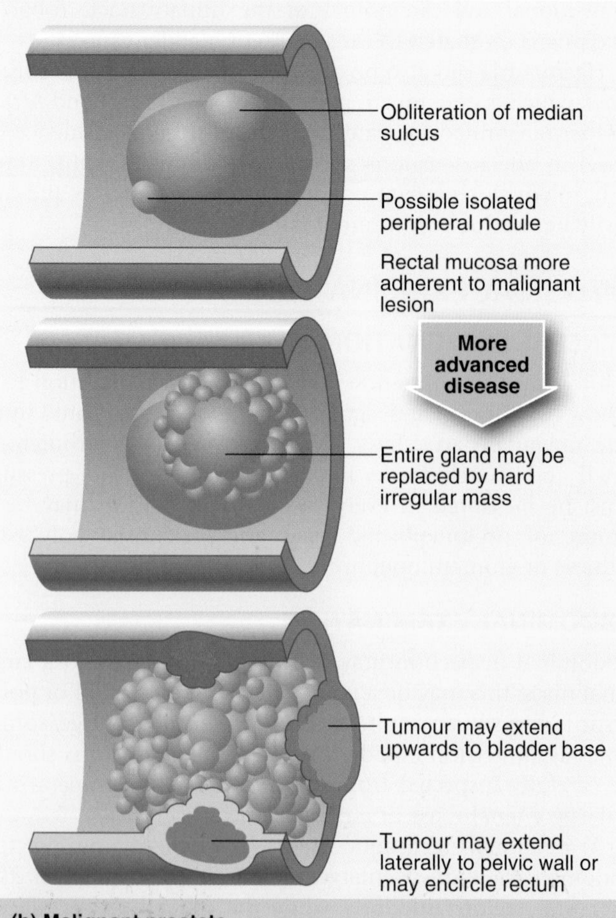

Fig. 34.3 Palpation characteristics of the prostate
(a) Benign. **(b)** Malignant

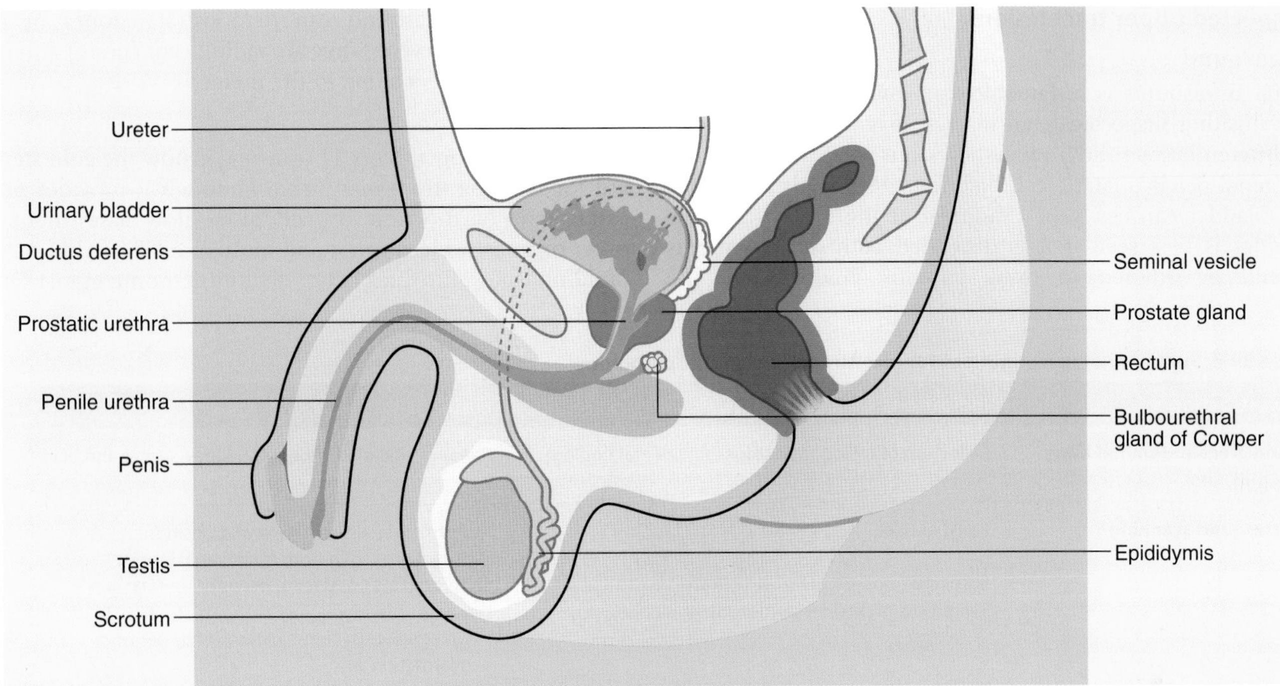

Fig. 34.4 Relationship of the prostate to the rectum and peritoneal cavity

Box 34.3 Blood tests useful in diagnosing urinary tract disease

Full blood count

- Hypochromic microcytic anaemia—chronic iron deficiency anaemia due to haematuria (rare)
- Normochromic normocytic anaemia—chronic renal failure (lack of erythropoietin), chronic inflammatory disorders, e.g. tuberculosis
- Polycythaemia—renal adenocarcinoma
- Leucocytosis—infection

Erythrocyte sedimentation rate (ESR) and C-reactive protein (CRP)

- Raised in chronic and acute infections, renal adenocarcinoma and retroperitoneal fibrosis

Urea, electrolytes and creatinine

- Impaired renal function in bilateral obstructive uropathy or chronic renal failure associated with hypertension, diabetes, etc.

Prostate specific antigen

- Raised in carcinoma of prostate. A normal level does not exclude prostatic carcinoma. Moderate elevations occur in benign disease, especially with acute retention of urine, urinary tract infection and following urethral instrumentation or prostatic biopsy

Alkaline phosphatase (bone isoenzyme)

- Raised in multiple bony metastases from any type of tumour

Calcium, phosphate, uric acid and parathyroid hormone levels

- Useful investigations in stone disease

bacilli and cultured. **Bacteriuria without significant pyuria** usually indicates contamination of the urine specimen. **Casts** found on microscopy suggest a nephritic (renal inflammatory) process. The presence of epithelial cells indicates perineal contamination of the specimen, a common problem in females and infants.

Urine cytology is a useful screening test for urothelial tumours in people at high risk, particularly those who have been exposed to industrial carcinogens. The test has a high positivity in carcinoma-in-situ and poorly differentiated tumours. Cytology needs to be performed on freshly voided urine. Some centres with an efficient local service use cytology for long-term follow-up of patients with treated bladder cancer.

WHERE IS THE LESION?

Investigations for localising urinary tract pathology are summarised in Table 34.3.

Suspected upper tract lesions

Ultrasound

Renal ultrasound is a valuable non-invasive technique for investigating suspected renal masses. It is particularly useful in differentiating solid from cystic lesions and for demonstrating renal pelvis dilatation. If bladder pathology is suspected, the bladder can easily be examined at the same time. The bladder is best seen if it is distended with urine; patients should be advised to drink copious fluids before the investigation. Ultrasound can demonstrate stones in the kidney or bladder even if they are radiolucent (urate), but can rarely demonstrate a stone in the ureter.

CT scanning

Computed tomography (CT) scanning is now the gold standard for imaging the urinary tract, although it provides poor assessment of function. It will also allow assessment of other organs. Modern spiral and multislice CT machines give rapid image capture and better definition; non-contrast CT is

Table 34.3 Summary of investigations for localising urinary tract pathology

Investigation	Indications	Findings
Plain erect abdominal X-ray ('KUB' film)	Follow-up of radiopaque stones (incidental finding)	Renal calcification; stones in kidney, ureter and bladder
Ultrasound scanning	Renal masses Suspected upper tract obstruction Symptoms of bladder outflow obstruction Transrectal ultrasound (TRUS) for assessing prostatic symptoms or enlargement Chronic renal disease and chronic urinary obstruction General investigation of urinary symptoms Investigation of urethral strictures	Abnormal renal size, shape and position Differentiates solid from cystic renal lesions Shows dilatation of renal pelvis or ureters Estimates bladder volume after micturition; bladder wall thickness; complications of upper tract obstruction Useful for assessing the size of the gland and guiding biopsy needles Thickness of renal cortex Morphology of upper tracts and bladder Definition of stricture and periurethral fibrosis
CT scanning (plus intravenous contrast)	Renal mass suspicious of tumour Palpable loin mass; differentiation of a pelvic mass from a prostatic or bladder tumour Loin pain (CT without contrast may be used specifically to detect renal and ureteric stones) (CQ)	Abnormal mass and blood supply typical of renal tumour Size, nature of lesions and extent of invasion Definition of cause particularly in calculous disease
Intravenous urography (with or without tomography)	Haematuria Suspected urinary tract stone	If tumour present, may show non-functioning part of cortex and/or distorted anatomy Back pressure effects of obstruction on upper tract; position of stone
Special contrast examinations of upper tract, e.g. retrograde or percutaneous (antegrade) ureterography	Obstruction of upper urinary tract not shown by other means	Site and perhaps nature of obstruction
Micturating cystography	Recurrent urinary tract infections or 'failure to thrive' in children	Severity of vesicoureteric reflux
Radionuclide renal scans	Definition of renal blood flow, function or morphology Diagnosis or follow-up of upper tract obstruction Vesicoureteric reflex	Renal morphology, excretory function (total and differential), presence and sites of obstruction Indirect evidence of vesicoureteric reflux
Radionuclide bone scans	Bone pain in (suspected or diagnosed) prostatic carcinoma	Bony metastases
Cystourethroscopy (with or without biopsy or bladder resection)	Haematuria Investigation of bladder neck obstruction and treatment, e.g. transurethral resection of bladder neck or prostate Treatment of bladder stones	Urothelial tumours of urethra or bladder Visual inspection of bladder neck and prostate Litholapaxy (stone crushing)
Ureteroscopy	Ureteric problems, particularly stones	Direct visualisation of ureter and guidance for instrumentation to destroy or retrieve stones

Table 34.3 Continued

Investigation	Indications	Findings
Urine flow rate	Measurement and charting of urinary flow in bladder outlet obstruction Poor flow indicates obstruction or poorly functioning detrusor	Assessment before and after prostatectomy or bladder neck incision
Cystometrography (usually video)	Investigation of incontinence Sometimes used in assessment of bladder outflow obstruction and results of treatment	Nature of incontinence To confirm bladder outflow obstruction in equivocal outflow obstruction To demonstrate overactive bladder (detrusor instability) in irritative voiding
Renal arteriography	Occasional use in renal tumours	Demonstrating abnormal tumour blood supply (rarely used nowadays) Therapeutic embolisation for bleeding or pain in inoperable tumours or prior to surgery

indicated for investigation of stone disease, particularly ureteric colic. CT with intravenous contrast helps distinguish renal malignancy from hamartomas and other benign diseases. It can also diagnose the rare **angiomyolipoma** of the kidney. In renal cell carcinoma, CT can demonstrate direct spread along the renal vein and into the inferior vena cava so that surgery can be better planned. Enlarged lymph nodes may be diagnosed and biopsied percutaneously and the liver examined for metastases. In bladder or prostatic cancer, CT can aid staging by demonstrating whether the disease is **organ-confined**.

Intravenous urography

In most centres, intravenous urography (IVU) has been superseded by CT for renal tract investigation. IVU involves intravenous injection of a contrast medium which is rapidly filtered by the glomeruli and excreted. This radiopaque solution opacifies the urinary system, demonstrating renal parenchyma, renal pelvis and the ureteric anatomy. The cortical concentration of contrast (**nephrogram**) gives an indication of the size, shape, thickness and bilateral symmetry of the renal cortex.

Cysts and tumours of the kidneys are usually revealed by the distortion of normal anatomy, but may be indistinguishable by this investigation. Tumours opacify with contrast to a variable extent and sometimes show a characteristic 'vascular blush'.

A dilated collecting system (renal pelvis, calyces and ureter) is usually easily seen on IVU and the level of an obstruction can often be demonstrated. When obstruction is almost complete, films may have to be taken at long intervals as back pressure delays cortical excretion.

Urothelial carcinoma may show as filling defects in the collecting system or bladder. If an abnormality is seen in the kidney or renal pelvis, **renal CT** is recommended to reveal more detail (see Ch. 5). If renal excretion is poor as in chronic renal failure, IVU yields poor images. In addition, the contrast material may lead to further impairment of renal function. Intravenous contrast is liable to precipitate acute renal failure in diabetic nephropathy. In such cases, retrograde pyelography may be a suitable alternative.

Special contrast investigations

Ascending ureterography, in which contrast is injected directly up the ureters via a cystoscope, is especially useful for defining ureteric tumours. Its use has radically declined as radiological experience and technologies have advanced.

Radionuclide scanning

Radionuclide scanning can be used to assess differential renal function and is particularly useful in monitoring function after relief of obstruction. Scans can demonstrate renal scars and are a non-invasive method of demonstrating vesicoureteric reflux in children.

Suspected lower tract lesions

Radiography and ultrasound

Ultrasound examination is the standard investigation. Modern high-resolution equipment can demonstrate tumours, cysts and other abnormalities of bladder and prostate shape and volume, but can seldom define lesions smaller than 5 mm. Ultrasonography can also define the size, shape and position of stones in the kidney, but is very operator dependent. It can also be used to estimate the bladder residual urine volume in outlet obstruction. **Transrectal ultrasound** can help assess the size of the prostate, enable directed biopsy of abnormal areas, or help achieve representative biopsies of all areas of the prostate.

Cystourethroscopy

Cystourethroscopy (cystoscopy), using rigid or flexible instruments, is an important diagnostic and therapeutic tool for disease of the urethra, prostate and bladder. Flexible cystoscopy can usually be performed under local anaesthesia on an outpatient basis.

A similar but longer rigid instrument, the **ureteroscope**, is used for retrieving stones from the ureter; a flexible ureteroscope allows passage to the kidney and treatment of calyceal stones by laser lithotripsy.

When a bladder tumour or urethral pathology is suspected, **cystoscopy** is the investigation of choice. Flexible cystoscopy allows direct visual examination, but if biopsy and immediate treatment are known to be required, rigid cystoscopy is usually performed under general or regional anaesthesia; this also permits deep bimanual palpation (EUA: examination under anaesthesia).

Other investigations

If clinical examination suggests local spread of a bladder or prostatic tumour, **CT** or **MRI scanning** can assess the extent of invasion. In carcinoma of prostate, **radionuclide scanning** is the most accurate non-invasive method for diagnosing and locating bony metastases.

In perineal injuries and pelvic fractures, **urethrography** is best for assessing suspected urethral rupture and may be combined with **suprapubic contrast cystography**. It is also used for urethral stricture examination. For suspected urethral obstruction, **contrast urethrography** or urethral ultrasound can localise the site of obstruction or stricture. If a colovesical fistula is suspected, **barium enema** may demonstrate the colonic lesion responsible (but rarely the fistula itself).

Urine flow rate provides a rapid assessment of the amount of outflow obstruction and can also assess response to treatment. It is easily measured and can be plotted on a graph as voiding progresses. The patient simply passes urine into a funnel leading to the machine, although volumes voided below 150 ml can be misleading. When incontinence and bladder overactivity are being investigated, **urodynamic studies** can assess the relationship between bladder pressure and volume. They are particularly useful in the case of high-pressure bladders with outlet obstruction and in diagnosing urge and stress incontinence.

Disorders of the prostate

35

INTRODUCTION

Benign hyperplasia and carcinoma are the most common prostatic disorders and have an increasing importance in an ageing population. Inflammation and infection of the prostate (**prostatitis**) is a less common condition that occurs in a younger age group and is rather poorly defined clinically.

ANATOMY

The normal prostate gland is about 3 cm long and 3 cm in diameter and weighs 10–15 g. The gland is situated immediately below the bladder neck so that the first 3 cm of the urethra lies within the gland (Fig. 35.1, p. 452) so the proximal urethral walls (the **prostatic urethra**) are composed of glandular tissue. The urethra then passes through the pelvic floor muscle that also constitutes the distal sphincteric mechanism. Prostatic hyperplasia or carcinoma may cause local urethral obstruction and carcinoma may invade and disrupt the sphincter mechanism.

The posterior aspect of the gland is palpable rectally (Fig. 35.1, pp. 450, 451) and a **median groove** can usually be identified. This groove is described as dividing the gland into two lateral lobes and tends to be obliterated in advanced prostatic cancer but is usually exaggerated in benign hypertrophy.

When the prostatic urethra is examined cystoscopically (see Fig. 35.3, p. 450), an important landmark is an elongated mound on the posterior wall known as the **veru montanum** (urethral crest), which can be variable in size and prominence. At its midpoint is a small depression, sometimes visible, into which the two **ejaculatory ducts** open. The posterior part of the gland above the ejaculatory ducts is known as the **median lobe**. If this becomes hypertrophied it may extend into the floor of the bladder (the surgical 'middle lobe'); this may act as a flap valve and obstruct the bladder outlet.

As seen in Figure 35.1, the bulk of the normal prostate consists of up to 50 peripheral **glandular lobules**. These converge into about 20 separate ducts opening into the prostatic urethra lateral to the veru montanum. As well as this glandular tissue proper, there is a zone of small para-urethral glands adjacent to the urethra, the **transition zone**. From middle age onwards, the transition zone tends to enlarge to cause **benign prostatic hyperplasia**. At the same time, the peripheral glandular tissue is compressed to form a fibrous outer 'surgical capsule'. In contrast, prostate cancer arises most often in the peripheral glandular tissue, tending to spread outwards into bordering structures more often than obstructing the centrally located urethra. Even after prostatectomy, cancer can arise in the residual peripheral zone.

The normal prostate gland is surrounded by a filmy **true capsule** of little surgical significance; external to this is a rich venous plexus which, in turn, is invested by a dense fascial sheath. During open or endoscopic prostatectomy, it is important not to disturb this venous plexus as it is a common source of bleeding during and after the operation. There are direct venous connections between the plexus and the vertebral extradural plexus which provide a direct route for blood-borne dissemination of prostate cancer. Posteriorly, the prostatic fascial sheath is fused with the dense **fascia of Denonvilliers**. This provides a barrier against direct spread of cancer from the prostate to the rectum and vice versa.

BENIGN PROSTATIC HYPERPLASIA

Benign prostatic hyperplasia (BPH) affects half of all men aged 50, and the proportion increases with advancing age so that BPH is almost universal at 70 years. Approximately half of those with BPH are asymptomatic or have only mild symptoms. In about 50% of men over 60, however, hyperplasia produces enough symptoms for treatment to be considered.

PATHOPHYSIOLOGY OF BENIGN PROSTATIC HYPERPLASIA

In pathological terms, the para-urethral transition zone glands undergo **nodular hyperplasia**. This causes progressive symmetrical enlargement of the gland up to several times its normal size (up to 150 g).

The prostate volume cannot be reliably estimated by digital examination and is best assessed by ultrasound. However, there is little relationship between prostatic volume and symptoms; the presence of a large prostate without symptoms is not an indication for treatment. Urine flow rate is determined by the calibre and length of the prostatic

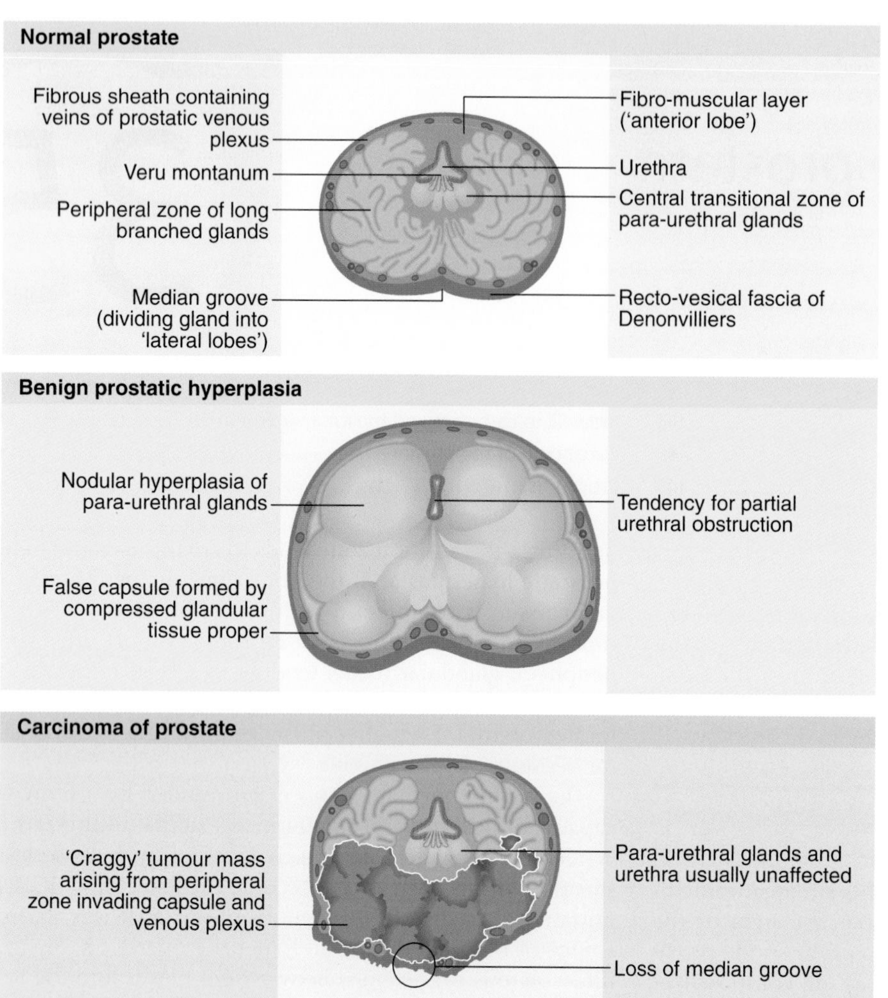

Fig. 35.1 Horizontal sections through normal, hyperplastic and malignant prostate glands

urethra and by detrusor contractility, not by prostatic bulk. Prostatic urethroscopy provides further anatomical detail but no functional information.

CLINICAL FEATURES OF BENIGN PROSTATIC HYPERPLASIA

Symptoms and signs of bladder outflow obstruction (summarised in Box 35.1) are usually gradual in onset. Benign causes are prostatic hyperplasia and the apparently independent disorder of **bladder neck hypertrophy and fibrosis**. **Acute retention** of urine may occur suddenly at any time and is commonly precipitated by bladder overfilling after excessive fluid intake. It is also a hazard of many general surgical or orthopaedic operations on older men and also of any pelvic or perineal operations after adolescence. In some patients, the severity of prostatic symptoms fluctuates from month to month (and even perhaps with the season), making it difficult to decide whether an operation is necessary.

COMPLICATIONS OF BLADDER OUTLET OBSTRUCTION

Prostatic obstruction can progressively interfere with the patient's ability to empty his bladder but only 20–30%

Box 35.1 Symptoms of bladder outlet obstruction

Symptoms formally assessed using the International Prostate Symptom Score (I-PSS). Each symptom is graded from 1 to 5 (up to 6 for nocturia) for the previous month. The total indicates the severity of symptoms: 0–7 = mild; 8–19 = moderate; 20–35 = severe

- Incomplete bladder emptying after urination
- Frequency—need for urination again after less than 2 hours
- Intermittent flow—stopping and starting during urination
- Urgency—difficult to postpone urination
- Weak stream—often made worse by a full bladder or by straining
- Straining to begin urination
- Nocturia—number of times needing to urinate per night

Other symptoms (not scored)

- Hesitancy, worse with a full bladder or at night
- Post-micturition dribbling
- Double micturition ('pis-à-deux')

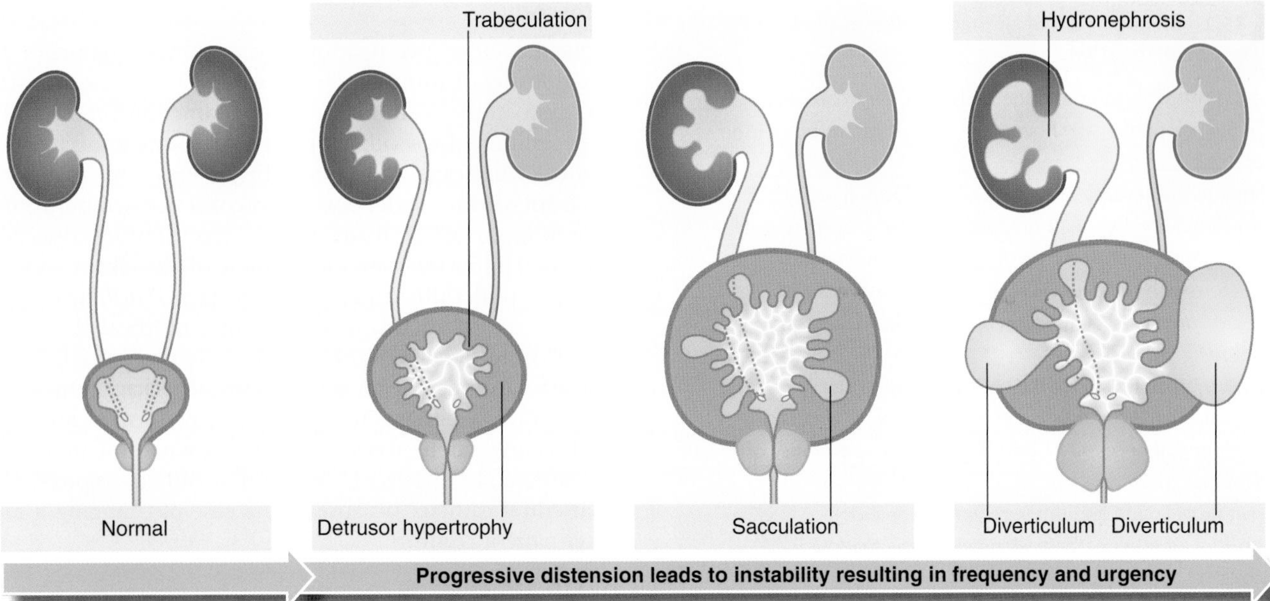

Fig. 35.2 Back-pressure effects of bladder neck obstruction

of patients have progressive symptoms and 50% remain unchanged over 5 years. In progressive cases, the volume of **residual urine** gradually increases over weeks and months (i.e. chronic retention) and in a minority leads to a rise in intravesical pressure. In the latter, the threshold for the voiding reflex is reached more quickly and calls to void become more frequent. The stagnant residual urine is prone to infection which exacerbates the symptoms. In chronic retention, the bladder becomes vastly distended and atonic, which can lead to **overflow incontinence**. In other cases, the detrusor muscle undergoes hypertrophy in an attempt to overcome the outflow obstruction. The normally smooth bladder lining then becomes trabeculated. Eventually, muscle fibre bundles are replaced by non-contractile fibrous tissue; this may explain why some patients fail to improve after obstruction is relieved. With a further rise in pressure, the depressions between the muscle bands deepen (sacculation) and eventually form **bladder diverticula**. Urinary stasis in the diverticula predisposes to stone formation (see Fig. 35.2).

A small proportion of patients with bladder outlet obstruction experience few local symptoms. In these, rising intravesical pressure can be transmitted back into the ureters and kidneys causing hydronephrosis and **progressive renal parenchymal damage**. Patients often present with systemic illness or symptoms such as anorexia, apparently of non-renal origin. The renal failure may be accompanied by anaemia, dehydration, acidosis and infection. Bladder outflow obstruction in these patients is easily overlooked unless the bladder is examined for distension and plasma urea measured.

MANAGEMENT OF BENIGN PROSTATIC HYPERPLASIA

The principles of management of bladder outlet obstruction believed to be due to benign prostatic hyperplasia are outlined in Box 35.2.

Diagnosis

A detailed history is first taken to assess the nature of the symptoms and how much they interfere with the patient's life. The International Prostate Symptom Score sheet helps in assessing the overall impact of symptoms in a standardised way (Box 35.1). This, and the patient's general condition, are the principal factors determining whether treatment is needed. The abdomen is examined for an enlarged bladder and the prostate palpated rectally. These clinical examinations, however, reveal only gross abnormalities.

The next step is to investigate the effects of outlet obstruction on the bladder by measuring **urinary flow rate** and estimating the **volume of residual urine** using ultrasound. This is reliable, quick, non-invasive, safe and cheap. When urinary symptoms are severe but residual volume is insignificant, the alternative diagnosis of an **overactive bladder** should be considered. Urodynamic studies are more complex and involve measuring the filling and emptying pressures of the bladder, but may be invaluable if diagnostic doubts remain.

Renal function is assessed by estimating plasma urea, creatinine and electrolytes. If these are abnormal, further metabolic investigations may be necessary and renal tract ultrasound is mandatory.

A **midstream specimen of urine** should be examined by microscopy and culture as urinary infection alone may be responsible for the symptoms or may have precipitated an episode of urinary retention. In addition, if surgery is intended, it is important that infection is eradicated to minimise risk of perioperative infection and secondary haemorrhage.

If the prostate feels nodular on palpation, cancer should be suspected, particularly if the serum **prostate specific antigen** (PSA) is elevated. Transrectal ultrasound scanning (TRUS) and needle biopsy should be performed even if prostatectomy is planned because a preoperative diagnosis of cancer is likely to alter the plan of management. Marked

Box 35.2 Management of chronic bladder outflow obstruction

- Assess the symptoms and the likely need for treatment from the history, particularly how much the symptoms bother the patient
- Estimate the severity of bladder outlet obstruction by ultrasound and by measuring urine flow rate (urodynamics)
- Investigate any disturbance of upper tract function and structure with renal function tests and ultrasound
- Exclude urinary tract infection by urine microscopy and culture
- Exclude prostatic carcinoma clinically, biochemically (prostate specific antigen) and by transrectal diagnostic ultrasound; if necessary, perform guided needle biopsy of abnormal areas
- Treat renal failure and other systemic problems
- Consider whether catheter drainage of the bladder is desirable
- Cystoscope the patient to rule out other pathology and to define the anatomical problem
- Discuss with the patient what can be offered and at what risk, i.e. drug treatment, transurethral resection of prostate (TURP), laser vaporisation or enucleation or, as a last resort, long-term catheterisation
- Implement appropriate non-surgical treatments

If operation becomes necessary, diagnose the cause and extent of obstruction by cystoscopy, then either:

- Resect benign prostatic hyperplasia, divide bladder neck hypertrophy transurethrally, or obtain biopsy material by TURP if carcinoma seems likely and prior confirmation has been negative

or

- Consider any other operative measures such as open prostatectomy or excision of diverticula where appropriate

elevation of serum PSA is diagnostic of prostatic cancer but a mildly elevated PSA may be due to benign disease or infection. A normal result does not, however, exclude cancer.

Relief of chronic retention and obstructive effects on the kidney

In chronic retention and a large volume of residual urine (750 ml or more), abnormal renal function or upper tract dilatation on renal tract ultrasound, the patient is usually catheterised to allow detrusor tone to recover over a few days. Drainage also allows any reversible component of renal failure to self-correct; it may take 3 weeks of catheter drainage to improve biochemical renal function tests, after which spontaneous improvement is unlikely. Initially, fluid and electrolyte balance is monitored and normalised if necessary by intravenous fluids. In patients with chronic outflow obstruction and obstructive renal failure, catheterisation may produce a **massive diuresis** and this should be anticipated and treated appropriately.

Cystoscopy

Despite the above investigations, the anatomical nature of the bladder outlet obstruction can be accurately assessed only by direct cystoscopic examination. At the same time, the bladder can be examined for other problems such as trabeculation, diverticula, tumours and stones. In patients with complications from bladder outlet obstruction or severe symptoms not responding to medical treatment, transurethral resection (TUR) or Holmium laser enucleation of the obstruction is performed under the same anaesthetic (see *TURP*, below). In elderly or unfit patients, placement of a **urethral stent** may be considered. However, these devices are prone to displacement, haemorrhage, local irritation and blockage. Only very occasionally are patients too unfit for some form of intervention. It is now rarely necessary to leave a patient with a long-term catheter; in this event a suprapubic catheter is preferable to a urethral catheter because of the ease of changing it and greater patient comfort.

Drug treatments

Finasteride and **dutasteride** block the enzyme 5-alpha reductase from converting testosterone to dihydrotestosterone and thus reduce the size of hyperplastic prostate glands. A 6-month trial of treatment is required; if successful, symptoms may improve to the extent that surgery can be delayed or avoided. Some herbal remedies such as **saw palmetto** contain naturally occurring 5-alpha reductase inhibitors.

Alpha-adrenergic A_1 receptors are present in the bladder neck and prostate and selective alpha-adrenergic blocking drugs may enable the prostatic urethra to open more readily, relieving symptoms. Newer drugs, e.g. tamsulosin or alfuzosin, have fewer side-effects than older drugs such as prazosin. Combination therapy with alpha-adrenergic blockers and 5-alpha reductase inhibitors may be more beneficial in patients with larger glands.

Transurethral resection of prostate (TURP) and other transurethral treatments

Transurethral prostatectomy has lower postoperative mortality and morbidity than open retropubic prostatectomy and requires a shorter hospital stay. **Holmium laser enucleation of prostate (HOLeP)** yields at least equivalent results to TURP with the added benefit of reduced blood loss. In addition, larger glands can be enucleated than could reasonably be resected, thus avoiding the need for open retropubic prostatectomy. **Laser ablation techniques** (using KTP-green light and holmium lasers) can be valuable in special circumstances, such as a patient on warfarin, and have shown promising results approaching those of TURP. Nonetheless, TURP remains the standard therapy, while other physical treatments have demonstrated lesser degrees of success. Cryoprostatectomy (freezing the gland), cold punch prostatectomy, microwave thermotherapy and transurethral needle ablation (TUNA) are obsolete procedures.

The aim of transurethral prostatectomy is to remove the bulk of the prostate but leave the compressed normal peripheral tissue. This protects the subcapsular venous plexus that might otherwise bleed catastrophically. In TURP, a series of 'chips' or strips of tissue are excised with a resectoscope using a cutting diathermy wire loop; the chips drift into the bladder. The enlarged gland is progressively sliced away as shown in Figure 35.3, taking great care to preserve the sphincter mechanism immediately distal to the veru montanum. The prostatic chips are always examined histologically and may reveal unsuspected carcinoma. A transparent isotonic irrigation solution is used during the process, which washes away blood and debris to allow continuous visibility. Since some irrigation fluid is inevitably absorbed, sterile **glycine solution** is most often used instead of water as it does not cause haemolysis. If large volumes are absorbed, this causes dilutional hyponatraemia and hyperammonaemia along with drastic plasma electrolyte changes, producing the **TUR syndrome**. Various isotonic sugar solutions can now be safely used as alternatives.

When obstruction is caused by bladder neck hypertrophy, the prostate is not usually resected but the bladder neck muscle is divided by making a longitudinal incision (bladder neck incision, BNI) using a diathermy point via the resectoscope. This operation is also effective where the obstruction is caused by a small prostate (<30 g).

Retropubic prostatectomy

Open prostatectomy, now rarely performed, is used mainly when the gland is so large that transurethral resection is not practicable, or occasionally when there are accompanying bladder diverticula or huge stones.

Complications of TURP and open prostatectomy

Prostatectomy usually disrupts the bladder neck mechanism that normally prevents semen entering the bladder during ejaculation. Patients therefore usually fail to ejaculate through the penis after prostatectomy (**retrograde ejaculation**), although the sensation of orgasm is unaffected. This affects 75% of patients. Maintaining fertility is not usually important in this older age group, but should the need arise, urine can be filtered to recover sperm for artificial insemination. **Erectile impotence** follows TURP in 5–10%, a rate similar to other major operations in the pelvis or perineal area. **Urethral strictures** develop in 1–10% of cases, reflecting the use of relatively large instruments and potentially harmful urethral catheters.

Minor **haematuria** can be expected during the first few weeks after prostatectomy. Secondary haemorrhage (due to infection or unsuspected cancer) can be more profuse and may cause **clot retention**, i.e. retention of urine caused by obstructing blood clot. Recovery of complete urinary continence is sometimes delayed following prostatectomy but permanent damage to the sphincter mechanism is rare.

Long-term catheterisation or stenting

Operation greatly improves the quality of life in most patients. Even in patients over 80, perioperative morbidity and mortality are acceptably low. Nevertheless, a small proportion of severely debilitated, immobile or demented patients are better managed by long-term suprapubic (or urethral) catheterisation, changed regularly by the family practitioner or as a hospital outpatient. In situ urethral stenting is an alternative, although it has a high rate of failure and other complications.

ACUTE URINARY RETENTION AND ITS MANAGEMENT

Acute urinary retention may occur in patients with longstanding symptoms of bladder outlet obstruction; indeed in the majority of men with chronic retention, acute retention is the first presentation. It is often precipitated by overfilling of the bladder, faecal loading or urinary tract infection. Acute retention is a common cause of emergency surgical admission and a frequent early complication after any major operation, especially in males; it may therefore occur at any age even without bladder neck hypertrophy or prostatic enlargement. Management of postoperative acute retention is described in Chapter 11.

DIAGNOSIS OF ACUTE RETENTION

In a patient with no urine output, acute retention must be distinguished from anuria. However, the diagnosis is not usually difficult—the patient in retention is acutely distressed with abdominal or perineal pain and a readily palpable bladder. A history of previous similar episodes, urological surgery or accidental injury should be sought in case special treatment is required.

CATHETERISATION

Acute retention is usually treated by urethral or preferably suprapubic catheterisation using an aseptic technique (Fig. 35.4). Urethral catheterisation may prove difficult in patients with a history of difficult catheterisation, prostatectomy or urethral stricture, or the finding of a non-retractile foreskin. If the problem appears complex, an experienced opinion should be sought early before risking urethral damage by unwise attempts at urethral catheterisation. Inserting a suprapubic catheter is quick and safe provided the bladder is palpably distended but should be avoided if there is a history of bladder tumour. A surgeon with urological training may elect to carry out cystourethroscopy and appropriate surgical treatment as a single scheduled procedure if catheterisation is not urgent.

EVALUATING THE UNDERLYING CAUSE AND ANY PRECIPITATING FACTORS

A catheter is usually left in situ for 1 or 2 days after relieving the acute retention until the patient has been fully assessed. At this point, the decision is whether to attempt a **trial without catheter (TWOC)**, i.e. test whether the patient can void urine satisfactorily when the catheter is removed, or clamped off in the case of a suprapubic, or whether to proceed directly with surgical or other treatment. Any urinary tract infection must be treated before any trial without catheter or operation.

'Trial without catheter'

If appropriate, the catheter should be removed either around midnight or very early in the morning so that a catheter can be replaced before the patient's bedtime if the trial is unsuccessful. Success is if the patient can pass reasonable volumes of urine with each voiding, i.e. more than about 100 ml. Even if passing good volumes, the patient must be examined at intervals to ensure that the bladder is not distending with

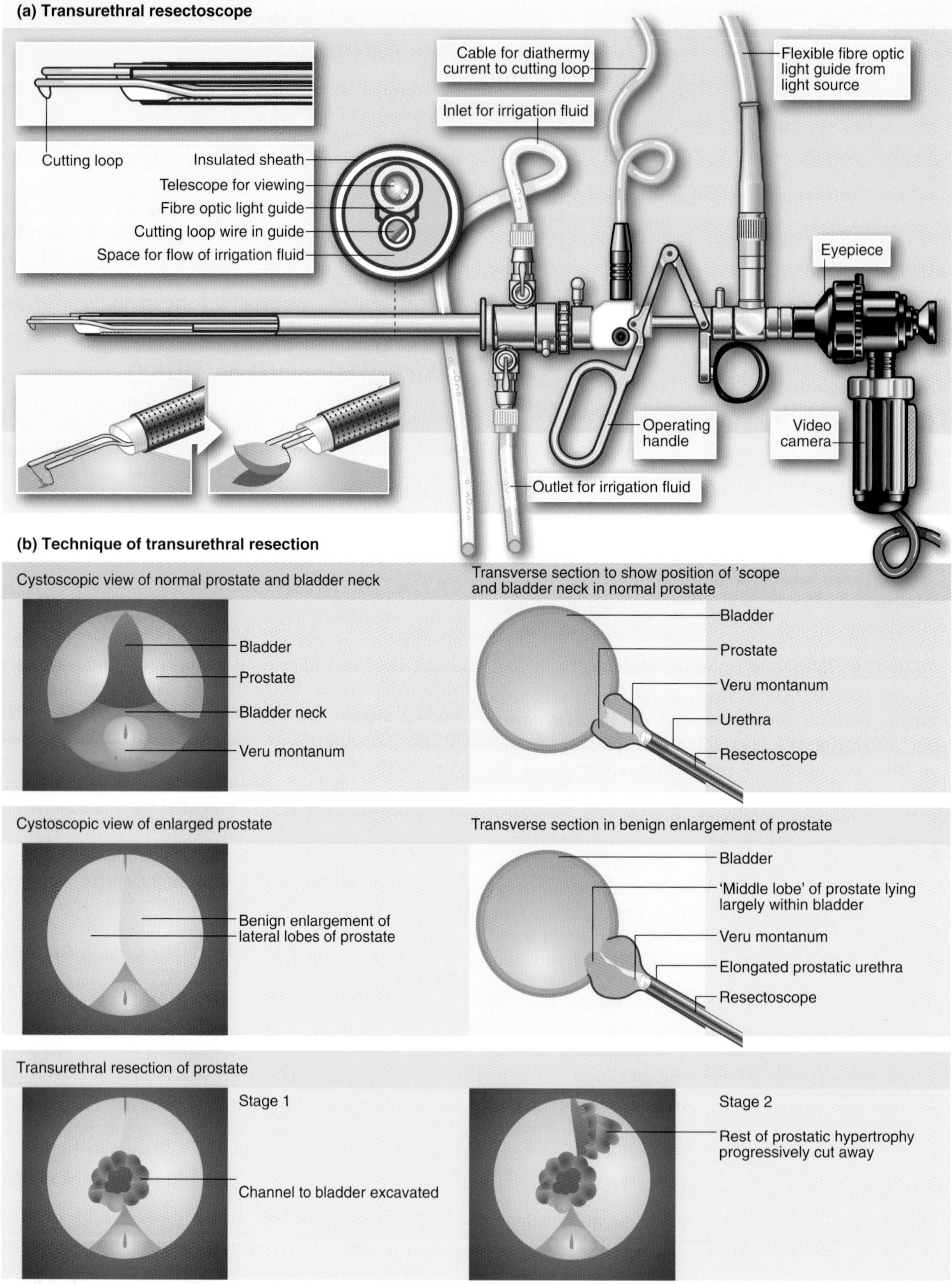

Fig. 35.3 Transurethral prostatectomy
(a) Transurethral resectoscope. 'Divots' or chips are cut by squeezing the handle towards the eyepiece while turning the diathermy current on. This 'cheese-wires' the cutting loop through tissue. **(b)** Technique of transurethral resection.

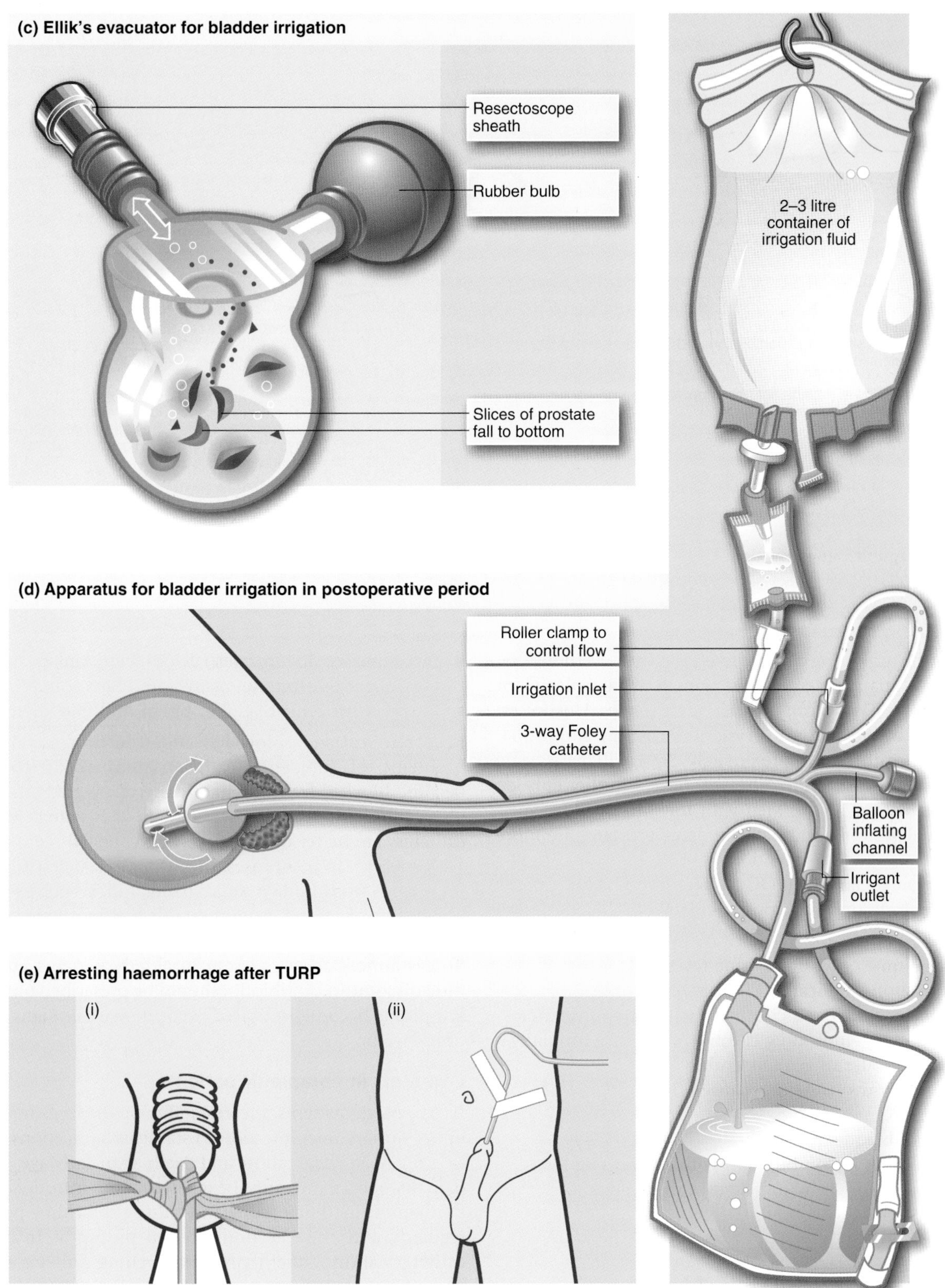

Fig. 35.3, Continued (c) Ellik's evacuator for bladder irrigation. The instrument is completely filled with irrigation fluid and then attached to the resectoscope sheath which is left in the bladder after withdrawal of the main instrument. Squeezing the bulb flushes fluid alternately in and out of the bladder, bringing the cut prostatic slices with it which then settle to the bottom of the container. **(d)** Apparatus for bladder irrigation in the postoperative period. The rate of fluid flow is adjusted to be fast enough to prevent clotting within the bladder. In practice the effluent should be pink rather than red. **(e)** Arresting haemorrhage after TURP. Excessive bleeding after transurethral resection can often be controlled by exerting traction on the catheter for 20 minutes (but not more). Tension is maintained by (i) tying a swab around the catheter, or (ii) attaching the catheter to the anterior abdominal wall with adhesive tape

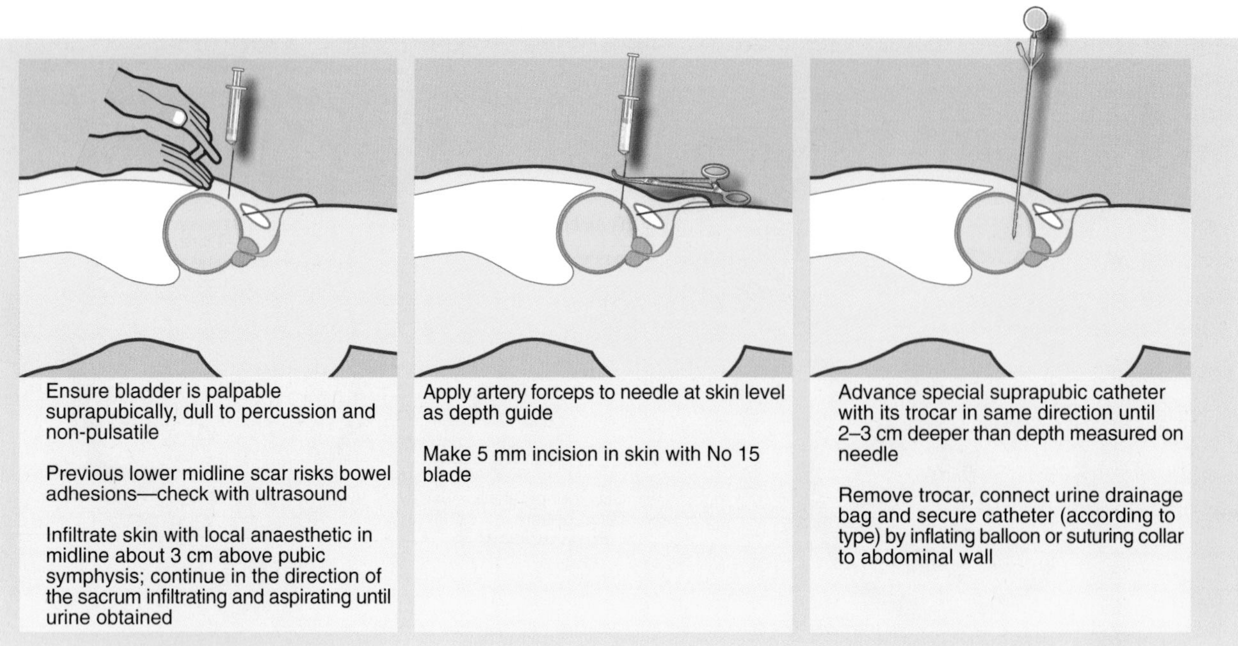

Fig. 35.4 Suprapubic catheterisation

retained urine indicating chronic retention with overflow. Prescribing an alpha-adrenergic blocker such as tamsulosin for 48 hours before TWOC can increase success rates. Unsuccessful TWOC is an indication for cystourethroscopy and probable surgical treatment. Approximately 50% will pass urine successfully, although up to 50% will have a further episode of retention within 1 year. Men with low urinary flow rates, large residual volumes and palpably large prostates are more likely to develop further retention.

In addition to failed TWOC, other common indications for cystourethroscopy and prostatectomy or bladder neck incision are:

- A huge volume of retained urine released by catheterisation—indicating chronic retention
- Raised plasma urea and creatinine which improve after catheterisation—indicating chronic obstructive uropathy
- Previous episodes of acute retention
- Bladder outflow obstruction caused by carcinoma of prostate
- Presence of bladder calculi
- Acute retention in combination with a history of lower urinary tract symptoms sufficient in themselves to warrant surgery

INDWELLING CATHETERS AND THEIR MANAGEMENT

Indications for permanent urethral or suprapubic catheterisation include:

- Patients unfit for prostatectomy
- Incontinent, elderly patients who are severely debilitated, demented or immobile
- Incontinence due to external sphincter damage caused by previous prostatectomy or invading carcinoma
- 'Sacral neurogenic bladder', e.g. in multiple sclerosis

Recurrent catheter blockage and **infection** are the major problems of long-term catheterisation. Catheters readily become blocked by epithelial debris or by gradual accretion of calculus. Modern silicone or silicone-coated 'long-term' catheters are better but must still be changed regularly every 10–12 weeks. In most cases, they can be changed at home by the GP or community nurse using full sterile precautions because if infection becomes established in the presence of a catheter, it is difficult to eradicate. However, low-grade infection is almost always present in elderly patients and causes little discomfort. Antibiotics should be prescribed only if local symptoms become troublesome or if systemic signs of infection develop.

Catheters in paraplegic patients

In paraplegic patients, ureteric reflux predisposes to recurrent upper urinary tract infections. Established infections can lead to progressive renal failure and death at an early age. For these patients, special care must be taken to avoid introducing infection, and urine microscopy and culture should be performed regularly and any infections treated promptly. **Intermittent catheterisation**, rather than an indwelling catheter, may be a better form of management provided it is performed correctly; in many cases, patients successfully perform this themselves.

CARCINOMA OF THE PROSTATE

PATHOPHYSIOLOGY OF PROSTATIC CARCINOMA

Carcinoma of the prostate is common after the age of 65 and is becoming increasingly common in the two decades before that. The rising incidence is partly explained by many more early cases discovered because of increasing public awareness, and screening using PSA testing, particularly in the USA. The rise may also be related to high meat and fat consumption: East Asians living on a predominantly vegetarian diet have the lowest incidence of prostate cancer.

Cancer usually arises in the **peripheral** prostatic glands rather than in the para-urethral tissue and thus is often slow to intrude on the urethra and cause obstruction. For the same reason, malignant change can occur in the **pseudo-capsule** of compressed peripheral glandular tissue after benign prostatectomy. Prostate cancers are nearly all **adenocarcinomas** with a variable degree of differentiation reflected in their behaviour and aggressiveness of local and metastatic spread. The exception is carcinoma of the prostatic ducts which is urothelial in origin and behaves similarly to bladder cancer.

Most adenocarcinomas are well differentiated and contained within the capsule, slowly invading adjacent prostatic tissue and sometimes involving the bladder neck or sphincter mechanism. In many cases, the prostate is already enlarged by benign hyperplasia. Prostate cancer metastasises to pelvic lymph nodes and via the bloodstream to bone (for which it has a particular affinity) and other organs. Tumour cells enter the subcapsular venous plexus then the spinal venous system which may explain the frequency of bone metastases in the pelvis and spinal column. The mean survival time after diagnosis of metastasis is about 2 years.

Most prostatic cancers secrete a glycoprotein, **prostate specific antigen** (PSA), detectable in the blood even when the tumour remains confined within the gland. More advanced tumours with greater tumour mass produce greater amounts and hence higher blood levels of PSA. Other prostatic conditions (e.g. hyperplasia, prostatitis) may cause elevation of PSA but levels over 10–15 nanograms/ml are likely to be caused by cancer, provided urinary infection can be eliminated as a cause. Specific markers for determining aggressiveness are under development.

The main prognostic indicators are the presenting PSA level, the PSA velocity (i.e. the rate at which it rises) and the histological grading. These factors have complicated the debate about the value of screening for prostatic cancer and the appropriateness of radical 'curative' surgery for localised asymptomatic disease. Prostate cancer screening has not been recommended in the UK or Australia. Even in the USA powerful national bodies have come out against it (see Ch. 6).

Many patients have asymptomatic, localised or dormant disease diagnosed incidentally at TURP for presumed benign disease. At autopsy, one-third or more of men over 50 and 90% of men over 90 dying of other causes have microscopic cancer in the prostate and it can be assumed that this is true for the population at large. The natural history of these occult cancers is unknown and many clearly do not progress to become clinically relevant. Even after characteristic local symptoms appear, the disease often pursues a prolonged course and many patients over 70 years of age die *with* their prostate cancer rather than *from* it. On the other hand, 50% of patients under 70 with moderately or poorly differentiated cancers will eventually die from the disease and a greater proportion will develop significant morbidity. Patients

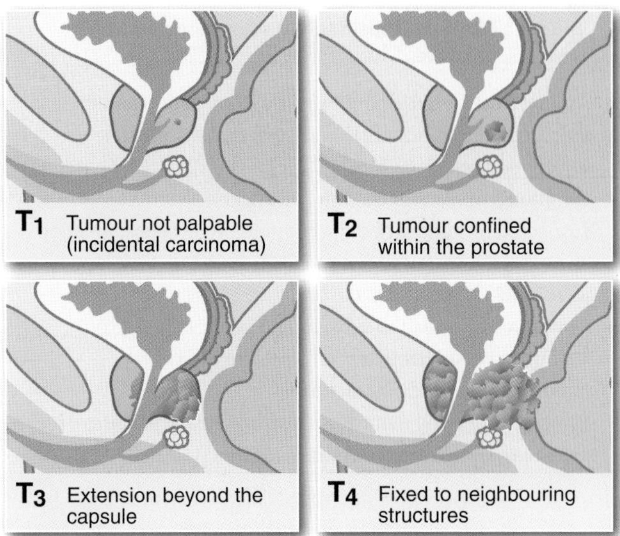

Fig. 35.5 TNM staging system for prostatic cancer

who suffer from other life-threatening co-morbid conditions should be offered an 'active monitoring' policy unless their metastases are symptomatic.

Symptoms and signs of prostatic cancer depend on the degree of local and systemic spread. Clinical staging is most commonly based on the TNM system (see Fig. 35.5). Incidence of pelvic lymph node involvement varies from 2% in T_1 tumours to 85% in T_5 tumours. The palpation characteristics of the malignant prostate are illustrated in Figure 35.1 (p. 446, 450).

SYMPTOMS AND SIGNS OF PROSTATIC CANCER

Patients with stage T_1 or T_2 tumours may be asymptomatic. They may be discovered incidentally or on a routine health check, or present with lower urinary tract symptoms equivalent to those of benign hyperplasia. Those with T_3 and T_4 tumours may present in the same way but many develop other local symptoms from advancement of the primary tumour, e.g. encirclement of the rectum or occlusion of ureters and presenting with renal failure. Patients with nodal disease (N^+) may have symptoms from local compression (swollen legs) and impaired lymphatic drainage (penile and genital oedema). Unfortunately, T_3 and T_4 lesions have often metastasised already by the time of presentation (M^+) and present with bone pain, pathological fractures (e.g., of the femur) or spinal cord compression. Thus older men presenting with **backache** should always have a rectal examination and PSA assay. In more advanced cases, non-specific symptoms of malaise, fatigue, weight loss and anaemia may develop and escape recognition for many months. Respiratory problems from pulmonary carcinomatous lymphangitis are an uncommon presentation.

Rectal examination can sometimes reveal the primary diagnosis. On palpation of a T_1 tumour, the prostate appears normal or smoothly enlarged by benign hyperplasia; stage T_2 typically presents with a nodular, asymmetrical surface, and stage T_3 with a large, hard, irregular gland with evidence of extension beyond the capsule or into the seminal vesicles. A

Box 35.3 Modes of presentation of carcinoma of the prostate

- Asymptomatic—screening by rectal examination and PSA
- Asymptomatic—incidental finding of nodular prostate on digital rectal examination
- Symptoms of bladder outflow obstruction—tumour suspected by finding nodular prostate on rectal examination or a suspiciously raised serum PSA or found on histology after TURP
- Symptoms of spread to surrounding pelvic tissues, e.g. change in bowel habit, loss of continence, recent impotence, ureteric obstruction
- Symptoms of bony metastases, e.g. bone pain, malaise, anaemia, pathological fractures

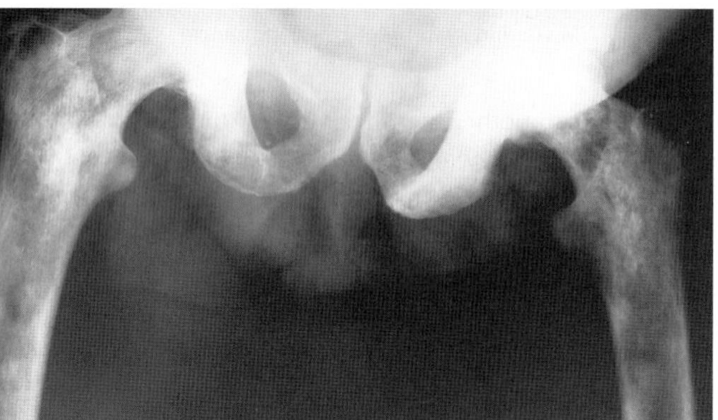

Fig. 35.6 Osteosclerotic bony metastases from prostatic carcinoma

tumour fixed to bone or adjacent pelvic organs is stage T_4. Local spread may involve the rectum (causing changes in bowel habit) or the bladder neck and ureters (causing incontinence, impotence or rarely obstructive renal failure). At this late stage, the tumour is obvious on rectal palpation. In very advanced cases where cancer has invaded laterally to involve the pelvic walls or encircle the rectum, the pelvis may appear 'frozen' solid with tumour. Some patients develop major deep venous thrombosis affecting the lower limb. Modes of presentation of carcinoma of the prostate are summarised in Box 35.3.

APPROACH TO INVESTIGATION OF SUSPECTED PROSTATIC CARCINOMA (Figs 35.6 and 35.7)

Unless the prostate feels malignant or there are obvious bony metastases, it may be impossible to distinguish clinically between benign disease and prostatic carcinoma. **Transrectal ultrasonography** is used to image the prostate irrespective of the findings on palpation and to guide transrectal needle biopsy if necessary. Serum PSA should be measured but results must be interpreted with caution, as modestly rising levels with advancing age are accepted as normal. A normal PSA result cannot exclude carcinoma confined to the gland; PSA is normal in 25% of these cases. Substantially elevated PSA usually indicates aggressive local disease or more often, metastatic disease, although false positive results can occur in

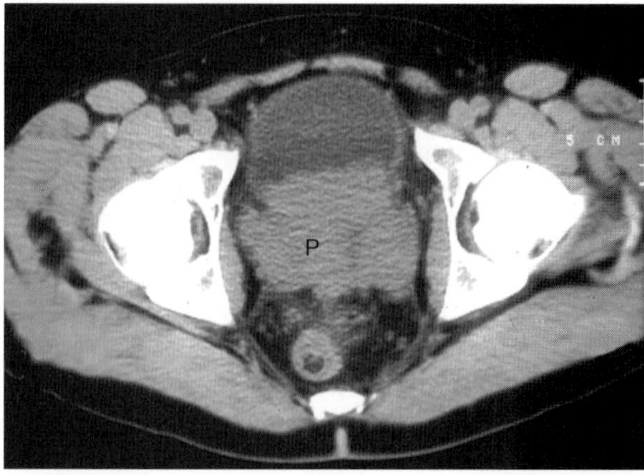

(a)

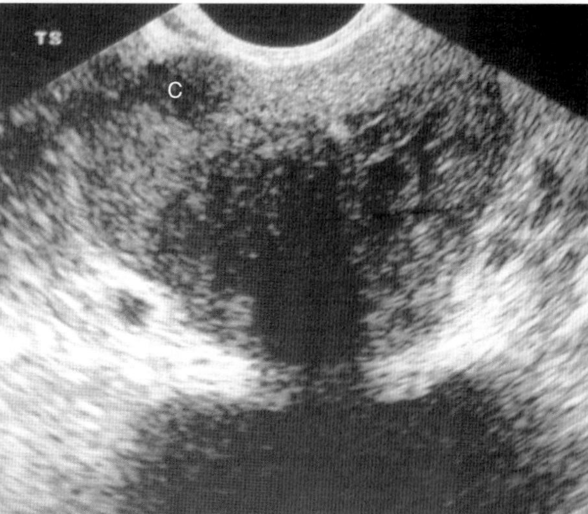

(d)

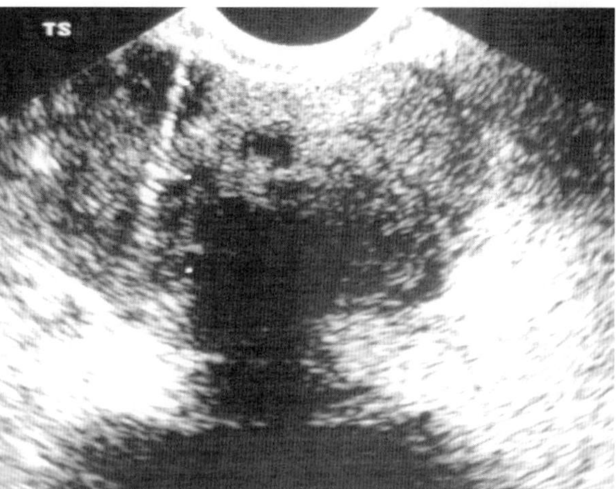

(c)

Fig. 35.7 Carcinoma of the prostate
(a) CT scan showing a large carcinoma of the prostate **P** invading extensively into the bladder anteriorly and posteriorly towards the rectum. This was a late and aggressive form of the disease and the patient lived less than 1 year. **(b)** and **(c)** Ultrasound guided biopsy. **(b)** Transrectal ultrasound scan of prostate showing a small cancer **C** within the peripheral zone and an acoustic shadow beyond it. The larger central zone is enlarged by benign hypertrophy. **(c)** After transrectal biopsy. The white line represents bubbles of air left after successful needle biopsy of the tumour

benign prostatic hyperplasia or inflammation (prostatitis). If carcinoma can be effectively excluded, any obstruction may be treated in the usual way by prostatectomy and the specimens examined histologically. At operation, carcinoma is suspected if the gland lacks the usual clear plane of cleavage.

If a patient has skeletal pain, X-rays and radionuclide bone scans are indicated. On X-ray, prostatic bony metastases are typically **sclerotic** or osteoblastic (i.e. dense, appearing white on X-rays) rather than **lytic** (as in most other bony secondaries), giving the characteristic patchy 'cotton-wool' appearance shown in Figure 35.6. Some lesions, however, are radiolucent. An isotope bone scan can reveal metastases even when a plain X-ray is normal.

MANAGEMENT OF PROSTATIC CARCINOMA

Early-stage disease (stages T_1 or T_2; N_0, M_0)

Radical prostatectomy or radical radiotherapy is potentially curative for organ-confined disease, i.e. disease confined to the prostate or 'true' stage T_1 and T_2, and there is enthusiasm for radical local treatment at specialist centres. If external beam radiation therapy is chosen, it is delivered so as to provide a high local tumour dose without adversely affecting the rectum. Cyber Knife radiotherapy claims greater precision. There is a revival in the use of radioactive seed implants (**brachytherapy**) as an alternative to external beam therapy; the seeds can be placed accurately under ultrasound control and provide the necessary high but localised dosage.

One treatment option for patients with low-grade, impalpable, organ-confined prostate cancer remains **active monitoring** until there is evidence of increased disease activity (rising PSA or detectable nodule on palpation). This gives outcomes equivalent to radical treatment for all patients and spares many the side-effects of radical treatment. There is, however, evidence of improved survival with radical treatment in patients with moderate to high-grade organ-confined disease compared to active monitoring although there is not yet any foolproof way of selecting these.

Radical prostatectomy entails risks such as incontinence or impotence, although complication rates are lower using advanced surgical techniques, including robotic-assisted radical prostatectomy (RARP); RARP or laparoscopic prostatectomy have become the operation of choice in many centres. Patient selection for radical treatment is important in terms of the cancer characteristics (staging, PSA level and tumour volume) as well as patient characteristics (co-morbidity, age, sexual function and patient preference). Patients must be fully counselled in the range of treatment options (including no treatment) and their complications.

Locally advanced disease (stages T_3 or T_4, N_0, M_0)

For patients presenting with bladder outlet symptoms, standard transurethral resection may relieve urinary symptoms; TURP may, however, risk permanent incontinence if the tumour has invaded the sphincter mechanism or the nerves controlling it. Further treatment then depends on local practice and patient preference. Locally advanced primary disease (stage T_3) is usually treated by **neoadjuvant** radiotherapy (before the principal therapy) or adjuvant radiotherapy, with or without hormone therapy.

Metastatic disease (stage N^+ and/or M^+)

Many patients still present with metastatic disease. In these, the aim of treatment is to control symptoms and to retard the progression of disease. For patients presenting with bladder outlet symptoms, standard transurethral resection or 'channel TUR' usually restores urinary flow.

Most prostatic cancers are androgen-dependent, at least initially, and hormonal manipulation is the mainstay of treatment of advanced disease. Local radiotherapy is frequently effective for treating painful metastases. Pathological fractures in the sclerotic metastases of prostatic cancer are much less common than in the lytic metastases of other cancers. This is fortunate since the dense bone is more difficult to cut and drill than normal bone should internal fixation be needed.

Hormonal therapy

Most cancers depend on the presence of male sex hormones for their growth and are rendered quiescent, at least for a time, by pharmacological or surgical castration. Three main treatment options are available:

- **LHRH agonists (LHRHa) such as goserelin**. These drugs need to be injected at 4–12 weekly intervals. Therapy causes initial **stimulation** of luteinising hormone (LH) release from the pituitary, which in turn causes increased testicular testosterone secretion for up to 2 weeks. This is followed by **inhibition** of LH release by competitively blocking the receptors, resulting in an 'anorchic' state. Hot flushes and sexual dysfunction are the major side-effects. Many patients experience a 'flare' of symptoms in the first 2 weeks, aggravating bone pain or spinal cord compression. For this reason, the first 2–3 weeks are usually covered by anti-androgen therapy (e.g. cyproterone acetate or flutamide)
- **Removal of both testes by subcapsular orchidectomy**. This is a quick and simple scrotal operation and removes about 95% of testosterone synthesised (the rest is from the adrenals), producing an immediate fall in plasma testosterone. The testicular capsules are left in situ and these fill with blood clot and preserve the scrotal contour. There are few side-effects other than hot flushes and sexual dysfunction, and no serious long-term sequelae
- **Anti-androgen drugs such as cyproterone acetate or flutamide**. These block the binding of dihydrotestosterone to its receptor at cellular level and, in contrast to LHRH agonists, block both testicular and adrenal testosterone. Flutamide may preserve the potential for sexual arousal for longer and may be the preferred treatment for younger patients with advanced disease

Almost inevitably, prostatic cancer eventually escapes its androgen dependency and becomes **refractory** to hormonal treatment. The mechanism is unknown but occurs at a mean of 2 years after commencing treatment in M^+ and 5 years in N^+ M^0 disease. When this occurs, secondary or salvage treatment with diethylstilbestrol may be of value. This is a synthetic androgen and suppresses LHRH secretion from the hypothalamus, but has a high rate of serious thromboembolic

Box 35.4 Management of prostatic carcinoma—summary

Histological diagnosis

- By ultrasound-guided transrectal biopsy (TRUS) or after TURP for symptoms of bladder outlet obstruction

Staging

- If radical treatment is contemplated—rectal examination, PSA, transrectal ultrasound, CT or MRI scanning for local spread and lymph node involvement

Treatment by stage

- At any stage, transurethral resection ('channel TUR') for persistent bladder outlet obstruction
- Stages T_1 and T_2—a choice of active monitoring or radical local treatment, i.e. prostatectomy or radiotherapy
- Stage T_3—radiotherapy, often with neoadjuvant or adjuvant hormonal therapy
- Stage T_4
  — anti-androgen therapies (e.g. bilateral orchidectomy) plus radiotherapy for painful bony metastases or spinal cord compression

  or

  — drug treatment with LHRH analogues

  or

  — drug treatment with anti-androgen drugs, e.g. cyproterone acetate, flutamide, bicalutamide

side-effects. Bone metastases can sometimes be palliated by intravenous radioactive strontium. Non-hormone chemotherapy has little to offer, and often only symptomatic and general palliative measures can be offered. The principles and techniques of palliative care are described in Chapter 13. The management of prostatic carcinoma is summarised in Box 35.4.

PROSTATITIS

Bacterial prostatitis is an uncommon inflammatory disorder of the prostate usually caused by coliforms, *Chlamydia* or *Neisseria*. Mycoplasma may also have a role. It occurs in acute and chronic forms. Urinary tract infection or instrumentation may be a predisposing factor.

ACUTE PROSTATITIS

Acute prostatitis is characterised by perineal pain and fever. Prostatic swelling may also cause bladder outflow obstruction and urinary frequency. The prostate is exquisitely tender on rectal examination and prostatic massage is inadvisable as it may precipitate bacteraemia.

Initial treatment is with intravenous antibiotics such as gentamicin until the patient is apyrexial and then an oral quinolone antibiotic for 6 weeks. Infective prostatitis may be the first presentation of diabetes mellitus.

CHRONIC PROSTATITIS

Chronic prostatitis presents with chronic, low-grade perineal and suprapubic pain. Symptoms and signs are often vague and the diagnosis is sometimes made on insufficient grounds. Around 5% of cases are due to chronic bacterial infection, most commonly by coliforms, whereas in 95%, no infective cause can be found. Other theories of causation such as autoimmunity and intraprostatic urinary reflux have been proposed.

Treatment is with appropriate antibiotics according to culture and sensitivity of prostatic fluid obtained after prostatic massage. Anti-inflammatory drugs may be used in addition to or instead of antibiotics, particularly in the non-infective cases; alpha-adrenergic blockers may also be employed.

Tumours of the kidney and urinary tract

36

INTRODUCTION

Two types of cancer arise from the renal parenchyma: renal cell carcinomas and nephroblastomas. **Renal cell carcinomas** (also known as renal adenocarcinomas and previously as hypernephromas) are confined to adults. **Nephroblastomas** (Wilms' tumours) are developmental in origin and present in infancy or early childhood (Ch. 51). Occasional benign renal tumours also occur, e.g. oncocytoma, adenoma and angiomyolipoma (see Box 36.1).

Tumours of the transitional cell epithelium lining the urinary tract (urothelium) are very common. They may arise anywhere in the tract, including the renal pelvicalyceal system, the ureters, the bladder and occasionally the urethra. Pelvicalyceal tumours are uncommon but occur frequently in some parts of the world, e.g. Balkan nephropathy. These **urothelial carcinomas**, previously known as **transitional cell carcinomas**, occur exclusively in adults and most commonly in the bladder. **Squamous cell carcinomas** sometimes occur in the urinary tract and probably arise from metaplastic squamous epithelium, caused by chronic irritation from stones or schistosomiasis. Squamous cell carcinomas also arise occasionally in squamous epithelium at the urethral meatus. Very rarely, an **adenocarcinoma** develops in the bladder from glandular epithelial remnants of the embryological **urachus,** or a **sarcoma** may develop from connective tissue elements.

RENAL CELL CARCINOMA

PATHOLOGY OF RENAL CELL CARCINOMA

Renal cell carcinoma accounts for about 3% of adult malignancies and is twice as common in males as females. It rarely develops before puberty but may occur at any age thereafter, with the peak incidence between 50 and 70 years. Renal cell carcinoma mainly occurs sporadically but there are rare familial forms such as von Hippel–Lindau disease. The only proven environmental risk factor is tobacco use.

Renal cell carcinoma originates in renal tubules. Tumour cells are characteristically large and polygonal, with clear cytoplasm representing accumulation of glycogen and lipid. For this reason, these tumours are sometimes known pathologically as **clear cell carcinomas**. In other variants, the cells are granular and stain more intensely.

Renal cell carcinomas vary in grade of malignancy. Small isolated tumours are often found incidentally at autopsy. Many pathologists regard tumours of less than 2 cm as virtually benign as they rarely display invasion or metastasis. Bilateral tumours are present in about 5%. Large tumours invade surrounding tissues and may metastasise to para-aortic lymph nodes. Advanced renal cell carcinoma characteristically extends into the lumen of the renal vein and into the inferior vena cava ('tumour thrombus'—see Fig. 36.1). Distant spread is typically to lung, liver and bone. Lung metastases are often typical discrete **'cannonball secondaries'**. Isolated metastases occasionally develop in the brain, bone and elsewhere.

STAGING OF RENAL CELL CARCINOMA

Stage I tumours are confined by the renal capsule; stage II tumours have penetrated the renal capsule but remain confined by Gerota's perinephric fascia; stage III tumours have renal vein involvement or nodal spread; stage IV have distant metastases.

CLINICAL FEATURES OF RENAL CELL CARCINOMA

The classic presentation is with the triad of **haematuria**, a **mass** and **flank pain**; although all three features only occur in about 15% of cases (see Fig 36.2), one is present in 40% of patients. Commonly, diagnosis is made **incidentally** by discovering a tumour on ultrasonography or CT scanning. Renal cell carcinomas often become large before diagnosis owing to their retroperitoneal position; unfortunately, tumours larger than 8 cm have an 80% chance of having already metastasised. Common and uncommon presenting features of renal cell carcinoma are summarised in Box 36.2.

APPROACH TO INVESTIGATION OF SUSPECTED RENAL CELL CARCINOMA

Ultrasound investigation reliably distinguishes simple benign cysts from solid masses most likely to be tumours, and can demonstrate tumour thrombus in the inferior vena cava. CT scanning is used to stage the disease by assessing invasion of perinephric tissues and by demonstrating regional lymph node or liver metastases (see Fig. 36.3).

Box 36.1 Histological classification of adult renal tumours of the Union Internationale Contre le Cancer (UICC)

A. Malignant

1. Conventional clear cell carcinoma (70–80%)
2. Papillary or tubulo-papillary renal carcinoma (10–15%)
3. Chromophobe renal carcinoma (5%)
4. Collecting duct carcinoma (rare)

B. Benign

1. Oncocytoma
2. Papillary or tubular adenoma
3. Angiomyolipoma (may be neoplastic or hamartomatous)

Box 36.2 Presenting features of renal cell carcinoma

Common presentations

- Frank haematuria
- Microscopic haematuria often discovered incidentally
- Loin pain
- Renal mass
- Incidental finding on imaging

Uncommon presentations

- Iron deficiency anaemia
- Polycythaemia due to erythropoietin production
- Hypertension due to renin production
- Hypercalcaemia due to parathormone-like protein production
- Pyrexia of unknown origin
- Elevated erythrocyte sedimentation rate
- Secondary lesions (e.g. 'cannonball' lesions on chest X-ray, pathological fractures)

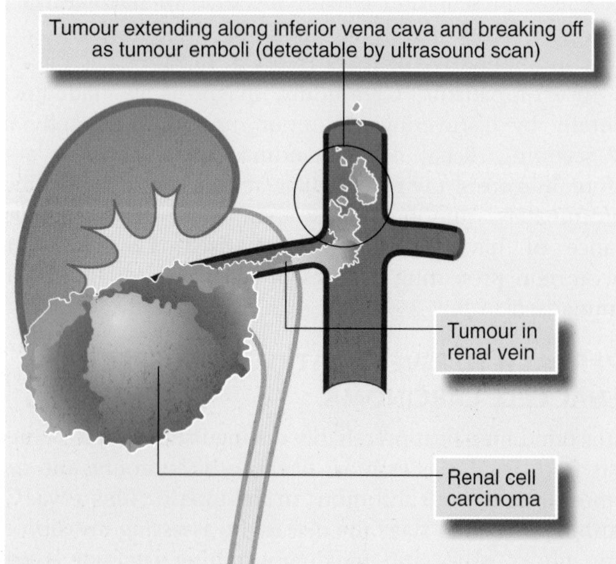

Fig. 36.1 Venous spread of renal cell carcinoma

Fig. 36.2 Renal cell carcinoma: plain radiography

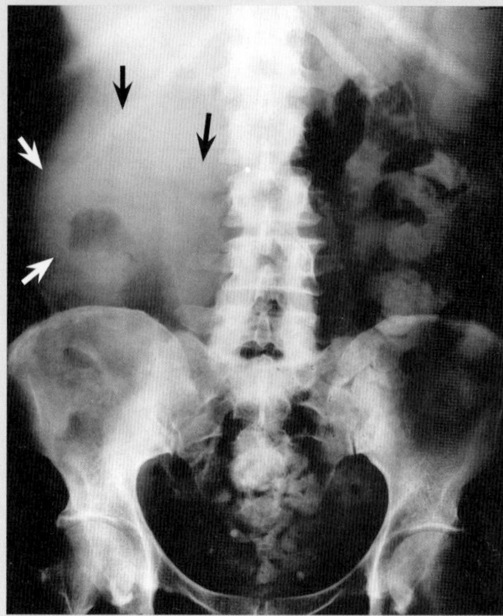

This 50-year-old man presented with painless haematuria. The plain abdominal film shows a large soft-tissue mass in the right loin which obscures the psoas shadow (arrowed). Later investigation showed this to be a renal cell carcinoma

Fig. 36.3 Renal cell carcinoma: CT scan

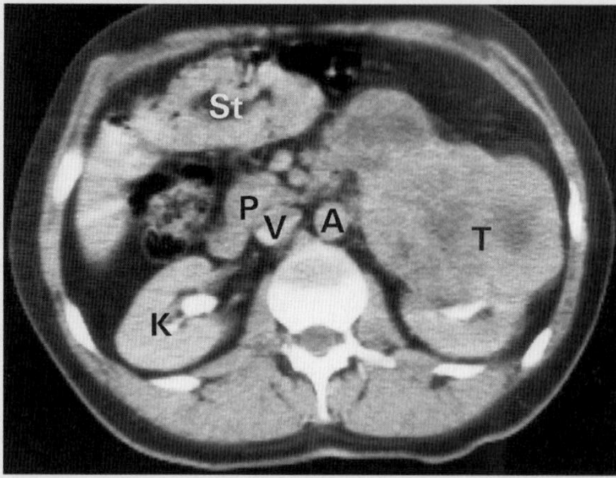

A 62-year-old man presented with left loin pain and a palpable loin mass. This CT scan shows a huge left renal tumour **T**; note the variable density of the tumour caused by areas of necrosis and haemorrhage. Note also the normal right kidney **K**, aorta **A**, pancreas **P**, inferior vena cava **V** and distal stomach **St**

Arteriography is still occasionally employed in the case of solitary unilateral or bilateral tumours to assess the prospects for segmental resection. Renal tumours have a characteristic circulatory pattern distinct from normal kidney (see Fig. 36.4a). Arteriography is also employed if therapeutic embolisation is being considered to reduce the vascularity of a tumour before surgery.

A full blood count is performed to look for anaemia or polycythaemia and a chest X-ray taken to look for pulmonary

Fig. 36.4 Renal cell carcinoma: arteriography and radiography

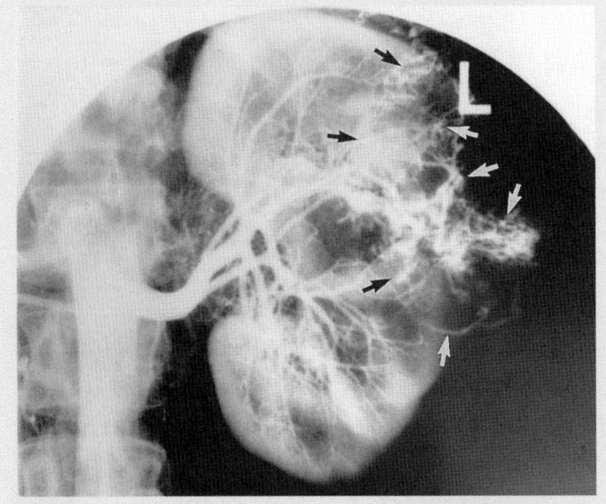

(a)

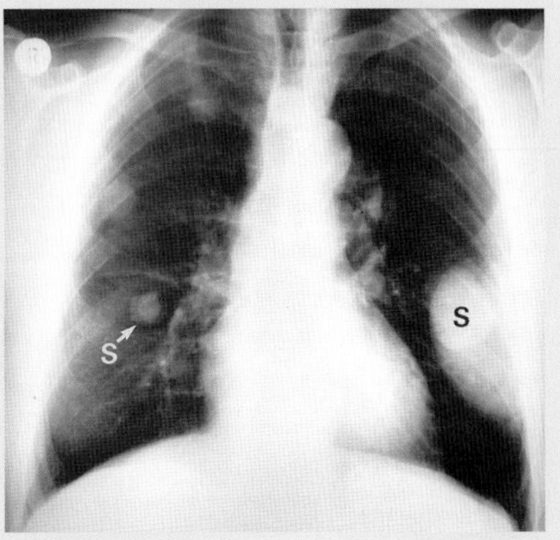

(b)

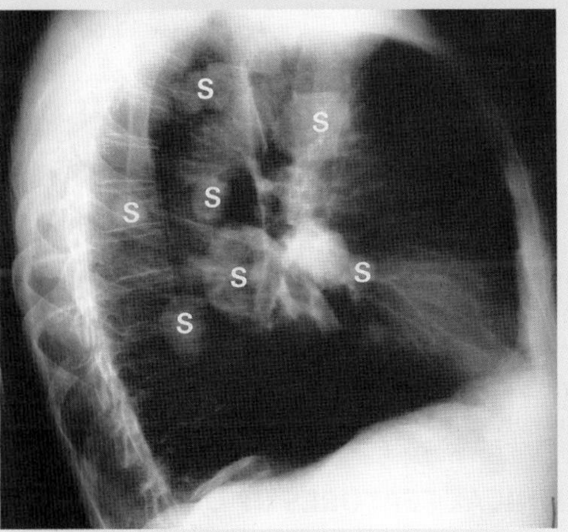

(c)

This 68-year-old woman presented with haematuria. A renal mass was demonstrated on intravenous urography. Before CT scanning was developed, renal arteriography was often used in the diagnosis of renal cell carcinoma and to display its arterial supply as an aid to surgery. **(a)** This left renal arteriogram outlines the normal renal vessels but also shows a large crescentic mass of abnormal vessels (outline arrowed in white) typical of renal cell carcinoma. Only the residual part of the tumour vasculature is demonstrated, the rest having been destroyed by necrosis within the tumour. Unfortunately, this patient had already developed pulmonary metastases, as shown in the chest X-rays **(b)** and **(c)**. **(b)** PA and **(c)** lateral chest X-rays showing multiple 'cannonball' secondary lesions **S** of various sizes. These are typical of renal cell carcinoma

metastases (see Fig. 36.4b, c). No other preoperative investigations are usually required.

MANAGEMENT OF RENAL CELL CARCINOMA

In most patients, the kidney involved by tumour is excised (**nephrectomy**). **Partial nephrectomy** has gained popularity in suitable cases in order to preserve as much renal function as possible. Most surgeons prefer an anterior transperitoneal approach which allows clinical staging, permits control of the inferior vena cava and provides access to the renal artery and vein during extensive resections. If the tumour is large, a postero-lateral thoraco-abdominal approach allows early access to the inferior vena cava and renal arteries. In radical nephrectomy, the kidney, perinephric fat and lymph nodes should be taken *en bloc* wherever possible. There is probably no role for radiotherapy, chemotherapy or hormonal therapy, although immunotherapy with interleukins or interferon may help, despite their toxicity. Tyrosine kinase inhibitors and anti-angiogenic drugs are also gaining popularity. Increasingly, nephrectomies are performed laparoscopically, allowing shortened hospital stay and earlier return to normal activity.

Renal cell carcinoma is unusual in that surgical removal of isolated pulmonary or cerebral metastases occasionally results in cure. These isolated metastases may present years after the primary surgery. For palliation of multiple metastases, chemotherapy or immunotherapy is sometimes used but treatment is generally ineffective.

UROTHELIAL CARCINOMA (TRANSITIONAL CELL CARCINOMA)

EPIDEMIOLOGY AND AETIOLOGY OF UROTHELIAL CARCINOMA

Tumours of urothelium are common. Histologically, they are nearly all urothelial carcinomas (UCs); other than rarities, the rest are squamous cell carcinomas (7%) or adenocarcinomas (1%). Most arise primarily in the bladder but they also occur in the pelvicalyceal system and ureters and rarely in the urethra. Urothelial tumours are uncommon below the age of 50 and the incidence increases with age. Men are affected three times more often than women. UC is at least four times more common than renal cell carcinoma.

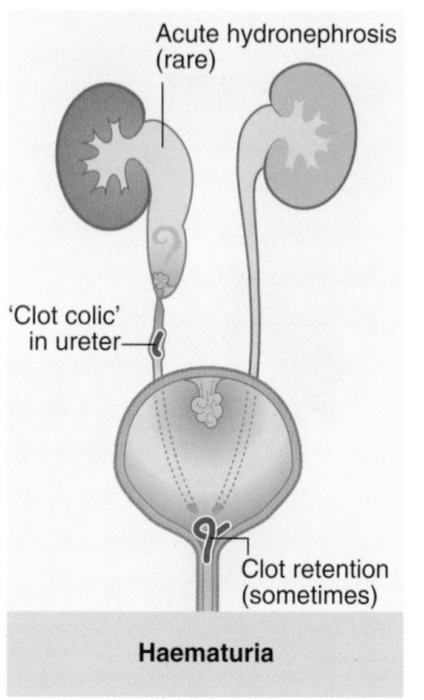

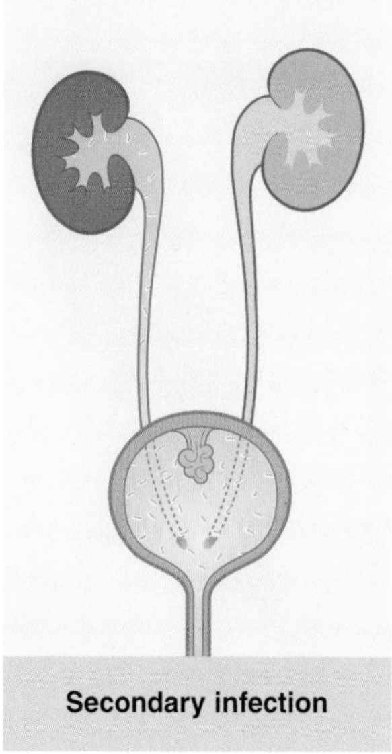

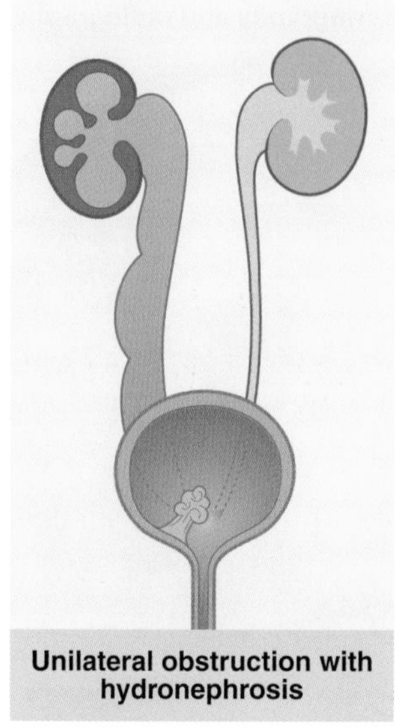

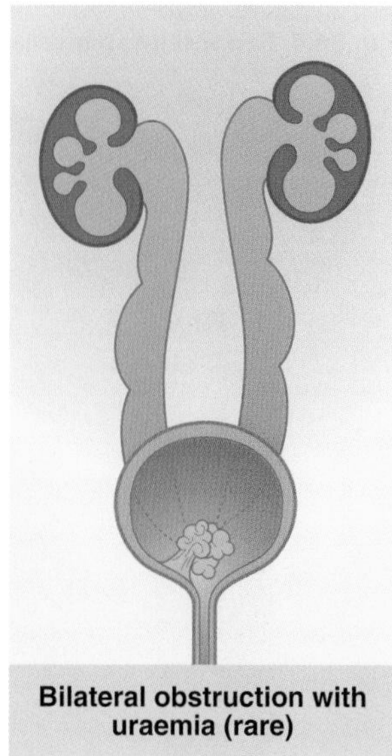

Fig. 36.5 Presenting features of urothelial tumours

Cigarette smoking is associated with a four-fold increase in incidence of urothelial tumours; this is probably mediated by urinary excretion of inhaled carcinogens. Urothelial cancers have been strongly associated with exposure to industrial carcinogens, once widely used in the rubber, cable, dye and printing industries. The likely carcinogens, benzidine, nigrosine and beta naphthylamine, are now banned in most countries but tumours can develop as long as 25 years after exposure and so a detailed occupational history should be taken in suspected cases. Prolonged exposure to carcinogens causes a 20–60 times increased risk of developing urothelial cancer. These carcinogens are excreted in the urine and the more prolonged presence of urine in the bladder compared with the rest of the tract probably explains why urothelial tumours most often arise in the bladder.

PATHOLOGY OF UROTHELIAL CARCINOMA

Well-differentiated UCs histologically resemble normal transitional epithelium. Less well-differentiated tumours become increasingly unlike their tissue of origin so that the most anaplastic tumours can only be classified as urothelial because they are known to have arisen in the urinary tract. The degree of differentiation tends to be reflected in the tumour morphology as visualised at cystoscopy. Well-differentiated tumours form papillary frond-like lesions, whereas more aggressive tumours form plaque-like lesions which invade underlying muscle and surrounding tissues.

Most aetiological factors act on the whole urothelium, predisposing it to malignant transformation. Consequently, urothelial tumours can be **multifocal** and there may already be multiple tumours at presentation. When the primary tumour is in the pelvicalyceal system or ureter, there is a high risk of tumours developing later in the urothelium distal to the primary. About 50% of patients with upper tract urothelial tumours will ultimately develop bladder urothelial tumours.

A sinister form of urothelial carcinoma is **carcinoma-in-situ**. This presents with frequency and dysuria, aptly named 'malignant cystitis'. These symptoms are often misdiagnosed as bacterial prostatitis in men. The lesions desquamate easily and have a high pick-up rate on urine cytology. Untreated, they infiltrate rapidly.

CLINICAL FEATURES OF UROTHELIAL CARCINOMA

urothelial carcinoma usually presents with painless haematuria (see Fig. 36.5). Very occasionally, an upper tract lesion may cause **ureteric colic** (clot colic) and long stringy clots are seen in the urine. If bleeding is gross, clots may cause ureteric obstruction. Rapid bleeding from a bladder tumour may cause **clot retention**, i.e. acute retention of urine due to clot obstruction. Bladder tumours arising near a ureteric orifice can obstruct one ureter, causing **hydronephrosis**. Rarely, bilateral obstruction causes uraemia. Bladder tumours also predispose to infection; unexplained recurrent urinary tract infections need investigating to exclude UC as a cause. Tumour invasion near the bladder neck may cause incontinence but this is usually preceded by haematuria or infection.

INVESTIGATION OF SUSPECTED UROTHELIAL CARCINOMA

Confirmed haematuria in the absence of infection must be investigated. Ultrasound examination may reveal hydronephrosis if there is ureteric involvement by UC. Contrast CT scanning will outline the upper tract as well as the renal parenchyma. IVU can also outline the upper tract, but is becoming obsolete (see Fig. 36.6). Imaging is followed by cystoscopy, the only reliable method of examining the lining of the bladder and urethra. If there is an upper tract tumour, cystoscopy may reveal blood emerging from a ureteric orifice.

Fig. 36.6 Urothelial tumours at different sites

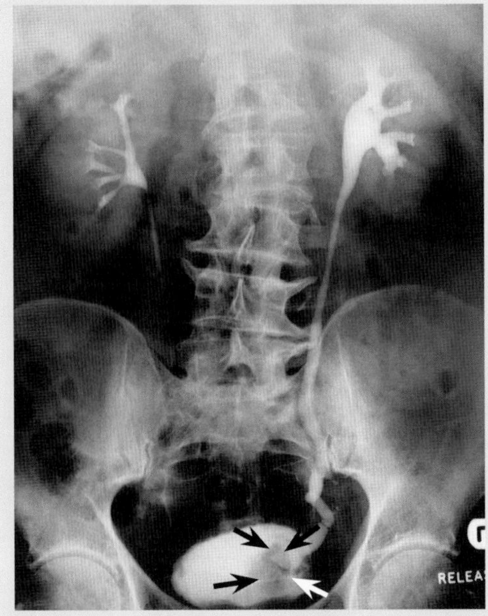

(a)

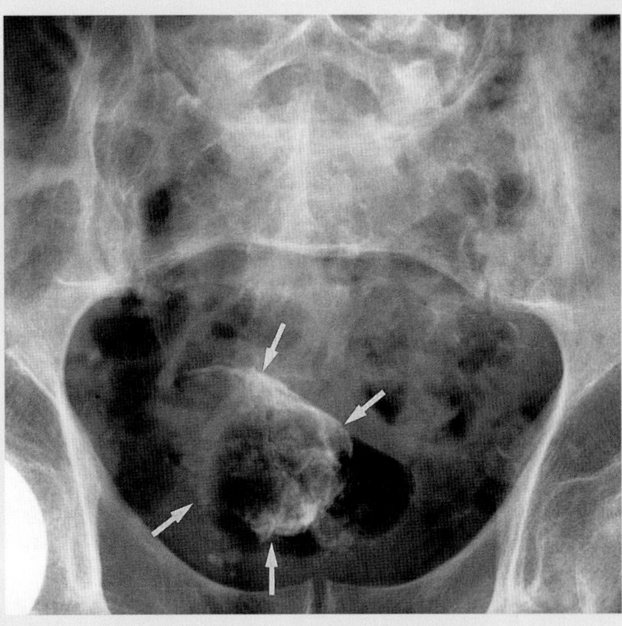

(b)

(a) This 67-year-old man complained of loin pain and haematuria. On the left side of this intravenous urogram there is hydronephrosis and ureteric obstruction caused by a bladder tumour visible at the vesicoureteric orifice (arrowed). **(b)** This 84-year-old man presented with recurrent urinary tract infections. This plain X-ray of the pelvis shows a huge calcified lesion in the bladder (arrowed), typical of calcification on the surface of a longstanding bladder tumour. In a woman, this appearance would more likely be due to a calcified uterine fibroid

STAGING OF UROTHELIAL TUMOURS OF THE BLADDER

Staging is achieved mainly by cystoscopic examination and palpation under anaesthesia, combined with histological examination of resected specimens. For small and superficial lesions, histology shows the extent of bladder wall invasion, degree of tumour differentiation and whether the tumour has been completely removed. Lesions near a ureteric orifice that appear to be superficial should be treated as having invaded underlying muscle. For larger or deeper lesions, palpation of the bladder under general anaesthesia bimanually between a finger in the rectum and a hand on the anterior abdominal wall should be performed before and after resection of the tumour. This gives an idea of the extent of bladder wall penetration and spread into the pelvis, but can be misleading, especially in the obese. CT scanning is a more reliable indication of spread into the bladder wall or beyond. Note, however, that CT scanning can also be misleading if performed soon after resection of a bladder tumour.

The TNM clinical system widely used in staging bladder tumours is illustrated in Figure 36.7 (the 'T' is the clinical stage of the tumour). In addition, some pathologists grade bladder tumours according to P and G pathological criteria. **The 'P' system** (small p for the biopsy specimen and capital P for the whole specimen) classifies the extent of invasion on gross anatomical and histological grounds. **The 'G' system** grades the lesion by degree of histological differentiation (G1 = well differentiated, G2 = moderately differentiated and G3 = poorly differentiated or undifferentiated). Thus, as an example, a pathologist may report a biopsy as pT_2, G3.

MANAGEMENT OF UROTHELIAL CARCINOMA

Bladder tumours

Urothelial carcinomas of the bladder display a variety of morphological types ranging from small, discrete, often multiple, frond-like lesions through to extensive papilliferous or flat tumours. The first type is usually at a very early invasive stage and such lesions were formerly known as papillomas before their malignant potential was fully realised. Four-quadrant biopsy of the rest of the bladder can help formulate a treatment plan and estimate prognosis. If papillary tumours coexist with carcinoma-in-situ (CIS), however, the long-term prognosis is ominous. These patients are usually treated by immunotherapy with a course of intravesical BCG to stimulate local immunity. However if CIS persists, then total cystectomy is the treatment of choice.

The initial management of bladder tumours is usually aimed at complete removal of tumour tissue by cystoscopic **transurethral resection of bladder tumour (TURBT)**, even with large lesions. Further management then depends on the stage of tumour spread determined by examination under anaesthesia, CT scanning and histological staging.

As shown in Figure 36.8, bladder tumours classified as T_a or T_1 can usually be completely resected. Single-dose **intravesical chemotherapy** with mitomycin C has been shown to reduce the recurrence rate after the initial TURBT

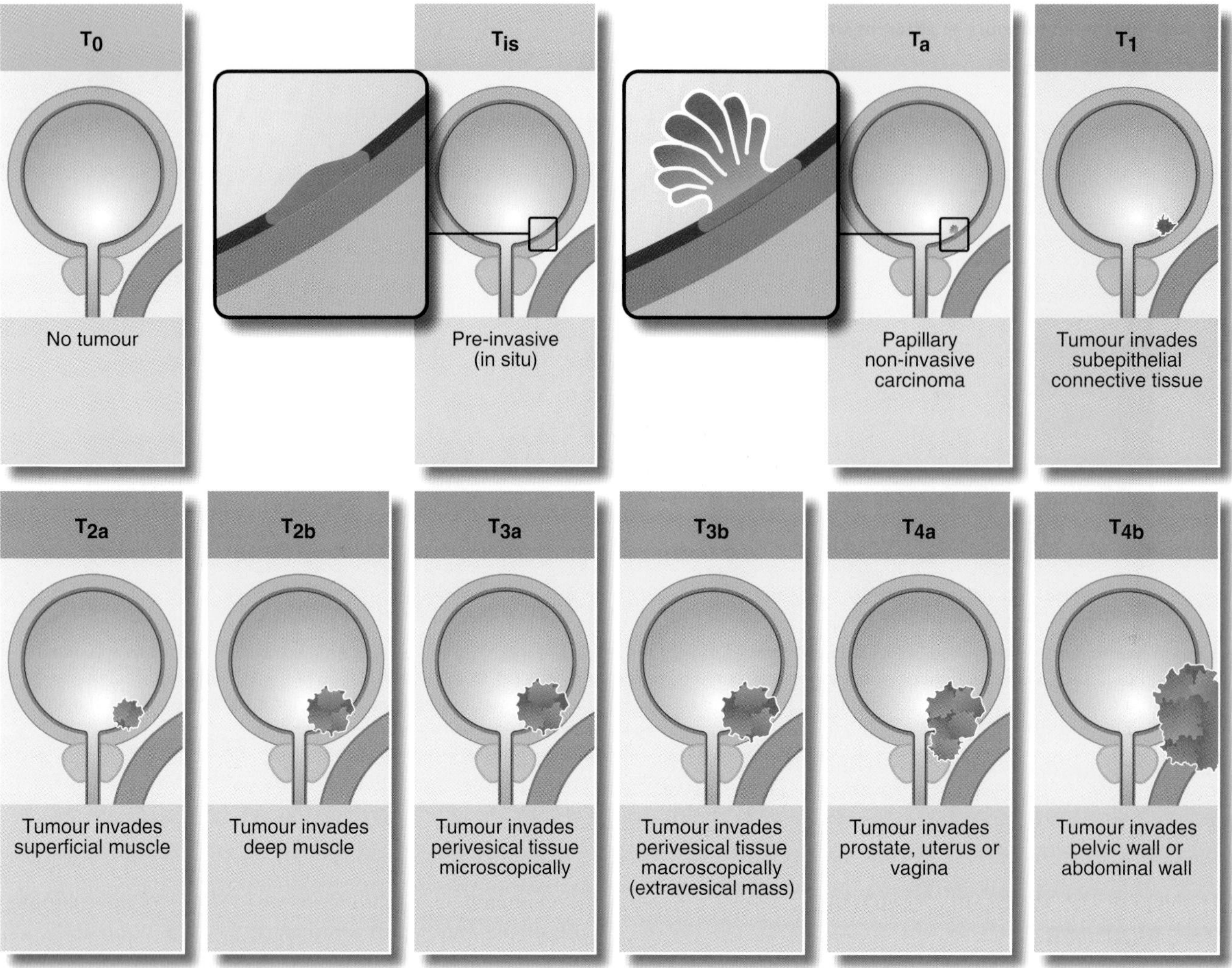

Fig. 36.7 UICC system for staging bladder tumours
Note that ureteric involvement usually classifies a tumour as T_{3a} or T_{3b}

in T_a or T_1 disease. T_1 lesions are notoriously recurrent and if they recur repeatedly, weekly courses of intravesical chemotherapy or BCG is the treatment of choice. For T_2/T_3 lesions, the preferred treatment in a fit patient is **radical cystectomy**. The tumour can sometimes be downstaged before surgery by neoadjuvant systemic chemotherapy. Radiotherapy is a good alternative for the unfit or older patient, in those unwilling to undergo cystectomy, or for relapse after initial cystectomy or initial systemic chemotherapy. There is no proven role for radiotherapy in superficial lesions.

When radical cystectomy is necessary, some method of **urinary diversion** is required. The classic operation involves isolation of a segment of ileum; both ureters are then anastomosed onto the ileal segment, creating an **ileal conduit**, whilst the other end is opened onto the abdominal wall as a urostomy. An earlier operation in which both ureters were diverted into the sigmoid colon has long been abandoned because of electrolyte disruption and a high risk of carcinoma at the ureterocolic anastomoses. Nowadays, most urinary diversions are into a **continent pouch** (a neo-bladder) usually constructed from a segment of ileum and anastomosed to the urethra.

T_4 tumours are usually incurable; even total cystectomy rarely eliminates the entire lesion. Radiotherapy offers palliation and is valuable for controlling pain and haematuria.

Urothelial tumours of the upper tract

UCs of the pelvicalyceal system and ureter are uncommon. Treatment usually requires excision of the whole upper tract on the affected side including kidney, ureter and a cuff of bladder wall surrounding the distal ureter. However, some small, isolated renal pelvic tumours can be dealt with endoscopically via a nephroscope passed percutaneously into the pelvicalyceal system or by laser ablation via a fibreoptic flexible ureteroscope.

Unusual urinary tract tumours

The uncommon **squamous cell carcinoma** of the urinary tract is diagnosed and treated along similar lines to urothelial

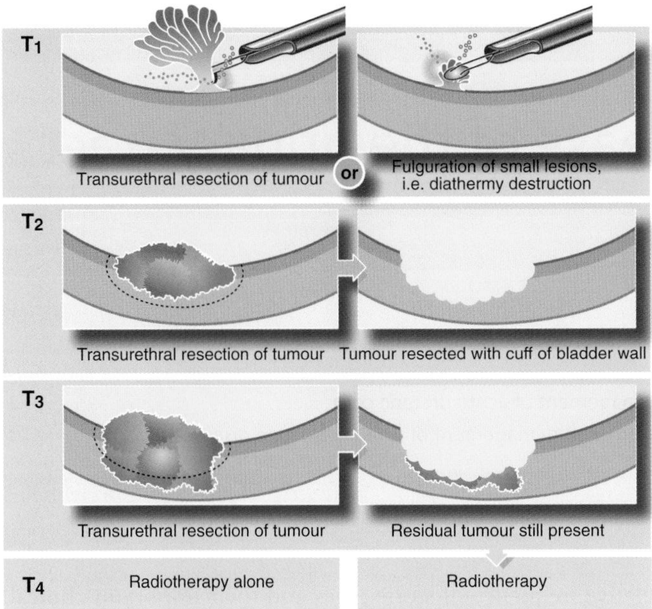

Fig. 36.8 Cystoscopic management of bladder tumours—summary

carcinoma. Many develop as a complication of schistosomiasis. Distal urethral lesions are managed in the same way as penile carcinoma (see Ch. 33). Adenocarcinoma is rare but can occur anywhere in the bladder, most often in a urachal remnant at the vault. Tumours of this type can often be removed by segmental resection of the bladder.

Follow-up and control of recurrent disease

Patients who have had potentially curative treatment for urothelial tumours (i.e. bladder stages T_1 to T_3 and all upper tract lesions) must be followed up for life. The goal is to detect recurrence of the original tumour and to diagnose new primary lesions at an early stage, bearing in mind that environmental factors that induced the initial lesion predispose the remaining urothelium to malignant change. It is not always easy to distinguish between small recurrences and new primaries; all tend to be labelled as 'recurrences'.

Follow-up involves regular 'check' flexible cystoscopies under local anaesthesia. Initially, these are performed at 3-monthly intervals and the interval is gradually extended to once a year if no further tumour is discovered. There is currently a vogue for using nuclear protein tumour markers which can pick up 50% of tumour recurrences; however, the reliability needs to be improved before it can replace existing methods. Urine cytology may also be used for screening normal individuals with a high occupational risk. Other urinary markers are also currently undergoing investigation.

Recurrent lesions are managed in the same way as the initial lesion, i.e. according to the stage of bladder wall invasion. The exception is when the initial treatment involved radiotherapy. For these patients, cure of recurrent cancer is improbable and palliative surgery ranging from TURBT to total cystectomy may be necessary to treat intractable problems such as severe haemorrhage.

37 Stone disease of the urinary tract

INTRODUCTION

Stone disease is second only to prostatic disease in the overall urological workload. Stones may occur in all parts of the urinary tract, including the pelvicalyceal system of the kidney, the ureter, the bladder and even sometimes the urethra. Stones most commonly provoke symptoms due to obstruction or by predisposing to urinary tract infections.

The pattern of stone disease has changed markedly over the last 150 years. Bladder stones were once common and were one of the few conditions successfully treated by surgery. 'Cutting for stone', or **lithotomy** (*lithos* = stone), was often performed by itinerant surgeons. They used a perineal approach, placing the patient in the manner still described as the **lithotomy position**.

Upper tract calculi are much more common than bladder calculi and the incidence is rising. Stones range from the uncommon **staghorn calculus** which fills the pelvicalyceal system, to small stones developing in the pelvicalyceal system that can migrate and obstruct the ureter. Acute ureteric obstruction causes severe pain and presents as the surgical emergency **ureteric colic**. Most stone disease is, however, asymptomatic or else presents non-urgently to the outpatient clinic.

In developed countries stone disease in childhood is now rare. It peaks in the 20s and 30s and declines slowly thereafter (Fig. 37.1). Males are affected two and a half times more often than females. There is also a high incidence of recurrent stones.

PATHOPHYSIOLOGY OF STONE DISEASE

CHEMICAL COMPOSITION

Stones are often formed from a mixture of chemical substances and minerals (e.g. calcium and oxalate) when their concentration exceeds their solubility in urine. Intermittent periods of super-saturation due to dehydration, following meals or medical conditions, can lead to the earliest phase of crystal formation. Lack of crystallisation inhibitors in the urine may also play a role in stone formation. Table 37.1 provides a simple chemical classification showing the relative frequency of stone types and their important clinical characteristics and aetiology. Calcium is present in approximately 80%, as oxalate or phosphate compounds or both. The aetiology of stone disease is multifactorial in most cases.

MECHANISMS OF STONE FORMATION

Calcium-containing stones

In patients with calcium-containing stones specific underlying abnormalities are rarely discovered. Some patients excrete excessive calcium (**idiopathic hypercalciuria**) without being hypercalcaemic; in these, there may be increased intestinal absorption of calcium leading to increased urinary excretion.

Stones caused by excessive urinary excretion of a stone constituent

A minority of patients have an underlying disorder responsible for excessive urinary excretion of the main constituent of the stone. Examples include **hyperparathyroidism** (calcium), **hyperoxaluria** (oxalate), **gout** (uric acid), **cysteinuria** (cysteine stones) and **xanthinuria** (xanthine stones).

Other predisposing factors

A specific predisposing factor can be detected in a further minority of cases. These include chronic infection, urinary stasis and foreign bodies, and are summarised in Box 37.1.

CLINICAL FEATURES OF STONE DISEASE

The clinical problem of discrete urinary stones should not be confused with calcification of the renal parenchyma, which can be a feature of tuberculosis and medullary sponge kidney. These and similar diseases can usually be diagnosed by their characteristic X-ray appearance.

The clinical presentation of stones depends on the size, morphology and site of the stone(s). Many cause no symptoms but represent a potentially serious problem. Other stones produce marked pathological effects which present with acute or chronic symptoms or are discovered incidentally on investigation of unrelated symptoms. The presentation of urinary tract stones is summarised in Box 37.2.

OBSTRUCTION OF URINARY FLOW

Pelvicalyceal obstruction

Obstruction of renal calyces causes local urinary obstruction (**hydrocalyx**) and typically leads to chronic or recurrent loin pain. Similar pain may also be caused by chronic, incomplete obstruction of the pelviureteric junction (PUJ) or ureter. The result is **hydronephrosis**, i.e. dilatation of the renal pelvis, both intrarenal and extrarenal. Severe obstruction may lead to

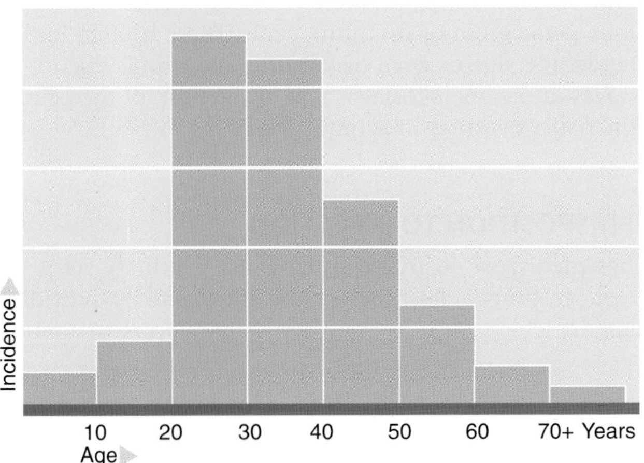

Fig. 37.1 Relative incidence of stone disease by age in developed countries

Box 37.1 Predisposing factors in stone formation

- Idiopathic (most common)
- Stasis of urine, particularly when associated with infection—e.g. congenital abnormalities, hydronephrosis, chronic obstruction (e.g. benign prostatic hyperplasia, neurogenic bladder)
- Chronic urinary infection (urea-splitting organisms, e.g. *Proteus*, cause alkaline urine and the development of magnesium–ammonium–phosphate stones, typically the 'staghorn' calculi of the renal pelvis—see Fig. 37.2)
- Excess urinary excretion of stone-forming substances—e.g. idiopathic hypercalciuria (calcium stones), hyperparathyroidism (calcium stones), hyperoxaluria (oxalate stones), gout (uric acid stones), cysteinuria (cysteine stones), xanthinuria (xanthine stones)
- Foreign bodies—e.g. fragments of catheter tubing, self-inserted artefacts, parasites (schistosome ova), fragments of diseased tissue (e.g. renal papillary necrosis)
- Dietary—e.g. over-consumption of dairy or high calcium content in water
- Multifactorial—e.g. prolonged immobility, children in the developing world, multiple fractures and paralysis (skeletal decalcification)

Table 37.1 Chemical composition, clinical features and aetiology of urinary tract stones

Chemical composition	%	Clinical features	Aetiology
Calcium oxalate	40	Three types of stone are described: — small smooth 'hemp-seed' stones — small irregular 'mulberry' stones — small spiculated 'jack' stones	Most cases are idiopathic; predisposing factors include urinary stasis, infection and foreign bodies Some are due to metabolic disorders which lead to excess urinary excretion of calcium or oxalate: — hyperparathyroidism — hyperoxaluria (rare inherited disorder)
Mixed calcium oxalate and phosphate stones	15	As above	Some are due to disorders associated with hypercalcaemia, e.g. sarcoidosis, multiple metastases, multiple myeloma, milk-alkali syndrome, overtreatment with vitamin D
Calcium and phosphate	15	As above	Some of these patients excrete abnormally large amounts of calcium possibly as a result of increased absorption (idiopathic hypercalciuria but without hypercalcaemia)
Magnesium ammonium phosphate (struvite/ infection stones)	15	Typically large 'staghorn' calculi of pelvicalyceal system and some bladder stones	Chronic infection with organisms capable of producing urease, typically *Proteus*. Urease splits urea, forming ammonia if the urine is alkaline
Uric acid	8	Stones tend to absorb yellow and brown pigments. Pure stones are radiolucent	Occur in primary gout and hyperuricaemia following chemotherapy for leukaemias or myeloproliferative disorders. Childhood urate bladder stones occur in some developing countries when urine pH is low
Cysteine or xanthine	2	Excess urinary excretion of cysteine or xanthine. Pure stones are radiolucent	Autosomal recessive inherited disorders

progressive renal parenchymal damage and impaired renal function; the patient may develop renal failure if both kidneys are affected.

Passage of stones into the ureter

If small renal stones pass into the ureter, there are several possible outcomes:

Box 37.2 Presentation of stones in the urinary tract

- Incidental finding on X-ray
- Loin pain
- Ureteric colic
- Painful passage of small stones via urethra
- Cystitis
- Pyelonephritis
- Haematuria
- Impaired renal function

Urinary tract stones produce their injurious effects in three main ways:

- By obstructing urinary flow
- By predisposing to infection
- By causing local tissue irritation and damage

- Stones may pass to the bladder and exit via the urethra causing minor symptoms. The patient may intermittently pass 'gravel' or 'sand' (see Fig. 37.2) and experience dysuria and sometimes haematuria
- Stones may pass into the bladder and act as a nidus for a larger bladder stone. Bladder stones occasionally cause bladder outlet obstruction and urinary retention
- A stone may impact in the ureter causing chronic partial obstruction and eventually hydroureter. This presents typically as loin pain but, surprisingly, may be asymptomatic
- A stone may impact in the ureter, causing sudden obstruction. The patient experiences extremely severe, unilateral colicky pain (**ureteric colic**) radiating from loin to the groin or tip of the penis. There is often loin tenderness due to renal distension. The pain is due to waves of ureteric peristalsis and at the peak of the pain, the patient writhes in agony

PREDISPOSITION TO INFECTION

Stones predispose to infection by causing urinary stasis, by preventing proper 'flushing' of the tract and by providing niches in which bacteria multiply. Pelvicalyceal or ureteric

CASE HISTORY

Fig. 37.2 Recurrent urinary tract stones

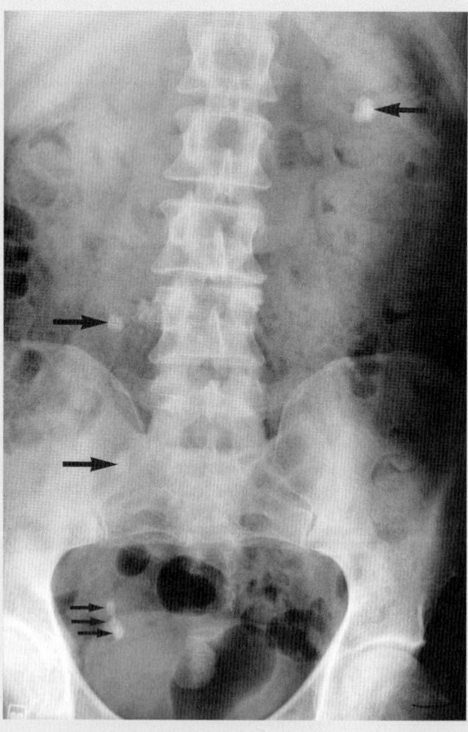

(a)

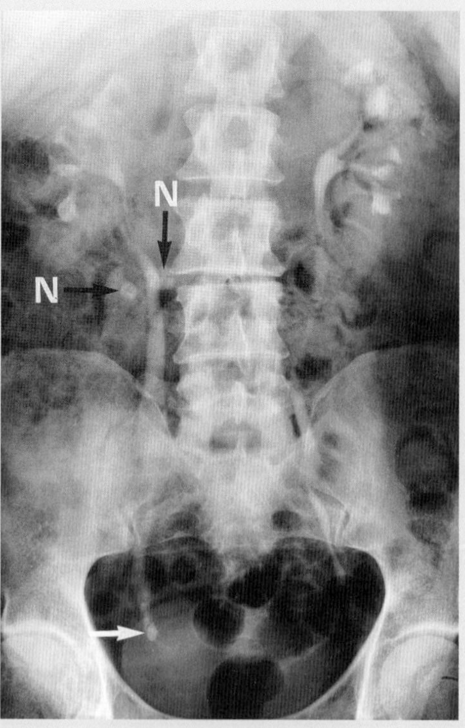

(b)

This man aged 40 had a 2-year history of passing small stones and 'gravel' in the urine. **(a)** Plain abdominal X-ray showing what appear to be several stones (arrowed) in the right ureter and in the upper pole of the left kidney. **(b)** Intravenous urogram (IVU) of the same patient showing partial obstruction at the lower end of the right ureter (arrowed); note that two of the radiopaque objects on the right side lie outside the area of contrast and thus probably represent calcified mesenteric lymph nodes **N** rather than ureteric stones; metabolic studies showed that this patient has idiopathic hypercalciuria

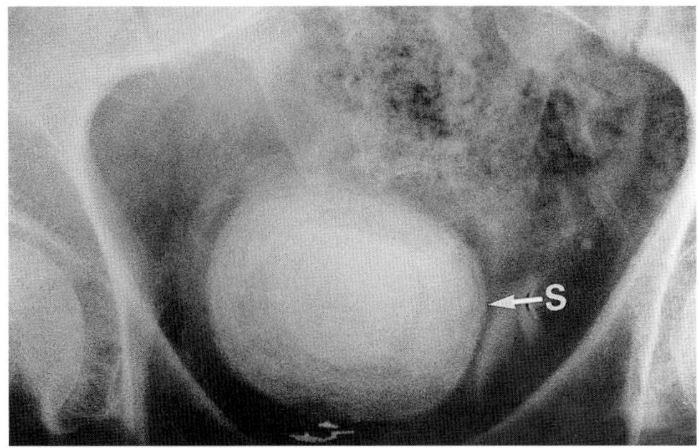

Fig. 37.3 Bladder stone
Plain X-ray showing massive bladder stone **S** in an 85-year-old man with benign prostatic hypertrophy and recurrent urinary tract infections; such stones are rare nowadays

stones can cause **acute pyelonephritis** and occasionally a **perinephric abscess**. Bladder stones predispose to cystitis and ascending infections (see Fig. 37.3).

LOCAL IRRITATION AND TISSUE DAMAGE

Stones may present as a result of their irritant effects on local tissues. Simple inflammation may cause bleeding and present as **haematuria**. Chronic inflammation may lead to fibrosis; if this occurs at a narrow part of the tract, typically the PUJ or ureter, a **stricture** may form. Prolonged irritation of the bladder mucosa by stones may cause **squamous metaplasia** and eventually **squamous carcinoma**.

Fig. 37.4 CT imaging in ureteric colic

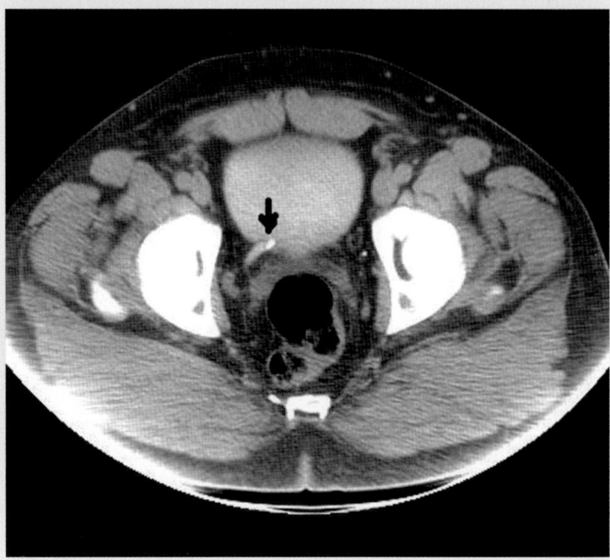

This 37-year-old man presented with right ureteric colic. The CT scan shows a stone at the vesicouretric junction, with a column of secreted contrast held up in the proximal ureter

Box 37.3 Indications for removal of urinary tract stones

- Obstruction of urinary flow
- Infection
- Persistent, recurrent or severe pain
- Stones likely to cause future obstruction or infection
- Small 'metabolic' stones likely to grow rapidly in size
- In patients where colic could be disastrous, e.g. airline or military pilots
- Patients with a solitary kidney

INVESTIGATION AND MANAGEMENT OF SUSPECTED URINARY TRACT STONES

APPROACH TO INVESTIGATION

When investigating a patient with urinary tract stones, the objectives are:

- To confirm a stone is present
- To locate the stone(s)
- To evaluate any deleterious effects of the stone(s) on renal function and urinary tract morphology
- To identify any structural disorders of the urinary tract acting as local predisposing factors
- To identify any metabolic predisposing factors

METHODS OF INVESTIGATION

In general, the objectives can be met by performing the following investigations. For convenience, they are conducted concurrently:

- Urine dipstick testing, microscopy, culture and sensitivities
- Tests of renal function, i.e. plasma urea, electrolytes and creatinine levels
- A 'KUB' (kidney, ureter, bladder) plain abdominal X-ray. Around 90% of stones are radiopaque because they contain calcium. Urate stones are radiolucent
- CT imaging of the abdomen and pelvis. In developed countries, this has become the standard modality for diagnosing loin pain and renal tract stones (Fig. 37.4)
- Intravenous urography (IVU). This consists of a pre-injection KUB and further films at 5–20 minutes after injection of radiopaque contrast and after micturition. Figure 37.2 shows an IVU with the effects of stone obstruction
- Renal ultrasonography. This demonstrates hydronephrosis as well as the stones

- Special contrast techniques. These are occasionally required when other techniques do not give the required information, e.g. percutaneous (antegrade) pyelography or ascending (retrograde) ureterography
- Biochemical analysis of any recovered stones
- Tests for metabolic disorders (for recurrent stones), i.e. serum calcium, phosphate, oxalate, uric acid and alkaline phosphatase; 24-hour urinary excretion of calcium, uric acid and cysteine

INDICATIONS FOR STONE REMOVAL (Box 37.3)

The finding of a urinary tract stone is not an automatic indication for its removal or destruction. The exception is in airline or military pilots in whom ureteric colic could prove disastrous. The usual indications for stone removal are summarised in Box 37.3. Small stones in the pelvicalyceal system often remain unchanged and asymptomatic for many years and can safely be monitored by annual radiography. Stones of 5 mm or less in diameter often pass right through the tract, although in doing so they may produce severe but short-lived symptoms of ureteric colic, haematuria or dysuria.

METHODS OF STONE REMOVAL

Stones can be removed by endoscopic methods, percutaneously or very rarely by open surgery. The choice of technique depends on the size, nature and site of the stone, the availability of expertise and special equipment, and whether there is a need to correct congenital or acquired structural abnormalities.

Cystoscopic techniques

Cystoscopic methods (Fig. 37.5) are suitable for most bladder stones and for impacted stones in the lower third of the ureter. Bladder stones can be broken into small fragments (**litholapaxy**) using a stone punch or **lithotrite**, a cystoscope incorporating stone-crushing jaws. The fragments are then washed out by irrigation. Stones can also be fragmented by directly applied pulsed ultrasound, laser or other energy sources via a cystoscope.

A rigid **ureteroscope** can be used to examine the entire length of the ureter and assist with stone removal (see Fig. 37.6a), as well as to apply energy via laser fibre, ultrasonic, electrohydraulic, or lithoclast probes directly onto the surface of a stone to destroy it. It can also help capture elusive stones via a Dormia basket (declining in popularity). **Flexible ureteroscopes** allow access to the renal pelvis and calyces so stone fragmentation can be achieved using holmium laser probes.

A **ureteric stent** may be placed after repeated instrumentation of the ureter to assist drainage. If an impacted stone is causing complete ureteric obstruction and leading to marked proximal dilatation, or if there is infection, a **percutaneous nephrostomy tube** should be inserted above the stone without delay (see Fig. 37.7, p. 470) to preserve renal function.

Open surgical methods

Open surgery was often required before current minimal access methods of removing or destroying stones. For the pelvicalyceal system **pyelolithotomy** was performed; for the ureter, **ureterolithotomy**; and for some bladder stones, **cystolithotomy**. 'Invasive' surgery is employed nowadays when the appropriate techniques are not available, are not indicated or have failed. Open stone removal is also indicated at the same operation if an elective correction of an anatomical abnormality which predisposes to stone formation is being performed. Examples are bladder diverticula, pelviureteric junction obstruction or ureteric stricture.

(a)

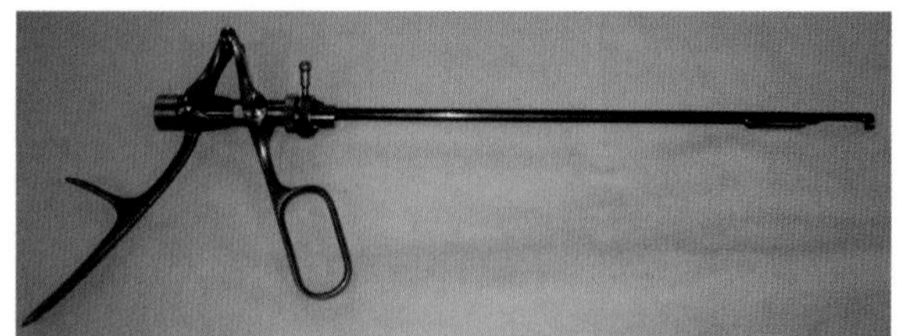

(b)

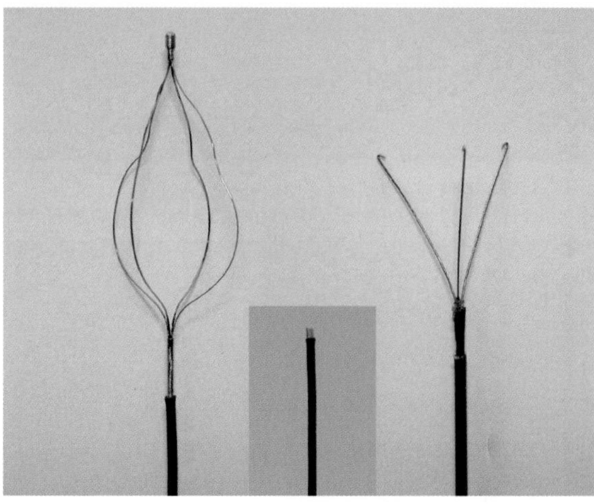

Fig. 37.5 Instruments for urinary stone removal
(a) Straight stone punch (lithotrite). A telescope fits through the centre of the lithotrite, allowing a direct view as the stones are crushed between the jaws. *Note*: the jaws are closed before passing the instrument into the bladder via the urethra. **(b)** Dormia basket and grasping forceps. The Dormia basket (centre and left) is advanced beyond the stone in the ureter and then opened by advancing the centre wire from the proximal end. When open (left), the whole instrument is gradually withdrawn until the stone lodges within the wire basket. The centre wire is then withdrawn further until the stone is firmly held within the basket and the whole instrument withdrawn complete with stone. The trident grasper (right) operates in a similar way, grasping the stone as the wire is retracted

Percutaneous techniques of stone removal

Direct percutaneous access to the renal pelvis can be obtained using radiological or ultrasound guidance. This allows a track to be created from the skin of the loin into the pelvicalyceal system (**nephrostomy**) under local anaesthesia, through which progressively larger instruments can be passed. Small stones can be retrieved using a basket or a steerable grasping tool. Larger stones can be broken into fragments with laser, ultrasonic, electrohydraulic or other probes, after which the

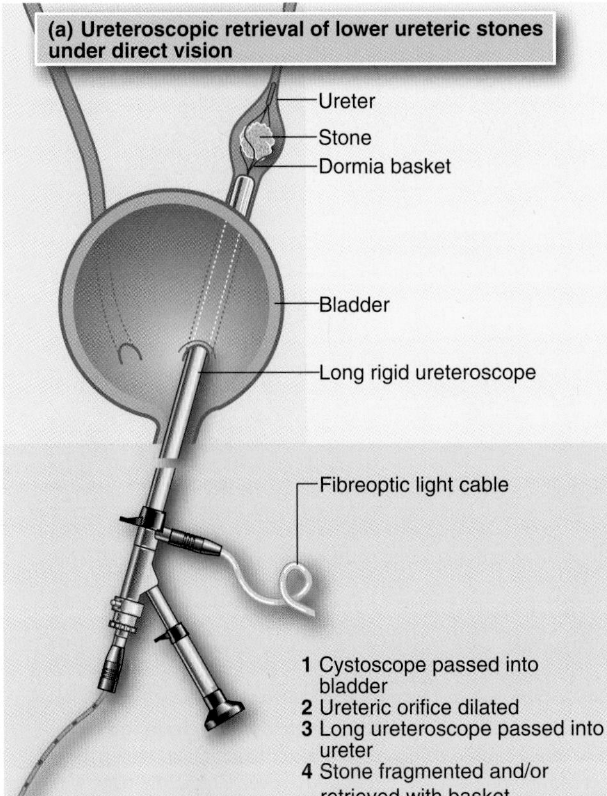

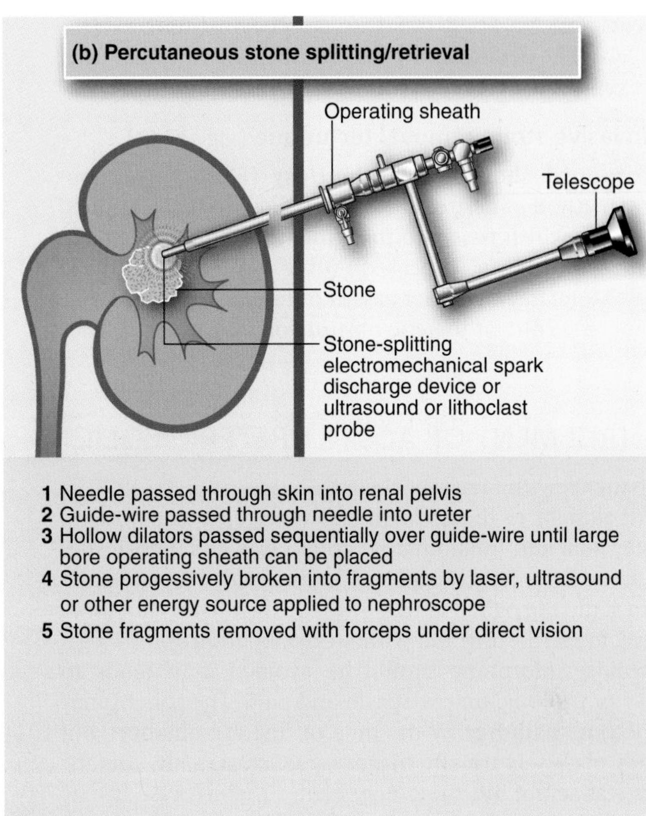

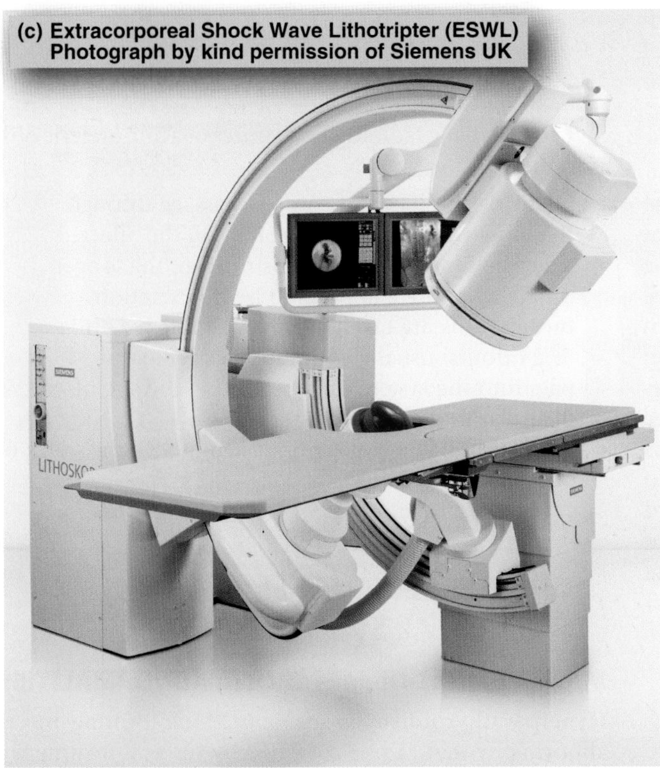

(c)

Fig. 37.6 Current methods of urinary tract stone removal

fragments can be lifted out with special instruments (see Fig. 37.6b). The nephrostomy track closes spontaneously after a short period.

Non-invasive stone removal technique (Fig. 37.6c)

Extracorporeal shock wave lithotripsy (ESWL) is a non-invasive method of destroying stones using externally applied shock waves which pass into the patient to shatter the stone. The ultrasound beam is focused on the stone by ultrasound or X-ray. Stone fragments are passed out in the urine and may cause ureteric colic or ureteric obstruction.

MANAGEMENT OF ACUTE URETERIC COLIC

Most patients with ureteric colic are seen urgently by a GP or brought straight to the accident and emergency department. Non-steroidal anti-inflammatory drugs given as suppositories or injection have largely replaced intramuscular opiate analgesia to settle the pain. NSAIDs (usually diclofenac) are more effective, longer-lasting and without risk of addiction or legal compromise. Morphine should be avoided as it tends to provoke or prolong ureteric spasm and pain. The patient may have become pain-free by the time of first examination, but the pain history is usually diagnostic. Occasionally, ureteric colic is less severe but more persistent, in which case it may mimic other acute abdominal conditions.

Many patients settle with a single analgesic dose but two or three doses may be required. In most cases, the stone gradually passes down the ureter and into the bladder. Each stage of movement may be accompanied by an attack of colic. If a stone is retrieved, it should be chemically analysed. If there is **complete obstruction** of the ureter, or infection above an obstructing stone, urgent intervention is usually required to prevent renal damage. Immediate treatment may involve placing a percutaneous nephrostomy tube to drain the renal pelvis (see Fig. 37.7), placing a stent beside the stone to allow drainage, or removing the stone endoscopically. After nephrostomy or stent placement, the stone sometimes passes spontaneously but more often further treatment is required. In cases with persistent pain not needing immediate intervention, plain abdominal X-rays usually record changes in the stone's position. Very large stones may have to be surgically removed. If a stone appears to be small enough to pass spontaneously, yet fails to progress, the patient can safely be allowed home provided criteria for urgent intervention are not fulfilled. The patient can be reviewed after a week or two with a plain abdominal X-ray and a decision taken then about any need for intervention.

INVESTIGATION OF URETERIC COLIC

Ureteric colic almost always causes **microscopic haematuria**, so the first investigation is 'dipstick' testing of urine for blood; if positive it should be confirmed on microscopic examination. A positive result reinforces the diagnosis. A CT scan or an IVU should then be performed urgently to confirm or refute the diagnosis (see Fig. 37.4, p. 467).

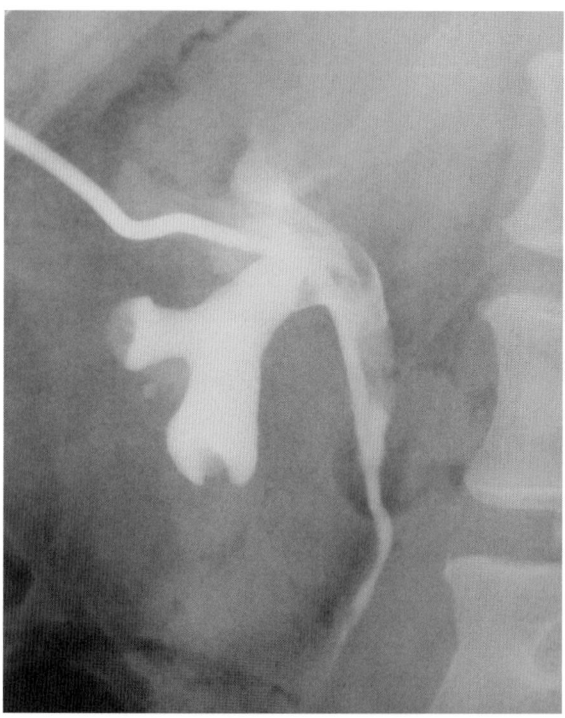

Fig. 37.7 Percutaneously placed nephrostomy drainage tube
A ureteric stone caused complete ureteric obstruction and the patient suffered continuing pain and developed a fever. Urgent drainage was required to prevent renal damage from a combination of obstruction and infection

Characteristic radiological features of acute ureteric obstruction on IVU are:

- **Delay** of all phases of contrast passage through the kidney and collecting system on the affected side; the more severe the obstruction, the longer the delay. If there appears to be no excretion, further films are taken every few hours for up to 24 hours; usually contrast will eventually pass into the system, demonstrating the site of obstruction
- **Dilatation** of the collecting system above the point of obstruction

LONG-TERM MANAGEMENT OF UROLOGICAL STONE DISEASE

MANAGEMENT OF METABOLIC ABNORMALITIES

Hyperparathyroidism is the only stone-forming metabolic abnormality that can be corrected by surgical treatment (parathyroidectomy). It is diagnosed by elevated plasma calcium, lowered plasma phosphate and elevated plasma parathormone levels. Most patients are also hypercalciuric.

Dietary hypercalciuria should be treated by reducing the intake of milk, cheese, butter, bread and pastry. Local tap water and bottled water imbibed by the patient should have its calcium level checked. **Idiopathic hypercalciuria** can be treated with thiazides. Urate stones dissolve in alkaline urine and treatment may involve alkalinising the urine with potassium citrate. **Primary oxaluria** is very rare; secondary oxaluria only occurs with huge intakes of tea, coffee, chocolate, strawberries or rhubarb.

The drug **allopurinol** may be given for hyperuricaemia (gout) and is routinely used during chemotherapy for leukaemia. Allopurinol inhibits xanthine oxidase, an enzyme involved in synthesis of uric acid. Allopurinol can be used in hyperuricaemia (see below) and may also prevent nidus formation in urine around which calcium crystals deposit during stone formation.

LONG-TERM FOLLOW-UP OF PATIENTS WITH URINARY TRACT STONES

For many patients, a symptomatic urinary tract stone manifests as an isolated episode with no apparent predisposing cause. Long-term follow-up for these patients is not usually required. Patients with stones that do not need removing or with recurrent stones need long-term follow-up with regular plain abdominal X-rays. Stones that enlarge during follow-up, that cause symptoms or obstruct need removing. Any patient with stone disease should be advised to increase fluid intake; dietary advice based on stone composition may also help. Drinking excessive fluids during a bout of ureteric colic, however, is misguided and is likely to cause increased pain.

38 Urinary tract infections

INTRODUCTION

Urinary tract infections are a common problem in surgery. They may be responsible for urinary tract symptoms presenting to a clinician for diagnosis or for abdominal pain that is not obviously urological. More often, urinary tract infections are a secondary problem. They can occur after operation, particularly if a urinary catheter has been employed, or may complicate surgical disorders of the urinary tract such as tumours or stones. Most infections are caused by common bacteria of faecal origin.

Urinary tract infections may also be caused by unusual organisms, in particular *Mycobacterium tuberculosis*. On a worldwide basis, other organisms are more important causes of infection, notably the trematode *Schistosoma*. One variety causes severe bladder disease in some developing countries.

Urethral infections are usually transmitted by sexual intercourse. Gonococci and *Chlamydia* are most commonly involved. A late result of gonorrhoea in males may be a fibrous **urethral stricture**. Urethral strictures are covered in this chapter, although most are traumatic and not infective in origin.

BACTERIAL INFECTIONS OF THE LOWER URINARY TRACT

PATHOPHYSIOLOGY OF LOWER URINARY TRACT INFECTIONS

Common urinary tract infections caused by faecal organisms involve the **bladder**, the **upper tract** (kidney, pelvicalyceal system and ureter) or both. The bladder is infected most often, with females being particularly susceptible. Probably half of all females are affected at some time. Infection rate rises with pregnancy and with increasing age. In females, the infecting organisms probably enter via the urethra, which is only 3 cm long. Organisms easily spread from perineal skin, particularly during sexual intercourse.

Normally, the bladder is flushed clean by the frequent passage of newly produced urine, preventing multiplication of bacteria. Stasis—such as incomplete bladder emptying, dehydration or immobility—interferes with this mechanism and predisposes to infection. Urethral instrumentation greatly predisposes to infection in either gender.

CLINICAL FEATURES OF LOWER URINARY TRACT INFECTIONS

Typical symptoms of bladder infection are **dysuria**, **frequency**, **urgency** and a sensation of **incomplete bladder emptying**. The term 'cystitis' is often used by patients to mean symptoms in this list; however, infection is not always involved and the term is best avoided. Even when infection is present, symptoms may be trivial or absent, making diagnosis difficult. Abdominal pain may be the only symptom so most patients with abdominal pain should have urine tested as a matter of course.

There are often no localising symptoms in the elderly or the very young, and the patient may be non-specifically unwell. In any ill patient in these age groups, urine must be sent for examination before antibiotics are given. Recurrent fever in a child can result from urinary infection. A sudden onset of **enuresis** or **urinary incontinence** in children or the elderly should also suggest bladder infection. Presentations of bladder infection are summarised in Box 38.1.

BACTERIOLOGICAL DIAGNOSIS OF LOWER URINARY TRACT INFECTIONS

Urinary tract infection is confirmed by examining a 'midstream' specimen of urine (MSU). If the specimen cannot be examined quickly, it should be refrigerated or it rapidly loses its diagnostic value. The specimen is examined microscopically for white blood cells ('pus cells') and bacteria, and cultured to identify the organism and determine antibiotic sensitivity. Bacterial contamination is common; a 'significant' infection is therefore defined as one with abundant pus cells (more than 100 000 (10^5) organisms per ml). Enteric organisms are almost always responsible, the usual culprits being *Escherichia coli*, *Proteus* spp., *Enterococcus faecalis* and *Pseudomonas* (the last in debilitated or catheterised patients).

Box 38.1 Presentations of bladder infection

- Dysuria with frequency and urgency of micturition (very common)
- Lower abdominal pain (common—usually children or young adults)
- Unexpected development of incontinence (common in the elderly)
- Development of enuresis (bed-wetting) in a previously 'dry' child
- Non-specific ill-health in previously well infants or the elderly (including pyrexia of unknown origin and systemic sepsis)

Staphylococcus saprophyticus is an important cause of uncomplicated bladder infection in young sexually active females.

Significant pus cells without bacterial growth most often result from patients taking antibiotics. If not, a stone, tumour, prostatitis or tuberculosis must be suspected and investigated. Infection often causes frank or occult haematuria but only warrants investigation if it persists after treating the infection. It must be noted that up to 10% of patients with infection have an underlying bladder cancer.

Some females experience symptoms typical of urinary infection but no evidence of bacterial infection of urine is found despite multiple MSUs. Non-specific urethral inflammation from the trauma of intercourse may be responsible (the 'urethral syndrome').

MANAGEMENT OF BLADDER INFECTIONS

Antibiotic therapy is the treatment for bladder infection, chosen on a 'best-guess' basis if treatment is urgent and changed if necessary. Treatment should be commenced only after an MSU specimen; this should be repeated if antibiotic treatment is ineffective or in complicated cases.

Patients who have had urinary tract infections should be encouraged to increase fluid intake. This is often effective with early or mild symptoms and probably allows mild infections to resolve without drugs.

In **pregnancy**, ureters and renal pelvis dilate under the effect of progestogens and become more susceptible to infection. Where bladder infection is suspected, significant bacterial growth should be treated with appropriate antibiotics, whether or not the patient is symptomatic. This is because of the risk of infection ascending to upper tracts and subsequent miscarriage. The antibiotic must be safe for use in pregnancy and non-teratogenic, e.g. a cephalosporin. Trimethoprim is also safe but may deplete folate. Standard texts such as the *British National Formulary* should be consulted on prescribing in pregnancy.

RECURRENT BLADDER INFECTIONS

Patients likely to suffer recurrent infections tend to fall into three groups:

- The elderly, debilitated and infirm
- Young and middle-aged women
- Patients with urinary tract abnormalities predisposing to infection

The elderly, debilitated and infirm

These patients often have multiple simple predisposing factors such as constipation, incontinence, an indwelling catheter, poor fluid intake and diminished resistance. Correction of these problems and good nursing care (e.g. regular changes of indwelling catheter) may break the pattern. Antibiotic-resistant bacteria are often a problem because of previous courses of antibiotics.

Young and middle-aged women

Many can be helped by simple hygiene measures. These include 'wiping from front to back' after micturition or defaecation, frequent and complete emptying of the bladder, increasing urine flow by raising fluid intake, and emptying the bladder soon after intercourse.

Patients with urinary tract abnormalities predisposing to infection

Abnormalities should be suspected in children or young men with a single episode of urinary infection if they fail to respond to simple measures, and anyone with recurrent urinary infections. These patients may have a structural abnormality or pathological condition which encourages bacterial proliferation and require investigation. Bladder stone or prostatic hypertrophy is commonly responsible and predisposing conditions can often be corrected surgically. In the rest no predisposing factor can be found. Some patients with recurrent infections may need long-term, low-dose antibiotics to prevent recurrence.

UPPER URINARY TRACT INFECTIONS

PATHOPHYSIOLOGY OF UPPER URINARY TRACT INFECTIONS

Infections of the pelvicalyceal system and renal parenchyma (**acute pyelonephritis**) arise by upward extension of a lower tract infection or via the bloodstream (haematogenous). **Ascending infections** are most common when there is an abnormality causing ureteric reflux or stasis such as ureteric obstruction, abnormal peristalsis (as in megaureter) and congenital incompetence of the cysto-ureteric antireflux mechanism. During pregnancy, ureters dilate under hormonal influences and this may increase the incidence of upper urinary tract infections.

With upper tract stasis, infection is often haematogenous. Common causes are stones in the renal pelvis or pelviureteric junction (PUJ) obstruction. In these, lower tract infection is a secondary phenomenon. Factors initiating renal infections are often unknown but pre-existing renal damage is a strong predisposing factor.

Pathological examination of an acutely infected kidney shows extensive neutrophilic infiltration of renal parenchyma, often with small abscesses. Usually only one kidney is involved and the causative organisms originate in the GI tract as in other urinary tract infections.

Box 38.2 Presenting features of acute pyelonephritis

- Unilateral loin pain and tenderness
- Poorly localised abdominal pain and discomfort
- Dysuria plus cloudy, strong-smelling urine
- Haematuria
- Pyrexia and tachycardia
- Systemic sepsis (especially young children and the elderly), often without urinary symptoms

CLINICAL FEATURES OF UPPER URINARY TRACT INFECTIONS

The classic clinical features of acute pyelonephritis are unilateral loin pain and tenderness (see Box 38.2). The patient is generally unwell with systemic features of infection, i.e. pyrexia and tachycardia. The urine is usually cloudy and there may be typical symptoms of bladder infection. Often the symptoms and signs are less specific, with unilateral abdominal pain or discomfort that may be mistaken for early acute appendicitis unless the urine is examined. Pyelonephritis may present without localising signs, especially in infants and the elderly, who may be more unwell and even develop signs of systemic sepsis.

MANAGEMENT OF UPPER URINARY TRACT INFECTIONS

Diagnosis is based on clinical symptoms, signs and urine examination. Blood is also taken for culture when there are systemic signs of infection. Treatment is with antibiotics, initially on a 'best-guess' basis, based on local microbiological advice. Dosage and route of administration depend on the severity of the illness; severe cases are treated with intravenous antibiotics.

Once the acute illness has been treated, further investigation may be indicated to search for predisposing factors. This is usually ultrasonography, CT, sometimes intravenous urography, and flexible cystoscopy. In children, investigation should include a contrast micturating cystogram or equivalent radionuclide scintigram to identify ureteric reflux (see Ch. 51).

COMPLICATIONS OF ACUTE PYELONEPHRITIS

(see Figs 38.1 and 38.2)

Pyonephrosis

Severe infections may be complicated by pelviureteric outlet obstruction, resulting in accumulation of pus in the renal pelvis. If untreated, this destroys the renal parenchyma. Treatment involves surgical or percutaneous drainage followed by correction of the obstruction.

Perinephric abscess

In severe infections, sometimes in the presence of a large 'staghorn' calculus, the accumulating pus may discharge through the renal capsule into surrounding fat, resulting in a perinephric abscess (Fig. 38.2). This presents as a slowly expanding loin mass, often with only low-grade local and systemic symptoms. The diagnosis should be considered in elderly patients with sepsis from an unknown source. Urine investigation will reveal pyuria, whilst ultrasound and radiology will show a non-functioning renal mass containing fluid-filled areas. A large renal calculus may also be seen. A perinephric abscess sometimes develops as a result of **haematogenous infection** of a traumatic perinephric haematoma. The treatment of perinephric abscess is drainage. If a perinephric inflammatory mass partially resolves, it can result in **xanthomatous pyelonephritis**, a solid mass often suspected of malignancy and hence removed surgically.

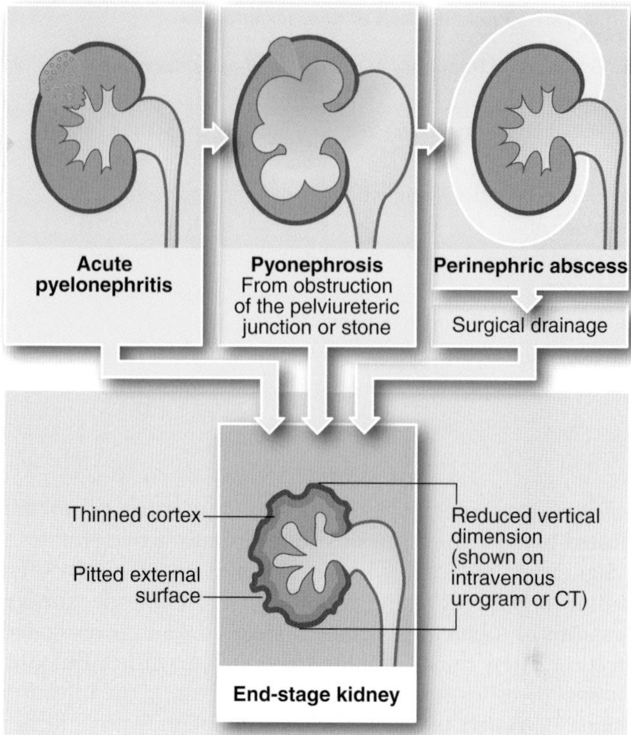

Fig. 38.1 Consequences of untreated renal infection

URINARY TRACT INFECTION IN THE CATHETERISED PATIENT

Even with the best of care, almost all catheterised patients eventually develop bacteriuria. To minimise the risk of generating antibiotic-resistant bacteria, antibiotic treatment should be employed only if there are systemic signs of infection.

GENITOURINARY TUBERCULOSIS

PATHOPHYSIOLOGY OF GENITOURINARY TUBERCULOSIS

About 4% of patients with tuberculosis have genitourinary involvement. Mycobacteria reach the kidney or epididymis via the bloodstream, causing typical centrally caseating granulomatous lesions which may later calcify. From the kidney, direct spread can occur to ureter (causing a fibrous stricture) or to bladder. Tuberculosis of the bladder usually begins around a ureteric opening and spreads to cause patchy ulceration of the bladder wall and later fibrotic contraction. Young adults are most commonly affected and there is a seriously

Fig. 38.2 Perinephric abscess

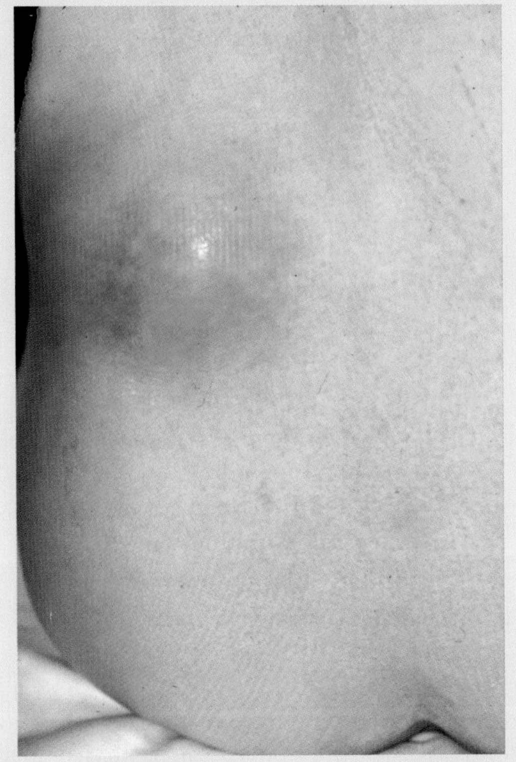

This woman of 55 presented with a 3-week history of left loin pain and 48 hours of rigors. The photograph shows a large abscess surrounding the left kidney, 'pointing' in the posterior loin. A plain abdominal film showed a staghorn calculus in the kidney and isotope studies showed no function in that kidney. The abscess was drained percutaneously and she was treated with antibiotics. The kidney was later removed

increased incidence among patients with acquired immune deficiency syndrome (AIDS). These and patients 'living rough' are poorly compliant with treatment and provide a reservoir of infection for others.

CLINICAL FEATURES AND INVESTIGATION OF GENITOURINARY TUBERCULOSIS

Urinary tract tuberculosis is often asymptomatic and is diagnosed during investigation of 'sterile pyuria', although painless urinary frequency, nocturia and haematuria are sometimes present. Systemic features may also be present, including weight loss, night sweats and respiratory symptoms if the lungs are affected.

When tuberculosis is suspected, at least three early morning urine (EMU) specimens must be sent to the laboratory to be stained and cultured for tubercle bacilli (also known as acid-fast bacilli, AFB). The entire volume of the first urine passed in the morning is collected and centrifuged to concentrate the small number of organisms. Culture usually takes 6–8 weeks but unfortunately a negative result does not exclude tuberculosis.

If there is a red patch around a ureteric orifice at cystoscopy, this can be biopsied and examined histologically for caseating granulomas and stained for tuberculosis organisms, thus accelerating the diagnostic process. Blood is tested for anaemia, lymphocytosis and elevation of the erythrocyte sedimentation rate (ESR), and for biochemical indicators of renal function. A chest X-ray is taken to search for pulmonary disease. Renal calcification may be seen on plain abdominal X-ray, while urography may show renal abnormalities or ureteric strictures.

MANAGEMENT OF GENITOURINARY TUBERCULOSIS

Drug therapy is the mainstay of treatment, as for pulmonary tuberculosis, with agents chosen according to the local prevalence of particular strains and the results of culture and sensitivities. Surgery may be required later to treat ureteric strictures or a contracted bladder, or to excise damaged kidney tissue (partial or total nephrectomy). For ureteric tuberculosis, corticosteroids are usually given along with antituberculous therapy to reduce the risk of stricture formation. Plasma urea and creatinine should be monitored during the usual 6 months of therapy and signs of upper tract dilatation sought with periodic ultrasound examinations.

SCHISTOSOMIASIS

Schistosomiasis (bilharzia) is the most important parasitic disease of the urinary tract. It causes chronic inflammatory lesions in the bladder that lead to severe fibrotic damage. Schistosomiasis also predisposes to stone formation and squamous carcinoma of the bladder.

Three *Schistosoma* species, *S. haematobium*, *S. mansoni* and *S. japonicum*, have a wide tropical distribution and are important human pathogens. The most destructive bladder disease is caused by *S. haematobium*, which is endemic to tropical and North Africa (particularly the Nile valley), and is also in some Middle Eastern and southern European countries. Effective treatment with **praziquantel** has dramatically reduced the reservoir of infection and the incidence of cases in Egypt, but treatment is relatively expensive and has so far made little impact in Sudan. Increasing worldwide travel makes it likely that the disease will be seen more frequently in travellers.

The schistosome has a sophisticated life cycle that depends on poor sanitation. Humans (the main definitive host) are infected by working or bathing in contaminated water. The free-swimming adult forms (**cercaria**) penetrate the skin and pass through the venous circulation and lungs to the systemic arterial circulation, which disseminates them throughout the body. In the portal veins, male and female worms mate. The females, crammed with fertilised ova, find their way via mesenteric veins to the venous plexuses of the pelvic viscera, notably the bladder, where ova are released. Aided by lytic enzymes, the ova then pass through the bladder wall into the urine and thence to the external environment. They then complete their life cycle via an intermediate host, a freshwater snail.

CLINICAL PRESENTATIONS OF SCHISTOSOMIASIS

Initial skin penetration may cause mild local inflammation. Soon afterwards, the phase of haematogenous spread may

Box 38.3 Clinical features of schistosomiasis

- Skin rash at site of cercarial penetration
- Low-grade systemic illness with eosinophilia
- Urinary frequency and terminal haematuria
- Chronic inflammation of the bladder
- Bladder fibrosis and contracture
- Bladder stones
- Squamous cell carcinoma (two-thirds of carcinomas) or transitional cell carcinoma (one-third) of the bladder

cause general malaise, low-grade pyrexia and eosinophilia. About 2 months later, ova invading the bladder mucosa cause local inflammation, and manifest as frequency, and haematuria at the end of micturition. The early symptoms may be trivial and may pass unnoticed.

The main bladder damage caused by schistosomiasis is due to an intense chronic inflammatory reaction to dead ova which have become sequestered in the urothelium. Granulomatous 'pseudotubercles' develop around each ovum and later become fibrotic and calcified. Heavy or recurrent infestations result in a variety of destructive lesions including **ulcers**, **papillomata**, **cysts**, **giant granulomata** and **severe bladder contracture**. All predispose to secondary bacterial infection and bladder stones. Squamous metaplasia is common and strongly predisposes to **carcinoma**: two-thirds of these are squamous and one-third transitional cell. The clinical features of urinary schistosomiasis are summarised in Box 38.3.

MANAGEMENT OF SCHISTOSOMIASIS

Bladder or ureteric calcification is almost diagnostic of schistosomiasis. Diagnosis is confirmed by microscopy of urine for ova or more reliably by cystoscopic biopsy of bladder lesions. Serological tests may also be of value in travellers from the developed world without previous exposure.

Treatment is with the drug **praziquantel** given in two doses of 20 mg/kg body weight on 1 day, 6 hours apart. **Metrifonate** is an alternative treatment. Surgery is occasionally needed later to correct or palliate residual lower urinary tract deformities.

About 5% of the world's population is affected by schistosomiasis and prevention must be the cornerstone of disease control. Effective treatment of affected individuals substantially reduces the pool of infection and the number of new cases, but better sanitation and clean water supplies are essential. Ironically, the rapid expansion of water conservation and irrigation schemes has spread the disease to previously unaffected populations.

URETHRAL INFECTIONS AND STRICTURES

URETHRAL INFECTIONS

The only clinically important urethral infections are sexually transmitted diseases. The most common are **gonorrhoea** and chlamydial infection. The acute condition usually presents with urethral discharge and dysuria. The surgical importance of urethritis, particularly gonococcal, is that it may lead, months or years later, to fibrous stricturing of the urethra. Fortunately, these strictures are becoming less common as effective antibiotic therapy is more available. However, in recent years multi-antibiotic-resistant strains have begun to emerge, particularly in the Far East.

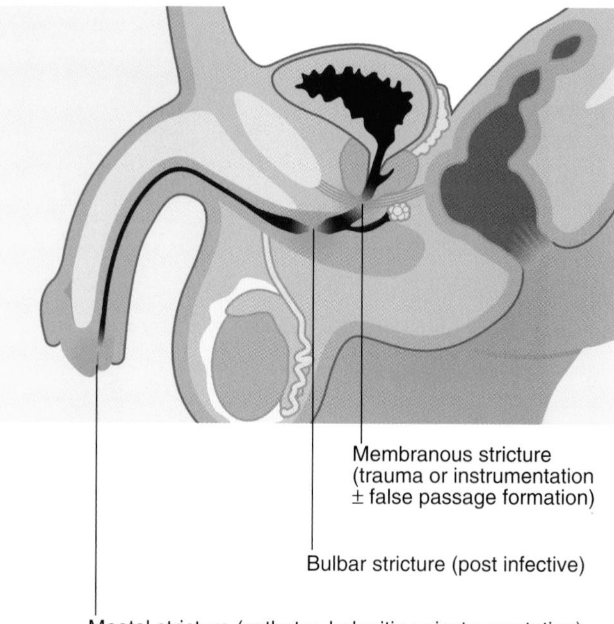

Fig. 38.3 Common sites of urethral strictures

Serological tests for gonorrhoea and *Chlamydia* are relatively unreliable and have largely been abandoned. The standard tests for diagnosis now involve molecular amplification (e.g. PCR) which can be done on urethral swabs and first-catch urine samples.

URETHRAL STRICTURE

Urethral strictures are now most commonly caused by inflammation resulting from **iatrogenic trauma**. Transurethral resection for prostatic surgery is the most common cause. Urinary catheterisation in patients with poor tissue perfusion is another common cause, particularly during cardiopulmonary bypass for cardiac surgery. Iatrogenic strictures involve the distal urethra or the meatus. Strictures may also be a complication of traumatic instrumentation, where the membranous urethra is most vulnerable (see Fig. 38.3). A few strictures result from urethral tearing or rupture following displaced pelvic fractures. These usually require open surgical reconstruction.

The characteristic symptom of urethral stricture is a progressive decrease in urinary stream. If there is also chronic urinary retention, there may be frequency and urgency, symptomatic of bladder outlet obstruction. Diagnosis is made by direct inspection using a cystourethroscope or by urethrography.

Strictures may be short, elongated or multiple. An effective treatment involves **stretching** the scar tissue by repeated self-dilatation. An alternative with tight strictures is to **cut the stricture** longitudinally with a urethrotome under direct urethroscopic vision, and follow this by repeated dilatation. Recurrence after treatment is almost to be expected, so skilled urological follow-up is needed. More complicated strictures may require **open surgical treatment**: for example, excision of a short stricture and end-to-end anastomosis of the urethra. For some, **inlays** of oral mucosa or post-auricular skin may prove successful.

Urethral strictures cause lifelong disability, and most can be avoided by extreme care of the urethra during catheterisation and urethral instrumentation. As a general rule, the urethra should not be catheterised or interfered with unless absolutely essential. Sick patients should be catheterised only with a silicone-coated urethral catheter or else a suprapubic catheter employed. Any catheter or other urological instrument should be placed gently and with minimal force or else under direct vision.

39 Congenital disorders and diseases secondarily involving the urinary tract

CONGENITAL URINARY TRACT DISORDERS

INTRODUCTION

Serious congenital disorders of the kidneys and urinary tract nearly all present at birth or in early childhood (see Ch. 51). The exception is **polycystic kidney** which presents more commonly in adulthood. Less common abnormalities of the upper tract may interfere with normal flow dynamics and predispose to infection, e.g. duplex systems or medullary sponge kidney. Asymptomatic abnormalities such as unilateral renal agenesis, renal cysts or horseshoe kidney may be discovered incidentally during investigation or during surgery. With advancing age, a large proportion of the population develops benign renal cysts; these are usually of no clinical consequence. A summary of congenital disorders that present after childhood is given in Table 39.1.

POLYCYSTIC KIDNEYS

Adult polycystic kidney disease (PCKD) is an autosomal dominant disorder characterised by bilateral multiple cysts of renal parenchyma (see Fig. 39.1). The cysts slowly expand, compressing the parenchyma, and may disrupt local control of blood pressure and eventually impair renal function. Polycystic kidneys have three main variants:

- A rare infantile form also affecting the liver; affected children often die young
- A serious adult form manifesting in middle age with hypertension or progressive renal failure. It is the commonest cause of inherited renal failure. Kidneys can appear normal on ultrasound scanning up to about the age of 20
- A less serious adult form usually found incidentally in later life with almost normal renal function. Patients are usually hypertensive

Thus, adult polycystic kidney may present with **hypertension** or progressive **chronic renal failure**. The enlarged kidneys may cause loin pain or be discovered incidentally on abdominal examination. These kidneys are vulnerable to even minor trauma, and **haematuria** and urinary tract infections are common presentations.

Some with polycystic disease also have multiple cysts in the liver and sometimes in the pancreas. They present with massive abdominal swelling due to gross liver enlargement. There is no specific treatment for polycystic kidney disease and despite good conservative management, about 50% will eventually require dialysis or renal transplantation.

MEDULLARY SPONGE KIDNEY

This is caused by cyst-like dilatation (**ectasia**) of the renal medulla collecting ducts and may affect one or both kidneys. Cysts tend to calcify, giving a characteristic radiographic appearance of streaky linear calcification of renal papillae (see Fig. 39.2). On excretion pyelography (IVU), tubular ectasia can be demonstrated as a 'flare' in the renal papilla. Marked degrees of medullary sponge kidney predispose to recurrent infection and stone formation because of intrarenal urine stasis but patients rarely present before adulthood. Minor degrees are often seen on IVU without causing symptoms.

DUPLEX SYSTEMS

The urinary collecting system may be duplicated to a greater or lesser extent. Duplication is usually complete proximally but may be incomplete distally. Lesser duplications are usually asymptomatic and discovered by chance on imaging. Complete duplex ureter is relatively common and may result in renal damage from infection, reflux or obstruction (see

Table 39.1 Congenital abnormalities of the urinary system presenting after childhood

Nature of abnormality	Presentation
Kidney	
Medullary sponge kidney Cystic dilatation of collecting ducts of one or more medullary pyramids (the subunits of the medulla) in one or both kidneys	May be found incidentally or during investigations for urinary infection. Cysts tend to become calcified and have characteristic X-ray appearance
Adult polycystic kidney Autosomal dominant disorder with multiple cysts throughout the parenchyma	Usually presents after age 30 with chronic renal failure, hypertension, haematuria or recurrent urinary tract infections
Renal cysts Can be simple or complex	Often an incidental finding. May present with loin swelling or pain
Horseshoe kidney Fusion of lower poles of kidneys preventing normal developmental ascent	Often found incidentally but may cause hydronephrosis due to pelviureteric obstruction. Sometimes found incidentally at operation for AAA, complication the procedure
Ectopic kidneys and abnormalities of rotation Due to failure of developmental ascent	Found incidentally or during investigation of complications such as pelviureteric obstruction
Pelvicalyceal system and ureters	
Ureterocoele Cystic dilatation of intravesical part of ureter due to stenosis of ureteric orifice	Incidental finding or may cause infection or symptoms of obstruction
Duplex systems Partial or complete duplication of a ureter	Often an incidental finding or cause of recurrent infection
Bladder and urethra	
Urachal abnormalities Cyst, sinus, abscess, secondary malignancy	Cysts and sinuses may present in adulthood as a result of persistence of urachal remnants. Adenocarcinoma sometimes develops in the urachal remnant

Fig. 39.3). The ureter draining the **upper renal pole** (upper moiety) is often inserted ectopically into the urethra (or vagina), resulting in continuous incontinence. Otherwise it joins the bladder ectopically **below** the orifice of the lower pole ureter. The orifice is often tightly stenosed, causing obstruction. This causes back pressure on the kidney and sometimes distal ureter dilatation known as a **ureterocoele**.

The ureter draining the **lower moiety** may have a defective distal antireflux mechanism, predisposing to infection and renal parenchymal damage. The typical IVU picture is of calyces that look like a 'drooping daffodil'.

RENAL CYSTS

Isolated renal parenchymal cysts are a common developmental abnormality and although rarely symptomatic, can be found in a fair proportion of the population in later life. They are usually recognised incidentally during imaging. Their importance lies in distinguishing them from solid tumours and hydatid cysts, which is usually easy with ultrasonography or CT scanning. Renal cysts can be simple or complex (containing blood, calcification or solid components). Occasionally simple cysts cause pain or swelling. For these, aspiration alone is of no value as the cysts rapidly refill. If intervention is required, cysts should be deroofed laparoscopically (in contrast to the treatment of polycystic disease).

HORSESHOE KIDNEY

This abnormality is caused by embryological fusion of the two developing kidneys at their lower poles. Normal renal ascent in fetal life is prevented by the inferior mesenteric artery at the abdominal aorta, so the isthmus of the kidney comes to lie across the aorta at the third or fourth lumbar vertebral level. The condition is usually a chance finding on imaging (see Fig. 39.4) or else at abdominal aortic surgery, when it may cause serious operative difficulties. Horseshoe kidney is sometimes associated with pelviureteric junction obstruction, the symptoms of which may prompt the diagnosis. Occasionally, a horseshoe kidney first causes problems during pregnancy.

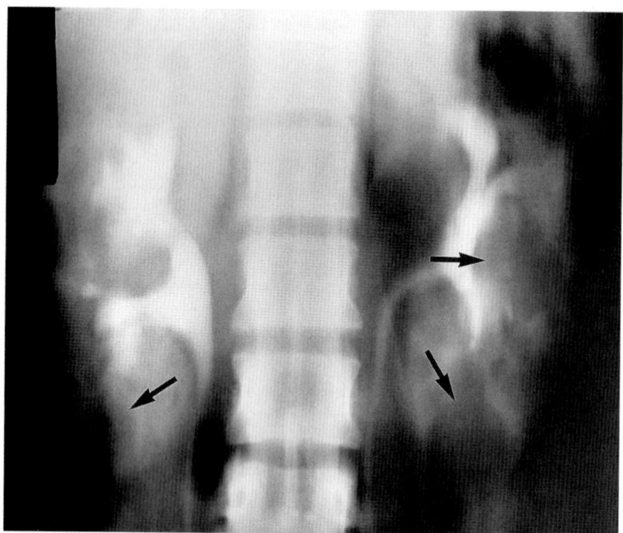

Fig. 39.1 Polycystic kidneys
IVU tomogram from a 52-year-old woman with hypertension and microscopic haematuria; both kidneys exhibit multiple lucent areas in the nephrogram representing cysts (arrowed) and the pelvicalyceal systems are slightly compressed

CASE HISTORY

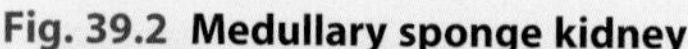

Fig. 39.2 Medullary sponge kidney

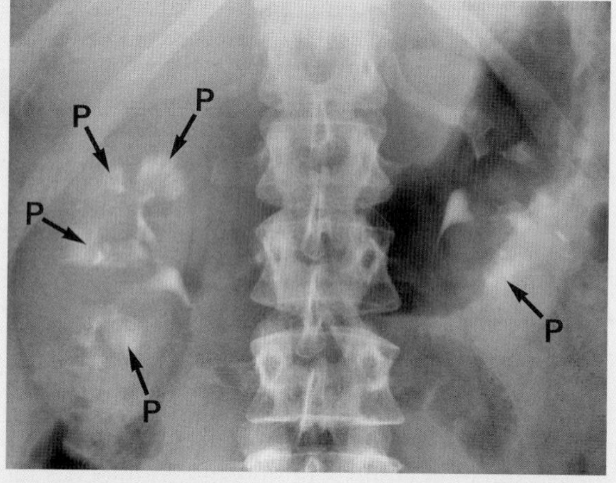

Bilateral medullary sponge kidney on an IVU from a 55-year-old woman with recurrent urinary tract infections; the renal papillae **P** has a typical 'flared' appearance and retains contrast because of the dilated collecting ducts. No radiopacity was visible on the control film although it can be seen in a considerable proportion of cases because of calcification in the ectatic ducts of the papillae

RENAL ECTOPIA AND OTHER RENAL ABNORMALITIES

Other renal abnormalities may be found incidentally. These include ectopic kidneys (see Fig. 39.5), rotational abnormalities, unilateral agenesis, aplasia or hyperplasia. These abnormalities may confuse the diagnosis and sometimes result in surgical mishap, e.g. excision of a pelvic kidney mistaken for an ovarian tumour. Note that transplanted kidneys are usually deliberately sited in the iliac fossa.

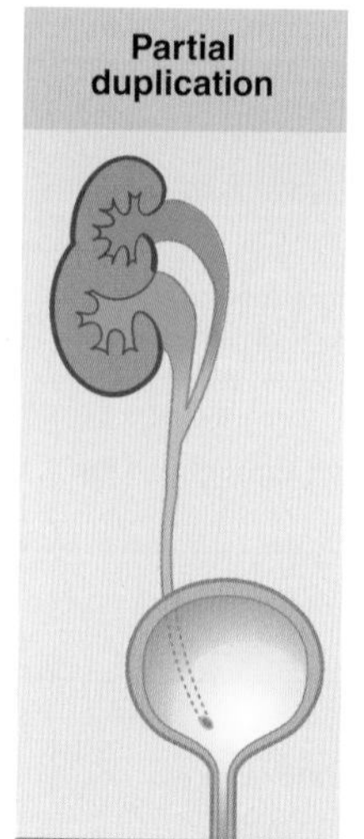

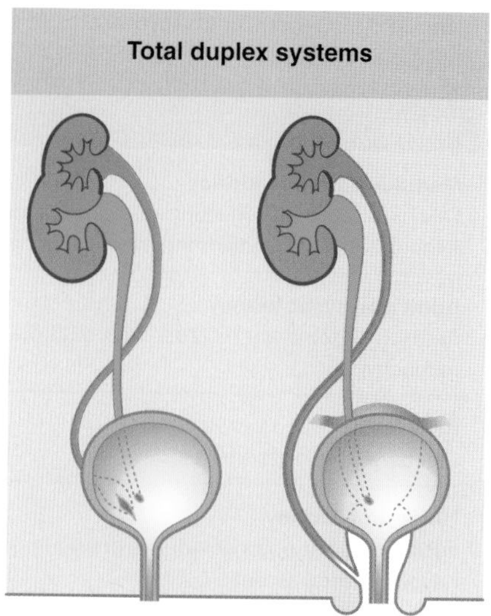

(a)

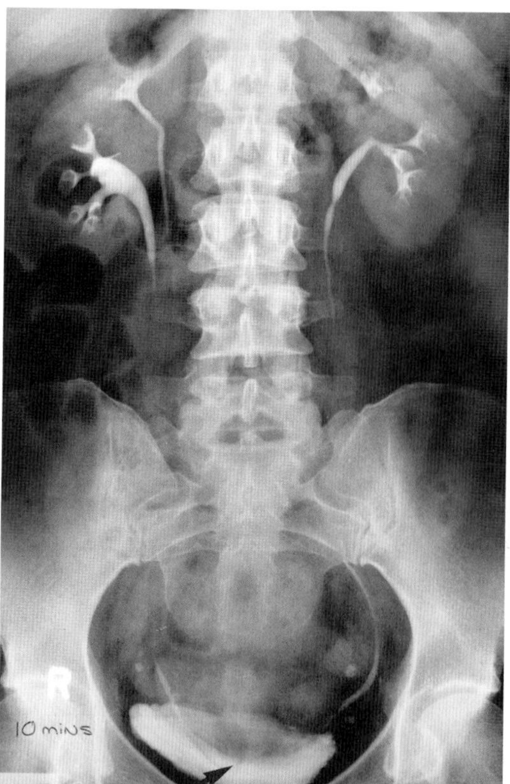

(b)

Fig. 39.3 Duplex systems
(a) Partial and total duplication. In a total duplex system (right), the ureter from the upper renal moiety may open into the urethra or vagina (i.e. wholly ectopic). Such an ectopic ureter causes continuous incontinence and presents early in life. Otherwise, it opens inferiorly in the bladder (centre). The orifice is often stenosed and a **ureterocoele** results (dilated lower end of ureter). Vesicoureteric reflux often occurs via the **upper** ureteric orifice back into the **lower** renal moiety. **(b)** Duplication of the ureters on the right side; only one ureter can be seen passing as far as the bladder. The vesicoureteric junction is associated with a small, elongated ureterocoele (arrowed)

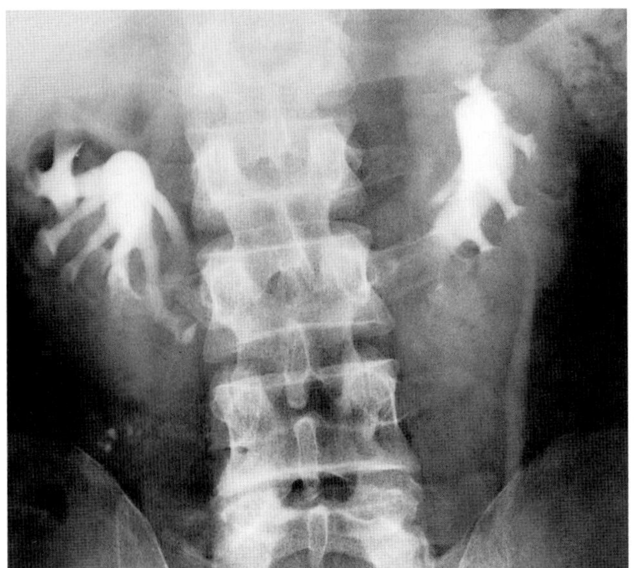
(a)

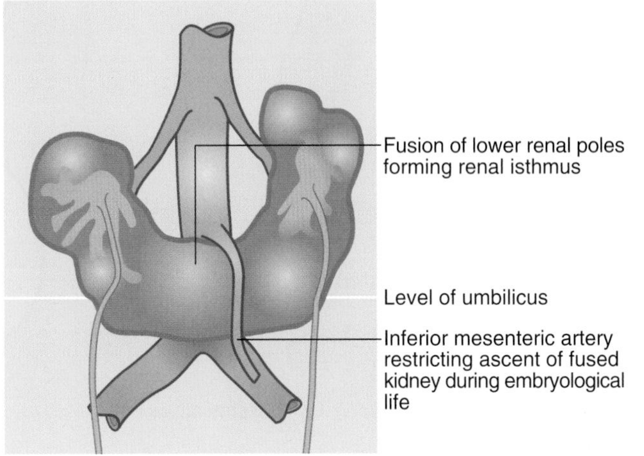

(b)

Fig. 39.4 Horseshoe kidney
Horseshoe kidney shown on IVU from a 51-year-old woman with recurrent urinary tract stones; the pelvicalyceal systems are oriented obliquely and converge inferiorly because the isthmus is stretched over the vertebral column. Each pelvis and ureter is more medially placed than normal and the whole renal mass lies much lower than would normal kidneys. The isthmus of a horseshoe kidney can rarely be demonstrated by IVU or ultrasound but can easily be imagined in this image

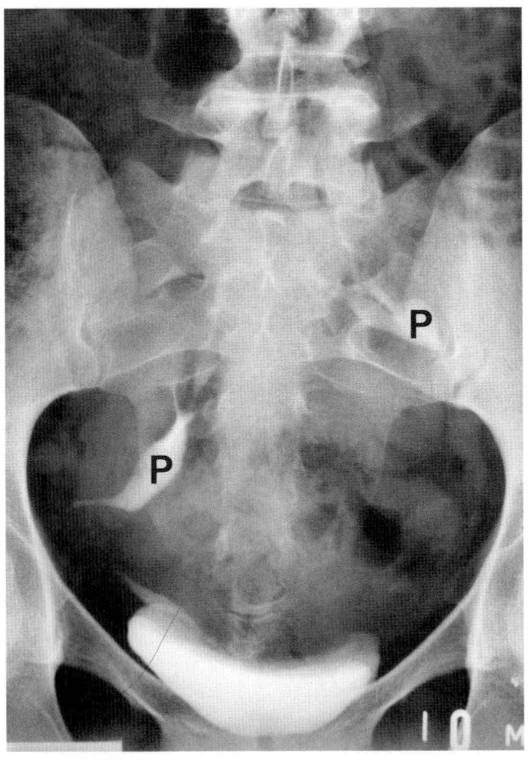

(a)

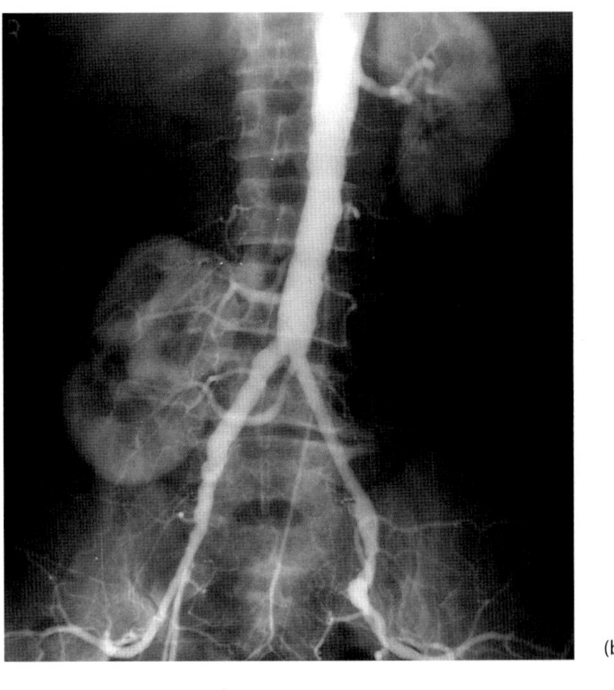
(b)

Fig. 39.5 Ectopic kidneys
(a) A 48-year-old woman with recurrent urinary tract infections; IVU shows abnormal pelvicalyceal systems **P** of bilateral pelvic kidneys. **(b)** Right pelvic kidney discovered incidentally during arteriography for severe claudication. Its blood supply can be seen to arise from the distal aorta and iliac artery. The patient needed an aortofemoral bypass but when faced with the technical difficulties, agreed to conservative management of her claudication

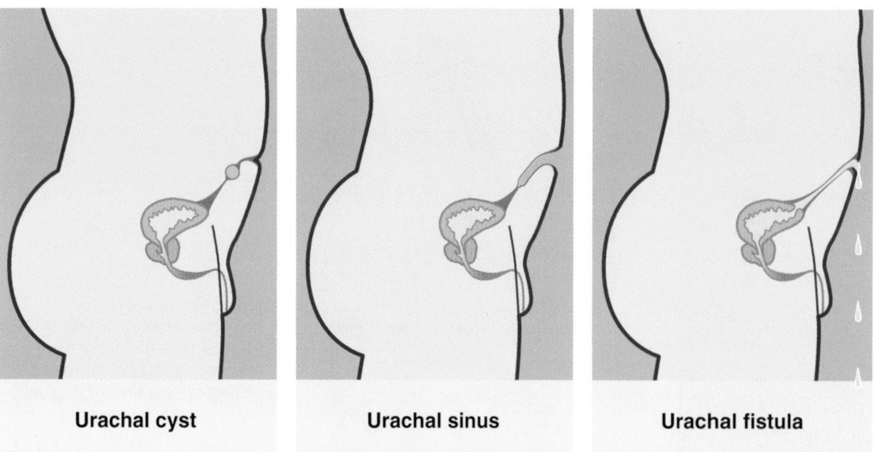

Fig. 39.6 Urachal abnormalities

URACHAL ABNORMALITIES (see Fig. 39.6)

During fetal development, the urogenital sinus communicates with the allantois via the urachus. Occasionally, this tract persists as a **fistula** between bladder and umbilicus. Sometimes the fistula does not open until adulthood. Similarly, a remnant may form a blind urachal **sinus** that opens at the umbilicus or result in a urachal **cyst** in the lower abdominal midline. These structural abnormalities may then become infected. Very rarely, an **adenocarcinoma** develops in a urachal remnant in the bladder vault or elsewhere.

DISEASES SECONDARILY INVOLVING THE URINARY TRACT

INTRODUCTION

Abdominal disorders such as tumours, inflammatory bowel disease, aneurysms and retroperitoneal fibrosis may secondarily involve the urinary tract, as may iatrogenic (surgical) damage. Any of these may affect the urinary tract by obstructing one or both ureters or occasionally by causing a fistula between bowel and urinary tract. Obstruction of one ureter alone may not be symptomatic although it may cause loin pain or predispose to infection; bilateral involvement usually presents with acute or chronic renal insufficiency.

TUMOURS AND INFLAMMATORY CAUSES

Of tumours outside the urinary tract, advanced **carcinoma of the uterine cervix** most commonly produces bilateral ureteric obstruction because of its close relationship to the ureters. This cancer may also ulcerate anteriorly into the bladder causing a **vesico-vaginal fistula**. This anatomical closeness also makes ureters vulnerable to trauma even at uncomplicated hysterectomy. Abdominal and particularly laparoscopic-assisted hysterectomy can be associated with damage to the ureter, causing stenosis and hydronephrosis or a uretero-vaginal fistula. An iatrogenic vesico-vaginal fistula can also be produced. Although carcinoma of the ascending or rectosigmoid colon rarely obstructs the right or left ureter respectively, most ureteric damage in relation to large bowel cancer results from colectomy operations.

Inflammatory disease that involves bowel serosa may extend to involve ureters and bladder and cause possible fistula formation. This is important in **Crohn's disease** and **diverticular disease**. A fistula between bowel and urinary tract presents as severe urinary infection, often with pneumaturia or faecuria.

An expanding abdominal mass can compress one or both ureters and cause symptoms from partial obstruction; sometimes **aortoiliac aneurysms** are responsible. An 'inflammatory' aneurysm near a ureter is likely to cause obstruction. This variant occurs in about 5% of aortic aneurysms. The cause is unknown but the effect is to produce retroperitoneal fibrosis across the anterior surface of the aneurysm. A much more common cause of ureteric dilatation is **pregnancy**, in which bilateral megaureter results from the effects of progestogens. The main significance of bilateral megaureter in pregnancy is predisposition to upper renal tract infection. Thus, significant bacteriuria in pregnancy, symptomatic or not, should be treated with antibiotics. Retention of urine can be caused by a pelvic mass such as a pregnancy of around 14 weeks or an ovarian lesion of similar size.

RETROPERITONEAL FIBROSIS (RPF)

This relatively rare and obscure condition is characterised by progressive, intense fibrosis of the connective tissue lying posterior to the peritoneal cavity. About 50% of cases are caused by retroperitoneal spread of malignant disease. In the remainder, the cause is unknown in many (i.e. idiopathic), but some rarely used drugs such as **methysergide** can induce the condition or it may be associated with an inflammatory aortic

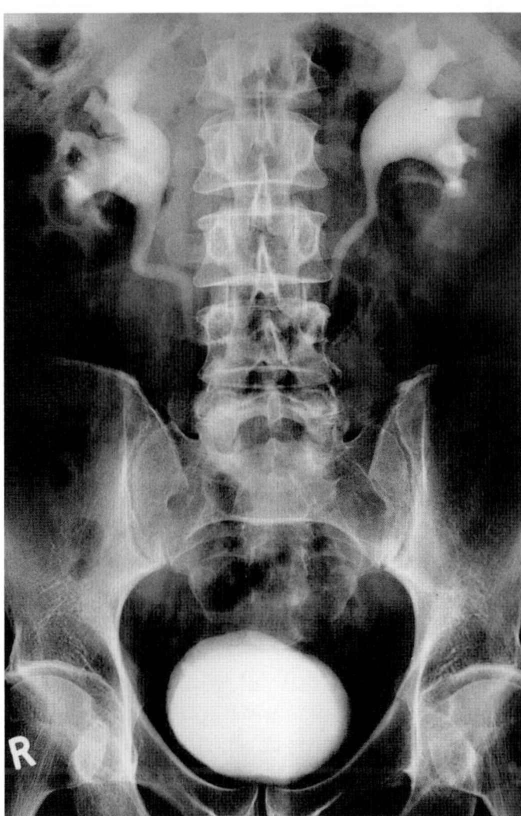

Fig. 39.7 Retroperitoneal fibrosis
This man of 62 presented with back pain. The IVU shows bilateral hydronephrosis due to ureteric compression; note how the ureters are tapered and characteristically drawn medially by the fibrotic process

aneurysm. Retroperitoneal fibrosis sometimes causes hypertension via its effect on the kidneys.

Retroperitoneal fibrosis compresses both ureters, causing bilateral hydronephrosis and eventually renal failure. It can also be associated with inferior vena cava obstruction. Diagnosis is usually made on IVU or CT scanning which shows bilateral hydronephrosis (see Fig. 39.7). The fibrotic process also draws the ureters closer together in the midline. The ESR is characteristically elevated.

Treatment usually involves a trial of high-dose steroids and insertion of **double-J stents** to maintain upper tract function whilst awaiting improvement. Surprisingly, ureters compressed by retroperitoneal fibrosis can usually be catheterised with ease. If medical treatment fails, the next step is usually dissection of the ureters from the retroperitoneal tissue (**ureterolysis**), which are resited within the peritoneal cavity in an attempt to prevent recurrent obstruction. A biopsy of the retroperitoneal tissue should be taken to exclude malignancy and confirm the diagnosis. If obstruction recurs, corticosteroid therapy may suppress the condition. Aortic grafting is indicated if a substantial aneurysm is present.

40 Pathophysiology, clinical features and diagnosis of vascular disease affecting the limbs

INTRODUCTION

The term 'peripheral arterial disease' (PAD) is often employed to mean obstructive ('obliterative') disease of major lower limb arteries causing ischaemia. However, a range of vascular disorders can cause symptoms in upper and lower limbs, and a broader term 'peripheral vascular disease' (PVD) includes any disease of arteries, veins or lymphatics outside the heart. This chapter concentrates on lower limb vascular-related problems as they are much more common; upper limb symptoms are outlined in Table 40.5 (p. 488).

Patients with PAD of the legs may have no symptoms, either because they do not walk far enough to claudicate or because the collateral circulation has developed to deliver enough blood to leg muscles. Patients with vascular limb disorders may present to any medical specialty and some require urgent action, e.g. acute limb ischaemia or a painful abdominal aneurysm. Thus all clinicians need to understand the principles of diagnosis and the scope and timing of treatment. This chapter covers the **pathophysiology** of limb vascular insufficiency, plus the details of **history taking** and **examining patients** with suspected vascular disease and the process of reaching a broad, 'first stage' diagnosis.

VASCULAR INSUFFICIENCY OF THE LIMB (Table 40.1)

Arterial insufficiency and venous insufficiency do not indicate any specific pathophysiology and either may be acute or chronic. Limbs vascular disorders are caused mainly by atherosclerosis, arterial thromboembolism, aneurysms, complications of diabetes, and thrombotic and varicose disorders of the venous system. Sometimes several causes interact.

Acute arterial insufficiency means inadequate arterial blood supply to a limb over hours or days. It may be caused by embolism into a normal artery, in which thrombus originating in the heart or other proximal site detaches and is swept distally until it lodges and obstructs the vessel. It can also occur by in situ thrombosis of an atherosclerotic plaque in lower limb arteries, by thrombosis of a popliteal aneurysm or by an aortic dissection extending into the lower limb vessels. Any disorder can manifest in several ways—see Table 40.2 for the various manifestations of popliteal aneurysm.

Chronic venous insufficiency means inadequate venous drainage for at least 2 weeks and often much longer.

SYMPTOMS AND SIGNS IN THE LIMB

An accurate initial diagnosis depends almost entirely on skilled and methodical clinical evaluation rather than on special investigations. Preliminary assessment notes obvious major risk factors (Table 40.3). Detailed history taking is covered in Table 40.4 and examination in Figure 40.1. In a suspected vascular case, the student or doctor tries to decide if the problem is arterial, venous or lymphatic, or has some other cause.

The principal symptoms and signs of vascular disease are pain, changes in skin texture, colour and temperature, tissue loss including ulceration, and swelling. The upper limb is affected by a largely different range of disorders with signs and symptoms with only a small overlap (see Table 40.5).

PAIN

Most limb pain is due to musculoskeletal disorders such as arthritis or trauma rather than vascular disease. Where lower limb peripheral ischaemia is the working diagnosis, a full cardiovascular workup is needed (see Table 40.4 and Fig. 40.1).

- **Lower limb**—patients may have itching and aching with varicose veins, or have exercise-related pain or severe and constant pain caused by obliterative arterial disease. Where the history is short, acute ischaemia may be the cause
- **Upper limb**—vascular-related pain is uncommon. Aching and swelling may be caused by subclavian vein

Table 40.1 Pathophysiology of arterial and venous insufficiency—the clinical consequences of vascular diseases affecting the lower limb*

Basic disease	Pathophysiological process	Clinical manifestations
Atherosclerosis and embolism causing ischaemia		
Atherosclerotic narrowing of large distributing arteries	Arterial supply inadequate to supply muscles during exercise Arterial supply inadequate even at rest, with relative ischaemia of all tissues. Risk of pressure ulceration. Healing severely impaired Limb is critically ischaemic; risk of limb necrosis in 6–8 hours unless urgently revascularised Thrombotic occlusion of atherosclerotic artery; clinical features as acute critical ischaemia	**Intermittent claudication**—muscle pain on walking, quickly relieved by rest **Chronic severe ischaemia**—rest pain in foot, worse at night. Onset sudden, or chronic over a few days or weeks. Skin pale/red/purple **Acute critical ischaemia**—often with patchy gangrene or ischaemic ulcers **Acute-on-chronic ischaemia**—sudden onset of acute ischaemia in patient with chronic ischaemia
Embolism arising from atherosclerotic lesions in carotid arteries	Atherosclerotic debris or platelet thrombi migrate distally and occlude cerebral arteries	**Transient ischaemic attacks** (TIAs) and strokes from carotid disease
Embolism from heart	Masses of thrombus detach and impact at arterial bifurcations, occluding flow	**Acute severe ischaemia** of upper or lower limb, brain or intestine. Often pre-existing atrial fibrillation or recent myocardial infarction
Diabetes mellitus		
The 'diabetic foot' (neuro-ischaemic foot)	Accelerated atherosclerosis and neuropathy in an unpredictable mixture. Loss of sensation predisposes to injury and ulceration Lesions often complicated by pyogenic infection	Foot lesions (often painless)—deep ulceration in pressure areas, necrotic toes. Assume atherosclerotic ischaemia unless foot pulses palpable. Infection spreads rapidly, causing limb-threatening necrosis and systemic sepsis. Needs early and vigorous treatment Resistance to infection impaired in diabetics
Venous disorders		
Thromboembolism **Acute deep venous thrombosis (DVT)** May be complicated by **pulmonary embolism**	Spontaneous thrombosis in deep veins of calf or thigh; may propagate to iliofemoral veins Obstructs venous return causing swelling and warmth. Venous gangrene in extreme cases	**Pain and swelling of calf and ankle**, often with calf tenderness, but often asymptomatic without clinical signs. Thigh swollen if iliofemoral veins thrombosed. Associated with risk factors, particularly immobility. Leg usually blueish or normal colour
Chronic venous insufficiency Post-thrombotic limb and venous eczema	Late complication of DVT Spontaneous recanalisation of occluded veins damages valves causing incompetence (reflux) and local venous hypertension Similar features in gross superficial venous insufficiency in varicose veins	**Chronic brawny oedema** of leg often with narrow ankle due to lipo-dermatosclerosis ('champagne bottle leg'). Skin atrophic, scaly and pigmented and gaiter area above ankle vulnerable to chronic ulceration after minor trauma

*Aneurysms are covered in Chapter 42 and varicose veins and thrombophlebitis in Chapter 43.

thrombosis. Claudication is rare and acute ischaemia is usually due to embolism. **Thoracic outlet syndrome** is also rare. The brachial plexus may be compressed as it passes between the clavicle and first rib (or extra cervical rib) causing nerve root symptoms. Even less commonly, the condition may cause arterial or venous obstruction at the thoracic outlet

INTERMITTENT CLAUDICATION

Chronic lower limb arterial insufficiency usually presents as muscular pain on walking. The history is characteristic: pain begins at a reproducible distance, is worse walking uphill and increases if walking continues; the patient usually begins to **limp**, accounting for the name 'intermittent claudication' (Latin: *claudicare* to limp), and the patient is forced to stop. Symptoms usually predominate in one limb. The pain subsides within a minute or two of stopping and recurs at the same walking distance. Pain is almost always in the calf, whatever level the arterial obstruction, but may extend into thigh or even buttock in aorto-iliac obstruction. If associated with impotence, this is known as **Leriche syndrome**.

After a thorough history, only **cauda equina claudication** or **pseudo claudication** might be mistaken for 'true' claudication. This is caused by compression of the cauda equina in the spinal canal by central disc protrusion or canal stenosis. Lower limb pain is also brought on by exercise but there are important differences—see Table 40.6.

CHRONIC ISCHAEMIC REST PAIN

With severe arterial obstruction, ischaemic pain occurs when the patient is in bed or even when sitting. Termed **rest pain**, this is usually felt in the skin of the foot and is very severe and burning. It occurs mostly at night because gravity assistance to arterial supply is lost, cardiac output falls at rest, and skin vessels dilate with warmth. The pain is characteristically relieved by hanging the leg out of bed or even walking around and is not fully relieved by any analgesics. Often, patients end up sleeping in a chair, causing lower limb oedema. Patients often present after tolerating this severe pain for several weeks. Only 10% of claudicants progress to rest pain.

There may also be skin changes or tissue loss such as gangrene and ulceration (see below). The term **critical ischaemia**

Table 40.2 Symptoms and signs of popliteal aneurysm—different clinical consequences of a similar underlying disorder

Clinical presentation	Pathophysiology
Asymptomatic—pulsatile swelling in popliteal fossa discovered by patient, by chance or during examination of patient with vascular problem	Often part of multi-aneurysmal disease Examine for other aneurysms—other popliteal fossa, abdomen, femoral arteries
Acute ischaemia	Thrombosis of aneurysm or distal embolisation of clot from within aneurysm
Chronic ischaemia	Gradual occlusion of aneurysm or arterial runoff by thrombus or atherosclerosis
Apparent deep venous thrombosis (DVT)—swelling, cyanosis of leg	Large aneurysmal swelling occludes popliteal veins. May lead to DVT
Rupture of aneurysm	Sudden pain and swelling behind knee; swelling and pain in leg; evidence of distal ischaemia

Table 40.3 Preliminary assessment of the vascular patient for obvious risk factors

Factors to assess first	Significance
Major risk factors for arterial disease—'GASD'	
Gender	Men affected by atherosclerosis and aneurysms 10 years earlier than women
Age	Peripheral atherosclerosis rare below 55 years—most common age 60–70. DVT unlikely below 20
Smoking cigarettes	Risk of atherosclerosis proportional to 'pack-years' smoked; PVD unlikely in people who have never smoked
Diabetes (especially type 2)	Premature and accelerated atherosclerosis, predominantly more distally in limb. 25% of PVD patients are diabetic compared with 2–3% of general population Peripheral neuropathies (sensory, motor and autonomic) Reduced resistance to infection
Other risk factors	
Hypertension	Predisposes to atherosclerosis, stroke and aneurysm expansion
Hypercholesterolaemia and hypertriglyceridaemia	Risk factors for atherosclerosis. Some inherited types have major adverse effects
Obesity and sedentary lifestyle	Difficult to quantify but likely to be significant factors

Table 40.4 History taking in suspected limb arterial or venous disease

History of presenting complaint—limb symptoms	Important features of the history
Symptoms and signs Pain Changes in skin texture Changes in skin colour (including gangrene) Changes in skin temperature Ulceration and tissue loss Swelling Loss of sensation	**Detailed history of each symptom:** **Where?** Upper/lower limb; one or both; which part of the limb; precipitating/relieving factors; extent of changes **When?** When did it start; sudden or gradual onset; progress—getting worse or better; worse during day or night **Initiating factors?** Preceding activity or event, e.g. trauma/excess exercise **Exacerbating factors?** e.g. exercise/posture **Relieving factors?** e.g. hanging leg out of bed/elevation/analgesics **Nature of symptoms?** Severity; periodicity, i.e. continuous or intermittent **Pain?** Site/severity/timing/precipitants/onset/radiation **Impact of symptoms?** What is the patient prevented from doing (working/walking/sleeping/sitting comfortably) **Disability?** e.g. impaired grip; heavy arm **Recent trauma to limb?** e.g. fracture and treatment, dislocation, soft tissue trauma

Table 40.4 Continued

History of presenting complaint—limb symptoms	Important features of the history
Past medical history	**Important features of the history**
General cardiovascular history	Venous or arterial thromboses; bleeding tendency
Peripheral vascular disease	
Arterial	Intermittent claudication; previous limb surgery—bypass operations; angioplasty; arterial thrombosis
Venous	Varicose veins/previous surgery; thrombophlebitis; DVT or pulmonary embolism; arm swelling; trauma + immobilisation, e.g. lower limb fracture/treatment/ligament injury (predisposing to silent DVT)
Related history	In claudication—back problems and surgery (possible cauda equina claudication) Cervical rib; hypothyroidism Pre-existing lymphatic disorder of limb (e.g. primary lymphoedema)
Cardiac disease	
Manifestations	Ischaemic heart disease; (angina, MI) Heart failure (chronic lower bilateral limb oedema) Hypertension; valvular disease; arrhythmias
Interventions	Medication/thrombolysis Coronary angiography/angioplasty /pacemaker Cardiac surgery, e.g. CABG; valve surgery
Cerebrovascular disease	
Manifestation	Ischaemic/haemorrhagic stroke; transient ischaemic attacks (TIAs)
Interventions	Medication; carotid artery surgery/angioplasty
Renal failure	Acute or chronic renal failure ± dialysis
Rheumatological disease	Collagen/vascular disease: Raynaud's; rheumatoid disease Systemic sclerosis/scleroderma; other connective tissue disorders; vasculitis
Miscellaneous contributing factors	
Lower limb paresis or deformity	Predisposes to pressure ulcers: stroke or congenital spinal problems, e.g. spina bifida
Haematological disorders	Thrombophilias, e.g. thrombocythaemia, factor V Leiden mutation, antithrombin III, protein C or S deficiency; polycythaemia vera
Drug history	
Is patient taking:	Antihypertensives (ACE inhibitors, beta-blockers, calcium channel blockers, diuretics); anti-platelet drugs (aspirin, clopidogrel, etc.) Anticoagulants (e.g. warfarin); a statin
Social history	
Smoking	Smoker/ex-smoker/passive smoker; how many pack-years
Exercise	Physically fit; regular exercise
Employment	Do symptoms impact on work; how does occupation impact on symptoms
Family history	
Hereditary cardiovascular disease?	Cardiac, PVD, aneurysm, arterial or venous thrombosis

implies that loss of part of the limb is inevitable unless it is revascularised. Beware of the trap in **diabetic patients** with neuropathy—**severe ischaemia may be painless**. Disruption of small vessel autonomic control may mean a severely ischaemic foot is warm and red rather than cold and white or blue. In the absence of palpable pulses, only arteriography will reveal the truth.

ACUTE CRITICAL ISCHAEMIA

This is of sudden onset, with pain similar to rest pain. However, if peripheral blood flow is very low, pain may be absent in the distal, most severely affected area, which becomes numb or has diminished sensation (paraesthesia) due to nerve ischaemia. Severe pain is present proximally where the tissue is less ischaemic. By this time, the patient has muscle

Table 40.5 Summary of signs and symptoms of vascular disease of the upper limb

Sign or symptom	Underlying disorder	Other clinical features
Swelling of arm and/or forearm		
	Axillary vein thrombosis Predisposing causes: Unaccustomed use of arm overhead, e.g. decorating Excess weight lifting Cervical rib or congenital bands obstructing vein Too narrow a space between first rib and clavicle	Blueness and heaviness of arm; later, prominent collateral veins over deltopectoral area. Symptoms usually abate spontaneously but early thrombolysis worth considering
Colour change		
Acute whiteness or blueness	Embolism (causes as lower limb) Trauma to brachial artery, e.g. supracondylar fracture	Acute ischaemia—hand cold, painful, loss of sensation and motor function
White finger(s)	Raynaud's disease (common): fingers go white then turn blue then red, often in response to cold. Due to vasospasm—pathogenesis unknown Secondary Raynaud's phenomenon (rare); underlying disorders include: Limited cutaneous scleroderma (CREST) Mixed connective tissue disease Sjögren's syndrome Systemic lupus erythematosus Vibration white finger due to power tool use	Recurrent symptoms especially in cold weather May lead to atrophy of finger tips but rarely major tissue loss As Raynaud's disease
Red painful fingers	Reflex sympathetic dystrophy post trauma following fracture, especially forearm	Pain, redness, disability in arm
Pain		
Vascular	Substantial subclavian arterial narrowing. Rarely symptomatic because of excellent upper limb collaterals Acute ischaemia—most commonly embolism of cardiac thrombus; sometimes acute-on-chronic thrombosis (see acute ischaemia above)	Muscle pain on exercise— arm 'claudication'. Low systolic pressure Acute pain of vascular origin plus other features of ischaemia—pulselessness, pallor, paralysis, loss of sensation
Neurovascular	Thoracic outlet syndrome— 95% neurological symptoms, 5% arterial—lower trunk symptoms affecting C8/T1 most common. Rare and difficult to diagnose	Chronic pain—usually musculoskeletal but may be due to thoracic outlet syndrome

Table 40.6 Comparison between cauda equina claudication and arterial claudication

Arterial insufficiency	Cauda equina syndrome
History	
'Fixed' claudication distance	'Variable' claudication distance
Pain exacerbated by walking uphill	Pain often absent when walking uphill; often better when cycling
No history of low back problems	History of low back problems
Pain disappears after 1–2 minutes rest	Pain takes 15–30 minutes to subside
Examination	
Absent peripheral pulses and low ankle pressure in affected limb	Pulses usually present and ankle pressure normal
No evidence of a lower motor neurone (LMN) lesion	Evidence of an LMN lesion such as diminished or absent lower limb tendon reflexes
Duplex ultrasound scan or arteriography shows arterial obstruction	CT or MRI scanning of the spinal canal is diagnostic, demonstrating a narrow spinal canal or disc protrusions impacting on the cauda equina

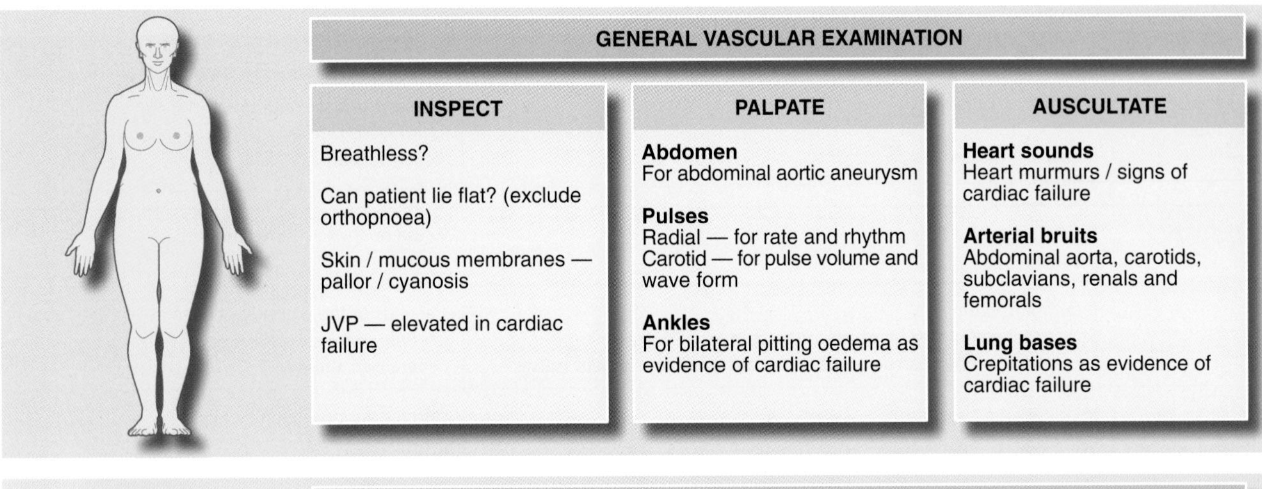

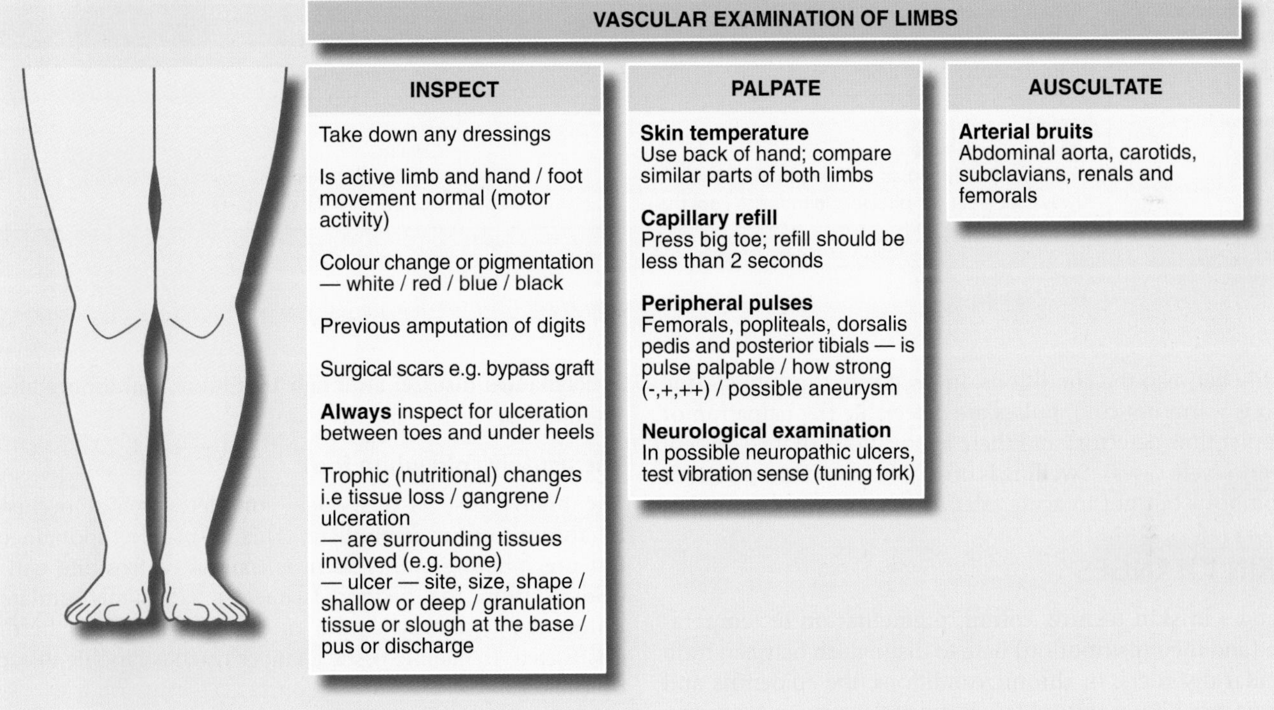

Fig. 40.1 Examination of the vascular patient

pain on moving the foot or paralysis due to muscle ischaemia. It is vital to recognise acute arterial insufficiency quickly as it rapidly progresses to irreversible necrosis without timely treatment.

The cardinal clinical features of acute critical ischaemia are:

- **Pain**—severe but variable in intensity; affects distal part of limb
- **Pallor**—the ischaemic area is initially white but later becomes mottled (marbling) due to stagnation of deoxygenated blood. If this blanches on pressure, the limb is still viable. If the mottling does not blanch (fixed staining) then the limb is non-viable
- **Pulselessness**— foot pulses are absent and popliteal and femoral pulses may be lost, depending on level of arterial occlusion
- **Perishing coldness**—most extreme at foot (or hand)
- **Paraesthesia** (reduced sensation) or **anaesthesia** of the periphery. This only occurs if ischaemia is severe
- **Paralysis** of calf muscles. The patient is unable to flex or extend toes or ankle. This only occurs if ischaemia is extreme. Pain may disappear at this stage

(As an *aide-mémoire*, these features are known as the six Ps: Pain, Pallor, Pulselessness, Perishing coldness, Paraesthesia, Paralysis. Not all are present all of the time; anaesthesia and paralysis are dire prognostic features and indicate that revascularisation is required immediately.)

DEEP VENOUS THROMBOSIS (ACUTE VENOUS INSUFFICIENCY)

In symptomatic DVT, swelling and heaviness are the usual presenting symptoms but pain is always less severe than in severe ischaemia. Physical examination usually distinguishes

Table 40.7 Interpretation of colour and temperature change in limbs

Colour of limb	Signs	Interpretation
White (see also Buerger's test, Fig. 40.4)	If cold with pulses If cold without pulses Asymptomatic	Physiological or vasospastic disorder Chronic ischaemia Acute ischaemia Constricted venules
Blue or cyanotic	Painful, absent pulses Swollen	Acute or chronic ischaemia DVT
Red	Intact skin, warm Superficial gaiter area ulceration, little pain Ulceration in foot or ankle plus severe pain; cold with absent pulses	Cellulitis or the diabetic ischaemic trap (see above) Chronic venous insufficiency Severe ischaemia
Brown	In gaiter area ± ulcer	Chronic venous insufficiency
Black	Toes or distal foot	Necrosis or gangrene
Temperature	**Other signs**	**Interpretation**
Cold	White (compare other limb)	See 'white' above
Warm or hot	Swollen Indurated, oedematous skin Ulcerated distally in diabetic + absent foot pulses Always hot—patient puts feet in fridge to cool them	DVT Cellulitis The diabetic ischaemic trap—do an arteriogram Erythromelalgia; unknown aetiology

readily between the conditions. In deep vein thrombosis, the limb is warm not cold, pulses are detectable (by palpation or Doppler flow detector) and there is no colour change (except in very severe cases). Swelling is often a feature of deep venous thrombosis but not in acute arterial ischaemia.

SKIN CHANGES

Changes in **skin texture**, **colour**, **pigmentation** or **temperature** (and their distribution) help to distinguish between limb vascular disorders. In chronic conditions, the epidermis and dermis may become atrophic because of deficient oxygenation and nutrition; these are termed **trophic changes**.

In arterial insufficiency, whatever level the obstruction, the trophic effects are most evident at the periphery, i.e. the foot and toes or hand. In contrast, the changes caused by chronic venous insufficiency are most severe around the medial ankle above the malleolus (the 'gaiter area'), almost never on the foot. Evidence of chronic venous disease includes venous eczema and haemosiderin deposition, progressing to lipodermatosclerosis (cutaneous fat around the ankle becomes thinned and indurated by fibrosis) and the characteristic 'champagne bottle' leg (marked sclerosis and narrowing at the ankle with oedema above—see Fig 43.1c).

CHANGES IN SKIN COLOUR AND TEMPERATURE

(see Table 40.7)

Many people, particularly the elderly, suffer from cold feet in cold weather; if both feet are pale or blueish when cold but are painless with normal pulses, this is normal. If pathological, the cause may be due to a **vasospastic disorder** such as Raynaud's disease, although this more commonly affects the hands.

The acutely cold white foot

The main cause is a sudden complete arterial occlusion by thrombosis or embolism. This is usually spontaneous but precipitating events such as trauma or frostbite will be evident from the history. Ischaemia is usually unilateral unless the abdominal aorta or both iliac arteries become obstructed. Ischaemic tissue changes reach a variable distance up the leg.

Colour change in venous thrombosis

Noticeable colour change is unusual in deep venous thrombosis but massive pelvic vein thrombosis may cause changes sometimes mistaken for arterial occlusion. Massive thrombosis was once more common, especially during late pregnancy. The condition was known as **white leg of pregnancy** or **phlegmasia alba dolens**. The whole lower limb is painful, pale and massively swollen. In contrast to arterial occlusion, the limb is warm and pulses are detectable despite the oedema. A more serious variant is **blue leg** or **phlegmasia caerulea dolens**, which represents incipient venous infarction.

The chronically cold foot

Blue toes

In severe claudication or rest pain, the onset of dusky skin in the foot suggests developing tissue necrosis (**pre-gangrene**). If finger pressure is applied to the skin, the rate of colour return gives some indication of skin perfusion (capillary refill). However, many elderly people with few symptoms have a slow refill time; these rarely have arterial disease and this can easily be excluded by Doppler ankle pressures.

Black toes

Necrosis in chronic ischaemia may be patchy and localised if there is a developed collateral circulation (Fig. 40.2). Such necrosis is usually confined to toes or part of the forefoot. The necrotic area slowly becomes hard, black and mummified (**dry gangrene**) and may eventually separate spontaneously from viable tissue. However, there is a risk that the necrotic area becomes infected. The tissue then becomes boggy and ulcerated and the infection and gangrene spread proximally, particularly in diabetics. This **wet gangrene** requires urgent treatment, often with a combination of revascularisation and amputation.

Redness

Skin redness indicates oxygenated blood is present in capillaries and implies there is no venous congestion or obstruction. With ischaemia, there is reactive dilatation of the microvasculature to hypoxia, a physiological attempt to extract the maximum oxygen from whatever blood is reaching the area. Thus severely ischaemic skin may feel cool but, paradoxically, be red—the so-called 'sunset foot'.

Buerger's test for severe ischaemia (Fig. 40.3) involves high elevation of the leg for a minute or two. If peripheral arterial pressure is inadequate to overcome gravity, the entire foot becomes white. When the leg is hung down, it gradually becomes blueish-red as blood flow returns. This test is easily misinterpreted—even in the normal limb, the foot will blanch somewhat with elevation.

The warm foot

Inflammatory dilatation of the microcirculation causes redness, and the skin is warm and slightly swollen because of enhanced blood flow. An example is low-grade bacterial **cellulitis** which may be seen in diabetes or chronic venous insufficiency or may arise unexpectedly. Note that if a severely ischaemic limb becomes infected, the usual signs of inflammation may not develop and the extent of infection may be underestimated. If blood supply is later restored, signs of inflammation appear.

Fig. 40.2 Necrosis from severe ischaemia

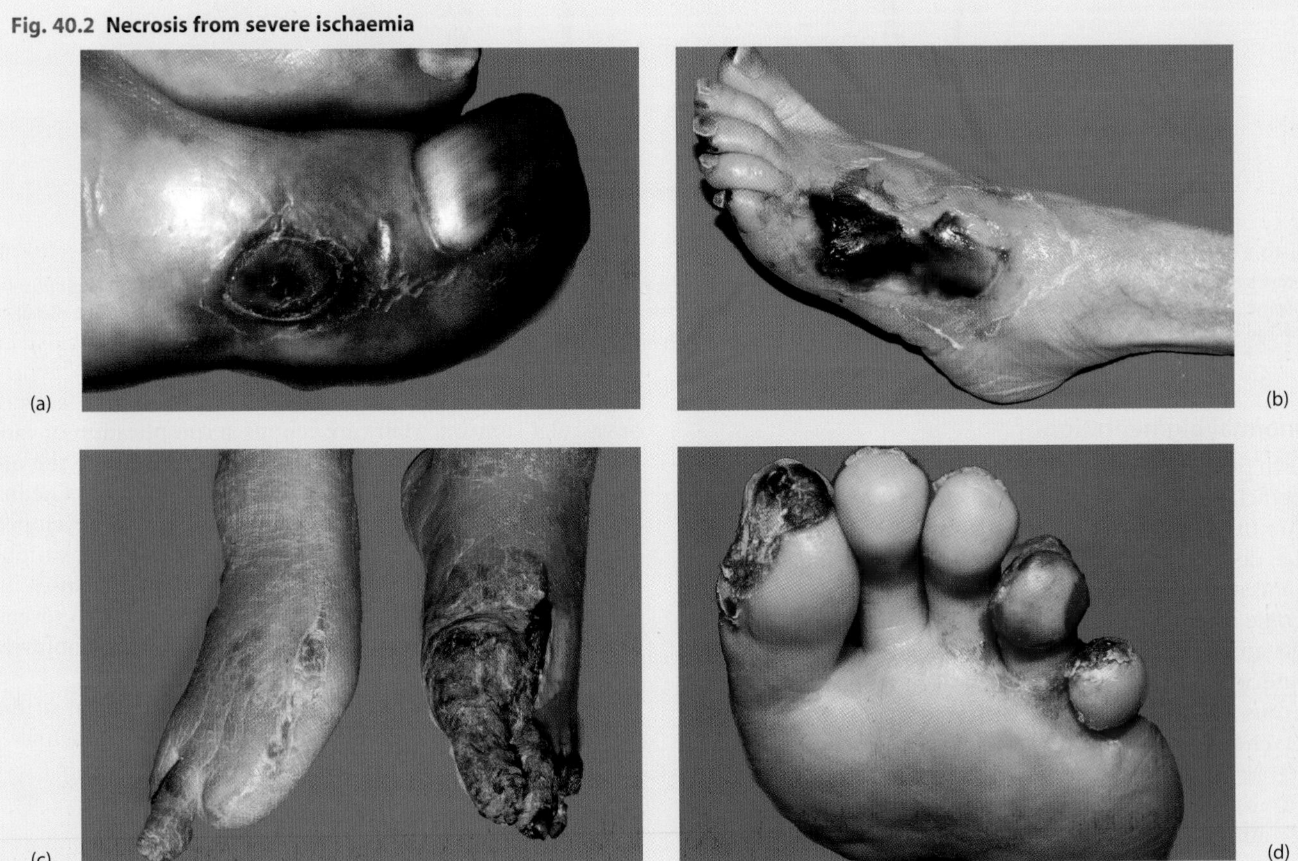

(a) Sudden thrombosis of an atherosclerotic superficial femoral artery ('acute-on-chronic' occlusion) led to acute ischaemia, manifesting as rest pain and necrosis of big toe. **(b)** Embolism of thrombus from left atrium into femoral artery led to severe ischaemia and necrosis of skin within 6 hours. Embolectomy was performed as early as possible. The photograph shows the resulting acute ischaemic ulcer of dorsum of foot. **(c)** Left foot shows signs of severe chronic ischaemia with dry gangrene. Right foot has healed following successful femoropopliteal bypass grafting and local amputation. **(d)** Typical patchy distal necrosis following spontaneous embolism of thrombus from within an abdominal aortic aneurysm

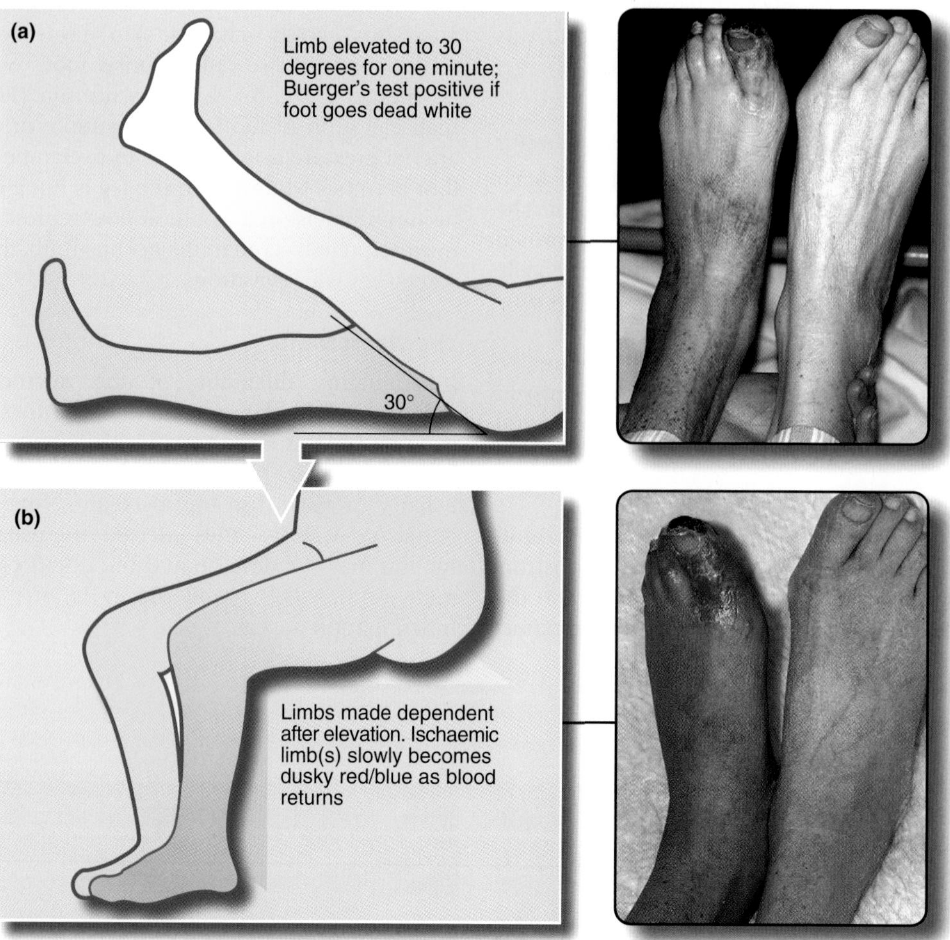

Fig. 40.3 Buerger's test in severe ischaemia of the lower limb
Buerger's test is only truly positive when limbs are severely ischaemic. This 78-year-old man had severe ischaemia of both legs with the left being critically ischaemic. **(a)** In the first stage, one or both feet are elevated. Both feet go pale but the right is dead white. The left big toe is seen to be necrotic distally. **(b)** In the second stage, with dependency, both feet go blueish red, most marked on the left

Abnormal pigmentation

Brown pigmentation around the gaiter area is often caused by superficial or deep **chronic venous insufficiency** due to gross reflux in varicose veins or a **post-thrombotic limb**. In the latter, deep vein valves have been disrupted by inflammation, organisation and recanalisation following DVT. Valves thus become incompetent and allow **deep venous reflux**. This prevents an effective muscle pump and leads to chronic venous insufficiency. In gross superficial or deep venous reflux, standing causes venous stagnation, increased venous pressure in the leg (**venous hypertension**) and chronic leg swelling. Red cells extravasate into the tissues and form haemosiderin deposits which cause brown pigmentation. This, accompanied by dry, scaly, atrophic skin, is described as **varicose** or **venous eczema** (see Fig. 40.4).

LOWER LIMB ULCERATION (Box 40.1)

Chronic ulceration is common, particularly in the elderly. These ulcers are usually managed by GPs and community nurses, with more difficult cases referred to a dermatologist or vascular surgeon. Many are venous, a complication of varicose veins or a late complication of DVT. Most of the rest are caused by arterial insufficiency or diabetic neuro-ischaemia and a few by vasculitis or ulcerating tumours. In developed countries, infection rarely plays a primary role but various tropical ulcers and tuberculosis are important causes in developing countries. Intractable cases may be due to several factors, e.g. local trauma, diabetic neuropathy and obliterative atherosclerosis.

Effective treatment depends on clinical evaluation of the patient's general condition first, then the following factors:

- History of the origin and evolution of the ulcer
- The site of the ulcer
- The characteristics of the ulcer
- The nature of the surrounding tissues
- Relevant regional findings

History of the ulcer

Details of the initial skin lesion and how it occurred may provide clues. **Minor trauma** or an insect bite may initiate it

CASE HISTORY

Fig. 40.4 Skin changes of chronic venous insufficiency

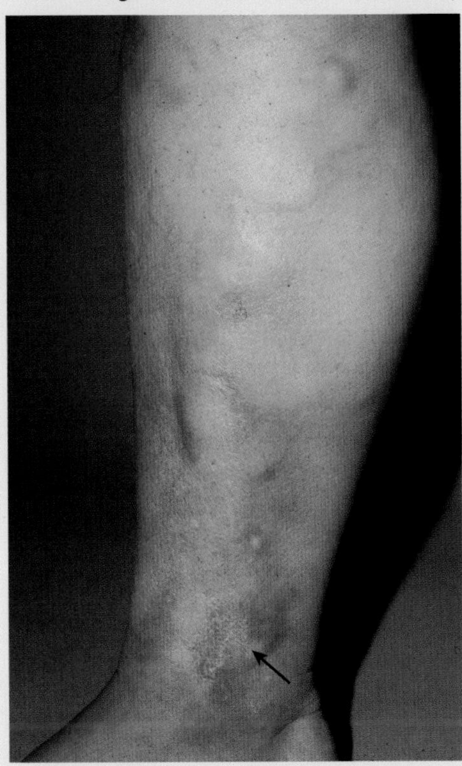

This 53-year-old woman suffered a deep vein thrombosis during her second pregnancy many years earlier. The leg is pigmented around the ankle and this tissue is woody on palpation (lipodermatosclerosis). The scar of a healed varicose ulcer is seen above the medial malleolus (arrowed)

but failure to heal can usually be attributed to abnormal skin nutrition. The common causes include chronic venous insufficiency, arterial ischaemia and diabetic neuropathy. The ulcer often begins insidiously with minor breakdown in a patch of atrophic skin. In venous insufficiency, the leg is often oedematous and the skin may 'weep' plasma.

The ulcer duration, its healing, and recurrences or change in extent or distribution give further clues. **Ischaemic ulcers** present early because pain becomes intolerable (except in diabetics with coexisting neuropathy and ischaemia)—see Table 40.8. In contrast, post-thrombotic and varicose ulcers are not severely painful and fluctuate between healing and breakdown. Very rarely, squamous carcinoma develops in a longstanding ulcer and is recognised by proliferative change at the ulcer margin. These are sometimes known as **Marjolin's ulcers** and were first described following burns which failed to heal (Fig. 40.5). Primary skin malignancies on the leg may ulcerate, but these usually begin as a cutaneous lump.

If the patient has claudication or rest pain, this suggests an ischaemic cause (Fig. 40.6). Neuropathic or mixed diabetic ulcers tend to be painless because of sensory neuropathy (which may be the main predisposing cause). Neuropathic changes to motor nerves affect small muscles of the foot, altering its shape and pressure areas, and autonomic dysfunction results in dryness, both predisposing to ulceration. A history or strong suspicion of previous deep venous thrombosis makes venous insufficiency the likely cause.

Site of the ulcer

Post-thrombotic and varicose ulcers typically arise just above the medial malleolus and may extend circumferentially

Box 40.1 Causes of chronic leg ulcers

- Chronic venous insufficiency
  - Previous deep venous thrombosis (post-thrombotic limb)
  - Varicose veins (superficial venous insufficiency)
  - Combined deep and superficial insufficiency
  - Congenital reflux—defective deep vein valves
- Chronic arterial insufficiency
- Diabetic neuropathy (often called neuro-ischaemia) or other sensory neuropathies
- Pressure sores
- Vasculitis, e.g. in rheumatoid disease and other collagen diseases
- Tropical ulcers involving bacterial or fungal infections, tuberculous ulcers. Ulcers common on feet of surfers—likely combination of trauma and infection
- Malignant tumours (Marjolin's transformation of a chronic ulcer, lymphoma, BCC, SCC, malignant melanoma)

Table 40.8 Main characteristics of ischaemic versus venous ulcers

	Ischaemic ulcer	Venous ulcer
Pain	Yes, unless neuropathic	Minimal; not intolerable
Duration	Less than 6 weeks	Often months or years
Past history	Cardiac ischaemia/coronary artery bypass graft common	DVT; severe varicose veins
Limb signs		
Swelling	Not swollen unless patient has been sleeping in a chair to relieve pain	Usually non-pitting plus pitting oedema unless effective bandaging in place
Temperature	Usually cold	Usually normal or warm
Pulses	Absent; low Doppler pressure	Present; normal Doppler pressure

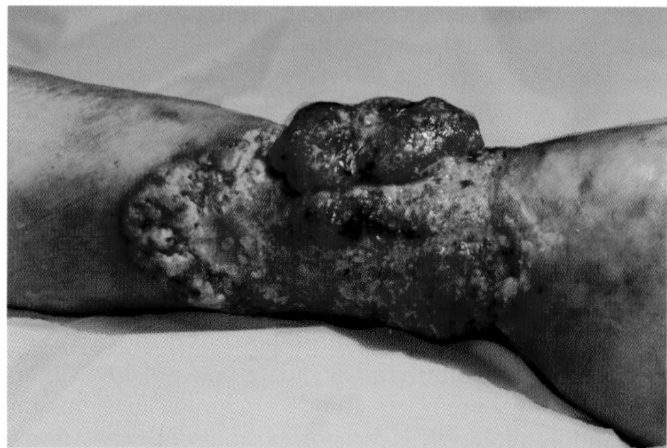

Fig. 40.5 Squamous carcinoma developing in a chronic venous ulcer
This very rare transformation, sometimes known as Marjolin's ulcer, followed 34 years of continuous venous ulceration. The leg was amputated below knee and the patient cured

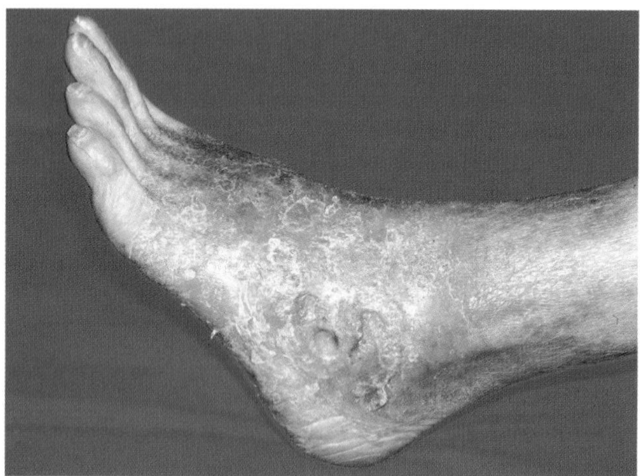

Fig. 40.6 Chronic ischaemic ulcers
This elderly man had intolerable pain in his foot, worse at night for 7 weeks. Note the foot is red and there are multiple ulcers over the lateral malleolus

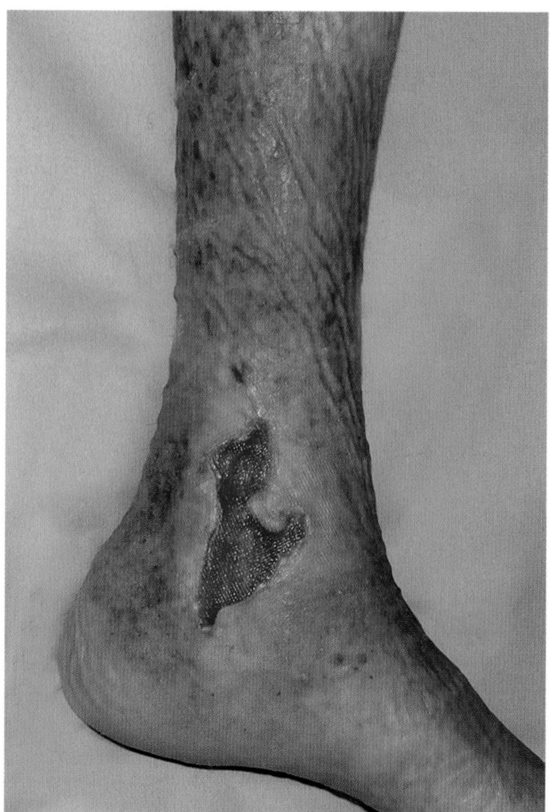

Fig. 40.7 Venous (varicose) ulcer
This longstanding ulcer is typical of venous ulceration by its site, the medial gaiter area of the ankle, its relative painlessness and the presence of venous eczema surrounding it. The visible corrugations in the skin above the ulcer are caused by four-layer compression bandaging

(Fig. 40.7). They rarely occur elsewhere. Diabetic neuropathic ulcers always occur on the foot either as perforating ulcers on the sole beneath metatarsal heads or at other bony prominences; these include the toes, the ball of the great toe and the malleoli (see Fig. 41.8, p. 507), but ischaemia must always be excluded first.

Arterial ulcers may occur anywhere below mid-calf. **Pressure ulcers** occur mainly in debilitated, elderly or unconscious patients, especially at the heel (see Fig. 12.8). Even a few minutes resting on a hard casualty trolley or operating table may initiate necrosis in an ischaemic limb. Pressure ulcers usually begin as a circumscribed patch of discolouration, becoming necrotic and later ulcerating. The heels of vulnerable patients should be nursed carefully and regularly inspected to avoid this. Treatment of pressure ulcers is difficult and prolonged and it is best to prevent them.

Characteristics of the ulcer

Most ulcers are shallow, involving only skin and subcutaneous fat. Diabetic ulcers tend to penetrate deeply into the foot, where there is necrotic and infected tissue. The base of any ulcer usually contains slough and fibrin but granulation tissue may be visible beneath. Slough should not be removed unless arterial insufficiency can be excluded. If there is proliferating tissue in the ulcer, this should be biopsied.

The edge of most chronic lower limb ulcers slopes towards the base with no diagnostic features, although epithelial proliferation growing inwards from the edge suggests healing. Diabetic foot ulcers have a characteristic 'punched-out' edge with abrupt transition from normal skin to the necrotic crater. On the sole, diabetic ulcers have a hyperkeratinised edge in response to excess pressure during walking caused by foot distortion and loss of sensation. Malignant ulcers may have a raised margin.

Nature of the surrounding tissues

The surrounding tissues indicate the background on which the ulcer has formed. These include colour, e.g. chronic venous pigmentation, texture, e.g. induration, and perfusion (shown by temperature, blanching response, venous filling and Buerger's test), as well as swelling.

Table 40.9 Causes of swelling of the lower limbs

Unilateral swelling	Bilateral swelling
a. Local causes	
	'Sluggish venous return', e.g. immobility, pregnancy, prolonged sitting in a chair, inefficient calf muscle pump (e.g. paralysis due to polio or hemiplegia) Lymphatic obstruction by filariasis (in tropical Africa and Asia)
Chronic venous insufficiency Destruction of valves in deep venous system following venous thrombosis (post-thrombotic limb)—superficial venous reflux Congenital lymphatic aplasia or hypoplasia, e.g. Milroy's disease Acute obstruction of venous return, e.g. deep venous thrombosis Chronic cellulitis (usually streptococcal)	May be bilateral May be bilateral
b. Regional causes	
	Left ventricular failure Venous obstruction by pelvic mass, e.g. advanced pregnancy, ovarian cyst, pelvic malignancy Lymphatic obstruction by malignant involvement of inguinal or more proximal nodes, or after block dissection or radiotherapy Lymphatic obstruction by Filiariasis (tropical disease) Inferior venal caval obstruction
c. Systemic causes	
	Congestive or right-sided cardiac failure Hypoalbuminaemia, e.g. malnutrition, nephrotic syndrome Fluid overload

Regional features

Regional examination should search for diagnostic clues, e.g. peripheral pulses, inguinal lymphadenopathy (infection or malignancy), varicose veins and deep or superficial venous thrombosis.

LIMB SWELLING

Lower limb swelling may be unilateral or bilateral. The causes are summarised in Table 40.9. If bilateral, this suggests a 'central' cause such as heart failure. Systemic causes, and conditions listed under 'sluggish venous return' cause bilateral swelling. Unilateral swelling is more likely to present to a surgeon. The other causes usually produce swelling of only one limb. Most causes of unilateral swelling are chronic and painless, except for acute deep venous thrombosis and cellulitis.

41 Managing lower limb arterial insufficiency, the diabetic foot and major amputations

INTRODUCTION

The specialty of **peripheral vascular surgery** has evolved over the last 50 years, with increasing cooperation between surgeons and interventional radiologists, ultrasonographers and vascular physicians. Peripheral atherosclerosis is well recognised as a marker for coronary and cerebrovascular atherosclerosis (approximately 30% 5-year mortality in intermittent claudication), and best medical therapy (antiplatelet agent, statins, optimal blood pressure treatment and diabetic control, smoking cessation, exercise) is often more important than dealing with the leg problem.

Chronic lower limb arterial insufficiency can be asymptomatic or picked up on screening (e.g. for diabetic foot), or cause mild to severe intermittent claudication or rest pain/ulceration/distal gangrene.

CHRONIC LOWER LIMB ISCHAEMIA

INTERMITTENT CLAUDICATION

SYMPTOMS

Intermittent claudication is the usual presentation of lower limb peripheral arterial disease (PAD). It more often affects men and is present in 5% of the male population over 65. The patient experiences cramping pain in leg muscles on walking which is relieved by rest. The calf is involved first because the superficial femoral artery is the most commonly affected with atherosclerosis. If arterial disease is also more proximal (i.e. iliac artery), the pain may ascend to the thigh or the buttock if walking continues. The distance before onset of pain is often reproducible and is reduced by walking uphill.

Symptom onset is usually insidious and often attributed to musculoskeletal causes. The patient seeks medical advice only when symptoms have lasted a few months without improving. Risk factors for intermittent claudication are as for any atherosclerotic disease and patients often have ischaemic heart disease (angina, previous MI, coronary artery bypass grafting) or cerebrovascular disease (previous stroke or transient ischaemic attack). Intermittent claudication is about twice as common in diabetic patients as in non-diabetics. Nearly all have smoked cigarettes at some stage. The severity of PAD increases with the number of cigarettes smoked, with heavy smokers having a four-fold risk of claudication. Non-smokers affected invariably have other risk factors; most are hypertensive, with a two and a half to four-fold age-adjusted risk of developing PAD, depending on gender. The presence of coexisting risk factors increases the risk exponentially, particularly cigarette smoking. Polycythaemia is a rarer causative factor. There is also some evidence of thrombotic risk factors clustering in healthy male relatives of men with PAD.

PHYSICAL SIGNS OF INTERMITTENT CLAUDICATION

Peripheral pulses are usually absent or reduced on the affected side but local examination is otherwise unremarkable. The dorsalis pedis, posterior tibial and popliteal pulses are almost invariably absent; the femoral pulse is weak or absent in about 30%. Trophic (nutritional) skin changes are rarely present. General systematic examination should seek other signs of atherosclerosis likely to bear on management and prognosis.

NATURAL HISTORY OF INTERMITTENT CLAUDICATION

The fate of the leg

The clinical course of intermittent claudication is largely benign. Three quarters of patients either stay the same or improve their walking distance. Only 5–10% with claudication will need endovascular or surgical intervention by 5 years for worsening claudication or severe limb ischaemia. Only 2% with claudication progress to needing major amputation. Smoking increases the risk of reconstructive surgery or major amputation. Patients with diabetes have a higher risk of major amputation in part due to small and distal vessel atherosclerosis.

The fate of the patient

Lower limb PAD is a marker of systemic atherosclerosis. The severity of PAD (as estimated by ankle brachial pressure index (ABPI) is associated with increasing coronary artery disease and the overall mortality rate. Some 10% of claudicants have a non-fatal cardiovascular event (myocardial infarction or stroke) within 5 years and the 5-year mortality rate is 30% with ¾ being cardiovascular. Smoking increases mortality rates amongst claudicants by 1.5–3.0 times.

SEVERE ISCHAEMIA

Severe lower limb ischaemia most commonly presents without claudication but sometimes manifests after a period of deteriorating claudication. In general, these patients are older and less physically active than typical claudicants.

The first manifestations of severe ischaemia develop in the foot and include:

- Intolerable rest pain initially at night, later becoming continuous during the day
- Trophic skin changes—atrophic shiny red skin of the leg; ischaemic ulcers between toes, in foot pressure areas or on the leg
- Patchy necrosis of the toes or skin of the foot
- Positive Buerger's test
- Failure of trivial injuries to heal
- Extreme vulnerability of feet to pressure sores

If untreated, a very small proportion improve and lose their pain, but most smoulder on with intolerable pain or progress to necrosis. Once the deep tissues of the foot become necrotic, local defences are overwhelmed and infection spreads widely in vulnerable ischaemic tissue, especially in diabetics. This causes wet gangrene and, ultimately, death from sepsis and multi-organ dysfunction. This sequence rarely runs its course since rest pain is so severe and signs of sepsis so obvious that vascular reconstruction or amputation becomes unavoidable.

Critical ischaemia

Critical ischaemia occurs when arterial insufficiency is so severe that it threatens the viability of foot or leg. This is formally defined by a European consensus document as follows: persistently recurring rest pain requiring regular analgesia for more than 2 weeks, or ulceration or gangrene affecting the foot, plus an ankle systolic pressure of less than 50 mmHg (*Note*: in diabetics, absent ankle pulses on palpation replace pressure as calcification may artificially elevate pressures).

MANAGING LOWER LIMB ISCHAEMIA

INVESTIGATION OF CHRONIC LOWER LIMB ARTERIAL INSUFFICIENCY

How far to investigate a patient with symptomatic ischaemia depends on the clinical picture (claudication vs. critical ischaemia) and, in claudication, whether it seriously impairs quality of life. Note that patient-reported claudication distance is unreliable and alone, is not an indication for treatment. All patients with critical limb ischaemia should be considered for revascularisation.

The ankle brachial pressure index (ABPI)

All claudication patients should have resting ankle systolic pressures measured in clinic to confirm the diagnosis, plus a full blood count to exclude polycythaemia and thrombocythaemia. Pressure is measured using a **Doppler ultrasound flow detector** (see Fig. 5.9, p. 72). Normal pressure is slightly above brachial systolic whilst patients with claudication usually range between 50 and 120 mmHg. Results are often expressed as a ratio, the **ankle brachial pressure index (ABPI)**, with normal values from 0.9 to 1.2. Note that Doppler pressures can be misleading; experience is needed in taking and interpreting measurements, and radical treatment should not be based on random pressure measurements. Values may be spuriously elevated in patients with diabetes owing to calcification in the arterial media which prevents cuff compression. In non-classical exercise-induced leg pain or those with a good history of claudication but normal resting ABPI, a treadmill test with pre- and post-exercise pressure or ABPI helps the diagnosis. A drop in ankle pressure after exercise gives an indication of arterial disease severity and the recovery rate an indication of collateral compensation.

Duplex ultrasonography

This combines greyscale ultrasound imaging (GSUS) and colour Doppler blood flow estimation. GSUS allows estimation of plaque narrowing and colour Doppler allows estimation of flow velocities, which increase in areas of stenosis. These methods provide a 'road map' of atherosclerosis in the arterial tree and are usually performed in a vascular laboratory by specialist ultrasonographers. It is non-invasive and rarely requires intravenous contrast media. There is substantial user dependency in the results.

Arteriography (see Ch. 5)

Arteriography should be reserved for patients thought to require angioplasty or reconstructive surgery. It maps the arterial system (see Fig. 41.1), showing sites and severity of stenoses and occlusions, the quality of inflow (arteries feeding the area of concern) and the runoff (arteries beyond the main obstruction, see Fig. 41.2). Arteriography is sometimes used wrongly by non-specialists to assess chronic arterial insufficiency but it cannot measure blood flow to the tissues or dynamic circulatory responses to exercise; it helps only with the mechanics of revascularisation. Traditional arteriography is performed via direct arterial puncture but carries risks of vessel trauma and high doses of contrast aggravating chronic renal impairment. It is being replaced by less invasive CT and MR angiography which use lower doses of intravenous contrast media.

APPROACH TO MANAGEMENT OF CHRONIC LOWER LIMB ARTERIAL INSUFFICIENCY

Treatment options range from conservative or 'expectant' treatment for most, to reconstructive procedures for the few with severe ischaemia. Treatments are summarised in Box 41.1.

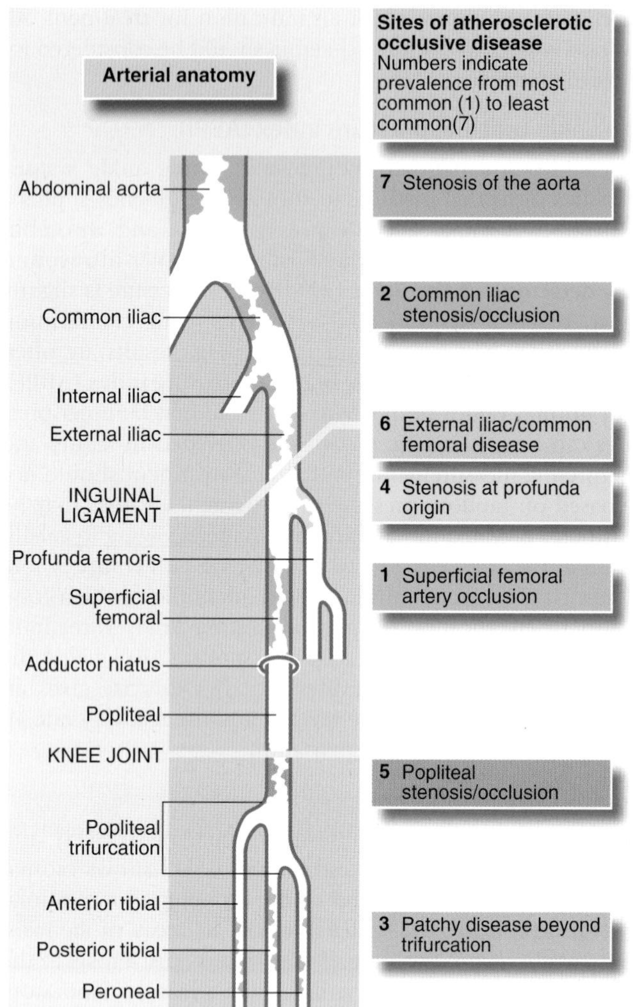

Fig. 41.1 Typical patterns of lower limb arterial disease

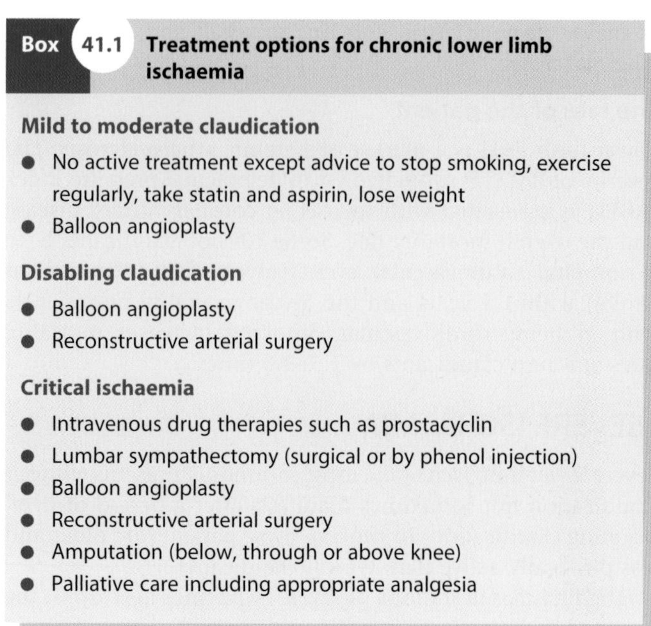

Box 41.1 Treatment options for chronic lower limb ischaemia

Mild to moderate claudication

- No active treatment except advice to stop smoking, exercise regularly, take statin and aspirin, lose weight
- Balloon angioplasty

Disabling claudication

- Balloon angioplasty
- Reconstructive arterial surgery

Critical ischaemia

- Intravenous drug therapies such as prostacyclin
- Lumbar sympathectomy (surgical or by phenol injection)
- Balloon angioplasty
- Reconstructive arterial surgery
- Amputation (below, through or above knee)
- Palliative care including appropriate analgesia

Conservative management

In intermittent claudication, management starts with **lifestyle measures** such as stopping smoking, attention to diet (reduced fat, more fruit and vegetables, weight reduction) and systematic exercise. Cigarette smoking is a primary risk factor in causing atherosclerosis and a secondary risk factor in causing deterioration, as well as causing occlusions or stenoses of angioplasty or graft after reconstruction. Symptoms are more likely to resolve (by collateral development) if the patient stops smoking. Giving up is difficult as nicotine is highly addictive but smoking cessation programmes can help as well as pharmacological aids such as nicotine replacement therapy, bupropion (Zyban) and varenicline (Champix). All family members need to give up together to reinforce the message.

Medical management is important, with blood pressure control and regular anti-platelet agents (usually aspirin) and a statin (even if cholesterol levels are normal). These measures aim to reduce mortality by treating systemic atherosclerosis, as well as encourage collateral vessels to develop. Treatment with the phosphodiesterase inhibitor **cilostazol** provides a small increase in walking distance but does have significant side-effects.

The degree of handicap in claudication is assessed clinically by careful history-taking and perhaps by walking with the patient. There is a marked trend towards conservative treatment these days, now we know many patients recover function and this recovery is more durable than intervention. The choice of active treatment depends on the handicap, the patient's willingness to give up smoking, the potential for treating the pattern of atherosclerosis and the patient's overall preference. Severe and critical ischaemia are clear indications for revascularisation (or amputation) since the symptoms cannot be tolerated in the long term.

Mild to moderate claudication

Most patients are optimally treated with best medical management and lifestyle advice. Symptoms often improve spontaneously over 6–18 months, especially if the patient stops smoking, exercises regularly and loses excess weight. Simple advice to walk more slowly and use a walking stick often greatly extends the claudication distance. Supervised exercise programmes produce a sustained increase in walking distance but need to continue for at least 3 months to show benefit—there is often a problem with compliance. These programmes are not yet offered in the NHS.

Disabling claudication

Disabling claudication usually requires treatment unless the patient is too unfit even for angiography. Symptoms may include severe exercise restriction in younger patients or markedly worsening symptoms, especially if proximal arterial obstruction is the cause (shown by absent femoral pulses), which is often easily treated by angioplasty. Reconstructive surgery is sometimes needed.

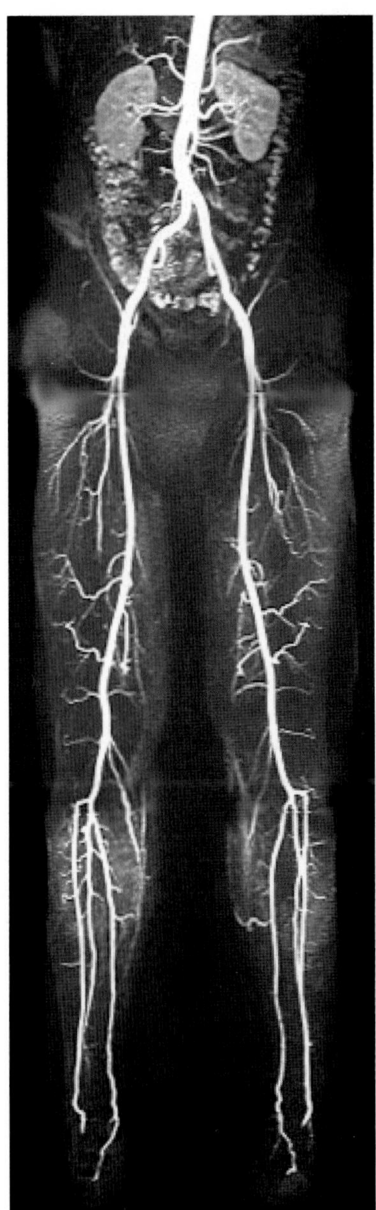

(a)

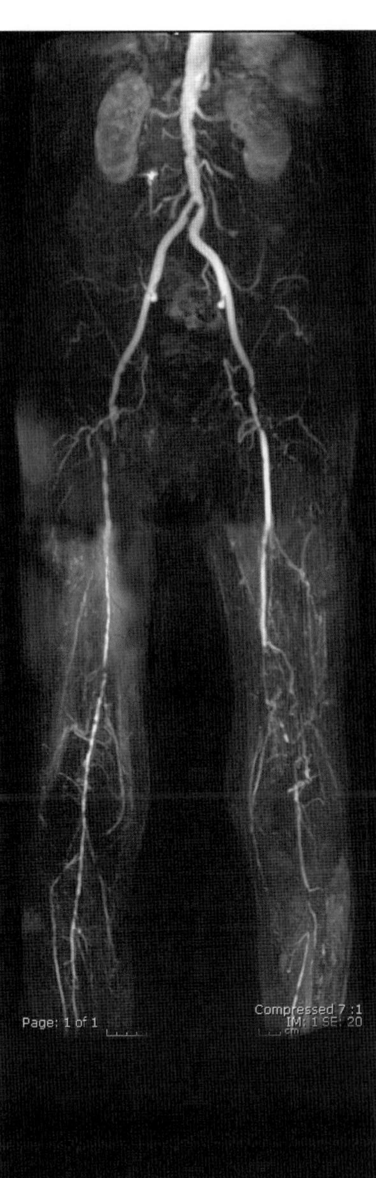

(b)

Fig. 41.2 Arteriograms comparing the normal with typical patterns of arterial obstruction affecting the lower limbs
(a) This magnetic resonance angiogram is entirely normal, showing smooth, regular arterial walls, all branches intact and three normal infra-inguinal arteries below knee on each side. **(b)** This composite subtraction arteriogram was performed because the patient suffered bilateral severe claudication. The aorta is irregular and narrowed by atherosclerosis from above the renal arteries to the bifurcation. The common, internal and proximal external iliacs are normal and smooth but the right external iliac is occluded and the left stenosed. Both profunda femoris arteries are occluded. The superficial femoral arteries are both diseased and occluded distally. On the left side, collaterals are visible around the knee area. The infrageniculate vessels are diseased on both sides with stenoses and occlusions. Reconstruction would have been extensive, difficult and risky, and hence conservative management alone was undertaken, in the absence of rest pain or tissue loss

TECHNIQUES OF REVASCULARISATION FOR CHRONIC ARTERIAL INSUFFICIENCY

Percutaneous transluminal angioplasty (PTA)

PTA involves cannulating an artery (usually the common femoral but occasionally the brachial), introducing a guidewire into this remote artery and advancing it to lie across the stenosis. A balloon catheter is passed over the wire and into position (see Fig. 41.3) and the balloon inflated to a high pressure (5–15 atmospheres), crushing the atheroma into the arterial wall to relieve the obstruction. Success is very operator-dependent and also depends upon the site, length and nature of the diseased artery. PTA is most effective for isolated short stenoses in iliac arteries. With increasing experience, longer stenoses and occlusions in smaller vessels can be tackled, avoiding the need for major surgery. The method is less successful for distal calf arteries. Angioplasty often provides symptom improvement for a few years but disease progression (and failure to modify lifestyle) is a limiting factor.

Arterial reconstructive surgery

Arterial reconstructive surgery began in the 1950s with open removal of atheromatous plaques and thrombus from the aorta and iliac arteries. This is known as **thrombo-endarterectomy**, and is technically difficult, bloody and time-consuming. It has been replaced by bypass grafting, except for carotid endarterectomy, which remains the standard operation for stenosis and for isolated common femoral artery occlusions.

Arterial bypass grafting was first developed during the Korean War to treat arterial trauma, using homografts from human cadavers. The initial results were excellent but grafts eventually suffered from aneurysmal dilatation and rupture. This led to the introduction of synthetic graft materials for

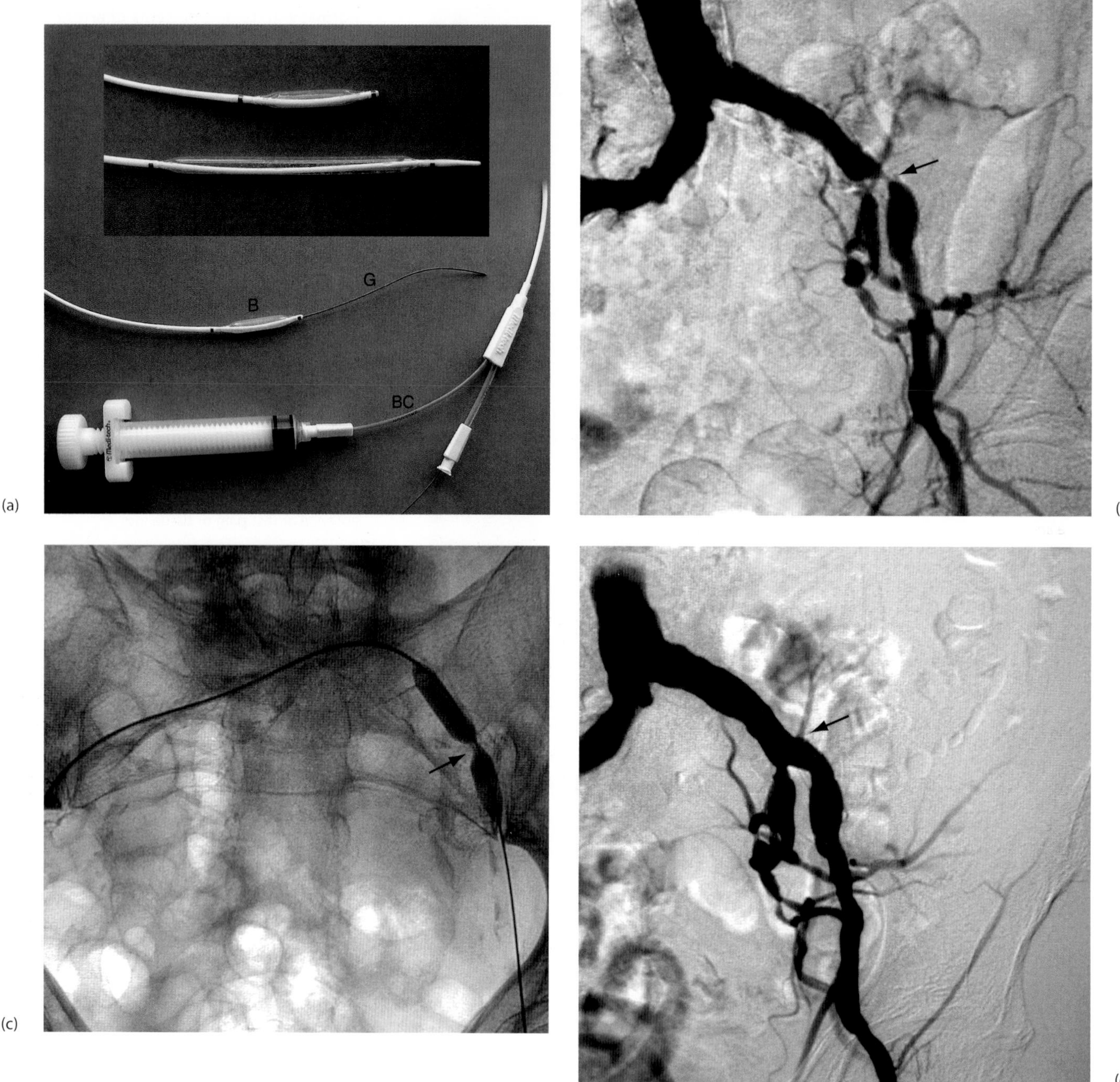

Fig. 41.3 Percutaneous transluminal angioplasty
(a) Balloon angioplasty equipment. This catheter is used for balloon dilatation of arterial stenosis. First, an artery some distance from the stenosis (usually the femoral) is punctured with a needle. A flexible guide-wire **G** is passed through the needle, along the artery and manipulated across the stenosis. The catheter is then threaded over the guide-wire until the distal balloon **B** (which is designed to only be inflated to a predetermined diameter) lies within the stenosis. The balloon is then inflated to high pressure using a special syringe attached to the balloon channel **BC**. Note the radio-opaque markers at each end of the balloon to allow it to be sited radiographically. **(b)** Arteriogram showing a tight stenosis at the distal end of the left common iliac artery (arrowed). **(c)** Catheter access proved impossible via the left femoral artery, so a guide-wire was passed from the right femoral, over the bifurcation and across the stenosis. An angioplasty balloon catheter was then guided across the stenosis. As it was inflated the 'waist' caused by the arterial stenosis became clearly visible (arrowed). With further inflation to 4 atmospheres pressure, the waist disappeared. **(d)** Appearance of the arteries post angioplasty. This procedure was completed in under an hour on a day-case basis under local anaesthesia and proved durable over several years

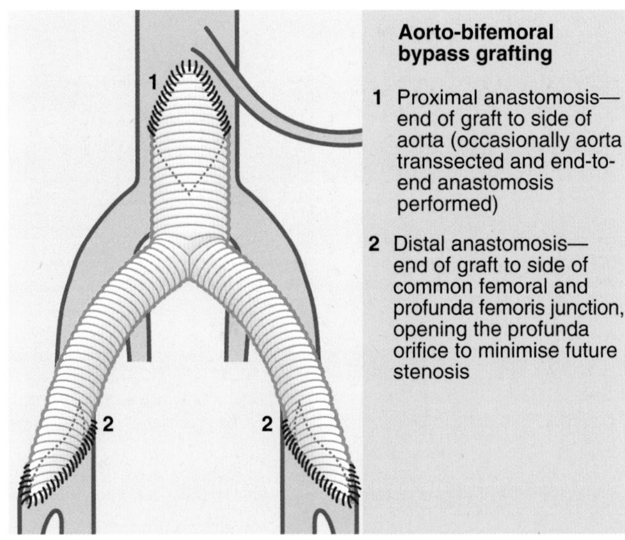

Fig. 41.4 Aorto-bifemoral bypass for aorto-iliac disease using a trouser or 'Y' graft
A Dacron bifurcation graft or prosthesis is used to bypass the aorto-iliac segment when it is occluded or stenosed, or to replace it when aorta and iliacs are aneurysmal. In the latter case, the distal anastomoses are to the iliac arteries not the femorals so as to maintain pelvic perfusion.

large arteries, now available in a variety of shapes, sizes and types of cloth. Knitted polyester (Dacron) is the most popular and is the standard material for aorto-iliac obstruction. Many grafts are now sealed with gelatin or other proteins to minimise porosity. For smaller arteries, autogenous **long saphenous vein** from the leg is the best conduit, provided it is large enough (usually >3 mm in diameter) and not damaged by thrombosis. Vein is also inherently resistant to infection, a useful attribute when treating infected lower limb wounds and ulcers.

Recognition that conservative management of claudication is often as good as intervention, and the availability and success of angioplasty, has meant that surgical reconstruction is now sparingly used and is largely reserved for severely ischaemic limbs, or when angioplasty is unsuitable or unsuccessful.

The most common procedures are synthetic 'trouser' grafting for aorto-iliac (supra-inguinal) disease and femoro-popliteal grafting using saphenous vein, for infra-inguinal disease (see Figs 41.4 and 41.5). However, a range of other bypasses and endarterectomy techniques sometimes have to be employed to cope with non-standard disease.

Aorto-iliac disease

The usual surgical procedure is a Dacron trouser or 'Y' graft (see Fig. 41.4), anastomosed to the side of the aorta below the renal arteries and to both common femorals below the inguinal ligament (aorto-bifemoral graft). This is a major operation, needing a laparotomy to access and cross-clamp the aorta and carries a mortality risk of about 5%. In patients with critical ischaemia but poor physiological reserve, legs can be revascularised using **extra-anatomic synthetic grafts** with a lower operative risk. Examples include a **cross-over graft** to supply blood from one femoral artery to the other or an **axillo-bifemoral graft**, supplying blood from one axillary artery to both femorals, tunnelling the graft subcutaneously along the lateral chest and abdominal wall.

Box 41.2 Complications of arterial surgery

- Complications of generalised arteriopathy: acute myocardial ischaemia, cerebrovascular accidents, renal failure, intestinal ischaemia—early or late
- Haemorrhage: arterial or venous—early
- Thrombosis of reconstructed vessels or graft leading to profound distal ischaemia (usually a technical fault)—early
- Embolism into limb vessels or renal vessels (particularly aneurysm surgery)—early
- Graft infection—early or late
- False aneurysm formation—late
- Progressive atherosclerotic lower limb ischaemia—late

Femoro-popliteal disease

The superficial femoral artery is the most commonly obstructed peripheral artery. If PTA is unsuitable, **femoro-popliteal bypass grafting** is employed using an autogenous vein graft. The long (great) saphenous vein (LSV) is dissected from groin to knee, its tributaries ligated and then reversed proximal to distal so the valves do not obstruct flow. An end-to-side anastomosis is performed at each end. If the LSV is unsuitable (i.e. diseased, small diameter or previously removed for CABG), the LSV from the other leg or veins from the arm can be used. An alternative technique leaves the vein in situ and destroys the valves with a **valvulotome**. As the vein tapers from proximal to distal, this allows bypasses to tibial, dorsalis pedis artery or smaller foot arteries for distal disease. These **infrapopliteal** or femoro-distal grafts are used only for severe ischaemia because of the higher risk of graft occlusion.

Synthetic materials (e.g. PTFE or Dacron) are much less satisfactory; these have lower long-term patency, particularly when crossing the knee joint, and are more prone to infection.

Complications of arterial surgery

These are summarised in Box 41.2.

OTHER THERAPIES FOR ARTERIAL INSUFFICIENCY

Intravenous and intra-arterial drug therapies

Drug therapy has no substantial effect in relieving claudication or severe ischaemia but recent research has examined gene therapy and local stimulation of angiogenesis (new blood vessel formation) in patients with critical limb ischaemia. However, the results are currently not yet robust enough to employ clinically.

Sympathectomy

Blood flow in the skin (but not muscle) is controlled by the sympathetic nervous system. Thus, early rest pain affecting the

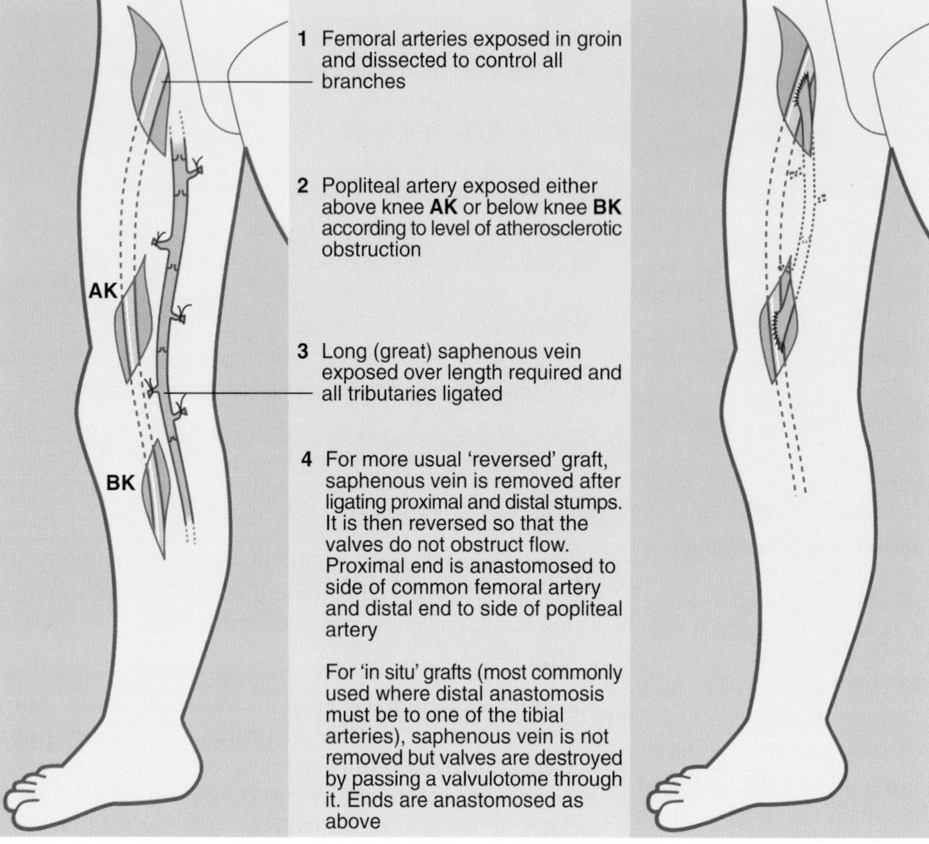

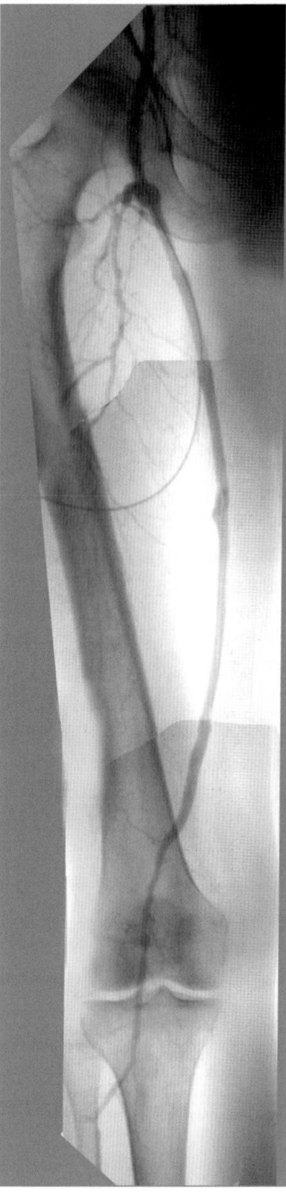

Fig. 41.5 Techniques of arterial bypass for femoro-popliteal grafting
(a) Technique of femoro-popliteal grafting. **(b)** Composite arteriogram showing patent femoro-popliteal bypass after operation

skin may sometimes be relieved by sympathetic blockade even if the overall arterial supply is inadequate. It is not beneficial in claudication.

Sympathectomy can be performed by excision of part of the lumbar sympathetic chain or, more commonly, by translumbar injection of 6% aqueous phenol. **Chemical sympathectomy** is performed under local anaesthesia with radiographic control. Only about 15% of patients obtain sufficient relief to avoid reconstructive operation or amputation and there is no way of selecting those likely to benefit; sympathectomy is certain to fail in the presence of tissue loss (gangrene) and is most likely to succeed in early rest pain. It may also help heal ulcers where moderate ischaemia coexists with chronic venous insufficiency.

ACUTE LOWER LIMB ISCHAEMIA

PATHOPHYSIOLOGY

The lower (or upper) limb can become acutely ischaemic from **embolism** or **thrombosis**.

Embolism

A large embolus impacting in a major distributing artery causes the distal blood supply to cease abruptly; since the distal arteries are not usually atherosclerotic, collateral networks have not developed and ischaemia is all the more severe. Most large emboli originate in the heart, as a result of **atrial fibrillation** or **mitral stenosis** or both (left atrial thrombus), or of **myocardial infarction** (mural thrombus). Emboli usually impact at branching points where the lumen abruptly narrows. Common sites are the aortic bifurcation (**saddle**

Fig. 41.6 Embolic occlusion of popliteal arteries

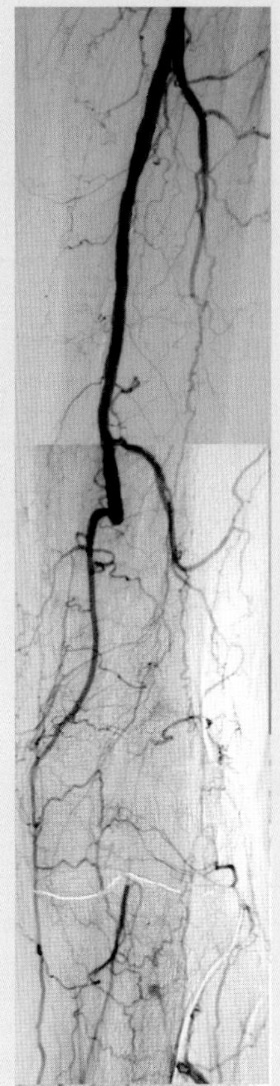

(a)

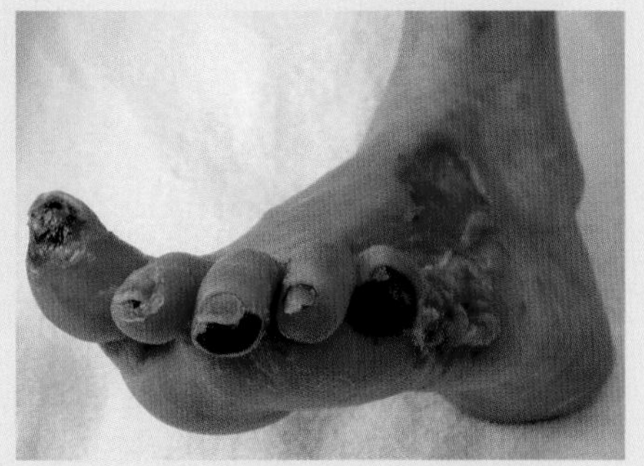

(b)

(a) Angiogram showing the thigh and upper leg arteries in a woman of 70 who presented with rest pain for 48 hours and necrosis of the dorsum of her foot and black toe tips for 24 hours. The left popliteal is occluded with a sharp cut-off typical of embolism. The patient was in atrial fibrillation and the likely source of the embolus was the left atrium. She underwent a successful embolectomy, but because of the delay, a below-knee fasciotomy was performed to prevent compartment syndrome. **(b)** The foot ulcer 3 weeks after revascularisation. The ulcer gradually healed completely

embolus), the common femoral bifurcation and the popliteal trifurcation. Aortic or popliteal aneurysms can be a source of embolism if thrombus accumulated in the sac travels distally (see Figs 41.6 and 41.7).

Thrombosis

Thrombotic causes include thrombosis of a **popliteal aneurysm** and acute occlusion of a previous bypass graft or angioplasty site. Occasionally, **widespread thrombosis** occurs in normal arteries causing acute ischaemia. This can be a complication of **blood disorders** including polycythaemia vera, thrombocythaemia or leukaemias, in nephrotic syndrome or in hyperosmolar hyperglycaemic states in diabetics.

Acute thrombotic occlusion causes catastrophic results when it occurs in critical sites, namely the popliteal artery (with few useful collaterals), the external iliac/common femoral arterial trunk (the axial blood supply of the limb) or the profunda femoris (if the superficial femoral artery is already occluded).

If an essential distributing artery narrowed by atherosclerosis becomes obstructed by secondary thrombosis or by rupture of an atherosclerotic plaque (**acute-on-chronic occlusion**) acute ischaemia may develop. The clinical presentation is often less severe because collaterals have developed to maintain distal circulation. This may allow time for less urgent investigation and management.

CLINICAL FEATURES OF ACUTE LOWER LIMB ISCHAEMIA (Box 41.3)

The condition usually presents as a sudden onset of pain, coldness and pallor, extending from the foot for a variable distance up the leg. If the blood supply is completely cut off, nerve ischaemia causes **loss of sensation** and then muscle **paralysis** after an hour or two (the **six Ps**—see Ch. 40, p. 489). Acute severe arterial occlusion must be recognised quickly as limb viability is in immediate danger and urgent steps are needed to revascularise it. Unfortunately, this urgency is not always appreciated by the patient, nursing staff or inexperienced doctors. Even with successful revascularisation, ischaemic changes may already be irreversible and with late intervention, there is a serious risk of muscle necrosis and permanent nerve injury from **reperfusion injury** and/or **compartment syndrome** (see Ch. 17, p. 235).

Later, tissue ischaemia becomes obvious when the affected area becomes mottled, dusky blue and discoloured. If the

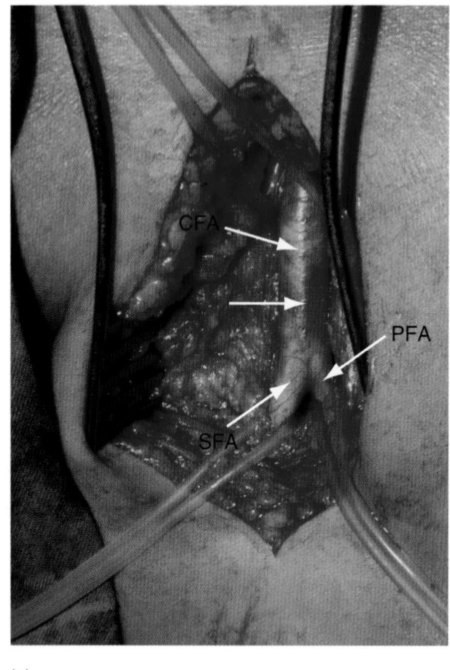

(a)

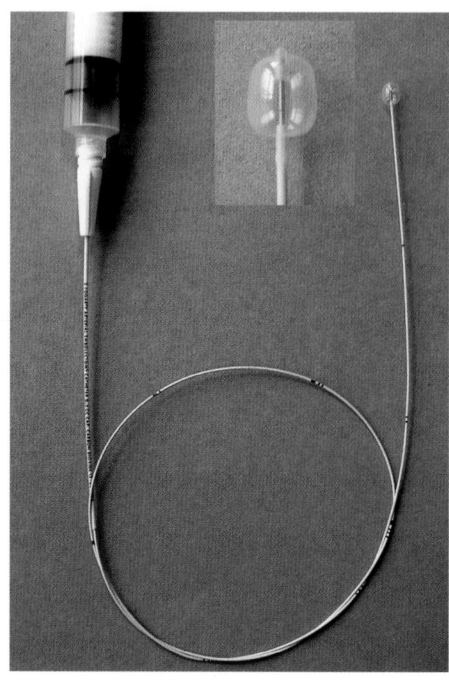

(b)

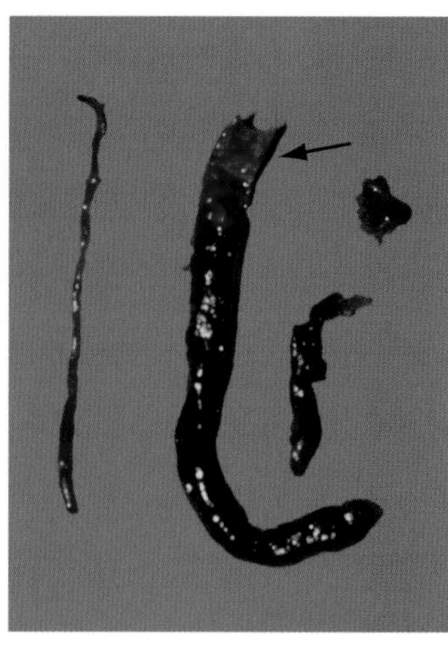

(c)

Fig. 41.7 Femoral artery embolectomy
(a) Surgical exposure of the femoral artery bifurcation, usually performed under local infiltration anaesthesia (but with full monitoring). The common femoral artery **CFA**, the profunda femoris **PFA** and the superficial femoral artery **SFA** are dissected cleanly and silicone slings placed around each artery. A transverse arteriotomy is made just proximal to the bifurcation (position arrowed). **(b)** A Fogarty balloon catheter is passed distally, the balloon is gently inflated and the catheter withdrawn to extract embolic and thrombotic material. This is performed in stages until the catheter can be passed to ankle level and back-bleeding occurs. **(c)** Embolic material removed at operation from the superficial femoral artery and beyond using a Fogarty catheter. Note the paler embolic material (arrowed) and the darker thrombus propagated beyond it

Box 41.3 Clinical features of acute severe lower limb ischaemia

Risk factors predisposing to embolism or thrombosis

- Recent chest pain or other evidence of myocardial infarction
- History of rheumatic heart disease
- History or finding of atrial fibrillation
- Previous arterial embolism
- History of intermittent claudication or other symptoms of peripheral arterial disease (thrombosis)
- Polycythaemia vera (prone to intravascular thrombosis)
- Popliteal aneurysm in contralateral limb (possible thrombosis or embolism in affected limb)
- Aortic aneurysm (possible source of embolism)

Symptoms suggesting acute lower limb ischaemia

- Sudden onset of continuous pain, usually in one periphery. *Note*: may be painless in diabetic neuropathy
- Sudden and persistent coldness, usually in one periphery
- Sudden numbness or paraesthesia, usually in one periphery

Signs of acute lower limb ischaemia

- Pallor or blueness of the periphery; in late cases, the fixed pigmentation of necrosis or skin blistering
- Unexpected coldness of the peripheral part of one or (less commonly) both legs
- Absent lower limb pulses (particularly if known to have been present before)
- Poor peripheral capillary return after pressure blanching
- Progressive paralysis and foot drop (late sign)
- Ankle pulses undetectable by Doppler or very low ankle systolic pressure

mottling still blanches, then the limb may still be saved but worsening ischaemia leads to fixed mottling and skin blistering; this is now irreversible and limb loss inevitable. These changes always involve the foot and may extend proximally (though rarely above the knee). At this stage, the upper limit of necrosis is usually well demarcated from proximal viable tissue.

PRINCIPLES OF MANAGING THE ACUTELY ISCHAEMIC LIMB

Management should be carefully planned at the outset. The window of opportunity before necrosis is short and delay or procrastination increases morbidity or mortality. Treatment is best carried out by cooperation between vascular surgical and radiological specialists so the full range of appropriate and timely treatment can be offered. As a first step, the patient should be anticoagulated with a bolus dose of 5000 U of **intravenous heparin** to prevent propagation of thrombus proximal and distal to the occlusion. If the diagnosis is later confirmed as embolism, oral anticoagulation is usually continued after surgery.

THROMBOSIS OR EMBOLISM?

Distinguishing clinically between thrombosis and embolism is unreliable, although the history may provide clues. Evidence of mitral stenosis, an arrhythmia or recent myocardial infarction suggests embolism, whereas a history of claudication or a prothrombotic blood disorder points to thrombosis. Examining the affected limb may not help distinguish but the other limb provides evidence of the state of peripheral arteries. If it is well perfused with good pulses and normal ankle pressure, then embolism is more likely. If there is arterial disease then in situ thrombosis is more likely; the severity of ischaemia may also be less profound. The popliteal fossa must always be palpated to exclude a **thrombosed popliteal aneurysm**. A large **saddle embolus** lodging at the aortic bifurcation often presents with severe ischaemia of both limbs extending into the proximal leg and thigh. This can be fatal, partly from the severity of ischaemia but also from intense reperfusion injury once limbs have been revascularised.

If clinical signs are strongly in favour of embolism, immediate surgical embolectomy can be undertaken with on-table **arteriography** if necessary. If there is doubt, urgent duplex scanning or angiography (usually CT angiography 'out of hours') is available, a definitive diagnosis can be rapidly determined and the best intervention delivered. This may be radiological rather than surgical.

In acute ischaemia, the speed of treatment is the key to success. Any patient with sensory loss affecting more than just the toes, especially with evidence of muscle weakness, requires immediate treatment with embolectomy, thrombectomy or bypass graft (see Fig. 41.4, 41.5, p. 502). In limbs that have been profoundly ischaemic, fasciotomies at the time are often required to prevent compartment syndrome. Thrombolysis is now rarely undertaken, except for unblocking a thrombosed bypass graft in a patient whose foot is predicted to remain viable for at least 12 hours.

EMBOLECTOMY

Embolectomy is often performed under local anaesthesia but the patient and theatre should be prepared for GA just in case; full monitoring should be applied. The patient has usually been anticoagulated with heparin. A groin incision exposes the femoral artery bifurcation, the vessels are all temporarily clamped and an incision (**arteriotomy**) made in the common femoral artery (Fig. 41.7) which may reveal the obstructing clot. A **Fogarty balloon catheter** is then passed gently into each main vessel in turn, proximally and distally for 10 cm or so, the balloon is inflated gently and the catheter drawn back to sweep out any obstructing clot. This is repeated 10 cm further each time until the distal limit is reached. The operation is successful if clot is retrieved and blood flows back (**'back-bleeding'**) from each vessel as it is unclamped. If the embolectomy catheter will not pass easily, this usually indicates acute-on-chronic thrombosis. Immediate arteriography and surgical treatment are required as delay carries a high rate of limb loss and death.

THE DIABETIC FOOT

The evolving epidemic of diabetes means that managing diabetic foot problems will become an increasing part of the surgical workload. Treatment should be delivered by a multidisciplinary diabetic team (vascular surgeon, diabetologist, podiatrist, orthopaedic surgeon and orthotist).

PATHOPHYSIOLOGY OF THE DIABETIC FOOT

Diabetic patients are prone to serious ulceration and infection of the feet. The underlying disorder is neuropathy, obliterative atherosclerosis or both together. Type 2 diabetic patients are at greater risk than type 1, but remember **there is no such thing as mild diabetes**. All diabetic patients should be screened for potential complications of diabetes.

Several factors may contribute to diabetic foot problems:

- **Neuropathy.** Microangiopathy probably causes peripheral neuropathies affecting motor, sensory and autonomic nerves. Affected **motor nerves** supply the small muscles of the foot and the consequent unmodified traction of the calf muscles distorts the morphology and weight-bearing characteristics of the foot. **Sensory neuropathy** lessens pain sensation and hence awareness of potential injury from ill-fitting footwear and foreign bodies in shoes. Damaged **autonomic nerves** disrupt vascular control and cause loss of sweating. Ulceration and infection in neuropathic feet are often painless and hence are often neglected by the patient

- **Arteriovenous communications.** These open beneath the skin, perhaps diverting nutrient flow away from it. Damaged tissue thus heals poorly and is vulnerable to infection, even if the injury or pressure damage is minor. This may also explain why an ischaemic diabetic foot can be warm and pink
- **Arterioles.** In a few cases, these become narrowed and restrict capillary perfusion
- **Impaired intermediary tissue metabolism** and a glucose-rich tissue environment. Both of these favour bacterial growth and spreading infection
- **Obliterative atherosclerosis.** Diabetics have a markedly increased predisposition to arterial insufficiency. Although 1–5% of the general population have diabetes, 25% of patients with lower limb ischaemia have diabetes. Atherosclerotic disease in diabetic patients follows the usual pattern (although often more distal) but tends to develop at a younger age

Identifying the causes of diabetic foot problems

Most diabetic foot problems can be identified as primarily neuropathic or primarily atherosclerotic but some have elements of both. The term 'neuro-ischaemic' foot is sometimes used but is not clinically precise. Typically, the **neuropathic foot** is painless, red and warm with strong pulses, whereas the **atherosclerotic foot** without neuropathy is pale, painful, cold and pulseless. However, when both occur together, **the diabetic trap** is that the limb can be seriously ischaemic yet painless, warm and pink. If the foot is neuropathic and pulseless, only **arteriography** or duplex scanning will properly demonstrate the arterial insufficiency.

Patients most at risk of neuropathic foot complications are elderly, poorly controlled, maturity-onset (type 2) diabetics and younger patients with longstanding type 1 diabetes. Similarly, patients with diabetic renal or retinal complications have an increased risk of foot problems. Recognising the **'at-risk' foot**, i.e. the neuropathic foot, before trouble strikes is fundamental, as virtually all neuropathic foot complications can be prevented with proper education, regular inspection and chiropody (podiatry) (Box 41.4).

Management of atherosclerotic ischaemia is similar in diabetic and non-diabetic patients. For mixed disease, the arterial insufficiency must nearly always be treated first if there is to be any hope of healing.

Box 41.4 The problem of the diabetic foot

- 'Diabetic gangrene is not heaven-sent but earth-born' (Joslin 1934)
- There is no such thing as 'mild' diabetes; all diabetics are potentially at risk
- Four out of five patients with diabetic foot problems have type 2 diabetes
- Foot problems are responsible for 47% of days spent in hospital by diabetics
- Diabetic foot problems are responsible for 12% of all hospital admissions in (internal) medicine
- In diabetics with new foot ulcers, 90% have peripheral neuropathy (compared with 20% in a diabetic control group), whereas only 14% have peripheral arterial disease compared with 10% in controls (Miami 1983–4)
- Patients with diabetic foot problems are incapacitated for an average of 16 weeks
- Diabetic foot problems are largely preventable
- Care and prevention of diabetic foot problems require specialist surveillance and management by a dedicated team; foot ulceration in diabetics represents a failure of medical management

Clinical presentations of diabetic foot complications

Foot complications of diabetic neuropathy present in four main ways (see Fig. 41.8):

- **Painless, deeply penetrating ulcers.** These usually develop in pressure areas caused by distortion of foot morphology, often beneath the first or fifth metatarsal head. The infecting organism is usually *Staphylococcus aureus*. Infection and necrosis spread through the plantar spaces and along tendon sheaths. Infection and local venous thrombosis appear to be the predominant factors causing tissue destruction
- **Chronic ulceration of pressure points** and sites of minor injury. Skin perfusion is otherwise adequate
- **Extensive spreading skin necrosis** originating in an ulcer and caused by superficial or deep infection. This develops very rapidly and spreads proximally, threatening limb and life
- **Painless necrosis of individual toes.** These first turn blue, then later become black and mummified, and may eventually be shed spontaneously. This usually occurs in mixed neuropathy and atherosclerosis and the management hinges on whether local amputations will heal or whether arterial reconstruction is needed

MANAGEMENT OF NEUROPATHIC FOOT COMPLICATIONS

CONTROL OF INFECTION

After excluding ischaemia, control of infection is the first priority in managing the diabetic foot. Minor foot lesions must always be taken seriously and treated early with **oral antibiotics (including cover for anaerobes)** and frequent local cleansing and dressing.

If there is any sign of spreading infection or systemic involvement (i.e. pyrexia, tachycardia or loss of diabetic control), the patient should be admitted to hospital for intensive treatment including parenteral antibiotics, elevation, excision of necrotic tissue and attention to blood glucose control. Pus in superficial or deep tissues is a medical emergency and

Fig. 41.8 Foot complications of diabetes

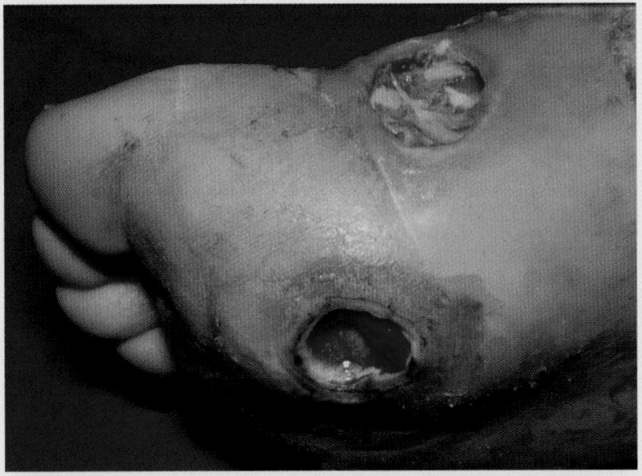

(a)

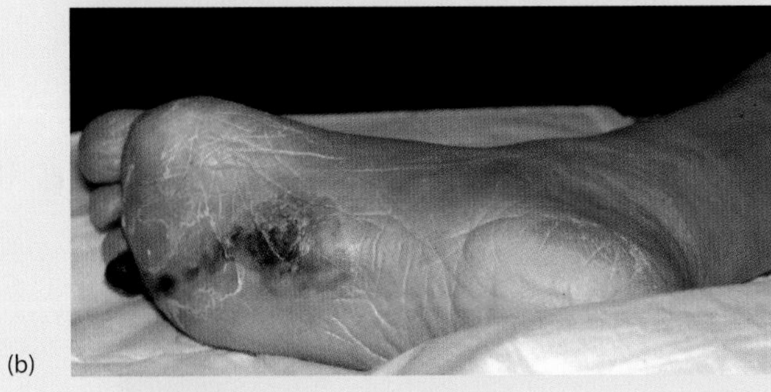

(b)

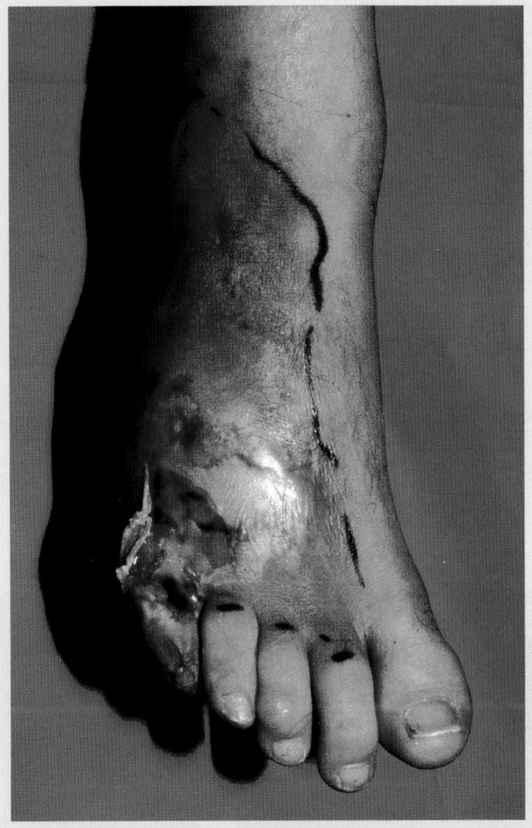

(c)

(a) Chronic penetrating ulcers in a 60-year-old man with maturity-onset diabetes. He had no evidence of major vessel disease but had signs of neuropathy. The deep ulcer beneath the head of the first metatarsal is characteristically surrounded with a thick keratin margin, and the ulcer on the medial side of the foot has an exposed tendon in its base. **(b)** This patient has a combination of neuropathy and arterial insufficiency. This foot was painless despite spreading necrosis and a collection of pus in the sole of the foot. He underwent femoro-popliteal bypass and local excision of dead tissue and healing was eventually complete. **(c)** This man of 34 presented with a neglected infection in his foot. He had severe neuropathy but no arterial disease. The entire dorsum of his foot was necrotic and he had to undergo a primary below-knee amputation. This complication would have been entirely avoidable had he sought and received treatment earlier

requires immediate drainage. This is difficult to diagnose clinically and foot imaging with MRI is required. Specialist management of blood sugar is often required as it is often grossly elevated.

REMOVAL OF NECROTIC TISSUE

Surgery may involve anything from simple **desloughing** of an ulcer to major amputation (see Fig. 41.9). If performed correctly, these result in complete and rapid healing. If good foot care is available, amputation of more than single toes is rarely required. Before debridement, arterial inflow must be assessed and the foot revascularised if necessary before debridement or digital amputation to maximise the chances of wound healing.

Osteomyelitis occurs in up to 20% with a diabetes-related foot ulcer. Diagnosis is clinically if an ulcer can be probed down to bone or else radiologically (plain X-ray or MRI). Treatment consists of long-term antibiotics (often parenteral), with a success rate of around 80%, or surgical excision. There is no current consensus on optimal treatment but prolonged antibiotics can increase the risk of *C. difficile* and emergence of multi-drug-resistant organisms.

PREVENTION OF THE DIABETIC FOOT

All clinicians dealing with diabetics should place the highest priority on prevention. All patients should be screened for peripheral neuropathy and those at risk given detailed advice on self-care and high-quality chiropody or podiatry. Foot ulceration occurs in about 15% of patients with diabetes and precedes 84% of all diabetes-related lower leg amputations; it **can** be prevented. Careful attention should be given to footwear to correct abnormal pressure patterns. Special insoles or special shoes may need to be made by an orthotist or surgical fitter. Careful follow-up and regular monitoring by a diabetic specialist nurse or clinic can successfully anticipate and prevent dire trouble.

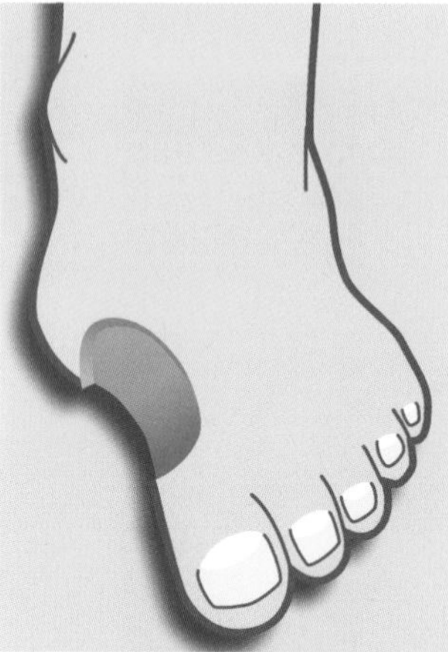

1 Excision of all necrotic tissue from ulcer, which is left to granulate

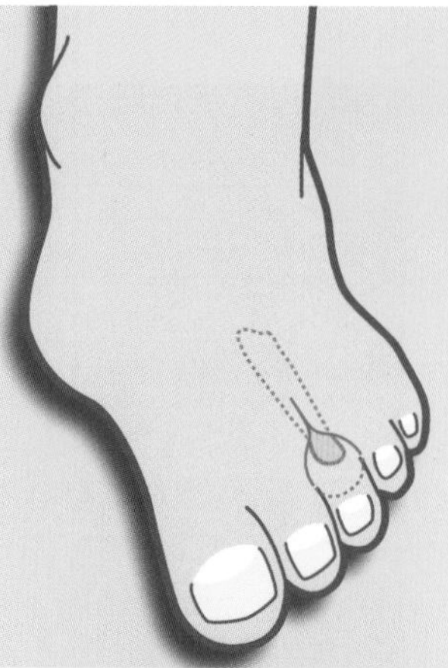

2 Digit amputation using racquet-shaped incision; toe is removed with both phalangeal bones and cartilage is nibbled from metatarsal (shaded)

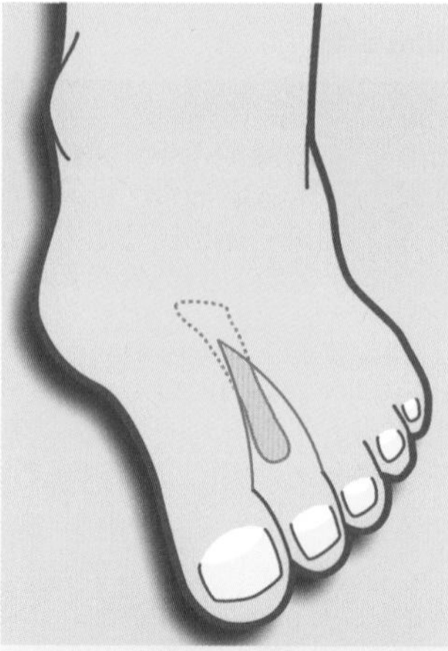

3 Filleting of digit and metatarsal if infection has spread more deeply. A cake-slice is taken out of the foot and the wound left unsutured to heal by granulation (see (b))

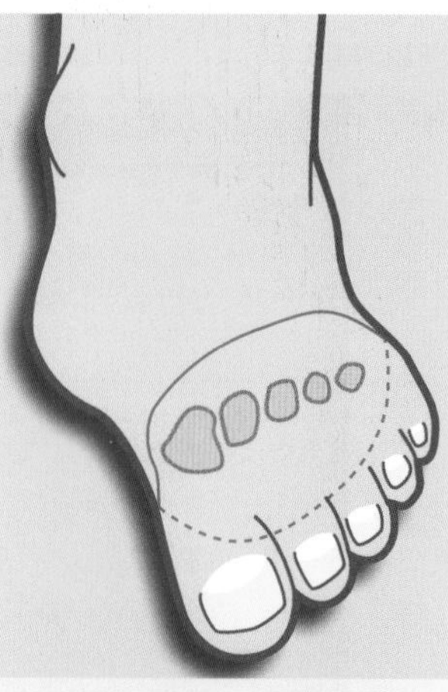

4 Transmetatarsal amputation

(a)

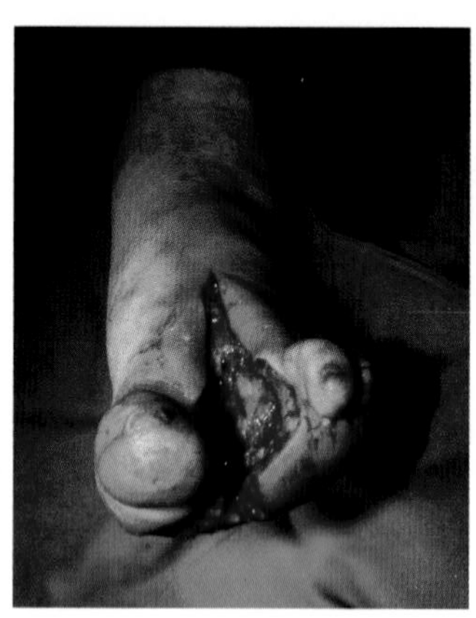

(b)

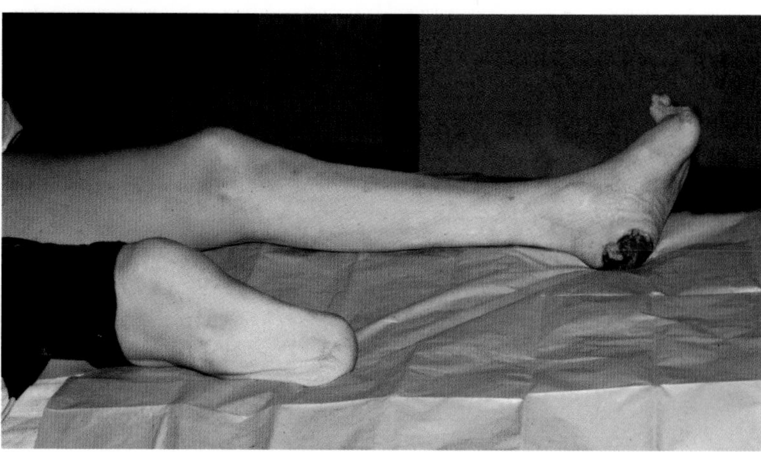

(c)

Fig. 41.9 Operations on the diabetic foot (a) Types of local amputation. **(b)** This patient had a neuropathic ulcer and necrotic toes but no arterial disease. The second and third metatarsals have been excised, together with all the necrotic tissue, in a 'cake slice' procedure. The wound was left open to heal by secondary intention, eventually giving a remarkably good functional result. **(c)** This elderly man suffered from a combination of neuropathy and obliterative atherosclerosis. He was blind as a result of diabetic retinopathy. The right leg was eventually amputated below knee because of spreading infection, but the left was saved by angioplasty of stenoses in the iliac and superficial femoral arteries, together with local surgery to remove necrotic tissue. Note the typical 'clawed foot' and distorted sole of motor neuropathy. Note also that the great toe has already been amputated. The heel has not yet been debrided

LOWER LIMB AMPUTATION

Strenuous efforts should be made to preserve ischaemic limbs by reconstructive surgery or interventional radiology. This is because the functional results of successful revascularisation are far better than even the best major amputation. Mobility with artificial limbs is disappointing, especially in the elderly or infirm. However, amputation cannot be avoided in patients where revascularisation is technically impossible (particularly in diffuse distal arterial disease), or if there is substantial tissue necrosis and a functionally useless foot, or deep spreading infection.

LEVEL OF AMPUTATION

Two principles guide the level of amputation (see Fig. 41.10):

- The amputation must be made through healthy tissue. If not, there is a high risk of wound breakdown and chronic ulceration, requiring further amputation at a higher level. When amputation is for (uncorrected) peripheral ischaemia, it is almost always necessary to amputate at mid-tibial level or above to ensure healing

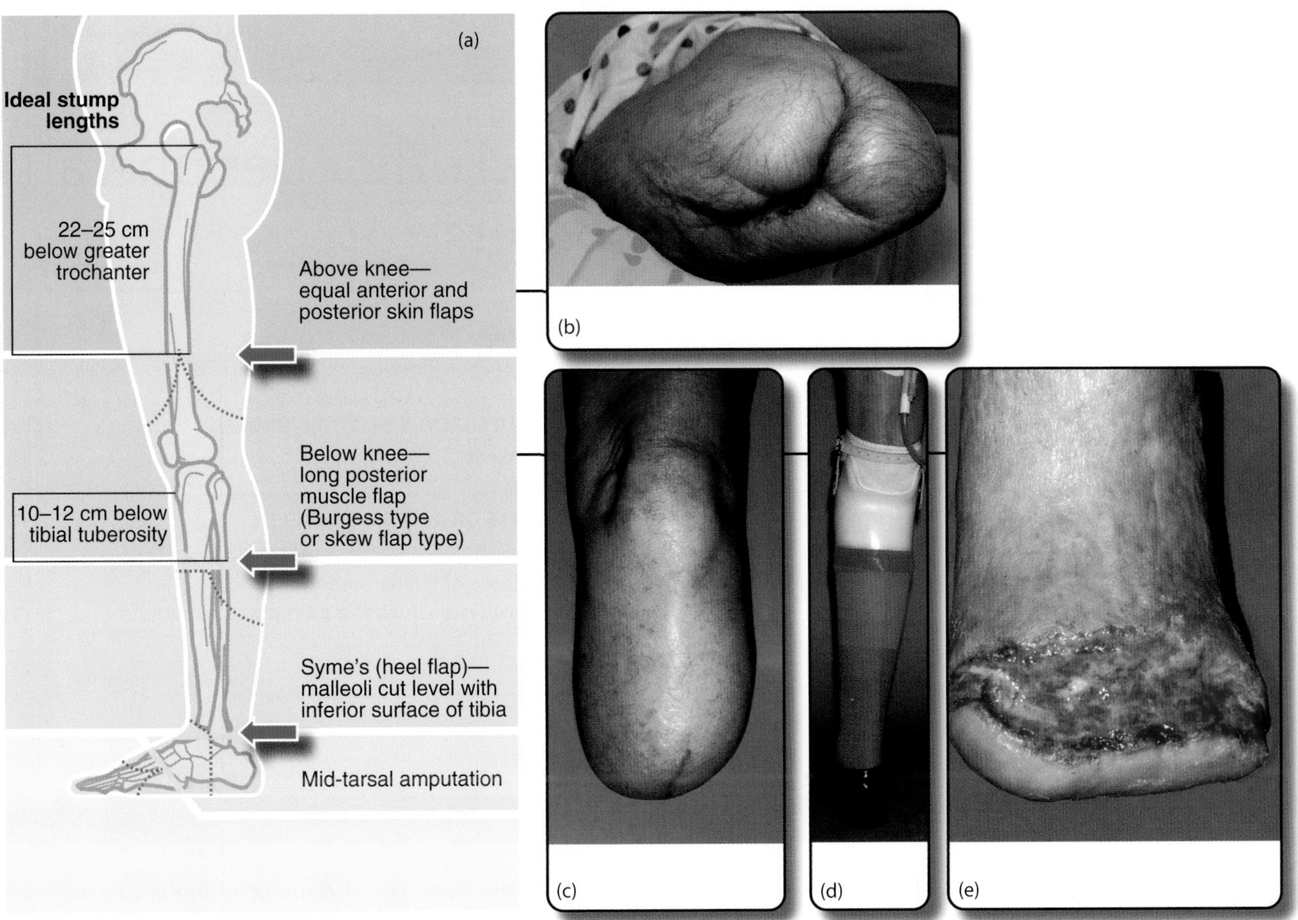

Fig. 41.10 Lower limb amputations
(a) Sites of election for lower limb amputations. **(b)** Above-knee stump in a diabetic patient. Unfortunately the original above-knee wound broke down and necrotic muscle had to be excised. The wound was left open and had nearly healed by secondary intention two months later. **(c)** A well-healed below-knee stump at 6 weeks. The operation used a long posterior muscle flap and equal length 'skew' skin flaps. **(d)** The same patient fitted with a modular below-knee prosthesis retained by a close-fitting socket and a small strap above the knee. Note the urinary catheter. **(e)** Breakdown of below-knee stump because of inadequate arterial blood supply

- The choice of amputation level must take into account the fitting of a prosthetic limb. For this purpose, the mid-tibia (**below-knee**) and lower femoral levels (**above-knee**) are preferred. If the knee joint can be saved, the functional success of a prosthesis is much better. With improved prostheses, through-knee amputation is possible but healing rates are poor; most surgeons and prosthetists prefer above-knee to through-knee amputation as it has a better healing rate and easier prosthetics

The traditional 'guillotine' amputation of the battlefield simply sliced off the limb, leaving the wound to heal by secondary intention. This reduced the risk of fatal gas gangrene or tetanus but the outcome for fitting a prosthetic limb was poor. There have been huge developments in amputation techniques in recent decades, particularly in the use of **myoplastic flaps**. For below-knee amputations, a long posterior flap of muscle and skin is wrapped forward over the amputated bone and sutured in place. This results in more reliable healing and a suitably shaped and cushioned stump. A variation, the Robinson **'skew flap'**, uses a long posterior muscle flap but equal skin flaps. The healing rate is no better but the stump is better shaped for earlier prosthetic fitting. With these techniques and in experienced hands, 70% or more of below-knee amputations for ischaemia will eventually heal even without revascularisation, preserving the knee joint and allowing reasonable walking. Modern below-knee prostheses are **modular** in construction and weight is borne mainly on the patellar tendon.

For above-knee amputations, myoplastic flaps are used in which the bony amputation level is proximal to the muscle/skin amputation level. This allows the muscles to be sutured over the exposed bone end. Short anterior and posterior skin flaps are then closed over the muscle.

42 Aneurysms and other peripheral arterial disorders

ANEURYSMS (see Table 42.1)

PATHOLOGY OF ANEURYSMS

An aneurysm is defined as a localised area of pathologically excessive arterial dilatation. For the abdominal aorta, an antero-posterior (AP) diameter of ≥3 cm is generally accepted as defining an aneurysm. In some patients with aneurysmal disease, all major arteries are wider (arteriomegaly) and one or more becomes truly aneurysmal. Aneurysms of the abdominal aorta and the iliac, femoral and popliteal arteries are often branded atherosclerotic but the primary disorder is **degeneration of the elastin and collagen** of the arterial wall. Atherosclerosis can be found within aneurysms but it is likely that the two pathologies share risk factors. Aneurysms are relatively uncommon; found mainly in males over 70 years of age, they are even less common in women in whom they present about 10 years later. At least a quarter of patients have more than one aneurysm.

Degenerative aneurysms are usually **fusiform**, slowly expanding in diameter. As it enlarges, the vessel wall thins, expansion accelerates and the risk of rupture increases. Most abdominal aortic aneurysms involve only the infrarenal aorta; some extend distally to involve common iliac arteries; sometimes there are separate aneurysms of internal iliac arteries (see Fig. 42.1). A few extend proximally to become **thoraco-abdominal aneurysms**.

CLINICAL PRESENTATION OF ANEURYSMS (see Table 42.1)

Aorto-iliac aneurysms are often found **incidentally**. The patient may notice a pulsatile abdominal mass or a pulsatile mass may be discovered on abdominal examination. An aneurysm may also be noticed incidentally on radiological investigation—as calcification on a plain abdominal X-ray, as an obvious aneurysm on CT or, most commonly, on ultrasound scanning for obstructive urinary symptoms (see Fig. 42.2). More recently in the UK, a national AAA screening programme has been approved, with the aim of offering all men an ultrasound scan of the abdominal aorta on reaching 65. Similar schemes are appearing in Denmark, Australia and other countries.

Despite this, nearly half the cases that reach surgeons present because of symptoms of retroperitoneal **leakage or rupture**. This carries a very high mortality. Several studies have shown that the total community and hospital mortality after rupture is more than 85% whereas elective treatment can have a mortality rate of around 5%. **Pain** is the most common symptom of a leaking aneurysm. The patient often gives a history of transient or persistent **cardiovascular collapse** (fainting, hypotension) which should alert clinicians to the probable diagnosis. The clinical picture ranges from an 'acute abdomen' to abdominal or back pain of up to a week's duration and the diagnosis is usually confirmed by finding a pulsatile abdominal mass. Sometimes the symptoms can mimic renal colic or back pain so an AAA must be excluded in all older men presenting with such symptoms. Intraperitoneal rupture and often extraperitoneal rupture are rapidly fatal and are frequently an unrecognised cause of **sudden death** in the elderly, with the cause often attributed to myocardial infarction.

Femoral and popliteal aneurysms are relatively uncommon and usually present as pulsatile masses. The larger they

Table 42.1 Clinical presentation and pathophysiology of aortic, iliac, femoral and popliteal aneurysms

Clinical presentation	Pathophysiology
Asymptomatic—discovered incidentally as pulsatile mass in abdomen, groin or popliteal fossa, on abdominal X-ray, CT or ultrasound scan	Progressive aneurysmal dilatation. May be self-limiting if hypertension and smoking controlled
Symptomatic—abdominal or back pain with tender aneurysm. Needs urgent surgery	Rapidly expanding aneurysms cause pressure on adjacent structures
Sudden death—acute, usually fatal, cardiovascular collapse. Often misdiagnosed as myocardial infarction	Sudden rupture of aneurysm only detected at autopsy or in the dissection room
Leaking/ruptured aneurysm—ill-defined back or abdominal pain often simulating ureteric colic or other abdominal emergency. Diagnostic if accompanied by transient collapse. Sometimes a history of recent similar episodes. Pulsatile abdominal mass palpable in 50%	Dilatation and thinning of the wall of an aneurysm leading to leakage of blood into retroperitoneal tissues—usually leads to catastrophic rupture within hours
Symptoms and signs of **acute severe leg ischaemia**; often pulsatile popliteal aneurysm on contralateral side	Sudden thrombotic occlusion of aneurysmal popliteal artery
Complete arterial occlusion—sudden distal ischaemia affecting lower limb due to embolism of thrombus from within aneurysm	Thrombotic occlusion of popliteal artery
Screening—discovered on population screening or opportunistic screening for aneurysm	

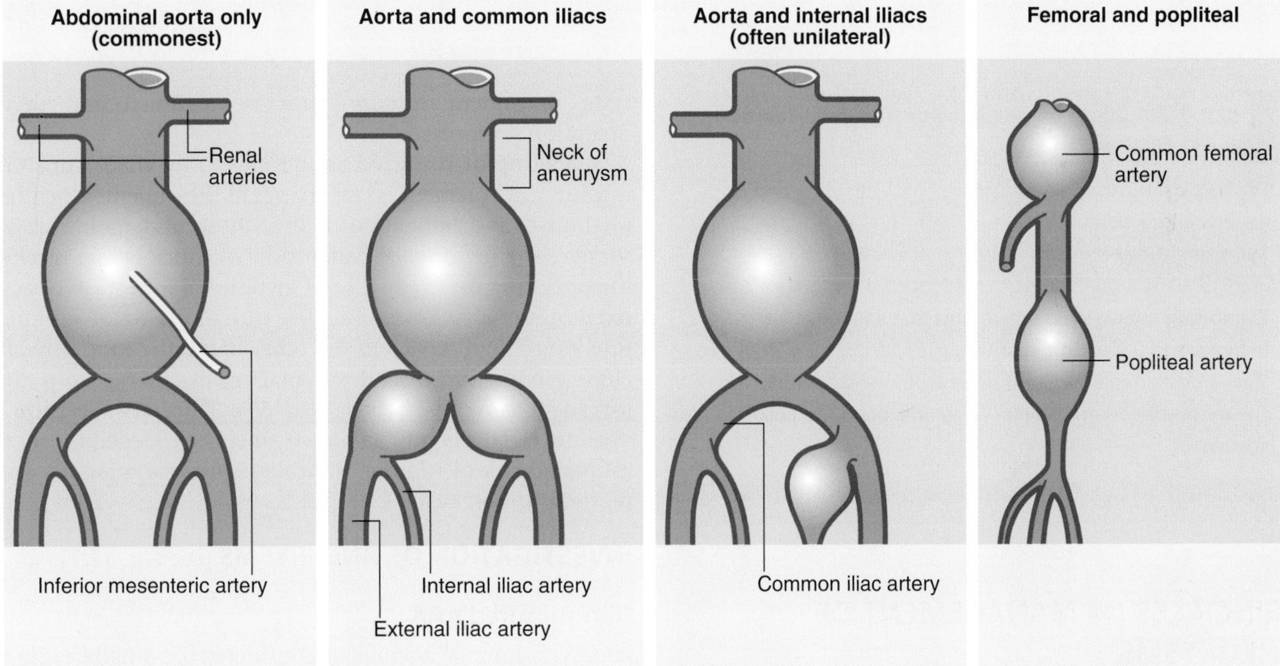

Fig. 42.1 Patterns of aneurysm formation
About 25% have more than one aneurysm either in continuity (common iliac, internal iliac, thoraco-abdominal) or not (femoral 10%; popliteal 20%; thoracic 5%). Abdominal aortic aneurysms rarely extend above the renal arteries. External iliacs are never aneurysmal

become, the more likely complications are to ensue. Femoral aneurysms occasionally rupture causing pain and massive swelling in the groin. Popliteal aneurysms are liable to undergo thrombosis or embolise, causing an **acutely ischaemic leg** (see Table 40.2). A thrombosed popliteal aneurysm carries a 50% risk of limb loss. In any patient presenting with an acutely ischaemic leg, it is vital to exclude this diagnosis as successful treatment often requires thrombolysis as well as surgery. Popliteal aneurysms can also rupture and cause a variety of other presentations listed in Table 40.2.

Fig. 42.2 Abdominal aortic aneurysm

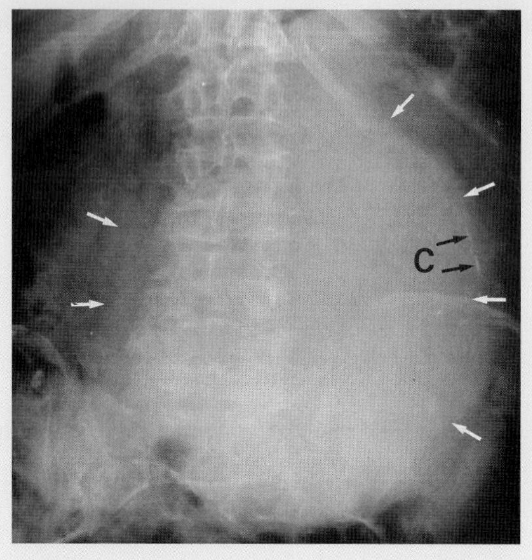

(a)

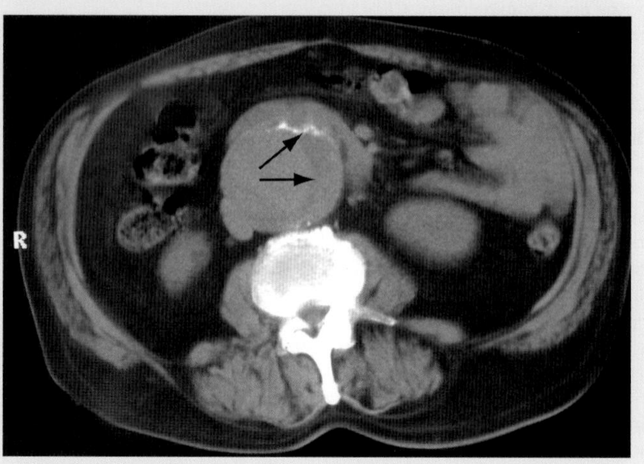

(b)

(a, b) This very obese 64-year-old man complained of continuous aching back pain for 2 weeks. **(a)** Plain abdominal X-ray showing huge abdominal aneurysm (outlined by arrows). Note calcification **C** along its left-hand aspect. **(b)** CT scan of a different patient with a 6 cm AAA. The thrombus lining the wall can clearly be seen (arrowed). Calcification is visible in the anterior wall where the third part of the duodenum is closely applied to it. Rarely, a primary aorto-duodenal fistula develops at this point

Box 42.1 Indications for operating on abdominal aortic aneurysms

- **Leaking or ruptured aneurysms**—if patient's state and general fitness permit
- **Symptomatic aneurysms**—aneurysms causing pain (particularly if tender), ureteric obstruction or embolism
- **Expanding aneurysms**—aneurysms that enlarge at a rate of more than 0.5 cm in 1 year
- **Size**—most arterial surgeons now recommend operation on aneurysms of 5.5 cm diameter or greater, or any saccular aneurysm

PRINCIPLES OF MANAGEMENT OF ANEURYSMS

INDICATIONS FOR OPERATION (see Box 42.1)

For **asymptomatic** aneurysms, the risk of rupture increases almost exponentially as the aneurysm dilates. Most vascular surgeons would consider operating on abdominal or thoracic aortic aneurysms of 5–5.5 cm or more or those that expand more than 0.5 cm a year; 6 cm is generally considered to be critical since 40% of such aneurysms can be expected to rupture over the following 2 years.

If there are **symptoms** such as back pain or abdominal pain, or signs of tenderness that can be attributed to the aneurysm, imminent rupture must be assumed and urgent operation performed.

A **leaking or ruptured** abdominal aortic aneurysm (AAA) is a surgical emergency. Less than half the patients reach hospital alive, and only about half of those undergoing surgery survive. The majority of patients die of shock before reaching the operating theatre or else of myocardial infarction or acute renal failure after operation. The true mortality of rupture is thus more than 85%. On the other hand, the mortality after elective operation or endovascular repair (EVAR, see p. 513) for aneurysm can be less than 5%. Thus, the decision to operate electively on a known aneurysm depends on the estimated risk of rupture. Indications for operation are summarised in Box 42.1.

INVESTIGATION OF ANEURYSMS (see Fig. 42.2)

Non-ruptured AAA

For asymptomatic aneurysms considered too small to warrant operation, ultrasonography is used for periodic **monitoring**, with referral to a surgeon once the size reaches an index diameter (usually 5 or 5.5 cm) or is seen to expand more than 0.5 cm in a year.

Where elective operation is planned, CT scanning is often used to show the relationship of the aneurysm to the renal arteries; the 5% of cases where the aneurysm extends above the renal arteries require a **thoraco-abdominal** operative approach and the operation carries a greater risk. CT can also show if iliac arteries are aneurysmal and if the aneurysm is **inflammatory** (i.e. has a thick layer of inflammatory tissue on its anterior surface that makes surgery technically difficult). Representative CT slices are usually taken through the chest to ensure the thoracic aorta is not aneurysmal; if there is a **thoracic aneurysm**, the management plan will have to accommodate it, according to size and position. If an aneurysm patient requiring surgery also has evidence of lower limb **ischaemia**, some form of arteriography is usually necessary in case a combined reconstruction is required.

Leaking or ruptured AAA

Any patient with a suspected leaking or ruptured AAA should be treated as a true surgical emergency but not necessarily by immediate transfer to the nearest operating theatre. There is good evidence that the survival rate increases when ruptured AAAs are treated by a specialist team of surgeons and anaesthetists, and this may mean transfer to a different centre. Over-aggressive blood pressure resuscitation of the hypotensive patient may convert a stable contained leak into a free rupture, and many clinicians support the use of **permissive hypotension** to facilitate transfer (see Ch. 15), i.e. not treating relative hypotension whilst the patient remains conscious and free from cardiac symptoms. This principle has increased the time available for transfer and/or further investigation.

Provided the patient with a leaking AAA is not demonstrating signs of cardiovascular instability, a CT scan can be valuable in helping to plan treatment. CT can demonstrate how the aneurysm relates to renal and visceral arteries and show any secondary iliac aneurysms; sometimes other abdominal pathology is shown that influences the decision to operate, e.g. liver metastases. In units equipped to undertake emergency endovascular repair (EVAR, see below), CT can show whether this is practicable.

Table 42.2 Comparison of conventional and endovascular therapy for aortic aneurysm

	Conventional surgery	Endovascular therapy
Mortality related to procedure	Approximately 5%	1.7%
Length of hospital stay	7–10 days	2–4 days
ITU/HDU care needed	Likely	Unlikely
Overall cost	£6500	£8000
Anatomical constraints	Distance between AAA and renal arteries can be less than 15 mm	Needs 15 mm of relatively normal aorta below renals
Past medical history	More difficult with previous surgery or peritonitis	Unaffected by previous abdominal surgery
Follow-up	Discharge at 3 months. Rescan after 5–7 years. Reintervention unlikely	Frequent CT and ultrasound for life. Reintervention rates high but improving

PRINCIPLES OF ANEURYSM SURGERY

The dilated aneurysmal segment is surgically corrected by means of a graft. Over recent years, there has been a trend towards treating AAAs using minimally invasive stent-graft placement (endovascular repair, EVAR) via the femoral artery. Many patients still, however, undergo traditional open surgery. The indications and relative merits of each technique are shown in Table 42.2. **Tube grafts** or **bifurcation grafts** of synthetic material (usually Dacron) are used for aorto-iliac and femoral aneurysms, whilst **autogenous saphenous vein** is preferred for popliteal aneurysms.

Open abdominal aortic aneurysm surgery (Fig. 42.3)

For abdominal aneurysms, the standard open approach is a long midline or a transverse abdominal incision. The aorta is usually reached via the peritoneal cavity or sometimes via an extraperitoneal approach. The patient is usually anticoagulated perioperatively with intravenous heparin to prevent distal thrombosis, and the iliac arteries and the infrarenal aorta are clamped (see Fig. 42.4). The aneurysm is incised longitudinally and any clot within it removed. Bleeding lumbar arteries opening into the posterior aortic wall are closed with sutures.

Proximally, the graft is sutured just above the upper limit of the aneurysm to (relatively) normal aortic wall within the aneurysmal sac, and to the native aorta at the bifurcation within the sac distally. Sometimes a bifurcated ('trouser') graft is used in aorto-iliac aneurysmal disease, with the distal graft ends sutured to an area of normal iliac artery. The aneurysm sac is left in situ and later closed around the graft. This is known as **inlay grafting**: it allows separation of the graft from the intestine, reducing the risk of an aorto-intestinal fistula arising later from the graft anastomoses.

Endovascular aneurysm repair (see Fig. 42.5)

Endovascular aneurysm repair (EVAR) is a minimally invasive technique employing combined stent-grafts. In the UK, NICE has approved it but recommends that clinicians ensure patients fully understand the long-term uncertainties and potential complications, including endovascular leaks, the possibility of secondary intervention and the need for lifelong follow-up.

Most cases are performed under general anaesthesia but many can be done under local anaesthesia. The procedure is performed in an operating theatre using a mobile X-ray image intensifier or in a specialist endovascular suite. The **stent-graft** consists of a self-expanding metal framework with a non-porous cloth covering; it is supplied in a constrained state and measures around 8 mm in diameter. When in situ, the main body of the device resembles a pair of trousers with one short leg.

Short transverse incisions are used to access common femoral arteries in the groin. The main device is passed into one femoral artery and guided proximally using radiological guidance to its position below the renal arteries. An

Fig. 42.3 Abdominal aortic aneurysm

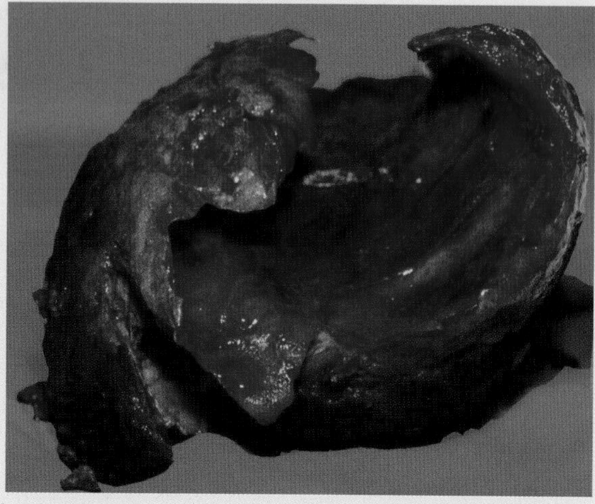

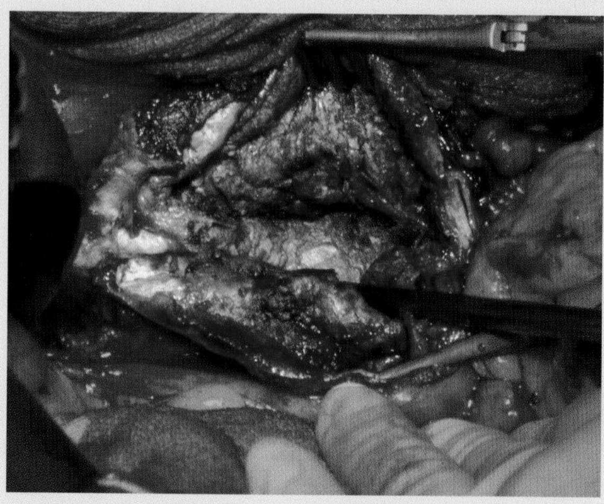

(a) A 70-year-old asymptomatic man in whom a pulsatile abdominal mass was an incidental finding. This cast of thrombus was removed from within the aortic aneurysm at operation; note the false lumen and concentric lamellae of thrombus progressively laid down as the aneurysm expanded over many months. **(b)** This shows the aneurysm sac opened at operation on a different patient who had complained of chronic back pain. The posterior wall of the aorta is completely deficient in part and the anterior longitudinal ligament is visible in its base

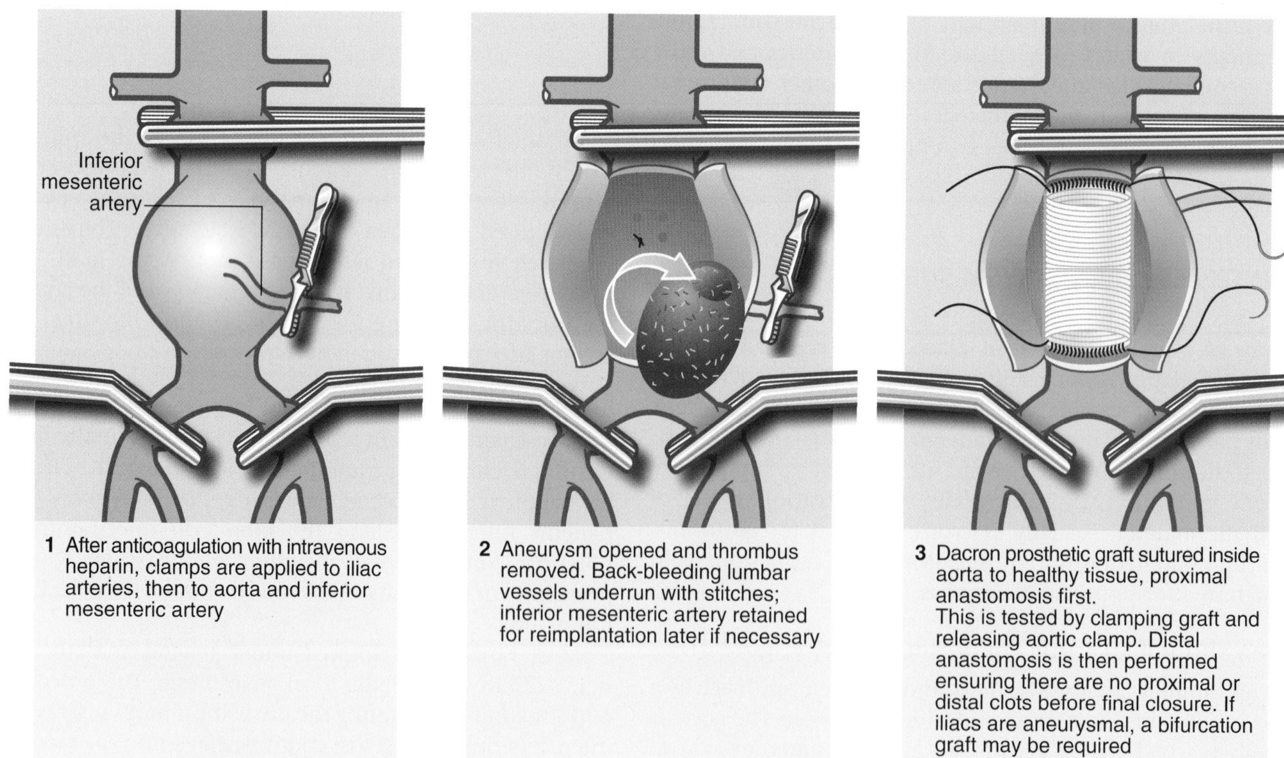

Fig. 42.4 Technique of abdominal aortic aneurysm surgery

angiogram checks the device can release below the renals. The constraining mechanism is then removed and the stent opens and expands against the vessel wall. The contralateral femoral artery is then exposed and a guide-wire passed proximally to enter the main graft body through the short leg. The second limb of the stent-graft is then completed by passing another covered stent over the guide-wire and securing it into the main graft body and the iliac artery. After completion, the device looks like a complete pair of trousers and extends from the renal arteries to the common iliacs.

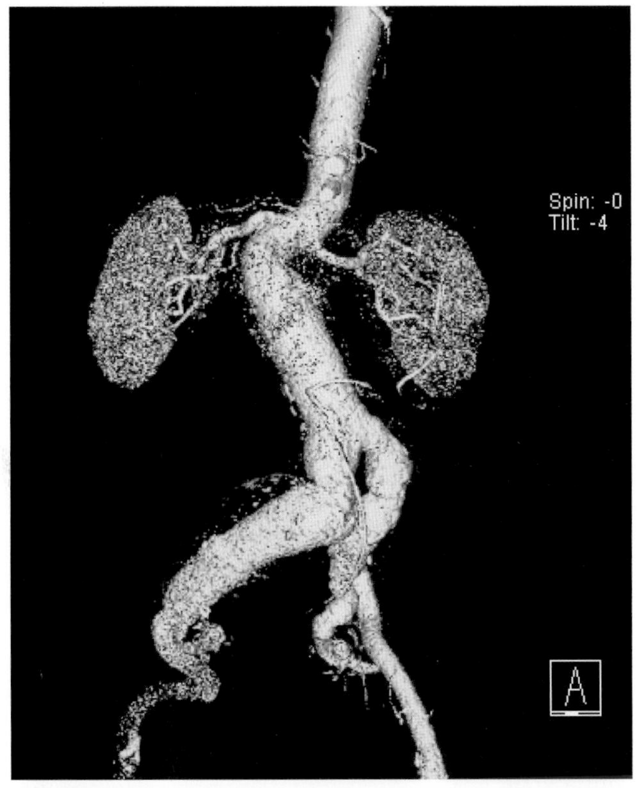

(a)

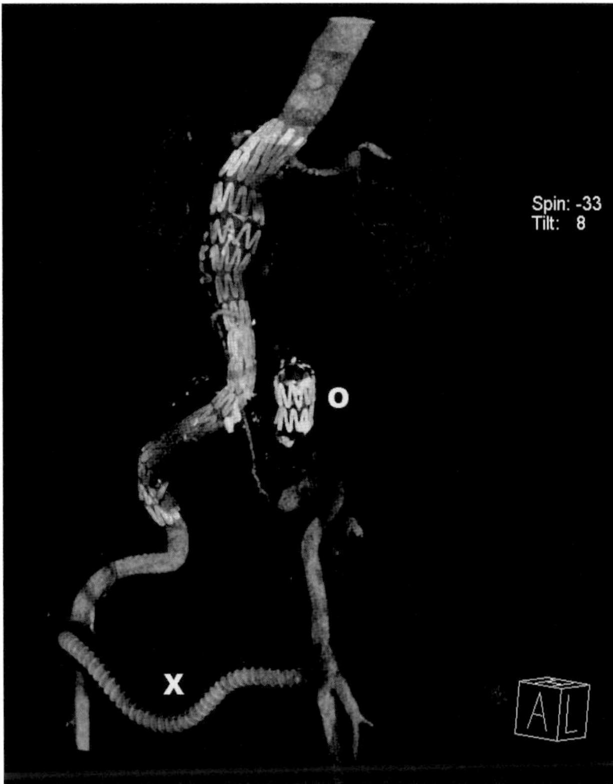

(b)

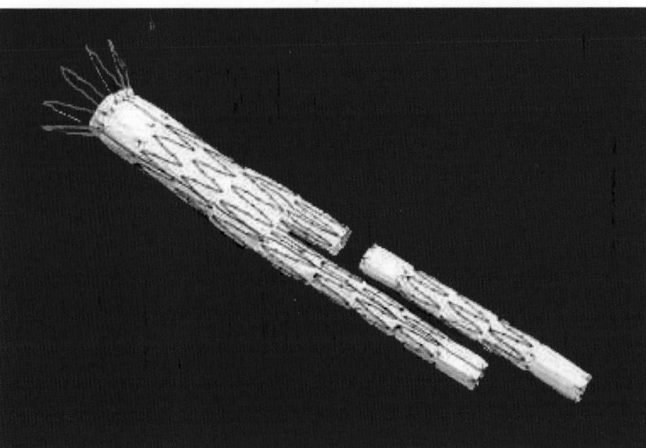
(c)

Fig. 42.5 Endovascular aneurysm repair
(a) Pre-procedure CT scan showing lumen of aorto-iliac aneurysm, suprarenal aorta and kidneys. On this view, the much larger diameter of the aneurysmal aortic wall is not visible. **(b)** Post-procedure CT scan showing the stent-graft in position extending from the right common iliac to just above the renal arteries. In this case, there were technical problems placing a bifurcation graft and so the left common iliac origin was deliberately blocked with an occluding stent **O** and the left lower limb was revascularised with a crossover femoro-femoral graft **X**. **(c)** Typical two-piece stent graft. Note the body and one limb are in one piece and the other limb is fitted afterwards. Note also the retaining wires at the proximal end

Other applications of EVAR

Open surgical repair of **thoracic aneurysms** carries a mortality of 10–20% and a high morbidity but many can be repaired by EVAR using just two small groin incisions. Even **ruptured aneurysms** (abdominal or thoracic) can sometimes be repaired using this technique, often using local anaesthesia. **Incomplete traumatic aortic transsections** have also been successfully treated with endovascular therapy. Advances continue to be made in EVAR technology so that more complex cases can be managed via this route.

UPPER LIMB PROBLEMS (see Table 40.5, p. 488)

UPPER LIMB ISCHAEMIA

Ischaemia of the upper limb is rare. This is because atherosclerosis is uncommon here and also because there is a rich collateral blood supply via scapular anastomoses that can bypass subclavian occlusive disease. Upper limb ischaemia usually occurs when the subclavian is compressed at the thoracic outlet or when emboli obstruct the brachial or more distal arteries. Occasionally, vasospastic disorders such as severe Raynaud's disease cause digital ischaemia. Embolic disease here has similar causes, presentation and treatment to embolism affecting the lower limbs (see Ch. 41 p. 502).

THORACIC OUTLET COMPRESSION

The subclavian artery and vein and brachial plexus pass through the space between the first rib and clavicle. If this becomes unduly narrow, neurological or arterial symptoms may appear; either can be part of **thoracic outlet syndrome**. Neurological symptoms are much more frequent but either variety of thoracic outlet syndrome is rare. Congenital causes include upward pressure exerted by a **cervical rib** lying above the first rib, or by fibrous bands. The gap may be encroached upon by acquired causes including a healed clavicular fracture, excess muscle development or other unknown means.

Neurological symptoms of thoracic outlet syndrome usually cause deficits in the T1 nerve root distribution (wasting and weakness of small muscles of hand; paraesthesia of inner forearm and hand). Symptoms of arterial compression include upper limb 'claudication' in people who habitually work with arms above their heads, as the artery becomes further compressed in this posture. In longstanding cases of subclavian artery compression, the artery beyond the stenosis may become dilated into an aneurysm (**post-stenotic dilatation**) which may collect thrombus. This can later embolise into the brachial artery causing acute ischaemia.

Occasionally arterial compression is diagnosed by finding a lower blood pressure in the affected arm, which varies with arm posture; obstruction can be confirmed by duplex ultrasonography or arteriography. Most cases are not so straightforward. Overall, the diagnosis of these syndromes is difficult and is best performed in specialist centres with input from neurologists, surgeons, radiologists and physiotherapists.

Operative intervention is becoming less common as conservative management improves. If indicated, treatment is by excising a cervical rib if present and/or excising the first rib, and dividing any obstructing bands. A post-stenotic subclavian aneurysm should be resected and replaced with a graft.

SUBCLAVIAN STEAL SYNDROME

This unusual syndrome is caused by stenosis or occlusion of the subclavian artery proximal to the vertebral artery origin. In consequence, the subclavian is fed by retrograde flow from the vertebral artery via the carotids and circle of Willis. This situation remains tenable and asymptomatic until there is excessive demand by the upper limb, when blood becomes diverted ('stolen') from the cerebral circulation causing transient cerebral ischaemia. Figure 42.6 illustrates a classic example. Treatment is by angioplasty or stenting of the subclavian disease or more rarely by bypass with a graft.

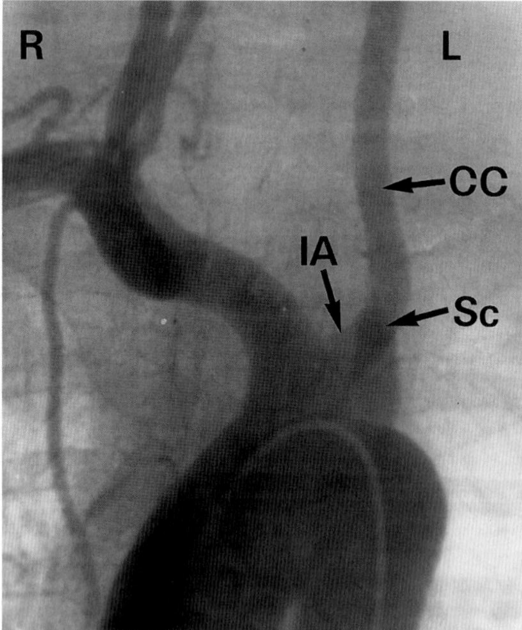

(a)

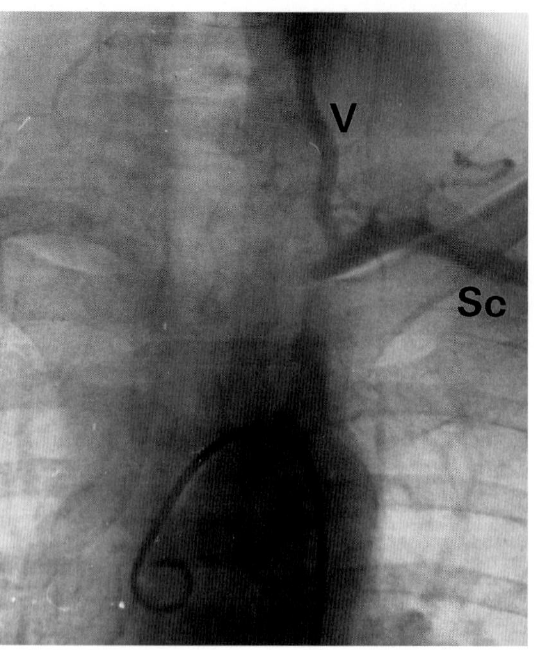

(b)

Fig. 42.6 Subclavian steal syndrome
Subtraction angiograms from a 55-year-old house-painter who complained of dizziness when painting walls and ceilings. **(a)** Aortic arch (with 'pigtail' arteriogram catheter visible) showing normal right innominate artery with its subclavian and common carotid branches. On the left, the arterial anatomy is anomalous, with the common carotid **CC** arising from a left innominate artery **IA** rather than direct from the aorta (a 'bovine arch'). The left subclavian artery **Sc** appears to be occluded beyond a short stump. **(b)** X-ray exposure taken 4 seconds later; the aortic arch and its branches are now clear of contrast, but contrast has appeared in the left vertebral artery **V**, flowing downwards from the circle of Willis. This has flowed onwards to fill the left subclavian artery **Sc** retrogradely. Thus there is complete obstruction of a segment of the left subclavian artery proximal to the origin of the vertebral artery, and the vertebral artery now supplies the left upper limb at the expense of the cerebral circulation. This results in episodes of transient cerebral ischaemia at times of high vascular demand from the left upper limb

EXTRACRANIAL CEREBRAL ARTERIAL INSUFFICIENCY

Strokes are common worldwide and about 1 million occur each year in the UK. Extracranial atherosclerosis is common and is probably responsible for about a quarter. The **common carotid bifurcation** is the area most affected by atherosclerosis, but can affect the distal internal carotid in the **carotid siphon**. Vertebral arteries are the next most commonly affected extracranial arteries. Less frequently, the orifices of the **great vessels** become obstructed where they branch from the aortic arch.

Atherosclerotic strokes are often heralded by a transient ischaemic attack (TIA) or a minor stroke. This recovers spontaneously without serious disability but the risk of recurrent stroke in recently symptomatic patients with severe carotid stenosis is as high as 28% over the course of the next 2 years.

CAROTID ARTERY INSUFFICIENCY

PATHOPHYSIOLOGY OF CAROTID ARTERY DISEASE

Carotid artery disease often results in **stenosis**, with cerebral blood flow becoming impaired when luminal narrowing exceeds about 70% (Fig. 42.7). Cerebral autoregulation of blood flow is able to compensate up to this point. Rough atherosclerotic plaques without gross narrowing may also be a source of **platelet emboli**. Small emboli may cause **transient ischaemic attacks** (including transient blindness, known as **amaurosis fugax**), with symptoms lasting less than 24 hours. In contrast, large emboli or embolism into critical areas cause major strokes. **Asymptomatic** stenoses may be discovered on investigation of **carotid bruits** or as part of general investigation before major arterial surgery elsewhere.

INVESTIGATION OF SUSPECTED CAROTID ARTERY DISEASE

A minority suffering transient ischaemic attacks or stroke are found to have a **bruit** on carotid auscultation. However, this does not indicate the extent of narrowing; a significant stenosis may be silent, as of course is complete occlusion.

Patients with strokes and transient ischaemic attacks should be investigated urgently for carotid stenosis by non-invasive means, ideally in a dedicated clinic. The preferred method is **duplex Doppler scanning**, which allows simultaneous imaging of carotid arteries and measurement of blood flow velocity. A measured rise in velocity allows the degree of stenosis to be estimated. In high-grade stenosis in symptomatic disease (i.e. over 70%), surgical intervention is the preferred

CASE HISTORY

Fig. 42.7 Carotid artery disease

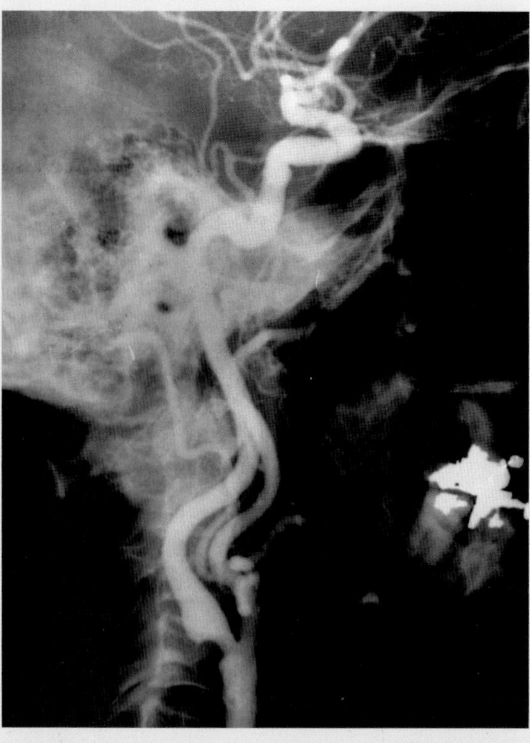
(a)

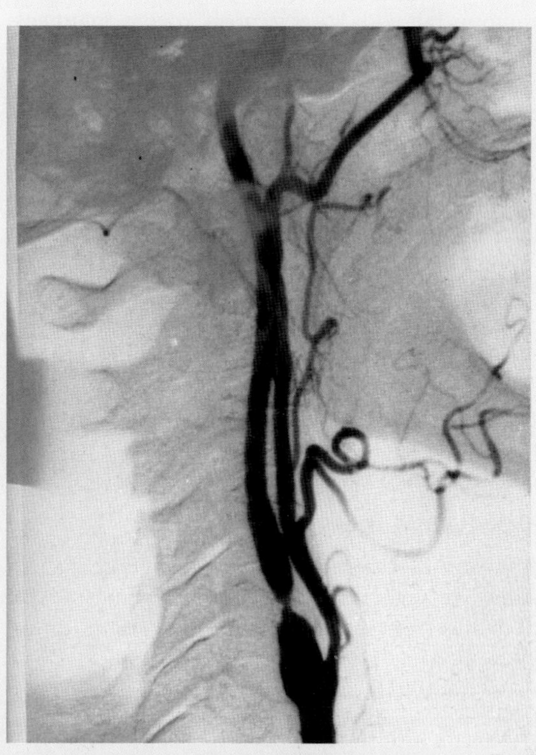
(b)

(a) This 71-year-old man suffered two transient episodes of left hemiparesis in 1 week ('TIAs'). Carotid angiography shows a localised 50% stenosis of the internal carotid artery just distal to the common carotid bifurcation; this degree of stenosis alone would not explain the symptoms. Note the typical post-stenotic dilatation immediately beyond the stenosis. The rest of the cerebral arterial system appears normal. At operation, an ulcerated atheromatous plaque was found, which was undoubtedly the source of the emboli that caused the transient ischaemic attacks. Endarterectomy was performed and the patient has been entirely well since. Studies in the USA and Europe have shown surgery is definitely better than medical management in patients with a 70% or greater stenosis. **(b)** Subtraction film from a carotid angiogram in a different patient. This shows a 90% stenosis in the internal carotid artery which is haemodynamically significant, causing cerebral ischaemia treatment. With skilled duplex examination, many surgeons feel that conventional **carotid angiography** is no longer necessary or desirable, particularly as this invasive technique carries a risk of stroke. Some centres now use magnetic resonance angiography as a less invasive form of imaging but it can overestimate the degree of stenosis.

TREATMENT OF CAROTID ARTERY DISEASE

Medical versus surgical or radiological intervention

The choice of treatment for symptomatic carotid artery stenosis consists of **medical** anti-platelet therapy (with aspirin 75–150 mg or clopidogrel 75 mg daily), surgical **endarterectomy** (i.e. removing the obstructing disease and thrombus) or, latterly, minimally invasive **stenting**. Carotid endarterectomy enjoyed an enormous uncontrolled vogue in the 1970s and 1980s for transient ischaemic attacks, completed stroke and asymptomatic carotid stenosis, particularly in the USA, but the role of surgery became much clearer after major randomised studies from Europe and the USA in 1998. These showed that surgery reduced stroke rate better than medical therapy only in patients with stenosis greater than 70%. In these high-grade stenoses, surgery reduced the annual stroke rate from about 6% in the 'medical' group to about 1.5%. However, the trials also showed a substantial risk of stroke or death from surgery of 6–8%.

Recent studies suggest patients with 50% or greater stenosis may benefit from surgery. Certainly, for patients suffering repeated symptoms but with lesser stenosis, cogent arguments can be made for intervention. Current risks of surgery include a stroke risk of about 2% and a myocardial infarction risk of between 1% and 2%. Unfortunately, surgery does not reduce long-term mortality from carotid artery disease even in high-grade stenosis. The mortality rate of about 5% per annum over 5 years is comparable in medically and surgically treated patients, taking the operative mortality of 2–3% into account.

Acute symptoms

There is good evidence that any symptoms referable to potential carotid disease, even a minor TIA, should be investigated urgently. This is because carotid endarterectomy is most effective at preventing threatened or future strokes if performed within 2 weeks of the herald symptoms. This benefit halves if patients are left untreated for 6 weeks or longer.

Asymptomatic carotid stenosis

The role of surgery in patients with **asymptomatic** carotid disease remains controversial. Recent trials indicate that even in the hands of surgeons with low complication rates, 15 asymptomatic stenoses need to be treated to prevent a single stroke. The figure for symptomatic disease is about six operations. There is also good evidence that the advent of best medical therapy (anti-platelet treatments, statins, strict blood pressure control and smoking cessation) has further reduced the risk of stroke in asymptomatic carotid disease.

Technique of endarterectomy

Currently, about 2000 carotid endarterectomies are performed annually in the UK. At present, seven males are treated for stenosis for every three females. The usual operation is **endarterectomy** and may be under general or local anaesthesia (studies have found no differences). The carotid bifurcation is incised longitudinally after clamping the carotid arteries and anticoagulating the patient. A temporary **shunt** is commonly used to maintain cerebral perfusion, with one end of the shunt in the common carotid below the stenosis and the other in the internal carotid above it, bypassing the operation site. The stenotic plaque is then dissected out and the carotid closed by direct suture (if the artery is large) or patched using vein or synthetic material to maintain the diameter. Carotid surgery carries an appreciable risk of mortality or cerebral complications such as stroke (around 3%) which needs to be taken into account when auditing individual results and when comparing patients treated medically or surgically.

Carotid angioplasty and stenting

Angioplasty with or without stenting is well established for treating peripheral and coronary artery disease but is relatively novel for carotid stenosis. Potential advantages include the lack of a neck incision, lower rates of haematoma formation and cranial nerve damage, and shorter hospital stays, but **disadvantages** include the risk of embolism during the procedure and possibly a higher rate of late restenosis. Recent meta-analysis suggests stenting causes more strokes in both the short and long term and endarterectomy is associated with cranial nerve injury and a higher cardiac event rate.

The technique of stenting involves passing a guide-wire from the femoral artery to the area of stenosis. A filter or basket at the end of the guide-wire is opened like an umbrella to catch debris to prevent it embolising to the brain and causing a stroke. A balloon-tipped catheter is then fed over the guide-wire to the target area and inflated to a high pressure to compress the plaque into the wall. The balloon is withdrawn and a self-expanding stent is guided to the area and released. The filter and balloon catheter are finally removed.

ARTERIAL INSUFFICIENCY IN OTHER ORGANS

MESENTERIC ISCHAEMIA

Blood supply to portions of the bowel may be compromised in four main ways:

- **Strangulation**. This is a mechanical problem presenting as bowel obstruction described in detail in Chapter 19 p. 271. It may be the result of a **hernia** (see Ch. 32), **volvulus** of small or large bowel or **fibrous bands** resulting from previous surgery (see Ch. 12 p. 172)
- **Acute thrombotic or embolic obstruction** (Fig. 42.8). This is analogous to acute thrombosis or embolism of

CASE HISTORY

Fig. 42.8 Acute mesenteric ischaemia

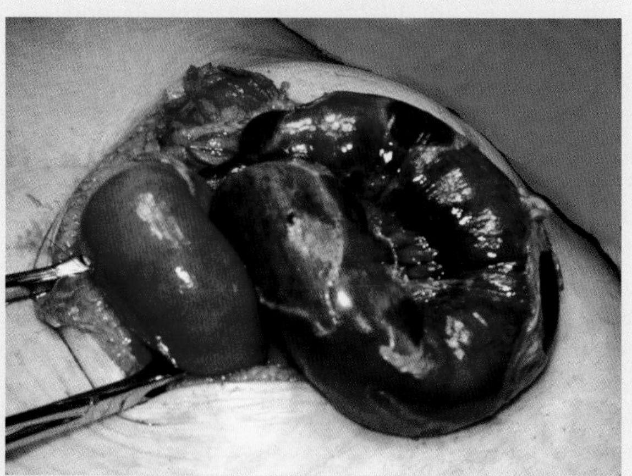

This woman of 77 presented with moderate abdominal pain and circulatory collapse requiring vigorous resuscitation. She was in atrial fibrillation and was acidotic. Mesenteric embolism was suspected and was confirmed at operation. Unfortunately, as often happens, the entire mid-gut territory, between a point 20 cm along the jejunum to the mid-transverse colon was necrotic and no beneficial procedure was possible

the lower limb described in Chapter 41. The cause is usually superior mesenteric artery occlusion and the condition presents as an 'acute abdomen' (see Ch. 19)
- **Transient ischaemia**. This presents as inflammation of the bowel characterised by abdominal pain and rectal bleeding. The condition is known as **ischaemic colitis** and is discussed at the end of Chapter 29
- **Chronic mesenteric artery insufficiency**. This rare condition presents with gross weight loss and abdominal pain following eating; it is analogous to intermittent claudication due to lower limb arterial insufficiency

CHRONIC MESENTERIC ISCHAEMIA

The rare condition of chronic mesenteric ischaemia or '**gut claudication**' occurs when the visceral blood supply is restricted to a point where it becomes inadequate during active digestion but remains adequate at rest. This occurs when there is gross atherosclerotic narrowing of all three main mesenteric vessels (coeliac, superior mesenteric and inferior mesenteric arteries). These patients present with severe epigastric pain on eating which causes '**fear of food**'. There is always **gross weight loss** and sometimes an epigastric bruit can be heard on auscultation.

Diagnosis is by arteriography with lateral views showing the origins of the three main vessels or CT angiography. Treatment is by stenting or surgical reconstruction of the origins of one or more mesenteric arteries.

RENAL ISCHAEMIA

RENAL ARTERY STENOSIS

Pathophysiology of renal artery stenosis

This relatively uncommon condition arises in two main ways. In children and young adults, the cause is **fibromuscular hyperplasia**. In older patients, **atherosclerosis** is the usual cause. Renal artery stenosis may present with hypertension (ischaemia of kidneys causes poor perfusion, activating the renin–angiotensin system) or functional renal impairment. It is sometimes discovered incidentally on urography as a non-functioning or poorly functioning kidney.

Treatment

Fibromuscular hyperplasia responds well to balloon dilatation, which often results in blood pressure returning to normal. Atherosclerotic disease may be treatable by angioplasty or reconstructive surgery but randomised trials have shown no improvement in blood pressure control or renal function. Renal artery stenosis needs to be recognised in patients having aortic reconstructive surgery, whether for occlusive or aneurysmal disease. This is because hypotension during the operation may initiate thrombotic occlusion of narrowed renal arteries and cause renal failure. These stenoses may need to be treated before operation by angioplasty, or by reconstruction at the time of the aortic operation.

COMPLICATIONS OF ARTERIAL SURGERY

Specific complications are summarised in Box 41.2 (p. 501). Local complications include **haemorrhage**, **embolism**, **thrombosis**, **graft infection** and **false aneurysm** formation.

SYSTEMIC COMPLICATIONS OF ARTERIAL SURGERY

Patients undergoing arterial surgery are subject to the usual complications of major surgery. In addition, they invariably have **generalised atherosclerotic arteriopathy**, rendering them vulnerable to serious or fatal cardiovascular complications. Patients with obliterative disease are more likely to have serious cardiac disease than those with aneurysms. For aortic and other major arterial operations, prolonged general anaesthesia, **aortic clamping** and heavy operative blood loss place extra stress on a compromised cardiovascular system.

Common systemic complications include myocardial infarction, cardiac failure, acute arrhythmias, strokes, renal failure and intestinal ischaemia. To minimise the risk, preparation for elective arterial surgery should include thorough preoperative cardiovascular assessment and sometimes treatment of cardiac abnormalities. Pre-existing medical conditions such as cardiac failure or hypertension should be stabilised under expert advice. Patients also require intensive monitoring during and after operation. Perioperatively, this usually includes central venous and peripheral arterial catheterisation for accurate pressure measurements. For patients with severe myocardial disease, transoesophageal ultrasound helps estimate cardiac output and guide fluid replacement. These and other high-risk patients should be closely monitored during the early postoperative period in an intensive care or high-dependency unit so that complications can be recognised and treated early.

LOCAL COMPLICATIONS OF ARTERIAL SURGERY (Fig. 42.9)

HAEMORRHAGE

During surgical access to affected arteries, nearby veins are vulnerable to tearing even when great care is taken in dissection. For example, iliac veins cross deep to the iliac arteries and are often adherent to them. Venous tears are more alarming than arterial ones because veins are very thin-walled, friable and difficult to repair. They are often inaccessible and thus lacerations can be difficult to identify and control; such tears often result in massive blood loss.

CASE HISTORY

Fig. 42.9 Complication of arterial surgery

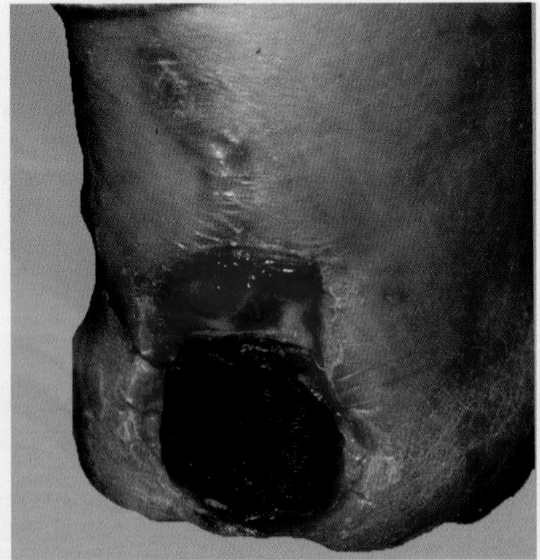

This patient was admitted to hospital with a ruptured aneurysm. He suffered arterial thrombosis of the lower limb during operation, and a thrombectomy to relieve it left him with an ischaemic foot. Poor attention to heel pressure relief during the early postoperative period led to this heel necrosis, which took several months to heal

Completing a satisfactory arterial anastomosis is demanding under the best of conditions, but it is made even more difficult if there are friable diseased vessels and calcified atherosclerotic plaques, as is so often the case. In the high-pressure arterial system, any defect is quickly revealed and blood sprays everywhere once clamps are released. Fortunately the arterial system can be remarkably forgiving and small leaks are quickly plugged by platelets if swabs are held in place for a few minutes. If blood loss is massive (10–25 units), platelets and coagulation factors are consumed and haemostasis is progressively impaired (**consumption coagulopathy**). Standard blood transfusions are of little help except as volume replacement, since stored blood lacks functioning platelets and clotting factors. In a deteriorating situation (and preferably in anticipation of it), expert haematological advice to infuse **platelet concentrates, cryoprecipitate (contains fibrinogen)** and **fresh-frozen plasma**, for example, provides the main answer. Where bleeding is difficult to control by sutures or packing, **organic-based glues** can be helpful in sealing bleeding areas. Patients are usually heparinised perioperatively before the arteries are clamped to prevent distal thrombosis. This does not usually interfere with haemostasis, but if necessary the effect can be reversed by injecting **protamine**.

There is a trend for the standard use of **cell-saving devices** intraoperatively to cope with anticipated heavy blood loss. These enable the patient's spilled blood to be collected, washed, concentrated and reinfused, minimising the use of stored blood. Inevitably, clotting factors are lost in the process.

Early postoperative haemorrhage is uncommon provided adequate haemostasis is achieved before completing the operation and closing the wound. When bleeding does occur, it usually results from a pinhole leak at the anastomosis or a slipped ligature. Haemorrhage is manifest by generalised signs of **hypovolaemia**, by progressive abdominal distension or, in the lower limb, by swelling beneath the wound. Postoperative haemorrhage occasionally stops spontaneously following transfusion of blood and clotting factors, but if blood loss continues, further operation must not be delayed.

EMBOLISM

In aneurysm surgery, embolism is usually caused by dislodging fresh or organised thrombus from within the aneurysmal sac. It is largely preventable by clamping the outflow vessels before the aneurysm is manipulated. Large emboli that lodge in femoral vessels can be retrieved with a Fogarty balloon catheter, but the more common case of fragmented distal embolism may cause infarction of digits or even the whole foot ('**trash foot**'). Infarction caused by this distal embolism is irreversible and usually necessitates amputation later. If embolism occurs during **carotid** artery dissection under general anaesthesia, the event is not usually apparent until the patient wakes up and is found to have suffered a stroke. Under local anaesthesia, embolic events may be immediately detectable.

THROMBOSIS

Thrombosis of reconstructed vessels is a major potential problem in arterial surgery. It rapidly leads to profound distal ischaemia and results in limb loss unless urgently corrected.

Sluggish flow leads to thrombosis and may arise for a variety of technical reasons as follows:

- Unrecognised stenosis or occlusion proximal or distal to the reconstruction causing poor inflow or runoff
- Faulty anastomotic technique causing stenosis or partial luminal obstruction
- Dissection of the layers of the distal vessel wall resulting in a loose flap of tunica intima and media which acts as a 'flap valve' occluding the lumen
- Twisting or kinking of a graft
- In situ thrombosis during arterial clamping

Thrombosis usually occurs in the first few hours after operation and becomes evident by deteriorating colour, temperature and pulses of the affected limb from the satisfactory state achieved at operation. Urgent reoperation is usually required. Judicious use of preoperative anti-platelet agents and/or inhibitors of the coagulation system can help prevent this complication. It is good practice to spend time at the end of the operation ensuring satisfactory flow in the reconstruction and good peripheral perfusion, as well as securing haemostasis. This can avoid the need for reoperation for a thrombosed graft or to arrest haemorrhage in the middle of the night.

GRAFT INFECTION

Infection of a synthetic graft is uncommon but can be a devastating complication. It can occur in the early post-operative period or at any time months or years later. The infecting organisms are usually from the patient's own intestine or skin, depending on the site of the graft. Infection is minimised by avoiding opening bowel, meticulous asepsis and haemostasis, and perioperative antibiotic cover. Antibiotics are normally given intravenously at anaesthetic induction and over the next 24 hours. A combination of gentamicin and flucloxacillin is usually suitable; where MRSA is prevalent, specific agents such as vancomycin are employed as well. In addition, protein-coated Dacron grafts can be soaked in an anti-staphylococcal antibiotic before placement, e.g. rifampicin or antibacterial silver impregnated grafts used.

Graft infection should be suspected if there is recurrent pyrexia and malaise or a persistently discharging wound sinus; occasionally, the wound breaks down, exposing the infected graft. Major graft infection, particularly when involving an anastomosis, has a bleak prognosis even when treated, the eventual outcome often being death from sepsis, or anastomotic breakdown with catastrophic bleeding. Standard treatment is to restore the distal circulation with an **extra-anatomic graft** (e.g. axillo-bifemoral) which bypasses the infected area, and remove the infected graft. Some units advocate use of the role of superficial femoral vein as a replacement conduit in the treatment of aortic graft infections. In early graft infection without anastomotic breakdown, prolonged graft irrigation with antibiotics can be successful on its own.

FALSE ANEURYSM FORMATION

A false aneurysm is the result of a slow anastomotic leak or a leak from an arterial puncture (e.g. a femoral artery puncture for coronary artery stenting) that is confined by surrounding tissues. A slowly expanding blood-filled cavity results, which can eventually rupture or undergo thrombosis. A false aneurysm usually presents as a palpable pulsatile mass. False aneurysms following a femoral artery puncture can be observed (if <2 cm diameter they can thrombose of their own accord), treated percutaneously with injection of thrombin, or repaired surgically. Patients are often taking dual anti-platelet therapy and have advanced coronary artery disease, the reason for the angiogram in the first place.

False aneurysms also can occur at an anastomosis (usually between a synthetic graft and artery). They used to be more common because of gradual breakdown of silk suture materials, but can still occur, sometimes as a consequence of low grade infection. They often require surgical reconstruction.

Occasionally a false aneurysm at an upper anastomosis of a graft with the abdominal aorta leaks into the overlying duodenum. This produces an **aortoduodenal fistula** and presents with major haematemesis. Aortoduodenal fistula may also result from graft infection.

LONG-TERM FOLLOW-UP AFTER ARTERIAL SURGERY

All patients with obliterative atherosclerotic disease are liable to disease progression and new ischaemic events. In fact, the risk of sudden cardiovascular death in claudication patients is the same as someone who has suffered a non-fatal myocardial infarction! Ideally patients should be on 'best medical treatment' for atherosclerosis, i.e. a statin, aspirin or clopidogrel, blood pressure control and, if diabetic, tight control of blood sugar. Effective advice regarding smoking cessation and exercise should be given.

Most patients are followed up long term after surgery or angioplasty to monitor deterioration, to detect new disease and to enable timely intervention if needed. Femoro-popliteal vein grafts can be examined at intervals using duplex Doppler scanning. Such **graft surveillance** can detect early graft

Fig. 42.10 Late formation of new aneurysm after aneurysm surgery

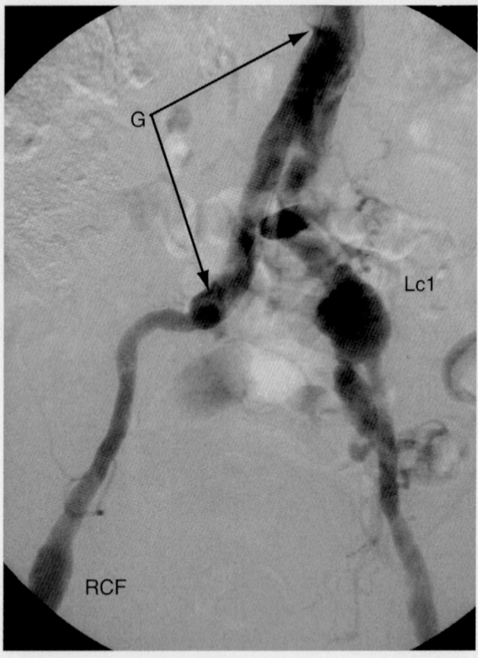

This arteriogram was performed for claudication 10 years after a trouser or 'Y' graft for abdominal aortic aneurysm. The trouser graft **G** is opacified and a new aneurysm has appeared in the left common iliac artery **LCI** beyond the graft. A small aneurysm is also seen in the right common femoral **RCF**. Neither was large enough to require surgery but periodic follow-up was continued using ultrasound. Obliterative disease responsible for the claudication was found in the superficial femoral arteries distal to this film

stenoses, enabling them to be treated and the graft preserved, although the efficacy of this is not proven. Aneurysm patients after open operation, on the other hand, can be discharged from regular follow-up 3 months after operation if there are no complications but should be rescanned by ultrasound at 5-yearly intervals for new aneurysms (Fig. 42.10). Stent-graft follow-up needs to be more rigorous as the devices are not as securely fixed as conventional grafts sewn in place. EVAR patients generally undergo CT scanning every 6 months to a year to look for leaks around the graft (**endoleaks**), but as devices have become more reliable there is a move towards 6-monthly ultrasound scans.

Venous disorders of the lower limb

43

VENOUS THROMBOSIS AND THE POST-THROMBOTIC LIMB

ANATOMY OF THE LOWER LIMB VENOUS SYSTEM

Blood is drained from the lower limb via two separate systems. The **deep venous system** drains the deep tissues of the foot and muscles of the lower leg and thigh. These deep veins lie within the mass of lower limb muscles and include the large **soleal venous sinuses**. Muscle contraction during walking and other exercise pumps blood back towards the heart against gravity (**the muscle pump**). Reverse flow is prevented by valves in the system.

The skin and other tissues superficial to the deep fascia drain into the **superficial system** with two main vessels, the **long (great) saphenous vein** and the **short (small) saphenous vein**. The long saphenous vein receives tributaries from the antero-medial aspect of the limb (and lower anterior abdominal wall), and penetrates the fascia lata in the groin to drain into the (deep) femoral vein (Figs 43.3). The short saphenous vein drains the posterior part of the leg and passes through the deep fascia into the popliteal vein of the deep venous system. There is a network of interconnecting superficial veins that drain blood from the limb if long or short saphenous veins are removed or ablated. The superficial system has no muscle pump to aid venous return but the valves normally prevent retrograde flow, particularly at sapheno-femoral and sapheno-popliteal junctions. Several **perforating veins** drain superficial blood into the deep system; valves on these normally ensure one-way flow. Most perforators lie medially on the calf above the ankle but there is a fairly constant '**Hunterian perforator**' in the medial mid-thigh.

PRESENTATION AND CONSEQUENCES OF VENOUS THROMBOSIS (Table 43.1)

Thromboembolic disease and its consequences are common and include acute deep vein thrombosis (DVT), pulmonary embolism and superficial thrombophlebitis ('phlebitis'). Deep venous thrombosis most commonly occurs as a complication of major surgery, lower limb fractures, myocardial infarction or other severe illness. About one-third of DVTs present with no apparent cause, though many of these patients have a detectable **prothrombotic state**. The risk factors, clinical presentations and management of acute DVT and pulmonary embolism are discussed in Chapter 12, p. 167.

Deep venous thrombosis is an acute local problem, and often causes major **long-term limb complications** but has the added risk of pulmonary embolism. The affected extremity is known as a **post-thrombotic limb** or, less accurately, a **post-phlebitic limb**. Often patients present with a post-thrombotic limb without a symptomatic or diagnosed DVT previously, though many have had major surgery or lower limb fractures.

PATHOPHYSIOLOGY OF POST-THROMBOTIC PROBLEMS

Following a DVT, the clot gradually undergoes **inflammation**, **organisation** and then **recanalisation** of the vein. During this process, valves are often damaged and become incompetent. This is because valve cusps fail to meet and interrupt the column of blood, allowing blood to reflux downwards causing increased pressure distally. This is **chronic deep venous insufficiency** and can take months or years to develop.

In the normal adult limb, ankle venous pressure while standing is about 125 cm of water. This falls markedly during walking as a result of the calf pump and valve function. In the post-thrombotic limb, where blood refluxes or veins remain occluded, ankle venous pressure remains high during walking. This leads secondarily to valve incompetence in perforating veins. Blood is forced into the superficial system causing local venous hypertension, disrupting normal vascular dynamics in skin and subcutaneous tissues. This may impair skin vitality and healing ability. Characteristic local

Table 43.1 A summary of lower limb venous disorders

Basic disease	Pathophysiological process	Clinical manifestations
Varicose veins— incompetent valves in veins connecting deep and superficial venous systems; often begins with sapheno-femoral valve incompetence	Failure of muscle pump means blood is forced from deep venous system to superficial system through incompetent valves causing slowly progressive tortuous dilatation of superficial veins Venous hypertension may cause chronic skin changes and sometimes ulceration. Women more often affected than men; varicosities often first appear during pregnancy	Slowly progressive development of prominent purple, dilated, tortuous superficial veins. Patient often complains of aching, especially after long period of standing. Patients may be distressed by cosmetic appearance or, if there is a family history, fear of progression or ulceration. Pain relieved by elevation. Dilated vessels are vulnerable to trauma and may bleed profusely
Superficial venous thrombosis (i.e. thrombophlebitis)—usually occurs in tortuous dilated varicose veins; more common in pregnancy. Occasionally affects normal veins in **thrombophlebitis migrans** occurring in patients with visceral malignancy	Spontaneous thrombosis in superficial veins; excites an inflammatory response in the vessel wall and surrounding tissues	Rapid onset of acute, highly localised pain and tenderness, associated with varicose veins. Overlying skin red and oedematous; underlying veins hard and nodular. Infection is not a feature so antibiotic treatment is illogical. Treatment is with non-steroidal anti-inflammatories. Occasionally ligation of the superficial vein at its junction with the deep vein is required to prevent thrombus propagating into the deep venous system
Deep venous thrombosis—predisposed to by previous DVT, pregnancy, oestrogen therapy, major surgery, trauma, obesity, abdominal or pelvic malignancy, immobility, a thrombophilia and increasing age. Long haul flying can be a factor may be complicated by pulmonary embolism	Thrombosis in deep venous system of calf; may propagate proximally into iliofemoral veins. Can obstruct venous return in both short and long term Spontaneous recanalisation may cause deep vein valvular incompetence, i.e. chronic venous insufficiency, and local swelling. Late complication is post-thrombotic venous hypertension. This obstructs capillary flow and inhibits metabolic exchange; leakage of red cells causes subcutaneous deposition of haemosiderin Combined effects cause atrophy of skin and subcutaneous fat, fibrosis, poor healing and predisposition to ulceration	Classic acute presentation is pain and swelling of calf and ankle with calf tenderness but is often asymptomatic. Dorsiflexion may cause pain (Homans' sign). Leg usually warm and normal in colour but pulses may be impalpable due to oedema. If iliofemoral veins involved, thigh also swollen. Late complication is post-thrombotic limb with chronic brawny oedema and narrow ankle due to lipodermatosclerosis. Skin atrophic, scaly and pigmented (varicose/venous eczema). Skin above medial malleolus most vulnerable to chronic ulceration after minor trauma

signs of a gross post-thrombotic limb are listed in Box 43.1 (see also Fig. 43.1).

The following factors contribute to the clinical features:

- Venous stagnation restricts arterial replenishment of capillary blood
- Arteriovenous shunts beneath the affected skin divert blood away from dermal capillaries
- Venous hypertension causes dilatation of local venules and the capillary network, allowing plasma proteins to leak into the interstitial spaces. Fibrin polymerises forming **pericapillary cuffs** which may interfere with metabolic exchange between blood and tissues

Box 43.1 Signs of a gross post-thrombotic limb

- Chronic lower leg **swelling** with brawny oedema
- **Varicose veins** with incompetent perforating veins
- Inflammation and haemosiderin **pigmentation** in the area above the medial malleolus (the 'gaiter' area) and other parts of the lower half of the leg. This is known as **varicose or venous eczema** and may be complicated by low-grade cellulitis
- Active or healed venous **ulceration** above the medial malleolus
- **Lipodermatosclerosis** around the ankle (replacement of soft subcutaneous fat with firm collagenous scar tissue). This causes the 'champagne-bottle leg' with oedema above and a narrow atrophic ankle below

INVESTIGATION OF VENOUS INSUFFICIENCY

Chronic venous insufficiency usually presents with a chronically swollen limb and/or typical skin changes of venous insufficiency around the ankle, and sometimes with ankle

Fig. 43.1 Post-thrombotic limbs and venous eczema

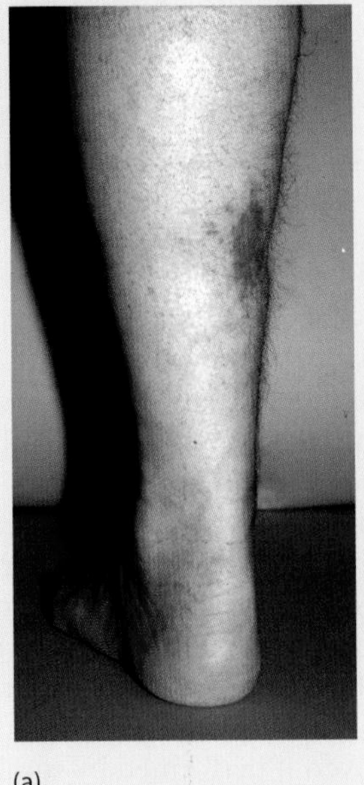

(a)

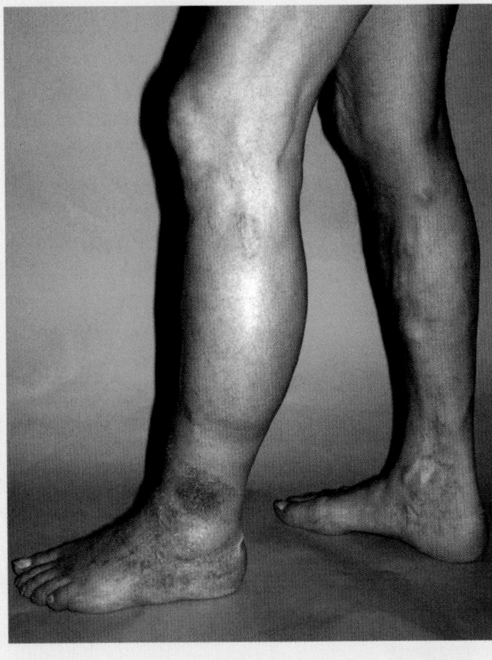

(b)

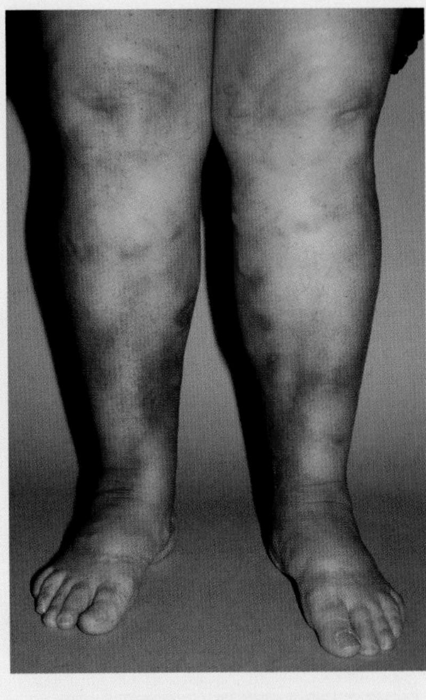

(c)

(a) Healed venous ulcer showing local loss of subcutaneous fat and surrounding pigmentation. **(b)** Man of 66 with no history of DVT showing marked swelling of the left leg with pigmentation in the lateral gaiter area representing venous eczema. The right leg has moderate varicose veins; the blue discolouration around both ankles is an age change due to dilated venules and is of no clinical consequence. On colour duplex ultrasound examination, there was evidence of deep venous thrombotic damage in the left leg. **(c)** Bilateral post-thrombotic limbs in a woman of 57 with gross venous eczema, fat atrophy, signs of healed venous ulceration and varicose veins

ulceration. This may be due to superficial or deep venous reflux (post-thrombotic or congenital absence of valves) or a combination of both.

The diagnostic pathway depends on responses to the following questions:

- Is the condition venous in origin? This is suggested by a history of DVT, prolonged bed rest in the past or lower limb fractures, or a finding of varicose veins or a '**champagne-bottle**' leg (i.e. proximal limb swelling due to oedema and distal narrowing due to fat atrophy and fibrosis). If the condition is not venous, another cause of ulceration and swelling should be sought
- If it is venous, is there superficial (Fig. 43.2) or deep venous insufficiency, or a combination of both?
- If a combination, how much is due to superficial venous insufficiency and therefore likely to respond to surgery (unlike deep venous reflux)

Patients should undergo a **colour-flow duplex Doppler ultrasound** investigation, now the 'gold standard'. This can give detailed information on the presence and severity of reflux in deep and superficial veins as well as determining whether there is venous obstruction. Functional detail will also be gleaned about the superficial system to enable targeted and appropriate treatment.

MANAGEMENT OF POST-THROMBOTIC PROBLEMS

The main post-thrombotic problems requiring active treatment are chronic venous ulcers and acute cellulitis.

Venous ulcers

Ulcers may develop spontaneously but are more commonly initiated by minor trauma which fails to heal, often complicated by secondary infection. Most venous ulcers can be healed by non-operative methods provided treatment is applied skilfully. Even if operative treatment is needed, conservative measures are used to prepare the limb. These include reducing swelling by multi-layer bandaging, removing necrotic tissue from the ulcer base and controlling cellulitis.

The systolic arterial pressure in the leg should be measured relative to the upper limb (i.e. ankle brachial pressure index (ABPI)—see Ch. 41, p. 497). If the ABPI is <0.8, the arterial circulation may be inadequate; it should be assessed and necessary treatment instigated before compression therapy as (a) poor arterial supply may be part of the reason for non-healing of an ulcer and (b) compression bandaging with low arterial pressure will make ulceration worse.

Properly applied support and compression of skin and superficial tissues is the mainstay of treatment, provided initially by elastic bandages and when healed, by correctly fitting

Fig. 43.2 Venous ulceration

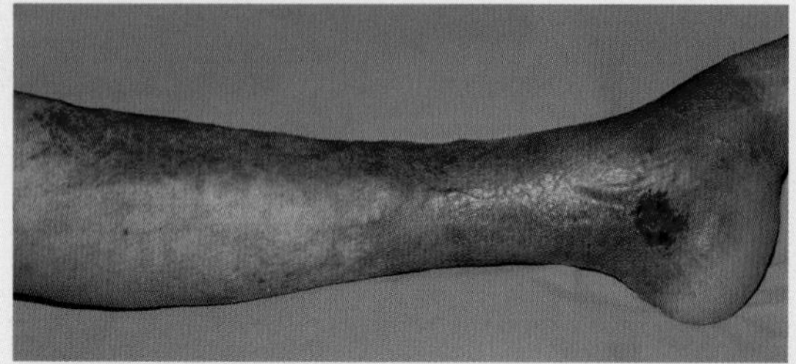
(a)

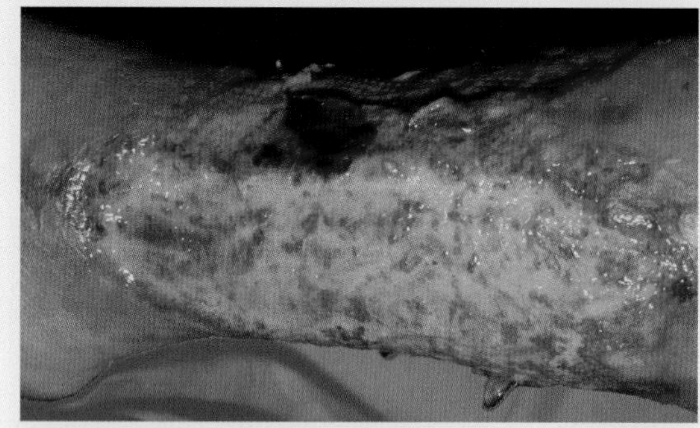
(b)

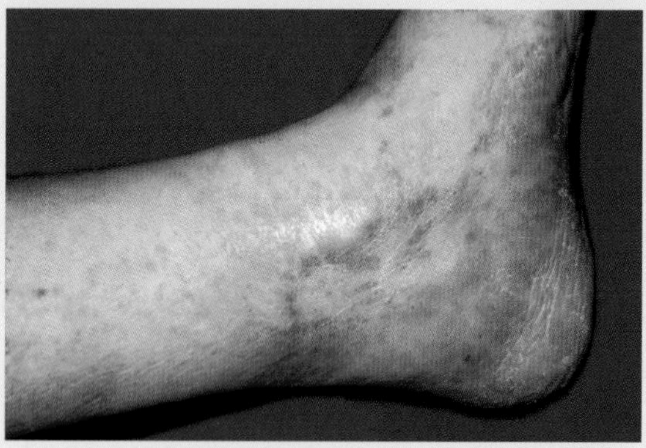
(c)

(a) Post-thrombotic limb with marked venous pigmentation and a chronic ulcer which heals and breaks down periodically. **(b)** Chronic venous ulcer in a post-thrombotic limb. The ulcer is virtually circumferential and represents a serious management problem. **(c)** Chronic ulcer that healed several years before, following a Cockett's operation, an open procedure for subfascial ligation of perforators, the scar of which is visible. This operation and endoscopic variations in the SEPS procedure are rarely performed nowadays

graduated compression stockings. In both cases, the aim is for pressure to be greatest at the ankle (up to 40 mmHg), reducing progressively up the limb. Great care must be taken that pressure does not cause ischaemia, or abrasions over tendons or bony prominences. Most venous ulcers can be healed rapidly whilst keeping the patient ambulatory by competent four-layer bandaging, avoiding the need for hospital care unless complications occur or skin grafting is required.

Spreading cellulitis should be treated with systemic antibiotics. Infection confined to the ulcer may be treated by saline soaks and perhaps excision of dead tissue; antiseptics are avoided as they may retard granulation tissue production and epithelialisation. Local antibiotics have no place in the management of ulcers.

Venous surgery may be indicated if there is superficial venous incompetence. Varicose veins should be ligated, treated endovenously or removed unless there is gross deep venous incompetence. Effective treatment of superficial venous reflux reduces the healing time for ulcers and halves the recurrence rate. Surgical disruption or ligation of incompetent perforating veins is of doubtful value, even if performed by subfascial endoscopic surgery (SEPS). Intractable or large ulcers may require skin grafting once the ulcer base is clean. Deep venous reflux is treated conservatively as there are no satisfactory surgical options that deliver long-term success.

Long-term care and prevention

As soon as a post-thrombotic limb is recognised, the patient should use graduated compression stockings and take care to avoid even minor trauma, especially to the gaiter area above the medial malleolus. Flaking and dryness of the skin should be treated with a moisturiser.

For minor venous insufficiency, well-fitting class I **elastic stockings** or tights provide suitable support. In more severe insufficiency, class II or III compression stockings may reverse tissue damage or arrest its progress. They also provide protection from minor trauma. Ideally they should be worn at all times except in bed. Correctly fitted stockings are vital; proximal constricting bands impair venous return and stockings sometimes need to be custom made. Effective elastic support will often be required for life but may not prevent further episodes of cellulitis or ulceration.

AXILLARY VEIN THROMBOSIS

Axillary vein thrombosis is uncommon and is the upper limb equivalent of DVT. It usually presents with a sudden onset of swelling of hand, forearm and arm, and aching pain in the whole arm. The limb often has a bluish tinge and sensation is preserved. The cause can be primary or secondary. A primary presentation often has no detectable cause but may be associated with visceral malignancy (**thrombophlebitis migrans**), or a thrombotic predisposition. **Paget–Schroetter** syndrome is also referred to as 'effort-induced thrombosis'. It usually occurs in younger people as a result of external compression of the subclavian vein between first rib and clavicle. The space may be congenitally narrow or physical activity such as weight-lifting may cause muscle hypertrophy or local trauma. Treatment options include anticoagulation to prevent propagation of thrombus and to encourage spontaneous clot lysis, or **thrombolysis** to restore vessel patency. Following successful lysis, patients may benefit from surgical excision of the first rib via an axillary or supraclavicular approach.

Secondary causes include long-term venous catheters, commonly employed in renal dialysis patients, and patients requiring long-term venous access for chemotherapy or parenteral nutrition. Catheter problems are usually managed with formal anticoagulation.

VARICOSE VEINS

Varicose veins are dilated, tortuous and prominent superficial veins in the lower limb (see Fig. 43.5). Varicose veins are common worldwide, being present in about 20% of people aged 20, increasing to 80% at 60 years. Nevertheless, only about 12% have symptoms or develop complications.

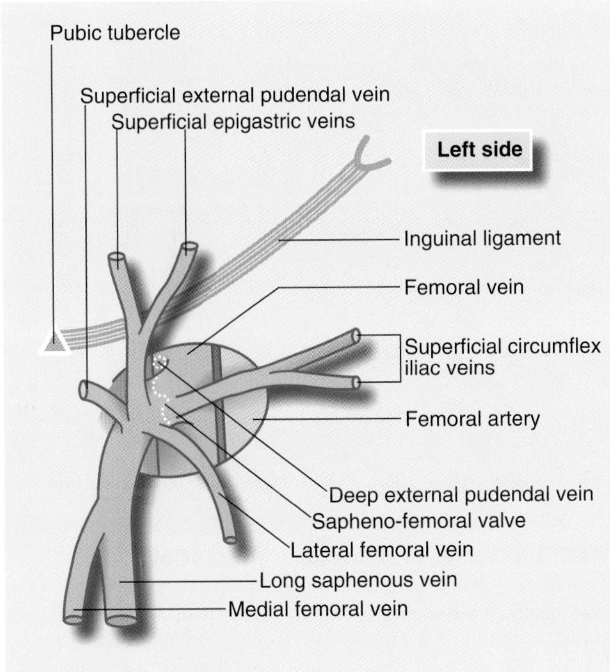

Fig. 43.3 Sapheno-femoral junction—anatomy

PATHOPHYSIOLOGY OF VARICOSE VEINS

Abnormal communication between deep and superficial venous systems is crucial in the development of varicose veins. The process probably begins with failure of the valve at the sapheno-femoral junction, leading to an uninterrupted column of blood from the heart which progressively dilates superficial veins down the limb (see Fig. 43.5a). Varicose veins usually develop slowly over 10–20 years, so surgical treatment is rarely urgent. The long saphenous system is involved in about 90% and the short saphenous in 25% (some have both systems involved).

Women are affected about six times more often than men, with most developing during or soon after the second or third pregnancy. An important factor is probably the high level of progesterone, causing changes in collagen structure (which may not fully recover), as well as smooth muscle relaxation. Pressure on the pelvic veins by the enlarging uterus may contribute by restricting venous return.

Hereditary factors appear to play a part in some patients, especially in men and in those who develop varicosities in their teens. Predisposing anatomical factors may include congenital absence of valves in iliac veins or abnormal vein wall elasticity. DVT plays little part in causing varicose veins. Rarely, multiple congenital arteriovenous fistulae (**Klippel–Trenaunay** and other syndromes) cause gross varicose veins. In these patients, there is gigantism of the lower limb and often venous ulceration (see Ch. 46). A technique of examining varicose veins is shown in Figure 43.6.

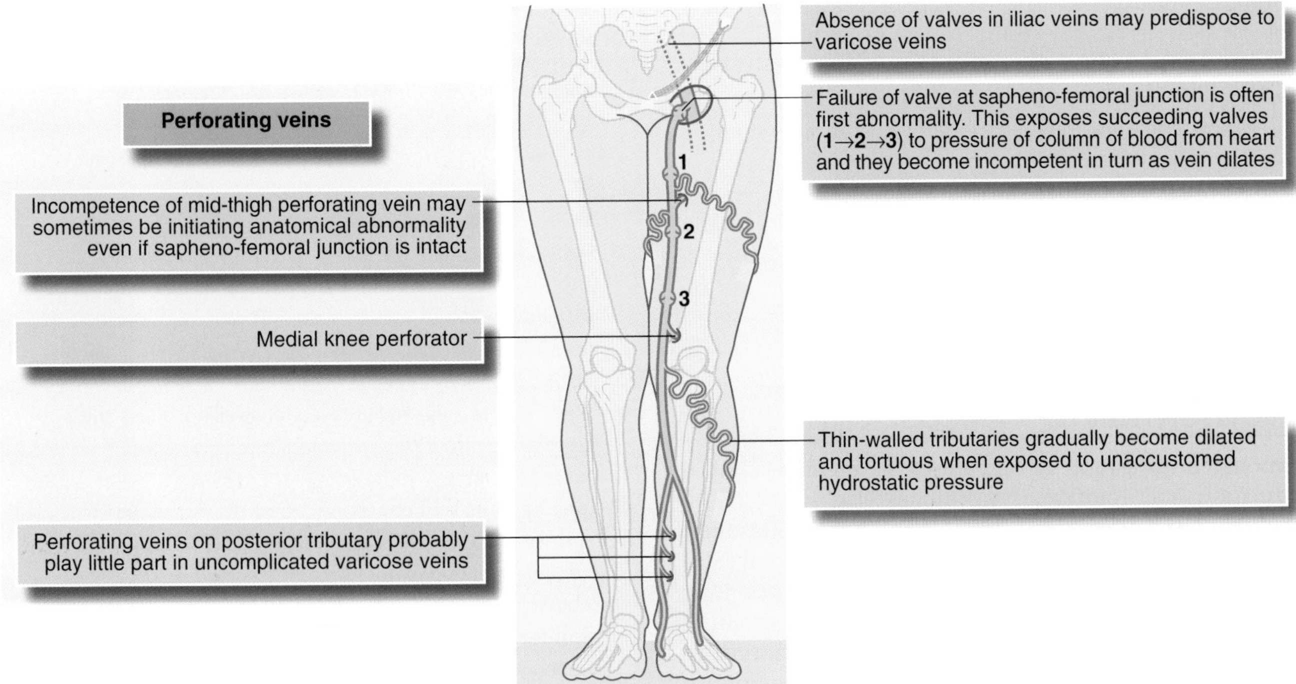

Fig. 43.4 Pathophysiology of varicose veins

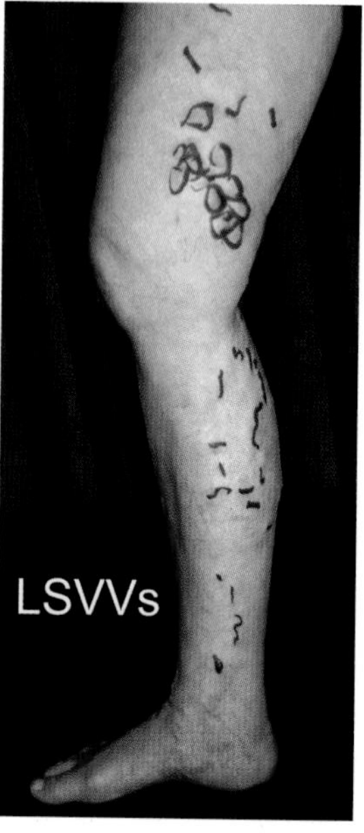

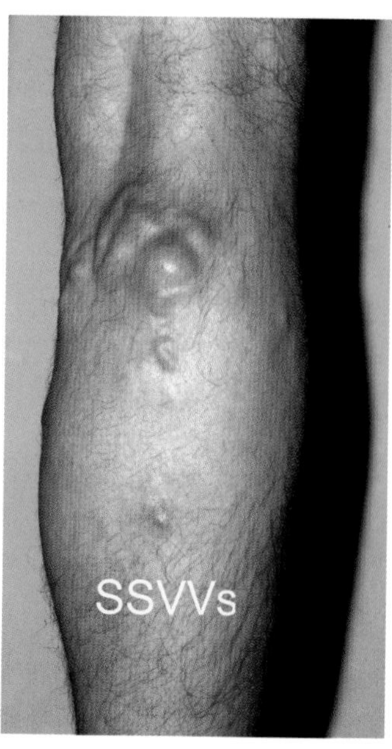

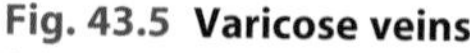

(a) (b)

Fig. 43.5 Varicose veins
(a) Typical varicosities in the long saphenous territory (**LSVVs**) evident both above and below knee and most prominent on the medial side of the limb. The indelible black markings were made immediately prior to surgery by the operating surgeon with the patient standing. **(b)** Typical short saphenous varicosities (**SSVVs**), which do not extend above the knee. These veins could not be controlled with an above-knee tourniquet and there was gross reflux evident on hand-held Doppler examination, confirmed on colour duplex Doppler scanning. The sapheno-popliteal junction (SPJ) has a variable position and should be marked before surgery using ultrasound so the surgeon knows where to site the incision

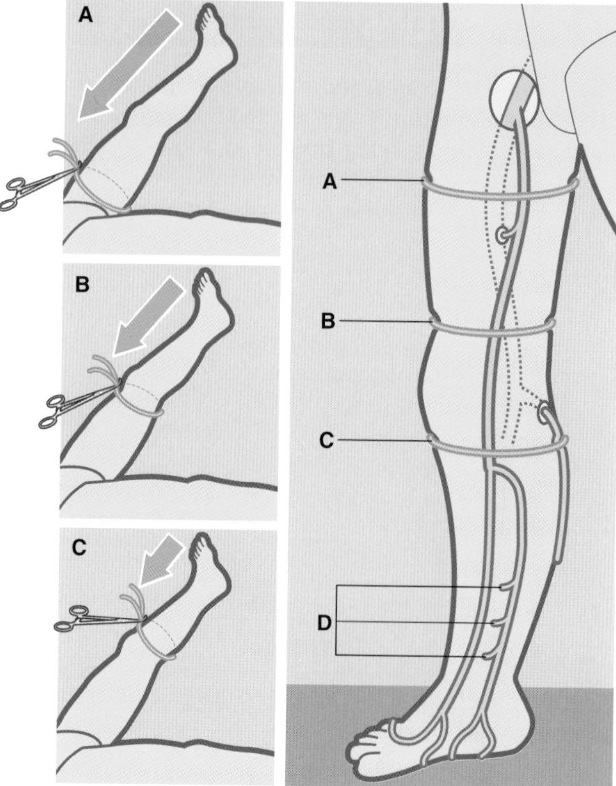

Fig. 43.6 A technique of examining varicose veins
Elevate limb and ensure veins are emptied by massaging distal to proximal. Apply tourniquet tightly around upper thigh **A** then stand patient up. Does tourniquet prevent veins filling and removing it cause rapid filling from above? If so, main communication is at the sapheno-femoral junction. If veins fill rapidly with tourniquet in place, repeat the test with tourniquet above the knee **B**. If this controls filling, then main communication is mid-thigh perforator. If this tourniquet fails to control filling, repeat below knee **C**. If this controls filling, communication is likely to be short saphenous-popliteal or medial knee perforator incompetence. If no tourniquet controls filling, communication is probably by one or more distal perforating veins, often post-thrombotic in origin **D**. Note that 80% of varicose veins involve the long saphenous system, sometimes with short saphenous incompetence as well.

SYMPTOMS AND SIGNS OF VARICOSE VEINS

The most common complaints related to varicose veins are:

- Aching legs, usually after standing all day
- Poor cosmetic appearance, especially in summer when the legs are exposed
- Fear of future leg ulcers ('like my mother had')
- Bleeding or worry about varicosities bleeding, particularly if traumatised
- Varicose eczema or ulcers
- Ankle oedema
- Recurrent superficial thrombophlebitis

INVESTIGATION OF VARICOSE VEINS

Traditional investigation of varicose veins includes clinical examination and tourniquet techniques (Fig. 43.6). As a screening investigation in clinic, hand-held ultrasound Doppler allows assessment of reflux at sapheno-femoral (SFJ) and sapheno-popliteal junctions (SPJ) and within the long and short saphenous veins. The probe is placed over either junction, the calf is pressed and the examiner can hear if there is significant reflux outwards through the junction on release of calf pressure. Formal duplex scanning is now advocated for

Box 43.2 Initial examination of varicose veins

- **Severity**—examine the extent and severity of varicose veins with the patient standing. Many patients attend with unsightly 'spider veins' which are not varicose. Others attend for advice because they are worried they will develop ulcers ('like my mother')
- **Skin changes**—examine the leg for swelling, ulcers and varicose eczema. If present, could indicate a post-thrombotic limb
- **Long or short saphenous**—examine the distribution of varicose veins. Are there varicosities above knee, indicating probable sapheno-femoral incompetence? Could these be short saphenous system varicosities, i.e. postero-lateral calf veins feeding towards popliteal fossa where short saphenous may be palpable

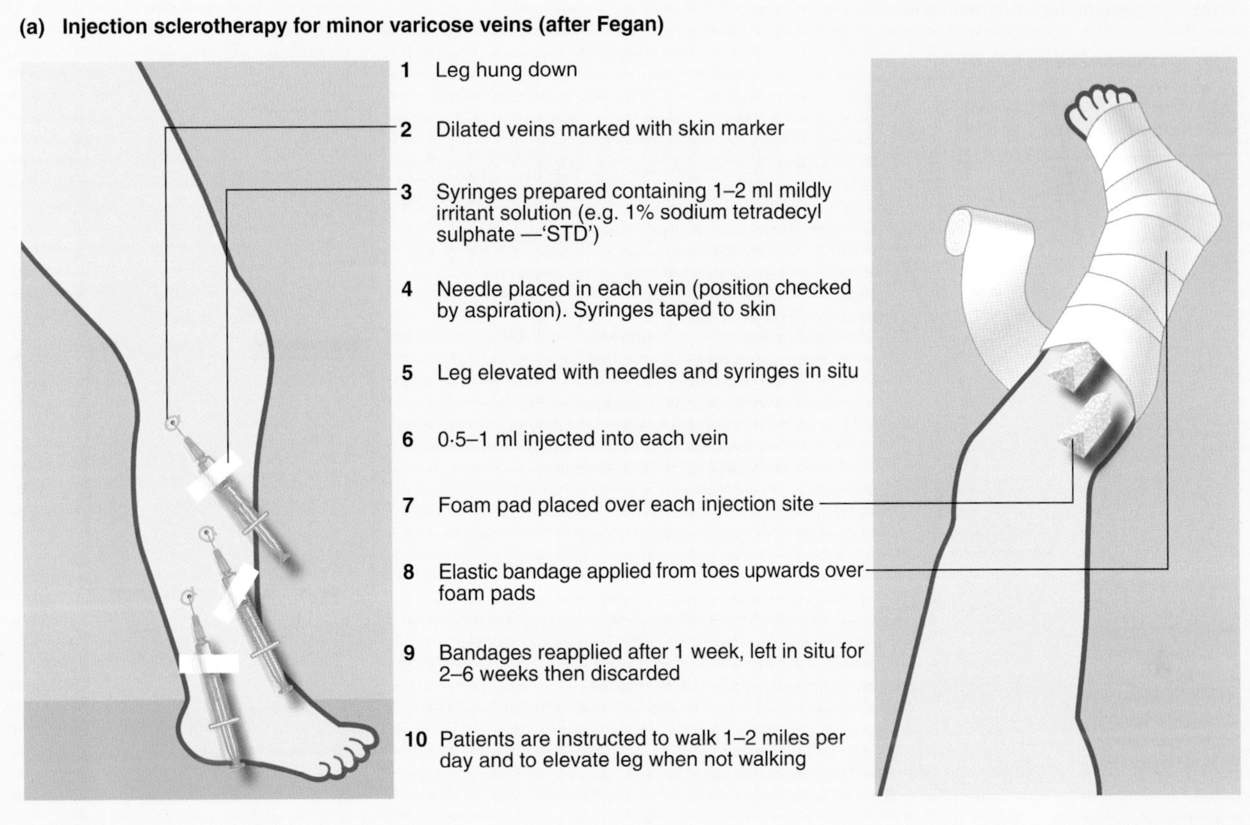

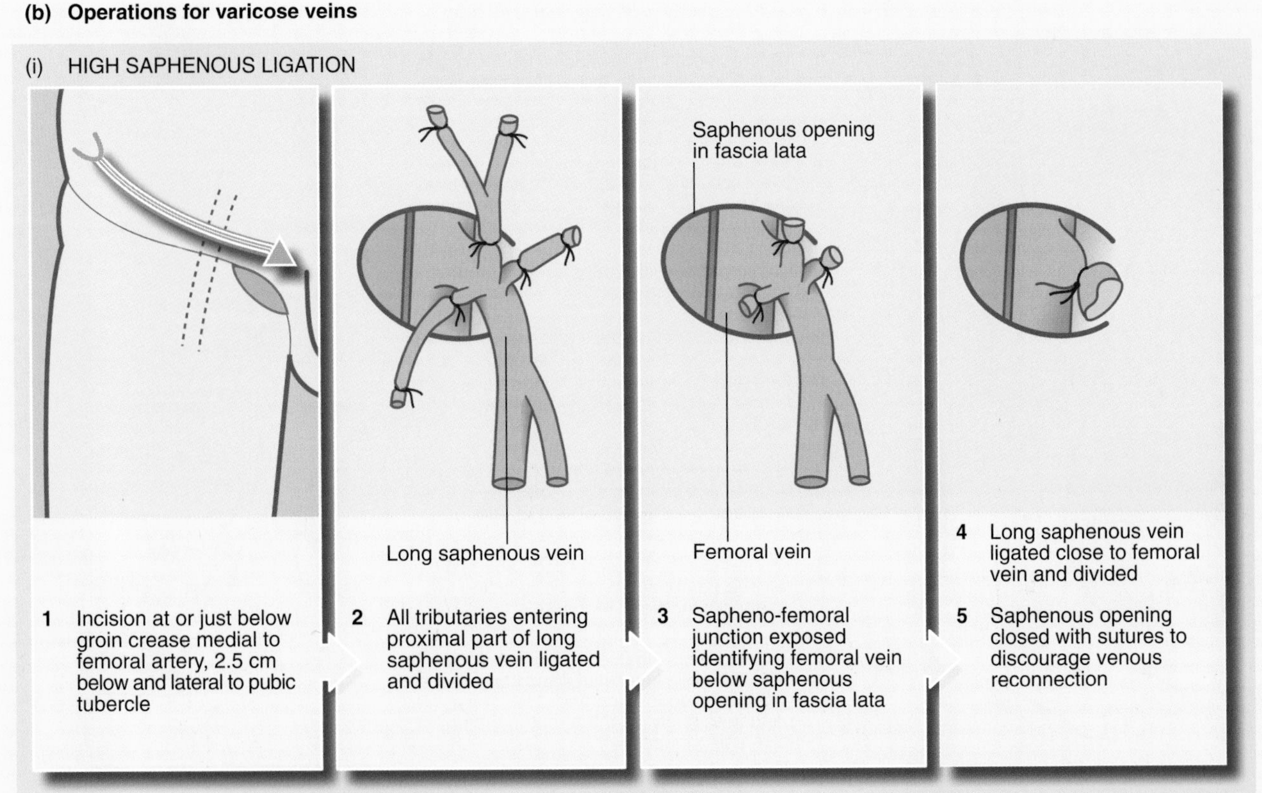

Fig. 43.7 **(a)** Treatment of varicose veins

(b) Operations for varicose veins

(ii) LONG SAPHENOUS STRIP

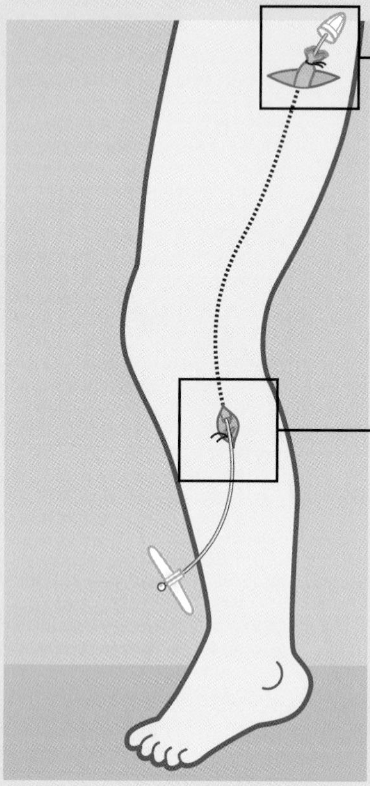

1 The stripper is a long flexible wire with a bullet-shaped knob on the 'business' end. The entry vein (proximal or distal, according to choice) is prepared as shown and the narrow end of the stripper passed down or up the long saphenous vein until it can be brought out to the surface within 15 cm below knee, not to the ankle as was done in the past

2 Stripping is usually downward. The vein is ligated to the wire at the bullet end and the narrow end is pulled smoothly and firmly, tearing off tributaries and any perforators on the way, emerging with the complete vein bunched up on the stripper

3 The wounds are closed and the limb firmly bandaged to minimise subcutaneous bleeding. Patients should be warned to expect postoperative bruising

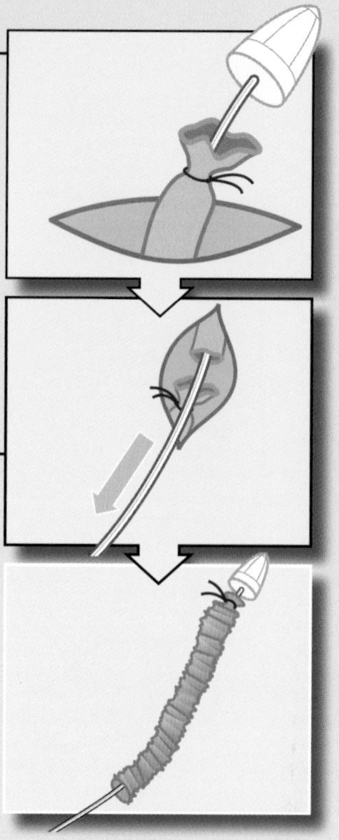

(iii) AVULSION OF VARICOSITIES

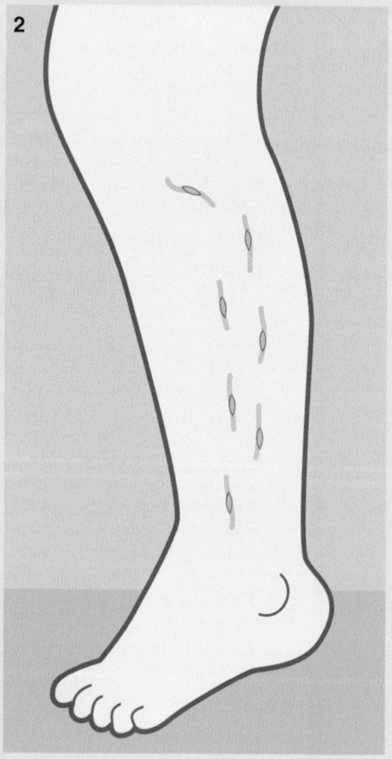

1 Before operation, all varicosities are marked by the surgeon with the patient standing, using an indelible spirit based fibre-tipped pen

2 Very small incisions are made over the marks in a longitudinal direction, or transverse around the knee. As much vein as possible is pulled out ('nick and pick') as follows:

(a) Vein grasped with artery forceps or special vein hook

(b) Second forceps applied and vein divided

(c) One end is drawn out of wound gently and further traction applied by means of another forceps

3 The vein will eventually break and bleeding is controlled by finger pressure. The process is repeated for the other end of vein

4 Forceps can be passed subcutaneously to retrieve nearby varices thus reducing the number of incisions required

5 Each wound is left open or closed neatly with 'steristrips' or a fine suture, and non-adherent gauze applied to each one. The limb is bandaged firmly from the foot to the upper thigh using crepe

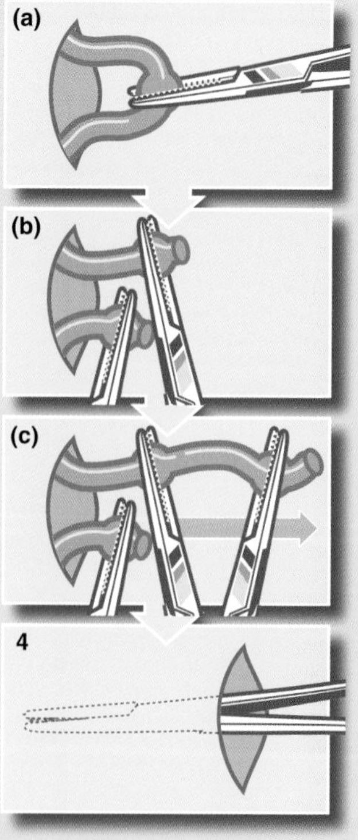

Fig. 43.7, Continued (b) Surgical treatment of varicose veins

all cases where intervention is planned. This gives accurate assessment of superficial and deep systems, determining anatomical areas of reflux and allowing appraisal for endovenous therapy.

MANAGEMENT OF VARICOSE VEINS

Most patients with longstanding varicose veins do not have venous complications. For these, surgical treatment is not usually necessary but advice can be given to elevate the legs when sitting and to wear supporting elastic stockings when standing for long periods.

INDICATIONS FOR SURGICAL TREATMENT OF VARICOSE VEINS

The main indications are **aching legs** after standing, relieved by elevation or when in bed at night (particularly with unilateral ankle oedema), **haemorrhage** from a varicose vein, **superficial thrombophlebitis** and **venous skin changes** due to superficial venous insufficiency. All of these can be treated with support bandages or stockings, but surgery is often preferable and more permanent.

Injection sclerotherapy (e.g. Fegan's technique) is used for treating small cosmetically unattractive varicose veins below the knee but is unsuitable for major varicosities, particularly in the thigh. This type of injection sclerotherapy and surgery for varicose veins is shown in Figure 43.7.

ENDOVENOUS TREATMENT OF VARICOSE VEINS

Newer endovenous treatments of main trunk varicose veins (i.e. LSV and SSV) have been introduced. These aim to ablate the main incompetent superficial vein using **foam sclerotherapy**, or **laser** or **radiofrequency ablation**. All can be performed under local anaesthesia without a groin incision, using ultrasound to give accurate guidance, and give a quicker return to normal activities.

Foam sclerotherapy involves injecting a sclerosant into a vein (e.g. sodium tetradecyl sulfate or polidocanol). It is first mixed with air or a physiological gas such as carbon dioxide in a syringe to create foam. Foaming increases the surface area of the sclerosant and ensures it displaces the blood, allowing it to act directly on the vein wall. For catheter ablation, the distal truncal vein is located by ultrasound and cannulated using a Seldinger technique to place a sheath into the vein. A laser fibre or a radiofrequency catheter is positioned just distal to the sapheno-femoral or sapheno-popliteal junction using ultrasound guidance. Before treatment, a tumescent mixture of local anaesthetic and normal saline is injected around the length of the vein for analgesia and to act as a heat sink. The vein is then heated internally by drawing the laser fibre or the ablation catheter along its length.

Results of all three techniques appear at least comparable with surgery but longer-term evaluation is in progress.

PERIOPERATIVE MANAGEMENT OF THE PATIENT HAVING VARICOSE VEIN SURGERY

Varicose veins must be marked out indelibly on the legs before operation, ideally by the surgeon doing the operation. The patient must stand first, often for some minutes, to allow veins to fill, and marking performed in this position. Most surgeons mark all prominent veins that are visible or palpable. Extra marks are often added for areas needing special surgical attention such as suspected perforating veins. Duplex scanning is often employed to assist marking of perforators or of the **sapheno-popliteal junction**, well known to have a variable anatomy.

Patients with a history of deep or superficial venous thrombosis should be prescribed **low-dose subcutaneous heparin,** as should those with other risk factors for DVT, especially obese patients. The first dose should be given 1–2 hours before operation.

Immediately after operation, the whole leg is bandaged firmly with an elastic bandage. The patient should then be mobilised and encouraged to walk about. All dressings can be removed 24 hours later, and the bandage exchanged for a graduated elastic stocking (class 2) which should stay on for a minimum of 2 weeks. On return home, patients should be encouraged to be active, walking several times a day for at least the first 2 weeks. The legs should be elevated when sitting, and the patient should get up and walk around about every half-hour. All these measures are designed to discourage venous stagnation and venous thrombosis. Most patients can drive a car 24 hours after operation and return to work after a week. The patient should be warned that the legs will be bruised when bandages are removed.

44 Cardiac surgery

INTRODUCTION AND CARDIOPULMONARY BYPASS

Surgery of the heart has long fascinated surgeons but only a very limited range of cardiac procedures was possible until cardiopulmonary bypass was successfully employed in 1953. For the first time, the systemic circulation could be sustained artificially, with the heart and lungs bypassed. The heart could be manipulated and lung ventilation discontinued, giving optimal conditions for operating on the heart. Since then, cardiac surgery has developed and expanded swiftly.

In keeping with the move towards minimal access in other areas, coronary artery bypass grafting and various valvular procedures can now be performed 'off-pump' via small incisions on the beating heart without bypass. However, most cardiac surgery is still carried out on bypass, with a bloodless field created by clamping the ascending aorta just proximal to where the aortic cannula returns arterial blood from the bypass machine (see Fig. 44.1). Without coronary artery blood flow, myocardial ischaemic damage has to be mitigated by reducing metabolic demands by inducing diastolic **arrest** with a high-potassium cardioplegic solution (16 mmol/L KCl) (Table 44.1) and **cooling** (to between 4 and 12°C).

Several problems may arise when blood is exposed to artificial surfaces in a cardiopulmonary bypass machine:

- Activation of the clotting cascade could occur, causing **intravascular coagulation**. This is prevented by anticoagulating with high-dose heparin (300 IU/kg) which is later reversed with **protamine sulphate** on coming off bypass
- Clotting factors and platelets are consumed in the extracorporeal circuit (mainly within the oxygenator) leading to a bleeding diathesis. Blood products may be needed to reverse this
- Activation of the complement cascade and other inflammatory mediators may result in systemic inflammatory response syndrome (SIRS) after bypass

ASSESSING RISK IN CARDIAC SURGERY

The complexity of cardiac surgery makes it potentially risky. In the UK, all cardiac surgical units have to undertake prospective audit including risk assessment and submit data to a national registry. Results of all units are published online, allowing suitable standards to be developed and maintained. This process will shortly be introduced in general surgery in the UK.

Several scoring systems have been devised to take patient factors into account in order to predict the risk of morbidity and mortality for an individual undergoing a particular operation, a process called **risk stratification**. Systems generally take account of the surgical procedure, its urgency and pre-existing co-morbidities. Online calculators for STS score and for EuroSCORE II are the latest tools and are based on actual outcomes in large numbers of the patients recently operated upon.

CONGENITAL CARDIAC DISEASE

TYPES OF CONGENITAL HEART DISEASE

Congenital heart disease occurs in about 2 per 1000 live births and falls into two main groups: those with and those without cyanosis.

CYANOTIC HEART DISEASE

Cyanotic heart disease exists when there is mixing of systemic arterial and venous blood through a predominantly **right-to-left cardiac shunt**. The most common examples are:

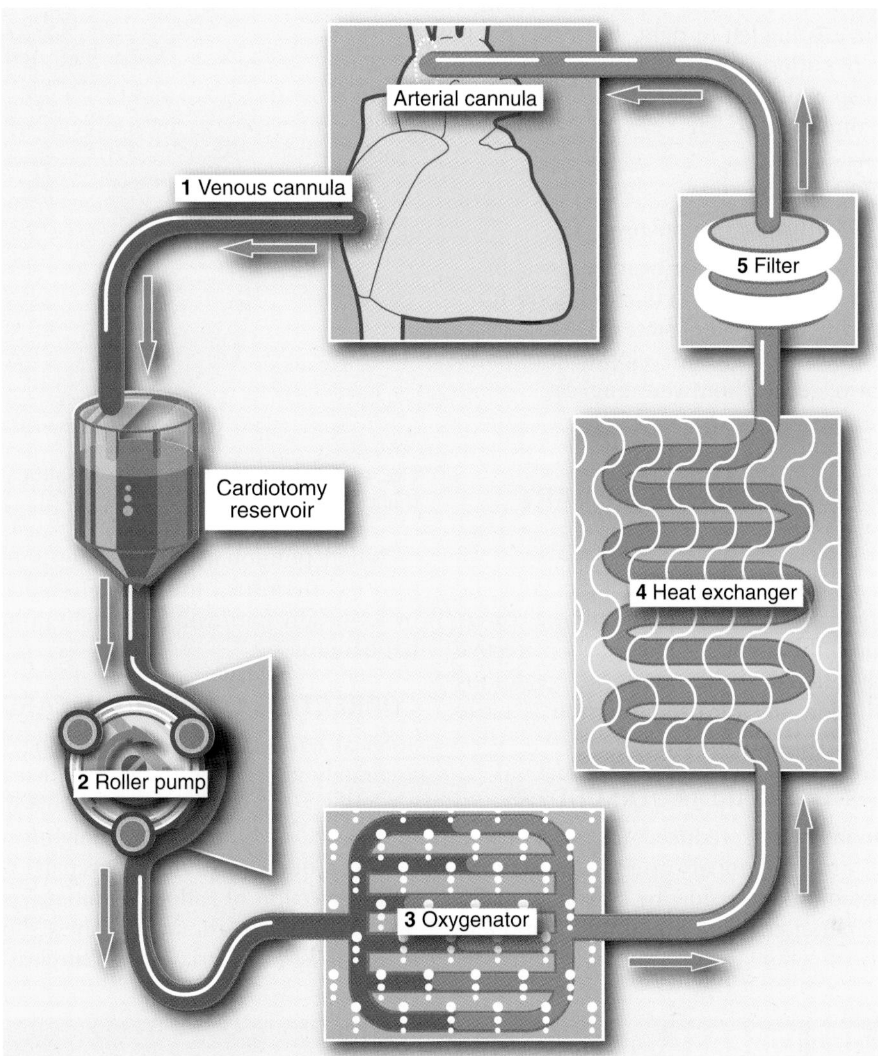

Fig. 44.1 The standard circuit for cardiopulmonary bypass

1. Systemic venous blood is siphoned into a reservoir by gravity from the right atrium (or from the superior and inferior vena cavae) via a venous cannula
2. Venous blood from the reservoir enters a roller pump
3. Blood is pumped under pressure through a membrane oxygenator
4. Oxygenated blood then passes through a heat exchanger to cool or rewarm the blood as necessary
5. The oxygenated and temperature-controlled blood finally passes through a filter and is returned to the systemic arterial circulation, usually via the ascending aorta by a roller pump

Note: If the right sides heart chambers need to be opened for surgical access (e.g. for atrial septal defect repair), the superior and inferior vena cavae are individually cannulated and snared to prevent air from entering the venous circuit and locking the gravity siphon

Table 44.1 Constituents of a typical infusate for cold cardioplegia (St Thomas's solution)

Constituent	Quantity
Sodium chloride	110.0 mmol/L
Potassium chloride	16.0 mmol/L
Magnesium chloride	16.0 mmol/L
Calcium chloride	1.2 mmol/L
Sodium bicarbonate	10.0 mmol/L
Procaine	16.0 mmol/L

- **Tetralogy of Fallot**—the four features are ventricular septal defect (VSD), pulmonary stenosis, right ventricular hypertrophy and an aorta which overrides the ventricular septum, receiving blood from both ventricles
- **Transposition of the great arteries**—the pulmonary artery arises from the left ventricle and the aorta from the right ventricle
- **Tricuspid atresia**—absence of a functional tricuspid valve
- **Truncus arteriosus**—the pulmonary artery and aorta fail to develop separately
- **Total anomalous pulmonary venous drainage**—pulmonary venous blood drains into the right side of the heart

- **Eisenmenger's syndrome**—increased pulmonary blood flow caused by a pre-existing left-to-right shunt (see next section) causes severe pulmonary hypertension later in life, which result in spontaneous reversal of the shunt so flow reverses to become right-to-left

ACYANOTIC HEART DISEASE

Acyanotic congenital heart disease may involve:

- A shunt from left to right sides of the heart (e.g. via an atrial or ventricular septal defect) or a ductus arteriosus which persists in its antenatal patent state (PDA)
- Failed or incomplete embryological development of parts of the heart or great vessels without shunting, e.g. coarctation of the aorta

MANAGEMENT OF CONGENITAL HEART DISEASE

In early cardiac surgery, palliation was often all that could be offered. Later, palliation was sometimes followed by a corrective operation when the child was larger. Nowadays, corrective procedures are usually offered at the outset, as operations have become more routine, myocardial protection is more predictable and operative risks are lower.

PALLIATING CONGENITAL CARDIAC DISORDERS

When pulmonary blood flow is **reduced** (as in tricuspid atresia, tetralogy of Fallot or pulmonary artery stenosis), palliation aims to increase pulmonary flow by creating a shunt between the systemic arterial circulation and the pulmonary artery (see Fig. 44.2).

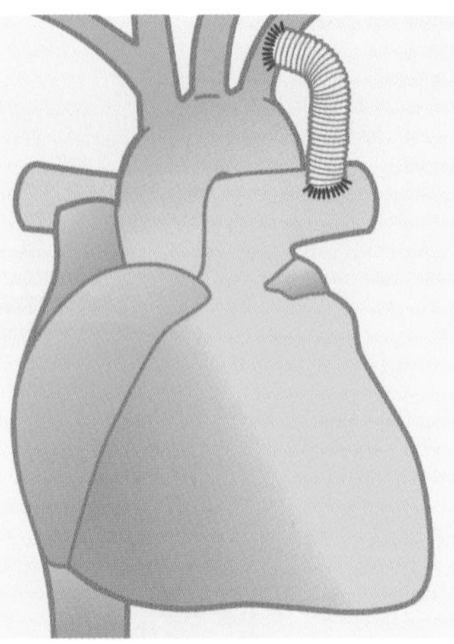

Fig. 44.2 Palliation of tetralogy of Fallot Modified Blalock–Taussig shunt

When pulmonary blood flow is **too great** (e.g. VSD or truncus arteriosus), the aim is to reduce the pulmonary flow by artificially narrowing the main pulmonary artery by external banding.

CORRECTING CONGENITAL CARDIAC DISORDERS

Surgical correction of congenital heart disease is based on accurately identifying the lesion or lesions, then performing procedures which restore the normal flow and functioning of the heart. Correction may be straightforward (e.g. PDA closure; resection of coarctation: VSD repair) or highly complex (e.g. total correction of Fallot's tetralogy; correction of anomalous pulmonary venous drainage). These should only be performed in specialist paediatric cardiac surgical units.

ACQUIRED HEART DISEASE

The types of acquired heart disease are listed in Table 44.2.

CORONARY HEART DISEASE

(see Table 44.3 for clinical presentations)

PATHOPHYSIOLOGY

Coronary heart disease (ischaemic heart disease) is nearly always atherosclerotic, with subintimal thickening caused by deposition of cholesterol-containing lipids, plus hyperplasia of media smooth muscle cells which migrate into the subintimal area. Together, these changes reduce the luminal diameter. Since resistance to flow is proportional to the fourth power of the radius (Poiseuille's Law), a small change in cross-sectional area causes a dramatic reduction in coronary blood flow. When assessed on angiography, a 50% reduction in coronary artery diameter shown in two planes is regarded as significant.

Acute coronary ischaemia is usually brought on by thrombosis of already narrowed coronary arteries, in some cases precipitated by haemorrhage into atherosclerotic plaques.

The worldwide distribution of coronary atherosclerosis is patchy. It is predominantly a disease of developed countries. Men are at greater risk than women, with 45% of men over 65 having some manifestation of it. Areas of historically high incidence include Scotland and Finland. The rates in some countries, notably the USA and much of Europe, have been falling in recent years, largely as a result of reduced cigarette smoking, control of hypertension and perhaps changes in diet and exercise.

Risk factors for coronary atheroma (and atherosclerosis elsewhere) include unfavourable cholesterol and lipid profiles (often hereditary), cigarette smoking, diabetes, hypertension, obesity and a sedentary lifestyle (and perhaps a life of severe unrelieved stress). The presentations of coronary heart disease are outlined in Table 44.3.

CONTROL OF PREDISPOSING FACTORS

The first step in treatment is usually to try to persuade the patient to modify risk factors known to contribute to disease progression. There are two purposes: if progression can be arrested, physiological development of collateral blood supply can proceed, which may make intervention unnecessary. Secondly, occlusion of any form of revascularisation is more likely if risk factors, particularly cigarette smoking, continue. On average, patients who continue to smoke gain no benefit from coronary artery bypass grafting (CABG). Smokers who

Table 44.2 Types of acquired heart disease

Type	Pathophysiology	Clinical presentation
Ischaemic heart disease	Usually caused by coronary atherosclerosis and rarely by spasm, embolism or trauma	1. Reversible ischaemia presenting as angina 2. Painless or silent ischaemia discovered incidentally 3. Myocardial infarction
Valvular heart disease, affecting aortic, mitral, tricuspid or pulmonary valves	1. Congenital valve disorders (e.g. bicuspid aortic valve) predisposing the valve to later malfunction, degeneration or disease 2. Rheumatic valvular heart disease—mitral valve most common; also affects aortic valve (occasionally follows rheumatic fever, causing thickening and tethering of leaflets, shortening of mitral valve chordae and valve calcification) 3. Secondary involvement of valves caused by disruption of nearby structures: —aortic dissection involving the aortic valve —myocardial infarction involving the papillary muscles —myocardial ischaemia leading to scarring and contraction of the papillary muscles —autoimmune disorders, e.g. Libman–Sacks endocarditis —'metabolic' defects, e.g. Marfan's syndrome 4. Infective endocarditis, usually on diseased valves	a. Disordered valve function —valve stenosis restricts blood flow —valvular incompetence causes reflux of blood b. Accumulation of 'vegetations' or thrombus which may embolise into the peripheral arterial tree c. Infection of vegetations or thrombus (bacterial endocarditis) —systemic symptoms (fever, anorexia, weight loss) —deteriorating valve function —infected systemic embolism to brain, kidneys, etc.
Disease affecting the great arteries		
Aorta	1. Aortic dissection within the media resulting from atherosclerosis or cystic medial necrosis 2. Aneurysm (connective tissue degeneration, syphilis, trauma, infection) 3. Traumatic transsection	a. Acute severe chest pain b. Acute severe hypovolaemic shock with collapse or sudden death
Pulmonary artery	Peripheral deep venous thrombosis detaches and passes through the heart to impact in the pulmonary arteries	a. Acute occlusion by pulmonary embolism—may be silent, symptomatic or 'massive' and fatal b. Recurrent embolism may cause pulmonary hypertension
Pericardial disease	1. Pericardial constriction (scarring or tumour)	Signs of constrictive pericarditis: systemic venous congestion with hepatomegaly and ascites; often atrial fibrillation
	2. Pericardial effusion	Retrosternal pressure; muffled heart sounds; cardiac tamponade if acute and severe

fail to improve thus suffer the risk and discomfort of surgery having squandered limited hospital resources. Nothing can yet be done about hereditary factors, but smoking, obesity and inactivity can be tackled. The benefits of lowering blood lipid levels are well established. Statins are widely used for this but have other beneficial effects including reducing arterial wall inflammation.

MANAGEMENT OF CORONARY ARTERY DISEASE

Coronary artery disease can be managed conservatively ('medical management') or by interventions employing percutaneous techniques or surgical bypass grafting. The anatomy of the coronary arteries is shown in Figure 44.3.

Percutaneous angioplasty techniques

Percutaneous techniques to dilate stenoses or recanalise occluded coronary arteries have progressed since the early 1980s; these are usually performed by cardiologists. The mainstay of treatment is **percutaneous transluminal coronary (balloon) angioplasty (PTCA)** and insertion of intra-coronary artery **stents**. Stents are expensive, particularly drug-eluting stents (e.g. sirolimus or paclitaxel coated stents) aimed at minimising in-stent restenosis. Indications for the various stents still need to be clearly defined by randomised trials.

When performed expertly, these techniques cause little disruption to the patient's life and recovery is rapid. However, set against this, there remains a definite early failure rate and a substantial medium-term restenosis rate (30% for bare-metal stents and about 10–15% for drug-eluting stents at 6 months). In addition, the patient has to be prepared to undergo an emergency operation if things should go wrong at angioplasty. With improving medium-term results, the main indication for PTCA is for first-time intervention for relieving symptomatic single or double coronary artery stenoses.

Coronary artery bypass grafting (CABG)

Coronary artery bypass grafting is usually indicated in two categories of patient:

Table 44.3 Presentation of coronary artery disease

Presentation	Secondary effects	Clinical effects
Ischaemic damage discovered incidentally in an asymptomatic patient	Potential risk of further MIs; developing complications of ischaemic heart disease; increased risk when performing an unrelated operation	Found incidentally, e.g. on ECG
A past history of myocardial infarction (MI)	Risk of further MIs; complications of ischaemic heart disease (IHD); risk during unrelated operation	History of typical pain (but note that 25% of MIs are painless)
Angina pectoris	Mortality/morbidity risks of unrelated operations increased	Typical pain brought on by exercise, anxiety or excitement
Complications of myocardial infarction	1. Rupture of part of the heart	Rupture of external wall of left ventricle Septal rupture causing a ventricular septal defect Papillary muscle rupture causing mitral or tricuspid regurgitation
	2. Fibrosis or scarring following myocardial infarction	Generalised fibrosis may cause cardiac failure through loss of contractile myocardium Localised fibrosis of an infarcted ventricular wall may cause a **ventricular aneurysm** Discrete fibrosis near a valve may cause tethering of a mitral leaflet resulting in mitral regurgitation Mural scars may disrupt the conducting system causing ventricular arrhythmias
	3. Mural thrombus may accumulate on a subendocardial infarct as an early response to injury	Thrombus may detach and cause systemic arterial embolism, e.g. to brain, lower limb or superior mesenteric artery; usually an early complication of myocardial infarction (1–6 weeks)

1. Those with symptomatic angina not relieved by medical therapy or who are intolerant of it. This is by far the largest group. Most are operated upon electively, but those with crescendo angina may need urgent or emergency surgery
2. Patients in categories believed to have a better prognosis after surgery than with medical therapy

Studies in the USA and Europe suggest improved survival after surgery is likely in patients with the following morphological characteristics:

- Stenosis of the left main stem coronary artery (before it bifurcates into anterior descending and circumflex arteries)
- Triple-vessel disease (i.e. disease of the right coronary, the left anterior descending and the circumflex arterial systems) plus impaired left ventricular contractility
- Two-vessel disease which includes a proximal stenosis in the left anterior descending coronary artery

The results of CABG are encouraging, with 85–90% relieved of angina without need for medication. A further 5% are substantially improved but require anti-anginal drug therapy.

Surgical technique (Fig. 44.4)

The aim of CABG is to bypass occlusive disease and provide a new source of inflow for patent distal coronary arteries. Occlusive disease is usually in the proximal third of the epicardial coronary arteries. This fortunate morphology enables the distal end of bypass grafts to be anastomosed to patent recipient arteries beyond the main disease. Saphenous vein bypass grafts are employed as conduits from the ascending aorta or else a nearby left internal mammary artery is mobilised and anastomosed to the distal coronary artery.

Prosthetic materials give poor results for CABG and are rarely used. Early conduits were exclusively reversed autologous long (great) saphenous vein. However, long-term patency is poor, with 50–70% occluding within 10 years of surgery. Long-term patency is better when the left internal mammary artery is grafted onto the left anterior descending coronary artery (see Fig. 44.4). This graft seems to be resistant to occlusion (90% patency at 10 years) and is the current choice for this site. Other arteries used for CABG including radial, right gastro-epiploic and inferior epigastric. A combination of left internal mammary grafting to left anterior descending artery and saphenous vein grafts to the other vessels remains the current surgical favourite.

In elective patients, the overall mortality risk of CABG surgery is close to 1%; in addition there is a 2% chance of stroke (especially with a previous history of stroke). Mortality rates for CABG are higher in patients with heart failure and those requiring emergency operations. The risk also rises with age.

To minimise the potentially damaging effects of cardiopulmonary bypass noted earlier, and also the cognitive deficit that probably follows all such operations, there is a vogue for revascularising without bypass. Operating conditions are more demanding which may adversely affect the accuracy of

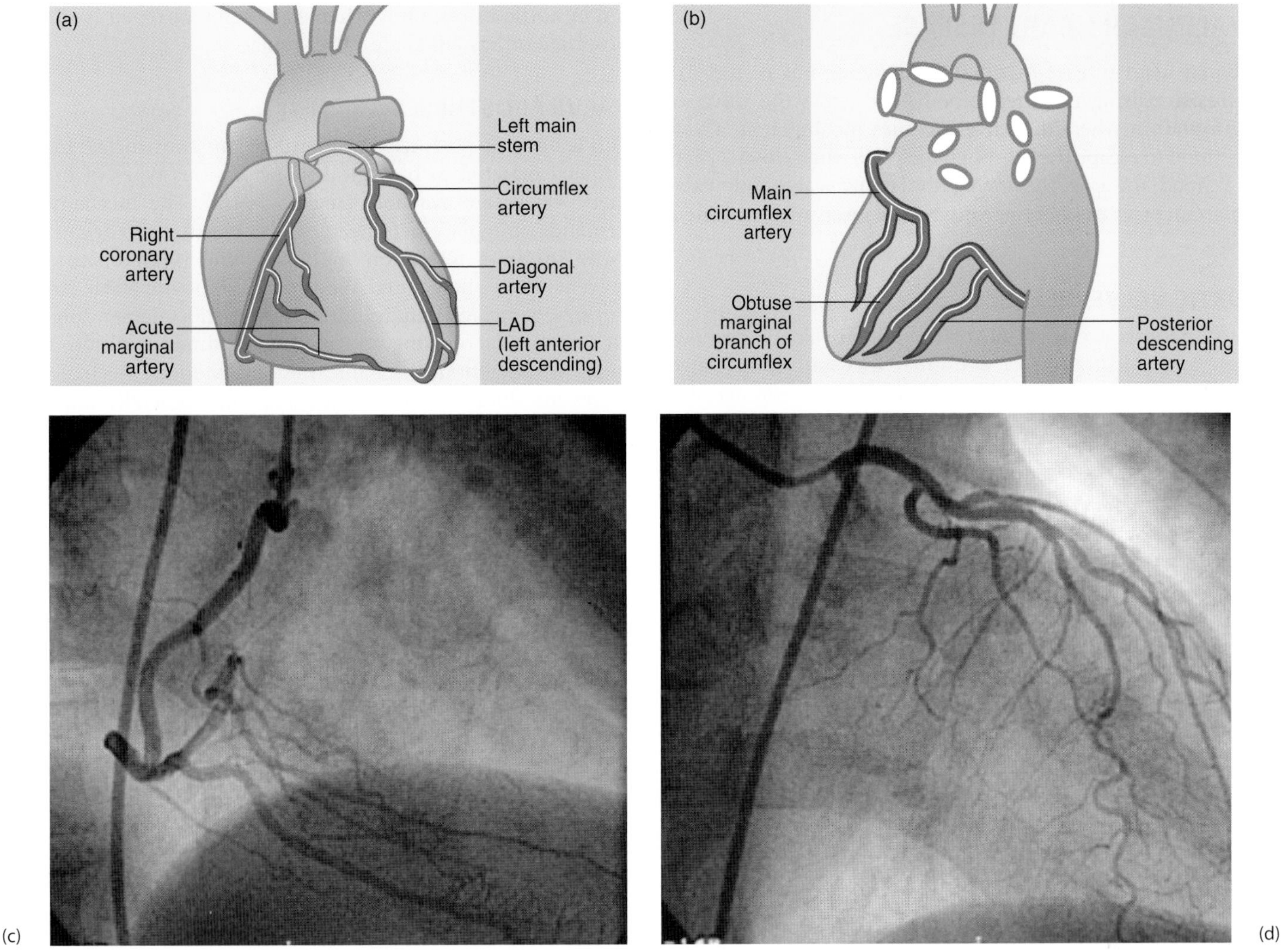

(a)
Left main stem
Circumflex artery
Right coronary artery
Diagonal artery
Acute marginal artery
LAD (left anterior descending)

(b)
Main circumflex artery
Obtuse marginal branch of circumflex
Posterior descending artery

(c)

(d)

Fig. 44.3 Anatomy of the coronary arteries (a) Anterior view of coronary arteries. **(b)** Posterior view of coronary arteries. **(c–d)** Selective coronary angiography (AP views as in **(a)**): **(c)** normal right coronary artery; **(d)** normal left coronary artery

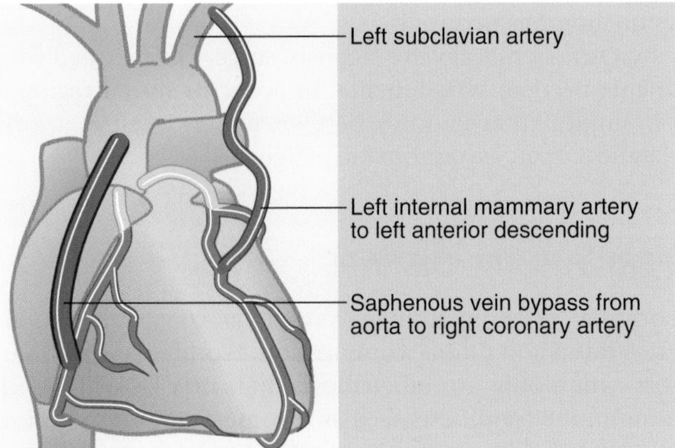

Fig. 44.4 Methods of coronary artery bypass grafting Note that an explanted autogenous radial artery may be used as a bypass graft instead of saphenous vein

anastomoses and increase the occlusion rate. So far, randomised studies comparing CABG on pump and off pump have failed to demonstrate significant benefit for off pump procedures.

Other types of surgery for ischaemic heart disease

Other forms of surgery in addition to CABG may be required for complications of myocardial infarction. These carry a higher risk than isolated CABG surgery and include:

- Excision of a left ventricular aneurysm—mortality about 5%
- Replacement or repair of a mitral valve leaking as a result of ischaemia—mortality 5–8%
- Surgical identification and ablation of a ventricular arrhythmic focus—mortality 10–15%
- Emergency repair of a post-myocardial infarction ventricular septal rupture—mortality 20–40%
- Post-CABG heart failure necessitating ventricular support (intra-aortic balloon pump) or cardiac transplantation—mortality about 15% at 1 year

VALVULAR HEART DISEASE

Valvular heart disease manifests with symptoms or signs of **stenosis**, causing restricted blood flow across the valve, or **regurgitation** where the valve becomes incompetent, allowing blood to escape back through the valve when closed. There is a trend towards conserving the native valve, but valve replacement is the alternative where conservative treatment fails.

AORTIC VALVE DISEASE

Aortic stenosis is caused most commonly by senile degeneration and calcification of a normal tricuspid aortic valve, affecting 2–4% of patients in their 6th to 8th decades. Bicuspid aortic valves are the most common valvular anomaly, affecting 1–2% of the general population, and may degenerate in the 4th to 5th decade of life. Aortic valve regurgitation may result from aortic leaflet abnormality (e.g. leaflet prolapse or perforation) and/or abnormal dilatation of the aortic valve annulus, a condition called **annulo-aortic ectasia**.

Severely stenotic aortic valves are usually treated by resection and replacement with a prosthetic valve. Some regurgitant valves are repaired but long-term durability is uncertain. A recent treatment for patients with aortic valve stenosis unfit for valve replacement (AVR) is a catheter technique via the left ventricular apex or femoral artery. It involves balloon dilatation of the stenotic valve and insertion of a stent-mounted prosthetic valve into the space. This transcatheter aortic valve insertion (TAVI) technique is less invasive than surgical AVR and is gaining acceptance across the Western world.

MITRAL VALVE DISEASE

Mitral stenosis following rheumatic fever can be successfully treated by **valvotomy** (separation of fused valve leaflets), if performed before calcification makes the leaflets immobile. In the early days of cardiac surgery, Cutler and Levine (1925) introduced semi-closed, blind mitral valvotomy, with mechanical dilatation of the valve via the left auricular appendage. With the heart beating, the auricle was opened, a finger or mechanical device inserted and the valve rapidly dilated. Symptomatic relief was usually reasonable, but the valvotomy was often incomplete, short-lived or caused splits in the leaflets rather than between them. Later, direct **open valvotomy** under cardiopulmonary bypass became popular. More precise and long-lasting results could be achieved by this method. More recently, there has been a return to closed valvotomy, with percutaneous trans-septal balloon dilatation of the stenosed valve.

In regurgitant valvular disease, surgical valve repair is possible in most patients but has been most successful for myxomatous or degenerate regurgitation. This conservative technique has a lower perioperative risk than valve replacement and better preserves left ventricular function. Thus, the overall functional result may be better than valve replacement. Repair techniques may also be employed for diseased tricuspid or aortic valves. Only where valvotomy or repair is inappropriate or has failed are valves replaced.

VALVE PROSTHESES (Fig. 44.5)

The leaflets of prosthetic heart valves are constructed from artificial material or biological tissue. Various types of prosthetic valves are available (see Fig. 44.5). The mechanical demands on replacement heart valves are extreme. They must cause minimal restriction to blood flow when open, yet prevent reflux when closed; they must be biocompatible, non-thrombogenic, resistant to infection and, most demanding of all, capable of opening and closing 70 times a minute for many years without mechanical failure. Modern mechanical valves are durable but thrombogenic and generally require lifelong anticoagulation. Anticoagulation carries its own risk with a mortality of about 2% over 5 years. Even with effective anticoagulation, there is still a small risk of arterial embolism.

Replacement tissue valves may be **homografts** (human) or **xenografts** (animal origin). Xenografts are most commonly made from bovine pericardium or porcine heart valves. In general, tissue valves are less thrombogenic (anticoagulation not necessary) but less durable through degeneration as time goes by. However, in patients over 60 years given an aortic bioprosthesis, 90% or more are free from structural valve degeneration at 10 years. Homograft (human) valves may be more resistant to degeneration and are preferred for young patients.

Infection of valve prostheses is devastating but fortunately rare. The risk is least for homograft valves. Prosthetic valve endocarditis carries a very high mortality and needs protracted antibiotic treatment, often requiring explantation (removal) of the infected prosthesis.

INDICATIONS FOR VALVE SURGERY

Valvular heart surgery is most successful when carried out at the right time, namely when risks of surgery are least and potential benefits greatest and before irreversible ventricular dysfunction has occurred.

In aortic or mitral valve stenosis, surgery is indicated when patients become symptomatic. In aortic or mitral regurgitation, surgical intervention is best when there is left ventricular dilatation in an asymptomatic patient.

PERICARDIAL DISEASE

Pericardial inflammation may result in constriction of the pericardium and cardiac compression. Worldwide, this occurs most commonly in tuberculosis but may also occur in autoimmune conditions such as rheumatoid arthritis, following pericardial trauma or mediastinal radiotherapy. Pericardial constriction impairs filling of the cardiac chambers causing equalisation of diastolic pressures in all four chambers of the heart. Clinical signs are those of pulmonary and systemic venous congestion together with a low cardiac output. Surgical treatment involves excision of the entire pericardium.

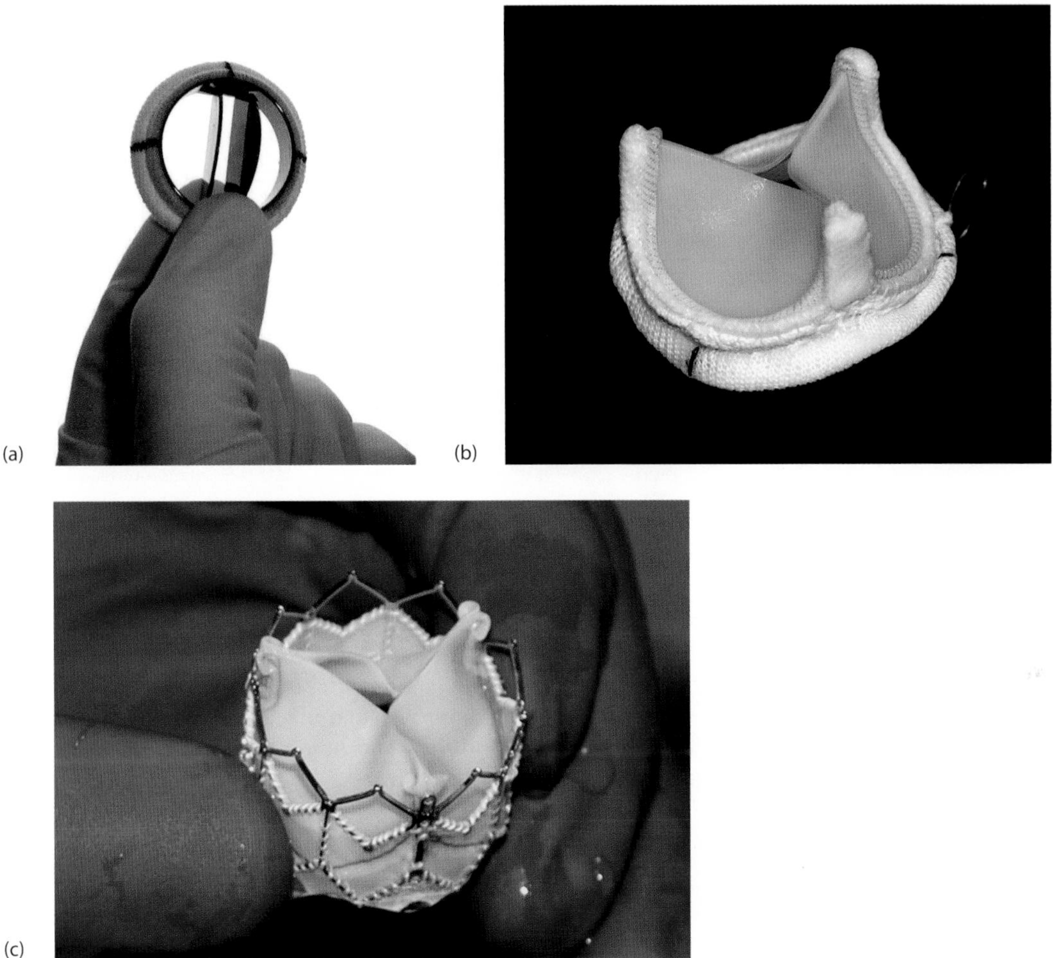

Fig. 44.5 **Prosthetic valves** Three commonly used prosthetic heart valve are shown here. **(a)** A St. Jude bi-leaflet mechanical valve—used in 90% of patients requiring a mechanical prosthesis. Lifelong anticoagulation is mandatory for all patients receiving mechanical valve prosthesis. **(b)** An Edwards Magna Ease bovine pericardial stent mounted bioprosthesis. **(c)** An Edwards SAPIEN transcatheter bioprosthetic valve.

DISEASE OF THE THORACIC AORTA

AORTIC DISSECTION

In aortic dissection, a breach in the luminal surface allows blood to leak out and split the media then flow along a false lumen for variable distances proximally and/or distally. The dissection flap may occlude any aortic branch and disrupt the aortic valve. The likely aetiology is degeneration of elastin and collagen in the media. Dissection occurs most often in the ascending aorta (65%), but also in the aortic arch (10%), or the descending thoracic aorta just distal to the ligamentum arteriosum (20%).

Dissection is classified according to the part affected; the most widely used method is the **Stanford system**. Type A indicates that only the ascending aorta is involved while type B is when any other part of the thoracic aorta is affected. An alternative classification method is that of DeBakey (see Fig. 44.6).

Without surgery, Stanford type A dissection carries an 80% mortality in the first month; with surgical management this falls to less than 20%. The operation involves resecting the ascending aorta and replacing it with a synthetic vascular graft. If the dissection reaches the aortic valve, it is likely to be disrupted causing acute severe regurgitation and perhaps occluding the coronary artery origins. In these cases, the valve will need resuspending or replacing.

Uncomplicated type B dissections have a 20% mortality at 30 days, and the outcome is similar whether surgically or medically managed. Medical management is by control of hypertension. Surgery is required in type B dissections complicated by aortic rupture, occlusion of vital branches, progressive dissection or, later, by aneurysm formation. Note that abdominal aortic aneurysms occur years later in about 50% after thoracic dissection.

THORACIC ANEURYSMS

Aneurysmal dilatation of the thoracic aorta may occur in the ascending part (Fig. 44.7), the arch or the descending part. There is a risk of rupture similar to abdominal aortic aneurysms and surgical intervention is usually recommended when the aneurysm reaches 6 cm diameter. Replacing the descending aorta, particularly when there is

Stanford type A (aortic valve may be involved)

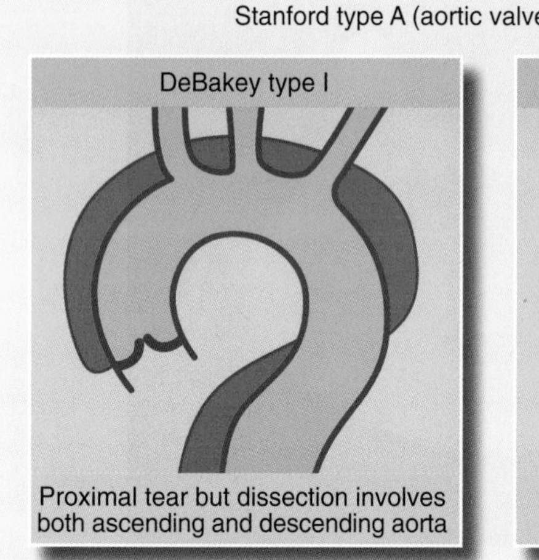

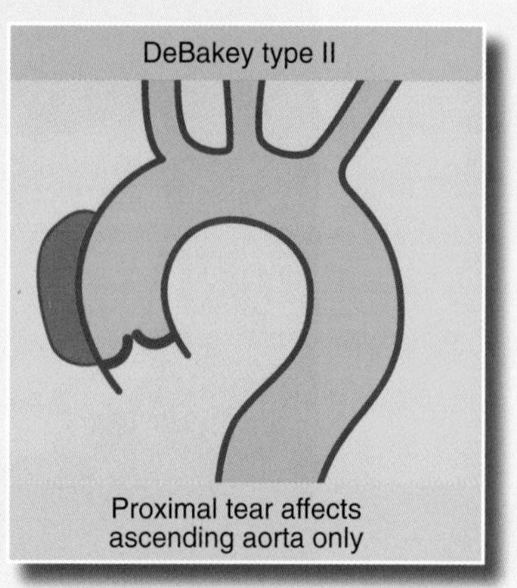

Stanford type B

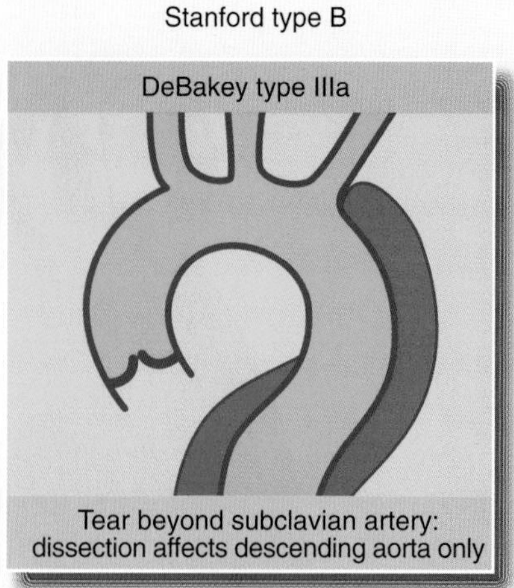

Fig. 44.6 Thoracic aortic dissection

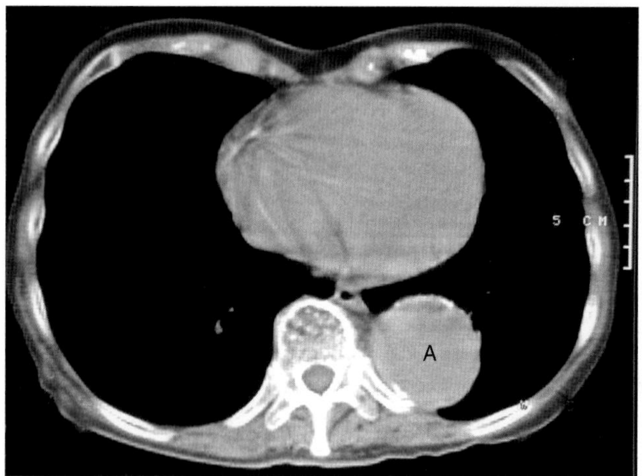

Fig. 44.7 Thoracic aortic aneurysm CT scan of chest showing a 5 cm aneurysm of the descending thoracic aorta **A**

thoraco-abdominal disease, threatens the main blood supply of the spinal cord (the artery of Adamkiewicz at about T10) so that paraplegia complicates 10–30% of these operations. There is a growing trend towards endoluminal stent-grafting for appropriate thoracic aneurysms with the promise of lower morbidity and mortality.

TRAUMA TO THE THORACIC AORTA

This may result from blunt or sharp injury. Blunt trauma is usually associated with severe deceleration as occurs in head-on impact in road traffic collisions. The common injury is a partial or complete transsection of the aorta at the junction between the arch and the descending aorta close to the ligamentum arteriosum. Complete transsection with free rupture is rapidly fatal; partial transsection with an intact adventitia and a contained haematoma is liable to rupture at any time and must be diagnosed to enable early emergency treatment. There is a trend towards treating these with intraluminal stent grafts via the femoral artery. Late aneurysm formation may also occur in those patients who survive an untreated occult aortic transsection.

PULMONARY EMBOLISM

Emergency surgical removal of a massive pulmonary embolism has become increasingly rare with the introduction of effective thrombolytic agents. Nowadays, there are few indications for emergency pulmonary embolectomy. These usually relate to situations where thrombolytic therapy might carry unacceptable risks, e.g. after recent surgery or during pregnancy. The operation is carried out under cardiopulmonary bypass.

In some patients with recurrent pulmonary embolism, the pulmonary vasculature becomes progressively obliterated causing **chronic thromboembolic pulmonary hypertension**. Life expectancy is substantially shortened when the mean pulmonary artery pressure exceeds 30 mmHg. This condition was previously treated by heart and lung transplantation but pulmonary endarterectomy is now being offered with superior immediate and medium term outcome.

Disorders of the breast

45

INTRODUCTION TO BREAST DISEASE

Virtually every woman with a breast lump, breast pain or discharge from the nipple fears she has cancer. The anxiety results from the unknown course of the disease, the threat of mutilation and the fear of dying. This has often prevented women from seeking medical advice, but publicity about self-examination and screening (see Ch. 6) and the potential benefits of early treatment has encouraged earlier presentation.

Anxiety may be heightened by friends' or relatives' experiences of breast cancer or a recent 'celebrity diagnosis'; for this reason, reassuring the 'worried well' is important. The effects of breast surgery on attractiveness and femininity must be considered; breast care nurses can provide psychological support throughout investigation and treatment.

Rates of referral to breast clinics have increased, reflecting easier access, widespread breast screening and public awareness of breast cancer. Despite the fears of those referred, in the UK less than 15% prove to have cancer. The rest include benign breast conditions and others within the normal range of anatomy and physiology (see Box 45.1).

ANATOMY OF THE FEMALE BREAST

The breast consists of 15–20 lobes containing lobules linked by ductules that combine to form ducts. The glandular tissue is supported by fibrous tissue connected by Astley Cooper's ligaments and lies over pectoralis major and minor. It is supplied by branches of the axillary and internal mammary arteries. Lymph drains primarily to the axillary nodes.

SYMPTOMS AND SIGNS OF BREAST DISEASE

Patients may present with symptoms or signs (see Fig. 45.1). Two-thirds complain of a discrete lump or lumpiness.

SPECIAL POINTS IN HISTORY TAKING

A detailed history can provide important clues to the pathology of a breast problem. Age alters the probability of different breast disorders (see Fig. 45.2); in particular, the risk of malignancy rises with age. The **duration of symptoms** should be established at the outset; cancers are usually slow-growing, whilst cysts can appear rapidly, sometimes almost overnight. Benign conditions such as fibroadenosis and fibroadenoma may present with lumps that **fluctuate with the menstrual cycle** or have decreased in size since first noticed. They are also more likely to be **painful and tender** than a malignant lesion.

A **previous history** of breast conditions, particularly malignancy, cysts or fibrocystic change, can be an indicator of the nature of a current breast problem. The greatest single risk factor for breast cancer is a previous history of the condition, however long ago (1% risk per year) (see Box 45.2). There is some evidence that patients with recurrent benign breast disorders are more liable to cancer.

Trauma from seatbelt injuries is common and patients should be asked whether bruising of the breast was followed by the appearance of a lump.

Drug history, particularly of the oral contraceptive pill (OCP) or hormone replacement therapy (HRT), should be recorded, including the duration and how recently the drug has been used. These drugs modulate the hormonal environment of breast tissue and tend to increase the risk of breast cancer. Other hormone-related risk factors for cancer include late age at first full-term pregnancy, lower parity (number of pregnancies) and early age of menarche and late age of menopause. Enquiry should be made about a **family history** of breast or ovarian cancer, including number of first- and

SYMPTOM OR SIGN	CLINICAL SIGNIFICANCE
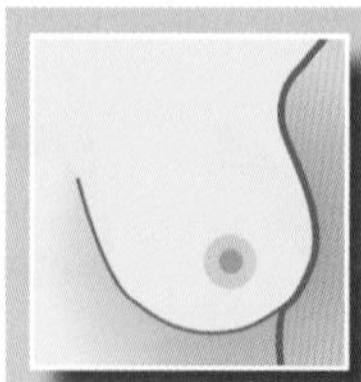 **1. Pain**	
Varying with menstrual cycle	Suggests a physiological cause such as premenstrual syndrome or fibroadenosis. Both are responsive to treatment
Independent of menstrual cycle **Refer non-urgently if pain not responding to treatment**	Not diagnostic but may occur in carcinoma, fibroadenosis or infection
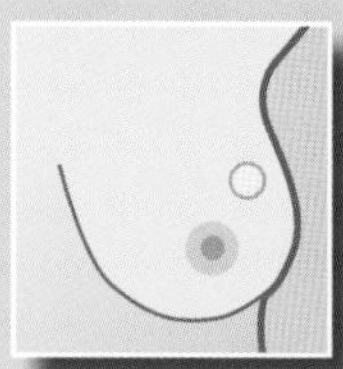 **2. Lump in the breast**	
Hard lump **Refer urgently**	A discrete mobile lump with a smooth surface is most likely to be a fibroadenoma or a fibroadenotic cyst. An ill-defined margin and any suggestion of tethering to superficial or deep structures strongly suggest carcinoma but are sometimes due to non-infective inflammation or fat necrosis
Firm, poorly defined lump or lumpiness **Refer urgently if:** **Lump enlarging or other features of malignancy** **Over 30 years of age and lump persists after next period** **Family history of breast cancer** **Post menopausal** **Previous breast cancer** **Males over 50, unilateral lump** **Refer non-urgently if:** **Under 30 years of age** **Unexplained persistent symptoms**	Suggests fibroadenosis, especially if outline is difficult to distinguish from normal breast tissue or if the breast is generally lumpy. Risk of malignancy small but see referral guidelines opposite
Soft lump	Usually a lipoma or occasionally a lax cyst
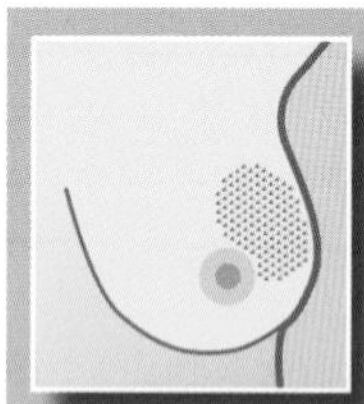 **3. Skin changes in the breast** **Refer urgently**	
Skin dimpling or tethering	Sometimes a subtle sign but highly suggestive of carcinoma
Visible lump	Cyst, carcinoma or phylloides tumour. Cysts can appear with alarming speed
Peau d'orange (appearance of orange peel)	Over a lump, this is virtually pathognomonic of carcinoma. It is due to tumour invasion of dermal lymphatics causing dermal oedema. However, it may occur over an infective lesion
Redness	Usually infection, especially if skin is hot. Sometimes a feature of mammary duct ectasia. Beware inflammatory carcinoma
Ulceration	Neglected carcinoma in the elderly (often slow-growing)
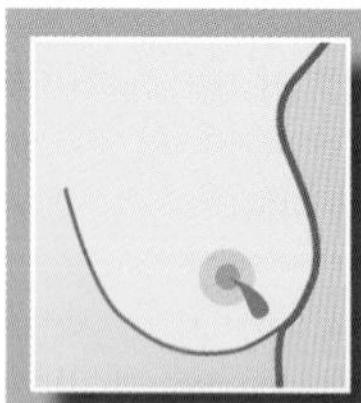 **4. Nipple disorders**	
Recent inversion or change in shape **Refer urgently**	Suggests a fibrosing underlying lesion such as a carcinoma or mammary duct ectasia but can be malignancy
'Eczema' (rash involving nipple or areola, or both) **Refer urgently if not responding to treatment**	If unilateral and persistent, this is the classic sign of Paget's disease of the nipple, a presentation of breast cancer
Nipple discharge	
Milky	Pregnancy or hyperprolactinaemia
Clear	Physiological
Green **Refer only if other signs or symptoms**	Perimenopausal, duct ectasia, fibroadenotic cyst
Blood-stained **Refer urgently**	Possible carcinoma or intraduct papilloma

Fig. 45.1 Symptoms and signs of breast disease (see also Figs 45.3 and 45.4)
UK NICE guidelines for urgent and non-urgent referral to a specialist are indicated on a pink background

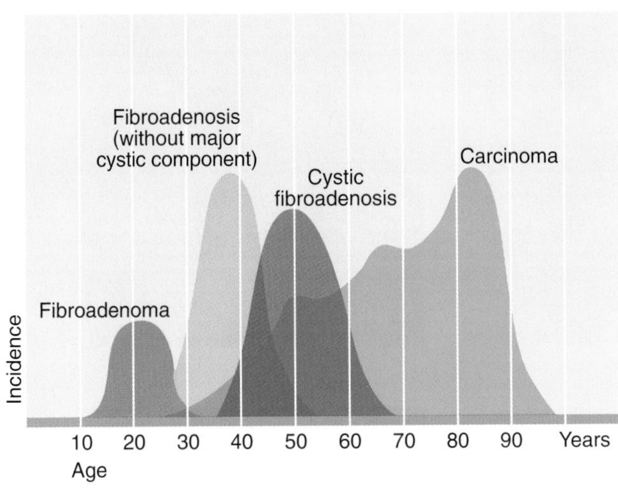

Fig. 45.2 Age incidence of common breast disorders

Box 45.1 Types of breast disease of surgical importance

Malignant neoplasms

- Ductal adenocarcinoma
- Lobular adenocarcinoma
- Sarcoma
- Metastasis from other tissues

Benign tumour-like lesions

- Fibroadenoma
- Intraduct papilloma
- Lipoma

Disordered physiological responses of breast tissue (abnormalities of normal development and involution, ANDI)

- Fibroadenosis (also known as fibrocystic disease, benign mammary dysplasia and chronic mastitis)

Mammary duct ectasia

- Chronic periductal inflammatory reaction due to retained duct secretions

Infections

- Cellulitis and breast abscess
- Subareolar abscesses in mammary duct ectasia

second-degree relatives, age of onset and bilaterality. Some families have mutations in the tumour suppressor genes *BRCA1* or *BRCA2*, which strongly predispose to breast and other cancers.

EXAMINATION OF THE BREASTS

There are several accepted methods for examining the breasts; one is shown in Figure 45.3. All areas of the breast must be examined, with particular attention to the axillary tail and retro-areolar regions. Breast examination involves six distinct manoeuvres:

- Observation with the patient sitting up
- Observation with the patient raising and lowering her arms

Box 45.2 Risk factors for breast cancer

- Increasing age
- Family history (number of first- and second-degree relatives, their age of onset and bilaterality, known BRCA1/BRCA2 mutations)
- Previous history of breast cancer or carcinoma-in-situ
- Early age of menarche (age <12 years)
- Late age of menopause (age >55 years)
- Late age at first full-term pregnancy (age <20 years protective)
- Nulliparity
- Previous breast biopsies showing non-malignant abnormalities
- Hormonal therapy—oral contraceptive pill or HRT
- Radiation at a young age (mantle irradiation for lymphomas, atomic bomb survivors)
- See also http://info.cancerresearchuk.org/cancerstats/types/breast/riskfactors/#reproductive

- Examination of the nipples
- Systematic palpation of each breast
- Palpation of axilla and supraclavicular fossa
- General examination for signs of distant metastases

During inspection, the signs to be looked for are listed in Figure 45.1.

Palpation may be done **circumferentially** using the flat of one hand, starting at the nipple then moving in progressively larger circles; **radially** from the nipple outwards like the spokes of a wheel; or by **sectors**, examining each quadrant in turn. Axillary lymph nodes are palpated whilst the examiner's other hand supports the patient's arm (Fig. 45.3g, h). This helps relax the muscles and aids assessment of the nodal groups (**medial, lateral, anterior, posterior and apical**). Note that clinical assessment of axillary nodes is unreliable, with a 30% false positive and a 30% false negative rate.

A history of **nipple discharge** can often be confirmed by pressure over the appropriate sector near the areola. Discharges not obviously blood-stained should be tested for blood using urinalysis dipsticks. In all cases, a smear preparation should be examined for cytological abnormalities.

Lumps

The differential diagnosis of a discrete breast mass is:

- Cyst
- Fibroadenoma
- Focus of fibrocystic change or fibroadenosis
- Fat necrosis (rare)
- Carcinoma

During the examination the patient needs to point out any lump she is worried about. The normal breast has a wide range of textures, from soft through nodular to hard, so the texture of the rest of the breast must be taken into account. When a lump is found, its characteristics should be defined (see Box 45.3), in particular whether it is discrete or dominant or whether it is an area of nodularity or 'thickening'. If there

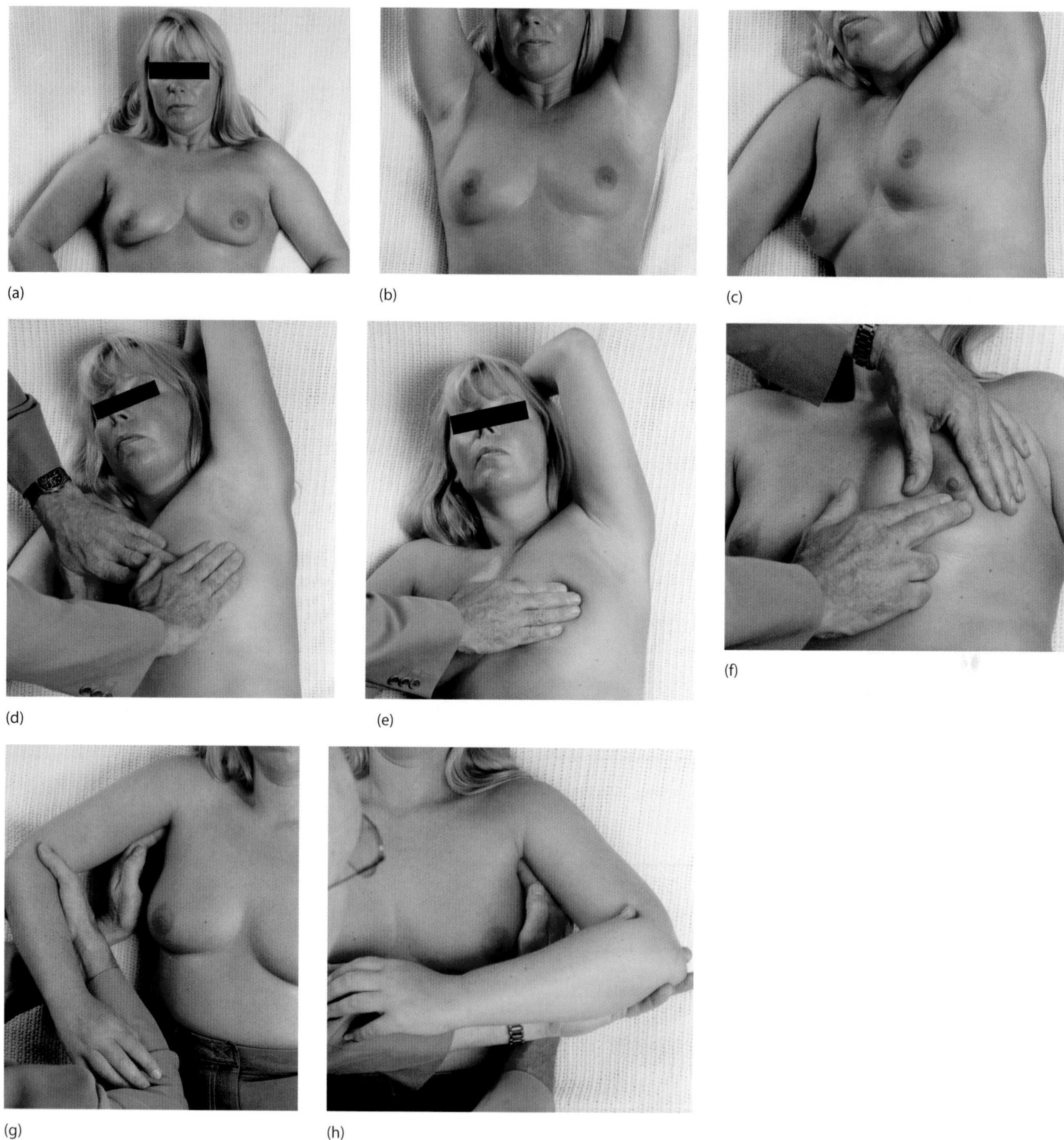

(a) (b) (c) (d) (e) (f) (g) (h)

Fig. 45.3 Technique of breast examination
Inspection: the breasts should be inspected for asymmetry, skin tethering and dimpling and changes in colour. This should be performed with the patient sitting comfortably, pressing hands on hips **(a),** lifting arms in the air **(b),** and pressing hands on top of the head. Palpation: the patient should sit on an examination couch as shown in **(c),** with the backrest at about 45° and rolled slightly to the contralateral side. The arm on the side to be examined should be elevated and the head rested on the pillow. The effect of these manoeuvres is to spread the breast over a greater area of the chest wall. The flat of the right hand is used to palpate the breast circumferentially by quadrants **(d)–(f).** The central part of the breast and the axillary tail must also be palpated. If there is a history of nipple discharge, the areola is pressed in different areas **(f)** to identify the duct from which it emanates and therefore the segment involved. Finally the axillary lymph nodes are palpated as shown in **(g)** and **(h)**. The left axilla is palpated with the right hand **(h)** and the right axilla is palpated with the left hand **(g).** It is important to relax the axillary muscles by supporting the weight of the patient's arm as shown. The fingers of the examining hand are firmly held in a curve, pressed high into the apex of the axilla against the chest wall and drawn downwards. The hand will then 'ride over' any enlarged axillary nodes

Box 45.3 Clinical characteristics of a breast lump

- Solitary or multiple
- Size—in centimetres
- Location—quadrant of breast or clock face
- Contour—smooth and round/ovoid (likely to be benign) or firm/hard (probable malignancy)
- Mobility—mobile (likely to be benign) or fixed (probable malignancy)
- Associated changes—skin/nipple retraction, skin tethering, bloody nipple discharge, erythema
- Axillary lymphadenopathy—enlarged and mobile or enlarged and fixed

is a discrete mass, does it appear benign or suspicious for malignancy? (Characteristic signs of cancer are shown in Fig. 45.4.) Note that even for breast specialists, clinical examination has a low sensitivity (i.e. ability to detect real abnormalities) of 65–80%. In one clinical evaluation system, increasing levels of suspicion are graded E1 to E5; an E3 designation may prompt a core biopsy even if radiological findings are not suspicious. Only 3% of breast cancers occur under the age of 30 but a discrete lump in a patient over 65 is a cancer until proved otherwise.

Skin tethering (as opposed to direct infiltration) can be a subtle sign and is accentuated by raising the arms to put the breast suspensory ligaments under tension. Deep fixation can be assessed by checking the mobility of the lump over pectoralis major with the muscle relaxed and then tensed.

CASE STUDY

Fig. 45.4 Carcinoma of the breast

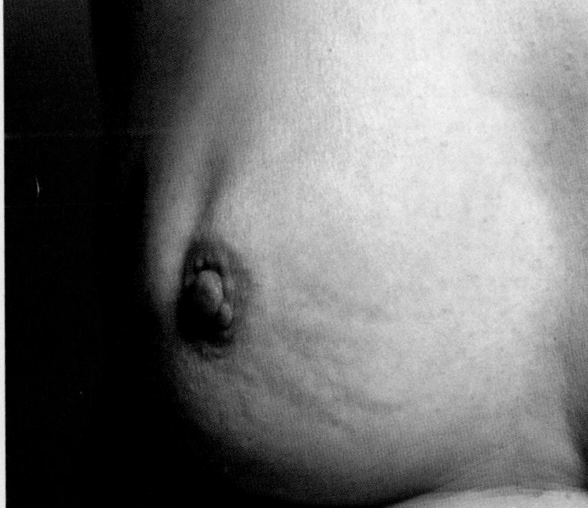

(a)

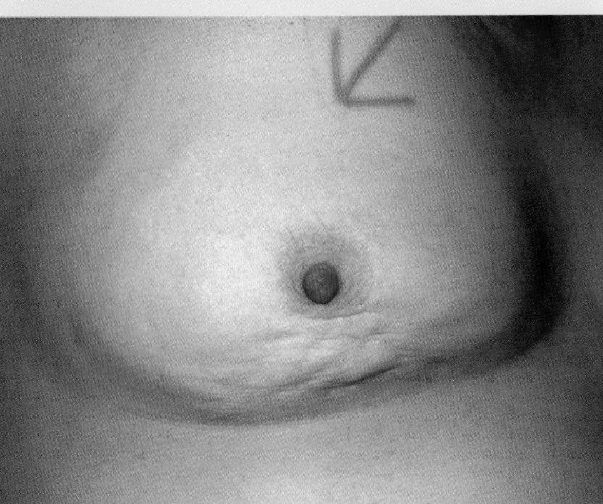

(b)

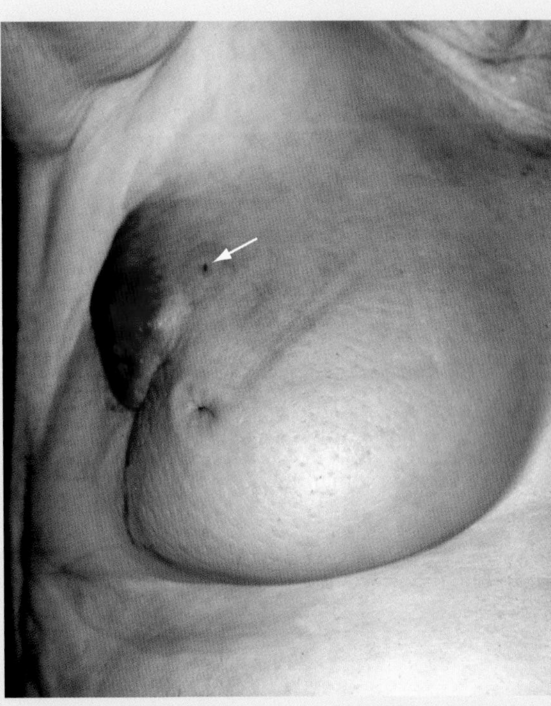

(c)

(a) and **(b)** Characteristic skin dimpling over breast carcinomas. This may be a subtle sign and only be visible in tangential light. **(c)** Nipple retraction and widespread 'peau d'orange' resulting from a large central breast carcinoma. Peau d'orange is caused by a combination of cutaneous infiltration by tumour and skin oedema (and occasionally by infection). Locally advanced breast cancer may cause distortion of the breast. The colour change and ulceration are uncommonly seen and only occur in neglected cases. Note also the puncture wound of a core biopsy (arrowed). There was no obvious axillary node enlargement

Paget's disease of the nipple

Some patients with breast carcinoma present with eczema-like reddening and thickening of the skin of the nipple and areola, together with fissuring and ulceration. This is more common in the elderly and is known as *Paget's disease of the nipple* (Fig 45.10).

INVESTIGATION OF BREAST DISORDERS

'One-stop' clinics allow rapid and comprehensive preliminary assessment. **Triple assessment** includes clinical examination, breast imaging and biopsy (when indicated) on the same day. This has an overall accuracy of 99.6% when performed by experienced personnel, meaning the chances of missing a cancer are less than 1%; patients shown not to have cancer can usually be discharged. If there is a clinically suspicious lump and needle biopsy is negative or equivocal, diagnostic **excision biopsy** should be performed. The discrete lump is completely excised and examined histologically.

IMAGING

Mammography (breast radiography) is an important method of radiological assessment of the breasts. In women over 40 years, it has a sensitivity of 88% for carcinoma. It is less sensitive in younger women because the breast tissue is denser, and is rarely performed below 35 years.

During mammography, the breast is compressed firmly in the machine. This spreads the tissue to an even thickness to give correct exposure for all the breast tissue to make it easier to detect any mass lesion. Radiological views are taken in two directions, medio-lateral oblique (MLO) and cranio-caudal (CC). Localised compression views can reduce the problem of superimposed structures simulating a mass. Focused magnified views can better display any abnormal area. Full digital mammography, which permits post-processing enhancement of the image, has nearly replaced film mammography.

Features looked for on a mammogram include:

- The presence of a mass lesion
- Microcalcification
- Architectural distortion
- Asymmetry
- Skin thickening
- Lymph nodes

A typical carcinoma appears as a **spiculated** mass lesion (dense centre with radiating lines) which may have malignant-type fine linear or granular microcalcification (Fig. 45.5). Fine granular microcalcification within a spiculate lesion is virtually pathognomonic of cancer. Tumours as small as 2–3 mm are sometimes detectable radiologically, long before they become palpable.

Benign-type microcalcification is coarse and 'chunky' (Fig. 45.6). Fine branching microcalcification is characteristic of **ductal carcinoma-in-situ (DCIS)**. Architectural distortion and asymmetry are subtle radiological signs but should be viewed with suspicion.

Ultrasound has long been used to distinguish solid lesions from cysts and has a specificity of 100% for this. Modern B-mode ultrasound demonstrates breast anatomy in great detail and is complementary to mammography. Benign lesions can be distinguished from malignancy with a sensitivity for cancer of at least 85%. Ultrasound can accurately measure the size of a cancer (Fig. 45.7) and can guide percutaneous needle biopsies and cyst aspiration (Fig. 45.8).

The strength of breast imaging comes from performing mammography and ultrasound together as the physical characteristics tested by the two techniques are different. The information acquired by mammography results from attenuation of the X-ray beam through breast structures whilst ultrasound tests the reflectivity of a pulsed ultrasound beam (of about 12 mHz) caused by subtle attenuation changes at tissue interfaces within the breast.

BIOPSY

Most palpable and all non-palpable image-detected masses are biopsied under image guidance, as are suspicious areas of calcification. **Fine needle aspiration cytology (FNAC)** specimens are rarely used for tissue diagnosis now (see Box 45.4). FNAC has a sensitivity of 95% for detecting malignancy but cannot distinguish between in situ and invasive cancers. By contrast, **core biopsy** has a sensitivity of 98%. The tissue architecture is preserved so that invasion can be confidently diagnosed on histology and tumours can be pathologically

CASE STUDY

Fig. 45.5 Carcinoma of the breast on mammography

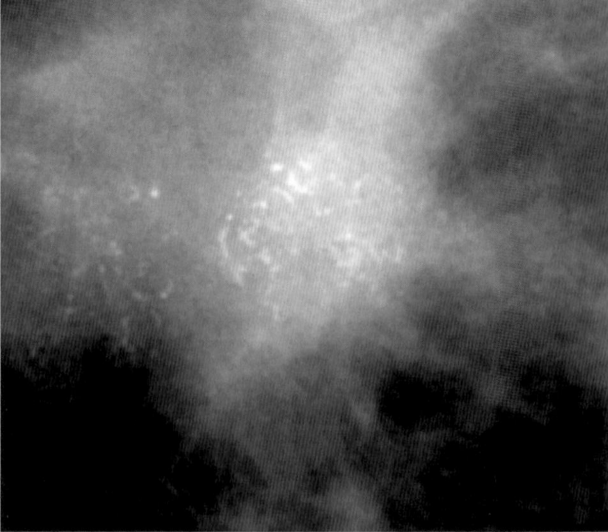

This 58-year-old woman presented with a 2-week history of a non-tender lump in the left breast. Clinical examination confirmed a hard irregular mass without skin dimpling, and a palpable left axillary node. Enlarged view of the carcinoma showing typical malignant-type microcalcification. This contrasts with the coarser calcification occurring in benign breast conditions (see Fig. 45.6c)

Fig. 45.6 Fibroadenoma of the breast

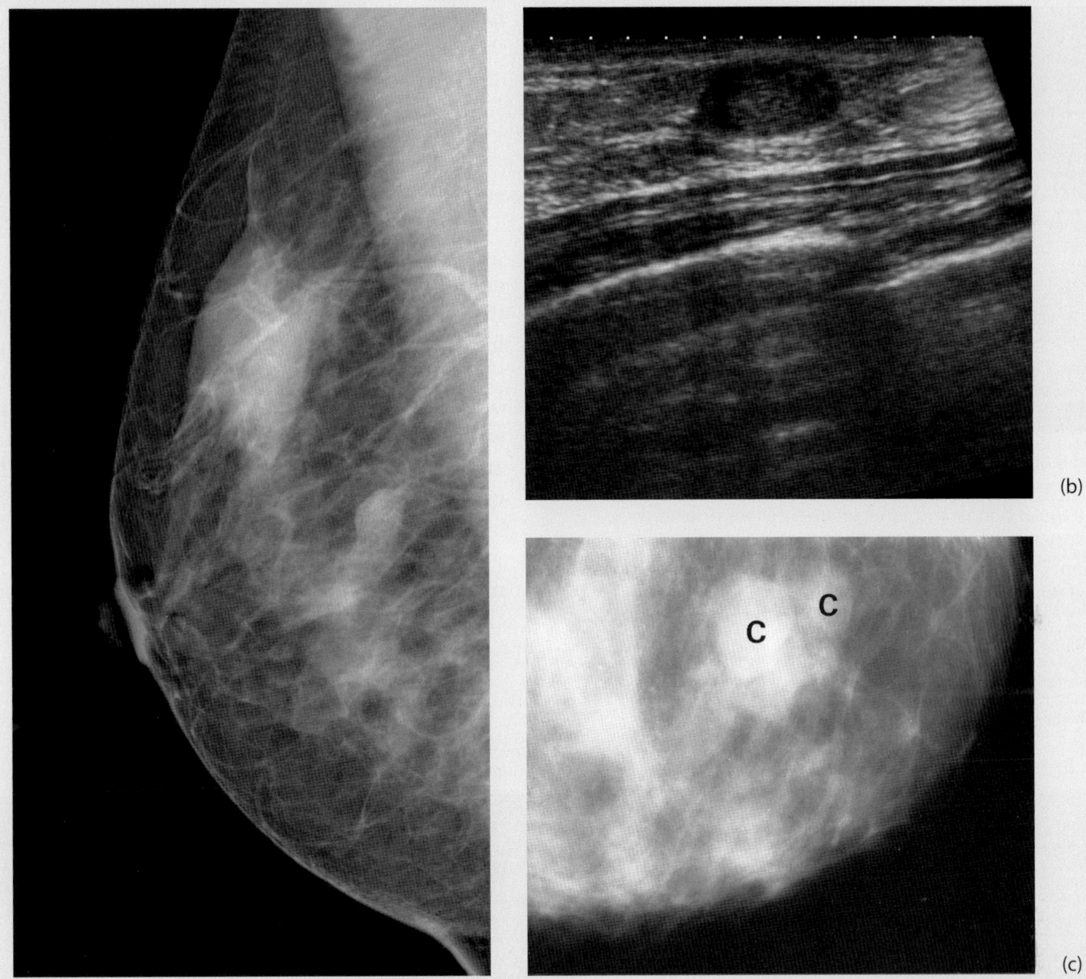

This 35-year-old patient presented with a 3-month history of a lump in the upper aspect of the left breast which was slightly tender at the time of menstruation. Clinical examination revealed a smooth round mobile mass which was firm and very mobile. **(a)** This mammogram shows simple lobulated mass lesion in the upper part of the breast with a well-defined border. These appearances are suggestive of a benign lesion (in this case a fibroadenoma). **(b)** This image shows the ultrasound appearances of the lesion in **(a);** it is a well-defined solid lesion with regular internal echoes and no posterior enhancement (compare with **Fig. 45.8b**). The lesion is 'broad' rather than 'tall' and is typical of a fibroadenoma. **(c)** An enlarged mammographic view of a different fibroadenoma in an older woman showing the much coarser calcification associated with benign breast lesions compared with carcinoma

CASE STUDY

Fig. 45.7 Carcinoma of the breast on ultrasound

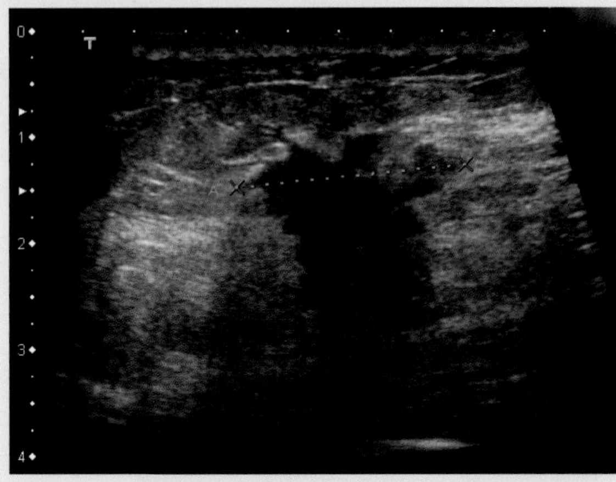

Ultrasound scan of the patient shown in **Fig. 45.5**. This shows a hypoechoic mass lesion extending the width of the blue dotted line. It has an irregular border and some internal echoes. The lesion is characteristically 'tall', i.e. deep, and there is acoustic shadowing deep to the lesion. This image should be contrasted with the appearances of a benign fibroadenoma (**Fig. 48.6b**)

Box 45.4 Reporting categories for fine needle aspiration cytology

C1—inadequate specimen
C2—benign
C3—suspicious but probably benign
C4—suspicious and probably malignant
C5—malignant

graded. After core biopsy patients need to return later for the results as the pathology has to be read after the specimen has been fixed. This has the advantage that any bad news can be broken in a phased manner. If needle biopsy is negative or equivocal, a discrete lump should be completely excised with a wide margin of apparently normal breast tissue and the specimen examined histologically. This procedure, **excision biopsy**, can also form the first step in controlling local disease.

Eczematous lesions suspicious for Paget's disease of the nipple can be 'punch' biopsied under local anaesthesia in the clinic.

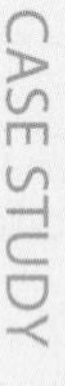

Fig. 45.8 Breast cyst

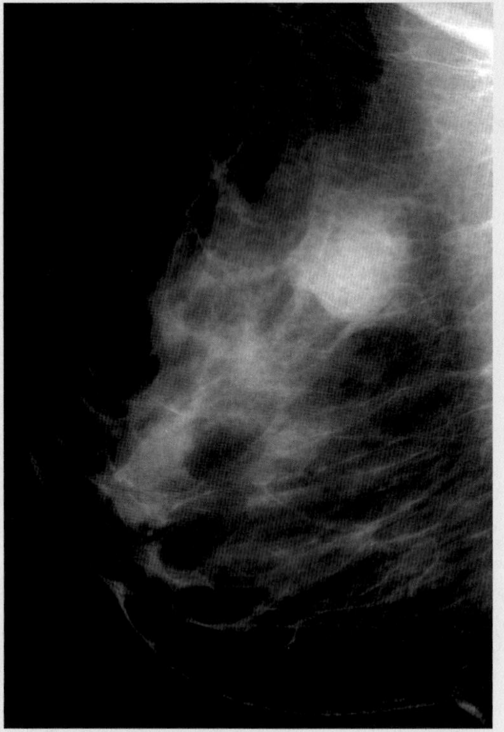

(a)

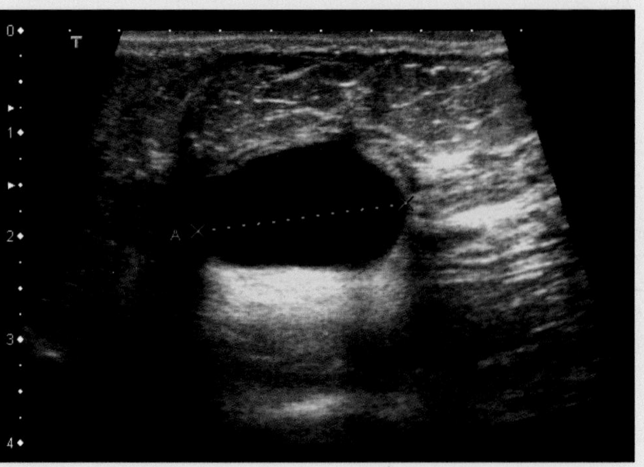

(b)

This 42-year-old woman presented with a tender lump in the superior aspect of the right breast. There was a previous history of breast cysts. Examination revealed a smooth, round and slightly fluctuant mass. **(a)** Mediolateral oblique view mammogram showing a well-defined lesion with circumscribed margins in the upper part of the breast. The appearances are of a benign lesion. **(b)** Complementary ultrasound examination reveals an anechoic mass with sharp, well-defined margins and posterior acoustic enhancement. This is diagnostic of a simple cyst

BREAST CANCER

INTRODUCTION

In Western societies, breast cancer is the leading cause of death in 35–55-year-olds. About 1 in 10 women will develop breast cancer (i.e. a lifetime risk of 10%) and 1 in 18 will die from it. In the UK, 25 000 new cases are diagnosed annually and 15 000 women die each year. Worldwide, there are about half a million deaths from breast cancer annually but despite an increasing global incidence, mortality rates have gradually fallen with earlier diagnosis and improved treatments, including advances in hormonal therapy.

RISK FACTORS

Age

Age is the greatest risk factor. Incidence rates rise from about 25, more steeply between 40 and 55, with a slight levelling off until about 70. After that, another fairly steep rise continues into old age (see Fig. 45.2). Breast cancer is the commonest cause of death in women aged between 40 and 50 years.

Genetic factors

The aetiology of breast cancer is multifactorial, with genetic factors being relatively more important in premenopausal women and environmental factors more so after the menopause. These play a small role in calculating the risk of breast cancer, but the risk is greater in women with a strong family history (two first-degree relatives, bilateral breast cancer or diagnosis before the age of 50). Such a family history accounts for 10% of cancers, with half due to genetic mutations, mainly BRCA1 (17q21) and BRCA2 (13q41) genes which are transmitted in an autosomal dominant fashion. A mutation in either of these leads to an 80–90% lifetime risk of developing the disease. The same mutations are also linked to ovarian cancers. Women with a BRCA mutation should be counselled about their individual risk of breast and ovarian cancer and the treatment options (ranging from surveillance to risk-reducing bilateral mastectomies, which reduce the cancer risk by more than 90% and oophorectomy).

Hormonal factors

Growth of most breast cancers is promoted by oestrogens, hence reproductive physiology and behaviour influence cancer risk. It has long been known that nulliparous women are at greater risk: Ramazzini commented in 1703 that breast cancer was common in Catholic nuns who as '*Vestalis Virgines*' were prone to '*horrendis mammarium canceris*'.

The interval between menarche and menopause is the **oestrogen window** and is an estimate of cumulative exposure to endogenous oestrogen; the longer the interval, the higher the cancer risk. Women who begin menses before the age of 12, or start the menopause after 55 are at an increased risk. A natural or a 'medical' menopause under 40 years reduces cancer risk by two-thirds. Nulliparity and a late age at first pregnancy increase risk and a first full-term pregnancy under 20 years halves the risk compared with one between 30 and 35 years or nulliparity, although the risk is still small.

Prolonged use of the **oral contraceptive pill** increases the risk of breast cancer by 20% and combined **hormonal replacement therapy** (HRT) for more than 10 years also increases the risk, although this falls when HRT is stopped.

Social and geographic factors

Breast cancer is more common in the Western world and in women in higher socioeconomic classes. Obese women are at a higher risk, possibly due to conversion of androgens to oestrogen in adipose tissue. Consuming more than 3 units of alcohol a day increases the risk by 50%.

EPIDEMIOLOGY

Breast cancer is not a new disease; it was recognised by the ancient Egyptians and mastectomy was certainly performed in Roman times. Nowadays, breast cancer is predominantly a disease of Western society but differences in incidence are more likely environmental than racial. The disease is uncommon in Japan, but Japanese immigrants to the USA acquire local incidence rates within two generations.

Breast cancer rates are rising fastest in Asiatic countries that have adopted Western lifestyles. The rise is most likely due to changes in reproductive practice, including deferring childbirth until past 30 years of age, smaller families, and prolonged use of the oral contraceptive pill.

Environmental factors

Exposure to irradiation in the teenage years may initiate some breast cancers which are then promoted by other factors years later. Female survivors of the atomic bombs of Hiroshima and Nagasaki have a high risk of developing breast cancer, as do those who have received mantle irradiation for Hodgkin's disease. Surprisingly, no link has been shown between smoking and breast cancer.

PATHOLOGY

Tumour types

Almost all breast cancers are adenocarcinomas and arise from the terminal duct/lobular unit. Over 85% originate from the ductal component and are designated invasive **ductal carcinomas** of 'no special type' (NST) (Fig. 45.9). About 8% arise from the lobules and are known as **lobular carcinomas**. These are similar in behaviour and prognosis to ductal carcinomas but can be difficult to see on mammography and often present late. Microscopically these tumours are characterised by linear arrangements of cells, so-called 'Indian filing' (Fig. 45.9b). A few invasive carcinomas have ductal and lobular features and are termed 'mixed' tumours.

The remaining 12–15% of cancers are known as '**special types**' (tubular, mucoid, medullary and papillary carcinomas). Special types are well differentiated and generally have a better prognosis.

In situ carcinoma

Breast cancers can develop from an in situ or non-invasive precursor known as **ductal carcinoma-in-situ** or **DCIS**. These

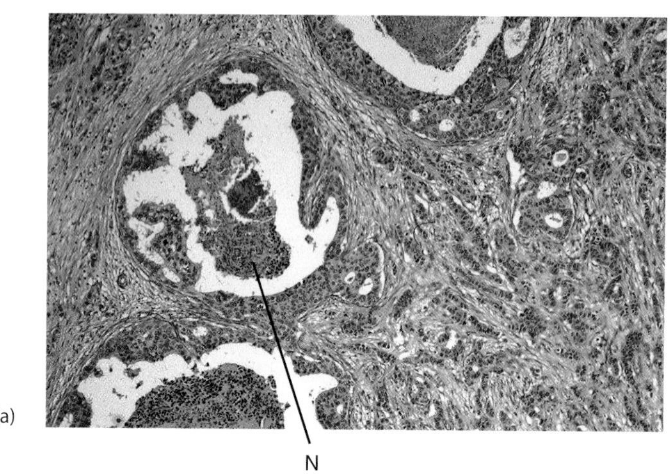

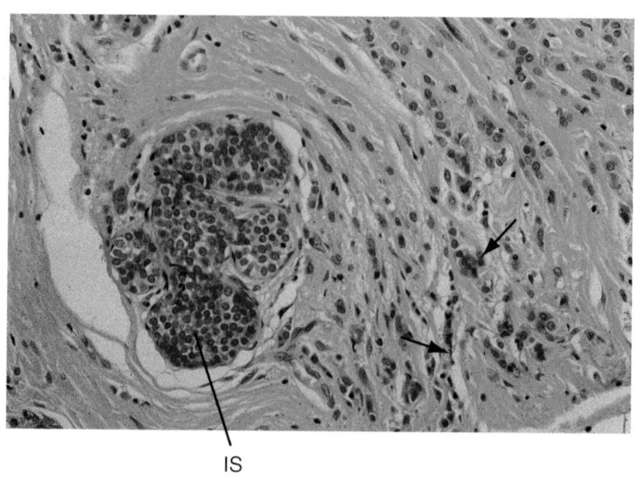

Fig. 45.9 Breast adenocarcinoma—histopathology
(a) Ducts to the left of the picture contain highly atypical epithelium, with central necrosis **N**, a type of in situ ductal carcinoma also known as comedocarcinoma. On the right of this micrograph is invasive ductal carcinoma composed of many small glandular structures diffusely invading breast tissue. **(b)** In situ **IS** and invasive lobular carcinoma. Malignant cells tend to be less atypical than in ductal carcinoma and do not form glands, but often invade in 'single-file' (arrowed). Intracellular mucin is also characteristic of this variant of breast carcinoma

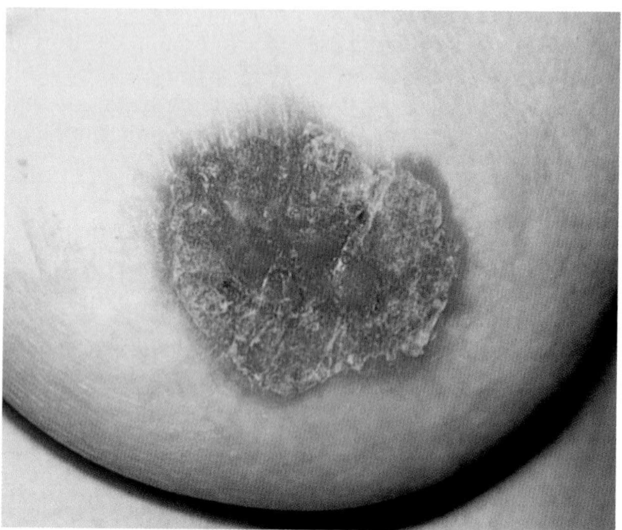

Fig. 45.10 Paget's disease of the nipple

are primarily detected through breast screening programmes as suspicious microcalcifications. Post-mortem studies suggest there is only a 20% chance of DCIS progressing to invasive cancer. DCIS ranges from low to high grade, and higher-grade lesions are more likely to progress if untreated.

Paget's disease of the nipple

In Paget's disease, the epidermis becomes infiltrated by neoplastic cells arising from an underlying ductal carcinoma. These reach the surface by intra-epithelial spread along mammary ducts (Fig 45.10).

Inflammatory carcinoma

Inflammatory carcinoma may be difficult to distinguish from infective conditions of the breast. It often develops without a palpable mass, and can be misdiagnosed as cellulitis. It should be suspected in older women with inflammation that does not respond to antibiotics. Mammogaphy and ultrasound are helpful in establishing the diagnosis although appearances can be similar as a breast abscess often contains necrotic debris simulating a solid mass on imaging. Chronic mastitis during pregnancy may mask an underlying inflammatory carcinoma and delay diagnosis.

Tumour grade

Breast carcinomas are graded histologically I–III according to degree of differentiation. Higher grade tumours tend to infiltrate blood and lymphatic vessels which increases the chance of lymph node and haematogenous metastases, and thus have a worse prognosis. Unfortunately, grade III tumours are more common in premenopausal women. Also, the larger the tumour, the worse the grade tends to be.

NATURAL HISTORY OF BREAST CANCER

Estimates of tumour doubling times suggest that many cancers have been present for 4–6 years before diagnosis. Individual breast cancers vary greatly in their behaviour. Some women present with advanced metastatic disease, others refuse treatment and live for many years, and yet others relapse 20 years or more after apparently successful treatment. Breast cancer tends to be more aggressive in young women and many have an early relapse after treatment. Once a metastatic relapse has been diagnosed, the median survival is 2 years.

There are two main theories about the biological dissemination of breast cancer. **Halsted** proposed in the 1880s that cancer spreads sequentially from a focus in the breast to regional lymph nodes and then into the bloodstream to produce haematogenous metastases. Thus, distant spread occurs only after lymph nodes have been invaded and their filtration capacity overwhelmed. On this basis, loco-regional control by radical mastectomy and/or radiotherapy would cure most patients. By contrast, **Bernard Fisher's** research between 1957 and 1970 challenged Halsted's concept (which mandated radical surgery) with evidence that breast cancer might already be systemic long before the primary is

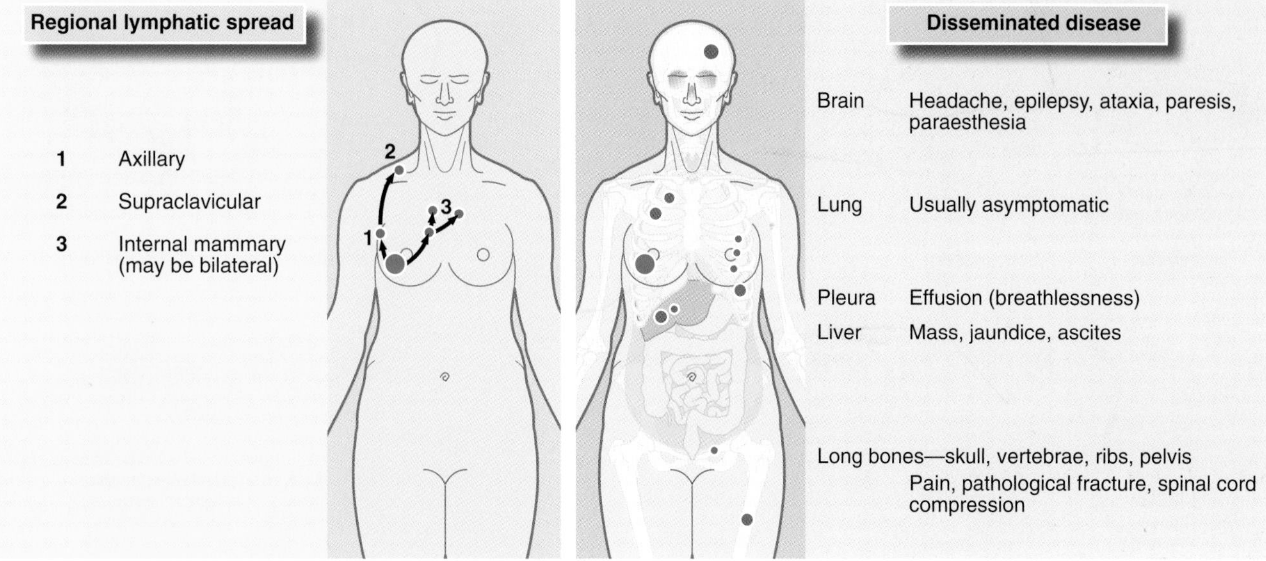

Fig. 45.11 Common sites of spread of breast carcinoma

Box 45.5 Primary treatment for breast cancer

Note that surgery and radiotherapy constitute loco-regional treatment

Surgery

- Mastectomy (radical, modified radical, simple)
- Breast conservation (lumpectomy, wide local excision, quadrantectomy)

Radiotherapy

- Breast radiotherapy (post breast conservation surgery)
- Chest wall (post mastectomy)

Systemic therapy

- Hormonal therapy
- Chemotherapy
- Biological therapy

Box 45.6 Principles of management of breast cancer

- Establish the diagnosis
- Control disease in the affected breast and chest wall
- Prevent and treat local and regional disease in early breast cancer
- Control advanced and disseminated disease

detectable. Furthermore, disseminated cancer cells could potentially metastasise throughout life and it is these that ultimately determine the patient's fate (Fig. 45.11).

In practice, both theories appear to apply in different situations, and breast cancers may show either biological behaviour. Poorly differentiated cancers in younger women are more likely to have distant micrometastases at the time of diagnosis and carry a higher chance of recurrence and death, hence screening would be useless. Conversely, cancers in older patients often have lower metastatic potential even when locally advanced and screening may detect them before systemic spread when they remain potentially curable.

PRINCIPLES OF MANAGEMENT OF BREAST CANCER (Boxes 45.5 and 45.6)

The overall prognosis for breast cancer patients has not changed substantially over the past few decades, but the duration of disease-free survival and to a lesser extent the survival rates have improved. Over the past 20 years, 10-year survival has increased from 55% to 74% and 20-year survival from 44% to 64%. Some of this improvement is due to earlier detection causing **lead-time bias**, but most of it is due to improved adjuvant therapy which acts on metastases as well as the primary.

Whilst the aim of treatment is generally cure, in practice, prolonging the disease-free survival or optimal management of metastatic disease may be a more realistic goal. Treatments have been evaluated in randomised trials and national and international guidelines for treatment have been formulated from these. For patients with advanced disease, palliation is the main objective, with particular emphasis on optimising quality of life.

STAGING

Once a diagnosis of cancer has been made, the disease should be staged to define the extent of spread. Staging begins with triple assessment of the breast and axilla (see above, p. 546). If there is no evidence of axillary nodal or distant involvement and the cancer is amenable to surgery, no further investigations are performed. Clinical signs that may preclude initial surgery are peau d'orange and inflammatory cancer, fixation to the chest wall and distant metastatic disease. These may be indications for **neoadjuvant** chemotherapy, i.e. in advance of surgery.

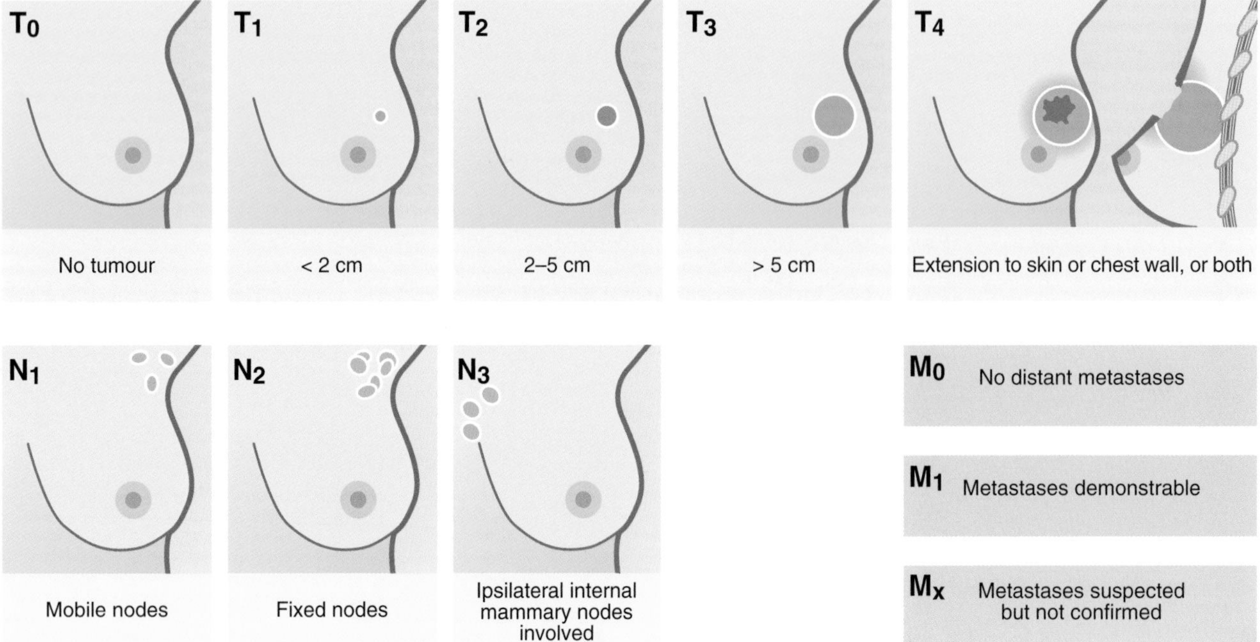

Fig. 45.12 Staging system for breast cancer using TNM classification

If there is evidence of axillary disease, this is a strong predictor of micrometastatic spread and a CT chest and abdomen and a bone scan are arranged to look for metastatic disease in lungs, liver and bone.

PROGNOSTIC STATUS

The TNM system (Fig. 45.12 and Table 45.1) classifies cancer according to the size of the primary *T*umour, the pathological *N*odal status and the presence or absence of distant *M*etastases. TNM grading is used to stage breast patients into four categories (see Table 45.1) and this correlates well with observed rates of disease-free survival at 5 years: 84% for stage I, 72% for stage II, 47% for stage III and 18% for stage IIIC tumours. For further details, see http://poptop.hypermart.net/brcastg.html. In addition to this traditional staging system, the Nottingham Prognostic Index (see http://nuhrise.org/2010/11/nottingham-prognostic-index-plus-npi-a-ground-breaking-tool-for-breast-cancer/) is widely used, which grades patients into six prognostic groups, based on tumour size, nodal status and histological grade.

Other factors used to assess prognosis are histological lymphovascular invasion and hormone receptor status.

Note that as a result of screening, the proportion of small tumours detected has increased but it is uncertain whether this brings an overall survival advantage.

Table 45.1 American Joint Committee on Cancer staging system based on TNM status (6th edition 2003)

T status	N status	M status	AJCC stage
Tis (in situ)	N_0		Stage 0
T_1	N_0		Stage I
T_0	N_1		
T_1	N_1		Stage IIA
T_2	N_0		
T_2	N_1		Stage IIB
T_3	N_0		
T_0	N_2	M_0	
T_1	N_2		
T_2	N_2		Stage IIIA
T_3	N_1		
T_3	N_2		
	N_0		
T_4	N_1		Stage IIIB
	N_2		
any T	N_3		Stage IIIC
any T	any N	M_1	Stage IV

LOCO-REGIONAL TREATMENT

The purpose of loco-regional treatment is to control disease in the breast, chest wall and axillary lymph nodes. For patients with small tumours of favourable grade and some screen-detected lesions, loco-regional treatment alone is potentially curative. These treatments involve surgery or radiotherapy or

Box 45.7 Selection criteria for breast conservation surgery

- Single lesion clinically and mammographically
- Tumour not larger than 3 cm (4 cm in larger breast)
- No extensive in situ component
- Tumours more than 2 cm away from nipple/areola
- Lesion of lower histological grade
- No extensive nodal involvement

a combination of the two. Complete removal of the breast (**mastectomy**) was the standard operation for invasive breast cancer, but over the past 30 years **breast conservation surgery** has become more prevalent. Each patient with breast cancer is best discussed at a multidisciplinary team (MDT) meeting involving surgeon, radiologist, histopathologist and others, and recommendations regarding surgery and further treatment made.

BREAST CONSERVATION SURGERY

This involves removing the tumour with a margin of surrounding breast tissue, followed by radiotherapy to the breast to minimise local recurrence; several long-term clinical trials have shown that overall survival is comparable with mastectomy. Despite this, some patients still opt for mastectomy even if suitable for conservation surgery, and patient choice is an important part of the decision-making process. In parts of the world where radiotherapy is unavailable or is feared, mastectomy remains the treatment of choice.

Selection criteria for conservative surgery are shown in Box 45.7. **Wide local excision** aims to remove the tumour with a 1 cm macroscopic margin of normal breast tissue. Skin is not usually excised unless there is tethering. It is possible to remove up to 20% of the breast volume and still achieve a reasonable cosmetic result. For impalpable tumours, excision can be directed by ultrasound-guided skin marking over the cancer or insertion of a hooked wire under mammography. A **quadrantectomy** is sometimes performed, which removes the tumour within a quadrant-shaped resection. However, this yields a poor cosmetic result.

Patients undergoing breast conservation surgery generally report better body image and sexual functioning than those undergoing mastectomy, but levels of anxiety and depression are similar.

MASTECTOMY

Mastectomy techniques have changed since the operation was first introduced. The **radical mastectomy** was devised by William Halsted in the 1880s in the USA. This operation involved removal of the breast, axillary lymph nodes and pectoralis major and minor muscles.

Patey later devised a less mutilating operation in which the pectoralis major was preserved but pectoralis minor was removed to facilitate lymph node clearance (**modified radical mastectomy**). Modern practice now preserves both pectoralis muscles and this **simple mastectomy** is now standard for invasive breast cancer. The cosmetic effects of mastectomy are of great psychological importance to patients and their families. Careful attention to this can alleviate distress and improve acceptance of disfigurement. Preoperative counselling by breast care nurses prepares the patient for treatment and after mastectomy, patients who do not undergo reconstruction should be fitted with a life-like breast prosthesis incorporated into the cup of a bra.

RECONSTRUCTIVE SURGERY

Patients having a mastectomy can now be offered breast reconstruction, either immediate or delayed. The aim is to restore the natural breast shape, re-establish symmetry and create a nipple-areolar complex. With **immediate reconstruction**, a **skin-sparing mastectomy** is first performed, removing all of the breast tissue via a periareolar incision. The simplest reconstruction option is with an implant or tissue expander, placed deep to the pectoralis muscle. Expanders are gradually inflated and later exchanged for a permanent implant. This is a relatively quick operation compared with tissue transfer techniques, with no donor site morbidity, but it is difficult to re-create larger, ptotic breasts with implants.

The second option to recreate the breast is to employ a myocutaneous flap, using skin, fat and muscle (if necessary). Tissue can be taken from the abdominal wall ('TRAM'—transverse rectus abdominis myocutaneous flap, or 'DIEP'—deep inferior epigastric perforator flap), or from the back ('LD'—latissimus dorsi flap) or from the buttock and inner thigh (Fig. 45.13). All of these can be augmented by implants. Tissue transfer produces a more natural-feeling and moving breast, but the operation takes a lot longer and there is substantial donor site morbidity. Most patients need additional procedures to augment or reduce the contralateral breast for symmetry and to create a new nipple. Immediate reconstruction aims to improve psychological well-being, but the effects of postoperative radiotherapy on the implant and reconstruction must be considered. Sometimes reconstruction is delayed due to the need for adjuvant chemo-radiotherapy, where wound healing problems could delay the treatment.

AXILLARY SURGERY

Axillary nodal status is the most important prognostic factor in breast cancer. Only 25% of patients present with involved lymph nodes and performing a clearance on every patient causes unnecessary morbidity and is no longer necessary unless nodes are involved. Axillary ultrasound at the time of initial assessment is becoming standard practice, according to NICE guidance. If suspicious nodes are located, a core biopsy or aspiration cytology specimen is taken. If this is positive for metastasis, the patient can then be offered a primary axillary clearance, so only one axillary procedure is necessary. If the biopsy is negative, the patient is offered a sentinel node biopsy.

Sentinel node biopsy

Lymphatic spread nearly always follows a predictable pattern, with a sentinel node the first to be affected, so the standard diagnostic procedure is now **sentinel lymph node biopsy** (Fig. 45.14). This node is identified using both a radioactive

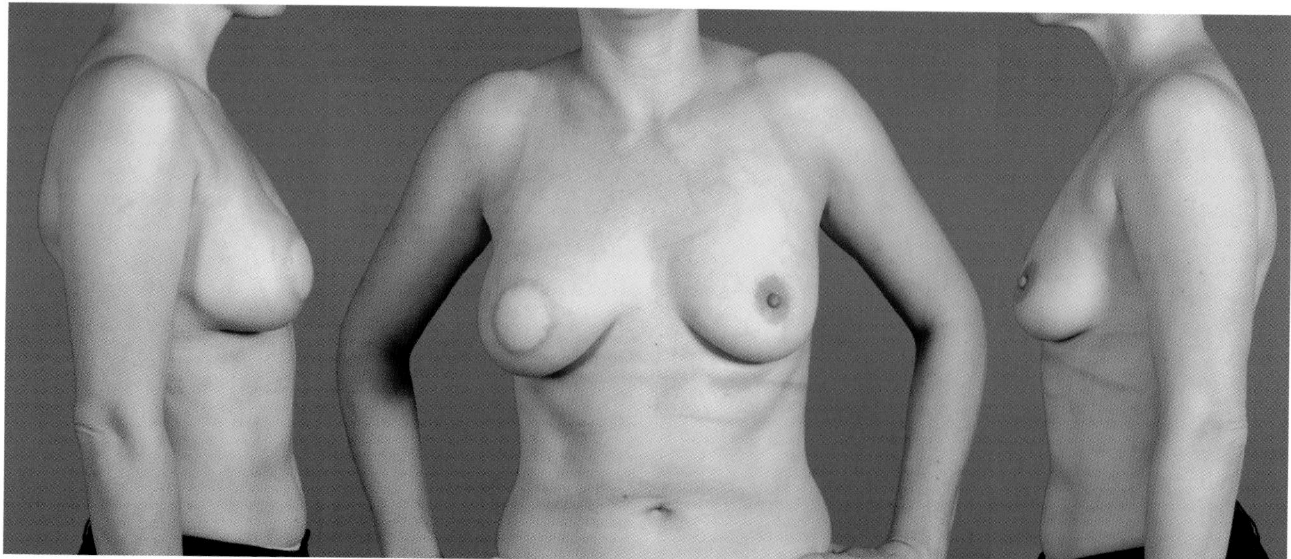

Fig. 45.13 Breast reconstruction following skin-sparing mastectomy using latissimus dorsi flap and silicone implant
Via a circumareolar incision, the entire breast tissue including the nipple–areolar complex is excised and the axillary node dissection performed. The latissimus dorsi muscle is mobilised as a pedicle flap together with an ellipse of overlying skin and tunnelled anteriorly to lie in the breast cavity. Excess skin is trimmed from the flap to leave a circular disc to replace the excised nipple. A silicone implant is sandwiched between the latissimus dorsi and pectoralis muscles to provide bulk and reshape the breast

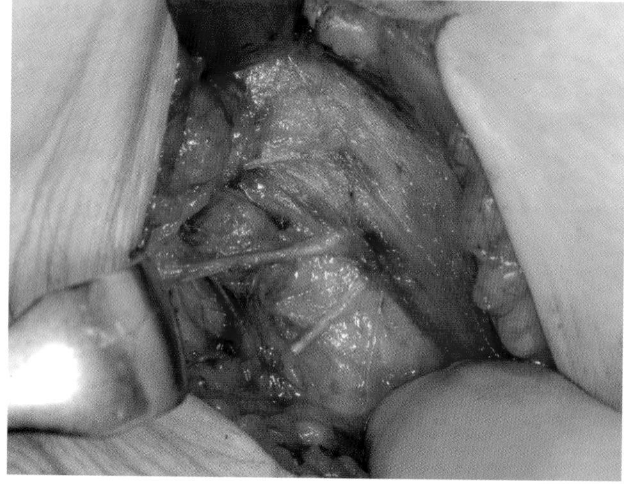

Fig. 45.14 Sentinel node biopsy
The sentinel node is usually the first axillary node to receive lymphatic drainage from the tumour. Before operation, a blue dye and a radiotracer are injected into subareolar area and at operation the sentinel node is identified visually and by using a device to detect radioactivity

isotope bound to albumin, injected next to the tumour 12 hours before surgery, and a blue dye injected into the periareolar area at the start of surgery. Radioactivity is detected at surgery and the visibly blue nodes are excised and examined by the pathologist. This can be done by immediate frozen section, and if the nodes are positive, an axillary clearance can be completed.

By detecting positive axillary nodes, sentinel node biopsy has reduced the morbidity associated with axillary surgery for 75% of patients.

Axillary clearance

Axillary surgery is performed both to fully stage the axilla and to treat proven axillary disease to improve local control and prevent recurrence. However, the indications for, and the extent of axillary surgery remain controversial. If axillary surgery is indicated, techniques need to keep the morbidity low to minimise lymphoedema and reduced shoulder function.

The **surgical levels** of axillary nodes are defined in relation to the pectoralis minor muscle. Most nodes are level I, below its lower edge. Level II is at the level of the muscle and level III is above it. Malignant cells generally progress from level I to level II to level III, with 'skip' metastases in only about 3% (i.e. involving higher levels without lower levels).

Most surgeons accept a level II clearance as optimising local control and staging; level III clearance causes higher morbidity with no survival benefit and should be performed only if higher nodes are palpable.

RADIOTHERAPY

Radiotherapy to the breast is mandatory after breast conserving surgery. It improves loco-regional control and reduces tumour recurrence by 65%; it is thought to reduce mortality from distant metastases by up to 5%. Treatment is by external beam irradiation (40–50 Gy over 3 or 5 weeks); patients with larger tumours or with a narrow margin of normal tissue in the excised specimen may receive a localised booster dose of 12–16 Gy.

Radiotherapy is also given to the 25% or so of patients who, after mastectomy, are shown to have large, poorly differentiated tumours with lymphovascular invasion and four or more involved nodes. In these, supraclavicular nodes and sometimes the internal mammary chain are also irradiated. Post-mastectomy radiotherapy reduces local recurrence by up

Table 45.2 Criteria for selection of adjuvant therapies*

Premenopausal			
Node negative	ER positive	Low risk Intermediate risk High risk, i.e. tumour >2 cm, grade III	No adjuvant therapy tamoxifen Chemotherapy + tamoxifen Consider ovarian ablation
	ER negative		Chemotherapy
Node positive	ER positive		Chemotherapy + tamoxifen Consider ovarian ablation
	ER negative		Chemotherapy
Postmenopausal			
Node negative	ER positive	Low risk Intermediate risk High risk, good general health	None or tamoxifen Tamoxifen ± chemotherapy Tamoxifen + chemotherapy
	ER negative		Consider chemotherapy
Node positive	ER positive		Tamoxifen/aromatase inhibitor + chemotherapy (calculate and discuss potential benefits)
	ER negative		Chemotherapy if general health good

* Low, intermediate and high risk refer to the chances of developing distant disease and relapse and are based on the criteria of tumour size, histological grade and nodal status

to 50% and is believed to improve survival by about 10% but it also increases the risk of arm lymphoedema.

ADJUVANT SYSTEMIC TREATMENT

The low cure rate for apparently early breast cancer is due to occult metastatic spread. The aim of systemic therapy is to delay or prevent these metastases. Some form of prognostic index is often used for planning systemic therapy (see Table 45.3, p. 558), although these are more reliable for predicting short-term than long-term survival. Patients in the best prognostic group are unlikely to have micrometastases and do not generally require systemic treatment. For the rest, the choice of adjuvant therapies (or none) often involves detailed discussion between patient and doctor about the balance of benefit and side-effects. Table 45.2 summarises current thinking about adjuvant systemic therapies for different categories of patient. An American web-based system called Adjuvantonline (www.adjuvantonline.com) is widely used internationally to estimate the benefits and side-effects of different therapies in individual patients and the likely risk of cancer-related mortality or relapse without adjuvant therapy. Data are entered about the patient and their cancer (e.g. age, tumour size, nodal involvement, histological grade) and estimates are then printed as graphs and texts to inform consultations.

CHEMOTHERAPY

Several pulses of systemic adjuvant chemotherapy improve survival in certain groups of patients. Some clinicians believe, however, that the benefit results from chemotherapy-induced ovarian ablation. Adjuvant chemotherapy certainly gives greater benefit in premenopausal women.

Short term toxicity of chemotherapy includes nausea, vomiting, alopecia, mucositis and neutropenia. Long-term complications include premature ovarian failure and induction of early menopause.

Combination chemotherapy is usual and most current regimens contain the alkylating agent cyclophosphamide. One of the first regimens, **CMF**, contained cyclophosphamide, methotrexate and 5-fluorouracil, and was used for many years. This has largely been superseded by regimens of cyclophosphamide plus an anthracycline. **Taxanes** are a newer class of agent which promote microtubule polymerisation leading to cell death. They work in a different way from anthracyclines and give extra response rates in metastatic disease of 50% plus.

Adjuvant chemotherapy is currently recommended for most premenopausal women with high-grade tumours and axillary nodal spread but without evidence of distant metastases. Treatment gives an average proportional increase in survival of approximately 30%, irrespective of nodal status. Systemic chemotherapy is used less frequently in node-negative patients and in postmenopausal women where the absolute benefits are less.

Neoadjuvant chemotherapy, i.e. given before surgery, is generally used in young women with large, high-grade tumours. One advantage is that the response of the cancer to treatment can be directly assessed. Neoadjuvant chemotherapy can also be used to downstage large tumours so that breast-conserving surgery might be possible.

HORMONAL THERAPY

Hormonal therapy for breast cancer includes ovarian ablation, selective oestrogen receptor modulators such as tamoxifen, and aromatase inhibitors.

Hormonal therapy only benefits patients with oestrogen receptor (ER)-positive tumours, in whom it can reduce mortality by up to 36%. The greatest benefit is in postmenopausal women, reducing 10-year mortality by 28%. Similar benefits occur in younger women but menopausal symptoms of oestrogen withdrawal may be troublesome. Hormonal therapy has been shown to reduce the risk of local and distant recurrences as well as the risk of a contralateral breast cancer.

Ovarian ablation yields benefits comparable to chemotherapy in oestrogen receptor-positive premenopausal women, and can be achieved with LHRH analogues or oophorectomy, the latter usually performed laparoscopically. Both improve disease-free survival in premenopausal women.

Tamoxifen is a selective oestrogen receptor modulator (SERM) that blocks the peripheral action of oestrogen in the breast by binding to the receptor. The main side-effects are menopausal symptoms such as vaginal dryness and hot flushes. In addition, the drug carries moderately increased risks of thromboembolism, endometrial cancer and visual disturbances. Treatment of ER-positive cancers with tamoxifen for 5 years reduces the risk of death from breast cancer by 20–30%. Tamoxifen has similar benefits in pre- and postmenopausal women, and its action is additive to chemotherapy.

Aromatase inhibitors (AIs) prevent oestrogen synthesis in peripheral adipose tissues by blocking the conversion of androgens to oestrogen by the enzyme aromatase. AIs significantly reduce peripheral oestrogen levels and block intratumoural synthesis of oestrogen. They can only be prescribed in postmenopausal women.

AIs decrease the risk of cancer recurrence and have fewer side-effects than tamoxifen but carry an increased risk of osteoporosis and fractures. NICE guidelines suggest postmenopausal women with low-risk tumours be offered tamoxifen whilst those with high-risk, ER+ tumours should be treated with AIs.

Patients who are elderly and unsuitable for surgery with ER+ tumours can be treated with primary endocrine therapy such as tamoxifen or letrozole, to slow disease progression.

BIOLOGICAL THERAPIES

These novel forms of therapy target growth factor pathways and are showing promise when used in combination with conventional therapies. **Trastuzumab (Herceptin)** is a humanised monoclonal antibody to the HER/neu (cerbB2) transmembrane receptor which is overexpressed in 30% of breast cancers and indicates a poor prognosis. Clinical response rates of about 35% in metastatic breast cancer have occurred in carefully selected cases. Trastuzumab has also shown striking effects when used as adjuvant treatment, with a 50% reduction of recurrence and a substantial survival benefit. Trastuzumab is given after surgery and chemotherapy at 3-weekly intervals for 1 year.

CONTROL OF ADVANCED AND DISSEMINATED DISEASE (Figs 45.15–45.18)

About two-thirds of breast cancer patients now survive for at least 20 years, but many eventually succumb from micrometastatic disease which later progresses to clinically evident metastases. Once metastases have appeared, treatment is palliative, but very worthwhile prolongation of life and improved quality of life can often be achieved. The commonest sites for metastases are **bones, liver, lung and brain. Bone metastases** are more likely in postmenopausal women with well-differentiated, ER-positive tumours. More than 90% of patients with metastatic disease have bone lesions. These are usually lytic and commonly affect ribs and vertebrae. They are very painful and can lead to pathological fractures (Fig. 45.17). Luckily, they often respond to palliative radiotherapy. **Lobular carcinoma** can metastasise to unusual sites such as skin (Fig. 45.18) and gastrointestinal tract.

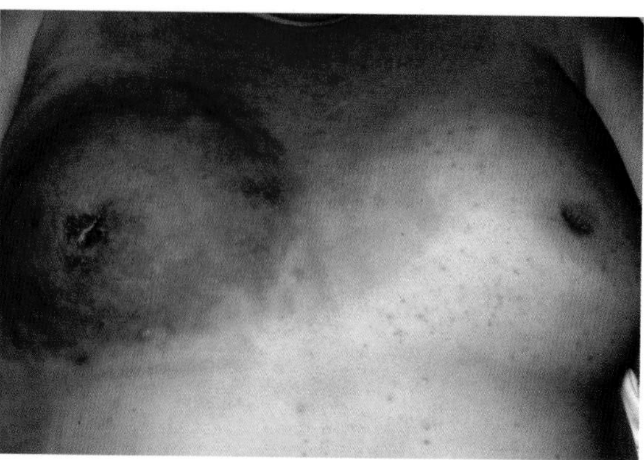

Fig. 45.15 Advanced breast cancer
This 60-year-old woman had been aware of a lump in her right breast for over a year before she could be persuaded to seek treatment. The whole breast is involved and malignancy has spread through the skin widely across the chest wall. Palliative treatment was given with radiotherapy and tamoxifen

Locally advanced breast cancer (stage III disease) often involves most of the breast tissue (see Fig. 45.15). The skin becomes infiltrated (peau d'orange or inflammatory cancer where dermal lymphatics are involved), and eventually ulcerates; the tumour can invade the chest wall. Ultimately much of the chest wall may become involved, when it is known as **carcinoma en cuirasse**. Locally advanced disease of breast and axilla may initially be inoperable but neoadjuvant hormonal or chemotherapy can downsize the cancer so a **toilet mastectomy** can be performed. Radiotherapy alone can be employed for palliation of advanced skin, breast, chest wall and lymph node disease.

Stage IV (metastatic cancer) typically presents in younger women with poorly differentiated tumours that have spread to viscera. Recurrent **pleural effusions** result from **pulmonary metastases** (Fig. 45.16) and are managed with aspiration or pleurodesis (obliterating the pleural cavity by instilling tetracycline or bleomycin) or performing surgical pleurectomy. **Ascites** occurs secondary to **liver** involvement, and patients can present with nausea, anorexia, weight loss and jaundice. **Lymphangitis carcinomatosa** (widespread dissemination in skin or lung lymphatics) and fulminant liver metastases may occur in the terminal stage of the disease. **Brain metastases** can present with headaches and neurological symptoms due to a rise in intracranial pressure.

In stage IV, the aim of treatment is palliation—to control the symptoms of the primary cancer and the metastatic

Fig. 45.16 Chest manifestations of metastatic breast carcinoma

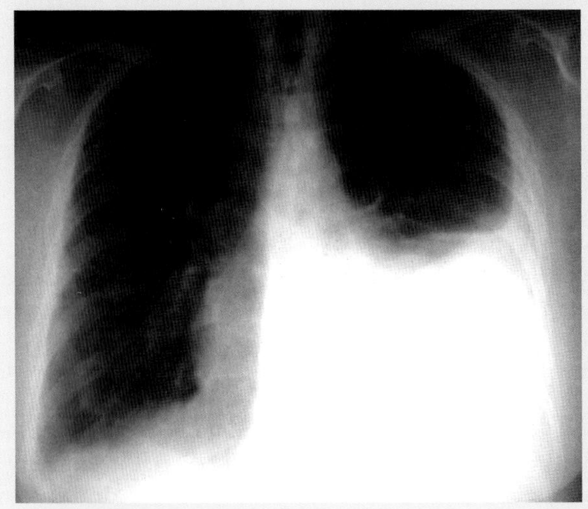

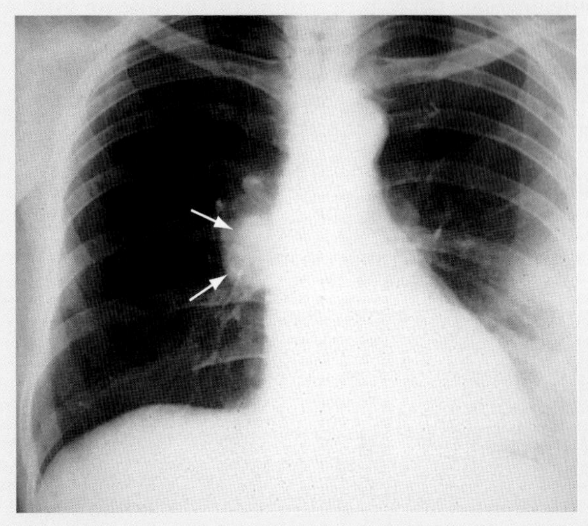

(a) (b)

(a) This 38-year-old woman had undergone a right mastectomy for ductal carcinoma 7 years before and presented with increasing shortness of breath. This chest X-ray shows a large left pleural effusion confirmed on cytology to be malignant. It was palliated by drainage and pleurodesis
(b) A different patient who had been treated 5 years before for lobular carcinoma of the breast. She presented with a chronic non-productive cough and was found to have a mass of lymph nodes at the right hilum (arrowed) and a right recurrent laryngeal nerve palsy due to invasion in the region of the carina

Fig. 45.17 Skeletal metastases from carcinoma of the breast

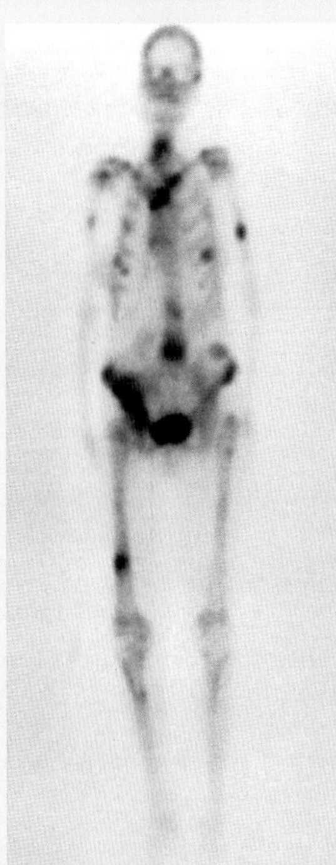

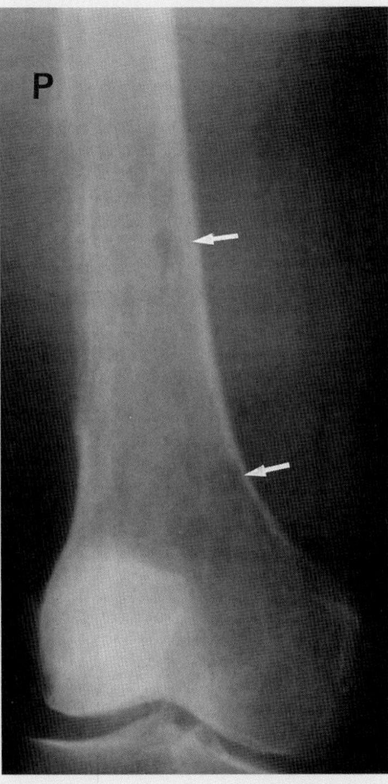

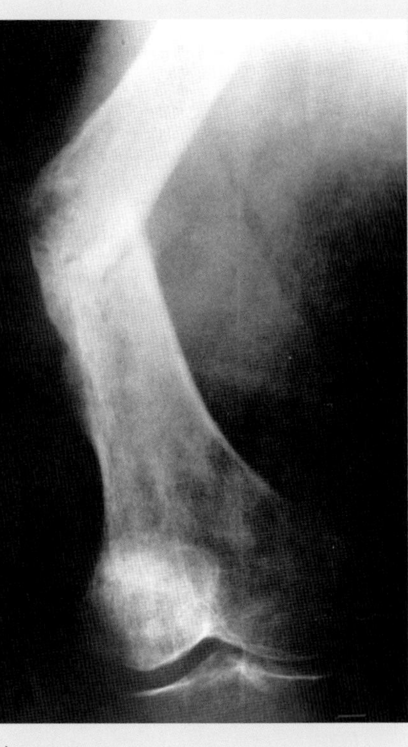

(a) (b) (c)

(a) Anterior view of radioisotope bone scan of a 48-year-old woman complaining of pain in the neck and right hip. She had undergone a mastectomy for carcinoma 8 years previously. The scan shows large metastatic deposits in the lower cervical and lumbar spine, right pelvis, right femur and left humerus as well as several smaller deposits in the ribs and elsewhere in the skeleton. **(b)** X-ray of the lower femur in a 79-year-old woman presenting with a fungating breast carcinoma and pain in the left knee. The X-ray shows radiolucencies (arrowed) in the distal femur and elevation of the periosteum **P** medially, indicating bony metastasis. Radiotherapy was arranged to alleviate the symptoms. **(c)** Some weeks later, despite treatment, the patient returned with this pathological fracture of the femur

burden, and to prolong worthwhile life wherever possible. Systemic therapy can delay progression of the disease and improves symptoms in 30—70% of patients. This can involve endocrine and traditional chemotherapy, together with radiotherapy and bisphosphonates for bony disease and hypercalcaemia.

LONG-TERM FOLLOW-UP

Women who have had one breast cancer have a 15% lifetime risk of developing a second cancer in the other breast. The risk is higher if the original lesion was a lobular carcinoma. Breast tissue in these women may have an increased susceptibility to cancer, or else breast cancer may have arisen at the same time in multiple foci. Thus patients with breast cancer should be followed up clinically and by mammography for 5 years after initial treatment, before returning to a screening programme (if within the screening age group). There is no evidence that more prolonged follow-up improves outcomes.

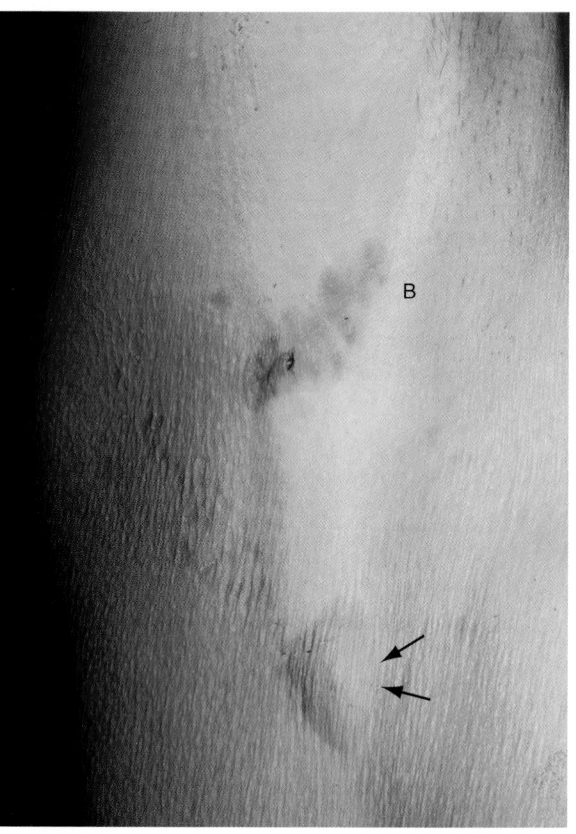

Fig. 45.18 Skin secondaries following simple mastectomy and radiotherapy
This patient presented with painless, slightly elevated nodules in the skin below the axilla 3 years after treatment for lobular carcinoma of the breast. In this photograph, the arm is elevated and one skin secondary can just be made out (arrowed); the site of excision biopsy of another is seen at **B**

LIFE EXPECTANCY AND PROGNOSIS

When long-term survival curves have been examined statistically, there is no evidence of 'cure' in the normally accepted sense (Fig. 45.19), although a 'personal cure' is achieved in about 50% of patients who die from some other disease. Micrometastatic foci can remain dormant for 35 years or more and become 'kick started' for unknown reasons into progressive metastatic disease and death. Loco-regional relapse often occurs within the first 5 years, but distant disease tends to occur much later.

Breast cancer survival estimates from prognostic scoring systems are meaningful only for about 10 years, and as estimates are based on group analyses, they are of doubtful relevance for any individual. A commonly used tool is the Nottingham Prognostic Index (NPI), which divides patients into five prognostic groups (see Table 45.3). **Adjuvantonline** is also popular for estimating prognosis.

Table 45.3 Nottingham Prognostic Index (NPI) for breast cancer*

Nottingham prognostic group	NPI score	Estimated 10-year survival
Excellent	≤2.4	95%
Good	≤3.4	83%
Moderate I	≤4.4	70%
Moderate II	<5.4	51%
Poor	>5.4	19%

* The NPI is calculated as follows: 0.2 × tumour size in cm + histological grade + lymph node status (node negative scores 1; one to three positive nodes scores 2, and four or more positive nodes scores 3)

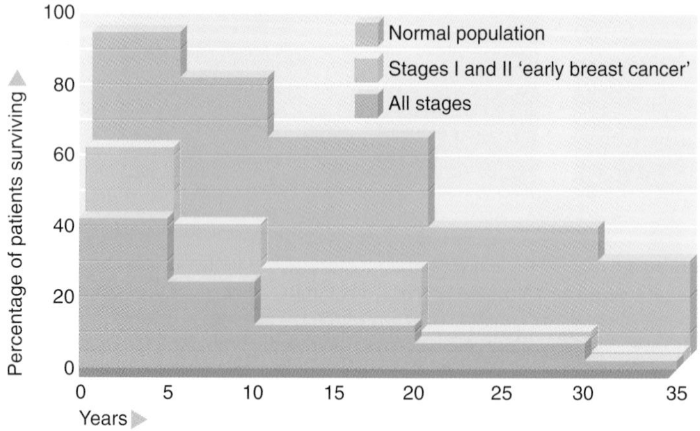

Fig. 45.19 Life expectancy after diagnosis of breast cancer (after Brinkley and Haybittle)
Note that 5- and 10-year survival has improved in recent years as a result of better diagnosis and treatment but it is uncertain that long-term survival will also improve

BENIGN BREAST DISORDERS

Most patients referred to breast clinics are found to have benign breast conditions. These include fibrocystic change or fibroadenosis (the most common), fibroadenoma, duct papilloma, fat necrosis, breast infections and mammary duct ectasia.

ABNORMALITIES OF NORMAL DEVELOPMENT AND INVOLUTION (ANDI)

PATHOLOGY

In women of reproductive age, breast tissue is constantly undergoing physiological changes in response to circulating hormones. This can produce a spectrum of proliferative and regressive changes in the breast parenchyma including distortion and overgrowth of the main structural components—the ducts, lobules and fibrous tissue. The concept of 'abnormalities of normal development and involution (ANDI)' thus encompasses a variety of clinico-pathological features which histologically include fibrosis, adenosis, apocrine metaplasia, epithelial hyperplasia and macro- and microcyst formation.

These changes together result in areas of general or focal **nodularity** associated with varying degrees of pain and tenderness. The term **fibrocystic change** or **fibroadenosis** has historically been applied to this condition. The main components are cyst formation, epitheliosis, fibrosis and proliferation of lobular acini, known as **adenosis**. Fibrosis may occur within areas of adenosis, splitting acini; this is known as **sclerosing adenosis**. Several of these features are often present within a single lesion, or in different areas of the same or the contralateral breast.

By definition, the hyperplastic element in ANDI is not histologically atypical and there is no increased risk of malignancy in this complex of benign breast changes.

CLINICAL PRESENTATION AND MANAGEMENT

Fibrocystic change (fibroadenosis) presents as either a single lump or areas of lumpiness which are painful and tender premenstrually, i.e. cyclically (see Fig. 45.20). These changes may be difficult to distinguish clinically from carcinoma, and florid fibrocystic change can mask a cancer both clinically and radiologically. Fibrocystic change is most common between the ages of 35 and 45 years.

Cyst formation is more prevalent over the age of 40 years and in perimenopausal women. Cysts may present symptomatically as single or occasionally multiple lumps. Cysts develop from lobules and are fluid-filled spaces. **Microcysts** are part of the involutionary process and may coalesce to produce a larger cyst which presents as a smooth, round palpable lump. Larger cysts may be tense, tender and fluctuant with the texture of a table tennis ball. Cysts can usually be diagnosed clinically and are readily confirmed with ultrasonography; they are usually recognisable on a mammogram. Simple cysts can be aspirated under ultrasound control or freehand. Provided the cyst fluid is not blood-stained, there is no residual lump post aspiration and there are no sonographically suspicious features, patients can be discharged without further follow-up, although cysts can recur or new cysts develop (see Fig. 45.21). Cysts are uncommon over the age of 60 years unless the patient is taking HRT. Under these circumstances it is important to exclude an intracystic papilloma, intracystic carcinoma or a cystic carcinoma.

MANAGING FIBROCYSTIC CHANGE

Once the patient has been reassured she does not have cancer, the symptoms of pain and tenderness associated with fibrocystic change can be treated. **Gamolenic acid (GLA)** in high doses may relieve cyclical symptoms in some women, but has to be used for a minimum of 3 months to see results. More than 90% of patients with mild to moderate breast pain can be satisfactorily managed with reassurance and simple analgesia. For those with moderate to severe cyclical pain, danazol

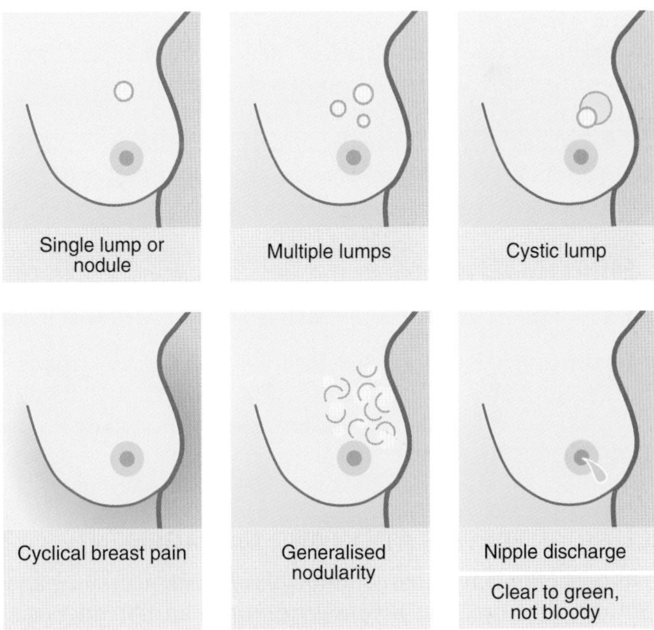

Fig. 45.20 Clinical presentation of fibroadenosis (fibrocystic change)

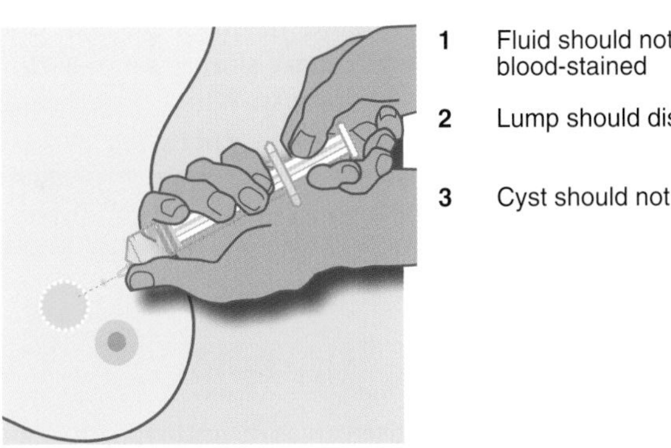

Fig. 45.21 Cyst aspiration and criteria for exclusion of cancer associated with a cyst

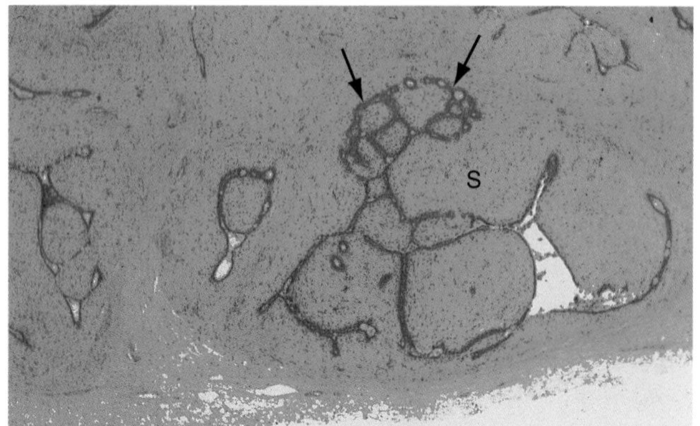

Fig. 45.22 Fibroadenoma—histopathology
This benign lesion shows proliferation of both glands (arrowed) and stroma **S**. In the variant illustrated, gland lumina are compressed by stroma. Fibroadenoma typically has a histologically well-defined edge.

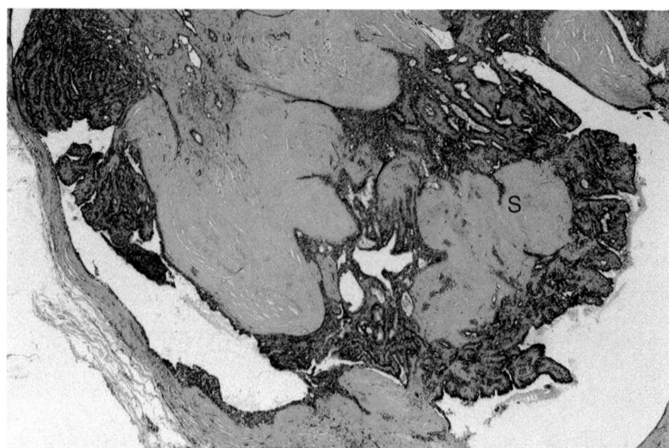

Fig. 45.23 Duct papilloma
This is essentially a localised form of epitheliosis. Papilloma in a larger duct must be distinguished from papillary carcinoma, which lacks the well-defined stromal cores **S**. Both lesions can present with blood-stained nipple discharge

or bromocriptine offers relief in 70% of women, but both these drugs have substantial side-effects which reduce compliance. Danazol inhibits pituitary gonadotrophin secretion and has androgenic side-effects of acne and hirsutism. Bromocriptine inhibits pituitary prolactin release and can produce dizziness.

FIBROADENOMA

PATHOLOGY

Fibroadenoma is a localised form of ANDI rather than a benign tumour. This lesion arises from a single lobule and is composed of epithelial and fibrous components (Fig. 45.22). Fibroadenomas undergo involution in the perimenopausal years but can persist into old age and become calcified.

CLINICAL PRESENTATION AND MANAGEMENT

Fibroadenomas are most common between the ages of 15 and 30 and thus occur in a younger group than fibroadenosis. They present as a single rounded mass which is smooth, firm and highly mobile. Smaller lesions are sometimes described as **breast mice** since they slip away from beneath the palpating fingers. Fibroadenomas are occasionally multiple and bilateral and are more frequent in an Afro-Caribbean population. Larger fibroadenomas should be distinguished from benign **phyllodes tumours** which have similar features clinically, radiologically and on core biopsy. Where suspicion of phyllodes exists or a fibroadenoma is enlarging, excision biopsy is indicated, otherwise the lesions regress spontaneously in 85–90% and do not require excision. Confirmatory tissue biopsy is unnecessary below 25, but is advisable over this age.

DUCT PAPILLOMA

Intraduct papillomas are localised areas of epithelial proliferation. They are villous lesions composed of a fibrovascular core covered by a double layer of epithelium. They usually occur as solitary lesions in the main lactiferous ducts close to the nipple but multiple papillomas can occur more peripherally. Papillomas are not premalignant (see Fig. 45.23). They present as spontaneous blood-stained or clear watery nipple discharge, often from a single duct; a retroareolar mass may be palpable. These lesions are best imaged with ultrasound and the diagnosis confirmed on core biopsy. Papillomas are treated by excision of the affected duct (microdochectomy) or a group of ducts (wedge resection). If the causative lesion cannot be found at operation, a subareolar excision of all the ducts may be necessary.

TRAUMATIC FAT NECROSIS

Trauma to the breast, either accidental or surgical, can produce an area of fat necrosis that can mimic carcinoma clinically and radiologically. There is an initial acute inflammatory response which can persist, provoking chronic inflammation and a fibrotic reaction. This gives a hard irregular lump which may have skin dimpling. Mammography may show a stellate area of distortion with calcification. Core biopsy distinguishes fat necrosis from carcinoma.

INFECTIONS OF THE BREAST

Breast infection is occasionally seen in neonates, but is commonest in premenopausal women. **Lactational mastitis** usually occurs during the first 3 months of breast feeding and can lead to septicaemia. Risk factors include a cracked nipple and poor feeding technique causing milk stasis. The organism responsible is almost always *Staph. aureus.* Patients present with pain, swelling and erythema. Treatment is with empirical antibiotics (such as flucloxacillin), together with continued feeding or milk expression. If the patient is septic, she may need intravenous antibiotics. If an abscess develops (see Fig. 45.24), this should be drained with repeated ultrasound-guided aspiration until resolution. Surgery is only indicated

CASE STUDY

Fig. 45.24 Breast abscess

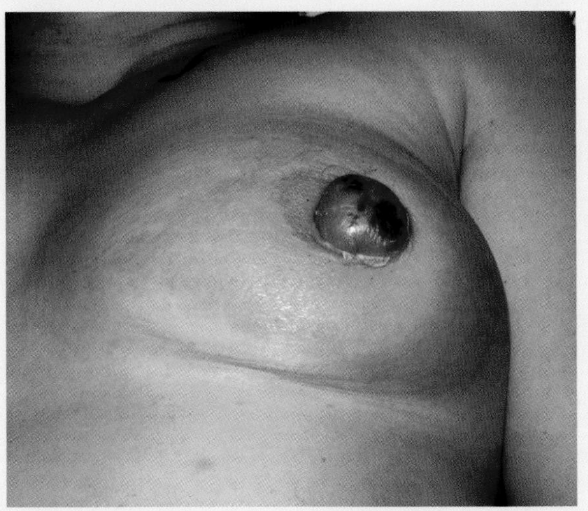

This woman of 40 presented with a neglected left breast abscess a few weeks after ceasing breast feeding. The abscess was drained at open operation but had destroyed much of the breast tissue. The organism was *Staph. aureus* as is commonly the case

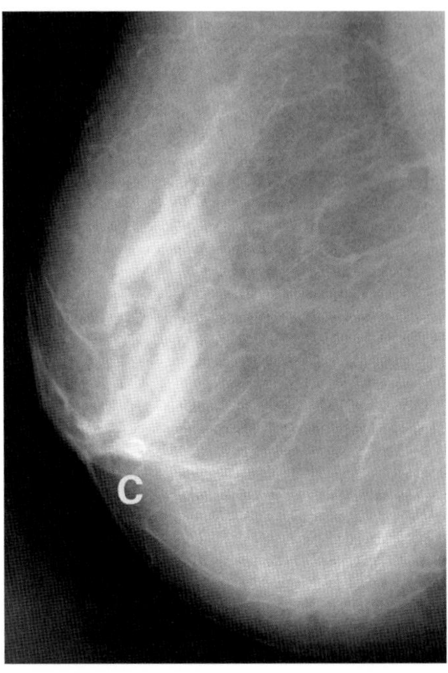

Fig. 45.25 Mammary duct ectasia Radiopaque mass of dilated ducts with no features of malignancy. Large duct calcification **C** is also seen. Note the skin indentation caused by fibrosis. Clinically, this condition can be mistaken for carcinoma

if the skin is threatened or necrotic. In this case, a small stab incision is made, and the abscess cavity is flushed until all the pus is drained.

Non-lactational mastitis is mainly periductal with active inflammation in non-dilated ducts, and should not be confused with duct ectasia. It is treated with broad-spectrum antibiotics with anaerobic cover (such as co-amoxiclav), and either aspiration or incision and drainage, although this risks a mammary duct fistula.

The diagnosis of an abscess is usually obvious, with local signs of acute inflammation, a tachycardia and fever. The affected segment of the breast is tender, red and warm. If the infection is inadequately treated, the abscess becomes fluctuant and eventually 'points' to the surface and discharges.

The early cellulitic phase is reversible if treated with appropriate antibiotics. Flucloxacillin is usually the antibiotic of choice on a 'best-guess' basis. The need for surgical drainage has declined in recent years because of prompt and appropriate antibiotic treatment, sometimes aided by needle aspiration.

DUCT ECTASIA

Mammary duct ectasia refers to dilatation and shortening of the major lactiferous ducts. It is a common involutional change appearing around the menopause. It presents with spontaneous cream, yellow or green nipple discharge, a palpable subareolar mass or nipple inversion. Plasma cells are a characteristic feature on histology; this may be described as **plasma cell mastitis**. Ducts can calcify and be seen on a mammogram (Fig. 45.25). Duct ectasia should be managed conservatively, unless radiological findings are suspicious for malignancy. Persistent discharge can be treated by subtotal or total nipple duct excision.

MALE BREAST DISORDERS

The two main breast conditions in males are gynaecomastia and cancer.

GYNAECOMASTIA (Fig. 45.26)

Gynaecomastia is a benign proliferation of the male breast which feels like a rubbery firm mass extending concentrically from the nipple. It results from an imbalance of oestrogens and androgens acting on the breast. Primary gynaecomastia is physiological and occurs in three phases: **infantile** gynaecomastia is present at birth in response to oestrogens crossing the placenta and resolves spontaneously over several weeks. In **puberty**, the condition is bilateral in 50–60%; the exact mechanism is unknown but most resolve spontaneously. **Senescent** gynaecomastia peaks at 50–69 years of age and is more likely in obese men.

Secondary gynaecomastia is either due to medication or pathological:

- **Medication**—drugs include spironolactone, digoxin, ranitidine, calcium channel blockers, together with anabolic steroids and cannabis use. Hormonal

CASE STUDY

Fig. 45.26 **Gynaecomastia**

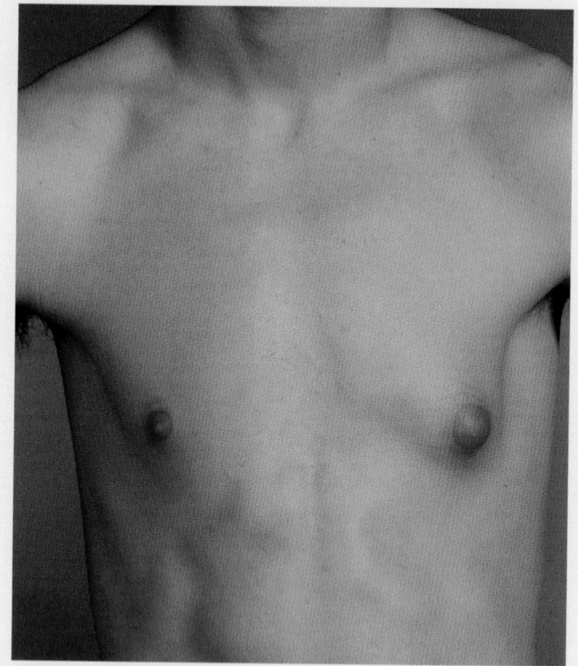

This 17-year-old was concerned about excess breast development on the left side. The breast tissue was removed via a subareolar incision

treatment for prostate cancer can also cause gynaecomastia

- **Pathological**—alcoholic cirrhosis interferes with the metabolism of oestrogens and decreases free testosterone and some testicular germ cell tumours may secrete oestrogens. Other predisposing illnesses include chronic renal failure, diabetes and hypogonadism

Adults with gynaecomastia should undergo triple assessment and have blood tested for prolactin, LH, oestrogen, testosterone and hCG to exclude hypogonadism and testicular tumours. Most men can then be reassured without treatment. Surgery is usually performed in younger males for cosmetic purposes.

MALE BREAST CANCER

Between 0.5 and 1% of breast cancers occur in males, who are an average of 10 years older than women at presentation. Male breast cancer is more common in carriers of *BRCA2* mutations and in states of hyper-oestrogenism such as liver disease and Klinefelter's syndrome. The patient may present late because the diagnosis has not been considered. Mastectomy is the usual surgical option and tamoxifen is prescribed for ER-positive tumours (80–90% are oestrogen receptor-positive). Stage for stage, the prognosis is similar for breast cancer in men and women; male breast cancer tends to behave like postmenopausal disease in women.

Disorders of the skin

46

INTRODUCTION

Only a small proportion of skin disorders is surgically important. These include unsightly lesions, lumps and possible malignant lesions. **Ulcers** of the lower limb are common and usually of vascular or diabetic neural and/or ischaemic origin. Some venous ulcers are managed by dermatologists, but many are managed by surgeons and specialist nurses; these are discussed in Chapter 43. Ulceration is also a characteristic of many malignant skin lesions.

The initial referral is usually made to a dermatologist but skin disorders still comprise about 15% of new outpatient general surgical referrals. Many require only excision biopsy under local anaesthesia. Others patients are referred for advice after a skin lesion has been excised by a family practitioner.

A small proportion has a potentially sinister course, particularly malignant melanoma which must be accurately diagnosed and treated. Suspected malignant skin lesions are often managed jointly by dermatologists or surgeons (including plastic surgeons) and oncologists.

Malignant melanomas comprise only 2% of skin cancers in Northern Europe but, like basal cell and squamous cell carcinomas, their incidence correlates with sun exposure and fair skin. Skin malignancies and premalignant stages are much more common in sunny countries like Australia where they have reached epidemic proportions; also the frequency of all skin cancers is rising with increasing foreign travel.

Finally, the nails, which are specialised skin appendages, pose surgical problems in the form of infected **ingrowing toenails** and **onychogryphosis**. The rare **subungual melanoma** is an important diagnosis which must not be missed.

STRUCTURE OF NORMAL SKIN (Fig. 46.1)

The skin has three main layers, **epidermis**, **dermis** and **hypodermis**:

- The epidermis has four layers—basal, prickle-cell, granular and keratin. Cell division normally occurs only in the basal layer
- The dermis consists of dense, tough interlacing collagen fibres; their orientation determines lines of skin tension known as **Langer's lines**. These are surgically important because incisions parallel to them heal with minimal scarring
- The deepest layer of the skin is the **hypodermis**, consisting of loose fibro-fatty tissue and containing skin appendages—sweat glands, hair follicles and associated sebaceous glands. The skin is generally mobile over deeper structures because the hypodermis is only loosely connected to the **superficial fascia**, but is tightly bound to fascia in the palms, the soles of the feet and the scalp.

SYMPTOMS AND SIGNS OF SKIN DISORDERS

The most common complaint is a lump. This may be tender or painful, and it may bleed, discharge or ulcerate. The lesion may be pigmented or have changed colour. It may have appeared suddenly or enlarged rapidly, or a longstanding lesion may have changed. Another reason for surgical referral is *hyperhidrosis* or excessive sweating.

The most frequent patient complaint is the ugliness or inconvenience of a lesion (e.g. in the way of a strap).

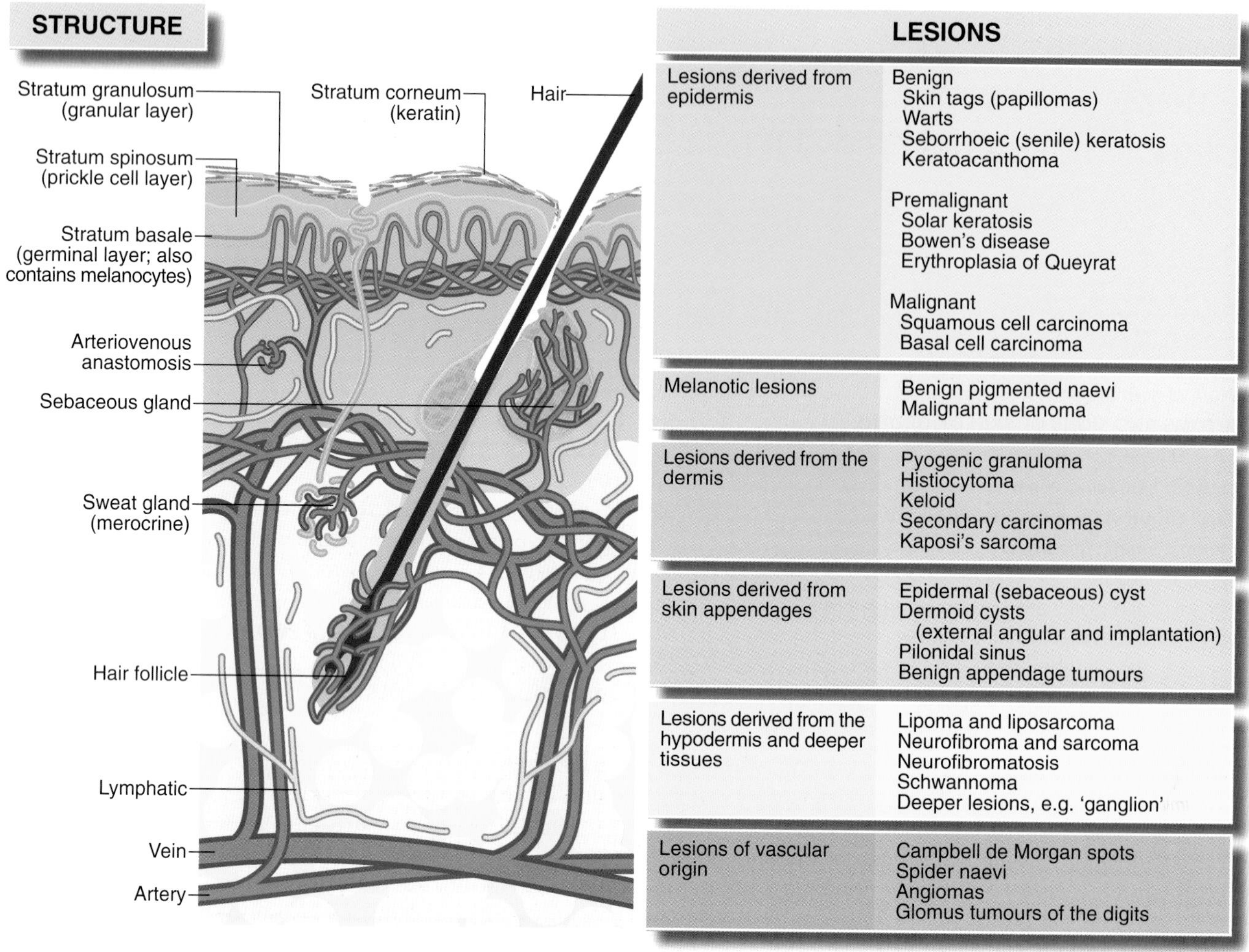

Fig. 46.1 Structure of the skin and lesions of surgical importance

Elderly patients often come reluctantly at the insistence of younger relatives. Some present late when a lesion is huge, while others present with trivial lesions. Either may fear malignancy.

In practice (and in clinical exams) skin lesion diagnosis rarely follows the pattern of history, examination and investigation. Rather, the lesion is thrust before the doctor's eyes and a 'spot' or differential diagnosis is made. History and examination then help confirm the diagnosis or narrow the possibilities. Table 46.1 summarises the clinical features of skin lesions and their diagnostic significance.

HISTORY AND EXAMINATION

As the patient describes the problem, the lesion is usually offered for examination which may guide the direction and emphasis of history taking. The patient should be questioned about sun exposure and about other similar lesions or any regional lumps. Detailed inspection and palpation follow, leading to a diagnosis or narrow differential diagnosis.

A **general history** must be taken to ascertain any relevant systemic symptoms (e.g. weight loss), concurrent disorders (e.g. diabetes predisposes to infection and influences surgical management), a history of previous similar lesions, surgical treatment or trauma to the area. For example, a history of rodent ulcers (basal cell carcinoma) makes this diagnosis more likely next time. Previous surgery or trauma can lead to *implantation epidermoids* or a chronic inflammatory response to a foreign body.

Family history is valuable in rare genetic disorders such as neurofibromatosis and tuberous sclerosis. **Social history** should include occupational details. For example, natal cleft pilonidal sinus is more common in truck drivers. Exposure to carcinogens such as lubricating oils persistently spilt on clothing may cause squamous carcinoma. Outdoor workers, especially in the tropics, are predisposed to all skin cancers. Chronic ulcers may be contracted during foreign travel, e.g. tropical ulcers, Madura foot, tuberculous or atypical mycobacterial ulcers. Patients sometimes deliberately injure themselves, producing odd chronic 'artefactual' lesions; a **psychiatric history** is valuable here, though rarely forthcoming.

Drug history is rarely relevant, though agents applied topically, e.g. silver nitrate stick, caustic agents and contact dermatitis to adhesive dressings can distort the clinical picture.

Table 46.1 Symptoms and signs of skin disorders

Symptoms and signs	Diagnostic significance
1. Lump in or on the skin Size, shape and surface features Revealed by inspection—is the lesion smooth-surfaced, irregular, exophytic (i.e. projecting out of the surface)?	Epidermal lesions such as warts usually have a surface abnormality but deeper lesions are usually covered by normal epidermis. A punctum suggests the abnormality arises from an epidermal appendage, e.g. epidermal (sebaceous) cyst
Depth within the skin Superficial and deep attachments Which tissue is the swelling derived from?	Tends to reflect the layer from which lesion is derived and therefore the range of differential diagnosis (i.e. epidermis, dermis, hypodermis or deeper)
Character of the margin Discreteness, tethering to surrounding tissues, three-dimensional shape	A regular shaped, discrete lesion is most likely cystic or encapsulated (e.g. benign tumour). Deep tethering implies origin from deeper structures (e.g. ganglion). Immobility of overlying epidermis suggests a lesion derived from skin appendage (e.g. epidermal cyst)
Consistency Soft, firm, hard, 'indurated', rubbery	Soft lesions are usually lipomas or fluid-filled cysts. Most cysts are fluctuant unless filled by semi-solid material (e.g. epidermal cysts), or the cyst is tense (e.g. small ganglion) Malignant lesions tend to be hard and irregular ('indurated') with an ill-defined margin due to invasion of surrounding tissue Bony-hard lesions are either mineralised (e.g. gouty tophi) or consist of bone (e.g. exostoses)
Pulsatility	Pulsatility is usually transmitted from an underlying artery which may simply be tortuous or may be abnormal (e.g. aneurysm or arteriovenous fistula)
Emptying and refilling	Vascular lesions (e.g. venous malformations or haemangiomas) empty or blanch on pressure and then refill
Transilluminability	Lesions filled with clear fluid such as cysts 'light up' when transilluminated
Temperature	Excessive warmth implies acute inflammation, e.g. pilonidal abscess
2. Pain, tenderness and discomfort	These symptoms often indicate acute inflammation. Pain also develops if a non-inflammatory lesion becomes inflamed or infected (e.g. inflamed epidermal cyst). Malignant lesions are usually painless
3. Ulceration (i.e. loss of epidermal integrity with an inflamed base formed by dermis or deeper tissues)	Malignant lesions and keratoacanthomas tend to ulcerate as a result of central necrosis. Surface breakdown also occurs in arterial or venous insufficiency (e.g. ischaemic leg ulcers), chronic infection (e.g. TB or tropical ulcers) or trauma, particularly in an insensate foot
Character of the ulcer margin	Benign ulcers—the margin is only slightly raised by inflammatory oedema. The base lies below the level of normal skin Malignant ulcers—these begin as a solid mass of proliferating epidermal cells, the centre of which eventually becomes necrotic and breaks down. The margin is typically elevated 'rolled' and indurated by tumour growth and invasion
Behaviour of the ulcer	Malignant ulcers expand inexorably (though often slowly), but may go through cycles of breakdown and healing (often with bleeding)
4. Colour and pigmentation *Normal colour*	If a lesion is covered by normal-coloured skin then the lesion must lie deeply in the skin (e.g. epidermal cyst) or deep to the skin (e.g. ganglion)
Red or purple	Redness implies increased arterial vascularity, which is most common in inflammatory conditions like furuncles. Vascular abnormalities which contain a high proportion of arterial blood such as Campbell de Morgan spots or strawberry naevi are also red, whereas venous disorders such as port-wine stain are darker. Vascular lesions blanch on pressure and must be distinguished from purpura which does not
Deeply pigmented	Benign naevi (moles) and their malignant counterpart, malignant melanomas, are nearly always pigmented. Other lesions such as warts, papillomata or seborrhoeic keratoses may become pigmented secondarily. Hairy pigmented moles are almost never malignant. Rarely, malignant melanomas may be non-pigmented (amelanotic). New darkening of a pigmented lesion should be viewed with suspicion as it may indicate malignant change

Continued

Table 46.1 Continued

Symptoms and signs	Diagnostic significance
5. Rapidly developing lesion	Keratoacanthoma, warts and pyogenic granuloma may all develop rapidly and eventually regress spontaneously. When fully developed, these conditions may be difficult to distinguish from malignancy. Spontaneous regression marks the lesion as benign
6. Multiple, recurrent and spreading lesions	In certain rare syndromes, multiple similar lesions develop over a period. Examples include neurofibromatosis and recurrent lipomata in Dercum's disease. Prolonged or intense sun exposure predisposes a large area of skin to malignant change. Viral warts may appear in crops. Malignant melanoma may spread diffusely (superficial spreading melanoma) or produce satellite lesions via dermal lymphatics
7. Site of the lesion	Some skin lesions arise much more commonly in certain areas of the body. The reason may be anatomical (e.g. pilonidal sinus, external angular dermoid or multiple pilar cysts of the scalp) or because of exposure to sun (e.g. solar keratoses or basal cell carcinomas of hands and face)
8. Age when lesion noticed	Congenital vascular abnormalities such as strawberry naevus or port-wine stain may be present at birth. Benign pigmented naevi (moles) may be detectable at birth, but only begin to enlarge and darken after the age of 2

Check if the patient is taking warfarin or aspirin since they may increase the risk of perioperative haemorrhage.

The lesion is examined in detail, looking for the points in Table 46.1. General clinical examination searches for other similar lesions, regional lymphadenopathy or a primary malignancy arising elsewhere and metastasising to skin. For example, if inguinal lymph nodes are enlarged, rectal and genital examination should be carried out to exclude concealed carcinoma. The lower limbs, including the soles of the feet, should also be examined for malignant melanoma.

PRINCIPLES OF MANAGING SKIN LESIONS

Many skin lesions can be diagnosed from the history and clinical examination, but where there is doubt, biopsy is needed, particularly if there is risk of malignancy. Excision biopsy is treatment if the lesion is small. Incision and excision biopsy techniques are illustrated in Chapter 10, p. 136 and Box 46.1 summarises surgical options for skin conditions.

For axillary **hyperhidrosis**, the most effective and least risky option is injections of botulinum toxin into axillary skin. This needs to be repeated at 6–9-monthly intervals. Local excision of axillary sweat glands is another popular surgical option. For palmar hyperhidrosis unresponsive to dermatological management, thoracoscopic destruction of upper thoracic sympathetic nerves is highly effective.

Box 46.1 Principles of management of 'surgical' skin lesions

Simple excision or other physical methods, e.g. electrocautery, laser therapy or cryotherapy—for small, obviously innocent lesions

Excision biopsy—if there is any risk of malignancy or the clinical diagnosis is doubtful (only for small lesions)

Biopsy—for large lesions. Definitive therapy is then planned according to the histology

Wide local excision with or without skin grafting—for malignant melanomas and sometimes for other large malignant lesions

Radiotherapy—an alternative to excision for basal cell carcinoma and primary squamous cell lesions. Also sometimes used if regional lymph nodes are involved in squamous cell carcinoma

Topical chemotherapy—with 5-fluorouracil cream for certain skin malignancies

Photodynamic therapy—for certain skin malignancies. Malignant cells absorb a photosensitising chemical which reacts with light of a particular wavelength to destroy the cells

Surgical lymph node clearance—if nodes are involved by malignant melanoma or squamous carcinoma

LESIONS ORIGINATING IN THE EPIDERMIS

BENIGN EPIDERMAL LESIONS

SKIN TAGS (SQUAMOUS CELL PAPILLOMAS)

Skin tags are small benign polypoid lesions up to 5 mm across consisting of loose connective tissue covered by normal, often pigmented, keratinised epithelium. Common in adults, they may occur anywhere, particularly the trunk, neck, axillae and groins; they may be irritated by clothing and bleed. Lesions are easily removed by cryotherapy (freezing), cautery or excision (under local anaesthesia), or by tying a fine thread around the stalk (also under local anaesthesia) which leads to ischaemic atrophy.

WARTS

Warts are small, virus-induced epidermal tumours characterised pathologically by irregular thickening of the epidermis with excessive keratinisation and exaggerated dermal papillae. The morphology depends on the location.

The **common wart** (verruca vulgaris), a papilliferous lesion up to 1 cm in diameter, is most often found on the fingers and back of the hands. In children, warts are often multiple and can occur on the face. Facial lesions are often less keratotic with a smoother, more dome-like shape. They are often called **juvenile or plane warts** (verruca plana juvenilis). Lesions on the sole of the foot, **plantar warts** (verruca plantaris), become very keratotic and flattened by pressure. They may extend deeply into the foot, causing pain. Warts may also occur on the genitalia, perineum and perianal area. These originate with papilloma virus infection and are usually spread by sexual contact. Genital warts sometimes grow to a large size and are then known as **condylomata acuminata**.

Warts are frequently seen in immune-suppressed patients. They grow and regress spontaneously over several months, but often require treatment to relieve pain, irritation or inconvenience or for aesthetic reasons. Keratolytic applications (salicylic acid or podophyllin resin preparations), cryosurgery (liquid nitrogen application) or topical imiquimod are often the first choice of treatment. If unsuccessful, electrocautery (with or without curettage) and simple excision can be used.

SEBORRHOEIC KERATOSIS

Seborrhoeic keratoses (**seborrhoeic warts**) are very common in elderly patients but occasionally appear in younger people (Fig. 46.2). They are most common on the trunk, face, neck and arms, often with many different sized lesions with varying pigmentation. They may be up to several centimetres in diameter. The lesions are slightly raised, sharply demarcated and plaque-like; they look and feel irregular and waxy. Darkly pigmented lesions cannot be distinguished clinically from superficial spreading malignant melanomas.

Histologically, a seborrhoeic keratosis is a localised proliferation of the epidermal basal layer. There is often hyperkeratosis in surface crypts, resulting in round keratin nests. Seborrhoeic keratoses are sometimes called **basal cell papillomas**, but are not true neoplasms and are unrelated to basal cell carcinoma.

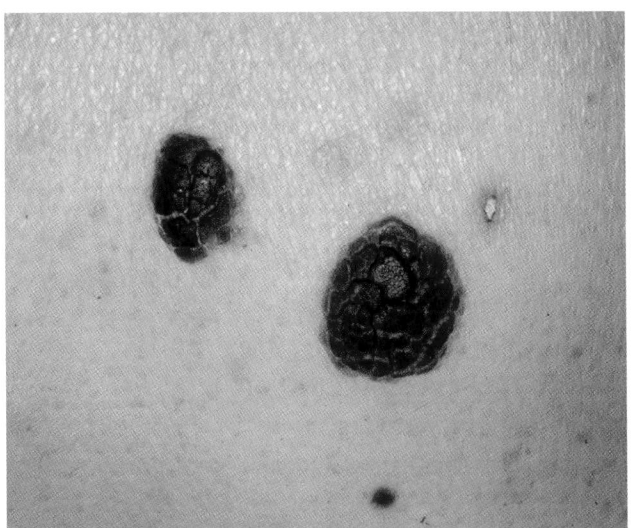

Fig. 46.2 Seborrhoeic keratoses

Treatment is only required for unsightly or easily traumatised lesions. As they are so superficial, they can be 'scraped off' with a curette or scalpel under local anaesthesia. Cryotherapy is used but caution is needed in patients with dark skin, since enthusiastic cryotherapy can lead to permanent loss of pigmentation.

KERATOACANTHOMA

Keratoacanthoma is a nodular, single skin lesion, up to 2 cm across (Fig. 46.3b, c). They have an irregular central crater containing keratotic debris. The histological lesion consists of localised tumour-like epidermal proliferation, with a thick prickle cell layer (**acanthosis**) and marked keratinisation. Some epithelial cells are large with atypical nuclei; the underlying dermis exhibits chronic inflammatory cell infiltration.

This benign lesion can be difficult to distinguish clinically or even histologically from squamous carcinoma. Keratoacanthomas, however, have a short life cycle, appearing rapidly and regressing spontaneously over 2–3 months, whereas squamous carcinomas continue to enlarge. Keratin horns may look similar but rarely regress. The cause is unknown but its behaviour suggests a viral origin.

Diagnosis and treatment is by local excision unless the lesion is obviously regressing. If there is diagnostic doubt, the patient should be followed up as for squamous carcinoma.

MELANOTIC LESIONS

Benign naevi

Deeper layers of the epidermis contain scattered melanocytes that synthesise melanin which is transferred to nearby epidermal cells where it is responsible for skin colour. Melanocyte concentration is similar in all races but pigmentation depends on the quantity of melanin produced. Although skin colour is determined mainly by genetic factors, it is enhanced by exposure to ultraviolet rays of sunlight (tanning).

Melanocytes originate from the neural crest and migrate to ectoderm during embryological development. Hamartomatous accumulations of melanocytes in the epidermis or dermis or both form raised, variably pigmented lesions known as **naevi** or **moles**.

Lesions range from about 3 to 30 mm in diameter. The surface may be smooth or irregular and may contain hairs. According to clinical and histological features, naevi can be subdivided into five types: **junctional, intradermal, compound, blue** and **Spitz or spindle cell (juvenile) naevi**. The first three are closely related pathologically. Their main surgical importance is distinguishing them from malignant melanoma.

Lentigo

Lentigines (the plural of lentigo) are benign pigmented lesions that feature in the differential diagnosis of melanotic lesions. They are large, heavily pigmented patches on the face and hands of the elderly. Melanocytes are numerous, and melanin

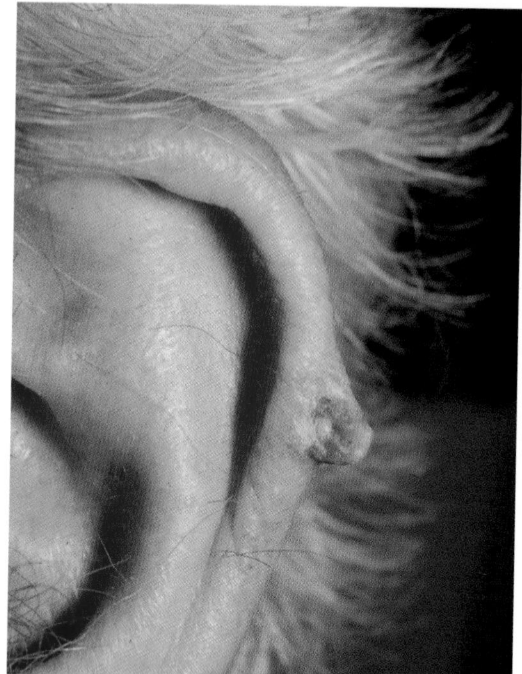
(a)

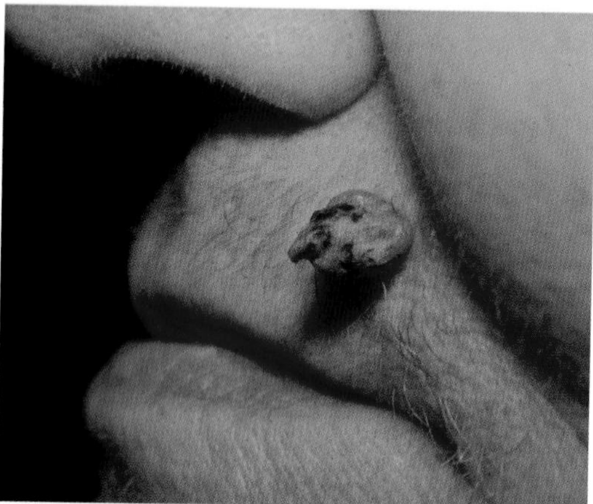
(b)

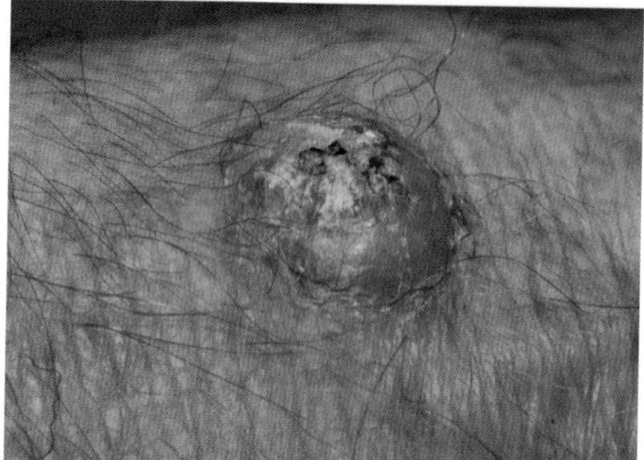
(c)

Fig. 46.3 Keratin horn and keratoacanthoma
(a) Keratin horn on the pinna of an elderly man. If untreated, these can grow large. **(b)** This alarming looking lesion is a benign keratoacanthoma. The central keratin plug is characteristic. Resolution is spontaneous after a few weeks. **(c)** Similar lesion on the back of the hand. Squamous and basal cell carcinoma need to be excluded

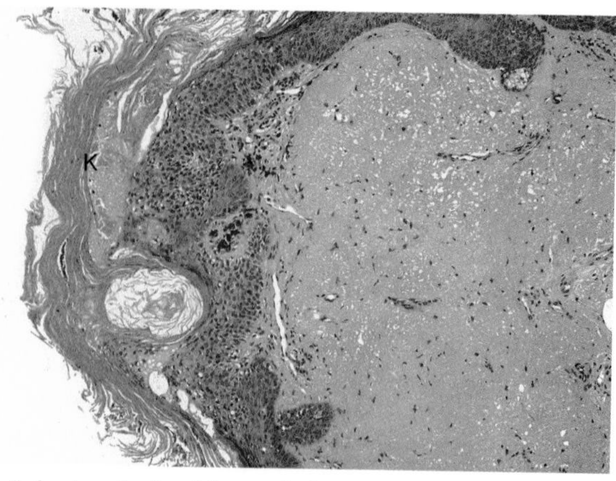

Fig. 46.4 Solar keratosis—histopathology
Occurring in sun-exposed areas, this lesion typically shows thickening of the keratin layer **K**. Epidermal cells can show a range of atypia, which may amount to squamous cell carcinoma-in-situ. The dermis shows severe solar damage

production is excessive but there is no accumulation of naevus cells. Lentigines are benign but predispose to superficial spreading malignant melanoma.

MANAGEMENT OF PIGMENTED LESIONS

People are more aware that pigmented lesions can be malignant, and large numbers now seek medical advice. Fortunately, only a small proportion has melanomas. With suspicion of malignancy, specialist dermatological opinion should be sought. A surgeon becomes involved if more than simple excision or biopsy is necessary.

It can be difficult to clinically differentiate different types of benign naevi, and to exclude malignancy; however, **dermoscopy** (dermatoscopy), i.e. examining the skin using surface microscopy, is useful in expert hands in distinguishing benign and malignant pigmented lesions. Note that if there is a recent change in a lesion or any doubt about its nature, excision biopsy is mandatory. In practice, if patient or doctor is worried about a pigmented lesion, no matter how benign it looks, it is usually removed. Lesions subject to chronic irritation (e.g. at the waist, neck or palm) or in a site that is difficult to observe (e.g. sole of foot or genitalia) should certainly be removed. A fusiform incision with a narrow margin of normal tissue (2–3 mm) removes the lesion, enabling the skin edges to be readily opposed. All excised pigmented lesions should be examined histologically because a few benign-looking lesions may turn out to be malignant.

PREMALIGNANT AND MALIGNANT EPIDERMAL CONDITIONS

SOLAR (SENILE) KERATOSIS AND INTRA-EPIDERMAL CARCINOMA

Pathology and clinical features

Solar keratoses are flat, well-demarcated, brown, scaly or crusty lesions with an erythematous base (Fig. 46.4). They bleed easily if traumatised or scratched. Solar keratoses are often multiple and are most common in later life on

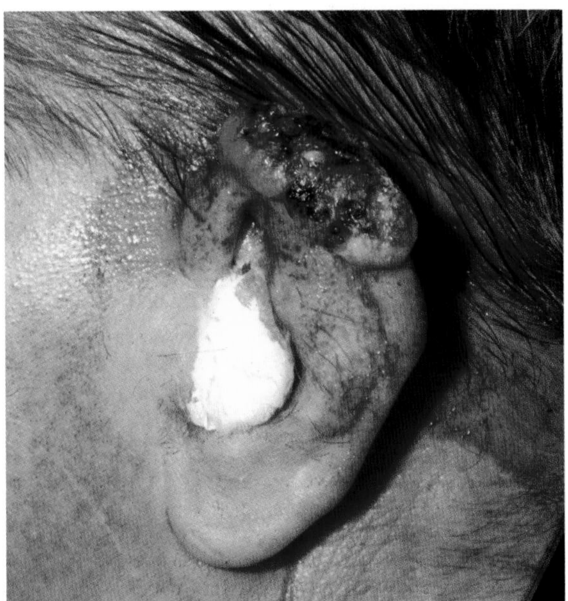
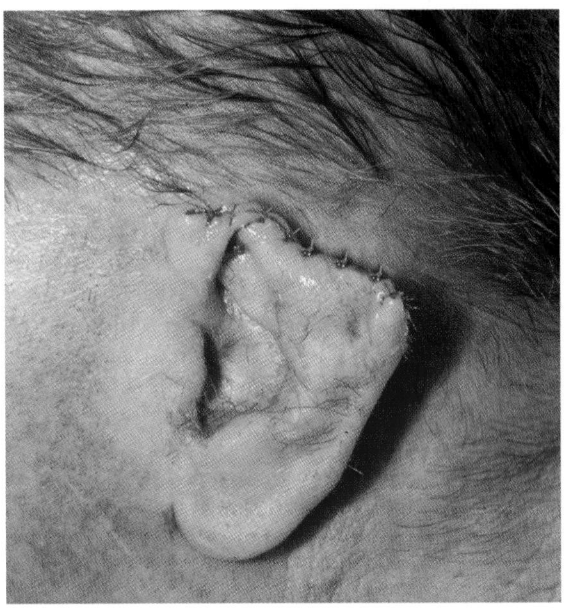

(a) (b)

Fig. 46.5 Squamous carcinoma (a) This 70-year-old farmer had worked in the fields exposed to the sun all his life. He presented with this obviously malignant lesion on the upper part of the pinna. It was confirmed on biopsy to be a well-differentiated squamous cell carcinoma **(b)** after local resection

sun-exposed parts such as face, neck, arms and hands. The incidence is higher in farm workers, fishermen and other outdoor workers. Solar keratoses are especially common in fair-skinned people living in tropical or subtropical regions like Australia or the southern USA.

Characteristic histological features are marked thickening of the keratin layer (**hyperkeratosis**) and prickle cell layer (**acanthosis**). There is a variable degree of dysplastic change and abnormal mitotic activity deep in the epidermis. These features suggest malignant transformation but, importantly, the basal layer remains intact.

The epidemiology and pathology of solar keratosis suggest it is a premalignant condition predisposing to squamous carcinoma. Lesions in which dysplastic changes extend from the basal layers to the surface (full thickness) are considered to be malignant and termed **carcinoma-in-situ** or **intra-epidermal carcinoma**. Clinically, these are larger and more erythematous than the common type and are described as **Bowen's disease**. Bowen's disease on the glans penis is known as **erythroplasia of Queyrat**.

Management

Management depends on number, size and distribution, age of the patient, and whether the skin type predisposes to cancer. Isolated lesions are best excised. For multiple keratoses, excision biopsy of representative lesions is performed initially to confirm the diagnosis, followed by topical 5-fluorouracil cream, diclofenac gel or imiquimod cream, or by excision biopsy, curettage or cryotherapy of suspicious lesions. Patients should be repeatedly advised to minimise exposure to UV rays by wearing protective clothing and hats and applying high factor total (UVA + UVB) sunscreen creams. Patients should be regularly examined for squamous cell carcinomas, basal cell carcinomas and melanomas, all more common with marked sunshine exposure.

SQUAMOUS CELL CARCINOMA

Pathology

Squamous cell carcinomas (SCCs, Fig. 46.5) occur anywhere on the skin or stratified squamous epithelium of the mouth, tongue, oesophagus, anal canal, glans penis or uterine cervix. Squamous cell carcinoma also occurs in metaplastic squamous epithelium in bronchus, oesophagus or bladder.

Skin SCCs usually occur in older age groups, in areas of skin exposed repeatedly to ultraviolet light. Often, they develop from pre-existing **solar (senile) keratoses**.

Rarely nowadays, squamous carcinoma develops in skin chronically exposed to **industrial carcinogens** such as ionising radiation, arsenic or chromium compounds, soot, tar, pitch or mineral oils. For example, carcinoma of the scrotum was common in chimney sweeps in the nineteenth century; recognising soot as the predisposing factor was a milestone in understanding carcinogenesis.

Chronic inflammation also predisposes to squamous carcinoma, which rarely develops at the margins of osteomyelitic sinuses or longstanding ulcers. These are common in developing countries where burns are poorly treated. A chronic burns ulcer in which carcinoma arises is known as a **Marjolin's ulcer**.

Histologically, squamous cell carcinomas of the skin are usually well differentiated, and tumour cells resemble normal prickle cells. Keratin pearls and individual cell keratinisation are common.

Clinical presentation

Squamous cell carcinoma usually presents as an enlarging painless ulcer with a rolled, indurated (hardened) margin. Other lesions have an exophytic (outward growing, proliferative) cauliflower-like appearance with areas of ulceration, bleeding or serous exudation. SCCs invade the dermis and deeper tissues such as bone or cartilage; further spread is usually to regional lymph nodes. Distant metastases are relatively uncommon.

Management of squamous cell carcinoma

Management involves first confirming the diagnosis by biopsy, then local radiotherapy or excision with a margin of normal tissue. For certain SCCs, including recurrences, at sites where conserving normal tissue is important for cosmetic or functional reasons, as well as for SCCs whose edges cannot be clearly defined, a special technique known as **Mohs' micrographic surgery** is often employed. Under local anaesthesia, this involves frozen section histology of sequential horizontal sections. If malignant cells remain, further sections are removed until clear of malignancy.

Infiltrated lymph nodes are treated with **radiotherapy** or sometimes **block dissection** (i.e. removing all regional nodes in a single block of tissue). In general, these tumours respond favourably to radiotherapy and recurrence is unusual.

Prognosis is less good for tumours larger than 2 cm, recurrent lesions, lesions arising in pre-existing scars, on the skin of the lips, ears and scrotum, and lesions with poor histological differentiation or perineural invasion. These patients are usually reviewed regularly for about 5 years after treatment.

BASAL CELL CARCINOMA (BCC)

Pathology and clinical features

Basal cell carcinomas are common and nearly always result from exposure to excess ultraviolet in sunlight. White-skinned people in tropical and sub-tropical regions have an extremely high incidence, with up to 50% affected at some time, often with multiple lesions. As with SCCs, basal cell carcinomas usually develop from middle age onwards, but incidence is rising in younger 'sun-worshippers'. Males are affected at least twice as often as females, reflecting greater occupational and recreational exposure to the sun.

Most BCCs arise on the upper part of the face (Figure 46.6), although any part of the skin can be involved. Most patients present early because lesions are so visible.

Basal cell carcinomas begin as small pearly-white nodules with visible telangiectatic blood vessels (Fig. 46.7). Early lesions may ulcerate, bleed and then heal again, but eventually they form irregular ulcers (**rodent ulcers**) with a pearly rolled margin. Although BCCs almost never metastasise they are definitely malignant, and will invade underlying bone and cartilage. Neglected lesions on the scalp or neck may even invade brain or spinal cord.

Histologically, tumour cells have strongly basophilic nuclei and little cytoplasm. Cells at the periphery are arranged in a palisade pattern reminiscent of normal basal cells.

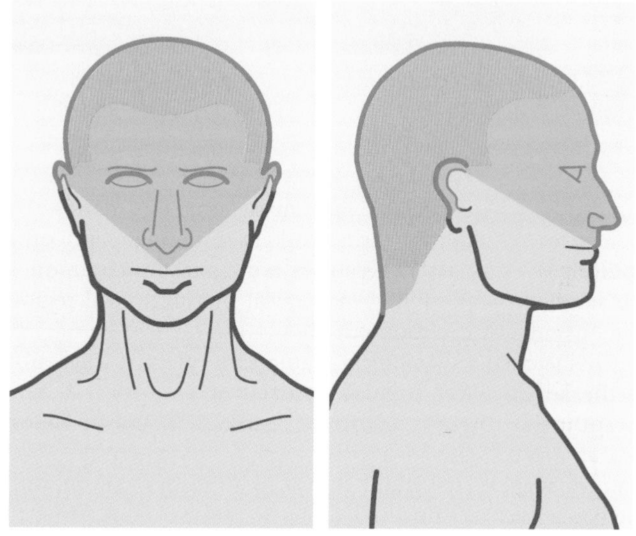

Fig. 46.6 Highest risk area for basal cell carcinomas shown in pink

CASE HISTORY

Fig. 46.7 Basal cell carcinoma (BCC)

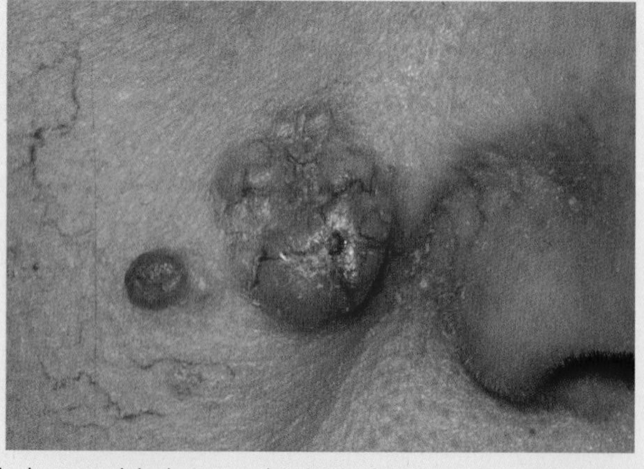

(a)

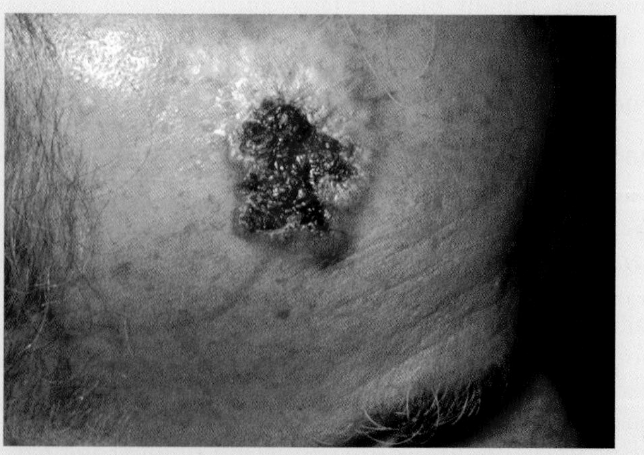

(b)

(a) The larger nodular lesion on the cheek of this woman aged 77 is a typical BCC. Note the pearly appearance of the lesion which is beginning to ulcerate. In this position, treatment with radiotherapy avoids distortion of the nasolabial fold. The smaller lesion lateral to the BCC is a benign naevus. **(b)** Large BCC on the scalp of an elderly farm worker. Again, the typical pearly edge can be seen. After confirming the diagnosis on an incision biopsy of the edge, this was treated with radiotherapy

Management of basal cell carcinomas

Small lesions are usually treated by cryotherapy without histology. Other treatments include topical chemotherapy with 5-fluorouracil or imiquimod cream, local radiotherapy or 2–3 cycles of curettage combined with electrocautery. Excision biopsy may be appropriate for isolated or suspicious lesions. Radiotherapy must be used with caution on nose or ear where cartilage is susceptible to radiotherapy damage and may undergo necrosis. Larger destructive lesions usually require reconstructive plastic surgery involving skin grafts or flaps.

Photodynamic therapy (PDT) employs topical **methyl amino-levulinate cream** and light therapy. The drug is selectively absorbed by cancer cells and converted into photoactive porphyrins. When cancer cells loaded with porphyrins are exposed to light of wavelength 570–670 nm, a molecular reaction destroys them. This selectively targets tumour cells whilst leaving normal cells unharmed. It is recommended for solar keratoses and basal cell carcinomas situated on the mid-face or ears, those on severely sun-damaged skin, particularly the lower legs of elderly patients, large lesions or recurrent lesions. Clinical trials have shown it gives cure rates at least as good as cryotherapy and surgery. It leaves minimal scarring and gives excellent cosmetic results.

As with squamous cell carcinomas, Mohs' micrographic surgery may be indicated for recurrent BCCs where conservation of normal tissue is important, or for BCCs where the edges cannot be clearly defined.

Fig. 46.8 Malignant melanoma

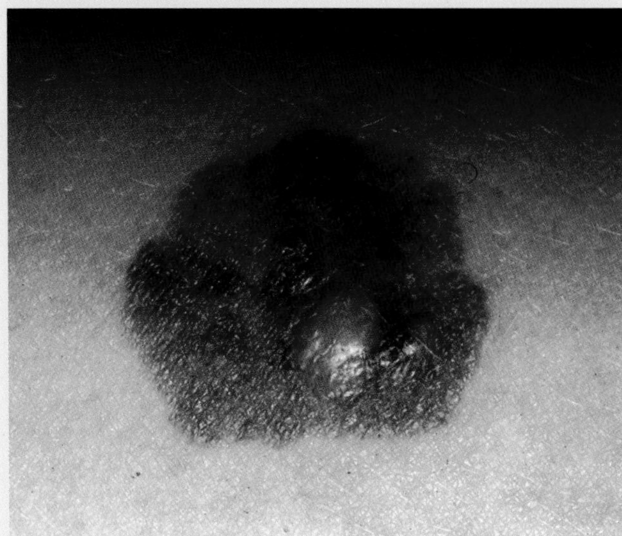

Pigmented lesion of the forearm in a 33-year-old woman. A small black lesion had been present for many years before starting to spread to reach its present diameter of 2.5 cm. Histologically, this proved to be a mixed type of malignant melanoma with both 'superficial spreading' and nodular elements

MALIGNANT MELANOMA

Introduction and pathology

Malignant melanoma (Fig. 46.8) arises by malignant transformation of melanocytes. Most are poorly differentiated, with numerous mitotic figures, and the presence of melanin is diagnostic. Suspected **amelanotic** (non-pigmented) **melanomas** may need to be confirmed by immunohistochemical tests.

Malignant melanoma is a common cancer with the peak incidence in the fourth decade of life. World incidence is rising substantially and in the UK, diagnosed new cases rose by 50% between 1990 and 2000. In 2008 around 11 770 new cases were registered, compared with 98 800 non-melanoma skin cancers. There have been improvements in 5-year survival for melanoma patients from about 40% in the 1940s to about 80% now. In 2008 in the UK, 2560 people died from skin cancer, around 2070 from malignant melanoma.

In particular, melanomas of less than 1 mm Breslow thickness (see later) have a 95–100% 5-year survival rate. Improved survival is due to greater public awareness, earlier detection and better treatment.

Risk factors

The epidemiology of malignant melanoma is fascinating. About 80% occur in white-skinned people and the disease is extremely common in albinos of all races. Until recently, malignant melanoma was rare in northern Europe but the incidence has risen sharply over the last three decades. About 1 in 100 Americans will be affected some time in their lives. The highest incidence is in northern and western Australia and it is certain ultraviolet radiation is the essential aetiological factor. Whilst cumulative sun is the main factor for other skin malignancies, short periods of intense exposure causing blistering sunburn appear to be more important for malignant melanoma. There is evidence that unaccustomed exposure to strong sunlight can suppress general immunological responses and, by implication, immunological tumour surveillance. This might explain malignant melanomas on skin not generally exposed to the sun, for example the soles of the feet or anal canal.

Other risk factors include a family history of malignant melanoma, freckling of the upper back, red or blond hair, blue or green or grey eyes and the presence of solar (actinic) keratoses. Each of these factors increases risk by about 3.5 times.

Melanoma subtypes

Melanomas may be classified as growing radially (**superficial spreading type**) or vertically (**nodular type**). About 80% are the superficial spreading type. These grow slowly and usually arise in pre-existing pigmented naevi. Lesions are flat with a variegated border, often with patches of regression. Nodular melanomas are more common in men. They demonstrate an early vertical growth phase and develop more rapidly and behave more aggressively; they tend to arise in normal skin. Five per cent of nodular melanomas are **amelanotic**.

Lentigo maligna melanoma is uncommon and presents as large (<3 cm) lesions on the face or neck of elderly women. It has a low metastatic potential but is locally invasive; it is distinct from **lentigo maligna**, its benign but precancerous counterpart.

Acral melanoma occurs on the palms or soles or under the nails. This is the only type found in dark-skinned individuals

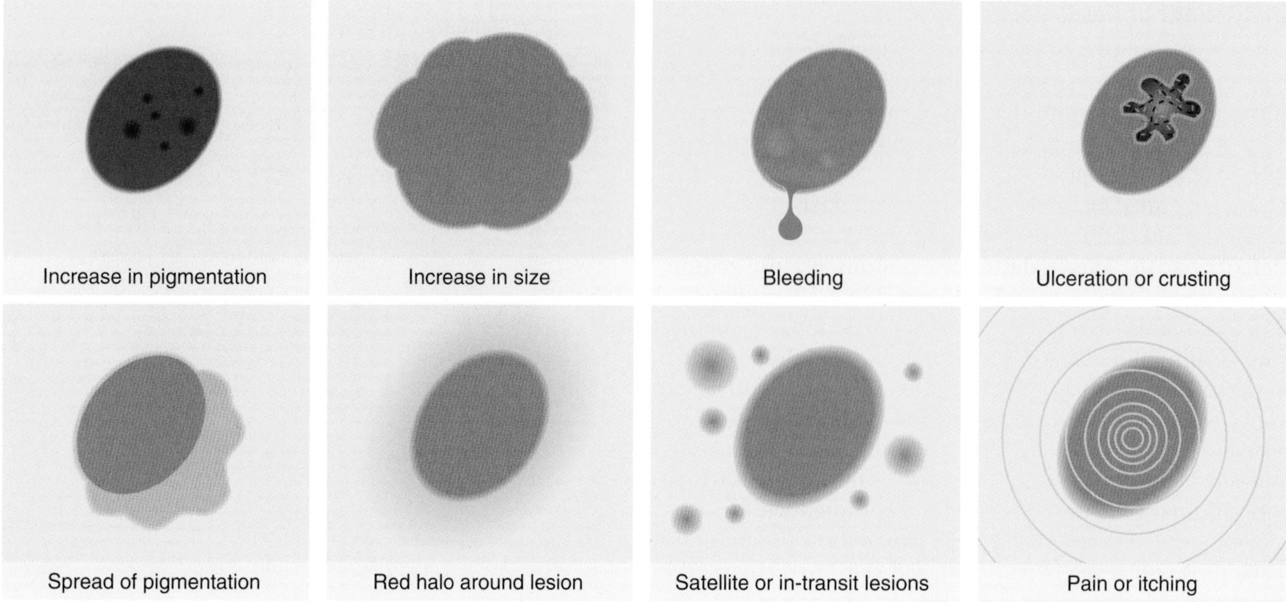

Fig. 46.9 Clinical features in a pigmented lesion that suggest malignant melanoma

and has a low incidence in white people. They occur at a mean age of 60 (see Fig. 46.19 below). Malignant melanomas in less obvious areas have a reputation for aggressive behaviour but this may be because of late diagnosis.

Mucosal melanoma occurs on any mucosal surface from mouth to anus, pharynx or paranasal sinuses or vagina. They tend to behave aggressively. **Ocular melanoma** arises from uveal melanocytes and is the most common ocular malignancy. It is unique in metastasising to the liver, often years after treatment of the primary lesion.

Clinical features of malignant melanoma

Most malignant melanomas are black or dark brown, flat or nodular lesions which may bleed or ulcerate. If a pre-existing or new mole enlarges, darkens, bleeds or becomes inflamed, ulcerated or itchy, it should be regarded with great suspicion (see Fig. 46.9). Superficial spreading melanoma can easily be mistaken for a pigmented seborrhoeic keratosis. In general, spread to regional lymph nodes occurs early. Lateral spread in dermal lymphatics may produce **satellite lesions** around the primary nodule and 'in transit' lesions may appear along the course of the lymph node drainage.

Haematogenous spread occurs later, involving lung, liver, bone, brain and other tissues. Behaviour of malignant melanoma in an individual is unpredictable, although lesions arising before puberty or in the elderly tend to be less aggressive. Rarely, disseminated lesions undergo complete spontaneous regression, signifying immunological factors are probably involved. Melanomas with marked lymphocytic infiltration on histology have a better prognosis.

Prognostic factors

Measured tumour thickness on histological examination (Breslow) is the most useful guide to prognosis (Table 46.2) and has proved more accurate than the older 'Clark's level of invasion'. Tumour thickness correlates well with the likelihood of regional and distant metastases (Table 46.2). Other factors affecting prognosis include:

Table 46.2 Risk of regional and distant metastasis in malignant melanoma according to Breslow thickness

Tumour thickness	Risk of regional metastases	Risk of distant metastases	10-year survival without nodal or distant metastases
Less than 1 mm	3–5%	3–5%	95%
1–4 mm	25–60%	10–20%	60–75%
More than 4 mm	>60%	70%	45%

- The presence of 'satellite lesions' around the primary or 'in transit' lesions between primary and lymph node field—make the prognosis worse
- Ulceration of the primary lesion—increases likelihood of metastases and reduces survival
- Site of primary—head lesions carry a worse prognosis
- Gender—with thick lesions, females fare better than males
- Pathological stage—nodal or distant involvement. The number and size of lymph node metastases affects survival—a single positive node is associated with a 40% 10-year survival, falling to 13% with two or more positive. If distant metastases are present, 2-year survival is only 25%
- Certain histopathological characteristics (e.g. high mitotic rate) indicate poorer prognosis

Management of malignant melanoma

The first aim with a pigmented lesion is to establish whether it is malignant. Unless malignancy is clinically obvious, small lesions should be removed by excision biopsy and more extensive lesions sampled by incision biopsy. As a result of controlled trials, there have been two major changes in managing the local lesion. Firstly, it is no longer necessary to excise the lesion with a 5 cm margin all around and, secondly, split skin grafting is no longer regarded as essential to achieve skin cover and provide early warning of local recurrence. For melanomas less than 1 mm thick, a clear margin of 1 cm is sufficient. For thicker melanomas (1.1–4 mm), excision with 2 cm clearance achieves optimum survival. For lesions thicker than 4 mm, a 3 cm clearance is believed desirable. Primary closure or the use of local rotational flaps can usually achieve skin cover.

As regards lymph nodes, **elective lymph node dissection** of palpable or ultrasonographically detected regional lymph nodes improves survival. There has been interest in sentinel node biopsy for lesions thicker than 0.75 mm. Lymphatic dye is injected to travel to and locate 'sentinel' nodes for frozen section biopsy, proceeding to node dissection if positive. However, a large controlled trial comparing this with 'watchful waiting' plus excision of nodes that become palpable showed no survival advantage.

Adjuvant therapy has improved with B-RAF inhibitors, e.g. vemurafenib. C-KIT inhibitors, e.g. imatinib, plus modified radiotherapy is under trial and may reduce local recurrence rates and even improve survival. Melanoma cells are sensitive to higher radiotherapy dose fractions than are usual (600 rad as opposed to 180 rad). Systemic cytotoxic chemotherapy gives disappointing results, but for locally advanced limb melanoma with 'in-transit' lesions and regional spread not amenable to surgical excision, hyperthermic local or limb perfusion chemotherapy may provide effective control (but not cure).

LESIONS ORIGINATING IN THE DERMIS

CYSTS

In pathological terms, cysts are epithelium-lined cavities; most represent ducts dilated by retained secretion, usually due to obstruction. In contrast, breast cysts may show epithelial hyperplasia, excessive secretion and structural distortion. Some cysts arise from ectopic epithelial remnants (dermoids) or as a result of central necrosis in a malignant epithelial mass. Cysts commonly require surgical removal (or drainage) for aesthetic reasons or to exclude malignancy.

Cysts are common in skin. Most arise from elements of hair follicles in the dermis and consist of an epithelium-lined cavity filled with viscous or semi-solid epithelial degradation products. These are **epidermal** and **pilar cysts**. Occasionally, cysts arise from developmental epithelial remnants (**dermoid cysts**) or by traumatic implantation of epithelial fragments (**implantation (epi) dermoids**).

Epidermal cysts

These are by far the most common skin cysts, and are often incorrectly described as '**sebaceous cysts**'. Usually solitary, they may be found anywhere on the body (except the palms or soles), most commonly scalp, trunk, face and neck. They range up to several centimetres in diameter. Epidermal cysts are smooth and rounded, and covered by normal epidermis in which a blocked duct (**punctum**) may be visible. On palpation, they have a doughy, fluctuant consistency and are not usually tender. An important clinical diagnostic feature is that since they originate in skin, they are attached to it but are mobile over deeper tissues. Multiple small epidermal cysts sometimes develop on the scrotal skin or areola and cause embarrassment.

Histologically, an epidermal cyst has a stratified squamous lining epithelium and is filled with keratin, consistent with derivation from a hair follicle. The cyst contents are thick and waxy, and were originally thought to be sebaceous material. This gave rise to the erroneous name.

Surgical removal (see Ch. 10)

Epidermal cysts are mainly removed because of recurrent inflammation. Others are removed for cosmetic reasons or sometimes because they interfere with clothing or hair combing. An incision is made over the cyst beside and around the punctum, taking care not to puncture the cavity. The cyst is enucleated by blunt dissection and delivered in its entirety. This ensures all lining epithelium is removed and prevents recurrence.

Inflamed epidermal cysts

Trauma to epidermal cysts (often unnoticed) may cause some contents to escape into surrounding tissues, eliciting an intense foreign-body inflammatory response. The patient may complain of pain, swelling, redness and even spontaneous discharge of liquefied cyst contents; this looks like pus but is sterile. These inflamed epidermal cysts are often described as 'infected' but this is rarely the case and antibiotic therapy is not indicated.

It is unwise to attempt removal of an acutely inflamed epidermal cyst because tissue planes cannot be recognised and some epithelial lining is likely to be left. If pain is severe, liquefied cyst contents should be drained by simple incision under local anaesthesia; this provides rapid symptom relief. Culture of this material rarely yields any growth. The residual smaller cyst should be excised later in the usual way as it is almost certain to flare up repeatedly if left.

Pilar cysts

Some individuals develop multiple epidermal cysts on the scalp known as pilar cysts. Multiple cysts are less common on the face or neck. Pilar cysts range from a few millimetres to many centimetres in diameter, but grow very slowly. They can easily be excised under local anaesthesia.

INFECTIVE LESIONS

PYOGENIC GRANULOMA

(*Note*: not infective in aetiology)

Pyogenic granuloma (Fig. 46.10) is a common inflammatory skin lesion that arises in response to minor penetrating foreign bodies such as splinters or thorns. It usually develops over about a week and rarely regresses spontaneously. Lesions are most common on the hands and feet but may occur on lips or gums. Pathologically, there is a mass of exuberant granulation tissue containing numerous polymorphs.

Clinically, these are solitary, reddish-blue fleshy nodules which may be polypoid. The surface may be ulcerated, making it clinically indistinguishable from amelanotic malignant melanoma. Pyogenic granulomas should be excised and the base curetted or cauterised to prevent recurrence.

FURUNCLE (BOIL) AND CARBUNCLE

A furuncle is a staphylococcal abscess that develops in a hair follicle in the dermis. Early lesions can be easily treated with topical fusidic acid. Diabetes mellitus can be a predisposing factor. The lesion rapidly enlarges and eventually 'points' at the surface, spontaneously discharging pus. The centre often contains a core of necrotic tissue. Once pus has discharged and the necrotic tissue shed, the lesion heals spontaneously; however, the necrotic core may need excising to speed healing. Drainage may be encouraged with poultices or dressings, such as magnesium sulphate paste, said to draw the pus to the surface by osmosis. Furuncles are most common in young men with acne, especially on the face, back of the trunk and lower limbs. Axillary furuncles are common in middle-aged females and tend to recur. Surgical drainage is necessary if a chronic abscess develops. A furuncle may be the source of systemic sepsis, especially in uncontrolled diabetes. **Cavernous sinus thrombosis** is a rare but very serious (and often fatal) complication of a furuncle on the lateral aspect of the nose or infra-orbital area. This area drains into the cavernous sinus via the facial vein and inferior ophthalmic veins (see Fig. 46.13).

A **carbuncle**, also staphylococcal, is larger than a furuncle and consists of a honeycomb of abscesses, often draining (inadequately) via multiple sinuses. The back (nape) of the neck is the usual site (Fig. 46.11); here the skin is tightly bound by interlacing bundles of fibrous tissue. Carbuncles are more likely to occur in diabetics, and may bring diabetes to light. Treatment is with anti-staphylococcal antibiotics such as flucloxacillin as early as possible. The aim is to minimise pus formation and necrosis that would lead to skin loss and delay healing. If pus has formed, thorough desloughing and drainage of the abscesses is required, usually leaving wounds open to heal by secondary intention.

NECROTISING FASCIITIS

This serious and alarming condition is usually a complication of surgery or traumatic wounds and is covered in Chapter 3.

CASE HISTORY

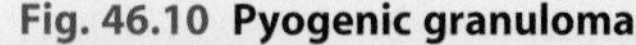

Fig. 46.10 Pyogenic granuloma

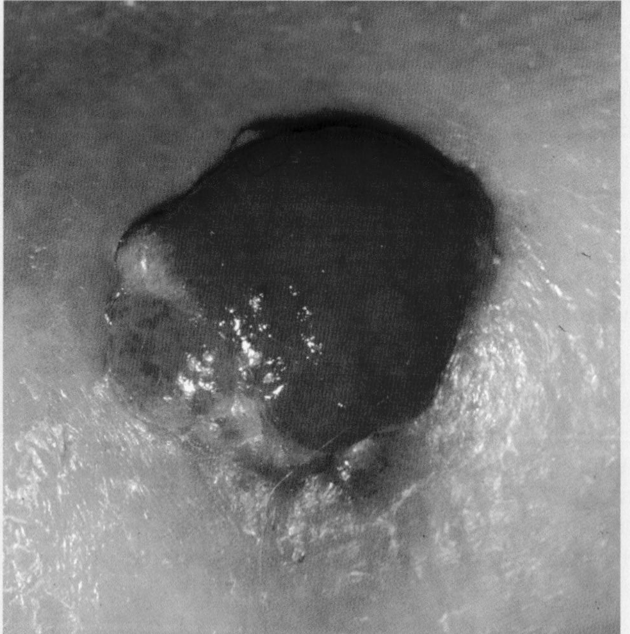

This man of 29 suffered a minor penetrating injury to his forearm from a piece of sharp metal. The wound did not heal as normal but produced this friable proliferative lesion. The appearance is typical of a pyogenic granuloma, composed largely of granulation tissue. It was removed by curettage under local anaesthesia and healing afterwards was uninterrupted

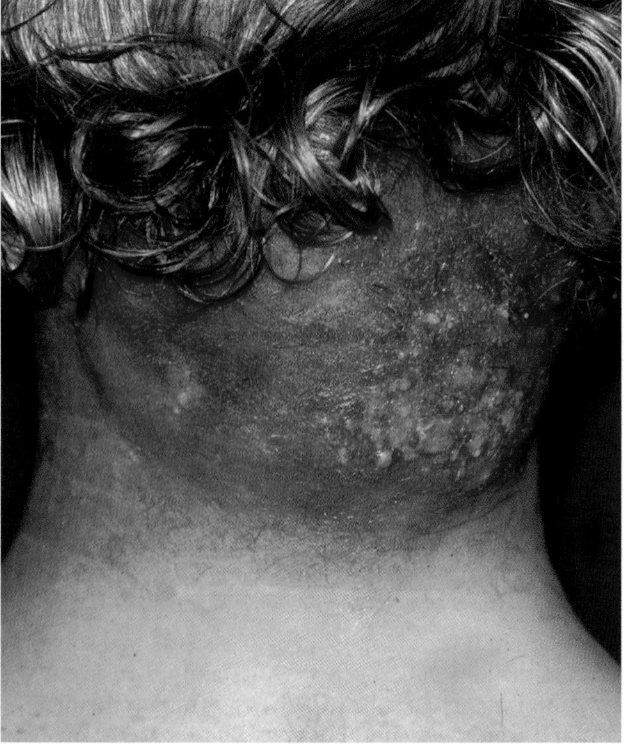

Fig. 46.11 Carbuncle on back of neck

MISCELLANEOUS LESIONS

SEBACEOUS HYPERPLASIA

Localised hyperplasia of sebaceous glands of the nose and in skin creases is common in men and women. Sebaceous glands are plentiful in this area. The condition probably reflects a mildly abnormal response to sex hormones. Apart from their unsightly appearance, these small nodular lesions may be clinically indistinguishable from basal cell carcinomas; diagnosis is made on histology after excision biopsy.

In **rhinophyma**, an extreme manifestation of sebaceous hyperplasia, the nose becomes enlarged and lumpy. It is mainly seen in older men, and is (unreliably) said to occur in heavy drinkers. Rhinophyma is treated by surgical correction, carbon dioxide laser or dermabrasion.

KELOID SCARS

Keloids are formed by excessive collagen deposition in the dermis during wound healing. The result is an elevated nodular lesion covered by normal epidermis. The chest and neck are particularly susceptible. The problem is much more common in black people.

Keloid formation may cause poor cosmetic results after injury, minor surgery, or even ear-piercing. Simply excising the lesion often makes scarring worse. Treatment is generally unsatisfactory; silicone gel under an occlusion dressing and/or intralesional steroids usually causes some regression. In extreme cases, excision of the scar followed by a low dose of local radiotherapy may suppress further keloid formation.

HISTIOCYTOMA

Histiocytomas (also known as **dermatofibromas**) are common painless skin lesions occurring mainly on the limbs. They are firm nodules, usually about 5 mm in diameter and deep reddish-brown in colour. They may be mistaken for malignant melanoma. Histologically, they contain numerous lipid-filled macrophages (**histiocytes**). One histological variant contains prominent vascular elements and has given rise to the confusing term **sclerosing angioma**.

DERMOID CYSTS

True dermoid cysts are pathologically similar to epidermal cysts, being lined by stratified squamous epithelium. As well as keratin, they can contain hair, sebaceous glands and other ectodermal structures. Dermoids are congenital lesions which arise from cystic change in epithelial remnants left at lines of embryological fusion. They are usually found in the midline of the scalp, neck and lower jaw and at the outer angle of the eyebrow (**external angular dermoid**). Treatment is by careful excision since some communicate with deeper structures and the tracts may need more extensive surgery.

IMPLANTATION (EPI)DERMOIDS

These small keratin-filled cysts arise from epidermal fragments implanted in the dermis by minor penetrating injuries. Though not derived from epidermal appendages, they are pathologically similar to epidermal cysts but may contain small foreign bodies. Implantation dermoids are most often seen on the fingers, often under the scar of a previous laceration.

MALIGNANT LESIONS

SECONDARY (METASTATIC) CARCINOMA

Metastatic tumour deposits may present as small hard painless skin nodules. They are usually located in the dermis and covered by normal epidermis. Visceral malignancy, e.g. pancreatic or colon cancer, rarely presents with a metastasis at the umbilicus (Sister Joseph's nodule). With skin metastases, there is usually a history of treated malignancy elsewhere. Lobular breast carcinomas are the most common cause, but carcinomas of stomach, uterus, lungs, large bowel and kidneys can also metastasise to skin. Occasionally, biopsy of a mysterious skin lesion leads to a diagnosis of occult malignancy.

True skin metastases are different from local spread or local implantation of cells during surgery. Laparoscopic surgery for malignancy initially acquired a bad reputation because of port sites recurrences, but improved techniques have virtually eliminated this.

Management of skin secondaries depends on the primary diagnosis but the overall prognosis is usually poor. Treatment is palliative, by local excision, radiotherapy or chemotherapy, depending on the severity of symptoms and the size, number and location of secondaries.

KAPOSI'S SARCOMA

This once rare condition has leapt to prominence as one of the most frequent presentations of **acquired immune deficiency syndrome** (AIDS). Kaposi's sarcoma (KS) is associated with human herpes virus 8. The condition appears as multiple blueish-red to brown nodules or plaques, all of which are primary tumours (Fig. 46.12). They most commonly occur on the limbs. Excision biopsy confirms the diagnosis. KS tumours are characterised by proliferating dysplastic fibroblasts, accompanied by chronic inflammation, endothelial proliferation and haemorrhage. Treatment varies: classical type KS usually does not need treatment but larger lesions respond to radiotherapy. Endemic KS is treated by chemotherapy, and AIDS-related KS is controlled by highly active antiretroviral therapy.

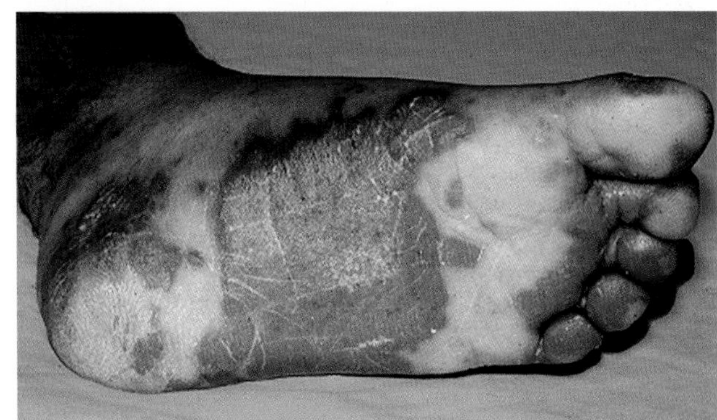

Fig. 46.12 Kaposi's sarcoma

LESIONS OF THE HYPODERMIS AND DEEPER TISSUES

CELLULITIS

Cellulitis is a diffuse spreading infection of subcutaneous tissues and deeper layers of skin. It may be acute or chronic. Beta-haemolytic streptococci, usually Lancefield group A (*Streptococcus pyogenes*), are commonly responsible. These bacteria produce fibrinolysins and hyaluronidase which break down intercellular barriers and promote spread of infection through tissue planes. Although an intense neutrophil inflammatory response develops, pus rarely accumulates. Rather, the tissues become red and oedematous. If the skin surface is broken, a serous exudate is released.

Any area of skin may develop cellulitis (Fig. 46.13), the organisms usually gaining entry via a traumatic or surgical wound, although a wound is not always found. Clinically, the skin is greatly thickened, tense, hot, red and painful; margins are fairly clearly demarcated from adjacent normal skin. Lymphatics draining the affected area become inflamed and **lymphangitis** develops. Inflamed lymphatics are visible as red streaks passing towards the regional lymph nodes, which are also swollen and tender (**lymphadenitis**). Systemic features such as fever and tachycardia indicate bacteraemia or even septicaemia.

Acute cellulitis was a serious infection in earlier times, not least as a complication of surgery. It is now readily treated with antibiotics.

CASE HISTORY

Fig. 46.13 Acute cellulitis of upper lip

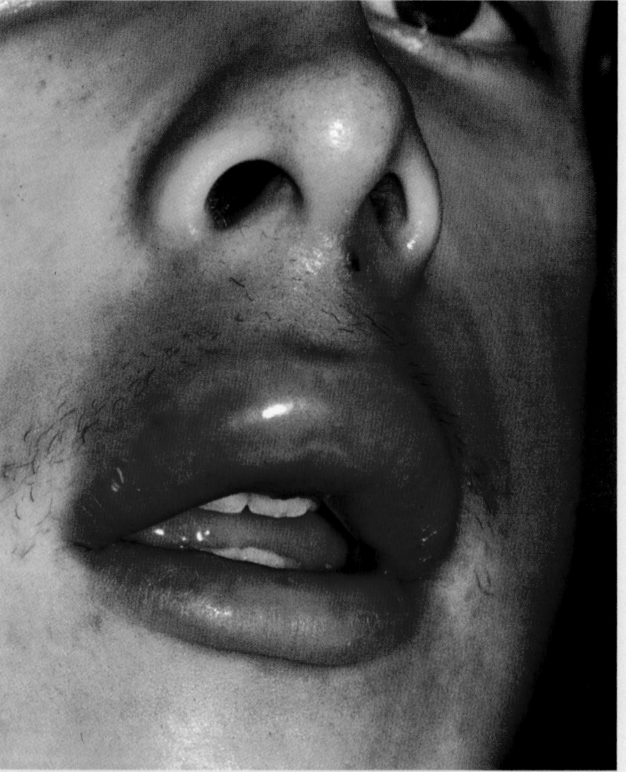

This 18-year-old presented with 4 days of increasing swelling and pain affecting the upper lip following 'picking' of an acne spot. This infection lies in the 'danger triangle' involving the nose and upper lip where serious infection can be complicated by cavernous sinus thrombosis. This patient responded rapidly to intensive antibiotic therapy. The organism proved to be *Streptococcus pyogenes*

CELLULITIS OF THE LOWER LIMB

Low-grade cellulitis can occur in the lower limb without evidence of any wound. This is usually in older women and presents as a localised, but not clearly demarcated, brawny inflammation of the leg, usually without regional lymph node involvement or systemic features of infection. Predisposing factors are lymphatic obstruction or oedema from any cause. These infections often recur and are difficult to document bacteriologically because there is no wound and no infected exudate. Nevertheless, they usually respond to antibiotics (such as tetracycline), rest, elevation of the limb, and compression stockings when the inflammation has settled. Recurrence is common at intervals of months or years.

A similar low-grade cellulitis may occur in the upper limb or chest wall as a result of lymphatic obstruction following lymph node excision or radiotherapy for breast cancer.

LIPOMA AND LIPOSARCOMA

Lipomas are benign tumours of fat. They occur anywhere fat is normally present, most often in the hypodermis of trunk and limbs. The aetiology is unknown, although mild trauma may be a factor. Typically, they present on the forearms (often multiple), in the supraclavicular fossa (Fig. 46.14), over the deltoid muscle or over the scapula. Lipomas can also be found within the peritoneal cavity, including the bowel submucosa, and within muscles or joints. They may also sometimes arise beneath periosteum.

Pathologically, lipomas consist of a multilobular mass of fatty tissue with thin fibrous septa. A tenuous fibrous capsule usually defines the lesion clearly from the surrounding tissue. Lipoma cells are histologically indistinguishable from normal adipocytes. Lipomas vary in size from about 2 to 20 cm and are shaped like a flattened dome. Overlying skin is normal. Their consistency is soft and almost fluctuant. Lipomas are removed if they are inconvenient or unsightly. If the margin is poorly defined at operation, recurrence is likely.

Liposarcoma is a rare malignant variant. It tends to occur in the retroperitoneal area and mediastinum rather than in the skin.

NEUROFIBROMA, NEUROFIBROMATOSIS AND SCHWANNOMA

Neurofibromas are benign tumours arising from the supporting fibroblasts of peripheral nerves. Tumour cells are loosely arranged in a gelatinous (myxomatous) intercellular material which often makes the lesion soft and pulpy to palpation. In the skin, neurofibromas may present as solitary sessile or

Fig. 46.14 Lipoma

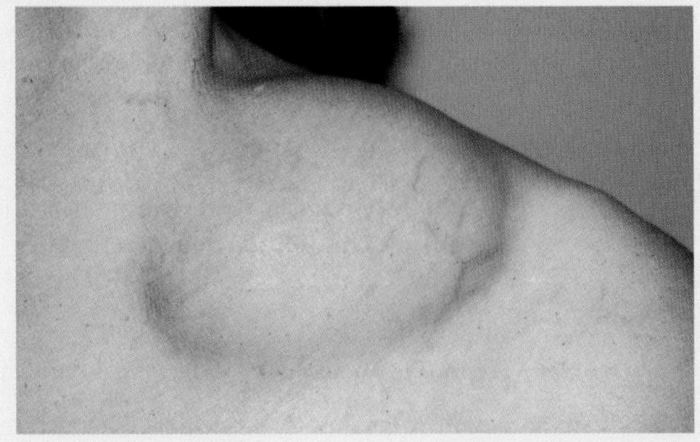

(a)

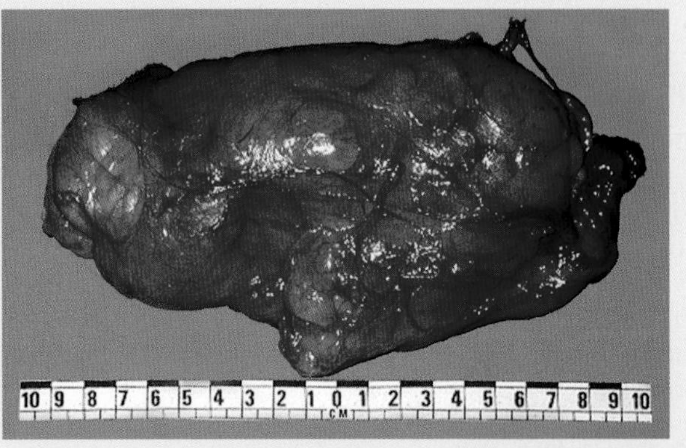

(b)

(a) Large soft lipoma overlying the supraclavicular fossa in a 46-year-old woman. This is a common site for lipomas. It had been present for many years but had recently started to enlarge. **(b)** The surgical specimen. Note that it is larger than its clinical appearance would suggest

pedunculated lesions near peripheral nerves. They are sometimes very tender.

The autosomal dominant inherited syndrome **neurofibromatosis** (von Recklinghausen's disease) is characterised by multiple neurofibromas and café-au-lait spots (coffee-coloured skin patches). Sometimes, neurofibromas are extremely numerous, and occasionally there is gross hypertrophy of subcutaneous tissues and skin folds. (This extreme variant was once thought to be the diagnosis of the famous 'elephant man' of Sir Frederick Treves; it is now believed, however, that he suffered from another inherited condition, Proteus syndrome.) A small proportion of neurofibromas undergo malignant change into sarcomas.

Schwannomas are benign tumours arising from the Schwann cells supporting peripheral nerves. They present as firm, nodular lesions tethered to a nerve, and pressure on the tumour may cause pain in the area of distribution of the nerve. Treatment is by careful excision, attempting to preserve the affected nerve. This requires an operating microscope and microsurgical manipulation.

GANGLION

This extremely common and inappropriately named condition is a cyst-like lesion derived from the lining of a synovial joint, tendon sheath or embryological remnants of synovial tissue. The 'cystic' space does not usually communicate with the associated joint or tendon sheath, and like synovial joint cavities, is not lined by epithelium. It contains a colourless, gelatinous fluid. Ganglia present as superficial lumps, usually about 1–2 cm in diameter, though sometimes larger. They are most common on the dorsum of the forearm and hand (Fig. 46.15) and around the ankle. They are rarely painful but sometimes cause mechanical problems or interference with footwear. Ganglia are easily recognised by their smooth, hemispherical surface, and firm but slightly fluctuant 'cyst-like' consistency. The overlying skin is normal and mobile and the ganglion weakly transilluminable.

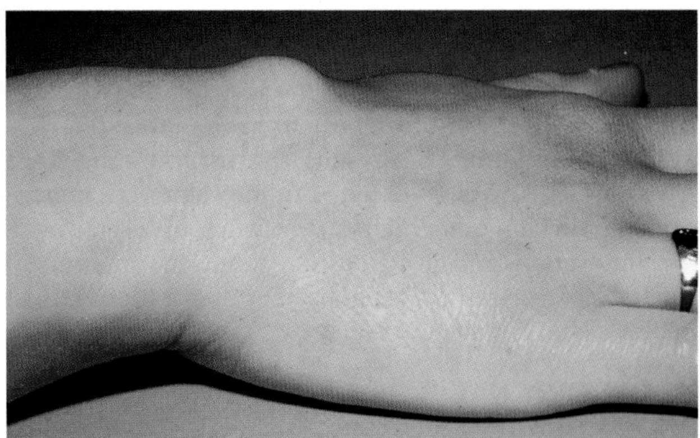

Fig. 46.15 Ganglion
This ganglion is in a common site, the dorsum of the hand

The age-old treatment for a ganglion was a sharp blow with a family bible, which dissipated the cyst contents into the tissues. Recurrence almost inevitably followed. Needle aspiration or surgical excision are the accepted methods of treatment now, but recurrence is still common.

LESIONS OF VASCULAR ORIGIN

CAMPBELL DE MORGAN SPOTS

Campbell de Morgan spots are small, bright-red spots which appear on the trunk, usually in older patients. They represent highly localised capillary proliferation and have no clinical significance except for titillation of bored examiners! Like other vascular lesions they blanch when compressed and then refill.

SPIDER NAEVI

Spider naevi or telangiectases are small red lesions consisting of a central arteriole from which radiate dilated capillaries. Isolated spider naevi may be found in normal individuals on trunk, neck and face. Their numbers markedly increase in chronic liver disease, especially cirrhosis, and occasionally in pregnancy. Treatment is rarely required but, when needed, laser therapy is probably the treatment of choice.

ANGIOMAS

Despite their name, angiomas are not true neoplasms but rather congenital hamartomas. They arise from localised excessive development of thin-walled blood vessels which may be of small diameter (**capillary haemangiomas**) or hugely dilated (**cavernous haemangiomas**). The histological appearance is often ambiguous, with most angiomas containing both elements, as well as arteriovenous or even lymphatic components.

'PORT-WINE STAINS'

The most common haemangiomas are port-wine stains. These occur anywhere, but especially on the face, neck and scalp, and cause cosmetic distress. They are present from birth and remain unchanged throughout life. Lesions are flat or slightly elevated and reddish-blue. They have an asymmetrical outline and range up to many centimetres in diameter. Trauma may cause bleeding or ulceration.

Surgical treatment, often urged by anguished patients, is rarely successful except for small lesions. Sclerosing agents can be injected to promote thrombosis, organisation and progressive devascularisation, but results are disappointing. Lasers such as the pulse dye laser, tuned to the colour frequency of haemoglobin, and other high-energy light sources are encouraging innovations and give promising results in some patients. Regrettably, the use of covering cosmetic preparations remains the best advice for most.

STRAWBERRY NAEVI

The strawberry naevus is a distinct type of angioma. These occur in early childhood as bright-red fleshy lesions and grow for a few years before involuting spontaneously. Almost all resolve without scarring. Large strawberry naevi causing complications, e.g. ocular occlusion, are treated primarily with oral propranolol. Surgery is not indicated except to deal with redundant skin left after involution.

CYSTIC HYGROMA

Cystic hygroma is a lymphangioma presenting as a lump in the neck, usually during childhood; it is described in more detail in Ch 47, p. 589. Characteristically, the lesion is highly transilluminable.

CONGENITAL SYNDROMES

Gross vascular malformations form part of several rare congenital syndromes. These include **Sturge–Weber syndrome** (angiomas of the face and intracranial contents) and **Klippel–Trenaunay syndrome**. The latter is characterised by the triad of port-wine stain, varicose veins and bone and soft tissue hypertrophy involving one lower limb; it may include the pelvis. Parks–Weber syndrome is probably another name for the same condition. The primary abnormality is probably multiple microscopic arteriovenous communications. These lead to hypertrophy of the limb (gigantism), which is warm to palpation. Venous abnormalities include gross varicose veins, deep venous abnormalities and persistent atypical veins often leading to venous ulceration.

GLOMUS TUMOUR

This is a benign tumour derived from glomus bodies, small arteriovenous communications normally found in the peripheries. Glomus bodies are thought to play a part in controlling local blood flow. Glomus tumours occur singly, usually in fingers and often beneath the nail. They are tiny (1–3 mm) red flat lesions, exquisitely tender to the touch. Treatment is by surgical excision.

LESIONS DERIVED FROM SKIN APPENDAGES

BENIGN APPENDAGE TUMOURS

Several benign tumours arise from skin appendages. The most common is the **cylindroma**, derived from sweat glands. Diagnosis is usually made only on histological examination of an excised nondescript skin lump.

Pilonidal sinus and abscess are described in Chapter 30.

DISORDERS OF THE NAILS

INGROWING TOENAIL

Pathophysiology

An ingrowing toenail (Fig. 46.16) occurs when the distal edge of the nail persistently cuts into the adjacent nail fold. The problem almost always affects the great toe. In effect there is a laceration which cannot heal because of the presence of a foreign body (the toenail). Superimposed infection by local bacterial and fungal flora complicates the picture. The combination of acute inflammation and attempts at repair produces exuberant granulation tissue around the laceration plus inflammatory swelling. Swelling aggravates trauma caused by the nail edge.

Ingrowing toenail is mainly confined to teenagers and young adults, particularly males. It probably results from a combination of inadequate hygiene, unsuitable footwear, cutting the nails too short at the corners and the macerating effect of sweat on the skin. High levels of circulating testosterone in adolescence may be an aetiological factor.

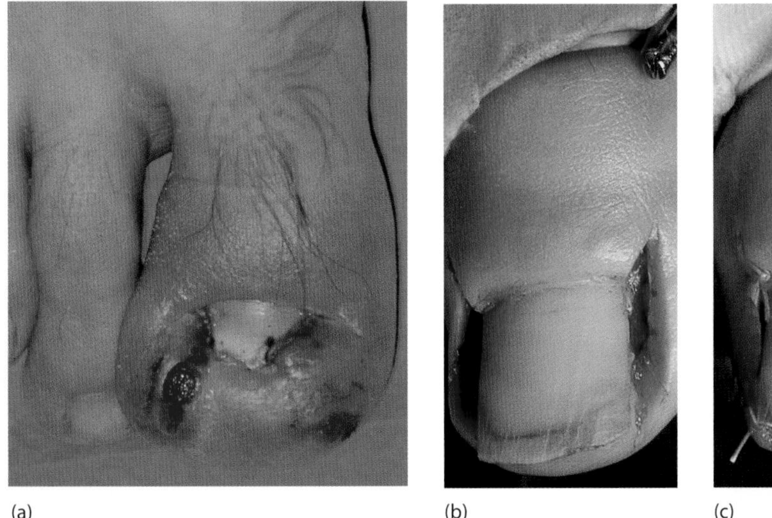

Fig. 46.16 Ingrowing toenail
(a) Inflamed ingrowing toenail affecting medial and lateral sides. There is a great amount of hypertrophy, making suitable footwear hard to find. **(b)** and **(c)** A different patient undergoing wedge resection and phenolisation of both sides of the nail. Note the use of a tourniquet

Removal of nail alone

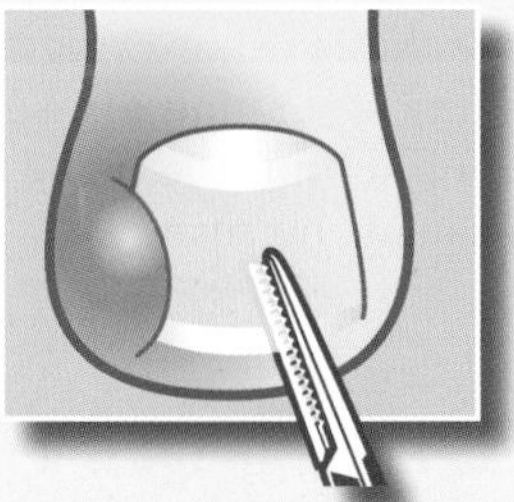

If badly infected and unresponsive to conservative treatment, 'first aid' is to remove the whole nail without disturbing the nail bed, under a local anaesthetic ring block
The nail can be lifted out by firmly grasping with artery forceps
Removal of the 'foreign body' allows inflammation to settle

Zadik's operation for permanent ablation of nail and nail bed

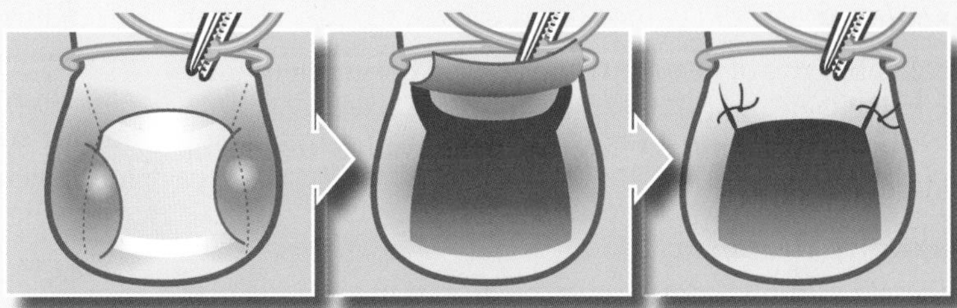

1. Nail and granulations removed and skin incised as shown (dotted lines)
2. Flap raised and full width of the germinal matrix treated by phenolisation as in 6 below
3. Flaps sutured back as shown

Wedge resection/phenolisation for permanent narrowing of nail

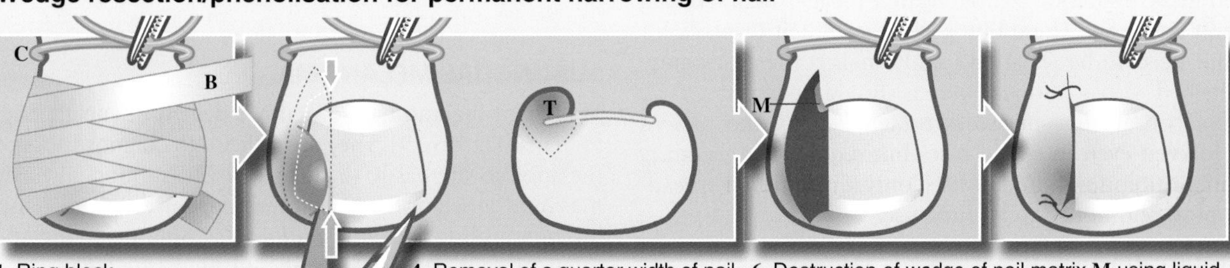

1. Ring block
2. Exsanguination of toe with 'mini-Esmark' bandage **B** (i.e. rubber bandage spirally applied)
3. Application of tourniquet **C** (e.g. thin rubber tube) around toe base before removing Esmark
4. Removal of a quarter width of nail using pointed scissors to cut from distal to proximal (between arrows) and lifting out fragment
5. Excision of a wedge of hypertrophic/inflamed tissue **T**
6. Destruction of wedge of nail matrix **M** using liquid 60% phenol. Undersides of the skin flaps are protected with paraffin jelly and a cotton pledget moistened with phenol placed on nail bed for 2 minutes
7. Skin closure with absorbable sutures if necessary
8. Pressure dressing. Leave toe tip visible and check for ischaemia. Non-adherent dressing and crepe bandage; then release tourniquet
9. Redress at 24 hours

Fig. 46.17 Operations for ingrowing toenail

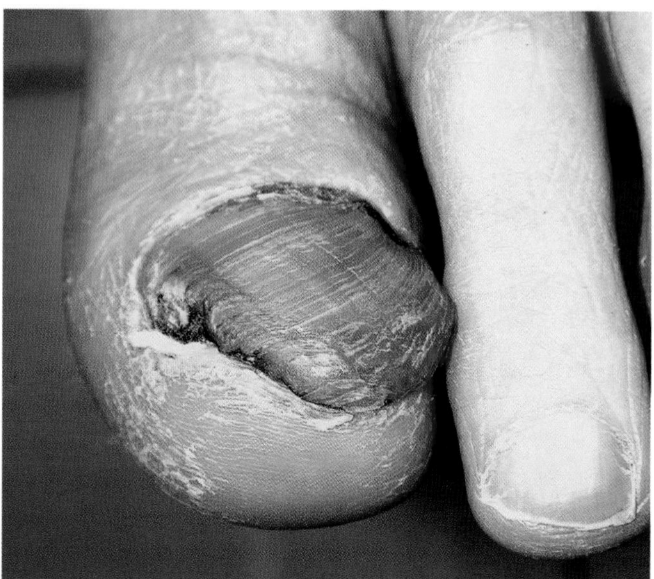

Fig. 46.18 Onychogryphosis.
Moderate degree of nail thickening and 'heaping up'

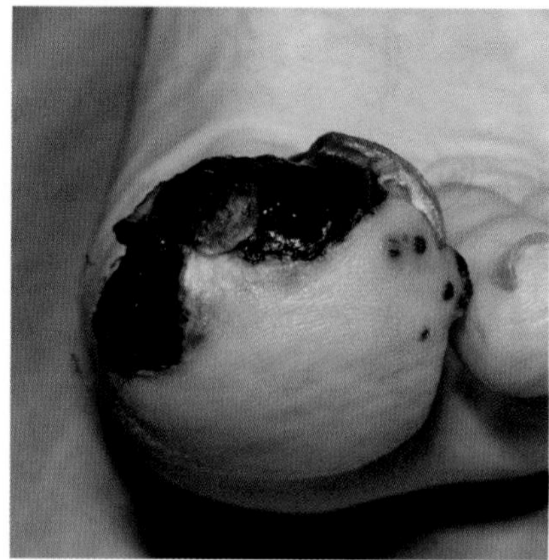

Fig. 46.19 Subungual malignant melanoma
Aggressive malignant melanoma arising from beneath the nail of the first toe. Note the large main lesion and the satellite lesions nearby. This patient died of melanomatosis 1 year after this picture was taken

Management

The main objective of treatment is to prevent persistent trauma by the nail edge. Surgical operations result in a week or more of discomfort and immobility, so conservative treatment should be tried first.

Conservative treatment

In all cases, simple conservative measures include regular bathing, frequent changes of socks (which should be cotton), avoiding tight or narrow shoes and avoiding trauma to the toe when inflamed, for example from kicking a football.

For an inflamed ingrowing toenail, foot soaks in warm saline should be carried out twice daily for at least 10 minutes. Surgical spirit applied twice daily may also help. A useful further measure, once inflammation is settling, is to pack a small pledget of cotton wool beneath the nail corner to lift it out of the laceration. At the same time, the nail fold can be pushed away by packing an elongated pledget between nail fold and nail edge. These tiny packs can be left in place for days but need to be expanded as the nail corner rises away from its bed. Loose fitting footwear should be worn.

These conservative measures undertaken by the patient often succeed even in severe cases but require perseverance. Systemic antibiotics should be used only if infection is spreading; topical antibiotics are of little use.

Surgical treatment

Urgent surgical treatment involves avulsing the whole nail, or removing one side of it. This immediately removes the 'foreign body' and permits rapid resolution. For recurrent ingrowing toenails, particularly if abnormal nail morphology is contributory, part of the nail bed is best removed. Popular procedures are illustrated in Figure 46.17. Operations are usually performed under local anaesthesia using a ring block and tourniquet. Local anaesthetic incorporating a vasoconstrictor such as adrenaline (epinephrine) must *never* be used in digits because of the risk of ischaemic necrosis.

ONYCHOGRYPHOSIS

Onychogryphosis ('ram's horn nail') (Fig. 46.18) is a gross abnormality of nail growth. It affects the great toenail, which becomes thickened and distorted and nail cutting with ordinary nail scissors becomes impossible. Onychogryphosis is usually seen only in elderly patients and probably results from previous nail bed trauma. The condition usually presents when it interferes with wearing shoes. A chiropodist (podiatrist) can treat onychogryphosis with grinding instruments at regular intervals. Surgical removal of the nail and ablation of the bed is sometimes performed.

SUBUNGUAL MELANOMA

Malignant melanomas sometimes develop beneath finger or toenails (Fig. 46.19). They are difficult to diagnose. Pigmented melanomas are easily mistaken for old subungual haematomas, and amelanotic melanomas appear even more innocuous, resembling pyogenic granulomas. Subungual melanomas often present early as a changing pigmented nail streak or **longitudinal melanonychia**. Advanced or clinically aggressive nail unit melanomas tend to present as a tumourous growth. Any suspicious lesion under the nail should be biopsied to avoid the disaster of missing a potentially curable malignant melanoma.

Lumps in the head and neck and salivary calculi

47

INTRODUCTION

Nearly all head and neck disorders reaching the general surgeon are lumps, including abscesses. Referrals are often made to exclude malignancy whilst some are for surgical treatment of a metabolic disorder such as thyrotoxicosis or hyperparathyroidism. There is a large overlap with other specialties in this area, particularly ENT, oral and maxillofacial surgery, plastic and reconstructive surgery and dermatology.

Thyroid swellings may be confused with other anterior neck swellings, so head and neck examination must include the thyroid area, described in Chapter 49.

Mouth problems are managed by oral and maxillofacial surgeons but patients often seek advice first from another clinician. Thus most doctors, particularly in an accident department, should understand the essentials of oral and dental disease and their management (see also Ch. 48).

HISTORY AND EXAMINATION IN THE HEAD AND NECK

Many different tissues are concentrated here, so there is a profusion of conditions causing lumps. Box 47.1 provides a simple classification.

Special points in the history and examination

As always, the history provides important clues to the diagnosis. The patient's age, the rate of growth of the lump and symptoms such as pain, discharge or swelling related to eating ('mealtime syndrome') may point to the diagnosis.

Most lumps are best examined with the patient sitting so the examiner can palpate from in front and behind. The examiner should establish the **characteristics of the lump** (Box 47.2) and determine how it relates to overlying or underlying structures. For example, a lump in the cheek may originate in skin, parotid, buccinator muscle, oral mucosa or parotid duct. In clinical exams, it is useful to describe the characteristics as if to someone who cannot see the patient.

With a lump or swelling, the whole of scalp, back of neck and skin behind and in the ears should be examined. Head and neck lymph nodes must be palpated. A simple method considers nodes lying in two planes, horizontal and vertical (Figure 47.1) which can be examined systematically. For lumps in the lower half of the face or submandibular region, the **oral cavity** should be examined to exclude salivary gland lesions, oral malignancies or sources of infection such as a dental abscess. For lumps in the parotid region, the integrity of the **facial nerve** should be tested since malignant tumours often cause neurological deficits. If the presenting complaint is **lymph node enlargement**, endoscopy of upper airways and pharynx may be necessary to exclude primary tumours or infected lesions.

Examination of the oral cavity

For many doctors, asking the patient to open the mouth represents the entire oral examination. The simple technique illustrated in Figure 47.2a–d, will enable most significant lesions to be seen without special instruments or lighting.

First, the patient should remove dentures. Then lips and their mucosal lining, and the lining of cheeks and gums are inspected. To do this, the lips are retracted by the examiner's gloved fingers or a wooden spatula and the mouth illuminated with a pen torch. Teeth are inspected for obvious decay and gum inflammation. A flap of gum over a partially erupted lower wisdom tooth can cause painful inflammation (Fig. 48.6).

If parotid disease is suspected, the duct papilla opposite the upper second molar should be identified and palpated. If the patient has dentures or irregular teeth, inspect for papillary scarring causing obstruction. The palate is best examined if the patient tilts the head backwards. Finally, the tongue and floor of the mouth are inspected for mucosal lesions. To assist, the patient first protrudes, then elevates the tongue.

Lumps in the floor of the mouth, submandibular area and cheeks should be palpated **bimanually** as shown in Figure 47.2d. Lumps in these areas are often mobile and tend to move away from examining fingers.

TUMOURS OF SALIVARY GLANDS

There are three pairs of major salivary glands, **parotid**, **submandibular** and **sublingual**. The parotid produces serous (watery) saliva, the submandibular a mixed seromucous saliva

Box 47.1 Causes of a lump in the head or neck

1. **Thyroid disorders** (classified in Table 49.1)
2. **Lymph node enlargement:**
   - Local inflammatory lymphadenopathy from acute infections of the head and neck
   - Inflammatory lymphadenopathy as part of a generalised lymphadenopathy, e.g. glandular fever or AIDS-related lymphadenopathy
   - Local inflammatory lymphadenopathy from chronic infections, e.g. tuberculosis
   - Lymphomas
   - Secondary tumour deposits (metastases)
3. **Congenital cysts**—thyroglossal, branchial and pre-auricular cysts, external angular dermoids and cystic hygroma (lymphatic malformations)
4. **Salivary gland disorders**—adenoma, carcinoma, stones, rare autoimmune disorders such as Sjögren's syndrome
5. **Lumps in the skin**—any skin lesion may occur in the head and neck but the main problem is one of differential diagnosis, e.g. lipomas and epidermal cysts
6. **Rare tumours**—carotid body tumours, carcinoma of the maxillary sinus (antrum), tumours and cysts of the jaw
7. **Actinomycosis** (very rare)

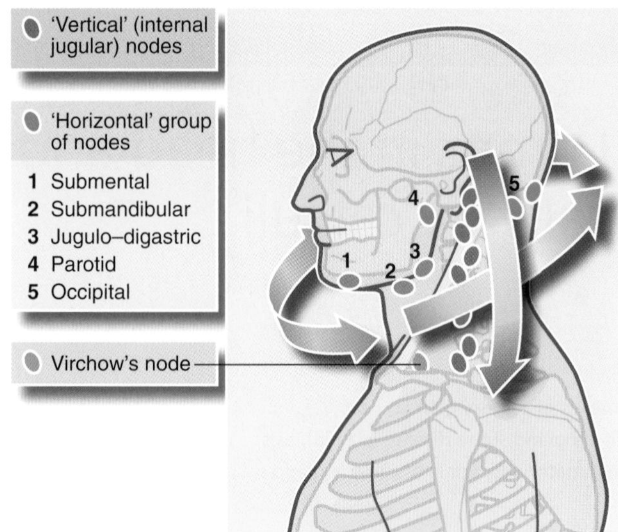

Fig. 47.1 Simple technique for palpating head and neck lymph nodes

Box 47.2 Characteristics of any lump on clinical examination

- Site
- Size
- Shape
- Surface characteristics
- Fixation (superficial and deep)
- Anatomical origin
- Consistency
- Fluctuance
- Pulsatility
- Temperature
- Transilluminability
- Bruit
- Local lymphadenopathy

and the sublingual a mucous secretion. The parotid and submandibular glands each drain into the mouth via long ducts, whereas the sublingual drains via small ducts into the floor of the mouth.

Surgical disorders of major salivary glands include benign and malignant tumours, stones, bacterial and viral infections and rare autoimmune disorders, all of which present as salivary gland lumps. The oral mucosa also contains numerous small 'minor' salivary glands which can undergo neoplastic change or form retention cysts.

SALIVARY GLAND TUMOURS

Pleomorphic adenoma

Pleomorphic adenoma is the most common lump in the parotid and by far the most common salivary gland neoplasm. In this gland, 80% are benign and of these 80% are pleomorphic adenomas. They present in middle age or later, and both sexes are equally affected.

Pleomorphic adenomas are derived from salivary gland epithelium and are benign but show variable differentiation. The name comes from the varied histological appearance. Columns and islands of neoplastic epithelial cells are separated by myxomatous connective tissue stroma, often with areas resembling immature cartilage. Some without myxomatous tissue are described as **monomorphic**.

Although they do not metastasise, pleomorphic adenomas are often poorly demarcated from surrounding tissue and have a 1% risk per year of undergoing malignant change. There is usually a well-defined thin capsule, but the surface is nodular, an important point when attempting removal.

Clinically, pleomorphic adenoma presents as a very slowly growing, painless lump (see Fig. 47.3). Most are in the parotid, some in the submandibular gland and a few are in minor salivary glands.

Most parotid tumours occur in the superficial part, external to the facial nerve plane. Occasionally, they occur in the deep part in intimate association with the facial nerve. In either case, the tumour can extend between the nerve branches, but being benign, it does not invade the nerve to cause facial palsy. Facial nerve damage is a risk during excision, especially of deeper lesions. Patients should be warned of this possibility before operation.

If an older patient has a slowly growing solid parotid lump without facial palsy, it is best to assume it is a pleomorphic adenoma or Warthin's tumour (adenolymphoma). Definitive

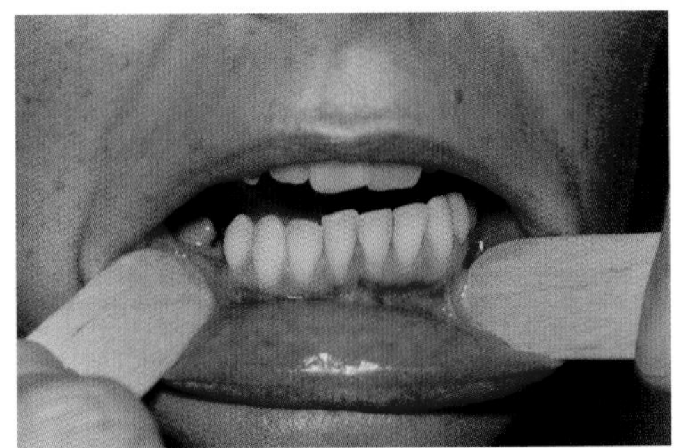
(a)

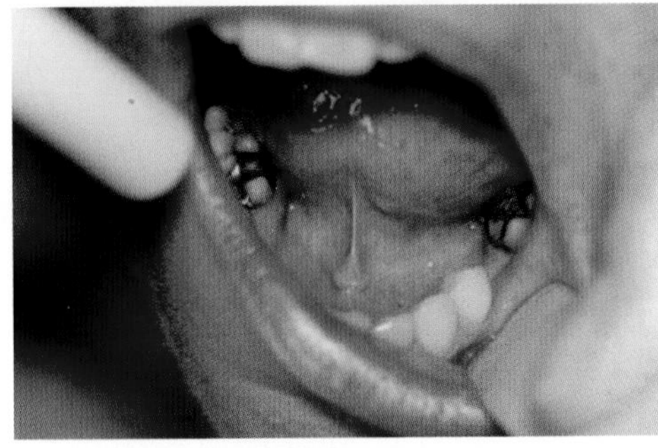
(b)

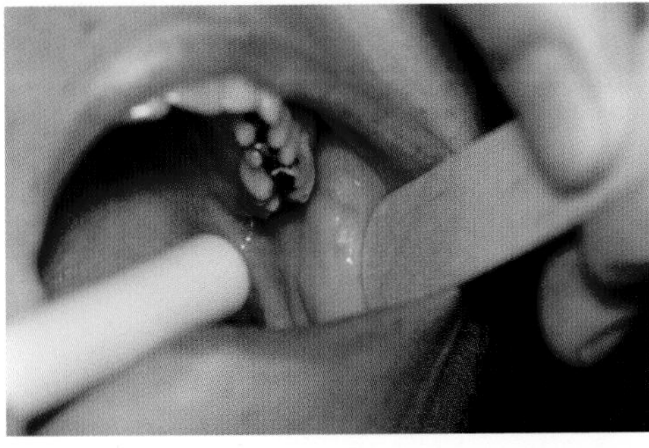
(c)

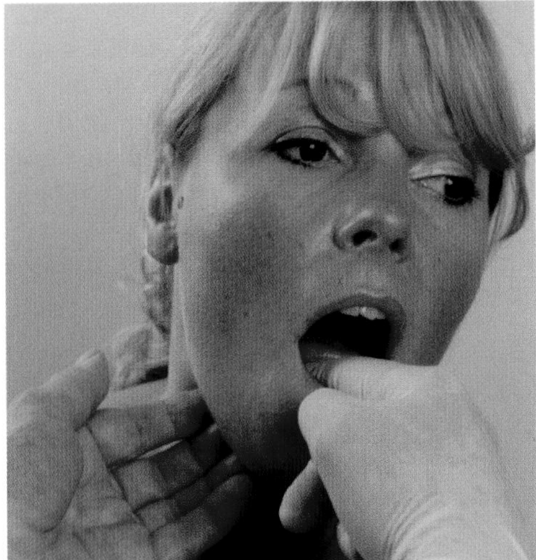
(d)

Fig. 47.2 Technique of oral examination
Teeth, gums and buccal sulci can be inspected by retracting the lips with wooden spatulas or fingers **(a).** The palate is inspected by tilting the patient's head back and retracting the lips, and the floor of the mouth and movements of the tongue examined as shown in **(b).** The parotid papilla is demonstrated in **(c).** Finally, bimanual palpation of the submandibular area, including the course of the submandibular duct, is performed with a gloved finger inside the mouth, as shown in **(d)**

diagnosis can usually be made by ultrasonography and fine needle aspiration cytology, and confirmed histologically after excision. If malignancy is suspected, CT scanning may be needed.

Treatment

Treatment is by excision. For superficial lesions, the standard operation has long been **superficial parotidectomy** to excise all glandular tissue superficial to the facial nerve, but nowadays many surgeons perform **extracapsular dissection** of the lump alone. In benign disease this cures the problem and carries a lower risk of side-effects, particularly facial nerve damage and **Frey's syndrome** of gustatory sweating (see below). Recurrence is uncommon with either procedure. For deeper lesions, an attempt should be made to excise the entire lesion, carefully identifying and preserving the facial nerve branches. Again, extracapsular dissection may be the safer option.

Complications of parotid surgery

The main complication is facial nerve damage. Damage to the temporal or upper zygomatic branches may prevent complete closure of the eye, leading to corneal drying and damage. Mandibular branch damage causes weakness at the angle of the mouth and embarrassing salivary dribbling. Nerve damage may also complicate submandibular gland excision: the mandibular branch of the facial nerve is vulnerable if the incision is incorrectly sited, and the lingual and hypoglossal nerves lie close to the deep surface of the gland. Damage causes unilateral tongue wasting and numbness respectively.

Salivary fistula is an occasional complication following parotid surgery, causing saliva to leak onto the face at mealtimes. The fistula usually resolves spontaneously after several weeks.

Frey's syndrome is a late complication of superficial parotidectomy in 25% or more cases but is virtually unknown after extracapsular dissection. It probably results from divided parasympathetic secretomotor fibres regenerating in the skin where they assume control of sweat gland activity. Facial sweating occurs in response to salivatory stimuli; known as **gustatory sweating**, this can be embarrassing. It is often managed by injection of botulinum toxin.

Adenolymphoma (Warthin's tumour)

This unusual benign lesion constitutes less than 10% of salivary neoplasms, and occurs almost exclusively in the parotid. They usually arise after middle age and there is a male predominance and a strong association with cigarette smoking. They sometimes occur bilaterally (up to 10%), at the same time or at different times.

Histologically, the tumour is composed of large glandular acini. The epithelium is embedded in dense lymphoid tissue with lymphoid follicles. Histogenesis is not understood, but the glandular part may be hamartomatous salivary duct tissue within a normal parotid lymph node.

Adenolymphomas are benign. They present as a parotid lump, clinically indistinguishable from pleomorphic adenoma. The diagnosis can sometimes be made by fine needle

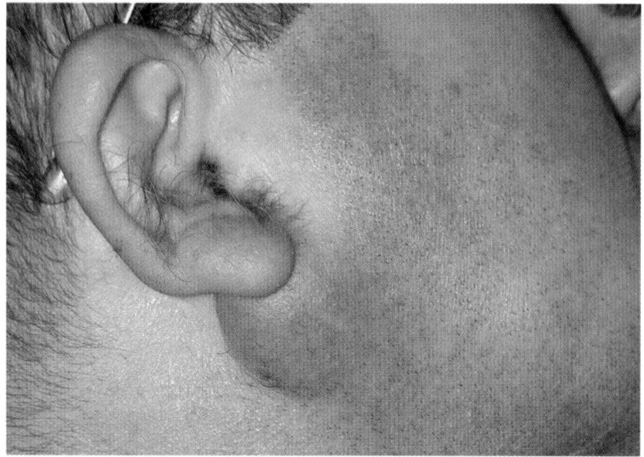
(a)

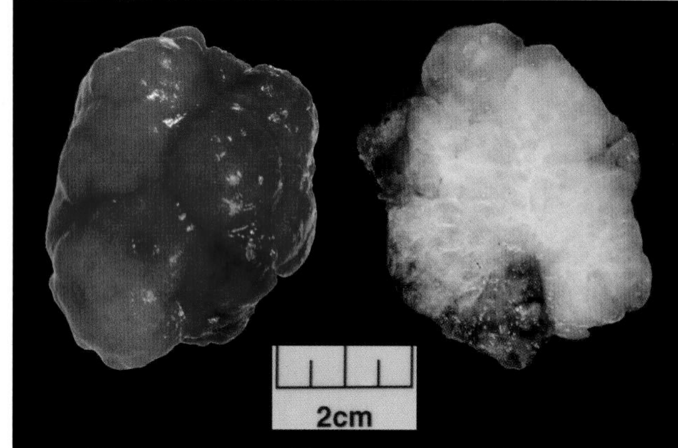

(c)

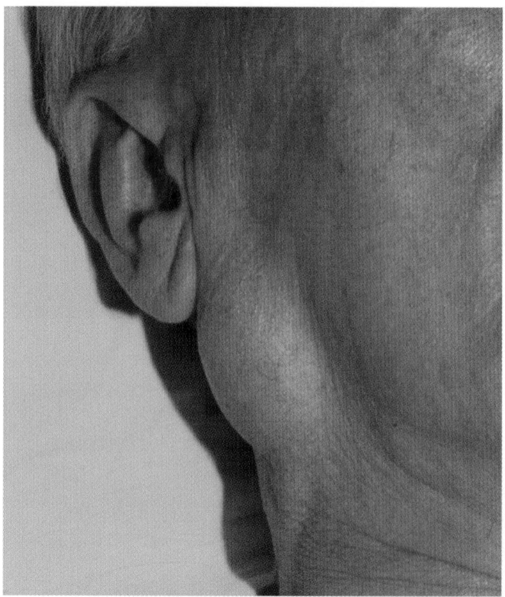
(b)

Fig. 47.3 Pleomorphic adenomas of the parotid
(a) Small lesion in the typical position below the ear lobe, between the posterior border of the ramus of the mandible and the upper end of the sternomastoid. **(b)** Larger lesion in an older man. This had been present at least 4 years before the patient presented. **(c)** Pathological specimen of large pleomorphic adenoma removed by extracapsular dissection. On the left the specimen has been freshly removed and shows the typical knobbly surface. On the right, the fixed and cut specimen shows the variegated and predominantly myxomatous appearance

aspiration cytology, then either enucleated or left alone. Adenolymphomas do not recur, but a satellite lesion may enlarge and present as another tumour.

Malignant primary salivary tumours

Malignant tumours are rare in major salivary glands but predominate in tumours of minor (accessory) salivary glands scattered throughout the oral mucosa. With parotid lumps, facial nerve weakness is diagnostic of malignancy. Most primary malignant tumours are **adenocystic carcinomas** (or less accurately cylindromas). The remainder include rare epithelial **acinic cell carcinoma** and **squamous cell carcinoma**. In Australia, the most common parotid tumour is malignant melanoma invading from skin. Overall, the commonest parotid malignancy is metastatic squamous carcinoma from a scalp primary.

Adenocystic carcinomas have a characteristic cribriform (sieve-like) microscopic appearance with small spaces in a tightly packed tumour cell mass. These are highly invasive with early regional and systemic metastasis. Treatment involves wide mutilating surgery which sometimes destroys the facial nerve. Unfortunately, recurrence is very common and may occur as long as 15 years after apparently successful eradication. The tumours are unresponsive to radiotherapy and prognosis is almost uniformly poor.

Secondary tumours in salivary glands

Lymph nodes within the parotid may become involved by metastases from face or scalp cancers. Similarly, secondaries from the mouth may develop in submandibular gland nodes. Finding a parotid or submandibular lump should therefore prompt a search for a primary locally, including the pharynx. Lymphomas, particularly arising from mucosal associated lymphoid tissue (MALT) also sometimes affect lymph nodes within salivary glands.

SALIVARY GLAND STONE DISEASE (SIALOLITHIASIS)

PATHOPHYSIOLOGY

The submandibular gland and duct are prone to form calcified stones (calculi) which obstruct salivary outflow and predispose to infection. Calculi also occur in the parotid duct but much less commonly. The aetiology is unknown, but the submandibular gland may be vulnerable because of its more viscid secretion and elongated duct.

Stones are not the only cause of obstruction causing gland swelling. In parotid and submandibular gland, duct orifice trauma may cause stenosis and salivary stasis.

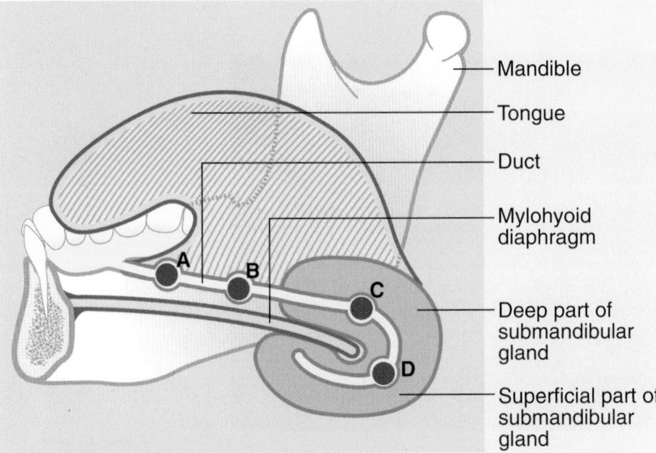

Fig. 47.4 Submandibular gland and duct showing common sites for stones

Submandibular stones may be found anywhere along Wharton's duct (Fig. 47.4), including its course within the gland. Stones vary from several millimetres to a centimetre in diameter. Those in the distal duct tend to have an elongated 'date stone' shape (see Fig. 47.5a).

CLINICAL FEATURES

Salivary calculi rarely cause complete obstruction but the patient usually experiences intermittent swelling or pain at mealtimes when salivary flow is high. The swelling then subsides over the next hour or so. Acidic foods such as lemon juice stimulate rapid salivary flow, and can be used as a test in clinic. Pain is not usually a prominent feature; rather, patients describe a sensation of fullness. Salivary calculi occasionally present with acute or chronic bacterial infection (**sialadenitis**). Secondary infection in the obstructed system leads to rapidly worsening symptoms and even spreading cellulitis of the floor of the mouth (**Ludwig's angina**, Fig. 47.6).

Most of the submandibular gland lies deep to the mandible and so there may be little to see on externally. In symptomatic stone disease, bimanual submandibular palpation usually confirms the gland is enlarged and firm. This involves a gloved finger palpating the floor of the mouth and the other hand below the jaw; any swelling can be felt between the two. This is the only clinical way to assess the gland size and may palpate a stone in the duct. Palpation is performed from the back towards the front of the mouth to avoid displacing a mobile stone backwards into the gland. On intraoral examination, a stone may be visible if impacted at the duct orifice.

MANAGEMENT OF SALIVARY CALCULI

Plain X-rays demonstrate most calculi. For the submandibular gland and duct, an **occlusal film** held between the teeth shows the floor of the mouth, and a lateral oblique gives a second viewpoint. For the parotid, AP and lateral views are often used. Contrast radiography of the ducts (**sialography**) is sometimes indicated if the history suggests stone disease yet no stone is palpable or visible on plain X-ray, although this has largely been replaced by ultrasound. Sialography (Fig. 47.7) requires cannulation of the salivary duct which may reveal a stenosis of the orifice and may relieve symptoms temporarily. Stenosis alone of any part of the duct may produce symptoms similar to calculus obstruction.

The anterior two-thirds of the submandibular duct lie in the floor of the mouth and calculi here are removed via an intraoral (Fig. 47.5a) approach. Immediately before operation, the stone should be confirmed to be present by palpation or X-ray. Operation may be performed under local or general anaesthesia. A longitudinal incision is made in the duct over the stone and the stone lifted out. If the stone is impalpable, the duct is incised from the orifice backwards and the stone removed with forceps. The incision is not sutured but left open to improve salivary drainage. Stones can also be removed endoscopically or destroyed by lithotripsy.

Less commonly, calculi lie within the gland where they are often multiple (Fig. 47.5c–e). The usual treatment is to excise the entire submandibular gland via an incision below the mandible, placed to avoid damaging the mandibular branch of the facial and avoiding the hypoglossal nerve.

Parotid duct stenosis may respond to dilatation and attention to the dentition causing trauma. If this fails, ductoplasty can be performed, although this is often unsuccessful.

INFLAMMATORY DISORDERS OF SALIVARY GLANDS

The salivary glands are subject to infection by viruses (such as mumps) and by bacteria. Mumps is rare outside childhood and young adulthood, is usually bilateral, and resolves spontaneously. It is rarely a surgical problem unless secondary bacterial infection occurs. The glands may also be affected by autoimmune disorders such as **Sjögren's syndrome**.

ACUTE BACTERIAL SIALADENITIS

Acute parotitis was once common in postoperative patients because of dehydration and poor oral hygiene but is now rare because of intravenous fluids and nursing attention to mouth care. It now usually occurs in elderly, dehydrated or debilitated patients, or in children, arising from a suppurating lymph node within the parotid capsule. Dehydration and reduced salivary flow encourage ascending infection with resident oral flora, usually *Streptococcus viridans* or pneumococci. The result is a painful, unilateral swelling and **trismus** (limited mouth opening), pyrexia and tachycardia. The parotid is tender and diffusely enlarged and a purulent discharge may ooze (or can be 'milked') from the duct orifice.

Fig. 47.5 Submandibular gland and duct calculi

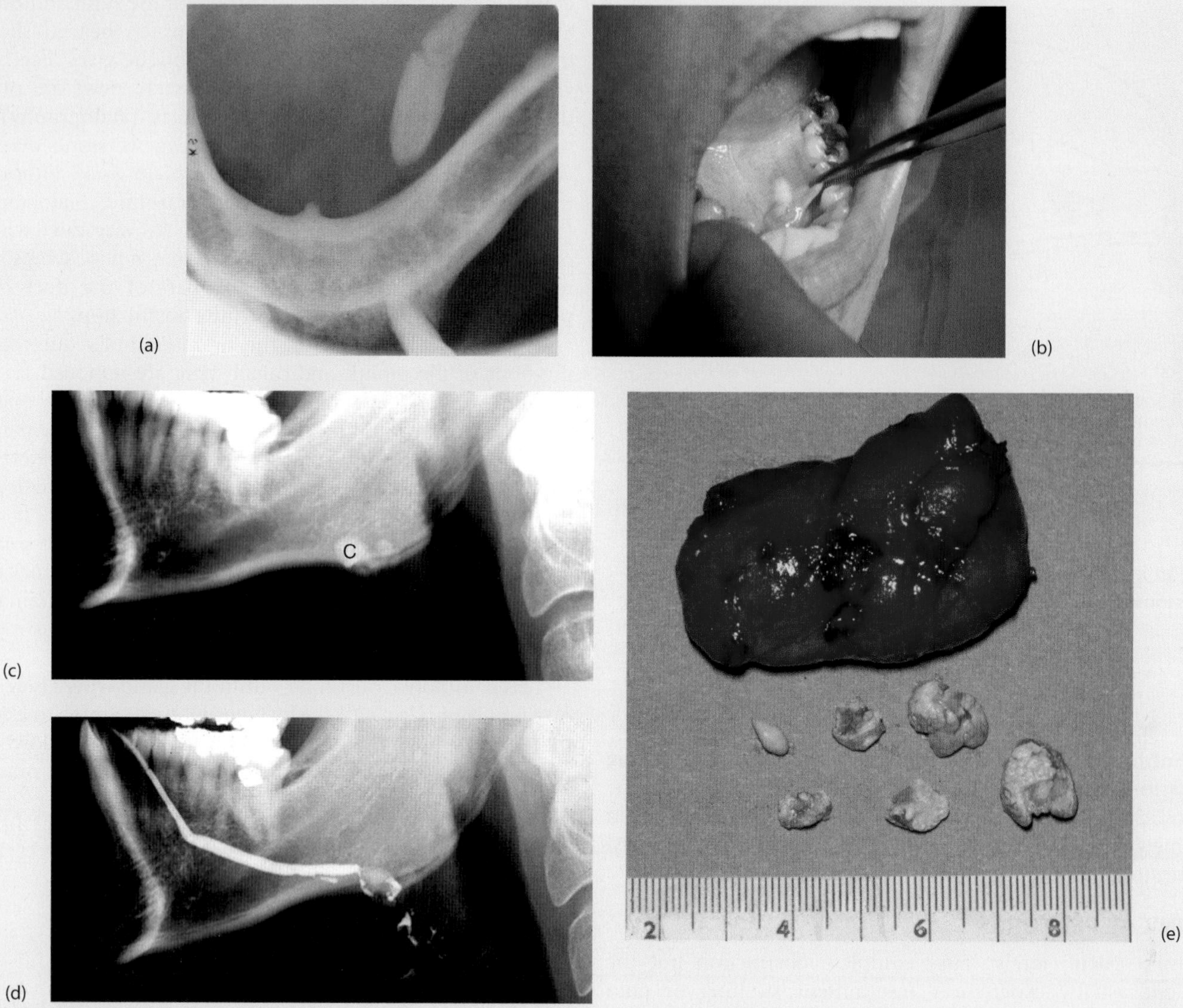

(a) (b) (c) (d) (e)

Submandibular duct calculus

(a) Occlusal X-ray showing large 'date stone' calculus in the left submandibular duct. This was easily palpable bimanually in the floor of the mouth and then removed via the oral route

Submandibular duct stone

(b) This photograph shows a stone visible in the anterior part of Wharton's duct; it was removed under local anaesthesia via a longitudinal incision in the duct

Submandibular gland stones

This 43-year-old man suffered chronic swelling and intermittent infection of the right submandibular gland. **(c)** Lateral plain X-ray showing calculi **C** within the gland. **(d)** Sialogram showing a normal Wharton's duct (note how rapidly it descends from the floor of the mouth). The stones within the gland are represented by filling defects in the contrast material. **(e)** The only means of dealing with the problem was excision of the gland via an extraoral (submandibular) approach. The gland contained six calculi

Bacterial sialadenitis should be treated promptly with antibiotics. If a parotid abscess has formed, external surgical drainage may be necessary.

CHRONIC SIALADENITIS

Prolonged calculus obstruction of a major salivary gland causes chronic inflammation. Glandular secretory elements progressively atrophy and are replaced by fibrous and adipose tissue. The duct system becomes dilated, fibrotic and infiltrated by chronic inflammatory cells. Chronic sialadenitis and salivary calculi usually involve the submandibular gland. The gland is swollen and there may be purulent duct discharge. The swelling is aggravated by eating. Treatment is by removing the duct obstruction; antibiotics may also be necessary. Glandular function may become irreversibly damaged, and the gland may require removal, although this is difficult because of fibrosis.

CASE HISTORY

Fig. 47.6 Ludwig's angina

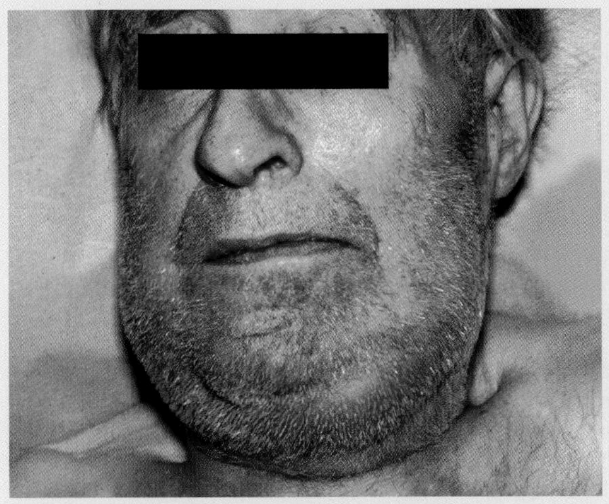

Spreading cellulitis of the submandibular region. This man of 70 had large obstructing stones of the left submandibular duct and this had led to infection in the duct and gland. This spread to the surrounding tissues. He was beginning to develop respiratory embarrassment as a result of laryngeal oedema but settled rapidly with antibiotics and removal of the stones from within the mouth

CASE HISTORY

Fig. 47.7 Parotid sialography showing stones

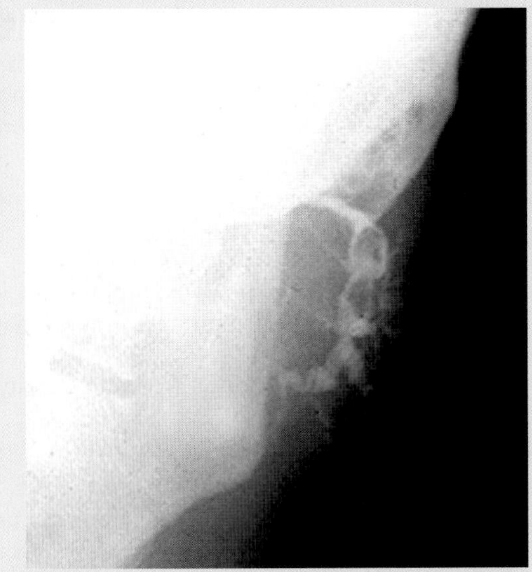

This man of 58 complained of intermittent swelling in the region of the left parotid gland, relieved on occasions by discharge of pus into the mouth. Contrast was injected into the orifice of the left parotid gland to outline the duct structure. The main duct is dilated and contains filling defects diagnosed as stones. This is an unusual finding as stones are much more common in the submandibular gland

RECURRENT SIALADENITIS

This uncommon condition may occur at any age and usually affects the parotid. One or both glands are subject to recurrent attacks of painful swelling. The cause is low-grade bacterial infection usually without duct obstruction. Recurrent attacks cause chronic swelling. Sialography shows dilatation of the duct system with terminal sacculation described as **sialectasis**. The cause is often a duct orificial stenosis, or stenoses of unknown origin proximally in the duct.

Immediate treatment includes antibiotics, chosen after culture of parotid duct discharge, as well as attention to oral hygiene. **Ductoplasty** to open the duct orifice is often successful. If sialography shows remote duct stenoses, these can sometimes be dilated using balloons similar to angioplasty devices.

AUTOIMMUNE SALIVARY GLAND DISORDERS

The salivary glands occasionally become involved in a chronic inflammatory process characterised by diffuse lymphoid infiltration and fibrosis. This is part of various poorly understood autoimmune disorders which also involve lachrymal glands and mucous glands of mouth and upper respiratory tract. The parotid and submandibular glands become diffusely and symmetrically enlarged, and salivary production is curtailed. The resulting dry mouth (**xerostomia**) causes discomfort and dysphagia and predisposes to rampant dental caries. Diminished lachrymal secretion results in **keratoconjunctivitis sicca** affecting the eyes.

In isolation, the condition is known as **primary Sjögren's syndrome**. It may also occur in rheumatoid arthritis and other connective tissue disorders when it is known as secondary Sjögren's syndrome.

SALIVARY RETENTION CYSTS

Large retention cysts sometimes develop in the floor of the mouth. A cyst of the sublingual gland can reach several centimetres and is known as a **ranula** (frog mouth). The ranula typically appears as a blue-grey dome-like swelling beneath the tongue. It may burst spontaneously, discharging its contents and collapsing, but it almost invariably recurs. The condition is painless but occupies space in the mouth. Excision is difficult because of the tenuous lining and because of the proximity to vital structures in the floor of the mouth; incomplete removal leads to recurrence. The usual treatment is excision of the sublingual gland, although **marsupialisation** is an option, i.e. de-roofing the cyst so that it opens into the floor of the mouth. Ranula may present as a lump in the neck, the so-called plunging ranula.

LYMPH NODE DISORDERS OF THE HEAD AND NECK

Patients are often referred to a surgeon for biopsy of an enlarged cervical lymph node, often with no other symptoms or signs. **Isolated lymph node enlargement** may be caused by local disease in its field of drainage. Examples of local disorders include tonsillitis or dental infection, tonsillar tuberculosis or a malignant oropharyngeal tumour. Nodes draining a bacterial infection may themselves suppurate, sometimes after the primary disorder has disappeared (see Fig. 47.8). Enlarged nodes may be part of a **systemic lymphadenopathy** caused by glandular fever, lymphoma or HIV. Thus, any patient presenting with an enlarged lymph node requires general examination as well as of the head,

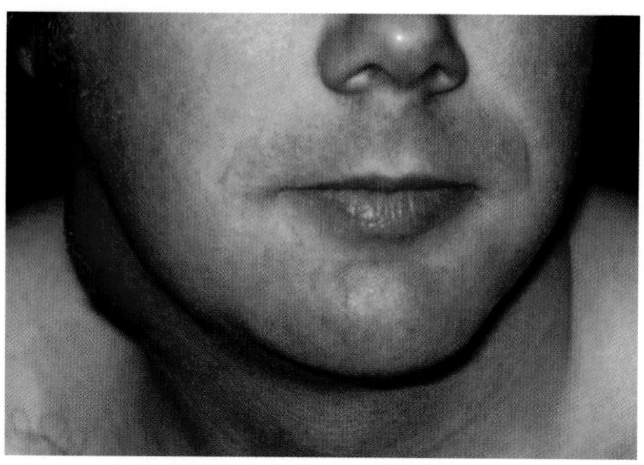

Fig. 47.8 Suppurating lymph node in the neck
This patient presented with a suppurating node in the neck which required external drainage. The primary site of sepsis was a dental abscess on a lower molar tooth

Fig. 47.9 Virchow's node

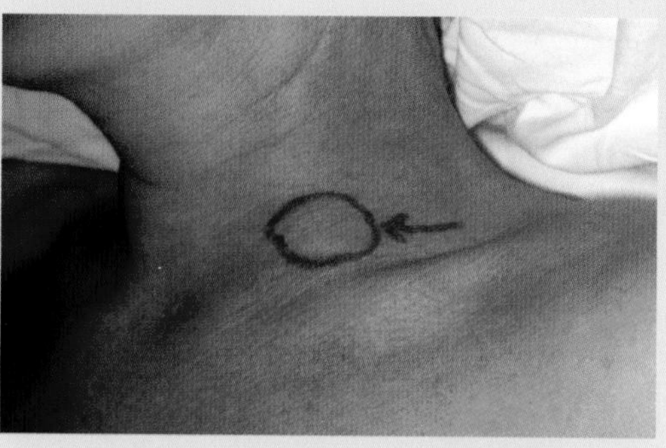

This 48-year-old woman noticed a painless lump in the left side of her neck. She had also lost a substantial amount of weight and had a poor appetite. Node biopsy revealed malignant adenocarcinoma cells and endoscopy showed that an advanced carcinoma of stomach was the cause. Palpation of a malignant node in this site is known as Troisier's sign, after the French physician who diagnosed gastric cancer in himself

neck and mouth. The latter often includes endoscopy of the pharyngeal area, usually by a specialist ENT surgeon (otorhinolaryngologist).

General clinical examination includes axillary and inguinal lymph nodes, liver and spleen. A chest X-ray may show enlarged thoracic nodes. If node biopsy is necessary, a fine needle aspiration or core biopsy under ultrasound control may suffice, although some pathologists are unhappy with needle biopsies in lymphoma. If excision biopsy is required, this should *always* be performed under general anaesthesia if practicable, since the operation is often unexpectedly troublesome because nodes are intimately related to many vital structures and preoperative palpation underestimates the size and extent of node involvement.

CERVICAL TUBERCULOSIS

Tuberculosis involving the cervical glands (**scrofula**) was once common, with the infection acquired by drinking milk from cattle infected with bovine tuberculosis. Cervical tuberculosis is now extremely rare in developed countries but may be seen in recent immigrants. The primary infection occurs in the tonsils but presents with secondary involvement of cervical nodes which become progressively enlarged and matted. In advanced cases, liquefaction of caseous material forms **cold abscesses**. If untreated, these eventually drain spontaneously onto the neck and leave disfiguring scars.

In the past, surgery was often required to drain and remove the affected glands. With modern chemotherapy this is rarely necessary and surgery is confined to diagnostic excision biopsy.

LYMPHOMAS

An enlarged cervical lymph node is a common presentation of non-Hodgkin lymphoma or Hodgkin's disease. The disease is often at an early stage without other clinical symptoms or signs. The diagnosis is made by histological examination of a biopsy specimen.

SECONDARY (METASTATIC) TUMOURS

Cervical lymph node metastases may originate from primary cancers in the head or neck, chest or abdomen. An enlarged node may be the first indication of a cancer or represent a recurrence following treatment.

Head and neck cancers usually metastasise initially to nodes in the submandibular region and upper anterior triangle, although disease lower in the neck at presentation is not unusual. The following head and neck tumours commonly metastasise to cervical lymph nodes:

- Squamous carcinoma or melanoma of the skin of neck, face, scalp and ear
- Squamous carcinoma of mouth and tongue
- Squamous carcinoma of nasopharynx, oropharynx, larynx and paranasal sinuses. Note the primary tumour may be exceedingly small
- Adenocystic carcinoma of major or accessory salivary glands
- Papillary (and occasionally medullary) carcinomas of the thyroid

In contrast, tumours from the chest or abdomen usually metastasise to the lower part of the posterior triangle, particularly to **Virchow's node** (Fig. 47.9), lying deeply in the angle between sternocleidomastoid and clavicle on the left side.

MISCELLANEOUS CAUSES OF A LUMP IN THE NECK

CONGENITAL CYSTS AND SINUSES

A variety of congenital cystic lesions occur in the head and neck and some may have an external sinus opening. All are uncommon except in clinical 'short-case' examinations! They can be subdivided into thyroglossal cysts, branchial cysts, fusion-line dermoid cysts, pre-auricular cysts and sinuses, and cystic hygromas (now termed lymphatic malformations). All are true epithelial cysts except for cystic

CASE HISTORY

Fig. 47.10 Branchial cyst

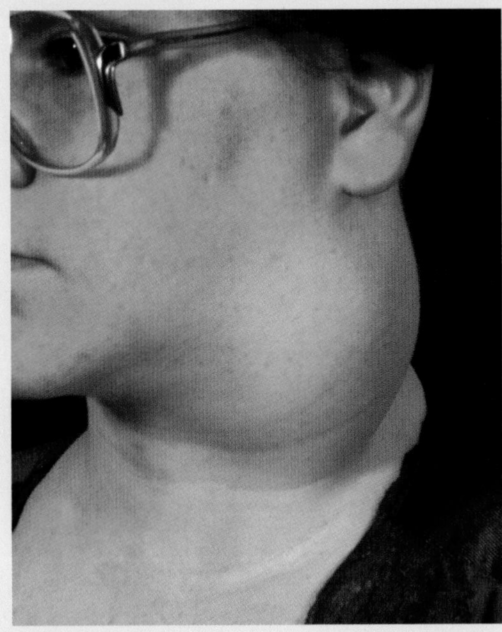

This 30-year-old woman reported the sudden appearance of this large swelling in her neck associated with moderate pain over the previous week. The swelling was non-tender and fluctuant. Ultrasound confirmed it contained fluid. It was aspirated several times but failed to resolve and was eventually excised. It is not known why branchial cysts often come to attention so suddenly

hygroma which is a hamartomatous lymphatic or lymphovascular malformation.

Branchial cysts, sinuses and fistulae

The embryological origin of these is disputed but they probably arise from remnants of the second pharyngeal pouch or branchial cleft. **Branchial cysts** usually present in early adulthood but sometimes later (Fig. 47.10). Such late presentation is unusual for congenital lesions generally. The patient typically complains of a painless swelling in the side of the neck which varies in size. Some present with a sudden painful red swelling due to inflammation of a previously unnoticed cyst.

The lump lies anterior and deep to the sternocleidomastoid, at the junction of its upper third and lower two-thirds. It protrudes into the anterior triangle of the neck and is soft and fluctuant. Provided it is not inflamed, the cyst usually transilluminates. Treatment is by surgical excision; percutaneous drainage is rarely permanent. Inflamed cysts may require urgent drainage.

Branchial sinus or fistula present as a discharging sinus near the lower end of the anterior border of the sternocleidomastoid. A **sinus** ends blindly on the lateral pharyngeal wall whereas a **fistula** communicates with the oropharynx near the tonsillar fossa. Surgical excision may be required.

Fusion-line dermoid cysts

Dermoid cysts of congenital origin arise from epithelial remnants along lines of embryological fusion in the head and neck. The most common are **external angular dermoids**, cystic swellings at the outer aspect of the supraorbital ridge usually noticed soon after birth. These cysts are tense and firm and do not transilluminate because of their thick keratinous contents. They are deeply fixed and immobile. External angular dermoids are usually removed for cosmetic reasons during childhood.

Midline dermoid cysts are described as teratoid cysts because they contain a mixture of ectodermal, mesodermal and endodermal elements (e.g. nails and teeth, glands, blood vessels). Rarely, dermoid cysts can arise in the midline of the head or neck, usually during the first year of life. They should be removed surgically.

Pre-auricular cysts and sinuses

Small cysts and sinuses may arise from developmental abnormalities of the first and second branchial arches that form the external ear. They become evident in early childhood, lying anterior to the tragus of the ear and present as a small lump or a tiny discharging sinus that occasionally becomes infected. There may be an obvious associated auricular abnormality. Treatment is usually by surgical excision.

Cystic hygromas (lymphatic malformations)

Cystic hygromas are not true cysts but lymphatic or lymphovascular hamartomas which form multilocular cyst-like spaces. They may be huge and disfiguring lesions present at birth. Smaller lesions may present in older children or adolescents as a painless lump in the neck below the angle of the mandible and are soft and fluctuant and highly transilluminable. Surgical excision may be difficult as they often extend deeply into cervical and orofacial tissues. Injection of sclerosants such as bleomycin are gaining popularity.

ACTINOMYCOSIS

Actinomycosis is a rare infection of the cervicofacial region caused by *Actinomyces israelii*, an anaerobic Gram-positive bacterium with a filamentous growth pattern similar to fungal mycelia. Actinomycosis is a chronic granulomatous infection which if untreated eventually forms multilocular abscesses that drain to the skin via multiple sinuses.

Actinomycosis is treated with a prolonged course (4–6 weeks) of high-dose penicillin. If necessary, the abscess network is surgically explored and drained. Actinomycosis also occurs in the ileocaecal area, gaining access from appendiceal perforation. Rarely, the infection is encountered in the pelvis, complicating intrauterine contraceptive devices.

48 Disorders of the mouth

DISORDERS OF THE ORAL CAVITY (EXCLUDING SALIVARY CALCULI)

The main oral disorders are **dental caries** (tooth decay) and its sequelae, inflammations of the gums and supporting bone (**periodontal disease**), **tumours** and premalignant conditions of mucosa (leukoplakia and squamous carcinoma) and **disorders of the accessory salivary glands** such as retention cysts. The main symptoms and signs are summarised in Box 48.1. Salivary gland disorders are covered in Chapter 47.

DENTAL CARIES

PATHOPHYSIOLOGY AND CLINICAL FEATURES

In developed countries, dental caries (dental decay) is a common bacterial disorder. First, the surface enamel of the tooth is breached by the demineralising action of lactic acid generated by commensal oral bacteria as a byproduct of carbohydrate metabolism, particularly of refined sugar. The most vulnerable sites for decay are just below the contact points of adjacent tooth crowns and the pits and fissures on the biting (occlusal) surface of molars and premolars. These sites are inaccessible to natural oral cleansing mechanisms and to tooth brushing.

Once enamel is breached, proteolytic bacteria enter the less calcified **dentine** beneath and cause progressive destruction. The enamel remains intact until the dentine is undermined and the enamel fractures. Thus, dental caries may be well advanced but invisible, even to a dental mirror and probe, and detectable only on X-ray. The decay process is asymptomatic until close enough to the dental pulp to cause inflammation and pain and, eventually, bacterial invasion and abscess formation. The pathological process and corresponding symptoms are outlined in Figure 48.1.

Once the pulp is **exposed**, inflammation and bacterial invasion usually destroy it, then spread to the periapical region forming an **abscess**. This causes painful oral and facial swelling, and if untreated, eventually drains into the mouth or occasionally onto the face. However, the initiating cause, the necrotic pulp, remains, so a chronic abscess flares up intermittently or continues with a persistent discharge.

The pain of dental caries is usually well localised and recognised as a 'toothache'. Dental pain is sometimes poorly localised and causes non-specific facial pain. In the upper jaw, this may simulate sinusitis. Dental caries should always be considered before rarer diagnoses. Overall, a surprising amount of dental caries, even with periapical infection, is asymptomatic.

MANAGEMENT OF DENTAL CARIES

Provided the dental pulp has not been invaded by infection (i.e. become 'exposed'), a dentist can usually drill out the carious enamel and dentine and restore it (Fig. 48.2) with synthetic resin, silver amalgam or gold, with a sedative insulating lining. Once exposed, the necrotic tissue must be removed by **endodontic treatment**, and the pulp cavity filled; this is 'root filling' (Fig. 48.2). In this way, the tooth can often be preserved.

MANAGEMENT OF DENTAL ABSCESSES

A periapical abscess is the most common manifestation of caries seen by general practitioners or casualty officers. Primary treatment, as for other abscesses, is drainage of pus. Extracting the offending tooth is most effective, but better to preserve the tooth by draining the abscess via the root canal then root filling it later. Patients with periapical abscesses should ideally be referred to a dentist.

Large acute abscesses 'pointing' within the mouth can be drained by incising at the site of greatest fluctuation. Oral penicillin should be prescribed for spreading infection.

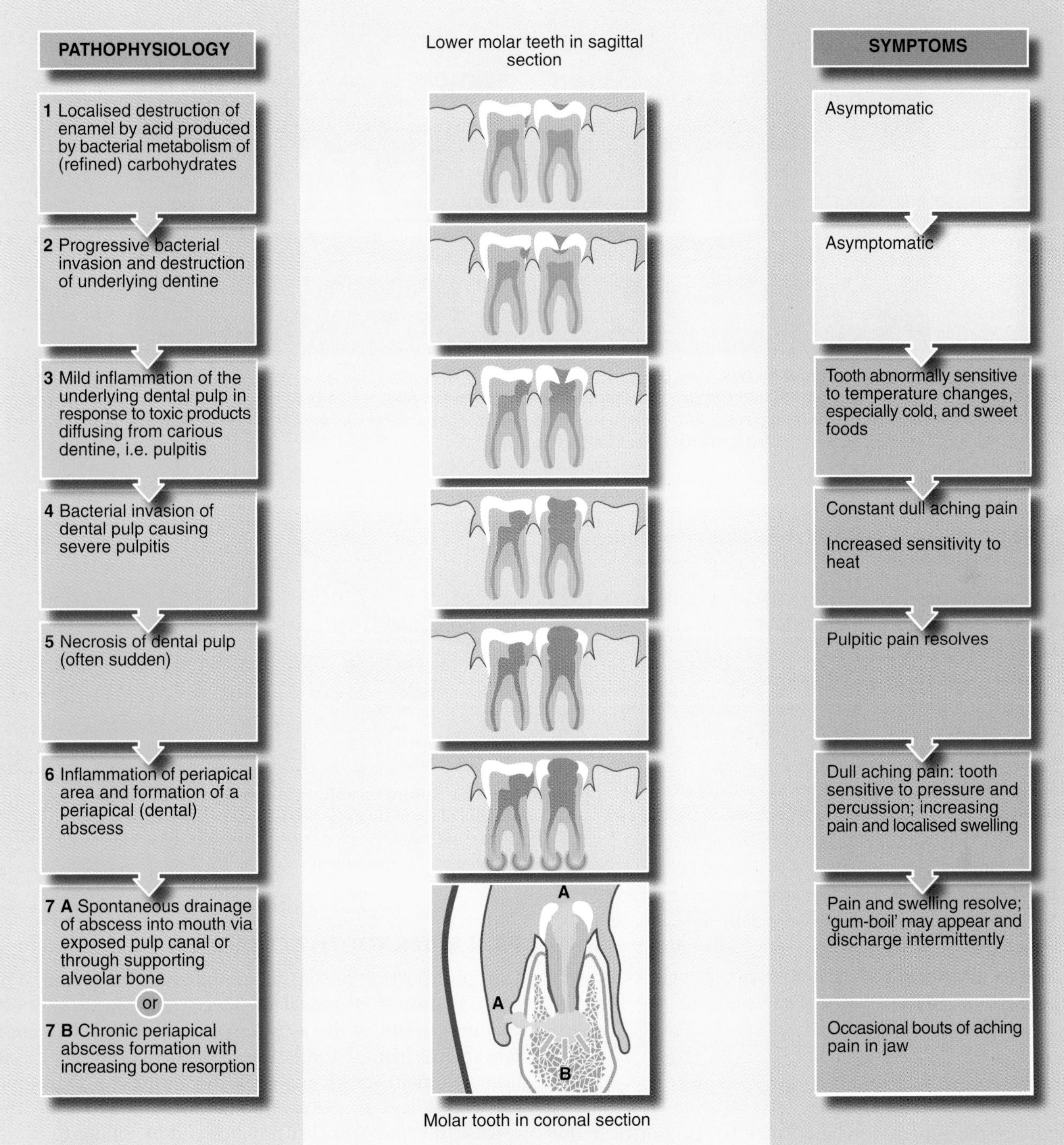

Fig. 48.1 Pathophysiology and symptoms of dental caries and its sequelae

Antibiotics have no part in managing toothache unless there is swelling or other signs of an acute abscess. A dental abscess occasionally presents on the face but usually settles with extraction of the offending tooth. Dental abscesses are rarely complicated by osteomyelitis.

TOOTH EXTRACTION AND POST-EXTRACTION PROBLEMS

Medical practitioners are rarely required to extract teeth except in isolated places. Caries prevention with fluoride toothpaste and modern restorative and endodontic techniques have made extraction much less common. Patients, however, often attend GPs or accident departments after tooth extraction or surgical tooth removal with bleeding, pain or swelling.

BLEEDING TOOTH SOCKET AFTER EXTRACTION

A small amount of blood mixed with saliva may look like severe haemorrhage. The extraction site should be inspected. A normal socket should be filled with firm clot with some

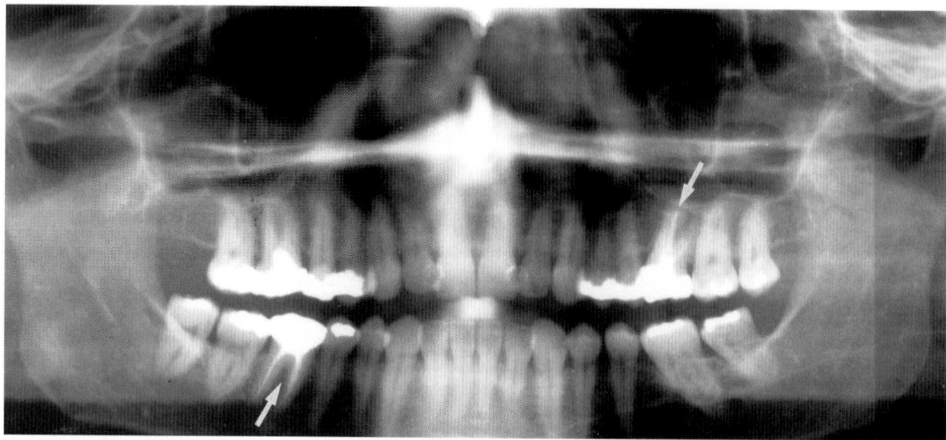

Fig. 48.2 Dental restorations and root fillings
This oral pantomograph (OPG) film shows silver amalgam restorations for caries in posterior teeth (shown as white radiopacities) and synthetic resin restorations in front teeth (relative radiolucencies in the upper incisors). In addition, the upper left first molar and the lower right first molar (arrowed) have radiopaque root canal fillings, necessitated by dental caries invading the pulp

Box 48.1 Symptoms and signs of oral disease and their main causes

- **Pain**—dental caries and its sequelae, acute gingival inflammation such as pericoronitis and Vincent's infection (acute ulcerative gingivitis)
- **Bleeding**—chronic gingival inflammation
- **Halitosis**—dental caries and chronic periodontal disease
- **White lesions**—epithelial dysplasia (leukoplakia), lichen planus and candidal infection
- **Oral ulceration**—aphthous ulcers, squamous carcinoma, retained tooth roots, chronic tooth or denture trauma, and rare epidermal disorders (e.g. lichen planus or Behçet's syndrome)
- **Discharging sinuses**—periapical tooth abscess ('gum boil')
- **Bony lumps in the jaws**—fibrous dysplasia, tumours, cysts, ectopic teeth
- **Salivary glands and duct-related lumps**—retention cysts, submandibular duct stones, tumours

ooze from the gingival margin. This is aggravated if the anxious patient disturbs the clot by rinsing or 'exploring' the socket with the tongue. Aspirin may also promote bleeding.

Oozing or minor bleeding is easily controlled by the patient biting on a small dry pack such as a folded gauze swab and maintaining pressure for 10–15 minutes. Persistent bleeding can usually be controlled by inserting sutures through the gingival margins across the socket (Fig. 48.3) then biting on a dry gauze pad. Suturing requires local anaesthesia infiltrated into the gingiva on each side of the socket. Absorbable polyglactin sutures are preferred as they do not leave irritating sharp ends and dissolve in 5–10 days. If bleeding continues after these simple measures, the patient should be investigated for a coagulation or platelet abnormality.

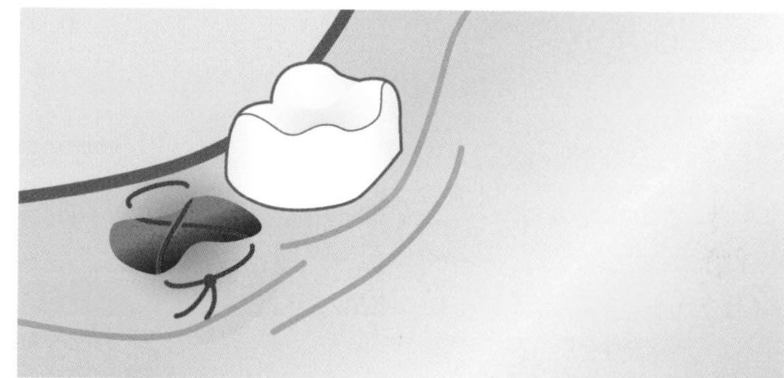

Fig. 48.3 Suture technique for bleeding tooth socket
A 'figure of eight' suture occludes bleeding gum edge on alveolar bone. The patient should bite for at least 10 minutes on a folded swab after suture to encourage clotting

PAIN AFTER TOOTH EXTRACTION

Forceps extraction or surgical tooth removal may lead to pain soon afterwards. Removal of lower molar teeth may cause **trismus** (spasm of the muscles of mastication), making jaw movements painful and restricted. If there is no sign of infection, treatment is with analgesia, not antibiotics. Pain appearing several days after extraction is usually due to a superficial osteitis of exposed socket bone caused by failure to fill with organised clot. This condition, known as a **dry socket**, is intensely painful and requires dental treatment. Antibiotic therapy is not helpful.

SWELLING AFTER TOOTH EXTRACTION

Soft tissue swelling is uncommon after extraction, with the exception of surgically removed teeth, especially lower third molars ('wisdom teeth'). Extraction of these often causes swelling around the angle of the mandible, with trismus and pain. This represents a normal inflammatory response plus interstitial haemorrhage rather than infection. The swelling subsides within a week or so and does not warrant antibiotic therapy.

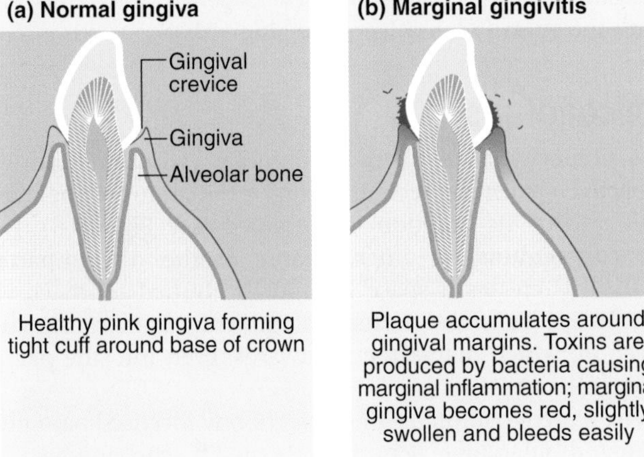

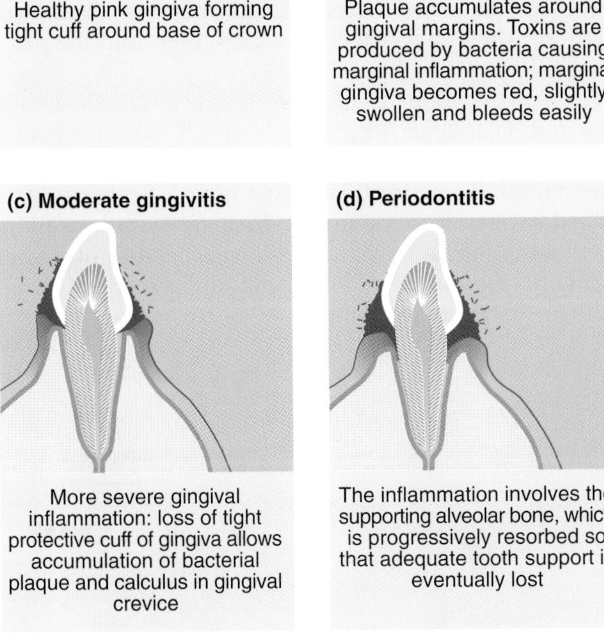

Fig. 48.4 Pathogenesis of periodontal disease

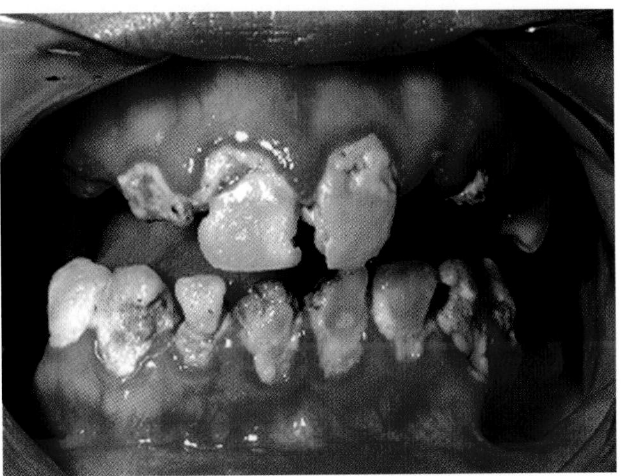

Fig. 48.5 Gingivitis and periodontitis
(a) Normal healthy gingivae. **(b)** Chronic gingivitis showing accumulated plaque and calculus around the gingival margins. At this stage, no alveolar bone has been destroyed and the inflammatory process is potentially reversible. Many of these teeth had to be extracted, however, because of rampant caries

INFLAMMATION OF THE PERIODONTAL TISSUES

GINGIVITIS AND PERIODONTITIS

Teeth are embedded in bony **alveolar ridges** in both jaws. A thin layer of **cementum** (a bone-like material) on the root connects to the socket bone by a tough **periodontal membrane or ligament**. Oral mucosa (**gingiva** or gums) is bound to the alveolar bone and normally forms a tight cuff around the tooth neck, protecting alveolar bone from bacteria and trauma. The **gingival crevice** extends down to the cemento-enamel junction where the tough stratified oral epithelium becomes a thin vulnerable layer.

If oral hygiene is inadequate, commensal bacteria colonise the gingival margin and form a white gelatinous **plaque** (Fig. 48.4). If allowed to persist, plaque becomes adherent to the tooth and becomes mineralised. This is known as **calculus**, and cannot be removed by tooth brushing. Bacterial toxins then cause gingival inflammation or **marginal gingivitis**. This appears as swelling and redness of the gums and bleeding during tooth brushing.

Figure 48.5 shows gingivitis causes eversion of the gingival margin. This encourages more plaque and calculus to form and results in greater gum trauma from food, both leading to more inflammation. If untreated, inflammation extends to deeper tissues causing progressive resorption of alveolar bone and destruction of periodontal membrane, known as **periodontitis**. By this stage, the gingiva is thickened and inflamed with a purulent discharge. This explains the old term 'pyorrhoea' or flowing of pus. Despite this, the patient is remarkably pain free, although **halitosis** is obvious.

As periodontal inflammation progresses, more alveolar bone is destroyed and gums recede. The root surface becomes exposed to view, giving rise to the expression 'long in the tooth'. Teeth gradually become more mobile until they fall out or can be extracted with the fingers! Periodontal disease is an insidious process commencing in early adulthood. It was once thought to be inevitable with advancing age, but is almost entirely preventable. In adults, **periodontitis** (not dental decay, as is commonly supposed) is responsible for most lost teeth. Inflammatory destruction of alveolar bone makes it difficult to construct satisfactory dentures for many of these patients, due to the lack of a retaining alveolar ridge.

Sometimes an acute **periodontal abscess** may complicate periodontitis.

Management of gingivitis and periodontitis

Gingivitis and periodontitis is preventable by thorough and regular tooth brushing and use of dental floss, plus periodic dental scaling to remove inaccessible plaque and calculus. Initial scaling and careful oral hygiene instruction and supervision cures gingivitis, which is reversible. During the early stages of improved oral hygiene, bleeding increases through brushing inflamed tissues but soon subsides unless further periodontal treatment is needed.

Once established, periodontitis requires meticulous oral hygiene after thorough cleaning of plaque and calculus. Lost bone is never replaced, and the gingival contour remains abnormal, making effective oral hygiene difficult. Surgical recontouring of the gingiva and underlying bone (**gingivoplasty**) may be appropriate. Antibiotics play no part in treating chronic gingivitis or periodontitis. Antibiotics are useful for acute gingival conditions such as pericoronitis and Vincent's infection (**acute ulcerative gingivitis**).

PERICORONITIS

This occurs when a lower third molar (wisdom tooth) is impacted against the second molar or the ramus of the mandible so that its eruption is prevented (see Fig. 48.6). If a flap (**operculum**) of gingiva partly overlies the impacted tooth, this creates a space around the buried tooth crown (Fig. 48.6b). Food and bacterial plaque collect and cause acute infection, which may extend outwards, even into the parapharyngeal area.

The patient complains of severe, poorly localised pain near the mandibular angle. Pain is aggravated by chewing because the opposing tooth bites on the swollen gingival flap. On examination, the pericoronal tissues of the affected tooth are red and swollen with a purulent discharge from beneath the flap. Oral examination may be difficult because of trismus. Externally, the submandibular and upper cervical lymph nodes are enlarged and tender.

CASE HISTORY

Fig. 48.6 Impacted lower third molars and pericoronitis

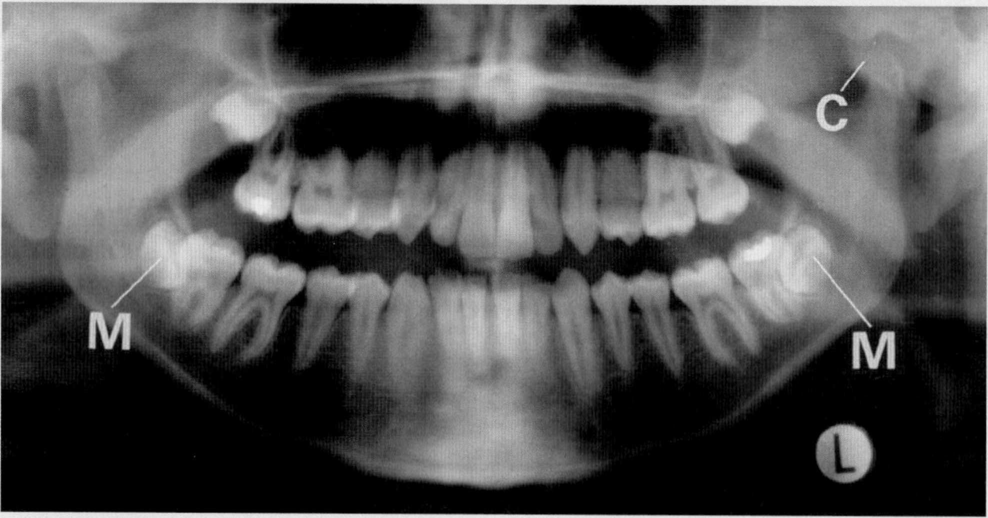

(a)

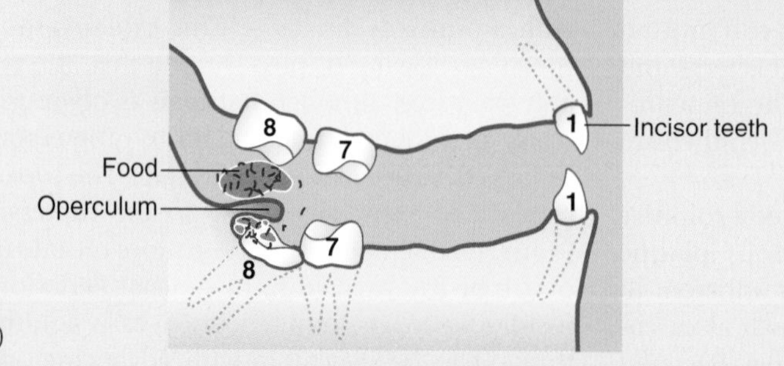

(b)

This OPG radiograph of a 16-year-old girl shows the whole lower jaw 'opened out'. Both lower third molars **M** are seen to be angled towards the second molars and impacted against them. The roots are not fully formed and there is little chance of these teeth erupting normally. These were an incidental finding, the X-rays having been taken to demonstrate a fracture of the neck of the left mandibular condyle **C**

Management of pericoronitis

Pericoronitis is cellulitis with incipient abscess formation caused by mixed organisms usually sensitive to penicillin or metronidazole. It is treated by irrigating beneath the flap with hydrogen peroxide and mouth washes several times daily with warm salty water. Rapid relief is obtained by removing the upper wisdom tooth if it impinges on the flap. Oral phenoxymethylpenicillin (penicillin V) and metronidazole are given if the patient is systemically unwell. If attacks are recurrent, the lower wisdom tooth may be removed surgically.

ACUTE ULCERATIVE GINGIVITIS (VINCENT'S INFECTION)

This is an acute inflammatory condition with necrotising ulceration of the gingival margin. It is caused by a mixture of Gram-negative organisms which are normal oral commensals. The most prominent are *Fusobacterium fusiformis*, *Borrelia vincentii* and *Bacteroides melaninogenicus*. Acute ulcerative gingivitis most commonly occurs in young adults who 'burn the candle at both ends' and become run down. Poor oral hygiene, pericoronitis and smoking may contribute. Acute ulcerative gingivitis is now uncommon, but was widespread in the First World War when it gained the name '**trench mouth**'.

There is an abrupt onset of gingival pain and bleeding, accompanied by a foul, often metallic taste and marked halitosis. Cervical nodes are enlarged and tender, and there may be fever, malaise and anorexia. Oral examination reveals characteristic ragged ulceration of the gingiva, especially between the teeth. In severe cases, the pharyngeal mucosa becomes inflamed and ulcerated (**Vincent's angina**). Acute ulcerative gingivitis is easily distinguished from **herpetic gingivostomatitis**, as the former is confined to the gingival margin, whereas herpetic ulcers are scattered all over the oral mucosa.

Management of acute ulcerative gingivitis

Vincent's infection rapidly responds to metronidazole tablets (200 mg t.d.s.), usually with full recovery of gingival morphology; penicillin is also effective. Tooth brushing is painful during an attack and the mouth should be frequently rinsed with warm water or weak hydrogen peroxide to keep it clean. Afterwards, careful attention to oral hygiene usually prevents recurrence.

TUMOURS OF THE ORAL MUCOSA

PATHOPHYSIOLOGY AND AETIOLOGY

The oral cavity and tongue is invested by stratified squamous epithelium. Oral squamous cell carcinoma (SCC) accounts for about 3% of all malignancies, and is the commonest cancer on the Asian subcontinent. Like their skin counterparts, these usually occur in older people, though this trend is changing as a result of human papillomavirus-induced SCC. Men are affected twice as often as women, but in HPV cancers the ratio is more even.

Tobacco products are the more usual cause, with pipe and cigar smokers and tobacco chewers at greatest risk in the West. The tongue and lower lip are the common sites, each accounting for about 25%. Chronic irritation by ill-fitting dentures, jagged tooth restorations or alcohol abuse may contribute to the aetiology.

In India, Sri Lanka, Papua New Guinea and other countries, the habit of chewing *paan*, a stimulant package of betel leaf, areka nut, cured tobacco and slaked lime, causes a very high incidence of buccal carcinoma, and submucous fibrosis which results in trismus and is itself pre-malignant.

Leukoplakia is a premalignant dysplasia found in 50% of patients with oral carcinoma.

CLINICAL FEATURES OF ORAL CANCER

Oral cancer usually presents as a slowly enlarging chronic indurated ulcer which fails to heal (Fig. 48.7b and c). An early lesion may present as a mucosal swelling. Lesions are usually painless unless secondarily infected, although advanced lesions may cause pain as they invade deeply. Carcinoma of the tongue, for example, may cause pain referred to the ear or pharynx via the lingual nerve or chorda tympani.

Oral SCC invades locally and usually metastasises initially to submandibular and upper cervical lymph nodes. Even small tumours can cause metastases. Spreading tumours of the posterior floor of mouth and tongue interfere with speech, mastication and swallowing and are particularly distressing symptoms.

MANAGEMENT OF ORAL CANCER

A chronic oral ulcer which fails to heal after removing aggravating factors (such as ill-fitting dentures) should undergo urgent incision biopsy to exclude cancer.

Oral cancers are excised with at least a 1 cm margin of normal tissue. This may not be possible anatomically or cosmetically and often necessitates major reconstructive surgery. Involved lymph nodes are removed by neck dissection, aiming to preserve vital structures such as the accessory nerve and great vessels.

Some cancers, particularly tongue base and oropharynx are best managed with radiotherapy. Induction chemotherapy is often used as a single modality but is never curative. Radiotherapy is usually via external beam, and rarely with radioactive implants. A disadvantage of radiotherapy is that it damages salivary glands, resulting in **xerostomia** (dry mouth) which can be debilitating. Apart from discomfort, this predisposes to salivary gland infection.

Carcinoma of the lip has the best prognosis. The crude 5-year survival rate of oral cancer is around 50%, with small tumours having the best prognosis. Regional node involvement reduces the chance of cure by half.

LEUKOPLAKIA

Leukoplakia means 'white plaque', and describes white patches on oral mucosa which cannot readily be scraped off (see Fig. 48.7a). This distinguishes them from candidal infections. White plaques may be caused by friction, oral lichen

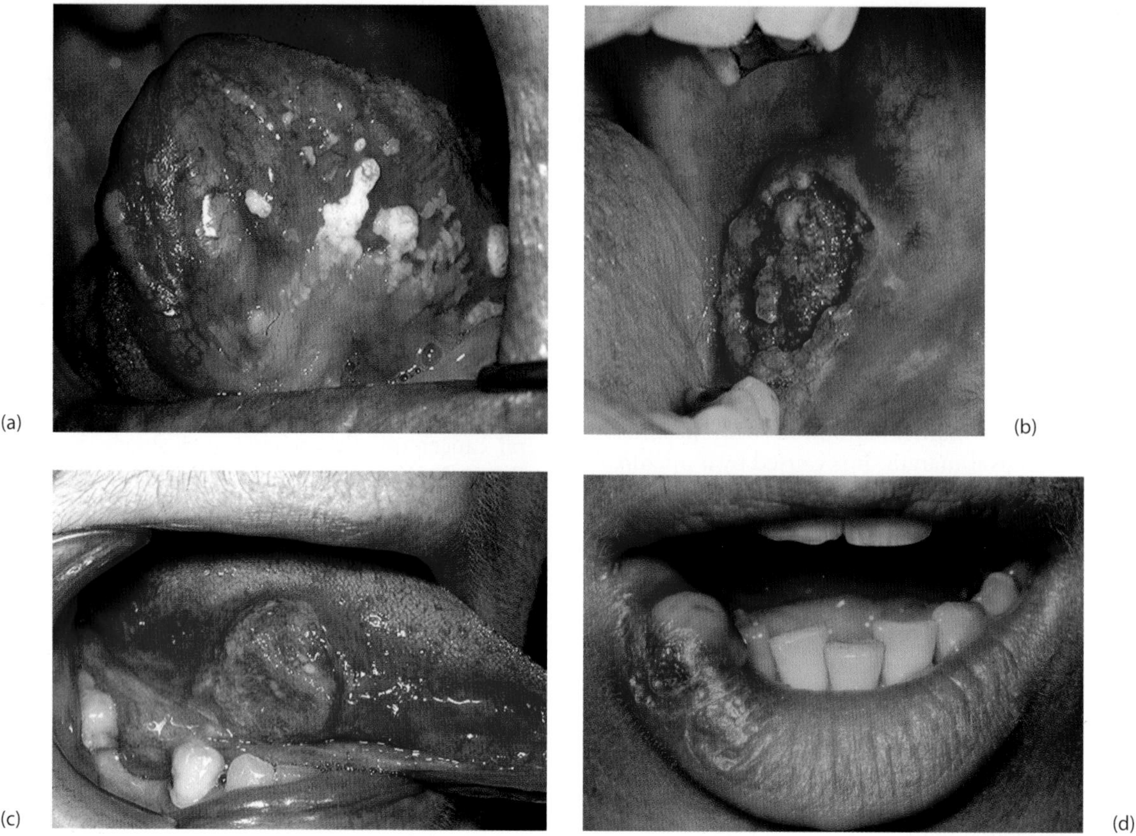

Fig. 48.7 Premalignant and malignant conditions of the mouth
(a) Leukoplakia under tongue. **(b)** Ulcerating squamous cell carcinoma (SCC) of the cheek. **(c)** Ulcerating SCC of the tongue. **(d)** Squamous cell carcinoma of the lip. This man of 60 had smoked a pipe most of his life. He tended to keep the pipe constantly in his mouth while he worked. He presented with a non-healing ulcer of the lip, proven to be a well-differentiated SCC on biopsy. A wedge resection of the lip was performed and produced a cure

planus or more rarely lupus erythematosus, but the main importance of leukoplakia is that it may represent epithelial dysplasia or even carcinoma-in-situ.

The cheeks and tongue are most often affected, although dysplastic patches may develop anywhere on oral mucosa. An innocent white line is often seen along the inside of the cheek; this corresponds to the biting surfaces of the teeth and is caused by frictional hyperplasia.

Severe or extensive leukoplakia should be referred for specialist maxillofacial opinion and biopsy. Areas of severe dysplasia require surgical removal, which may necessitate grafting.

EPULIS

An epulis is a benign, localised gingival swelling. Two types are recognised: fibrous epulis and giant cell epulis.

A **fibrous epulis** is simply a benign fibrous tissue tumour arising from periodontal membrane or nearby periosteum. It forms a smooth, firm, slowly growing lump, covered with normal gingiva. A fibrous epulis usually emerges between two teeth, which may be pushed apart by pressure. Treatment is by excision with curettage of the origin to prevent recurrence (Fig. 48.8).

A **giant cell epulis** arises in a similar location but grows much faster. It forms an irregular red fleshy mass which ulcerates and bleeds. The lesion consists of numerous giant cells in a vascular stroma, which may invade local bone. Treatment involves extracting associated teeth and excising and curetting bone to avoid recurrence (Fig. 48.8).

Pyogenic granulomas may occur on gums or oral mucosa of the lips. They look like pyogenic granulomas of skin and often occur in pregnancy (see Ch. 46, p. 574).

Fig. 48.8 Lumps and bumps around the mouth

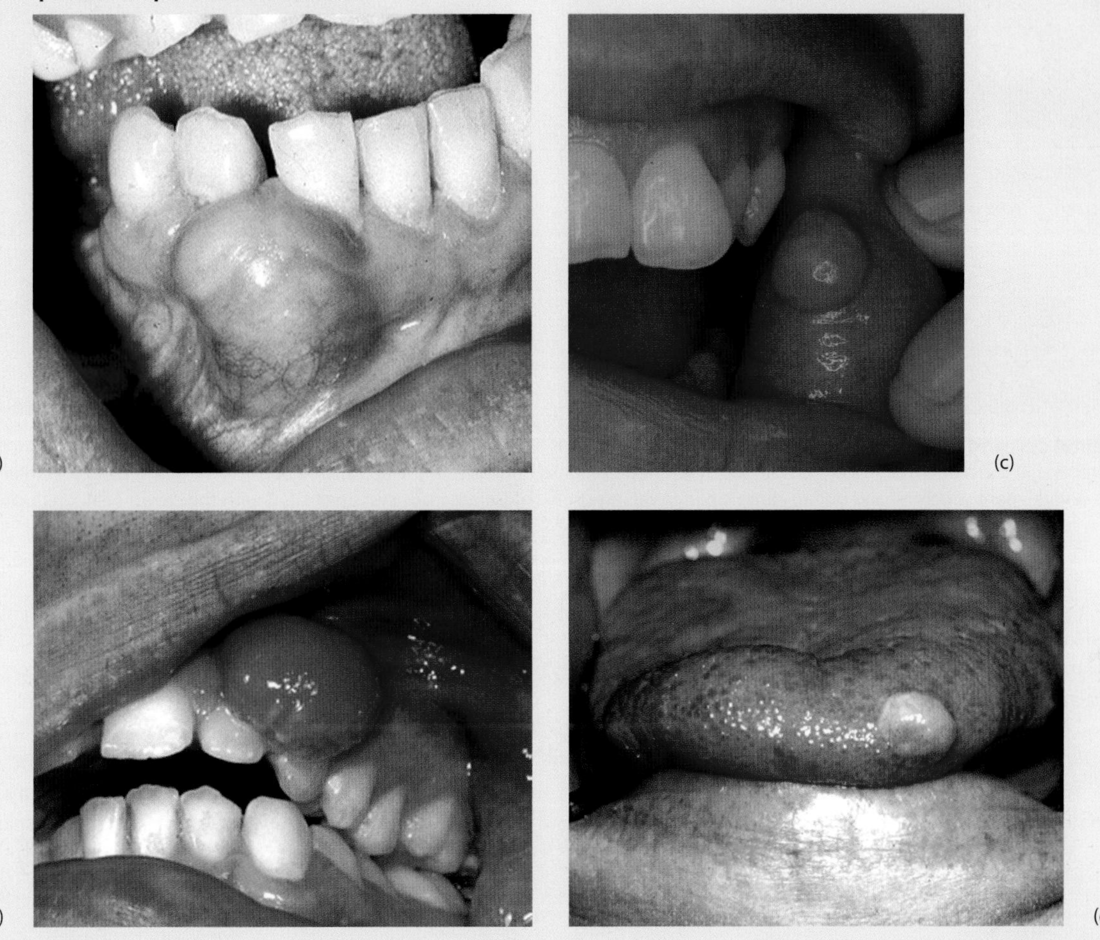

(a) Fibrous epulis. This can be seen to be moving the nearby tooth out of alignment. **(b)** Giant cell epulis. Both of these are in typical interdental location. The fibrous epulis is the same colour as the gum, while the giant cell epulis is a deeper red. **(c)** Fibroepithelial polyp inside cheek. These lesions are common and are probably initiated by minor biting trauma to the cheek or lip. They are often inadvertently chewed upon and gradually become larger. Excision is usually straightforward. **(d)** Pyogenic granuloma of the tongue. These are probably initiated by injury and maintained by an excessive healing response. They can occur on the gum or anywhere else in the mouth

MISCELLANEOUS DISORDERS CAUSING INTRAORAL SWELLING

RETENTION CYSTS OF ACCESSORY SALIVARY GLANDS

The oral mucosa contains numerous accessory mucous and serous salivary glands. Small retention cysts probably develop as a result of duct trauma. Most retention cysts are smaller than 1 cm in diameter. They commonly occur in the lower lip mucosa where they are irritating and are readily traumatised. Retention cysts are blue-grey and are soft to palpation. They often rupture spontaneously but usually reform. Small retention cysts can usually be enucleated under local anaesthesia; larger ones may need marsupialisation. Swellings in the upper lip are almost always neoplastic and are malignant until proven otherwise.

TUMOURS OF ACCESSORY SALIVARY GLANDS

Tumours occasionally arise in accessory salivary glands. These are often malignant **adenocystic or muco-epidermoid carcinomas**. They present as small, firm lumps in the oral mucosa, upper lip or posterior palate, and are often discovered before invading deeply or metastasising. Treatment is by wide excision but the prognosis is often poor.

BONY EXOSTOSES

Local outgrowths of jaw bones are common and produce an intraoral lump which may be suspicious of neoplasia to the uninitiated doctor. The common site is the middle of the hard palate, known as a **torus palatinus**. A similar exostosis, usually bilateral, occurs on the lingual (tongue) side of the mandible, opposite premolar teeth and is known as **torus mandibularis**.

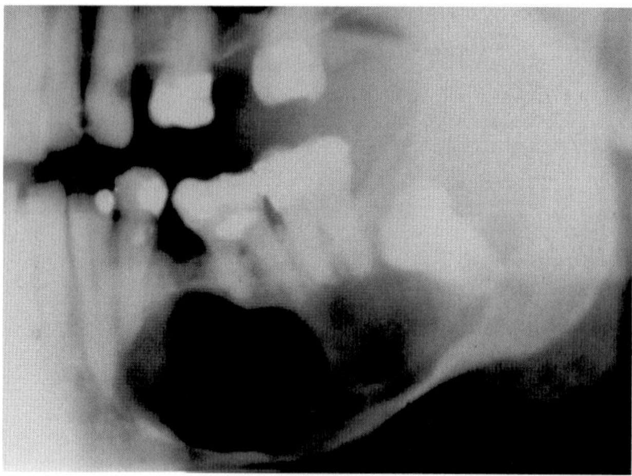
(a)

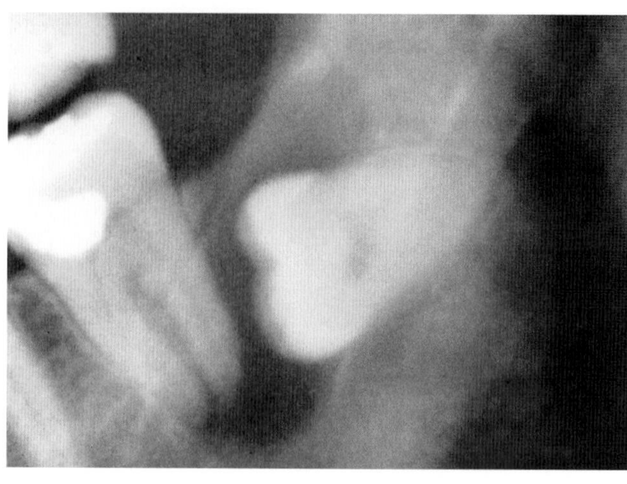
(b)

Fig. 48.9 Dental cyst and dentigerous cyst
(a) Large dental cyst in the mandible. This arose from tooth-forming epithelial remnants in the apical area of the lower left second premolar tooth which was extracted several months beforehand due to chronic periapical infection. **(b)** Dentigerous cyst associated with the crown of an unerupted lower third molar. These cysts originate from epithelial remnants of the tooth bud

These lesions are bony hard and are covered by normal oral mucosa. Excision is rarely needed unless there are problems in wearing a removable denture.

CYSTS AND TUMOURS OF THE JAWS

Various cystic lesions and tumours arise in the jaws. Many are abnormalities of tooth-forming epithelium, developmental or acquired. Figure 48.9b shows a mandibular dentigerous cyst, a developmental cyst. They are rare and can usually be diagnosed radiologically. The jaws are occasionally the site of benign or malignant bone tumours such as osteosarcoma and osteoclastomas. They can also be affected by metastatic tumours from breast or prostate. Bony growth disorders such as fibrous dysplasia and Paget's disease may also affect the jaw.

Disorders of the thyroid and parathyroid glands

49

INTRODUCTION

Patients with thyroid disorders presenting to a surgeon usually have a **neck lump**, often asymptomatic but the patient may fear malignancy. In some, the mass may be causing pressure symptoms or cosmetic deformity. A discrete thyroid lump may be found or the whole gland may be enlarged. A large thyroid swelling is known as a **goitre**, from the Latin for throat '*guttur*'. Most patients are clinically euthyroid (i.e. normal hormone activity) and thyroid function tests are normal. Occasionally patients are referred with **hyperthyroidism** when medical treatment has failed, radioisotope treatment is unsuitable or there is an overactive nodule. All may require some form of thyroidectomy.

Patients with **parathyroid disorders** usually attend because of symptomatic or biochemically detected **hypercalcaemia** caused by excess parathormone, treatable only by surgery for a solitary adenoma, multi-gland hyperplasia or, very rarely, carcinoma.

THYROID DISORDERS

Pathophysiological and clinical features of the various disorders are summarised in Table 49.1, except for thyroid malignancy, outlined later in Table 49.2.

MAIN CLINICAL PRESENTATIONS OF THYROID DISEASE IN SURGICAL PRACTICE

DIFFUSE OR GENERALISED ENLARGEMENT OF THE THYROID

The term **goitre** is often used for any thyroid enlargement. Most large thyroid swellings in developed countries are simple **colloid goitres** i.e. idiopathic diffuse or multinodular hyperplasia. **Multinodular goitres** usually develop from diffuse goitres after some years.

Iodine deficiency is the usual cause of *endemic* goitres (often in isolated, mountainous regions such as Nepal), preventable by adding iodine to the diet. These are often asymmetrical, soft and composed of hyperplastic nodules, and can reach enormous sizes (see Fig. 49.1). Although unsightly, endemic goitres cause surprisingly few symptoms and the patient is usually euthyroid.

Anaplastic carcinomas may cause thyroid swellings in elderly patients (see Fig. 49.2), usually with symptoms of invasion including **hoarseness** (recurrent laryngeal nerve), and **stridor**, particularly at night, with tracheal invasion. The gland is hard on palpation. The uncommon thyroid **lymphomas** also present with diffuse enlargement.

In **Graves' disease** (primary hyperthyroidism) there is usually some smooth thyroid enlargement, often increased by drug treatment but almost never the presenting feature. Similarly, in **Hashimoto's** thyroiditis, the thyroid may be moderately enlarged but firm and finely nodular on palpation.

SOLITARY THYROID NODULE

A clinically solitary thyroid nodule is common but 50% are multinodular on imaging (Fig. 49.3). When small, these nodules are found incidentally, often noticed when the patient swallows. Less than 10% of true solitary nodules are malignant although this rises to about 40% after neck irradiation. Almost all thyroid nodules in **childhood** are malignant. Fallout from the Chernobyl nuclear meltdown caused many thyroid cancers in children. Malignancy should be excluded in any solitary nodule, and FNA cytology or core needle biopsy is the first step.

A solitary nodule is usually idiopathic hyperplasia which if discrete, is a **thyroid adenoma**. **Thyroid cysts** are fairly common. Both fall within the description '**simple or multinodular colloid goitre**'.

Table 49.1 Benign diseases of the thyroid

Condition (relative frequency in developed countries)	Pathophysiology	Clinical features
1. Developmental abnormalities		
a. Thyroglossal cyst *(uncommon)*	Cyst formation anywhere along the midline thyroglossal tract. This marks the line of embryological descent of the thyroid from the foramen caecum via the hyoid bone to the normal position in the neck	Smooth, rounded swelling in midline of neck anywhere between the submental area and isthmus of thyroid. Usually found in children and young adults
b. Thyroglossal fistula *(rare)*	Incision into or incomplete removal of a thyroglossal cyst can cause a fistula	Fistulous (or sinus) opening near midline of neck. Intermittently discharges clear fluid or becomes infected and discharges pus
c. Ectopic thyroid *(uncommon)*	Part or all of the thyroid lying anywhere along the thyroglossal tract	Usually symptomless but may present as an unusual swelling near foramen caecum at junction of anterior two-thirds and posterior third of tongue
2. Inflammatory and autoimmune disorders		
a. Hashimoto's thyroiditis *(common)*	Diffuse lymphocytic infiltration of thyroid gland with progressive destruction of thyroid follicles. Over a period of years, leads to progressive atrophy and fibrosis. Various anti-thyroid antibodies usually present in plasma in high titres. Polygenic inherited disorder which may be associated with other autoimmune disorders, e.g. pernicious anaemia. Focal lymphocytic thyroiditis is probably a milder variant of the same condition	Presents in adulthood with mild, diffuse, sometimes tender thyroid enlargement. Often the thyroid is not enlarged. Patient usually euthyroid or hyperthyroid at outset, but later becomes hypothyroid. Affects females much more frequently than males
b. Graves' disease *(fairly common)*	Diffuse thyroid hyperplasia due to the action of a circulating immunoglobulin 'long-acting thyroid stimulator' (LATS). This binds to thyroid acinar cells mimicking the effects of TSH and producing excess thyroid hormone	Diffuse thyroid enlargement, sometimes with a bruit, but main feature is marked hyperthyroidism (thyrotoxicosis) causing weight loss, heat intolerance, tachycardia, hyper-reflexia, tremor and sometimes exophthalmos
c. De Quervain's acute thyroiditis *(uncommon)*	Diffuse inflammation of thyroid gland, probably viral in origin. Neutrophilic and later lymphocytic and histiocytic infiltration of gland occurs	Very tender, diffuse moderate thyroid enlargement, with or without systemic symptoms. Episodes last weeks to months and are often recurrent. Patient usually euthyroid but may be hyperthyroid in acute phase
d. Riedel's thyroiditis *(very rare)*	Dense fibrosis of thyroid gland. Possibly an autoimmune process	Extremely hard ('woody goitre') often asymmetrical thyroid mass suspicious of tumour. Sometimes produces symptoms of compression
3. Hyperplastic and metabolic disorders		
a. Simple non-toxic colloid goitre *(very common)*	Benign, diffuse or multinodular hyperplasia of thyroid follicles. Cause is unknown but possibly minor abnormality of thyroid hormone synthesis	Diffuse or sporadic multinodular thyroid enlargement or single 'adenomatous' nodule or cyst. Patient clinically euthyroid and all thyroid function tests normal. Affects females much more than males
b. Endemic goitre *(very rare in UK)*	Diffuse hyperplasia of thyroid follicles due to dietary iodine deficiency or goitrogenic foods. Endemic in inland, developing countries, especially in mountainous areas	Diffuse, often massive thyroid enlargement which may later become nodular. T4 is low or normal and TSH tends to be elevated
c. Drug-induced goitre *(uncommon)*	Diffuse thyroid hyperplasia secondary to interference with thyroid hormone synthesis. Drugs causing this are anti-thyroid drugs used in therapy (e.g. carbimazole) or others like lithium and aminoglutethimide	Diffuse thyroid enlargement. Patient usually euthyroid. Can be prevented by using replacement dose of T4 concurrently with blocking drugs ('block and replace')
d. Dyshormonogenesis *(very uncommon)*	Diffuse thyroid hyperplasia caused by a variety of uncommon genetic (recessive) defects affecting thyroid hormone synthesis	Presents at birth or in childhood with thyroid enlargement and severe hypothyroidism (cretinism). In developed countries, these defects are usually diagnosed at birth by neonatal screening tests before any goitre has developed
e. Physiological *(common)*	Diffuse thyroid hyperplasia often associated with pregnancy and puberty	Mild diffuse thyroid enlargement. Patient euthyroid

Table 49.2 Malignant diseases of the thyroid

Condition (relative frequency in developed countries)	Pathophysiology	Clinical features
Adenocarcinomas		
a. Papillary carcinoma *(relatively common—two-thirds of all thyroid carcinomas and 90% in children)*	Papillary adenocarcinoma forms a complex branching structure with a fibrous stroma (papillary pattern) and **psammoma** (sand grain) bodies. Variable degree of dysplasia. Commonly metastasises to cervical nodes but distant metastases rare	Slowly growing firm thyroid lump or cervical lymph nodes or both. Occurs in adults and sometimes children, 3F:1M. Excellent prognosis even with local metastases—90% survival at 10 years
b. Follicular carcinoma *(relatively uncommon)*	Tumour forms a well-developed follicular pattern reminiscent of normal thyroid. Generally well differentiated but metastasis is usually distant, e.g. lungs and bone	Similar presentation to papillary carcinoma but does not involve cervical nodes. Affects slightly older age group than papillary carcinoma, 3F:1M
c. Anaplastic carcinoma *(relatively uncommon)*	Aggressive tumour rapidly spreading beyond the confines of the gland	Diffuse, hard thyroid enlargement, often with symptoms of tracheal or recurrent laryngeal nerve involvement. Affects elderly patients. Very poor prognosis
d. Medullary carcinoma (*very uncommon*)	Well-differentiated tumour derived from parafollicular calcitonin-secreting cells (C-cells). Tumour contains deposits of amyloid	Stony hard thyroid lump, possibly with secondaries in cervical nodes. Often associated with MEN II. Poor prognosis. Calcitonin in blood is a tumour marker
Lymphoma (rare)	Diffuse lymphoid infiltration of thyroid gland	Diffuse thyroid enlargement. Patient euthyroid. Usually occurs in Hashimoto's disease

CASE HISTORY

Fig. 49.1 Endemic goitre

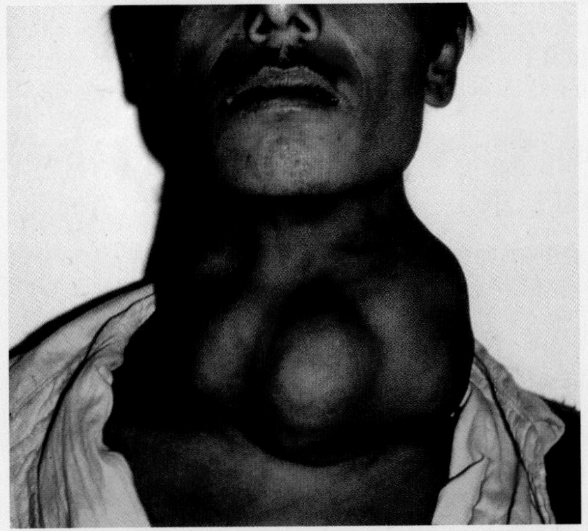

This condition, caused by iodine deficiency, is extremely common in isolated mountain regions. The thyroid can reach an enormous size, yet the patient suffers only minimal symptoms and is usually euthyroid. This typical example in a Nepalese man is only of moderate size by local standards!

CASE HISTORY

Fig. 49.2 Anaplastic carcinoma

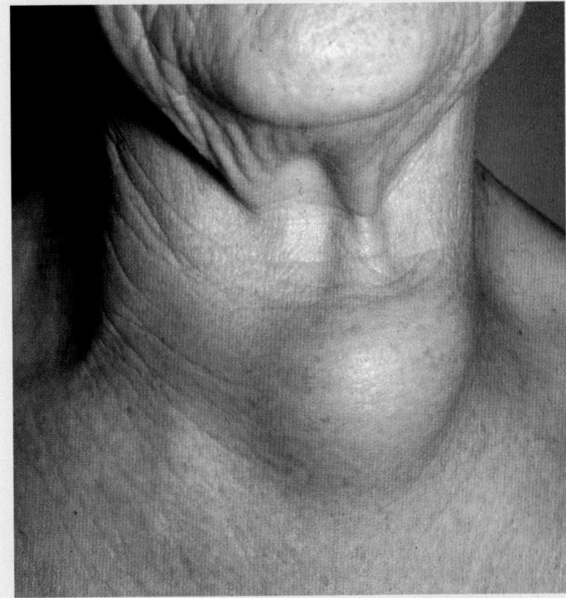

Rapidly enlarging hard thyroid mass in an elderly woman. The mass was firmly tethered to strap muscles and deeper structures. Treatment was purely palliative as this tumour does not respond to any current therapy

OTHER FEATURES ASSOCIATED WITH THYROID ENLARGEMENT

A new area of enlargement in an existing goitre may result from haemorrhage into a cyst or nodule, enlargement of a hyperplastic nodule or a developing carcinoma. If the gland extends into the anterior mediastinum behind the sternum (see Fig. 49.6, below), the trachea may be compressed or displaced by this **retrosternal goitre** and cause **stridor**, often only obvious when the neck is in certain positions, for example, sleeping on one side. Hoarseness or stridor may also

CASE HISTORY

Fig. 49.3 Multinodular goitre

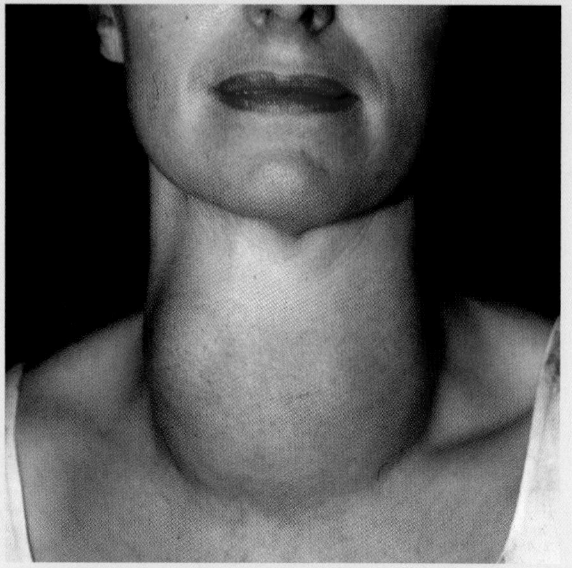

Longstanding multinodular goitre in a woman of 40 with a strong family history of thyroid disorders. The thyroid is multinodular on palpation, and on ultrasound there are multiple nodules of various sizes plus some small cysts. Any change in a multinodular goitre may herald malignancy

CASE HISTORY

Fig. 49.4 Hyperthyroidism

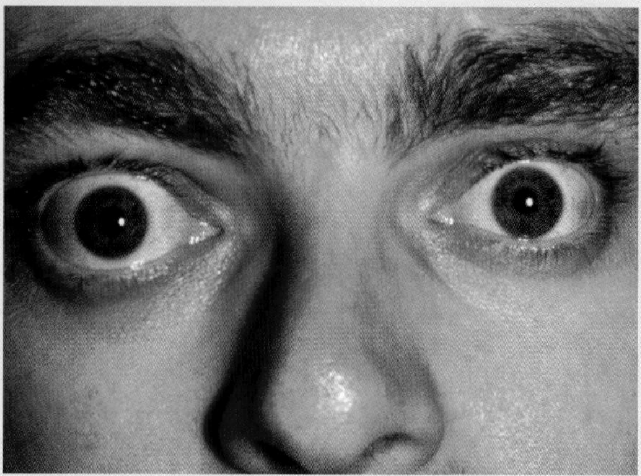

Exophthalmic eye signs of hyperthyroidism in 43-year-old man with 6-month history of hyperthyroidism. His family had noticed his increasingly staring eyes. He had proptosis and lid lag

Box 49.1 Clinical manifestations of thyrotoxicosis

- **Metabolic**—heat intolerance, increased appetite with weight loss, diarrhoea, menorrhagia
- **Cardiovascular**—palpitations, tachycardia even while asleep, atrial fibrillation
- **Neuropsychiatric**—hyperkinesis, insomnia, emotional instability, tremor, proximal myopathy
- **Ocular**—exophthalmos including proptosis, lid retraction and eventually ophthalmoplegia (see Fig. 49.4)
- **Cutaneous**—pretibial myxoedema

result from **invasion** of trachea or recurrent laryngeal nerve by anaplastic carcinoma.

Pain and tenderness are uncommon presenting features, but characterise the rare infective **de Quervain's thyroiditis**. Sometimes the thyroid is painful and tender in Hashimoto's thyroiditis.

HYPERTHYROIDISM

Clinical manifestations of hyperthyroidism are summarised in Box 49.1 (see also Fig. 49.4). Excessive thyroid hormone is a feature of Graves' disease. Mild hyperthyroidism also occurs in the early stages of Hashimoto's thyroiditis, burning out later with the patient becoming hypothyroid. A solitary adenomatous nodule may produce excess thyroid hormone causing hyperthyroidism. This is known as a **toxic or hot nodule**.

HYPOTHYROIDISM

Hypothyroidism is usually the late result of primary thyroid atrophy or Hashimoto's thyroiditis, or treatment for hyperthyroidism. In any case, the gland is small and fibrous. Hypothyroidism is a late complication in up to 25% of patients after subtotal thyroidectomy and even more after radioiodine therapy for thyrotoxicosis, and is inevitable after total thyroidectomy. Hypothyroidism should be considered in surgical patients presenting with constipation and has also been implicated in aortic thrombosis in middle-aged women.

SPECIAL POINTS IN EXAMINING A THYROID SWELLING

The patient should be seated in a chair (Fig. 49.5) with space to palpate from behind and have a glass of water available to swallow. General examination should look for signs of hyperthyroidism (tachycardia, atrial fibrillation, fine tremor, sweaty palms and hyper-reflexia) and for signs specific to Graves' disease (exophthalmos and ophthalmoplegia). Next, the front of the neck is inspected while the patient swallows; the characteristic rise of a thyroid swelling results from its investment in **pretracheal fascia** attached to the larynx above. A normal thyroid is not visible even on swallowing, and is not normally palpable.

The thyroid area is next palpated from behind. This is best for examining the size, shape and consistency of the gland. It also allows the lower edge of a swelling to be palpated to identify retrosternal extension. The thyroid lobes wrap around the larynx and lie deep to the sternomastoid muscles which tend to conceal thyroid enlargement and make it tricky to examine the whole gland.

The jugular chain of **lymph nodes** should be palpated for metastases. In thyrotoxicosis, auscultation may reveal a **bruit** of increased vascularity.

If there is suspicion of recurrent laryngeal nerve palsy because of **hoarseness**, vocal cord function tests should be

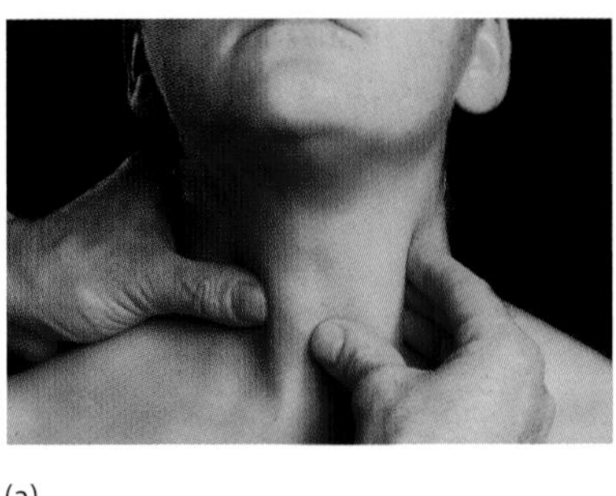

(a)

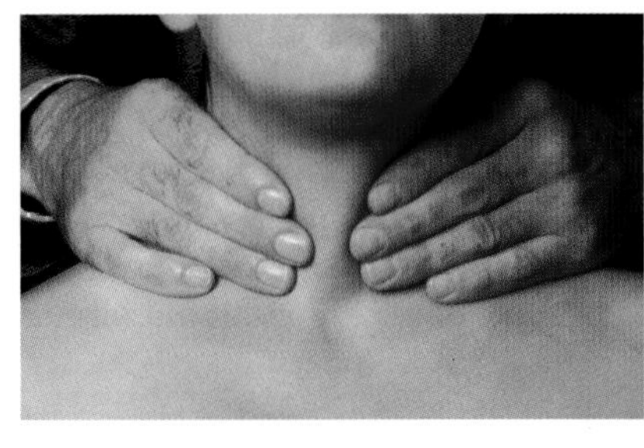

(b)

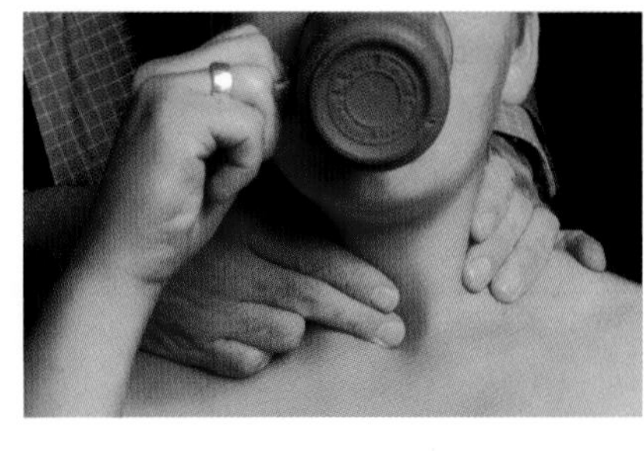

(c)

Fig. 49.5 Examination of the thyroid gland
The patient should be sitting upright in a chair with room for the examiner to approach from behind. **(a)** Gentle palpation from the front with slight sideways pressure from the left hand whilst palpating with the right. This is repeated for the right side of the gland. **(b)** General palpation of the gland from behind. Is there enlargement? Is it a single nodule or multinodular? How big is it? **(c)** Palpation of the gland while the patient swallows. Does the gland rise with swallowing? Is there retrosternal extension?

Box 49.2 Principles of investigation of a thyroid mass

- **General thyroid status**—thyroid function tests and thyroid autoantibodies
- **Morphology of the gland**, i.e. size, shape and physical consistency, effects upon surrounding structures—ultrasound, plain X-rays of thoracic outlet, CT scanning
- **Tissue diagnosis**—fine needle aspiration cytology or needle biopsy, incision or excision biopsy

performed. The patient is asked to cough and to pronounce the sound 'ee'; both are likely to be abnormal if there is nerve damage. In this case, or if surgery is contemplated, assessment of cord function should be performed by indirect laryngoscopy, usually in an ENT department.

APPROACH TO INVESTIGATION OF A THYROID MASS

The questions during investigation are summarised in Box 49.2 and described in detail below. Patients who have undergone previous neck radiotherapy should be considered at high risk of thyroid carcinoma.

GENERAL THYROID STATUS

First establish whether the patient is **euthyroid**, **hyperthyroid** or **hypothyroid**. Initially, this is clinical but estimations of free thyroxine (fT4) and TSH are usually performed. Thyroid-binding globulin is elevated in pregnancy and puberty; using free thyroxine level corrects for this and avoids misinterpretation. If the patient is clinically hyperthyroid but the fT4 is normal, tri-iodothyronine (T3) levels are occasionally measured. TSH level is usually low in hyperthyroidism and elevated in hypothyroidism. Some laboratories prefer to measure just the TSH level initially and perform detailed tests if this is abnormal.

Thyroid autoantibodies are assayed if autoimmune disease is a possibility. Although not usually measured clinically, the presence of long-acting thyroid stimulating factor (LATS) is diagnostic of Graves' disease. Hashimoto's thyroiditis is characterised by elevation of anti-thyroid antibodies such as anti-thyroglobulin or anti-mitochondrial antibodies (anti-thyroid M).

MORPHOLOGY OF THE GLAND

Ultrasound scanning is useful to establish morphology and diagnose cysts. It can also indicate retrosternal extension. CT scans of neck and thoracic outlet are taken if malignancy is suspected or if there appears to be tracheal displacement or compression (Figs 49.6).

TISSUE DIAGNOSIS

Tissue diagnosis using fine needle aspiration cytology (FNAC) or core needle biopsy is usual for solitary nodules or recently enlarged nodules in multinodular goitres. This can be performed without ultrasound, but ultrasound gives a fuller picture and guides biopsies. Given a competent and involved thyroid cytologist, 90% of thyroid nodules can be categorised this way. Needle core biopsy gives larger specimens with a greater diagnostic potential. If a **colloid nodule** is diagnosed, excision is not necessary unless it causes compressive symptoms or cosmetic deformity. Obviously malignant lesions require operation. These include **papillary**, **medullary** and early **anaplastic carcinomas**. Most **lymphomas** are inadequately sampled by FNAC or core biopsy and **follicular carcinomas** cannot be distinguished cytologically from **benign follicular adenomas**; both display sheets of follicular cells. Lesions with this appearance should be removed, although most will be benign.

Incision biopsy at open operation is occasionally used for diagnosing generalised thyroid enlargement where the chances of malignancy are low, or lymphoma is suspected.

FUNCTIONAL ACTIVITY OF GLANDULAR TISSUE

Injected radionuclides of iodine are avidly taken up by functioning thyroid tissue and used to be widely employed for thyroid scanning. The increasing use of ultrasound and needle cytology and knowing that only 10% of cold nodules are

Fig. 49.6 Retrosternal goitre

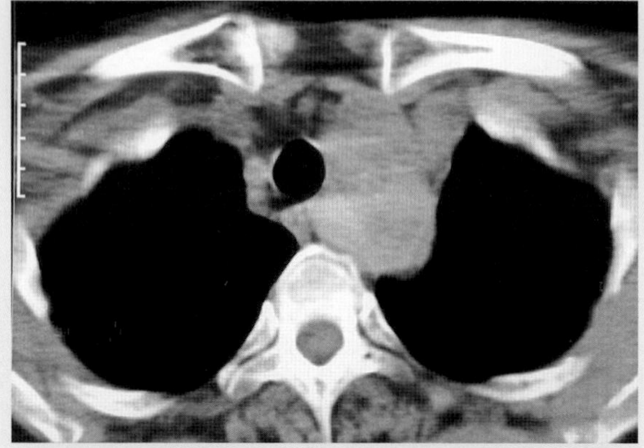

(a)

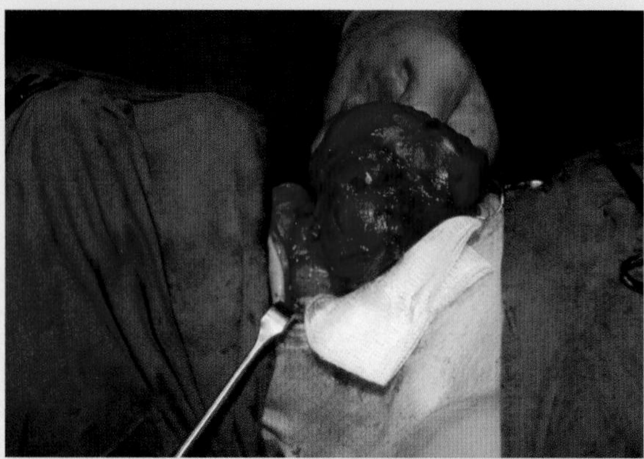

(b)

This 38-year-old woman had suffered stridor at night for several months. On palpation, the thyroid was not particularly large but the trachea was markedly deviated and the thyroid did not rise on swallowing, both providing evidence of substantial retrosternal extension. **(a)** CT scan at the level of the clavicles showing enlargement of the left side of the thyroid gland with moderate deviation but no compression of the trachea. **(b)** At operation, this huge retrosternal extension was drawn up out of the anterior mediastinum. As this was a multinodular goitre, a total thyroidectomy was performed. Histopathology confirmed a benign multinodular goitre

malignant have greatly reduced the need for radionuclide scanning.

When scanning is employed, the gland is imaged after isotope injection to identify the distribution of isotope activity. This may fall into one of four patterns:

- **Diffuse, homogeneous uptake**—found in normal glands or in diffuse hyperactivity, e.g. Graves' disease
- **Generalised but patchy uptake**—in multinodular goitre where hyperplastic nodules are less active than the surrounding normal tissue
- **The cold nodule**—an area devoid of uptake indicates non-secreting tissue, i.e. tumour, inactive adenomatous nodule or cyst and requires tissue diagnosis
- **The hot nodule**—or toxic adenoma. This represents an autonomous focus of excess T4 secretion. Secretory activity of the thyroid is suppressed. The patient is usually euthyroid but sometimes thyrotoxic ('toxic nodule')

Very occasionally, **thyroid malignancies** secrete thyroid hormones and show up as warm or hot nodules on isotope scanning. Isotope scanning can also identify and localise **ectopic thyroid tissue** (in the tongue or along the course of the thyroglossal duct), **retrosternal extension** of a thyroid swelling and **metastases** of functioning thyroid carcinomas, provided the thyroid has been removed or ablated.

SPECIFIC CLINICAL PROBLEMS OF THE THYROID AND THEIR MANAGEMENT

HYPERTHYROIDISM (THYROTOXICOSIS)

Two percent of women and 0.2% of men in the UK have hyperthyroidism. Untreated, it causes weight loss, anxiety, tachycardia, palpitations and increased risk of cardiovascular death. Most are caused by Graves' disease, some by toxic multinodular goitre and a few by toxic adenoma. Carcinoma is a very rare cause, occasionally diagnosed incidentally when a hot nodule is examined histologically. Graves' disease is an autoimmune disorder in which circulating antibodies bind to TSH receptors in the thyroid and stimulate follicular cells to secrete thyroid hormones independent of pituitary feedback. Hashimoto's thyroiditis may produce mild hyperthyroidism in its early stages but is self-limiting. If in doubt, the aetiology can be determined by radioisotope scanning.

Treatment of hyperthyroidism

There are three main options: **anti-thyroid drugs**, **radioisotope destruction** of functioning thyroid tissue and **subtotal (or total) thyroidectomy**. Anti-thyroid drugs are the first-line except in the elderly and unfit; also patients with arrhythmias, angina and osteoporosis are usually treated with radioiodine from the outset. A randomised trial of all three treatments showed that of those treated with drugs, 34% developed recurrent hyperthyroidism. In the radioiodine group, half needed more than one dose but all became hypothyroid within a year. In those treated surgically, 8% recurred and needed further therapy. All groups reported 95% satisfaction with no differences in quality of life.

Thyrotoxic eye disease

Half of thyrotoxic patients develop eye signs known as thyrotoxic ophthalmopathy which can arise or regress independently of thyroid function. Eye disease does not occur in multinodular or adenoma thyrotoxicity. Eye disorders range from minor inflammation of conjunctiva with mild prominence of the globe to severe, debilitating and disfiguring eye disease that occurs in 3–5% of thyrotoxic patients.

Radioactive iodide therapy

Radioactive iodide (^{131}I or ^{125}I) is given by mouth as capsules or solution in doses 100 times higher than for diagnostic scanning (see Fig. 49.7). This is appropriate for middle-aged or elderly patients but is contraindicated in pregnancy because of the risk of fetal thyroid damage and genetic disruption. Iodide is avidly taken up by the gland, and beta particle emission destroys the most active thyroid tissue over a period of weeks or months. Note that anti-thyroid drugs usually need to continue until radioiodine achieves its greatest effect. After

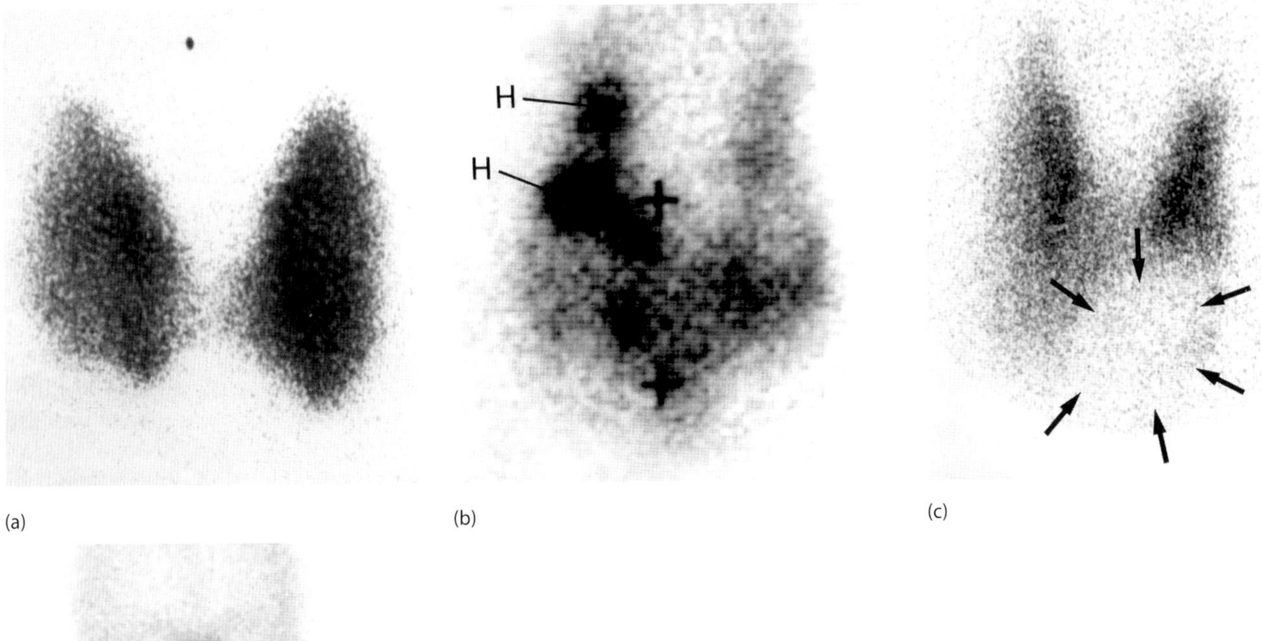

Fig. 49.7 Radioisotope thyroid scans
(a) This enlarged thyroid shows homogeneous tracer uptake typical of a simple colloid goitre. **(b)** Heterogeneous tracer uptake in a multinodular colloid goitre. The dark areas **H** are 'hot nodules'; to maintain the euthyroid state, the rest of the gland exhibits diminished uptake. The + signs indicate the positions of the thyroid cartilage and the suprasternal notch. **(c)** Solitary 'cold' thyroid nodule. The area of low uptake (outline arrowed) at the lower left pole of the thyroid corresponds with a palpable nodule. In the case of a solid lesion (as confirmed by ultrasound), a cold nodule may indicate malignancy. **(d)** Solitary 'hot' thyroid nodule. The area of high uptake in the lower part of the right lobe corresponds to a palpable mass. This patient was hyperthyroid and the lesion could be described as a 'toxic nodule'. Activity of the rest of the gland is suppressed by pituitary-mediated negative feedback from the high serum thyroxine level. The rectangle marked **BG** measures the background radiation in order to quantify the thyroid uptake

treatment, the rest of the isotope is excreted via the kidney, faeces, sweat, saliva and breath. Gamma rays are emitted from the patient's body and may be absorbed by others nearby. Patients should avoid pregnancy for 6 months afterwards.

Different radioiodide doses are used in different units, with higher doses giving a better chance of eliminating hyperthyroidism but giving higher rates of hypothyroidism. Between 10% and 20% need a second dose but once treatment is effective, recurrence is unlikely. Most patients eventually become hypothyroid (about 2–3% each year), especially older patients, those treated with anti-thyroid drugs or those given a high dose. Many units now aim electively to make patients hypothyroid within 6 months and routinely provide levothyroxine replacement. This eliminates the risk of missing hypothyroidism years later and may lower the cardiovascular death risk in euthyroid patients after treatment. There is also a theoretical risk of radioiodine inducing malignancy and so treatment is not advisable in the young. Toxic multinodular disease and toxic adenoma also respond to this treatment; these patients rarely become hypothyroid afterwards.

Unwanted effects

There is a risk of exposing others to radiation during treatment. Current advice is that patients should keep 1 m away from anyone over 5 years for 11 days, from children aged 3–5 for 16 days and from those under 3 for 21 days.

Radioiodine tends to make thyrotoxic ophthalmopathy worse whereas anti-thyroid drugs and surgery do not affect its course. There is no increase in overall cancer death rate in treated patients.

Anti-thyroid drugs

Most thyrotoxicosis patients are initially managed with anti-thyroid drugs to block hormone synthesis. This treatment is not suitable for nodular toxicity because hyperactivity inevitably recurs. **Carbimazole** is the most popular drug and is generally well tolerated. Carbimazole restores plasma hormone levels to normal over 4–8 weeks and treatment is continued for 12–18 months. Unfortunately, hyperthyroidism recurs in about half within 2 years. Between 5% and 10% develop a rash and there are rare cases of agranulocytosis, usually reversible. The white blood count should be monitored during treatment; a sore throat or other infection should alert the patient and doctor to this possible complication. **Propylthiouracil** is an effective anti-thyroid drug without these side-effects but poor control, frequent relapses, other side-effects and non-compliance lead to eventual referral for definitive treatment in up to 40%. In unstable patients with hypothyroidism alternating with hyperthyroidism, a **block and replace** regimen may succeed. Patients are given a higher dose of carbimazole to completely block thyroid hormone production, together with a standard replacement dose of thyroxine.

Beta-adrenergic blocking drugs such as **propranolol** rapidly control the distressing and dangerous effects of thyrotoxicosis. These drugs may be used initially in extremely toxic patients until anti-thyroid drugs take effect, or if a patient urgently needs to be stabilised before thyroidectomy.

Surgical management

Indications for surgery

Surgery for thyrotoxicosis may be indicated as follows:

- When a quick and effective cure is desired that avoids long-term drug therapy. It is often the best treatment for Graves' disease, particularly in younger patients, where the disease is unlikely to burn itself out for years
- When anti-thyroid drugs have proved unsatisfactory and radioiodide treatment is unsuitable
- In toxic multinodular goitre. Response to drug treatment is variable, and surgery also deals with the cosmetic deformity
- Toxic solitary nodules ('hot nodules') may be best excised to allow the suppressed normal thyroid to recover

Preoperative assessment and management of thyrotoxicosis

For all thyroid operations, preoperative assessment often includes **laryngoscopy** to demonstrate vocal cord function. This evaluates recurrent laryngeal nerve function should there be a question of operative damage later. Even without demonstrable cord damage, there is often a subtle change in voice quality after thyroidectomy, sometimes due to external laryngeal nerve damage. Patients should be warned of this before operation, especially if they are singers or politicians!

Wherever possible, thyroid function should be normalised before operation. The thyrotoxic state carries anaesthetic risks, especially of cardiac arrhythmias. Furthermore, manipulation of the gland may provoke massive release of thyroid hormone, precipitating a potentially lethal **thyrotoxic crisis** or 'thyroid storm'. Control is usually achieved with anti-thyroid drugs in the weeks preceding operation. If this fails, or if operation is very urgent, beta-adrenergic blockade can be used.

Anti-thyroid drugs increase the vascularity and this may add to surgical difficulty in toxic enlargement. It is standard practice to administer **Lugol's iodine** solution orally for 10 days before operation while continuing anti-thyroid therapy. This is believed to reduce vascularity and increase the firmness of the gland, making the operation easier.

Subtotal thyroidectomy

Surgery (Fig. 49.8) for hyperthyroidism aims to remove enough thyroid tissue to render the patient euthyroid whilst preserving enough to prevent hypothyroidism. For Graves' disease or toxic multinodular goitre, about 5–8 g of the gland is left intact. The technique of **subtotal thyroidectomy** leaves the posterior rim of each lobe in situ, minimising the risk of parathyroid or recurrent laryngeal damage. However, the risk of permanent hypoparathyroidism is 1–4% and of permanent recurrent laryngeal nerve damage 1–5%. Patients need to be warned of these risks before giving their consent to operation. A low transverse collar incision along a skin crease gives the best cosmetic result. Meticulous care is required in ligating the **inferior thyroid artery** (after identifying the recurrent laryngeal nerve) and the **upper pole vessels**. Primary or reactionary haemorrhage is a serious complication causing major blood loss and laryngeal compression. To avoid suffocation from a postoperative bleed, instruments for emergency reopening of the wound should be kept at the patient's bedside after operation. The potential complications of thyroidectomy are summarised in Box 49.3.

THYROID MALIGNANCIES (Table 49.2)

Thyroid malignancies are uncommon, comprising less than 1% of all malignant tumours. Nearly all originate from thyroid follicular cells and form distinct pathological entities: **papillary**, **follicular** and **anaplastic carcinomas**, each with a characteristic pattern of behaviour and prognosis. Papillary and follicular carcinomas are usually well differentiated with low metastatic potential, whereas anaplastic carcinomas behave aggressively. With rare exceptions, none of these secrete thyroid hormones.

About 7% of thyroid carcinomas arise from calcitonin-secreting APUD C-cells. These are known as **medullary carcinomas**. **Lymphomas** occasionally involve the gland, usually in pre-existing Hashimoto's disease.

Exposure to ionising radiation during childhood predisposes to thyroid cancer. This includes radiotherapy (once popular for treating 'status thymolymphaticus' and other benign disorders) and radioactive fallout. Many people exposed at the Hiroshima and Nagasaki bombings and the Bikini Atoll nuclear tests developed thyroid cancers and, more recently, children exposed to the Chernobyl fallout had a high rate. In most cases of thyroid cancer no aetiological factor is identified.

Papillary carcinoma

Papillary carcinoma constitutes about two-thirds of thyroid malignancies in adults and nearly all in children. Females are affected three times more than males and the peak incidence is 30–45 years. Histologically, the tumour forms a complex branching papillary structure with a fibrovascular stroma, often containing characteristic calcified '**psammoma bodies**'. Epithelial dysplasia ranges between apparently benign and obviously malignant but all tumours grow slowly. Papillary carcinomas are microscopically multicentric in about 80% and about one-third affect both lobes; this is important in planning treatment. The tumour occasionally invades locally into trachea or oesophagus.

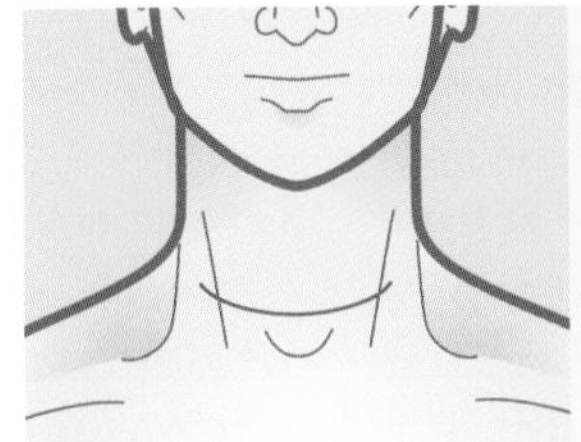

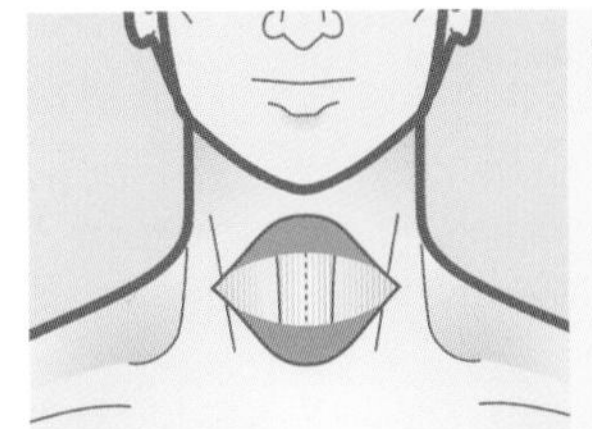

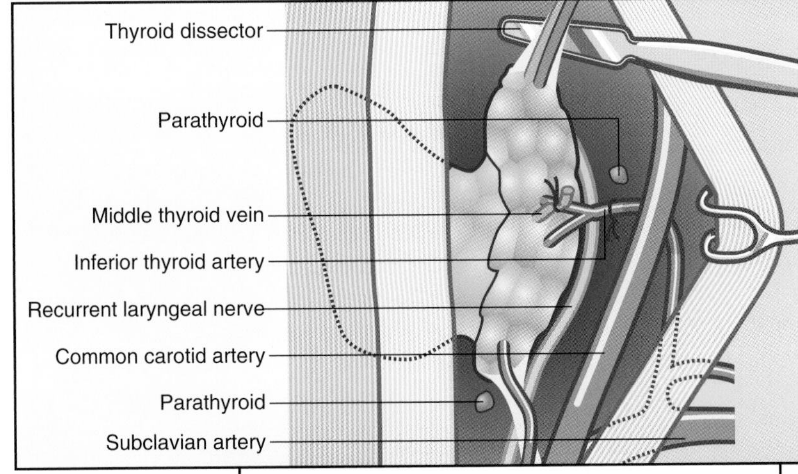

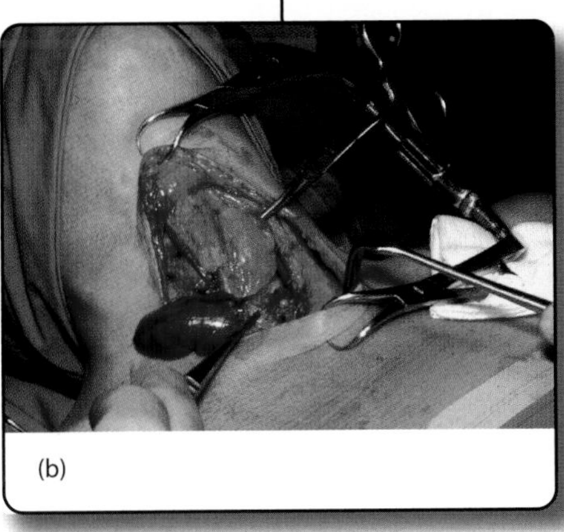

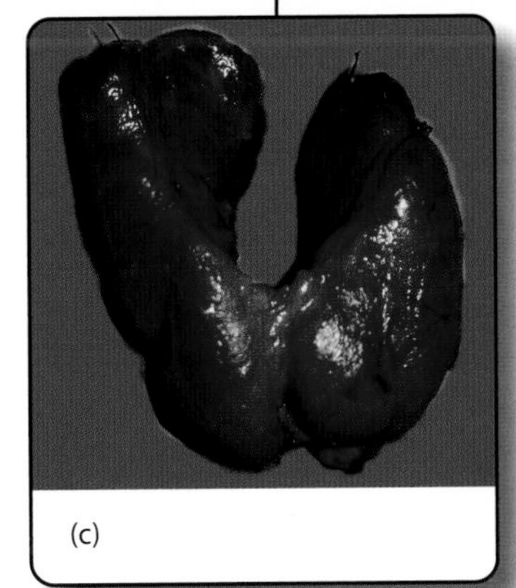

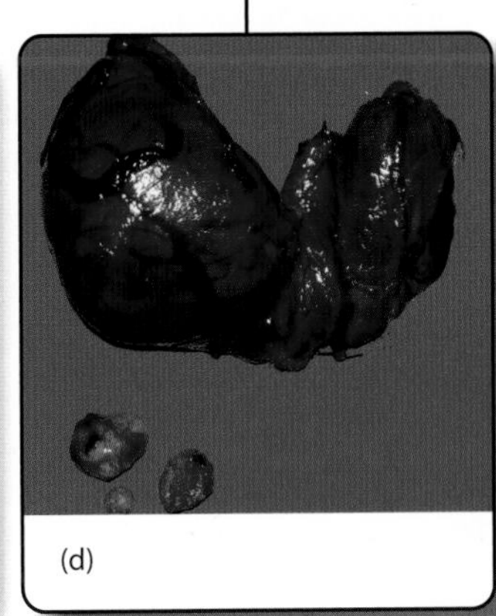

Fig. 49.8 Thyroid and parathyroid operations
(a) The drawings show the standard neck exploration approach to thyroid and parathyroid operations, and the structures at particular danger—the recurrent laryngeal nerve and parathyroid glands. In the photographs, **(b)** shows neck exploration for hyperparathyroidism. A collar incision has been made and upper and lower flaps are held apart with the specially designed Joll's retractor. A single large parathyroid adenoma is clearly visible.
(c) Subtotal thyroidectomy specimen after operation for hyperthyroidism. **(d)** Total thyroidectomy specimen after operation for right-sided medullary carcinoma. Involved lymph nodes were 'cherry picked' and are also shown

Metastasis is to central and later lateral cervical **lymph nodes** and only rarely to distant sites such as lung or bone. At presentation, lymph nodes are involved in about 40% (90% in children). Node enlargement is often the sole presenting feature and the histology is so close to normal that at one time this was known as '**lateral aberrant thyroid**'. The prognosis is the best of all thyroid carcinomas with only about 10% of patients dying of it by 10 years (of remote metastases); it is remarkable that survival is hardly prejudiced by node metastases. The prognosis is even better for '**minimal papillary carcinoma**', defined as a single tumour less than 1 cm in diameter in a young patient with no local invasiveness or metastases.

Symptoms and signs

Clinically, papillary carcinoma presents as a slow-growing solitary thyroid or an enlarged lymph node close to the gland. The patient is euthyroid. Isotope scanning shows no uptake in the nodule. Sometimes, other tumour foci in the gland are large enough to manifest as 'cold nodules' too. The diagnosis is usually made nowadays by FNAC. A patient presenting with just an enlarged cervical lymph node may be diagnosed unexpectedly after excision and histological examination.

Management

The standard management is **total thyroidectomy** because of the high risk of other foci in the gland. Palpable cervical nodes

Box 49.3 Complications of thyroidectomy

Complications during operation

- Uncontrollable haemorrhage—uncommon, usually results from a slipped ligature on the upper pole vessels which then retract
- Unilateral or bilateral recurrent laryngeal nerve damage—bilateral nerve damage presents as laryngeal obstruction after tracheal extubation and necessitates immediate tracheostomy. Unilateral damage causes hoarseness and a weak voice and impairs coughing, see below
- Inadvertent damage to other structures—tracheal or oesophageal perforation or damage to laryngeal muscles or nerves

Early postoperative complications (within the first 12 hours)

- Major haemorrhage—presents as rapid swelling of the neck or a large volume of blood loss via the wound drain. This requires emergency surgical exploration of the wound to release the clot (to prevent laryngeal oedema) and then achieve haemostasis
- Mediastinal haemorrhage—presents with hypovolaemic shock
- Laryngeal oedema—presents as stridor, rapidly progressing to respiratory obstruction. This requires endotracheal intubation
- Thyrotoxic crisis—presents with abrupt onset of extreme agitation and confusion, hyperpyrexia, profuse sweating and rapid tachycardia or other arrhythmia. This requires emergency beta-adrenergic blockade, intravenous hydrocortisone and potassium iodide therapy. The mortality of thyrotoxic crisis is 10% from coma, pulmonary oedema or circulatory collapse. The condition is very rare if the patient has been rendered euthyroid before operation by drug treatment
- Tracheomalacia—removal of a longstanding lesion compressing the trachea may lead to tracheal collapse and stridor

Later postoperative complications

- Hypoparathyroidism due to inadvertent parathyroid damage—presents with muscle cramps, paraesthesiae and tetany within 36 hours of operation. Treatment is with calcium and vitamin D analogues
- Unilateral recurrent laryngeal nerve damage—presents with hoarseness of voice and defective cough
- External laryngeal nerve damage—changes the quality of the voice

Long-term complications

- Hypothyroidism—often overlooked because it develops insidiously. Features are loss of energy, weight gain, depression and intellectual deterioration and intolerance of cold weather
- Recurrent thyrotoxicosis—insufficient gland removed

are removed at the same operation. Total thyroidectomy is also recommended because recurrent local disease, lymph node or distant metastases can then be treated effectively with radioiodine (^{131}I); this requires a very high TSH level which only occurs if no normal thyroid tissue remains. A further advantage is that plasma thyroglobulin can be used as a **tumour marker** to detect recurrent disease.

After treatment, oral thyroxine replacement is always necessary at levels appropriate for keeping TSH close to zero. This minimises the risk of stimulating any residual malignant cells; the treatment rarely causes problems. Tumour recurrence in cervical nodes is treated by excision and even this does not adversely affect prognosis. External radiotherapy may be employed for local recurrence, or chemotherapy with doxorubicin for remote metastases.

Since papillary carcinomas progress so slowly and only about 15% develop contralateral lobe recurrence, some surgeons prefer to retain one thyroid lobe if the primary tumour is small and there are no palpable or isotope-detectable nodules. Their reasoning is that further tumours can be removed later without reducing life expectancy.

Follicular carcinoma

Follicular carcinoma is another well-differentiated malignancy. Histologically, neoplastic cells form a well-developed **follicular pattern**, impossible to distinguish from benign adenomatous hyperplasia on FNAC and even on histology of the surgical specimen. Malignancy may be difficult to diagnose unless there is evident capsular or vascular invasion. Unlike papillary carcinoma, multicentricity is far less common. The peak incidence is 40–50 years, older than papillary carcinoma, but it is three times commoner in women. Generally, follicular carcinoma grows slowly and metastasises late. In contrast to papillary carcinoma, metastasis occurs via the bloodstream to lungs, bone and other remote sites rather than local nodes.

Since follicular carcinoma is rarely multicentric, management depends on local invasion. A tumour with only micro-invasion of the capsule has a very good prognosis and only requires removal of the tumour-containing lobe. If there is gross capsular or vascular invasion (or known remote metastases), total thyroidectomy is performed to enhance the radioiodine uptake of metastases for diagnosis, or for treatment with high-dose radioiodine.

Prognosis for the primary can be predicted by the degree of capsular and vascular invasion. Without invasion, 10-year survival is close to 100% but falls to about 30% if there is extensive local invasion.

Anaplastic carcinoma

Anaplastic carcinomas are extremely aggressive with an appalling prognosis and are found almost exclusively in the elderly.

Most other cancers are less aggressive in older age groups. Most patients die within a year of diagnosis.

Anaplastic carcinoma consists of sheets of very poorly differentiated cells which proliferate rapidly. The result is a diffuse, hard thyroid enlargement. The tumour soon invades surrounding structures, causing tracheal and oesophageal obstruction and recurrent laryngeal nerve damage. There is also early dissemination to regional lymph nodes and haematogenous spread to lungs, skeleton and brain.

Anaplastic carcinomas respond poorly to radiotherapy and chemotherapy. The distressing symptoms of tracheal obstruction can sometimes be relieved by placing a luminal metal tracheal stent which avoids the need for surgery but does nothing to slow tumour growth.

Medullary carcinoma

This uncommon malignancy arises from parafollicular or C-cells. The tumour often secretes abnormal quantities of **calcitonin**, a marker of tumour recurrence after excision. Tumours may also secrete other peptides and amines such as **serotonin** and **ACTH-like peptide**. Medullary carcinoma usually arises sporadically but may be transmitted genetically in **multiple endocrine neoplasia syndrome type II (MEN II)**. This is an autosomal dominant trait with 50% penetrance and is associated with other APUD cell tumours, particularly **phaeochromocytoma** and **parathyroid adenomas**. Thus patients with medullary carcinoma should be examined for these before surgery as a phaeochromocytoma would take operative precedence.

Medullary carcinoma is of pathological interest because the stroma contains extensive **amyloid** which makes the tumour mass stony hard. Medullary carcinoma grows relatively slowly, metastasising first to regional lymph nodes and later to lungs, bone, liver and elsewhere. The tumour does not take up radioiodine and is resistant to radiotherapy; hence an aggressive surgical approach is required. Standard treatment is total thyroidectomy and clearance of involved anterior cervical and superior mediastinal lymph nodes. Without metastases, operation is often curative but when nodes are involved, 10-year survival falls to about 50%. During follow-up, calcitonin levels are monitored and raised levels indicate tumour recurrence. Surgical re-exploration of the neck may be undertaken to remove involved nodes.

Thyroid lymphoma

Thyroid lymphomas are rare and usually arise in pre-existing autoimmune (Hashimoto's) thyroiditis. Most are non-Hodgkin lymphomas. Diagnosis can only be made histologically, by core needle biopsy or open biopsy, as FNA is inadequate. Treatment is with radiotherapy, and survival depends on whether spread has extended beyond the thyroid capsule. For lesions within the capsule, 5-year survival is 85%, falling to 40% when local spread has occurred.

GOITRES AND THYROID NODULES

Several hyperplastic and metabolic disorders cause diffuse or nodular thyroid enlargement (see Table 49.1).

Idiopathic non-toxic hyperplasia

In developed countries, most goitres referred to surgeons are simple, idiopathic hyperplasia of thyroid follicles. The condition probably begins with diffuse micronodular enlargement; later nodules become heterogeneously enlarged to form a **multinodular colloid goitre**. Within the same spectrum are **solitary hyperplastic nodules** (often adenomas) and **thyroid cysts**, which are huge colloid-filled follicles or else contain straw-coloured fluid.

The aetiology of simple thyroid hyperplasia is unknown, but is probably related to disordered sensitivity to TSH. The patient is usually euthyroid with normal thyroid function tests. Sometimes, hormone secretion escapes from hypothalamic control so the patient becomes hyperthyroid and occasionally thyrotoxic.

Secretory activity within the gland is patchy, explaining the patchy distribution of radioiodine uptake on scanning. Overall hormone secretion may still be within the euthyroid range. Diffuse or multinodular idiopathic goitres develop slowly and cause little trouble until present for many years.

The reasons patients reach surgeons with thyroid enlargement are:

- A goitre has become so large as to be cosmetically unacceptable
- A localised lump has appeared in the thyroid region. This may be a solitary adenomatous nodule, a cyst or, in 10%, thyroid cancer. The apparent solitary lump may be part of an asymmetrical multinodular or multicystic enlargement
- A pre-existing multinodular goitre has undergone rapid asymmetric change
- The patient has become hyperthyroid
- The patient has developed stridor from tracheal compression caused by enlargement of a retrosternal extension

Surgical management of goitre

The indications for surgery in idiopathic goitre are:

- A lump suspicious of malignancy
- A retrosternal thyroid causing compression
- A solitary toxic nodule
- Toxic multinodular goitre
- Cosmetic deformity

In principle, only enough thyroid tissue is removed to achieve the objective, but in multinodular goitre, recurrence is likely and best treatment is total thyroidectomy with lifetime thyroxine replacement.

Patients presenting for cosmetic reasons with moderate thyroid enlargement have often been treated with thyroxine. The theory is the gland may shrink to an acceptable size when TSH is suppressed. Unfortunately, clinical trials have shown this is ineffective. In hyperthyroidism caused by idiopathic thyroid hyperplasia, this is unresponsive to anti-thyroid drugs and ineffectively treated with radioiodine; hence surgery is required if treatment is needed.

Thyroid cysts are diagnosed as fluid-filled lesions on ultrasound or by aspiration. Cytology should be performed to exclude malignancy. Large or recurrent cysts are best treated surgically.

Congenital thyroid disorders

Embryology

The thyroid originates as a midline diverticulum between the first two branchial pouches. Its origin is represented in the adult by the **foramen caecum**, visible at the junction of the anterior two-thirds and the posterior third of the tongue. The thyroid diverticulum forms the **thyroglossal duct** which extends caudally through the developing tongue. It passes down in relation to the hyoid bone (in front of, through or behind it) to reach its normal position below the larynx. By this time, it has become a bilobed structure with the lobes connected by a narrow central **isthmus**. The thyroglossal duct later degenerates. The calcitonin-secreting C-cells originate from the **ultimobranchial body** of the fifth pouch.

Thyroglossal cyst and 'fistula'

Part of the thyroglossal duct may persist and become cystic. A thyroglossal cyst presents in children and occasionally adolescents as a smooth, rounded, midline swelling in the neck. Most thyroglossal cysts occur below the hyoid, although rarely they occur in the submental region. A diagnostic feature is that the cyst rises when the patient swallows or protrudes the tongue. Most thyroglossal cysts are asymptomatic but they are prone to inflammation which causes pain and swelling. If an inflamed cyst is surgically drained, it may become an intermittently discharging sinus, often incorrectly described as a **thyroglossal fistula** (Fig. 49.9).

Thyroglossal cysts are usually excised along with the thyroglossal tract up to the base of the tongue. This requires removing the middle third of the hyoid bone (**Sistrunk's operation**). A persistent sinus or a recurrent cyst is likely to complicate incomplete excision.

Fig. 49.9 Thyroglossal 'fistula'

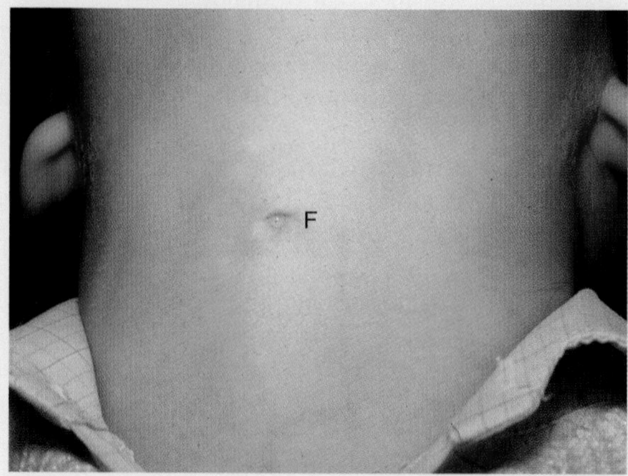

This photograph shows the front of the neck in a 14-year-old boy. An attempt had been made to remove a thyroglossal cyst several years previously. The inevitable result of incomplete surgical removal was an intermittently discharging fistula **F** in the midline of the neck

Ectopic thyroid tissue

An ectopic thyroid is a rare congenital abnormality resulting from interruption of normal descent. It may present like a thyroglossal cyst or as a lump in the tongue. As this may be the patient's only thyroid tissue, isotope scanning should check if there is thyroid tissue in the normal position before proceeding to excision.

DISORDERS OF PARATHYROID GLANDS

HYPERPARATHYROIDISM

Hyperparathyroidism is characterised by excessive secretion of PTH, a polypeptide hormone containing 84 amino acids. Primary hyperparathyroidism (PHPT) is caused by excessive production. It usually occurs in adults and is slightly more common in females. Increased parathormone increases osteoclastic activity, causing reduced bone density and hypercalcaemia. Many cases remain undetected but estimates from 'routine' calcium estimations suggest that about 1% of the adult population has primary hyperparathyroidism. About 80% of these are due to benign parathyroid adenoma. Most of the rest are due to hyperplasia of multiple parathyroid glands and less than 1% are due to parathyroid cancer.

SYMPTOMS AND SIGNS

Hyperparathyroidism is the most common clinical disorder of the parathyroids. Patients are usually referred to a surgeon after discovery of hypercalcaemia during investigation of **musculoskeletal pain** or **recurrent urinary tract calculi**. About half the affected people are likely to have the classical clinical features of hypercalcaemia in addition to non-specific muscle weakness, thirst, polyuria, anorexia, weight loss and constipation. Classical features of hypercalcaemia are bone pain (sometimes with radiological changes of osteomalacia or osteitis fibrosa cystica), urinary tract stones, abdominal pain (caused by peptic ulcer or recurrent pancreatitis), and mental changes such as confusion, depression or even psychosis. These can be remembered by the *aide-mémoire* **bones, stones, abdominal groans and psychic moans**.

In multiple endocrine neoplasia type I (MEN I), primary hyperparathyroidism may be associated with other hyperplastic endocrine disorders such as pancreatic islet cell tumours secreting insulin or gastrin or pituitary tumours. In MEN II, it may be associated with medullary carcinoma of the thyroid and/or phaeochromocytomas.

Hypercalcaemia is frequently found incidentally on biochemical screening and if patients have raised parathormone levels, hyperparathyroidism can be diagnosed. Many of these apparently asymptomatic patients turn out to have suffered non-specific fatigue and malaise for years or have signs of hypertension or renal failure.

Secondary hyperparathyroidism occurs in renal failure and vitamin D deficiency (see below). In addition to osteomalacia and osteitis fibrosa cystica, these patients also develop ectopic calcification, for example around joints and in arteries.

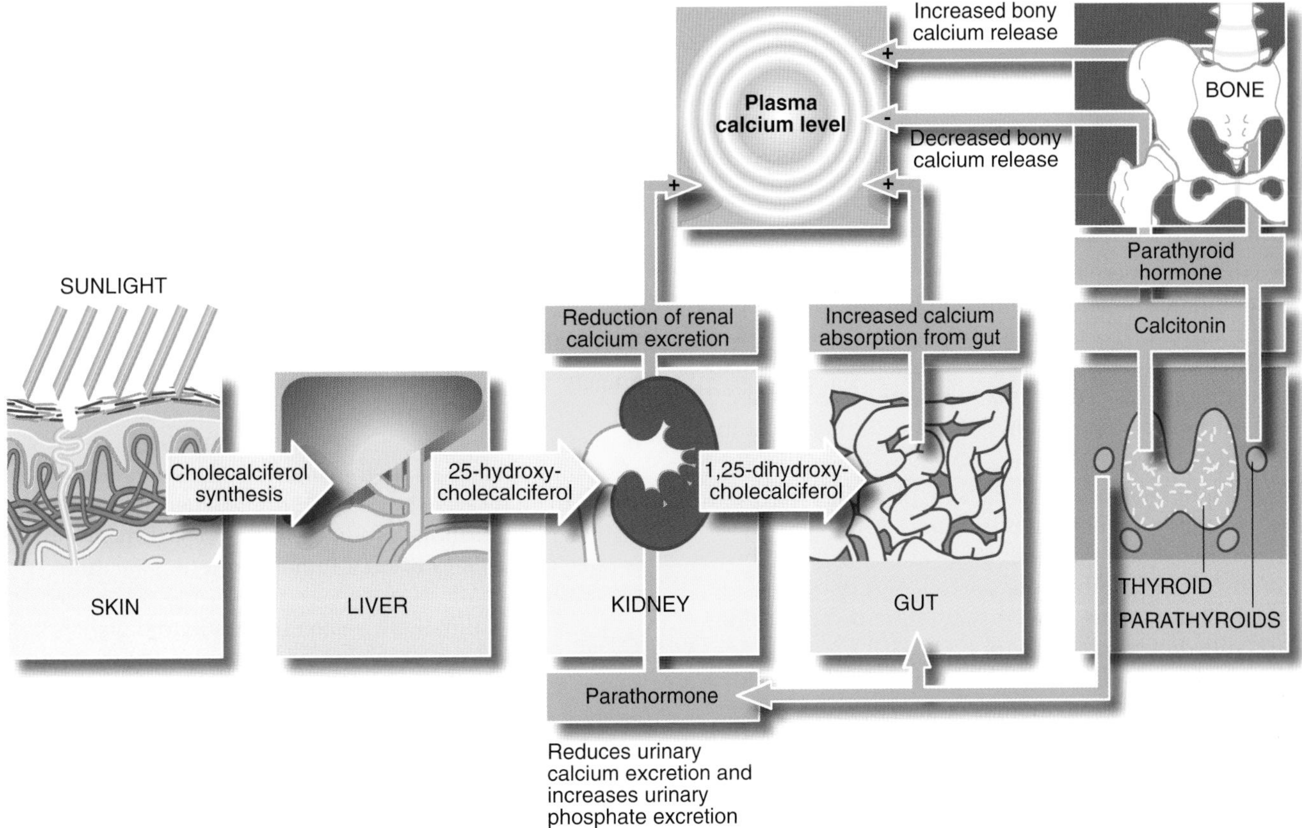

Fig. 49.10 Main control mechanisms for plasma calcium

Raised plasma calcium levels cannot be tolerated for long without causing serious systemic problems or damage to bone. From Figure 49.10, it might seem paradoxical that urinary tract calculi are a common presenting feature of hyperparathyroidism, since parathormone *reduces* urinary calcium excretion. The probable reason for stone formation is the excess phosphate excretion. This is associated with increased urinary alkalinity, which predisposes to precipitation of calcium salts.

CONTROL OF PLASMA CALCIUM (Fig. 49.10)

The plasma calcium level is maintained within a very narrow range by the combined effects of parathormone and vitamin D. Parathormone secretion rate is governed directly by the plasma concentration of ionised calcium. If parathormone is overproduced, this raises the plasma calcium and causes phosphaturia, thereby decreasing serum phosphate.

Parathormone raises plasma calcium levels in the following ways:

- Increases osteoclastic activity and release of calcium from bone matrix, liberating calcium into the circulation
- Enhances renal tubular reabsorption of calcium and diminishes reabsorption of phosphate, thereby increasing the renal clearance of phosphate
- In the presence of vitamin D, it promotes calcium absorption from the small intestine

Vitamin D (as cholecalciferol) is produced by the action of sunlight on cholesterol derivatives in skin. Cholecalciferol is then converted to 25-hydroxycholecalciferol in the liver, and is further hydroxylated by the renal tubules to the active compound **1,25-dihydroxycholecalciferol**. This active compound is required for intestinal absorption of calcium. Calcitonin, produced by C-cells of the thyroid gland, probably plays little part in normal calcium homeostasis.

Calcium homeostasis is thus dependent on normal functioning of parathyroids, liver and kidney, together with adequate dietary intake of calcium and suitable quantities of vitamin D from diet or exposure to sunlight.

TYPES OF HYPERPARATHYROIDISM

Hyperparathyroidism is classified as follows:

Primary hyperparathyroidism

a. Single parathyroid adenoma

The most common cause of primary hyperparathyroidism, found in 80% of cases. One of the four parathyroid glands becomes replaced by an enlarged benign neoplasm which secretes parathormone in excessive amounts. Secretion by the other parathyroids is suppressed.

b. Diffuse parathyroid hyperplasia

This is an uncommon cause of primary hyperparathyroidism. The secretory cells of two or more of the glands undergo idiopathic hyperplasia, resulting in excess hormone production.

c. Parathyroid carcinoma

This is extremely rare (1% of primary hyperparathyroidism) and involves only one of the glands. These tumours are often palpable and cause gross elevation of plasma calcium.

Secondary and tertiary hyperparathyroidism

In **secondary hyperparathyroidism**, there is an abnormal chronic stimulus to parathormone production and the glands undergo **diffuse hyperplasia**. This occurs most often in chronic renal failure (including nearly all patients on dialysis to some degree) but also occurs in vitamin D deficiency. The altered calcium/phosphate physiology in chronic renal insufficiency includes:

- Damage to the glomerulus causing phosphate retention which leads to hyperphosphataemia
- Hyperphosphataemia inhibits calcium absorption by the gut, reducing absorption of calcium to a minimum
- Renal tubular injury leads to reduced renal production of 1,25-dihydroxycholecalciferol (1,25-DHCC)
- The low blood calcium causes the negative feedback system to increase elaboration of parathormone. This promotes osteoclastic activity, restoring calcium levels but causing the bone disorders of osteomalacia and osteitis fibrosa cystica
- The raised product of calcium and phosphate in the blood leads to ectopic calcification in abnormal sites

After renal transplantation, hyperparathyroidism may persist if the hypertrophied parathyroid glands fail to return to normal. The glands continue to over-secrete in an autonomous fashion with normal or even elevated serum calcium levels. This is described as **tertiary hyperparathyroidism** with clinical effects similar to secondary hyperparathyroidism.

MALIGNANT HYPERCALCAEMIA

Hyperparathyroidism is only one cause of hypercalcaemia; the other main cause is malignant diseases. In 70%, this is due to secretion of **parathormone-related protein (PTH-rP)** and in the rest to widespread bone destruction from **lytic bone metastases**. The most common tumours to secrete PTH-rP are squamous cell carcinoma of lung, renal cell carcinoma and bladder cancer. Tumours causing hypercalcaemia by bone destruction include breast cancer, leukaemias and multiple myeloma.

MANAGEMENT OF HYPERPARATHYROIDISM

Corrected plasma calcium levels are elevated but precise diagnosis was difficult before immunoassay for parathormone (PTH). Modern techniques use polyclonal antibodies marked by radioactive, luminescent or enzyme labels to recognise the PTH molecule. Elevated plasma calcium and PTH levels confirm the diagnosis of hyperparathyroidism in virtually all patients who do not have renal failure or metastatic disease.

In primary hyperparathyroidism, an **adenoma** can often be identified by radioisotope scanning using **sestamibi**, which is 2-methoxy isobutyl isonitrile labelled with technetium-99m. This is taken up by thyroid and any active parathyroid tissue but persists longer in the parathyroid, enabling an adenoma or sometimes a carcinoma to be localised. Normal or even hyperplastic parathyroids are so small that they are not detected by this method. In practice, ultrasound is usually employed in addition. **Diffuse hyperplasia** is best dealt with by surgical exploration of the neck and examination of all four parathyroid glands. Preoperative localisation can also be valuable prior to re-exploratory operations for recurrent hypercalcaemia.

Surgical management

Surgery is the only definitive treatment for primary and tertiary hyperparathyroidism. Secondary hyperparathyroidism is managed by treating renal failure and giving phosphate absorbing agents, although parathyroidectomy may be necessary if there is severe bone resorption. Hypercalcaemia due to ectopic parathormone production is managed medically as it is rarely possible to resect a tumour secreting parathormone-like protein.

There are normally two pairs of parathyroid glands, superior and inferior on each side, lying close to the thyroid. The superior pair usually lie close to where the inferior thyroid artery enters, near the middle of the gland. The inferior pair are usually located below the lower poles of the thyroid or sometimes within the thymus gland retrosternally. They may be located elsewhere in a variety of sites including as low down as the aortic arch.

Parathyroid surgery is exacting and time-consuming, often interrupted by histological examination of frozen section biopsies during the operation. Surgical access is as for thyroidectomy. The likely anatomical position of each parathyroid is then meticulously explored. Although the parathyroids have a characteristic yellow-brown colour, they are often difficult to distinguish from thyroid, especially if the tissues have been traumatised.

If one of parathyroid gland is enlarged and the others are normal, the diagnosis is **parathyroid adenoma** or, rarely, **adenocarcinoma**. In either case, the abnormal gland is completely removed and the others left in situ. If an adenoma can be localised before operation, there is a trend to minimal surgery, simply removing the enlarged gland without exploring the rest of the neck.

If no individual gland is disproportionately enlarged, a diagnosis of diffuse hyperplasia is made. In this case, there is a trend towards total parathyroidectomy rather than incomplete removal, now that plasma calcium can be better controlled medically. Some surgeons remove three and a half glands, while still others remove all the parathyroid tissue and reimplant tissue in a forearm muscle pouch. If hyperparathyroidism persists, this parathyroid tissue is more readily removed than from the neck. The main problem in diffuse hyperplasia is that some parathyroid tissue may remain unidentified, however meticulous the surgery. In some units, plasma PTH is measured intraoperatively to ensure the operation is complete.

Complications of parathyroidectomy are similar to those of thyroid surgery (see Box 49.3 earlier). Hypoparathyroidism is more likely and plasma calcium must be carefully monitored in the early postoperative period and treated if abnormally low.

HYPOPARATHYROIDISM

The most common cause of hypoparathyroidism is surgical removal or devascularisation of the parathyroids during thyroid or parathyroid surgery. Autoimmune hypoparathyroidism also occurs occasionally.

Hypoparathyroidism presents clinically with the effects of hypocalcaemia. A fall in plasma calcium level increases neuromuscular excitability causing cramps or even **tetany** in severe cases. An early symptom is paraesthesia, especially around the lips. After thyroid or parathyroid operations, patients should be asked if they have experienced tingling around the mouth, and plasma calcium estimations should be performed the morning after operation, and 24 hours later.

Clinical tests for hypocalcaemia include tapping over the parotid gland. This provokes transient contraction of the facial muscles and is known as **Chvostek's sign**. A further test involves inflating a sphygmomanometer cuff on the upper arm to above systolic pressure. This induces carpal spasm within about 3 minutes (*'main d'accoucheur'* or obstetrician's hand).

Early postoperative hypocalcaemia is treated with intravenous calcium gluconate. Persistent hypocalcaemia is controlled by oral administration of high doses of calcium and vitamin D.

50 Acute surgical problems in children

INTRODUCTION

A **neonate** is a newborn less than 28 days old, an **infant** is less than a year, a **child** is 1–18 years old and an **adult** is 18 or older. In the UK, those between 13 and 18 are increasingly being managed in adolescent units, where their needs are better met. Many children are treated by general surgeons with a paediatric interest, but surgical problems in infants, major congenital abnormalities and malignant tumours are usually managed in regional centres by specialists. The range of surgical conditions in children differs from adults and varies between age groups, particularly for emergency presentations. Paediatric emergencies are considered here by age group, i.e. **newborn** (the first few days of life, including premature babies), **infants and young children** (up to about 2 years) and **older children** (up to puberty). During puberty, the disorders merge with those of adulthood. Non-emergency and urogenital disorders are less age-specific (see Ch. 51).

PHYSIOLOGICAL DIFFERENCES BETWEEN INFANTS AND ADULTS

Infants are not small adults and successful surgical management depends on managing the physiological differences between neonates, infants, children and adults. For example, the **basal metabolic rate** is very high in the newborn, with an oxygen demand of 5–8 ml/kg/min. This falls in older children and adults to 2 ml/kg/min. The **blood volume** in a baby is 80 ml per kg body weight, a much higher volume to weight ratio than an adult, but the total blood volume is very small (typically around 250 ml in a full-term newborn infant), so operative technique needs to be meticulous to minimise loss. In an adult, losing 100 ml is negligible but can be life-threatening to a small child; even small losses need to be accurately measured and replaced if necessary during surgery.

FLUID AND ELECTROLYTE PROBLEMS

Fluid deficiency and **electrolyte imbalances** occur rapidly because each compartment has such a small fluid volume and paediatric fluid requirements are relatively greater than adult because the kidneys have less concentrating ability and obligatory urine output is greater. Faecal fluid losses are higher, particularly under 2 years. In severe diarrhoea, dehydration and electrolyte disturbances occur with frightening speed. Signs of fluid depletion are also different from adults. Young fluid-depleted children are often lethargic or drowsy and may even be comatose. The eyes and anterior fontanelle may be sunken but skin turgor is not lost. Tachycardia is usual, but hypotension is a late sign because of compensatory mechanisms. Urine output is likely to be low—normal output should be at least 1 ml per kg body weight per hour.

BLOOD GLUCOSE

Hypoglycaemia readily occurs because a baby's glycogen stores are meagre; there needs to be a regular supply of glucose by feeding or intravenous infusion. Adrenergic responses to trauma and stress also increase glucose requirements. Hypoglycaemia is likely to occur when a baby is fasted before surgery but not given intravenous dextrose, or when a blood transfusion temporarily replaces i.v. dextrose. All small children undergoing surgery need close monitoring of blood glucose to prevent hypoglycaemic brain damage.

TEMPERATURE REGULATION

Temperature regulation in infants is less robust and **hypothermia** a real hazard. Infants have a relatively large surface area, poor vasomotor control of skin vessels and are unable to generate heat by shivering. These differences are more marked in premature neonates, who are poorly adapted to life ex utero. A controlled, heated environment is essential for operating on and nursing newborn infants. For those under 1 kg, the temperature is set between 34.5 and 35.5 °C, and for those over 3 kg, between 31.5 and 34.5 °C. The infant is placed on a heated mattress and all parts of the body kept insulated. Intravenous fluids and skin cleansers are warmed and anaesthetic gases humidified and warmed.

LIVER FUNCTION

Liver function is immature in the newborn. Physiological jaundice caused by high levels of unconjugated bilirubin is common because the immature liver cannot synthesise the enzyme **glucuronyl transferase**. There is also reduced ability to detoxify analgesic drugs, and many drugs cross the blood–brain barrier more readily and hence are more likely to cause cerebral side-effects. Drugs must often be used in greatly reduced doses after checking a paediatric formulary. A further consequence of liver immaturity is reduced **prothrombin** production. Prophylactic vitamin K should be given after the baby's birth, or intravenously in the perioperative period.

IMMUNITY

Infection can be rapidly fatal in small babies, particularly premature and small-for-dates babies likely to have impaired immunological defences. Infection can be minimised by good surgical technique, meticulous haemostasis to avoid haematomas, and prophylactic antibiotics where appropriate. Vigilance for perioperative infection is essential.

MANAGING SURGERY IN INFANTS

Survival of babies undergoing complex surgery has steadily improved as their specific problems are better understood and managed, with surgeons and paediatricians working together. Examples include effective **total parental nutrition** to prevent babies dying from malnutrition whilst waiting for paralytic ileus to resolve, and better understanding of how to manage mechanical ventilation. Specialised understanding of fluid and electrolyte balance, drug effects and nutritional demands is necessary for safe pre- and postoperative care of these small patients. The successes of neonatal surgery over the past 30 years have depended upon advances in neonatal care.

ABDOMINAL EMERGENCIES IN THE NEWBORN

The widespread use of **antenatal ultrasound** means many congenital abnormalities needing surgical correction can be diagnosed before birth. Typically two scans are carried out during an uncomplicated pregnancy—the first is a dating scan around 12 weeks and the second an 'anomaly scan' at 20 weeks. Detectable abnormalities that will need surgical correction soon after birth include diaphragmatic hernia, abdominal wall defects such as gastroschisis and exomphalos, and congenital pulmonary airway malformations (CPAM). Once forewarned, parents can be counselled and preparations made for organised perinatal management. This is often best achieved via consultation with a tertiary paediatric centre, with a multidisciplinary team of fetal medicine consultants, neonatologists, midwives and paediatric surgeons. Very few conditions such as malrotation, gastroschisis or a tracheo-oesophageal fistula in a ventilated baby need truly urgent surgery. For these, delivery should take place where the surgery will be carried out. Less urgent cases can safely be left until the next day if born during the night, and posterior urethral valves may simply need a bladder catheter before being investigated.

The more common neonatal abdominal emergencies are summarised in Box 50.1. All are congenital with the exception of necrotising enterocolitis.

INTESTINAL OBSTRUCTION

Intestinal obstruction is the underlying phenomenon in most neonatal abdominal emergencies and occurs about once in 1500 live births. Most causes are not detectable by antenatal ultrasound. Complete obstruction, particularly of the proximal portion of the intestinal tract, prevents the fetus from swallowing amniotic fluid and may result in **maternal polyhydramnios**. Just as in adults, intestinal obstruction presents with vomiting, constipation and abdominal distension.

In a baby, signs pointing to intestinal obstruction include poor feeding, failure to pass meconium and bile-stained vomiting. Abdominal distension may not occur in upper GI obstruction. In lower GI obstruction, distension may not be noticed unless the baby is completely undressed. Meconium is passed within the first 24 hours in 80% of babies and delay is a cause for concern. Vomiting small amounts of milk (**posseting**) is normal and simply reflects an immature gastro-oesophageal valve mechanism; however, **green vomiting** should be treated seriously. In a premature baby, bile is normally golden but eventually turns green when mixed with gastric juice. It is a sign of gastric stasis caused by mechanical

Box 50.1 Main non-urological abdominal emergencies occurring in the newborn

- Incarcerated or strangulated inguinal hernia
- Gastrointestinal atresias and stenoses
- Midgut malrotation with volvulus
- Anorectal abnormalities
- Meconium ileus and other problems with meconium
- Hirschsprung's disease
- Congenital diaphragmatic hernia
- Deficiencies in the abdominal wall (gastroschisis, exomphalos and ectopia vesicae)
- Necrotising enterocolitis

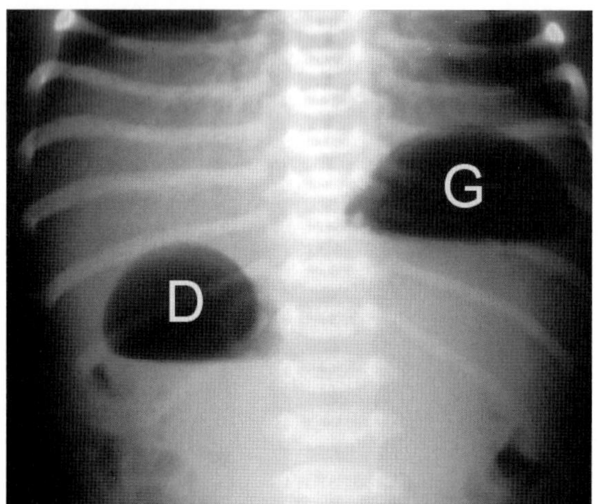

(a)

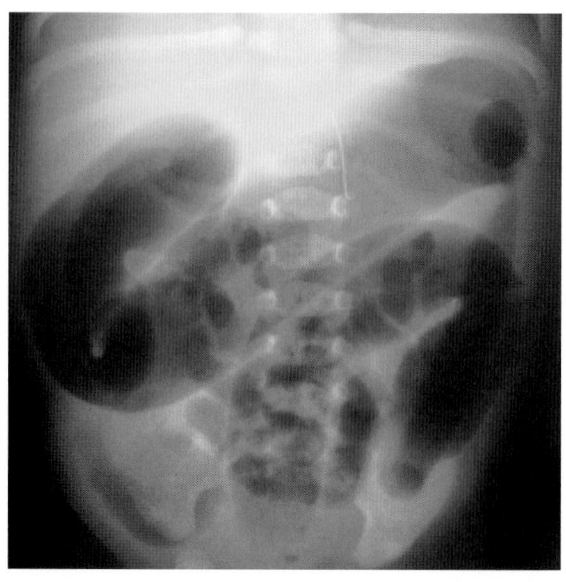

(b)

Fig. 50.1 Intestinal obstruction (a) Erect plain abdominal X-ray of a baby with 'high' intestinal obstruction, showing the typical 'double bubble' appearance of gas in the dilated stomach **G** and the first part of the duodenum **D**. The differential diagnosis includes duodenal atresia, malrotation with volvulus obstructing the duodenum and a very high jejunal atresia. Fluid levels are seen in this erect film. **(b)** Abdominal X-ray of a baby with a 'low' intestinal obstruction, showing several dilated loops of bowel. The differential diagnosis includes Hirschsprung's disease, meconium ileus and ileal atresia

obstruction, paralytic ileus or immaturity of the gut. Sepsis in babies from any source may cause paralytic ileus.

The important causes of upper intestinal obstruction in babies are **duodenal atresia** and **malrotation with volvulus**. Causes of low obstruction include **Hirschsprung's disease** and **meconium ileus. Small bowel atresia** may affect jejunum or ileum, causing high or low obstruction respectively. Plain abdominal X-rays usually confirm intestinal obstruction. When obstruction is high, there is a lack of distal intestinal gas (Fig. 50.1a); when low, there are dilated loops of bowel (Fig. 50.1b). If malrotation is suspected, an upper GI contrast study can determine the abnormal position of the duodeno-jejunal flexure. Other causes such as incarcerated inguinal hernia or imperforate anus can be detected by clinical examination. A plan for managing babies with suspected obstruction is outlined in Fig 50.2.

If transfer to a specialist paediatric centre is necessary, the infant must be placed in a portable incubator. Oxygen and suction must be available, and frequent gastric aspiration via a nasogastric tube reduces the risk of inhalation pneumonitis. Endotracheal intubation is vital for infants with respiratory insufficiency. In the UK, specialist neonatal transport teams are now used to transfer neonates across networks.

GASTROINTESTINAL ATRESIAS AND STENOSES

Atresia is defined as complete obliteration of a segment of the GI tract, which is thus totally obstructed. A **web** sometimes partially or completely occludes the lumen. A **stenosis** is an indistensible narrowing causing partial obstruction. These are most common in the oesophagus, the small intestine, and in the colon following necrotising enterocolitis.

Oesophageal and duodenal atresias and anorectal malformations are true embryological abnormalities, often associated with other congenital abnormalities. For example, major cardiac, vertebral or renal abnormalities are found in 40% of babies with oesophageal atresia, and 30% of duodenal atresias are found in infants with trisomy 21. In contrast, small bowel atresias probably result from intrauterine **mesenteric vascular accidents** or failure of canalisation of the bowel and are rarely associated with other abnormalities.

Oesophageal abnormalities

Potentially lethal oesophageal abnormalities occur in 1 in 3000 live births and there is associated **polyhydramnios** in nearly 30%. Oesophageal atresia with a distal tracheo-oesophageal fistula (TOF, Fig. 50.3) accounts for 90% of these, pure oesophageal atresia without a fistula for 5% and other variations for the other 5%. Babies with oesophageal atresia may have other abnormalities as part of a spectrum of disorders, the **VACTERL** association. This may include one or more V—vertebral, A—anorectal, C—cardiac, T—TOF, E—'(o) esophageal' atresia, R—renal and L—limb abnormalities.

Oesophageal atresia may be suspected before birth if there is an absent gastric bubble on ultrasound scan together with polyhydramnios but these are unreliable signs. If a newborn infant has excessive frothy saliva around the mouth, this diagnosis must be excluded before feeding to prevent choking or cyanotic attacks with fluid entering the lungs by aspiration from the blind upper pouch or by regurgitation of acid from the stomach via the fistula. Aspiration pneumonia is a serious complication. The diagnosis of atresia is made by passing a nasogastric tube (10 F gauge) through the mouth. If gastric contents are not aspirated, a plain X-ray showing the tube lodged in the upper pouch confirms the diagnosis. If the oesophagus is obstructed but there is gas in the stomach, there must be a fistula between distal oesophagus and trachea.

Operation is performed soon after diagnosis and after excluding other abnormalities, particularly cardiac, which may interfere with anaesthesia or intrinsically have a very poor prognosis. Most are corrected by dividing the fistula and

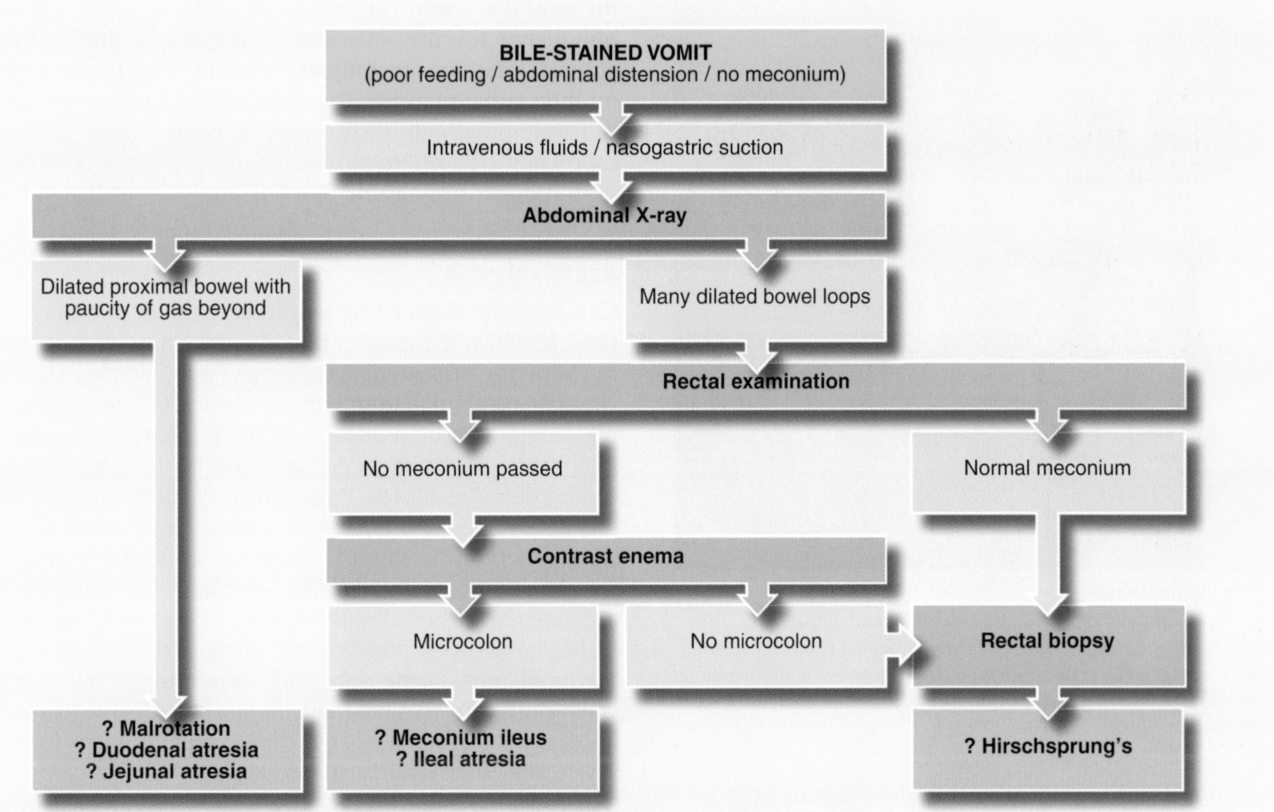

Fig. 50.2 Plan for investigating and managing babies with suspected intestinal obstruction

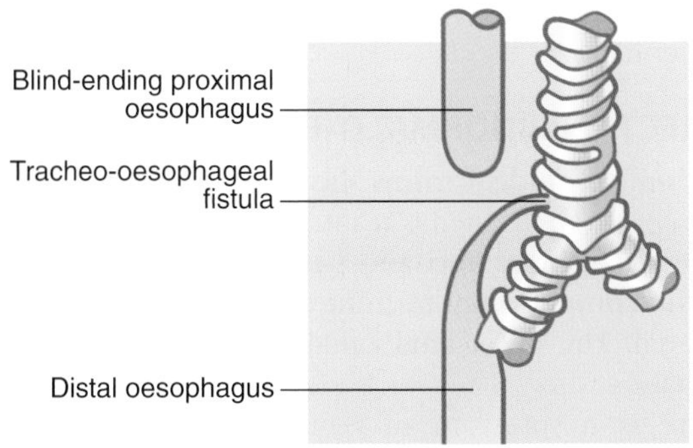

Fig. 50.3 Oesophageal atresia with tracheo-oesophageal fistula
This is the most common variant of oesophageal atresia, found in 90% of cases. Air enters the gastrointestinal tract via the fistula and may be seen on plain X-ray. 'Frothy' breathing may occur because the mouth and pharynx are full of saliva

primary oesophageal anastomosis. Oral feeding can usually be started a few days after surgery.

Dysphagia commonly occurs following technically successful reconstruction, with boluses sometimes sticking and causing obstruction because the peristaltic wave is uncoordinated. It can be managed with a diet of finely chopped food until the child learns to chew food thoroughly, often after the age of 4 years. Anastomotic strictures can occur and need dilatation. Most patients after oesophageal atresia wean slowly, are slower eaters, and need to drink more during meals.

In pure **oesophageal atresia without fistula** there is usually a wide gap between upper and lower oesophagus. Reconstruction is by delayed primary anastomosis at 4–6 weeks or by using a gastric, colonic or small bowel conduit when the baby is bigger. Until then, feeding is via a gastrostomy. The upper end of the pouch is usually brought out as an oesophagostomy; the baby is given **sham oral feeds** when receiving gastrostomy feeds, so swallowing can be learnt.

Duodenal obstruction

Duodenal atresia causes obstruction of the second part of the duodenum, usually just below the common bile duct entry resulting in **bile-stained vomiting**. The anomaly is a web across the lumen or complete separation of the bowel ends. If the web is incomplete, there is initial poor feeding and failure to thrive until a milk curd impacts, causing obstruction. Plain abdominal X-ray shows a **double bubble**, with one air–fluid interface in the stomach and another in the duodenum (Fig. 50.1a).

Provided there is no malrotation or volvulus, surgery can be delayed. This involves joining proximal duodenum to duodenum distal to the obstruction as a duodeno-duodenostomy. The ends can easily be brought together without tension so bypass procedure is not necessary. Previously, gastrojejunostomy was performed but often led to bacterial colonisation of the defunctioned loop causing failure to thrive, stomal ulceration and gastrointestinal bleeding. Recovery after duodeno-duodenostomy is often slow because the proximal

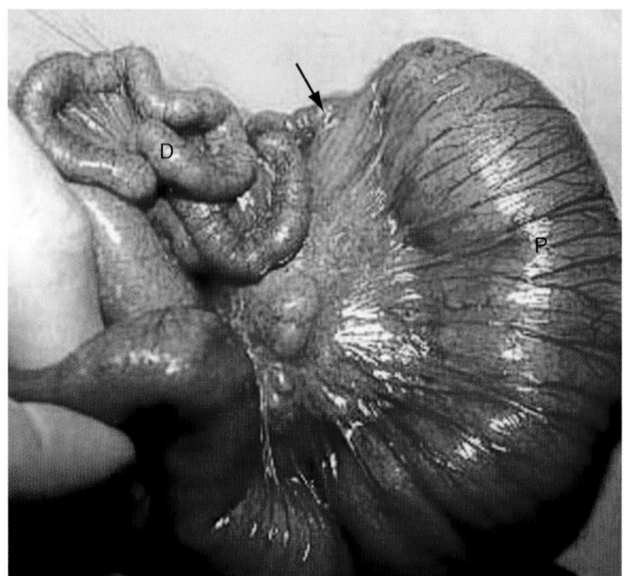

Fig. 50.4 Jejunal atresia
Findings at laparotomy on a neonate presenting with intestinal obstruction. The proximal jejunum **P** is greatly dilated whilst the distal jejunum is collapsed **D**. In between is an atretic segment without a lumen (arrow). This was resected and the bowel ends joined. The infant thrived soon afterwards

duodenum is atonic and peristalsis slow to start. Almost all patients need perioperative total parenteral nutrition.

Jejuno-ileal atresias

Jejunal or ileal atresias are similar to duodenal atresia, with a gap between bowel ends or an intraluminal web. A gap is often the result of a mesenteric vascular accident in utero. Obstructions occur at any level and are sometimes multiple. Bile-stained vomiting and abdominal distension are often associated with **visible peristalsis** and hypertrophied proximal bowel. The diagnosis is usually evident from the abdominal X-ray.

Obstruction may be present from birth or delayed a few days if a web is incomplete. Presenting signs depend on the level of obstruction: high jejunal obstruction presents like duodenal atresia or malrotation with bile-stained vomiting and a lack of gas on X-ray (Fig. 50.1a); low ileal obstruction presents like meconium ileus or Hirschsprung's disease, with failure to pass meconium, poor feeding, abdominal distension and dilated intestine on X-ray. Small bowel atresia is sometimes associated with cystic fibrosis, and patients should have a genetic screen and a sweat test to exclude it.

Surgery involves resecting the web segment or the blind ends and end-to-end anastomosis. Return of intestinal function may be slow, but may be accelerated if the most dilated and atonic proximal bowel is resected too (Fig. 50.4).

MIDGUT MALROTATION WITH VOLVULUS

Pathophysiology

The midgut develops outside the abdomen during early embryological development. By the end of the third month, it normally returns, rotating 270° anti-clockwise, giving a normally sited duodeno-jejunal (DJ) flexure and the caecum in the right iliac fossa. The midgut mesentery is wide, stretching obliquely across the posterior abdominal wall, preventing volvulus. If rotation is **incomplete**, the DJ flexure lies right of the midline rather than left; the mesenteric fixation to the posterior abdominal wall is narrow and volvulus may occur. At one time **Ladd's bands** (peritoneal folds across the duodenum) were thought responsible but it is now known that volvulus is the usual cause.

Acute volvulus

Children with malrotation may undergo **acute volvulus** at any time, in which the mass of bowel twists on its axis, occluding the superior mesenteric (midgut) vessels, causing intestinal ischaemia and infarction. This is a surgical emergency presenting as high intestinal obstruction with bile-stained vomiting. Plain radiographs show features similar to any other high obstruction (Fig. 50.1a). Previously well children who present acutely with sudden duodenal obstruction, particularly with signs of peritonitis, should have very urgent surgery to prevent midgut infarction. At operation, the bowel is untwisted and any gangrenous bowel resected. Surgery also involves dividing Ladd's bands. This broadens the mesenteric base by moving the duodenum to the right and caecum to the left. A stable situation is thus created, reducing the risk of recurrent volvulus. If there is insufficient small bowel remaining, **short bowel syndrome (intestinal insufficiency)** is likely.

Intermittent obstruction

If an older child has a history of intermittent bile-stained vomiting, an upper gastrointestinal contrast study can demonstrate an abnormal position of the duodeno-jejunal flexure. Elective surgery may then be needed to broaden the mesenteric base.

ANORECTAL ABNORMALITIES

The primitive hindgut forms the **cloaca** in the early embryo and a septum then divides it into an **anterior compartment**, forming the urinary tract and part of the genital tract, and a **posterior compartment** forming rectum and upper part of the anal canal. The lower anal canal develops from ectodermal invagination.

There is a spectrum of congenital anorectal disorders (imperforate anus) that has led to complex classifications. However, clinically, it is sufficient to separate imperforate anus into **high or low** according to whether the bowel terminates above or below levator ani. In nearly all, there is a fistula from the end of the bowel. When the malformation is low, the fistula opens to skin anterior to the sphincter complex and meconium may emerge from it; because of this, the abnormality may not be immediately recognised (Fig. 50.5). Newborn babies need to be carefully examined to ensure the anus is situated correctly. In high malformations, there is usually a fistula to the urethra in the male or vagina in the female. Patients with a urethral fistula require prophylactic antibiotics to prevent UTIs. **Urinary tract malformations** and lower vertebral anomalies are commonly associated with anorectal abnormalities and should be sought.

In suspected anorectal abnormalities, the perineum is carefully examined for a fistula. If one is not found, it is worth

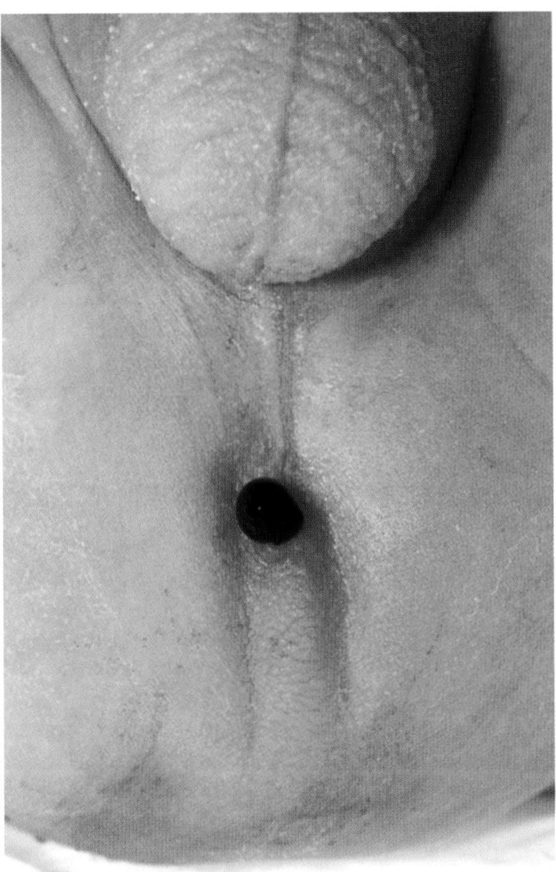

Fig. 50.5 Low imperforate anus
This shows an infant's perineum with an anterior fistula through which meconium has passed; the sphincter complex lies posterior to the fistula. The presence of visible meconium makes the diagnosis easy to miss

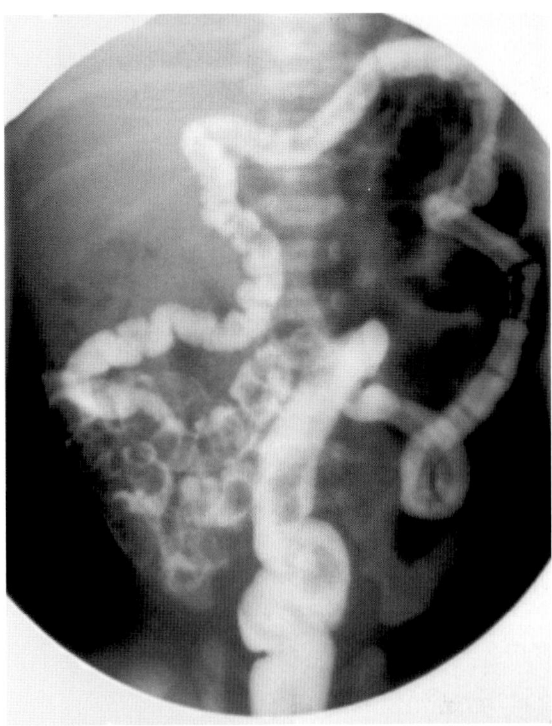

Fig. 50.6 Gastrografin enema in meconium ileus
Gastrografin enema X-rays in a baby with meconium ileus, showing the microcolon and the filling defects caused by abnormal meconium obstructing the distal ileum

waiting 24 hours and then examining the perineum under anaesthesia for one. If one is not found, the anomaly is treated as high and a colostomy performed as a first stage.

Treatment depends on the level of the distal pouch. In **low lesions**, the main pelvic muscle of continence (puborectalis) is well formed and operations via the perineum are often sufficient. An **anoplasty** or a limited posterior-sagittal anorectoplasty (mini-PSARP) is performed, increasing the fistula calibre and importantly, moving the opening into the sphincter complex. **High lesions** require a preliminary colostomy to allow the baby to empty the bowel and feed, followed by complicated reconstructions later; these involve mobilising the bowel end and reconstructing the sphincter mechanism around it. The essence is accurate apposition and repair of the levator muscles and external anal sphincter. Long-term faecal continence and bowel control is imperfect in many children with either low or high anomalies, and constipation is usually a problem.

FAILURE TO PASS MECONIUM

MECONIUM ILEUS

In meconium ileus, the distal ileum is obstructed by abnormal thick, viscid meconium and mucus plugs. About 95% of babies with this have **cystic fibrosis** and all babies with meconium ileus must be tested for it. The colon and rectum distal to the obstruction are of very small calibre. This microcolon results from the fact that no bowel contents have passed down it rather than any inherent abnormality (Fig. 50.6).

The condition presents soon after birth with lower intestinal obstruction; the diagnosis is suspected when rectal examination reveals a patent but very narrow rectum. A Gastrografin enema may demonstrate inspissated meconium in the distal ileum and may also break up the material by a detergent-like action, relieving the obstruction. Laparotomy is required for unrelieved obstruction or any with signs of peritonitis. In most cases, the maximally dilated loop of ileum containing the inspissated meconium is resected and a primary anastomosis performed.

Babies with cystic fibrosis have abnormal mucus-secreting glands which cause secondary changes in the lungs, liver, pancreas and small bowel. Pancreatic enzymes which normally liquefy meconium are deficient. Pancreatic enzyme supplements are given to prevent malabsorption and to prevent the equivalent of meconium ileus in older children. Regular physiotherapy is given to help prevent pulmonary complications.

HIRSCHSPRUNG'S DISEASE (CONGENITAL AGANGLIONOSIS)

Hirschsprung's disease (Harald Hirschsprung 1830–1916) is a congenital abnormality of distal intestine which affects all

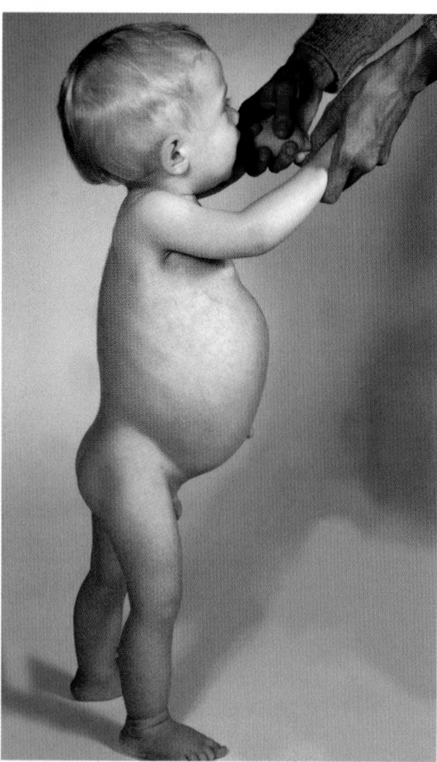

Fig. 50.7 Hirschsprung's disease
A historical photograph of a 3-year-old child with neglected Hirschsprung's disease demonstrating failure to thrive with buttock wasting and a dilated abdomen

of the intramural autonomic nerves and causes functional intestinal obstruction. Ganglion cells are absent from the inter-myenteric and submucosal plexuses, and the parasympathetic and sympathetic nerves are scattered in a disorderly way throughout the layers of the bowel wall. The aganglionosis always involves the rectum, extending into the sigmoid in 80% and reaching the small bowel in 5%. The pathology is continuous without 'skip' lesions.

Peristalsis is deficient in the affected bowel and the internal anal sphincter does not relax. The baby therefore has a **functional obstruction** that usually presents soon after birth with intestinal obstruction; in patients with long-segment disease, it can present in later childhood with constipation and failure to thrive (Fig. 50.7). About 80% of normal babies pass meconium within the first 24 hours but about 80% of babies with Hirschsprung's disease do not, and this is a diagnostic pointer.

Rectal examination may cause an explosive release of air and meconium. Rectal biopsy is the definitive investigation and should be carried out in all children where a diagnosis of Hirschsprung's disease is entertained. Contrast radiology may help determine the level of disease, particularly if performed prior to rectal examination, but often unhelpful. Mucosal biopsies show absent ganglion cells in the myenteric plexus and an increase in cholinesterase-positive (parasympathetic) nerves. A severe form of enterocolitis (Hirschsprung's enterocolitis) may occur in infants where the diagnosis of congenital aganglionosis has been delayed, and death may result from circulatory collapse. This enterocolitis can also occur after definitive surgery. Parents should be warned of the danger of this occurring during a viral illness, which may result in anal sphincter spasm with acute obstruction. The danger of these episodes diminishes as children get older.

Definitive surgery for Hirschsprung's may be carried out any time after birth but has traditionally been delayed until the baby reaches 10 kg. Initially, a colostomy can be sited in normal bowel to allow the baby to feed and grow, although more often nowadays conservative management is employed with frequent rectal washouts at home by parents after training. Definitive surgery involves removing the entire length of aganglionic bowel and joining normal bowel to rectum at the dentate line. After 4–6 weeks, the patient is readmitted electively for a primary 'pull-though' operation, typically performed with laparoscopic assistance.

CONGENITAL DIAPHRAGMATIC HERNIA

The diaphragm develops from a complex of structures including septum transversum mesoderm, lateral pleuroperitoneal folds and the dorsal mesentery of the embryo. The **phrenic nerve** arises in the cervical region. Fusion of the various segments takes place round about the eighth week of gestation.

Failure of the **pleuroperitoneal canal** to close results in the most common type of diaphragmatic hernia (Fig. 50.8b) which is postero-lateral. The incidence is 1 : 3500 live births and 80% are on the left side. Abdominal viscera lie in the chest, displacing the mediastinum. Lung development is abnormal, with fewer branching events during development causing variable pulmonary hypoplasia (Fig. 50.8a), which may be so severe as to be incompatible with life.

Diagnosis is now frequently made at antenatal screening. Soon after birth, the infant develops respiratory distress; survival depends on adequate residual lung volume and function. Cyanosis, mediastinal shift and an 'empty' (scaphoid) abdomen are the classic signs and the diagnosis is confirmed on chest X-ray following passage of an orogastric tube. Cardiac malformations are commonly associated.

Initial treatment is orogastric decompression to prevent air entering bowel in the chest to minimise pulmonary compression. Gentle assisted ventilation with permissive hypercapnoea and low airway pressures is the mainstay of treatment to prevent secondary pulmonary damage. Pulmonary hypertension and right-to-left shunting can occur and vigilance is required to prevent early deterioration and a potential fatal outcome. In pulmonary hypertension, extracorporeal membrane oxygenation (ECMO) can maintain systemic oxygen saturation; other medical therapies include inhaled nitric oxide and oral sildenafil.

Urgent surgery is usually delayed until the baby is stable and requiring minimal ventilation. At operation, the diaphragmatic defect is closed via an abdominal incision. A complete diaphragm can often be fashioned by suturing diaphragmatic remnants together. Large defects may require a prosthetic patch or a flap of abdominal wall muscle. **Midgut malrotation** is present in 25% so the position of the DJ flexure needs to be assessed and corrected if necessary.

Despite advances in care, overall mortality remains between 60 and 70%, and is 50% for those diagnosed antenatally.

(a)
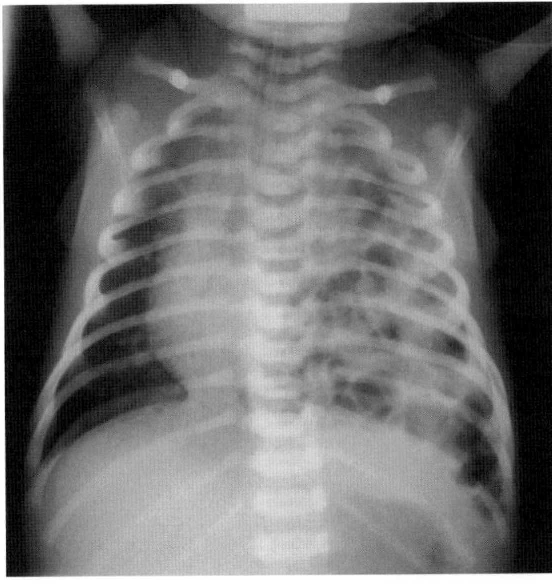

(b)
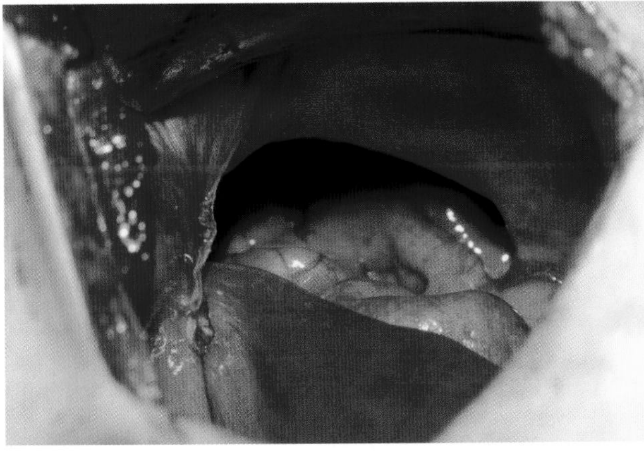

Fig. 50.8 Congenital diaphragmatic hernia
(a) Plain chest X-ray showing air-containing loops of bowel in the left chest and displacement of the mediastinum to the right. Note the endotracheal tube in place to allow assisted ventilation. **(b)** An operative picture viewed from the abdomen, showing the pleuro-peritoneal canal defect in the diaphragm. Some of the intestine had already been reduced from the thorax

Fig. 50.9 Gastroschisis

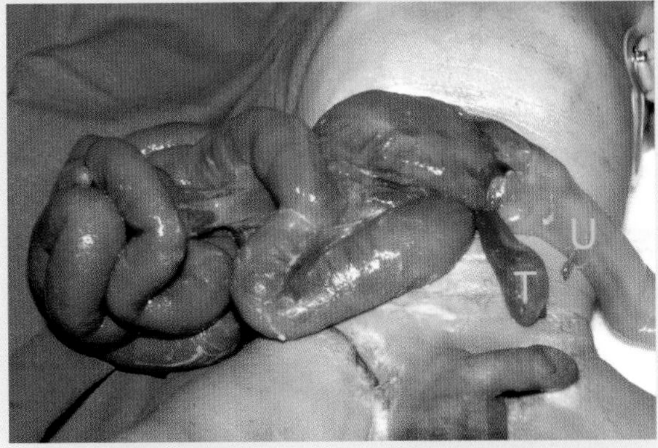

Gastroschisis in a newborn infant. The defect in the abdominal wall is small, lying to the right of the umbilicus. The intestine has no covering and loops are somewhat matted together by fibrinous adhesions. A testis **T** can be seen lying outside the abdomen on the left. The umbilical cord **U** is also visible

Survival for those who come to operation has improved steadily over recent years to around 90%.

OTHER SURGICAL CONDITIONS CAUSING RESPIRATORY PROBLEMS IN THE NEWBORN

VASCULAR RING

This is caused by a persistent double aortic arch or by abnormal configurations of vessels arising from the aortic arch. Either abnormality encircles the trachea and oesophagus causing compression. Symptoms include noisy breathing during the first few weeks and sometimes acute apnoeic events with cyanosis. Sometimes there are persistent respiratory symptoms without frank stridor, often treated as asthma or bronchiolitis. Surgery is necessary in children with severe symptoms. Mild symptoms may improve spontaneously with growth. Oesophageal symptoms include vomiting, choking or dysphagia and tend to occur in older infants and children or even into adulthood.

CONGENITAL PULMONARY AIRWAY MALFORMATIONS

Congenital pulmonary airway malformation (CPAM), previously known as 'congenital cystic adenomatoid malformation' is a rare abnormality of the lower respiratory tract affecting around 1:5000 live births. Patients may be discovered antenatally or present with neonatal respiratory distress or may remain asymptomatic until later life. Surgical resection where necessary is definitive treatment.

CONGENITAL LOBAR EMPHYSEMA

This usually affects an upper lobe of right or left lung. A weakness in a lobar bronchus allows air to enter the lobe, but bronchial collapse during expiration prevents deflation. Progressive lobar expansion compresses normal lung and leads to deteriorating respiratory function. Surgical excision of the emphysematous lobe is relatively straightforward and curative.

ABDOMINAL WALL DEFECTS

Major deficiencies in the anterior abdominal wall are dramatically obvious antenatally on ultrasound and at birth. They originate from a midline abdominal wall defect so much of the bowel (and sometimes other viscera) lies outside the abdominal cavity, with or without a membranous covering. In **exomphalos (or omphalocoele)**, the viscera are invested with a layer of amnion whereas in **gastroschisis** (Fig. 50.9) coils of bare gut are exposed. **Ectopia vesicae** (bladder exstrophy) is the rarest of the major defects and is more common in boys. It presents as a defect between the rectus muscles and pubic bones with failed development of the entire anterior wall and neck of the bladder and urethra.

EXOMPHALOS

In exomphalos, the abdominal wall defect may be large (**major** > 5 cm diameter) or small (**minor** < 5 cm). Babies may also have congenital cardiac problems, neural tube defects (spina bifida or anencephaly), chromosomal abnormalities or Beckwith–Wiedemann syndrome (gigantism, exomphalos, macroglossia, risk of neonatal hypoglycaemia and predisposition to intra-abdominal tumours, especially Wilms' tumours).

In **exomphalos major**, part of the abdominal wall is missing. The defect may be up to 20 cm in diameter and can affect most of the abdominal wall. At birth the bowel is covered with a sac of amnion and peritoneum; this can rupture spontaneously in utero and present as gastroschisis. Rupture after birth is rare in Western countries but may occur in developing countries where exomphalos is likely to be treated conservatively. Rupture allows evisceration of bowel, predisposing to infection and sepsis. Treatment is described below, along with gastroschisis.

Exomphalos minor represents herniation of the umbilical cord. The bowel can be easily reduced and the abdominal wall repaired as a primary procedure. Exomphalos major and exomphalos minor are associated with chromosomal abnormalities and/or other congenital abnormalities and these determine the prognosis. Paradoxically, exomphalos minor is associated with more chromosomal abnormalities.

GASTROSCHISIS

This abdominal wall defect is characterised by bowel herniation through a slit-like defect right of the umbilicus. There are few associated congenital problems, although babies may be small and are often premature. The defect is usually about 3 cm long and the bowel has no covering membrane (Fig. 50.9). A narrow defect may impair the intestinal blood supply in the fetus causing **small bowel atresias**. **Malrotation** or non-rotation is usually present. Antenatal exposure to amniotic fluid can cause adhesions and shortened oedematous bowel loops which may lead to intestinal insufficiency.

Treatment of exomphalos major and gastroschisis

The aim is to reduce the viscera and close the abdominal wall. In gastroschisis, primary abdominal wall closure is often possible. In exomphalos, part of the abdominal wall is missing and the abdominal cavity never reached its normal capacity so primary closure would cause diaphragmatic splinting and IVC compression. In these, a **silo bag** covering the intestine can be placed and the bowel progressively reduced by putting tucks into the silo, expanding the intra-abdominal volume. Repair is performed when this is complete. Intravenous feeding is usually needed until normal bowel activity returns. The mortality rate for even large lesions requiring a silo is low except when associated with cardiac malformations.

ECTOPIA VESICAE (BLADDER EXSTROPHY)

This is a very rare and complex abnormality present at birth, with bladder mucosa exposed on the abdominal wall and penile epispadias in boys. Pubic bones may be widely separated, causing posterior hip joint rotation. Treatment involves closing the defect, aiming to achieve urinary continence without back-pressure on the kidneys. Initially, the exposed bladder mucosa is covered with cling-film or a silicone dressing to prevent damage to the fragile urothelium, followed by early referral to a specialist centre for continuing management. Two main operations are practised in the UK: a soft tissue closure or 'Kelly' procedure, or the use of posterior osteotomies to facilitate soft tissue closure.

NECROTISING ENTEROCOLITIS

Necrotising enterocolitis (NEC) is the most common condition needing intra-abdominal surgery in newborn babies. The incidence is 0.7–3.0/1000 live births, with mortality between 20% and 40%. It may run a relatively benign course or may be rapidly fatal. Babies affected are almost invariably premature, small-for-dates or seriously ill in special care baby units. The pathophysiology is poorly understood but involves reduced blood flow to the intestine causing relative ischaemia. The bowel wall then becomes invaded by gas-producing bacteria causing transmural inflammation, necrosis and perforation. It can affect small or large bowel and may be part of a generalised illness with multisystem failure. The diagnosis can be made clinically if a neonate has bile-stained vomiting, passage of blood per rectum and abdominal distension and is confirmed on X-ray by finding intramural gas (pneumatosis intestinalis). Necrotising enterocolitis may progress to bowel necrosis, perforation and generalised peritonitis. Bell's staging can be of use, with patients with suspected NEC in group I, with definite NEC in group II and those requiring surgery forming group III.

Treatment involves vigorous resuscitation with intravenous fluids, nasogastric decompression and broad-spectrum antibiotics. Laparotomy and probable surgical resection is indicated if medical treatment fails or if bowel perforates and free intraperitoneal gas is seen on X-ray. Unfortunately mortality and long-term morbidity remain high in severe cases. Rates of NEC continue to rise as advances in neonatal intensive care mean more sick neonates survive the early neonatal period.

ABDOMINAL EMERGENCIES IN INFANTS AND YOUNG CHILDREN

INCARCERATED INGUINAL HERNIA

PATHOPHYSIOLOGY

The description **incarcerated** means a hernia has become acutely irreducible, whereas the term **strangulated** implies there is also impairment of the blood supply to its contents. Strangulation can follow incarceration but luckily is uncommon in young children, unlike in adults (Fig. 50.10).

Incarcerated inguinal hernia is a common cause of acute surgical admission in boys (and sometimes girls) below the age of 2 years and may occur at any time from birth onwards. There is invariably a congenital **patent processus vaginalis**,

Fig. 50.10 Strangulated inguinal hernia

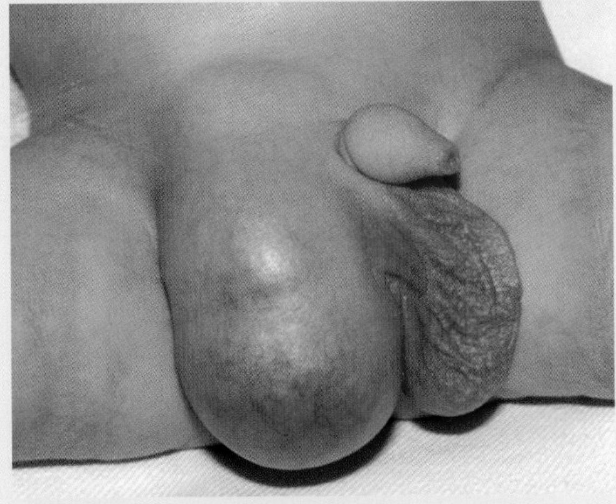

(a)

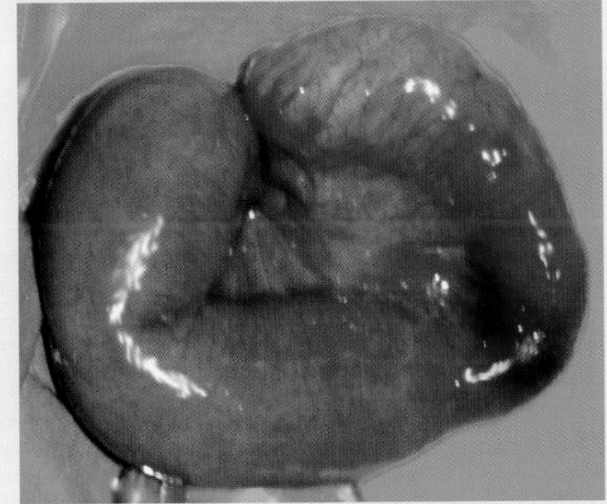

(b)

(a) Strangulated inguinal hernia in an infant. **(b)** At operation, an ileal loop trapped in the sac had undergone ischaemic necrosis and had to be resected

i.e. the hernia is indirect, although an actual hernia may not have been evident before the acute presentation. There is a high incidence of incarceration in premature babies; 40% of hernias in the neonatal period are discovered because they become irreducible but the risk declines as a child becomes older. The high incidence of incarceration in young children is a strong argument for operating upon any hernia in this age group soon after discovery, with the need greatest in the very young.

CLINICAL FEATURES

When a hernia incarcerates it becomes painful, tender and irreducible. Classically, a mother discovers a firm lump in the groin in her crying (usually male) child. He may have vomited but the diagnosis is usually made before intestinal obstruction becomes established. The child is usually well with an obvious, irreducible lump in the groin (Fig. 50.10) sometimes extending into the scrotum. If bowel becomes obstructed, vomiting follows, causing fluid depletion and electrolyte disturbances. The blood supply of the incarcerated segment of intestine may become obstructed (strangulation) causing bowel infarction (Fig. 50.10b). Pressure on the spermatic cord at the external ring may cause testicular vascular obstruction, and rapid treatment is needed to prevent testicular infarction and irreversible damage.

MANAGEMENT

There is usually a painful, acutely tender groin swelling. The child is not systemically unwell and the hernia is neither tender nor red. At this stage, it is very unlikely that bowel has become infarcted. Emergency surgery is best avoided if possible, except in the unwell child with signs of intestinal obstruction, as the friable hernia sac makes surgery difficult and recurrence likely. Treatment involves actively reducing the hernia and performing elective herniotomy 48 hours later when oedema has resolved.

Active reduction is by gentle manipulation with the child sedated with intravenous opiates; it succeeds in about 80% but competent technique and experience are needed. The testis and hernia should be drawn towards the opposite, descended testicle, with the external ring held open with the other hand. This results in narrowing of hernial contents, allowing them to pass back through the ring with a satisfying gurgling. It is often said to be impossible to reduce necrotic bowel in a hernia, but this is untrue so it is important to carefully monitor a child for clinical deterioration after a difficult reduction, including respiratory rate and oxygen saturation. The hernia must be fully reduced; if there is doubt, or if it proves irreducible, urgent surgery should be performed. No child is too small to have surgery provided the team has been trained in paediatric surgery and anaesthesia. Note that failed reduction of an incarcerated hernia is associated with a high rate of testicular atrophy (up to 40%).

CONGENITAL HYPERTROPHIC PYLORIC STENOSIS

PATHOPHYSIOLOGY

This common condition of unknown aetiology commonly occurs between 2 weeks and 2 months of age. It presents with a gradual onset of progressive pyloric obstruction over days or even a week or two, with projectile vomiting of milk following feeds. The cause is hypertrophy of mainly circular pyloric muscle, progressively occluding the gastric outlet. It occurs in about 1 in 400 normal babies with a male predominance of 4:1. Hereditary factors play a part since it is often found in siblings. It is also common for a parent or other close relative to have had congenital pyloric stenosis, with the risk highest in a male with an affected mother.

Prolonged vomiting results in fluid depletion and characteristic electrolyte disturbances. The loss of hydrochloric acid causes **hypochloraemic alkalosis**. In severe cases **hypokalaemia** may occur as a result of renal hydrogen/potassium exchange, in which potassium irons are sacrificed to conserve hydrogen ions. There is usually a paradoxical **aciduria** as dehydration causes the kidney to conserve plasma tonicity at the expense of hydrogen ions, the loss of which compound the metabolic alkalosis.

CLINICAL FEATURES

Typically, the infant thrives for the first 3 or 4 weeks and then begins to vomit after every feed. This characteristically becomes **projectile**, i.e. the vomit clears the baby's chin. The vomitus is not bile-stained, readily distinguishing it from duodenal stenosis or atresia. The child appears well and is eager for further milk. With sustained vomiting, however, the child becomes progressively dehydrated and electrolyte depleted and loses vigour and becomes reluctant to feed. Standard examination often reveals no abdominal abnormality.

DIAGNOSIS

Persistent vomiting leads to hospital admission, where the child's response to feeding is observed. Diagnosis is made by carrying out a test feed, i.e. feeding the baby and palpating the abdomen at the same time. It is important to decompress the stomach first by nasogastric tube, as a dilated stomach often displaces the pylorus to lie under the liver edge. If pyloric stenosis is present, a firm mass about 2 cm in diameter (often described as olive-like) is usually palpable deeply below the liver and disappears after the feed. The condition can be detected by ultrasound, but requires a skilled operator. If the diagnosis remains in doubt, an upper gastrointestinal contrast study can reveal the typical narrow pylorus and little contrast in the duodenum.

TREATMENT

The natural history without surgery is for the hypertrophy to gradually resolve over several months. However, most children would die from electrolyte disturbances or malnutrition before this happened. Treatment is surgical, by **Ramstedt's pyloromyotomy**—Figure 50.11—described in 1912 (Conrad Ramstedt, 1867–1963). However GA in an unprepared neonate with alkalosis and an immature respiratory drive would often result in prolonged postoperative ventilation and all its attendant risks. Operation should be performed only on a stable baby after correcting dehydration responsible for the metabolic alkalosis. The stomach should be emptied by nasogastric aspiration and washed out with normal saline to prevent further vomiting.

In the classical operation, operation is via an incision lateral to the umbilicus. Nowadays the procedure is carried out via a periumbilical incision or laparoscopically. The hypertrophied pyloric muscle is incised longitudinally and then split without breaching the mucosa (Fig. 50.11). Postoperative recovery is rapid, with full-strength milk feeding started immediately afterwards. Babies typically tolerate sufficient feeds to be discharged within 24 h. Babies with a prolonged preoperative course may develop gastritis, which may itself lead to postoperative vomiting; this may be helped by ranitidine.

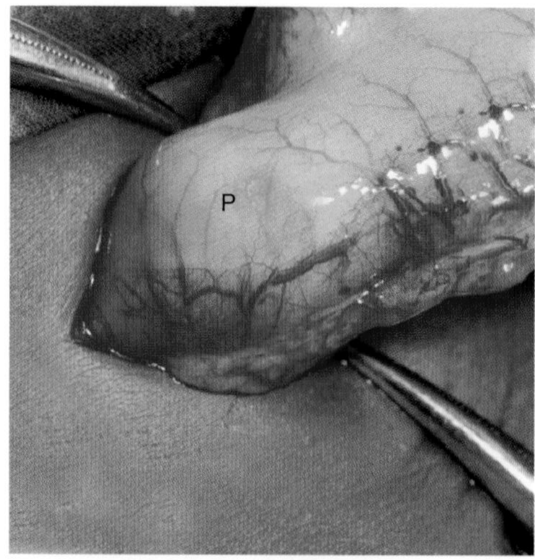

(a)

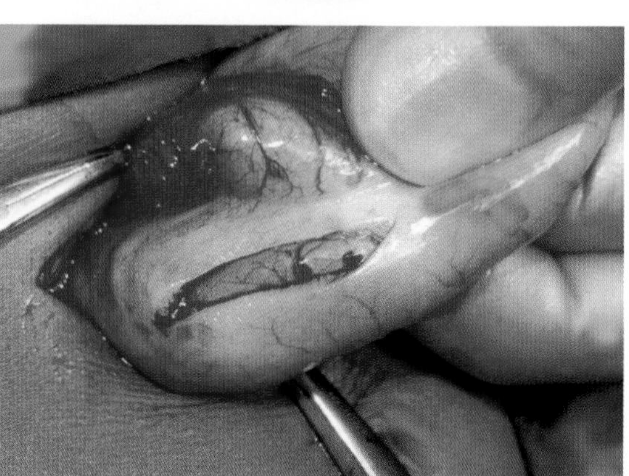

(b)

Fig. 50.11 Hypertrophic pyloric stenosis—Rammstedt's operation **(a)** A small supra-umbilical incision has been made and the stomach and pyloric 'tumour' **P** delivered. **(b)** The serosa over the tumour has been incised and the hypertrophic muscle split with forceps. The mucosa is seen bulging through the muscle split

INTUSSUSCEPTION

PATHOPHYSIOLOGY

Intussusception is an acquired disorder most common between the ages of 6 weeks and 2 years. There appears to be a seasonal increase in the spring and autumn. Up to 40% of children with intussusception have adenovirus infection, commoner at these times of year. Intussusception arises when a proximal segment of bowel becomes telescoped or prolapsed into the bowel immediately distal to it (Fig. 50.12). The lead point (intussusceptum) is commonly a thickening of bowel wall caused by non-specific or viral hypertrophy of Peyer's lymphatic patches. The invaginated segment progressively elongates as it is propelled distally by peristalsis. **Ileocolic intussusception** is the usual variety and it commonly extends well into the transverse colon and sometimes even prolapses from the anus.

Intussusception presents with severe colicky abdominal pain. If untreated, the affected segment may undergo **venous infarction** over a period of hours or days. Pathology other than Peyer's patch hypertrophy may initiate intussusception, and should be suspected in a child presenting outside the usual age range or if it recurs after radiological reduction. Ten per cent of patients have an anatomical abnormality termed a pathological lead point (PLP). In older children or adults, the initiating factor may be a bowel wall tumour or polyp. Meckel's diverticulum or even a lymphoma may also present in this manner. Children with Henoch–Schönlein purpura

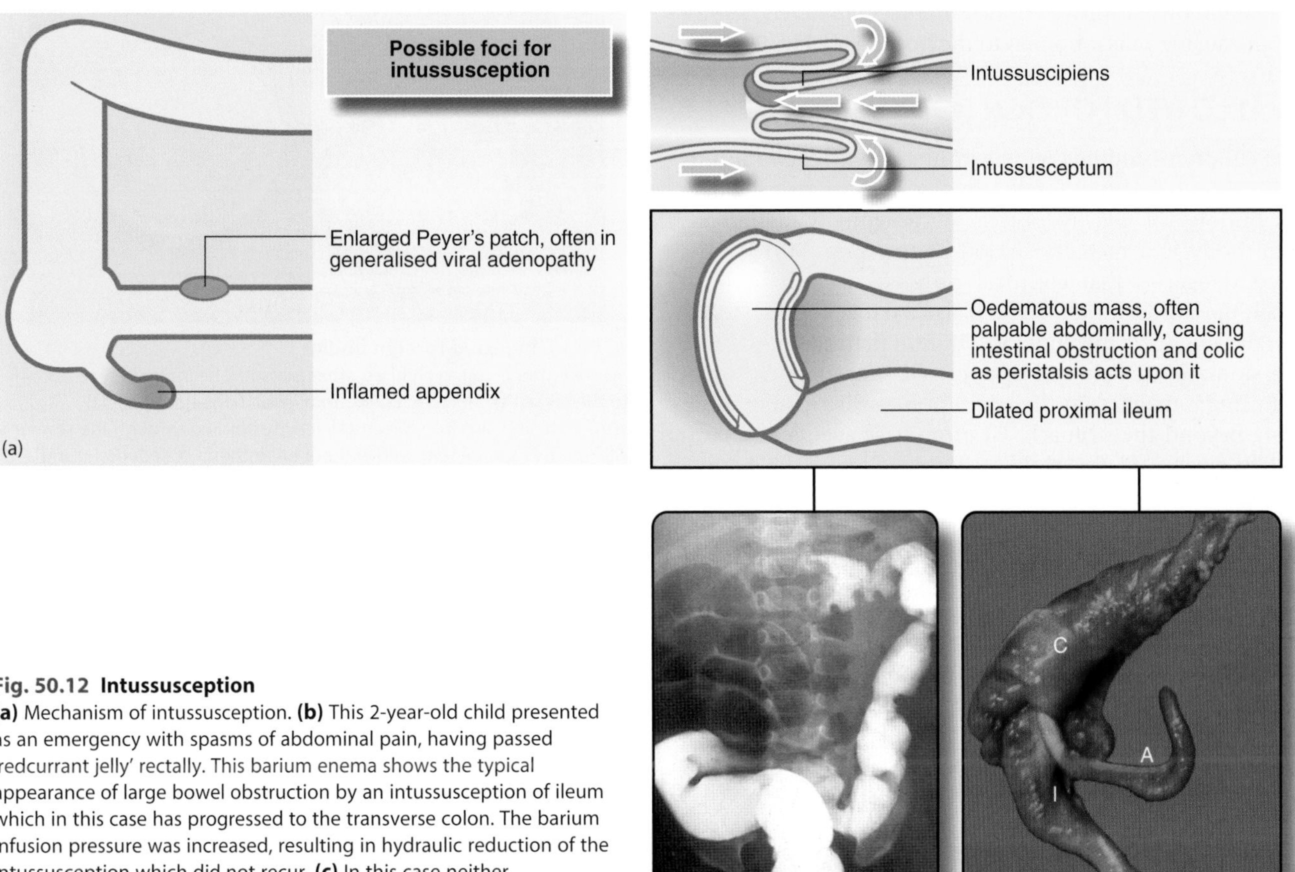

Fig. 50.12 Intussusception
(a) Mechanism of intussusception. **(b)** This 2-year-old child presented as an emergency with spasms of abdominal pain, having passed 'redcurrant jelly' rectally. This barium enema shows the typical appearance of large bowel obstruction by an intussusception of ileum which in this case has progressed to the transverse colon. The barium infusion pressure was increased, resulting in hydraulic reduction of the intussusception which did not recur. **(c)** In this case neither preoperative barium enema nor manual attempts at reduction were successful so the terminal ileum **I** and ascending colon **C** were resected. Note the appendix **A**

(characterised by a purpuric rash on the extensor surface of the legs and buttocks and microscopic haematuria) may sometimes develop ileo-ileal intussusception.

CLINICAL FEATURES

Intussusception classically presents with bouts of severe colicky abdominal pain lasting for minutes during which the child is doubled up and screaming. Episodes are separated by periods when the child appears entirely well. Within the first few hours, the child often passes a small amount of jelly-like blood per rectum described as **redcurrant jelly stool**, which is almost pathognomonic when the other clinical features are present. Vomiting begins later, consistent with distal small bowel obstruction, but there may be profound fluid depletion even without complete obstruction. Some children with intussusception may be very drowsy, only partly explained by fluid depletion.

Diagnosis should generally be made on clinical grounds. A sausage-shaped mass is often found in the upper right quadrant with a scaphoid (hollowed) appearance in the right iliac fossa (*Dance's sign*). The rectum is empty but may contain a little blood. Ultrasound may detect an intussusception and in skilled hands has a high sensitivity and specificity, but a normal result does not exclude it. An air enema and plain X-ray is quick to carry out and reliably demonstrates the condition provided it has reached the colon. Intussusception is potentially life-threatening so a definitive diagnosis must be made urgently with a view to treatment, even in children who appear initially well.

MANAGEMENT

Treatment needs to be prompt and active. Intravenous access should be secured early as deterioration may be imminent. Fluid resuscitation is vital even before attempting to diagnose or reduce an intussusception in an often isolated radiology department. Patients are usually given a fluid bolus of 20ml/kg of suitable crystalloid and an empirical broad-spectrum antibiotic therapy before transfer to the radiology department. The intussusception can usually be reduced using an air enema with carefully controlled pressure, performed under X-ray screening (Fig. 50.12b). Reported rates of successful reduction are as high as 90%. Radiological reduction is inappropriate if the child is unwell; in these, rapid resuscitation should be followed by laparotomy. At operation, the intussusception is reduced by gentle manipulation. Resection with primary bowel anastomosis becomes necessary if the intestine is ischaemic or if it proves impossible to completely reduce without causing major trauma to the bowel (see Fig. 50.12c).

SWALLOWED FOREIGN BODY

Young children examine their environment with their mouths and frequently swallow foreign bodies such as coins, safety pins, buttons or plastic objects. A potentially dangerous foreign body is a mercury button battery (Fig. 50.13). The greatest danger is that electrical currents allow it to burn through the stomach wall. There is also a danger of disintegration, releasing toxic mercury salts. Button batteries remaining in the stomach are removed by upper GI endoscopy or sometimes using a magnet on the end of a nasogastric tube. After passing beyond the stomach, GI propulsive agents and laxatives are given and the child is admitted until the battery passes out.

Foreign bodies commonly arrest at the lower end of the pharynx or in the lower oesophagus. All should be removed by endoscopy. Surprisingly, sharp foreign bodies rarely cause trouble but exceptionally penetrate the bowel wall causing peritonitis. Sharp foreign bodies in the stomach can usually be managed conservatively, but are often removed by endoscopy. Blunt foreign bodies require intervention only if they obstruct bowel, usually at the terminal ileum or the pylorus.

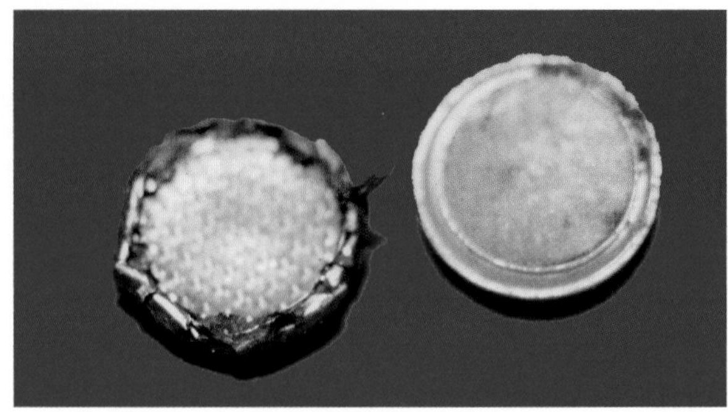

Fig. 50.13 Ingested foreign bodies
Mercury battery. Young children often put small hearing aid-type batteries into their mouths. They are at risk from inhalation and bronchial obstruction, and also from electrical activity burning through the stomach wall. Batteries can be removed without anaesthesia or sedation using a magnet on the end of a nasogastric tube

Coins in the stomach are not removed but parents are instructed to inspect the stools and to return quickly if signs of bowel obstruction or abdominal pain develop. If the coin has not been found a week later, a further X-ray is taken and the coin removed if still present. Portable metal detectors can locate intra-abdominal coins without need for X-rays.

ABDOMINAL EMERGENCIES IN OLDER CHILDREN

THE ACUTE ABDOMEN

DIFFERENTIAL DIAGNOSIS (Box 50.2)

From childhood to adolescence, acute abdominal pain is a common cause of surgical admission. **Appendicitis** is usually suspected (see Ch. 26). Major differential diagnoses are acute non-specific abdominal pain (common), closely followed by **mesenteric adenitis** (Box 50.2). Mesenteric adenitis sometimes causes a higher fever than appendicitis and signs and symptoms usually settle within 24 hours; there is often a recent history of viral upper respiratory tract infection, and enlarged cervical lymph nodes may be palpable.

Less commonly, acute abdominal pain in this age group is caused by extra-abdominal causes such as:

- **Lower urinary tract infection** (urinary symptoms are usually present)
- **Basal pneumonia**, usually right sided
- **Ear, nose or throat infection**
- **Torsion of the testis**—sometimes presents solely with abdominal pain; genitalia must always be examined in boys with abdominal pain
- **Meningitis**

PRINCIPLES OF MANAGEMENT

If acute appendicitis is diagnosed when the child is first seen, operation should be performed after necessary resuscitation and giving empirical antibiotics. More commonly, the diagnosis is uncertain. In these children, urinary tract infection should be excluded by dip stick testing and the child should be re-examined at intervals and a worsening or improving trend soon becomes apparent.

ACUTE APPENDICITIS (see also Ch. 26)

Acute appendicitis is uncommon in children less than 2 years of age. Anorexia is usual, although this may be absent in adolescent males, and vomiting often starts after the onset of pain. Children with appendicitis find that movement exacerbates pain. If asked to hop or jump, some children bluntly refuse, and others complain of pain. An inflamed pelvic appendix may cause secondary inflammation of rectum or bladder, causing diarrhoea or urinary symptoms. Pus cells may be found in the urine.

A full general examination must include an ear and throat assessment, chest examination, testicular examination and a search for rashes and neck stiffness. Otitis media, pharyngeal inflammation, basal pneumonia, testicular torsion or even meningitis can cause abdominal pain in children. Mesenteric adenitis can mimic appendicitis; a high fever and widespread lymphadenopathy suggest this diagnosis.

On examination the child's breath may be foul (foetor oris) and there may be signs of dehydration or shock. The child may be pyrexial but a temperature of more than 38.5 °C suggests a cause other than appendicitis, unless there is generalised peritonitis. The abdomen is often tender in the right iliac fossa with localised guarding—the cardinal feature of appendicitis. Appendiceal perforation can lead to generalised peritonitis, with guarding over the whole abdomen. Unlike

Box 50.2 Differential diagnosis of acute abdominal pain in pre-adolescent children

- Acute non-specific abdominal pain
- Acute appendicitis
- Mesenteric adenitis
- Extra-abdominal causes

adults, children often present with peritonitis, and children under the age of 5 usually have a perforation or a gangrenous appendix at operation.

A definitive diagnosis of appendicitis often cannot be made initially. Investigations are of little help other than to exclude urinary tract infection and the child may find them frightening. The white blood count and CRP are unhelpful as these are raised in other inflammatory conditions. Ultrasound has some positive predictive value but cannot exclude appendicitis, and a CT scan involves a substantial radiation burden, particularly in small children, and is not normally performed. Laparoscopy gives a precise diagnosis, but requires general anaesthesia; the procedure is better avoided if the appendix is not inflamed, as most children would agree.

In the equivocal case, the best way to diagnose appendicitis is **active observation**. The child is admitted and allowed to eat (because fasting ameliorates the physical signs and delays diagnosis). The child is examined every 2 hours or so, preferably by the same doctor, including abdominal palpation. By the second or third examination it is usually clear whether physical signs are getting better or worse. This approach may be used in family practice and during surgical admission. It reduces psychological trauma and the rate of unnecessary operations and ensures appendicitis is not missed until peritonitis has become all too obvious. The argument that this risks perforation, pelvic infection and infertility in girls is not borne out by fact. Active observation can select out those children with acute non-specific pain without detectable pathology and who need no active treatment, least of all surgical invasion of their peritoneal cavity.

TORSION OF THE TESTIS

Torsion can occur when there is a congenital abnormality of testicular fixation (termed the 'bell-clapper' testis) that predisposes to twisting on its vascular pedicle. The diagnosis must be considered in any male less than 25 years of age presenting with acute testicular pain. Torsion may present with iliac fossa pain alone, without testicular pain. Torsion must not be missed as the testis undergoes necrosis within 4–6 hours. Predisposition to torsion is usually bilateral and both testes are at risk; thus the non-torted testis should undergo fixation at the same time as the torted testis (see Ch. 33).

Intrascrotal pathology that can mimic testicular torsion includes **torsion of a hydatid of Morgagni** and **epididymitis**. Palpating individual scrotal structures is often impossible because of extreme tenderness and sometimes oedema, but a non-tender testis with an acutely tender epididymis (behind the testis) indicates epididymitis. Very localised tenderness at the superior pole of the testis is sometimes found in torsion of a hydatid of Morgagni.

Duplex ultrasound monitoring may help where the clinical picture makes torsion unlikely, as it is reassuring to know there is good blood flow. However, ultrasound can delay surgery and may compromise survival of the testis. Furthermore, ultrasound does not exclude intermittent torsion. It is seldom a useful investigation except in the most skilled hands and where it is readily available.

When a diagnosis of torsion cannot be excluded, the only safe option is to carry out urgent surgical exploration. If torsion is present and the testis is viable, it should be untwisted and fixed to prevent re-torsion. A non-viable testis should be removed and the contralateral testis should be fixed at the same time since predisposition to torsion is usually bilateral and both testes are at risk (see Ch. 33).

51 Non-acute abdominal and urological problems in children

INTRODUCTION

The acute conditions described in Chapter 50 are largely congenital disorders presenting in the neonatal period, whereas non-acute conditions present across the whole of childhood. The most common referrals are hernias and associated problems, abnormalities of testicular descent and foreskin problems. Less often, surgeons manage chronic or recurrent abdominal pain, chronic constipation, rectal bleeding, an abdominal mass or rectal prolapse. Many children present first to a paediatrician and are referred to a paediatric or general surgeon.

Finally, a range of **urological problems** occur in infancy and childhood. Most are unique to young patients and are usually dealt with by paediatric urologists. Congenital urological abnormalities are often diagnosed by ultrasound in the antenatal period.

PROBLEMS WITH THE GROIN AND MALE GENITALIA

EMBRYOLOGY

The indifferent gonad (i.e. ovary or testis) begins to develop at the fifth week in the **gonadal ridge**, part of the mesodermal urogenital ridge that will also form the kidney, ureter and genital ducts in the male or uterus and uterine tubes in the female. At the lower pole of the putative testis, a strand of mesenchyme becomes the cord-like **gubernaculum**. In the eighth week, a prolongation of peritoneum, the **processus vaginalis**, appears beside the gubernaculum (or round ligament), and extends into the labioscrotal fold. The testis then migrates distally along the peritoneal canal.

HERNIAS AND ASSOCIATED PROBLEMS

The processus vaginalis normally closes spontaneously soon after birth. Persistence causes three common problems in boys: patent processus vaginalis (PPV), hydrocoele and inguinal hernia, which may all present as inguinal or scrotal swellings, usually in babies and pre-school children (Fig. 51.1).

PATENT PROCESSUS VAGINALIS (PPV)

This term should be reserved for hydrocoeles communicating with the peritoneal cavity via a remnant too narrow to admit bowel. Children with these **communicating hydrocoeles** present with scrotal swelling that increases during the day as peritoneal fluid accumulates and subsides at night. They are seen up to the age of 3 years. Treatment is excision of the peritoneal remnant as in herniotomy after the age of 2 (see below). Before this age, most settle spontaneously.

HYDROCOELE

Non-communicating hydrocoeles are mostly seen in neonates and young babies (Fig. 51.2). The usual type is a scrotal swelling resulting from incomplete reabsorption of fluid within the tunica vaginalis after closure of the processus vaginalis. There may be a separate hernia present. These so-called '**primary hydrocoeles**' sometimes appear following a viral illness. Rarely, a **secondary hydrocoele** results from testicular trauma or torsion, epididymitis or a testicular tumour.

On examination, there is a fluid swelling surrounding a normal testis; the sac transilluminates brightly and the testis can be felt posteriorly (but note that neonatal bowel is thin and may also transilluminate brightly in a hernia). If this cannot be achieved, investigation needs to exclude a secondary hydrocoele. In inguinal hernia the examiner cannot 'get above' the swelling, i.e. the swelling originates in the groin; this is the cardinal feature. Hydrocoeles also occur in the

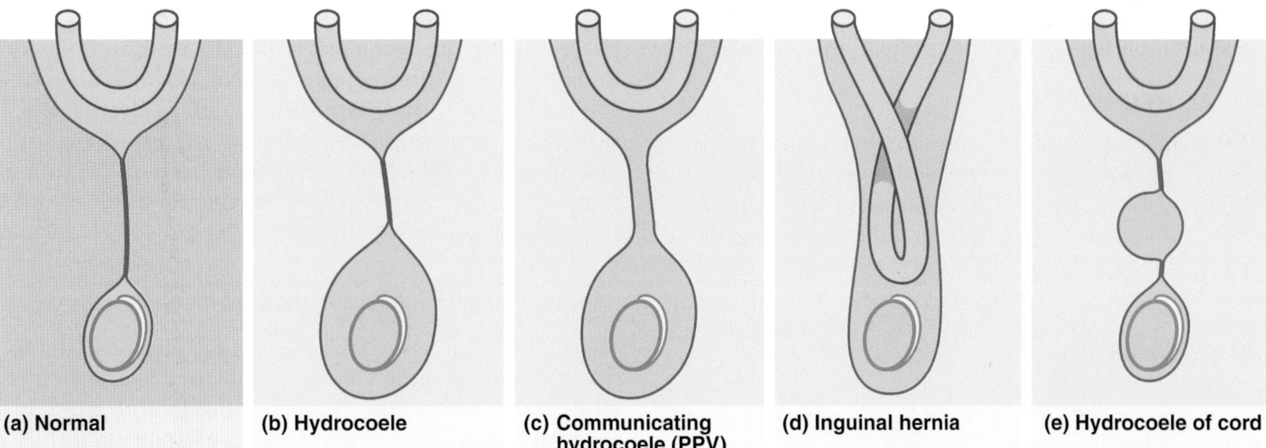

Fig. 51.1 Abnormalities associated with the processus vaginalis

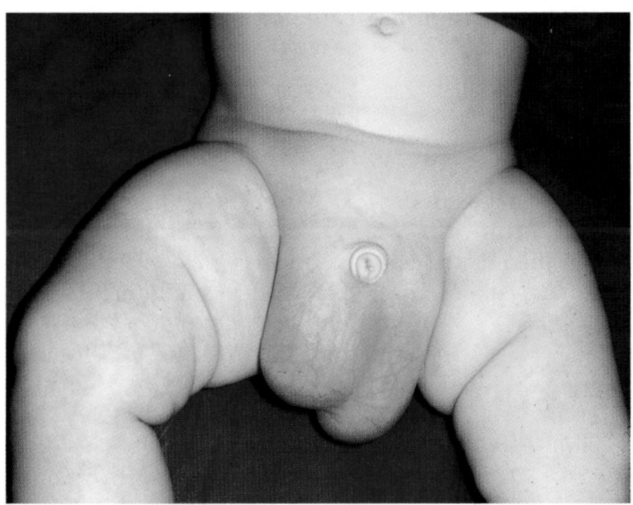

Fig. 51.2 Hydrocoeles
This 11-month-old boy had an enlarged scrotum confirmed by transillumination to be the result of hydrocoeles

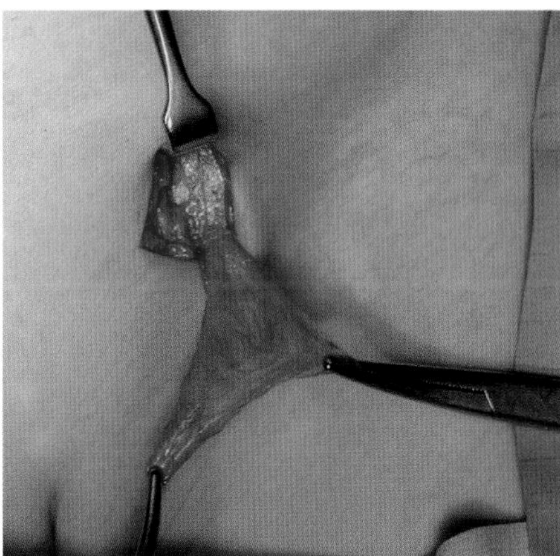

Fig. 51.3 Operation for inguinal hernia
At operation, the peritoneal sac is being held out before it is excised. No other procedure was necessary in this 4-year-old child. Unusually, the patient was female

spermatic cord (hydrocoele of the cord) or in the round ligament in girls where they are known as **hydrocoeles of the canal of Nuck**. Most hydrocoeles resolve between 18 and 24 months of age. A hydrocoele persisting beyond the age of 2 or appearing later may require surgery.

INGUINAL HERNIA

Inguinal hernias in children arise because the processus vaginalis fails to close after testicular descent; they are true congenital abnormalities. Anatomically, they are the same as indirect inguinal hernias in adults (see Ch. 32) but without a substantial abdominal wall defect. The incidence in infants ranges from 1% to 4.4%, with a male preponderance of 4:1; 98% are indirect. The incidence in **premature neonates** is 30% and the overall incidence is increasing in line with the number of premature neonates surviving.

A hernia usually presents as a lump at the external inguinal ring, when the child cries or strains at stool, but then reduces spontaneously. When seen electively, there is often no abnormality, but most surgeons accept a parent's clear history of a hernia and arrange surgery. With larger defects, a lump is constantly present and expands during crying. The urgency of hernia repair is governed by age; the older, the less likely it will become incarcerated (acutely irreducible). Infants at home should have hernias fixed on the next available operating list. Neonates and pre-term infants in hospital should have them fixed before discharge. Older children without episodes of incarceration can have hernias fixed electively.

Inguinal hernias may become **acutely irreducible** and painful, sometimes with obstructive symptoms such as vomiting (see Ch. 50). In these cases, there is a real risk of testicular necrosis and/or strangulation of the hernia contents, e.g. bowel or ovary (see Fig. 50.10). In known hernias, parents should be instructed to bring the child to hospital for urgent herniotomy if it becomes incarcerated to prevent these risks.

The standard operation is **inguinal herniotomy**, a common general paediatric operation. In babies and children, this involves separating the peritoneal sac from the cord (or round ligament), ligating it at the external ring and removing it. There is rarely any need to perform a repair (herniorrhaphy); see Figure 51.3. The incidence of an undiagnosed contralateral hernia in boys is between 1:8 and 1:13 but contralateral groin exploration is no longer performed in the UK.

FEMORAL HERNIA

Femoral hernias are much less common than inguinal hernias in children and are located lower and more medially in the groin. Enlarged lymph nodes can also occur here. Operation includes removing the sac and suturing the medial part of the inguinal ligament to the pectineus fascia to narrow the femoral canal.

UMBILICAL HERNIA

Many newborn babies have umbilical hernias, particularly if premature (Fig. 51.4), but the defect usually cicatrises and resolves during the first 2 years of life; they are common in Afro-Caribbean babies and can run strongly in families. Small umbilical hernias may undergo spontaneous closure up to 4–5 years of age. Rarely, they become incarcerated or strangulate. Indications for repair are symptoms, persistence beyond 5 years and perhaps social pressure to prevent teasing. The size of the abdominal wall defect should be determined; large defects (>2 cm) are less likely to close spontaneously, although very large swellings may have small abdominal wall defects likely to close spontaneously. It is important to differentiate umbilical hernias from epigastric hernias which do not close spontaneously. At operation, a small subumbilical 'smile' incision allows emptying and ligation of the peritoneal sac and placement of a few absorbable repair sutures. The umbilical skin is usually sutured to the repair to restore its normal recessed appearance.

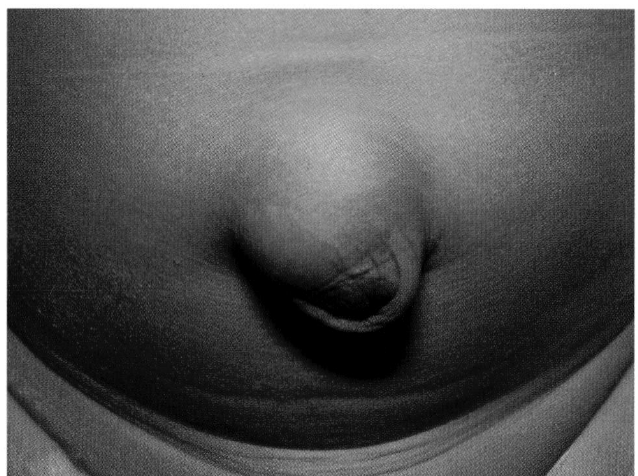

Fig. 51.4 Umbilical hernia in a 14-month-old boy This was repaired surgically but smaller ones usually resolve spontaneously

TESTICULAR MALDESCENT

There are several terms for testes not fully descended into the scrotum; **undescended** is inaccurate in that most missing testes started along the normal pathway and arrest in the inguinal region, a few descended to the wrong place and a few are missing altogether. The terms **maldescended** or **incompletely descended** cover all but the truly absent testis. Clinically, one or both testes fail to reach the scrotum in 3% of full-term newborn males, but much higher rates with prematurity. Full descent has occurred in most boys by the age of 3–6 months, leaving about 1.6% with maldescended testes and these rarely descend later because androgen levels are highest in the first few months and then fall to very low levels until puberty.

The normal mechanism of descent is not fully understood but does occur in two phases. Migration from the gonadal ridge to the internal inguinal ring depends on shortening of the gubernaculum, driven by Müllerian inhibiting substance (MIS). This phase is not androgen-dependent, unlike the second phase of descent from internal ring to scrotum. A maldescended testis may arrest anywhere on its path of descent. About 20% lie within the abdomen but 80% lie in the groin area, in the inguinal canal or usually outside the external ring in the **superficial inguinal pouch** or upper scrotum. In addition, 1% of testes are deflected and lie ectopically. Second phase maldescent can result from the testis being structurally abnormal, rather than any abnormality being caused by maldescent. The common sites of incomplete descent or ectopia are shown in Figure 51.5.

The main concerns with maldescended testes are the risks of malignancy, subfertility, and torsion or trauma in an abnormal position; cosmetic appearance and psychological impact of cryptorchidism has a bearing in later life:

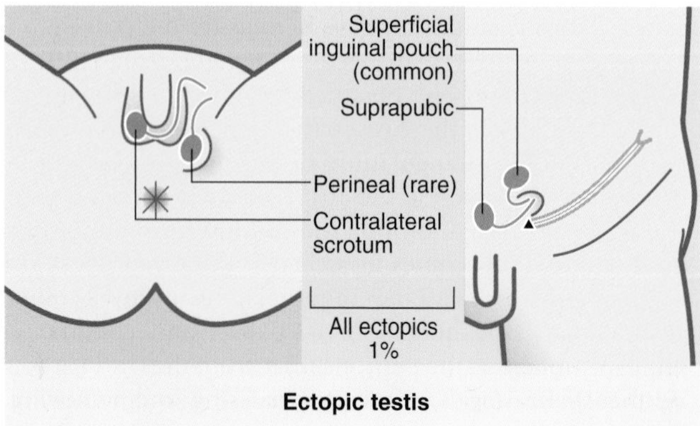

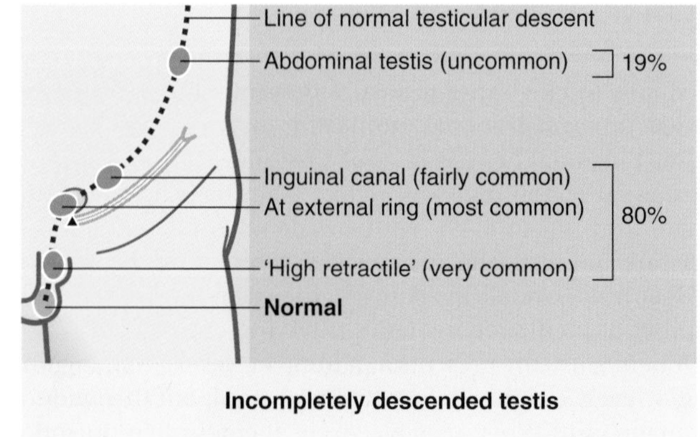

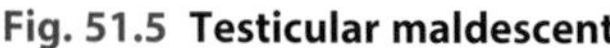
Fig. 51.5 Testicular maldescent

- **Neoplasia**—carcinoma-in-situ is present in 2% of undescended testes and maldescent has up to 10 times the normal risk of testicular malignancy (although the risk is still small); if surgical correction is done sufficiently early, it may reduce this risk but the principal purpose is for the patient to perform self-examination and report lumps in later life. Long-term follow-up after orchidopexy is desirable. Seminomas are the most common tumour (60%) and usually present between 20 and 40 years of age. It is important to inform the parents of the increased risk of malignancy and to reinforce the importance of testicular self-examination in adult life
- **Subfertility**—maldescended testes exhibit incomplete maturation of seminiferous tubules, leading to sperm abnormal in quantity, form or motility. This may be by virtue of being at normal body temperature instead of at least 1° cooler in the scrotum. Early orchidopexy helps maturation of the tubules and spermatogenesis, ideally between 6 and 12 months of age. Patients with unilateral maldescent have more subfertility and lower sperm counts. Those with bilateral intra-abdominal testes have the most subfertility
- **Torsion**—incompletely descended testes are abnormally mobile. Torsion of the testis, actually torsion of the spermatic cord, causes strangulation of blood supply, testicular necrosis and later atrophy. Torsion sometimes occurs during **intrauterine life** but may happen at any age. Intrauterine or neonatal torsion occurs proximal to the reflection of the tunica vaginalis (i.e. **extravaginal**). Infarction results in atrophy and loss of the testis so that at laparoscopy, only blind-ending testicular vessels and vas deferens are found. The condition occurs bilaterally in up to 30%
- **Psychological**—normal genitalia are important in the development of body image, gender acceptance and personality in adolescence. Orchidopexy at an early age provides reassurance to the child and parents

Boys should be examined regularly from birth right through school age to identify maldescent and allow timely **orchidopexy**. Periodic examination is needed because unequivocally descended testes can later ascend and parents and doctors should be alert to this possibility. There may be a fibrous band within the processus vaginalis preventing elongation of testicular vessels as the boy grows. The resulting 'stationary' testis appears to ascend, and no longer comes comfortably into the scrotum.

With a history of a missing testis, the chief point is whether the testis is palpable. If palpable at the scrotal neck, it should be gently manipulated into its correct position. If it then stays put, it is **retractile** and needs no treatment provided it become less retractile as the boy grows. If the testis immediately retracts, it is maldescended and needs treatment.

If the testis is impalpable, investigations should be undertaken to locate it. Laparoscopy is the investigation of choice; the testis may be found intra-abdominally or the cord may be seen entering the deep ring; in either case, the testis is mobilised and placed in the scrotum. Alternatively, a blind-ending spermatic cord may be found indicating the testis is missing, probably as a result of intrauterine torsion. No action is needed if this is unilateral but if bilateral, genetic screening is required and possible hormonal treatment and testicular prostheses.

SURGERY FOR TESTICULAR MALDESCENT

The optimum age for operation is 6 months to 1 year so fertility is not compromised. The usual technique of orchidopexy involves mobilising the testis and spermatic cord through a groin incision, separating and excising the processus vaginalis and placing the testis in a subcutaneous pouch outside the dartos muscle via a separate scrotal incision. For intra-abdominal testes, the operative technique is a laparoscopic staged Fowler-Stephens procedure. In the first stage, the testis is mobilised by dividing the testicular artery and vein intra-abdominally. Six months later the testis is mobilised on the vas with its attendant artery and delivered into the scrotum laparoscopically. This approach has improved the success rate for intra-abdominal testes to almost 90%.

FORESKIN PROBLEMS

At birth the foreskin or prepuce is adherent to the glans penis and undergoes gradual separation between birth and puberty. Parents should not attempt to retract an adherent foreskin as this may provoke fibrosis. Note that some adhesions may perfectly normally persist into adolescence. The prepuce protects the glans from ammoniacal dermatitis when the child is in nappies. By the time continence is achieved, 95% of boys have a retractile foreskin.

PHIMOSIS

In phimosis, a tight fibrotic ring develops at the end of the foreskin preventing retraction. **Primary phimosis** presents with chronic foreskin irritation or 'spraying' on micturition. 'Ballooning' on micturition is just a sign of a non-retractile foreskin and is not necessarily pathological. There is often a history of recent or recurrent **balano-posthitis** (infection beneath the foreskin). Most boys with primary phimosis do not require circumcision; careful attention to hygiene (avoiding forcible retraction) allows the prepuce to retract normally in time. Attempts to dilate the phimosis under anaesthesia are unsuccessful as this causes further scarring and rapid relapse.

Circumcision may be indicated in cases of recurrent infection particularly in boys with upper renal tract abnormalities or other congenital problems such as posterior urethral valves and may help to reduce the incidence of UTIs in these boys. In young men, a non-retractile foreskin may cause sexual problems. For these, the lesser operation of **preputioplasty** may suffice if the phimosis is not too tight. This involves dividing the tight band longitudinally and suturing it transversely, increasing the meatal calibre to allow easier retraction.

Secondary phimosis is usually due to **balanitis xerotica obliterans** (BXO) which is characterised by a thickened, whitish, fibrotic non-retractile foreskin. Plaques are formed on the deep surface which adhere to the glans and may cause meatal stenosis. The peak incidence is around 8 years and the condition is a definite indication for circumcision.

PARAPHIMOSIS

Paraphimosis sometimes occurs in children, especially in phimosis. The tip of the foreskin forms a tight band when retracted and becomes trapped in the coronal sulcus behind the glans. The band inhibits venous return and causes swelling of the glans, making return of the prepuce even more difficult. Paraphimosis is painful and requires urgent reduction. This can sometimes be achieved using EMLA cream (local anaesthetic) or a penile block. Manual compression of the glans often allows reduction but if this fails, general anaesthesia is needed. Sometimes the band needs dividing with a **dorsal slit**. Circumcision is usually performed later once oedema has settled.

RENAL, VESICAL AND URETHRAL ABNORMALITIES

About a third of all congenital anomalies affect the genitourinary tract. These include abnormalities of kidney, renal calyces or pelvis and ureters. Anomalies of the bladder and urethra complete the spectrum of paediatric urogenital problems, which may present at birth but need long-term follow-up, often into adulthood. Around 90% of renal tract abnormalities can now be detected at an antenatal 12- or 20-week scan, allowing parents to be prepared for postnatal management. The most common ones are hypospadias, pelviureteric junction (PUJ) obstruction and vesicoureteric reflux (VUR). Renal parenchymal disorders are less common. Some disorders present later, including unilateral renal agenesis, horseshoe kidney and polycystic kidneys (see Table 39.1).

RENAL DYSPLASIA

Incomplete or abnormal differentiation during development causes renal dysplasia. Dysplasia is classified into **agenesis** (absent), **hypoplastic** (underdeveloped) kidney and **multicystic dysplasia.** Bilateral agenesis is incompatible with life. Unilateral agenesis has an incidence of 1 in 1000 with a male preponderance. The contralateral kidney is usually normal and the disorder is not usually diagnosed until adulthood.

A kidney affected by **multicystic dysplasia** contains many cysts of different sizes. The kidney is non-functional and there is ureteric atresia. Most multicystic kidneys spontaneously involute (atrophy) without complication but nephrectomy is sometimes needed.

In **renal ectopia** (see Fig. 39.5), the kidney lies in an abnormal position in the pelvis, or abdomen. Renal ectopia can be discovered incidentally or associated with other anomalies such as anorectal malformations.

Abnormal fusion of the developing metanephric masses during the first two months of fetal life results in a **horseshoe kidney** (see Fig. 39.4). This may cause hydronephrosis by PUJ obstruction or be discovered incidentally at any age. Skeletal and cardiovascular abnormalities occur in at least a third; girls with Turner's syndrome often have a horseshoe kidney.

NEONATAL HYDRONEPHROSIS

Fetal urinary tract abnormalities occur in about 1% of pregnancies, and hydronephrosis accounts for half. Management depends on severity and whether unilateral or bilateral. Antenatal hydronephrosis may be caused by PUJ obstruction, vesicoureteric junction obstruction or reflux, multicystic kidney, primary obstructive megaureter or posterior urethral valves. The urgency and type of investigation depends on the size of the hydronephrosis. Small unilateral hydronephrosis requires no action, whereas larger lesions require ultrasound, micturating cystography and perhaps isotope renal scans repeated at intervals to decide if surgery is needed. Early investigation is essential in bilateral severe hydronephrosis, particularly in boys, to exclude bladder outlet obstruction secondary to posterior urethral valves.

VESICOURETERIC REFLUX (VUR)

Any anatomical or functional urinary tract abnormality predisposes to infections. This is particularly true in children, where the commonest predisposing abnormality is **vesicoureteric reflux**, i.e. retrograde flow of urine from bladder to kidneys. This exposes the upper tracts to the greater range of pressure variation of the lower tract and to ascending infections. The causes are complex but in essence there is a faulty mechanism at the junction of ureter and bladder (vesicoureteric junction), see Box 51.1. Reflux is classified severities ranging from I to V (see Table 51.1).

Neonatal VUR is caused by anatomical abnormalities, with both sexes equally affected. Later, the condition appears predominantly in girls where **voiding disturbances** play a large role. Dysfunctional voiding refers to abnormal storage of urine or an abnormal emptying phase of micturition and involves urgency, frequency, incontinence and urinary tract infections. A vicious circle may develop, with reflux leading to infection, then bladder instability and further dysfunctional voiding.

Box 51.1 Causes of vesicoureteric reflux

Primary, i.e. maldevelopment of vesicoureteric junction

- Short submucosal tunnel
- Delayed maturity of vesicoureteric junction

Secondary

- Posterior urethral valves
- Duplex system and ureterocoele
- Ectopic ureters
- Congenital megaureters
- Detrusor instability
- Neurogenic bladder
- Surgical procedures to the lower end of the ureter

Table 51.1 International classification of vesicoureteric reflux (VUR) and clinical classification

Grade of VUR	International classification	Clinical classification
I	Reflux into lower ureter on voiding	Mild non-dilating VUR on micturition
II	Reflux into ureter and renal pelvis on voiding but without dilatation	
III	Reflux into the ureter and renal pelvis on voiding with mild dilatation	
IV	Constant reflux with upper tract and ureteric dilatation	Constant severe dilating VUR
V	Constant reflux with blunted calyces and grossly dilated tortuous ureters	

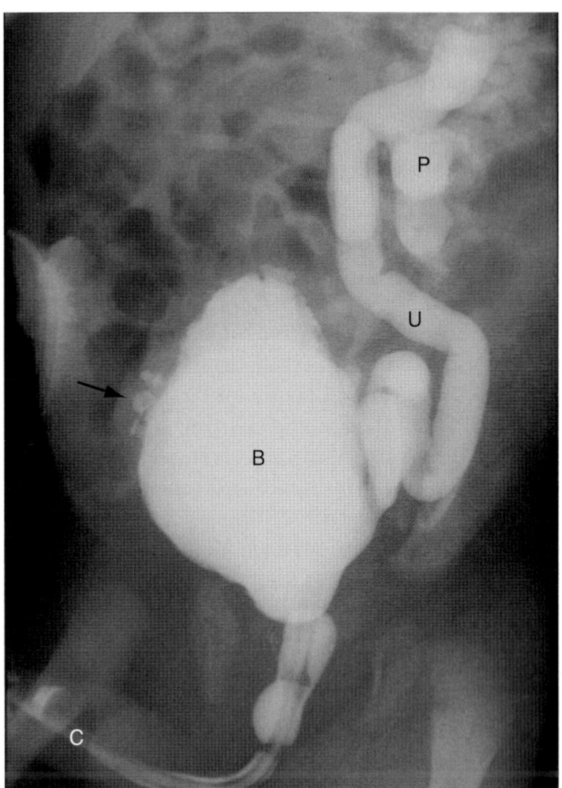

Fig. 51.6 Vesicoureteric reflux
Micturating cysto-urethrogram (MCUG) in a child with recurrent urinary tract infections. The bladder **B** is trabeculated (diverticula arrowed). On voiding, the left ureter **U** and pelvicalyceal system **P** filled with contrast as a result of severe dilating vesicoureteric reflux. This is defined as grade V reflux

PATHOPHYSIOLOGY

In the normal individual, the distal ureter passes obliquely through the bladder wall so as bladder pressure rises, the ureter is flattened, acting as a sphincter preventing urine from refluxing ('flap-valve' **anti-reflux mechanism**). This prevents transmission of intermittent high bladder pressures. **Primary vesicoureteric reflux** is most common and usually results from a minor (often familial) abnormality of ureteric insertion or from ectopic or duplex ureters or congenital megaureter (a peristaltic abnormality). **Secondary VUR** may be caused by bladder outlet obstruction, neuropathic bladder or surgical procedures to the lower end of the ureter.

Ascending infection of the upper tracts begins with bacteria reaching the bladder via the urethra and colonising it. Infected urine refluxes into upper tracts but cannot be cleared effectively from it, infecting the upper tract. Lower tract infections can also cause inflammation at the VUJ, preventing it from closing, aggravating reflux.

Reflux of sterile urine into the pelvicalyceal system during early childhood probably causes impaired renal development and function. Mild, non-dilating VUR (grades I to III; see Table 51.1) causes little damage but severe (dilating) VUR (grades IV and V) may cause renal scarring and reflux nephropathy, which may progress to irreversible renal damage if untreated (Fig. 51.6). If both kidneys are involved, this eventually results in renal insufficiency and hypertension. Scarring typically occurs apically in the kidneys. Loss of the normal conical shape of the papillae allows intrarenal reflux, which in the presence of infection results in pyelonephritis and renal scarring.

CLINICAL PRESENTATION AND INVESTIGATION

During antenatal screening, VUR can be detected as urinary tract dilatation. Another common presentation is one or more urinary tract infections at any age. Girls are more prone than boys after the first year, because of a short urethra and its proximity to the anus. Note that infants or young children with urinary infections may not exhibit urinary symptoms or signs; the diagnosis is often made on investigation of vomiting, fever or failure to thrive. Older children typically present with incontinence, frequency or dysuria, or abdominal pain and tenderness (mimicking appendicitis). In **symptomatic urinary tract infections**, the prevalence of vesicoureteric reflux is as high as 50% in neonates, and 30% in those aged 2–18 years.

In a child with urinary tract infection, clinical examination seeks evidence of abnormal external genitalia, spina bifida and impaired perineal innervation (sensation and anal sphincter tone). To demonstrate reflux, the sequential investigations are ultrasound scan, micturating cystography, and isotope scans using DMSA and MAG3, coupled with indirect radionuclide cystography. **Micturating cystography** should only be used in selected cases (Fig. 51.6); there is a 1% risk of pyelonephritis and the test is stressful for child and parent. It is the gold standard for demonstrating VUR and excluding posterior urethral valves but involves instilling contrast into the bladder via a urinary catheter which is then removed and X-rays taken during voiding. The radiological grades of severity are shown in Table 51.1 and provide a useful guide to the likelihood of future renal damage. Severe dilating VUR requires **isotope studies**: ^{99m}Tc DMSA, bound to renal tubules, shows differential renal function and scarring within renal parenchyma. In older children, an excretion MAG3 scan and indirect radionuclide cystogram shows differential function, reflux and sites of urinary tract obstruction.

MANAGEMENT OF VESICOURETERIC REFLUX

With no other anatomical abnormalities and an undilated ureter (i.e. grades I and II), there is an 85% chance of resolution of reflux as the child grows. In the meantime, the risk of urinary infection should be minimised by encouraging high fluid intake, avoiding constipation and maintaining perineal hygiene, plus medical management of bladder dysfunction. The child is maintained on continuous **antibacterial chemotherapy** (such as trimethoprim) and followed-up regularly with serial ultrasound scans and charting growth and development, blood pressure and plasma creatinine.

Surgical correction becomes indicated when there are recurrent infections, deterioration of upper tract function or non-compliance with medical management. Otherwise, surgery is reserved for severe dilated VUR with complications and for other obvious anatomical abnormalities. Newer treatments include injection of Deflux into the submucosa of the ureter at the junction with the bladder; success rates of up to 90% are possible. Less commonly operations aim to **reimplant the ureter** so that a length of it lies deep to the bladder mucosa; during voiding this is flattened restoring an anti-reflux mechanism.

Without renal scarring, the child can be discharged from follow-up after operation. With unilateral scarring, blood pressure should be monitored lifelong for hypertension. In bilateral scarring, renal function must also be monitored.

PELVIURETERIC JUNCTION DYSFUNCTION

PATHOPHYSIOLOGY

Obstruction at the pelviureteric junction (PUJ) may be unilateral or bilateral, and can present between birth and the end of the fourth decade. It affects both sexes equally. PUJ dysfunction is a congenital condition that manifests as dilatation of the renal pelvis and calyces (**hydronephrosis**) and incomplete or intermittent obstruction of the PUJ. Usually a functional abnormality, there is an aperistaltic segment of ureter that lacks muscle. Aberrant lower pole vessels may cause mechanical obstruction in older children. A normal PUJ prevents urine reflux into the kidney when the ureter contracts, but in PUJ obstruction, urine accumulates and dilates the pelvicalyceal system. This increases pressure in the renal collecting system which may cause deterioration of renal function. Stasis may also predispose to infection and stone formation.

CLINICAL PRESENTATION AND DIAGNOSIS

PUJ dysfunction is now most often diagnosed antenatally. Management is regular postnatal follow-up with ultrasound. Those with persistent or progressive hydronephrosis are investigated for VUR, renal function and renal drainage effectiveness and treated appropriately.

Many with PUJ dysfunction go undetected. Others are discovered by chance on ultrasound or urography for an apparently unrelated condition. Symptoms may be intermittent: some patients complain of aching in the renal area; others suffer bouts of severe abdominal or loin pain (renal colic), some with urinary tract infection or haematuria (which may be induced by exercise). Symptoms can be exacerbated by drinking large volumes of fluid precipitating a Dietl's crisis, or by sudden changes in posture.

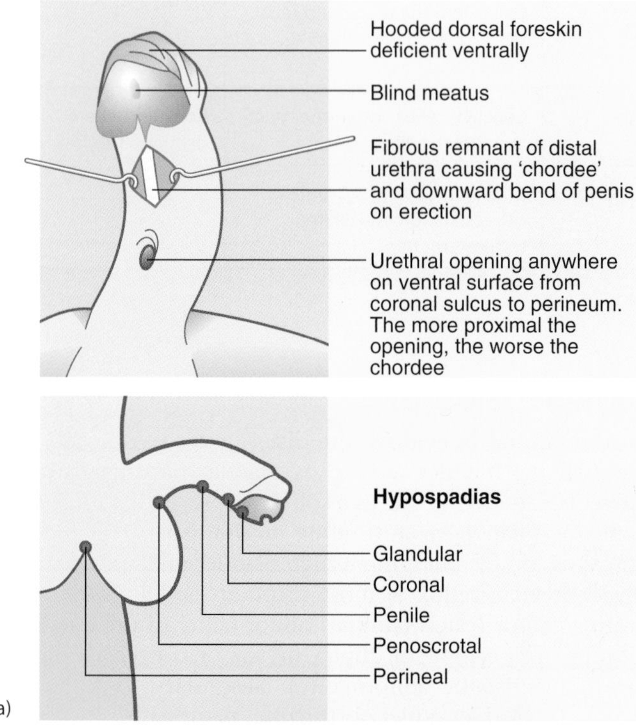

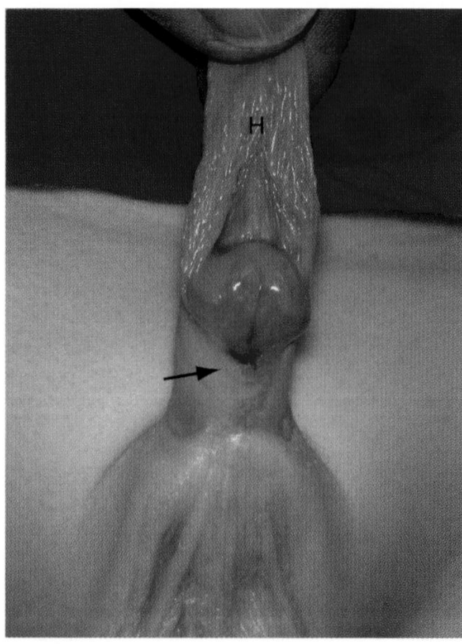

Fig. 51.7 Hypospadias
(a) Hypospadias **(b)** Distal coronal hypospadias. The urethral meatus is arrowed and **H** indicates the hooded foreskin. Chordee, a marked downward bend of the penis, was prominent in this case but is not visible here

The initial diagnosis is by ultrasound, with detection of a dilated renal pelvis. The next step is to distinguish between static non-obstructive dilatation with preserved renal function and genuine PUJ obstruction causing stasis, dilatation and deteriorating function. **Radionuclide diuretic renography (^{99m}Tc MAG3 scan)** is the investigation of choice and in classical PUJ obstruction, gives a characteristic non-excretion curve.

Indications for operation include a loss of differential renal function >10%, or more commonly an increase in the anterior–posterior diameter of the renal pelvis to >35 mm.

MANAGEMENT

PUJ dysfunction with obstructive symptoms, stone formation, recurrent infections or progressive renal impairment, together with an obstructed isotope excretion curve, are indications for intervention. Pyeloplasty is indicated unless the kidney has less than 10% of total renal function, in which case nephrectomy may be indicated. Minimal invasive techniques include percutaneous antegrade endopyelotomy and laparoscopic pyeloplasty. Standard operations have a high technical success rate and usually prevent deterioration of renal function.

HYPOSPADIAS AND EPISPADIAS

Hypospadias is a common congenital abnormality of penis and urethra. It occurs in 1 in 125–300 male births and is increasing in incidence. The distal urethra fails to develop normally, so the urethral meatus lies somewhere along the ventral surface of the penis between glans and perineum (see Fig. 51.7). The urethral remnant distal to the meatus is fibrotic, often causing the penis to bend downwards or sideways on erection, known as **chordee**. The more proximal the meatus, the worse the chordee. In addition, the ventral part of the foreskin is absent, giving a hooded appearance. Distal hypospadias is more common, accounting for about 85%, with the urethral opening between glans and the mid-shaft with minimal chordee.

Surgical correction is a highly specialised procedure performed for function and cosmesis. Functional correction enables voiding in forwards and forward ejaculation later. Since surgical repair utilises the foreskin, circumcision should **never** be carried out without specialist advice. The ideal age for surgery is 6–12 months.

Epispadias is rare and may be associated with other genitourinary abnormalities. In epispadias, the urethral meatus is on the dorsal aspect of the penis.

POSTERIOR URETHRAL VALVES (PUV)

Urethral valves are congenital mucosal folds in the posterior urethra of a boy that impede or occlude urinary flow. Antenatal ultrasound screening usually detects the characteristic signs of oligohydramnios, a small thick-walled bladder and bilateral hydronephrosis and hydroureter. If not diagnosed antenatally, complete obstruction becomes apparent soon after birth, but partial obstruction may be overlooked.

Severe oligohydramnios caused by this can be associated with pulmonary hypoplasia, which is incompatible with life. Neonates born with bladder outlet obstruction require urgent assessment. Urethral catheterisation facilitates accurate fluid management in the immediate postnatal period but management of post-obstructive diuresis and electrolyte abnormalities can be difficult and is best done in a specialist unit. Ultrasound scan and micturating cystography confirm the diagnosis.

Definitive treatment involves ablating the valves by diathermy or cold-knife using a paediatric resecting cystoscope. Long-term follow-up is imperative, as renal function may deteriorate to the point of renal replacement therapy or transplantation in about 50%. Sometimes a low-capacity, high-pressure bladder persists, requiring drainage or a bladder augmentation procedure.

ABDOMINAL PROBLEMS

CHRONIC AND RECURRENT ABDOMINAL PAIN

Chronic or recurrent abdominal pain is common in children of school age but no cause is usually discovered and the problem gradually resolves (Box 51.2). Children may be referred to a surgeon if an organic problem seems likely, but psychological factors are fairly common. The common organic causes are constipation, hydronephrosis, inflammatory bowel disease and gallstones associated with haemolytic anaemia.

CHRONIC CONSTIPATION

Chronic constipation is a very common problem in children; it may present as **faecal soiling**, i.e. faecal overflow incontinence. A detailed history including socio-psychological factors may reveal a cause but in most the aetiology is unknown. The problem should not be neglected as it may lead to lifelong problems. Early constipation usually responds to simple measures such as a high-fibre diet, increased fluid intake, regular attempts at defaecation and combinations of osmotic and stimulant laxatives (e.g. lactulose or senna derivative or Movicol).

Box 51.2 Organic causes of chronic or recurrent abdominal pain in children

- Chronic constipation—common
- Lower urinary tract infection—common
- Hydronephrosis—uncommon
- Sickle cell crises—uncommon
- Recurrent appendicitis—rare
- Crohn's disease
- Recurrent volvulus of small bowel—rare
- Gallstones—rare, sometimes associated with haemolytic anaemia
- Peptic ulceration—rare

In severe constipation, it is important to investigate for **cystic fibrosis, hypothyroidism** and **Hirschsprung's disease** (Ch. 50, p. 619). If these can be excluded, the child may require an operation such as anterior resection for redundant non-functional rectum or the creation of a conduit into the colon to allow antegrade enemas.

GASTROINTESTINAL BLEEDING IN CHILDREN (Table 51.2)

UPPER GASTROINTESTINAL BLEEDING

In neonates, apparent vomiting of blood may result from swallowed maternal blood. In older infants, gastritis may be the cause. Less common causes are bleeding disorders and coagulopathy.

LOWER GASTROINTESTINAL BLEEDING

Rectal bleeding in neonates is most often due to anal fissure, necrotising enterocolitis or malrotation with volvulus. Rectal bleeding is a common problem in older infants and children; the causes are summarised in Table 51.2 and include perianal abscess and fistula, anal fissures, large bowel polyps, rectal prolapse and Meckel's diverticulum.

Anal fissure

Anal fissure occurs at any age during infancy and childhood and is probably initiated by straining to pass a large hard stool. This splits the anal mucosa in the midline posteriorly or anteriorly. Anal fissures can also develop after severe diarrhoea. The main symptoms are pain at defaecation and a small amount of bright red blood on the stool or leaking out immediately after defaecation. The condition is readily diagnosed when digital rectal examination is found to be impossible because of extreme tenderness; the posterior end of the fissure may sometimes be seen by parting the buttocks. Treatment is conservative, with medical treatment of constipation and management of painful defaecation. Anal skin tags often develop following healing of an anal fissure.

Polyps

A **juvenile hamartomatous polyp** is a common cause of rectal bleeding. These are nearly always solitary and usually occur in the rectum or sigmoid colon. Polyps may present with intermittent rectal bleeding in a child without constipation; as pain on defaecation without an anal fissure; or by prolapsing through the anus. The polyp may be palpable on digital examination and is confirmed on proctoscopy; it can then be suture ligated and resected. If no polyp is visible, colonoscopy is performed and identified polyps removed by snare. Juvenile polyps are almost never malignant, nor do they recur. **Familial adenomatous polyposis** may present in childhood with rectal bleeding. As described in Chapter 27, polyps of this type inevitably turn malignant from about the age of 16.

Table 51.2 Common causes of gastrointestinal bleeding in children

Age	Upper gastrointestinal	Lower gastrointestinal
1–12 months	Oesophagitis Gastritis	Anal fissure Intussusception Necrotising enterocolitis Malrotation with volvulus Perianal abscess and fistula
1–2 years	Peptic ulcer disease associated with: Burns (Curling's ulcer) Head trauma (Cushing's ulcer) Malignancy Sepsis	Anal fissure Polyps Rectal prolapse Meckel's diverticulum Perianal abscess and fistula
2–15 years	Oesophageal and gastric varices Portal hypertension with cirrhosis	Polyps Inflammatory bowel disease Trauma Sexual abuse Gastroenteritis—*Campylobacter* Arteriovenous malformations Miscellaneous lesions

Rectal prolapse

Transient rectal prolapse is a common and alarming childhood problem, usually during the first 2 years. The common cause is excessive straining during defaecation. Prolapse may be a presenting feature of cystic fibrosis because there is less mucus in the bowel and the mucus is thick and sticky. In addition, thick mucus often obstructs exocrine pancreatic secretion, impairing fat digestion. Most prolapses can be gently manipulated back without pain although they frequently recur unless the stool is kept soft and the child can open the bowels without straining. If the problem is persistent or recurrent, proctoscopy and sigmoidoscopy are indicated. A rectal polyp is occasionally responsible. If simple stool-softening measures fail to prevent recurrence, submucosal injections of hypertonic saline or phenol in oil have been used

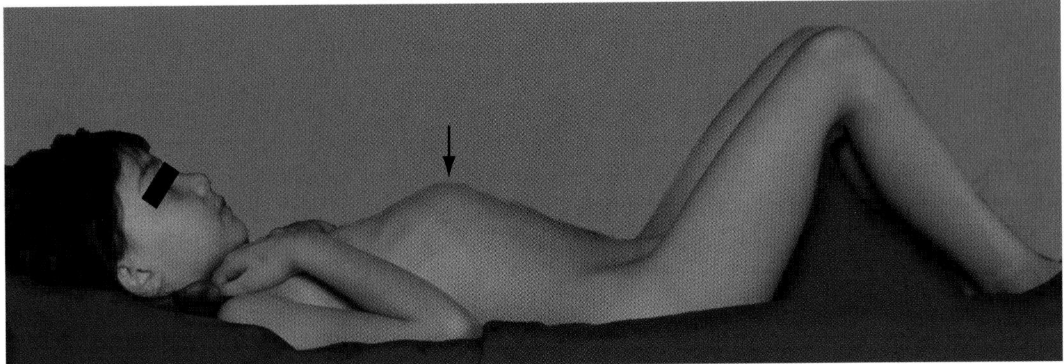

Fig. 51.8 Nephroblastoma
This 9-year-old girl presented with a large unilateral mass (arrowed), which was later confirmed to be arising from the left kidney (Wilms' tumour or nephroblastoma)

to induce fibrosis. In the rare event of failure, a subcutaneous circumanal suture may be inserted.

Perianal abscess

This is common in infants and results from infection of an anal gland, as in adults. The abscess points 1–2 cm from the anal verge. Drainage alone would convert this into a **fistula** so correct treatment involves opening the tract entirely under general anaesthesia, as in adults.

Meckel's diverticulum

A Meckel's diverticulum is present in less than 2% of the population. It represents the embryological remnant of the **vitello-intestinal duct** which joined the fetal midgut and the yolk sac. It is situated on the antimesenteric border of the distal ileum about 60 cm from the ileocaecal junction. They are usually asymptomatic.

Meckel's diverticula often contain a variety of gut-related tissues. These include **ectopic acid-secreting gastric mucosa**, which may cause inflammation and peptic ulceration. In children below 2 years, this is an important cause of rectal bleeding which may require transfusion. In older children, the gastric mucosa more often causes chronic occult bleeding leading to iron deficiency anaemia. Much less commonly, **peptic ulceration** results in **perforation** which presents with signs of peritonitis.

If a Meckel's diverticulum is suspected in rectal bleeding, a radionuclide Meckel's scan may be positive but the test has a low negative **predictive value** and a laparoscopy or laparotomy often has to be performed to examine the bowel directly.

A Meckel's diverticulum with a narrow neck may become inflamed like appendicitis and cause similar symptoms and signs (see Fig. 26.4, p. 345); the diagnosis is only made at operation. As with appendicitis, the complications are perforation and peritonitis. Meckel's diverticulitis is uncommon in children under 10 years.

At operation, the diverticulum should be resected, together with 2 cm of normal ileum on each side, and primary ileo-ileal anastomosis performed. This is because ectopic gastric mucosa can extend beyond the diverticulum.

INFLAMMATORY BOWEL DISEASE

(see Ch. 28 for adult disease)

The incidence of Crohn's disease in children is increasing and can involve any part of the GI tract. Perianal disease is common, with chronic indolent abscesses and fissures. These fissures are often lateral, suggesting the diagnosis. Crohn's disease varies greatly in its presentation and this may cause delay in diagnosis. As in adults, there may be a history of recurrent abdominal pain and weight loss. The first presentation in adolescents may be faltering growth or delayed onset of puberty.

Ulcerative colitis presents with diarrhoea, malaise and weight loss; perianal disease and proctitis is uncommon. Management of both conditions is similar to that in adults. A need for surgery is uncommon in childhood and is best managed in a specialist centre.

ABDOMINAL MASS

An abdominal mass is an uncommon reason for surgical referral in children. It may be caused by a malignant embryonal tumour, most often a **nephroblastoma** (Wilms' tumour). Other causes include **hydronephrosis** and **post-traumatic pancreatic pseudocyst**.

NEPHROBLASTOMA (WILMS' TUMOUR)

Nephroblastoma presents in early childhood, with 80% presenting before the age of 5, at a median age of 3.5 years. The tumour arises from embryonal renal tissue in the kidney. Tumours are locally invasive and metastasise to regional nodes, liver, lungs and bone. Often, a large abdominal mass is noticed by the mother as the child is bathed (see Fig. 51.8). The mass is sometimes so large as to obscure its site of origin. Less common presenting features include haematuria, classically after trivial trauma, anorexia, weight loss, pyrexia and hypertension. Diagnosis is by clinical examination, and tumour size and characteristics are shown by ultrasonography or CT scan. The diagnosis is confirmed by Trucut biopsy.

Treatment is by neoadjuvant chemotherapy via Hickman line followed by surgery (usually a radical nephrectomy with lymph node sampling). In the UK all children with Wilms' tumour are managed by strict protocol by a multidisciplinary team. When surgery was the only treatment, the cure rate was about 10%, but the modern combination of neoadjuvant chemotherapy, surgical resection and sometimes radiotherapy gives a good chance of complete cure even when distant metastases are present.

NEUROBLASTOMA

This embryonal tumour occurs in early childhood. It is highly malignant and arises from embryonal sympathetic nervous tissue in the adrenal gland or sympathetic chain. Standard treatment is a combination of surgical resection, chemotherapy and radiotherapy, but the prognosis is poor. A less aggressive variant is the **neuroganglioblastoma**. This sometimes presents as an abdominal mass but the usual presentation is failure to thrive.

Index

Page numbers ending in 'b', 'f' and 't' refer to Boxes, Figures and Tables respectively. 'GA' stands for 'general anaesthesia'.

A

C

D

E

F

G

H

I

J

K

L

M

N

O

P

Q

R

S